COMPLETE GUIDE TO PRESCRIPTION & NON-PRESCRIPTION DRUGS

By H. WINTER GRIFFITH, M.D.

Technical consultants:
John D. Palmer, M.D., Ph.D.
William N. Jones, B.S., M.S.

NEW!

UPDATED FOR 1986
NOW INCLUDES
4000 BRAND NAMES!

HPBooks®

Publisher: Rick Bailey
Executive Editor: Randy Summerlin
Editor: Judith Wesley Allen
Editorial Assistance: Roberta Janes
Art Director: Don Burton
Production Coordinator: Cindy J. Coatsworth
Typography: Michelle Carter
Director of Manufacturing: Anthony B. Narducci
Cover Photo: Balfour Walker

HPBooks, Inc.

P.O. Box 5367
Tucson, AZ 85703
602-888-2150

ISBN: 0-89586-404-5
Library of Congress Catalog Card Number: 85-81840

12th Printing; New & Updated for 1986
Printed in U.S.A.

Notice: The information in this book is true and complete to the best of our knowledge. The book is intended only as a guide to drugs used for medical treatment. It is not intended as a replacement for sound medical advice from a doctor. Only a doctor can include the variables of an individual's age, sex and past medical history needed for wise drug prescription. This book does not contain every possible side effect, adverse reaction or interaction with other drugs or substances. Final decision about a drug's safety or effectiveness must be made by the individual and his doctor. All recommendations herein are made without guarantees on the part of the author or HPBooks. The author and publisher disclaim all liability in connection with the use of this information.

Contents

About the Author

H. Winter Griffith has authored several medical books, including the *Complete Guide to Symptoms, Illness & Surgery,* published by The Body Press. Others are *Instructions for Patients, Drug Information for Patients, Instructions for Dental Patients, Information and Instructions for Pediatric Patients* and *Pediatrics for Parents.* Dr. Griffith received his medical degree from Emory University in 1953. After 20 years in private practice, he established a basic medical-science program at Florida State University. He then became an associate professor of family and community medicine at the University of Arizona College of Medicine.

Technical Consultants

John D. Palmer, M.D., Ph.D.

Associate professor of pharmacology, University of Arizona College of Medicine
Associate professor of medicine (clinical pharmacology), University of Arizona College of Medicine

William N. Jones, Pharmacist, B.S., M.S.

Clinical pharmacy coordinator, Veterans Administration Medical Center, Tucson, Arizona
Adjunct assistant professor, Department of Pharmacy Practice, College of Pharmacy, University of Arizona

Drugs and You

My first day of pharmacology class in medical school started with a jolt. The professor began by writing on the blackboard, "Drugs are poisons."

I thought the statement was extreme. New drug discoveries promised to solve medical problems that had baffled men for centuries. The medical community was intrigued with new possibilities for drugs.

In the 30 years since then, many drug "miracles" have lived up to those early expectations. But the years have also shown the damage drugs can cause when they are misused or not fully understood.

As a family doctor and teacher, I have developed a healthy respect for what drugs can and can't do. I now appreciate my professor's warning.

A drug cannot "cure." It aids the body's natural defenses to promote recovery.

Likewise, a manufacturer or doctor cannot guarantee a drug will be useful for everyone. The complexity of the human body, individual responses in different people and in the same person under different circumstances, past and present health, age and sex influence how well a drug works.

All effective drugs produce desirable changes in the body, but a drug can also cause undesirable adverse reactions or side effects in some people.

Despite uncertainties, the drug discoveries of the last 40 years have given us tools to save lives and reduce discomfort.

Before you decide whether to take a drug, you or your doctor must ask, "Will the benefits outweigh the risks?"

The purpose of this book is to give you enough information about the most widely used drugs so you can make a wise decision. The information will alert you to potential or preventable problems. You can learn what to do if problems arise.

The information is derived from several expert sources. Every effort has been made to ensure accuracy and completeness. When information from different sources conflicts, I have used the majority's opinion, coupled with my clinical judgment and that of my technical consultants. Drug information changes with continuing observations by clinicians and users.

Information in this book applies to generic drugs in both the United States and Canada. Generic names do not vary in these countries, but brand names do.

BE SAFE! TELL YOUR DOCTOR

Some suggestions for wise drug use apply to all drugs. Always give the following information to your physician, dentist or other health-care professional. They must have complete information to prescribe drugs safely for you. This information includes your medical history, your medical plans and progress while under medication.

MEDICAL HISTORY

Tell the important facts of your medical history dealing with drugs. Include allergic or adverse reactions you have had to any medicine in the past. Name the allergic symptoms you have, such as hay fever, asthma, eye watering and itching, throat irritation and reactions to food. People who have allergies to common substances are more likely to develop drug allergies.

List all drugs you take. Don't forget vitamin and mineral supplements, skin, rectal or vaginal medicines, antacids, antihistamines, cold and cough remedies, aspirin and aspirin combinations, motion-sickness remedies, weight-loss aids, salt and sugar substitutes, caffeine, oral contraceptives, sleeping pills or "tonics."

FUTURE MEDICAL PLANS

Discuss plans for elective surgery, pregnancy and breast-feeding.

QUESTIONS

Don't hesitate to ask questions about a drug. Your doctor, nurse or pharmacist may be able to provide more information if they are familiar with you and your medical history.

YOUR ROLE

Learn the generic names and brand names of all your medicines. Write them down to help you remember. If a drug is a mixture, learn the names of its generic ingredients.

TAKING A DRUG

Never take medicine in the dark! Recheck the label before each use. You could be taking the *wrong* drug! Tell your doctor about any unexpected new symptoms you have while taking medicine. You may need to change medicines or have a dose adjustment.

STORAGE

Keep all medicines out of children's reach. Store drugs in a cool, dry place, such as a kitchen cabinet or bedroom. Avoid medicine cabinets in bathrooms. They get too moist and warm at times.

Keep medicine in its original container, tightly closed. Don't remove the label! If directions call for refrigeration, don't freeze.

DISCARDING

Don't save leftover medicine to use later. Discard it on the expiration date shown on the container. Dispose safely to protect children and pets.

REFILLS

All refills must be ordered by your doctor or dentist, either in the first prescription or later. Only the pharmacy that originally filled the prescription can refill it without checking with your doctor or previous pharmacy. If you go to a *new* pharmacy, you must have a new prescription, or the new pharmacist must call your doctor or original pharmacy to see if a refill is authorized. Pharmacies don't usually transfer prescriptions.

If you need a refill, call your pharmacist and order your refill by number and name.

Use one pharmacy for the whole family if you can. The pharmacist then has a record of all of your drugs and can communicate effectively with your doctor.

LEARN ABOUT DRUGS

Study the information in this book's charts regarding your medications. Read each chart completely. Because of space limitations, most information that fits more than one category appears only once.

Take care of yourself. You are the most important member of your health-care team.

Guide to Drug Charts

The drug information in this book is organized in condensed, easy-to-read charts. Each drug is described in a two-page format, as shown in the sample chart below and opposite. Charts are arranged alphabetically by drug generic names, and in a few instances, such as **ADRENOCORTICOIDS, TOPICAL**, by drug class name.

A *generic name* is the official chemical name for a drug. A *brand name* is a drug manufacturer's registered trademark for a generic drug. Brand names listed on the

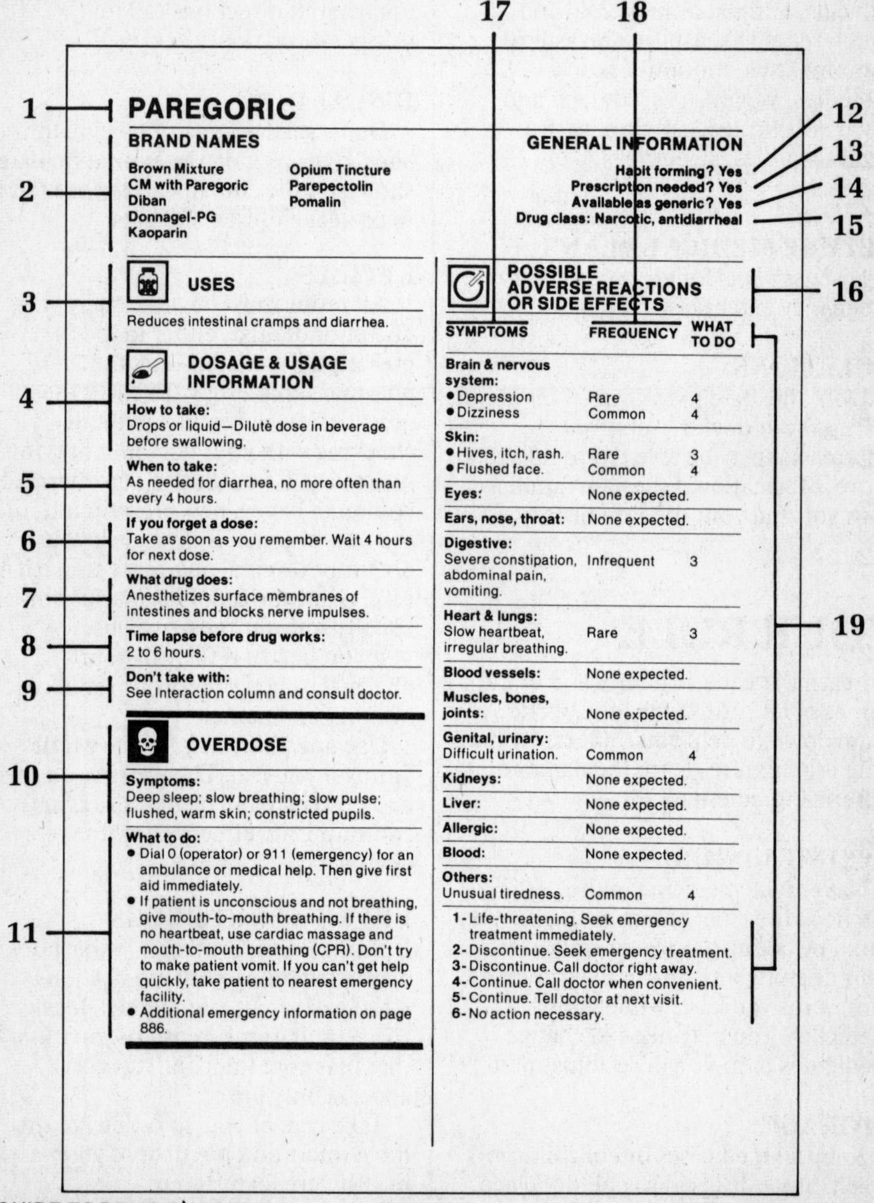

17
18
1
PAREGORIC
2
BRAND NAMES
Brown Mixture
CM with Paregoric
Diban
Donnagel-PG
Kaoparin
Opium Tincture
Parepectolin
Pomalin
GENERAL INFORMATION
Habit forming? Yes
Prescription needed? Yes
Available as generic? Yes
Drug class: Narcotic, antidiarrheal
12
13
14
15
3
USES
Reduces intestinal cramps and diarrhea.
4
DOSAGE & USAGE INFORMATION
How to take:
Drops or liquid—Dilute dose in beverage before swallowing.
5
When to take:
As needed for diarrhea, no more often than every 4 hours.
6
If you forget a dose:
Take as soon as you remember. Wait 4 hours for next dose.
7
What drug does:
Anesthetizes surface membranes of intestines and blocks nerve impulses.
8
Time lapse before drug works:
2 to 6 hours.
9
Don't take with:
See Interaction column and consult doctor.
10
OVERDOSE
Symptoms:
Deep sleep; slow breathing; slow pulse; flushed, warm skin; constricted pupils.
11
What to do:
• Dial 0 (operator) or 911 (emergency) for an ambulance or medical help. Then give first aid immediately.
• If patient is unconscious and not breathing, give mouth-to-mouth breathing. If there is no heartbeat, use cardiac massage and mouth-to-mouth breathing (CPR). Don't try to make patient vomit. If you can't get help quickly, take patient to nearest emergency facility.
• Additional emergency information on page 886.
16
POSSIBLE ADVERSE REACTIONS OR SIDE EFFECTS
SYMPTOMS
FREQUENCY
WHAT TO DO
Brain & nervous system:
• Depression Rare 4
• Dizziness Common 4
Skin:
• Hives, itch, rash. Rare 3
• Flushed face. Common 4
Eyes: None expected.
Ears, nose, throat: None expected.
Digestive:
Severe constipation, abdominal pain, vomiting. Infrequent 3
Heart & lungs:
Slow heartbeat, irregular breathing. Rare 3
Blood vessels: None expected.
Muscles, bones, joints: None expected.
Genital, urinary:
Difficult urination. Common 4
Kidneys: None expected.
Liver: None expected.
Allergic: None expected.
Blood: None expected.
Others:
Unusual tiredness. Common 4
19
1- Life-threatening. Seek emergency treatment immediately.
2- Discontinue. Seek emergency treatment.
3- Discontinue. Call doctor right away.
4- Continue. Call doctor when convenient.
5- Continue. Tell doctor at next visit.
6- No action necessary.

charts include those from the United States and Canada. A generic drug may have one or many brand names.

To find information about a generic drug, look it up in the alphabetical charts. To learn about a brand name, check the index first, where brand names are followed by their generic ingredients and chart page numbers.

The chart design is the same for every drug. When you are familiar with the chart, you can quickly find information you want to know about a drug.

On the next few pages, each of the numbered chart sections below is explained. This information will guide you in reading and understanding the charts that begin on page 18.

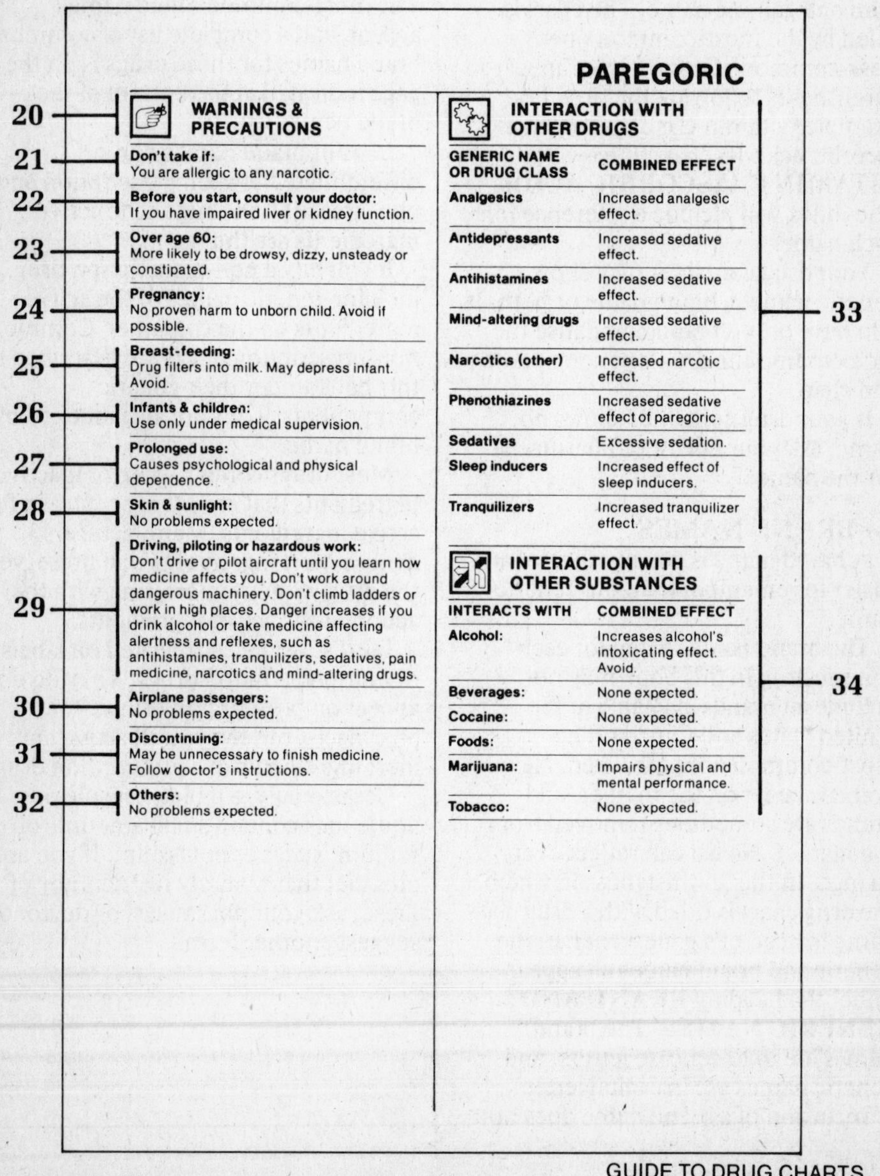

PAREGORIC

20 **WARNINGS & PRECAUTIONS**

21 **Don't take if:** You are allergic to any narcotic.

22 **Before you start, consult your doctor:** If you have impaired liver or kidney function.

23 **Over age 60:** More likely to be drowsy, dizzy, unsteady or constipated.

24 **Pregnancy:** No proven harm to unborn child. Avoid if possible.

25 **Breast-feeding:** Drug filters into milk. May depress infant. Avoid.

26 **Infants & children:** Use only under medical supervision.

27 **Prolonged use:** Causes psychological and physical dependence.

28 **Skin & sunlight:** No problems expected.

29 **Driving, piloting or hazardous work:** Don't drive or pilot aircraft until you learn how medicine affects you. Don't work around dangerous machinery. Don't climb ladders or work in high places. Danger increases if you drink alcohol or take medicine affecting alertness and reflexes, such as antihistamines, tranquilizers, sedatives, pain medicine, narcotics and mind-altering drugs.

30 **Airplane passengers:** No problems expected.

31 **Discontinuing:** May be unnecessary to finish medicine. Follow doctor's instructions.

32 **Others:** No problems expected.

INTERACTION WITH OTHER DRUGS 33

GENERIC NAME OR DRUG CLASS	COMBINED EFFECT
Analgesics	Increased analgesic effect.
Antidepressants	Increased sedative effect.
Antihistamines	Increased sedative effect.
Mind-altering drugs	Increased sedative effect.
Narcotics (other)	Increased narcotic effect.
Phenothiazines	Increased sedative effect of paregoric.
Sedatives	Excessive sedation.
Sleep inducers	Increased effect of sleep inducers.
Tranquilizers	Increased tranquilizer effect.

INTERACTION WITH OTHER SUBSTANCES 34

INTERACTS WITH	COMBINED EFFECT
Alcohol:	Increases alcohol's intoxicating effect. Avoid.
Beverages:	None expected.
Cocaine:	None expected.
Foods:	None expected.
Marijuana:	Impairs physical and mental performance.
Tobacco:	None expected.

GUIDE TO DRUG CHARTS

1—GENERIC NAME

Each drug chart is titled by generic name, or in a few instances, by the name of the drug class, such as **DIGITALIS PREPARATIONS**.

Sometimes a drug is known by more than one generic name. The chart is titled by the most-common one. Less-common generic names appear in parentheses following the first. For example, vitamin C is also known as ascorbic acid. Its chart title is **VITAMIN C (ASCORBIC ACID)**. The index will include a reference for each name.

Your drug container may show a generic name, a brand name or both. If you have only a brand name, use the index to find the drug's generic name and chart.

If your drug container shows no name, ask your doctor or pharmacist for the name.

2—BRAND NAMES

A brand name is usually shorter and easier to remember than the generic name.

The brand names listed for each generic drug in this book may not include all brands available in the United States and Canada. The most-common ones are listed. New brands appear on the market, and brands are sometimes removed from the market. No list can reflect every change. In the few instances in which the drug chart is titled with a drug class name instead of a generic name, the generic and brand names all appear under the heading **BRAND AND GENERIC NAMES**. The brand names are in lower case letters, and generic names are in capital letters.

Inclusion of a brand name does not imply recommendation or endorsement. Exclusion does not imply that a missing brand name is less effective or less safe than the ones listed. Some generic drugs have too many brand names to list on one chart. The most-common brand names appear, and a complete list of common brand names for those drugs is on the page indicated at the bottom of the brand names list.

Lists of brand names don't differentiate between prescription and non-prescription drugs. The active ingredients are the same.

If you buy a non-prescription drug, look for generic names of the active ingredients on the container. Common non-prescription drugs are described in this book under their generic components. They are also indexed by brand name.

Most drugs contain *inert,* or inactive, ingredients that are *fillers* or *solvents* for active ingredients. Manufacturers choose inert ingredients that preserve the drug without interfering with the action of the active ingredients.

Inert substances are listed on labels of non-prescription drugs. They do not appear on prescription drugs. Your pharmacist can tell you all active and inert ingredients in a prescription drug.

Occasionally, a tablet, capsule or liquid may contain small amounts of sodium, sugar or potassium. If you are on a diet that severely restricts any of these, ask your pharmacist or doctor to suggest another form.

3—USES

This section lists the disease or disorder for which a drug is prescribed.

Most uses listed are approved by the U.S. Food and Drug Administration. Some uses are listed if experiments and clinical trials indicate effectiveness and safety.

Other uses are included that may not be officially sanctioned, but for which doctors commonly prescribe the drug.

The use for which your doctor prescribes the drug may not appear. You and your doctor should discuss the reason for any prescription medicine you take.

You alone will probably decide whether to take a non-prescription drug. The Uses section may help you make a decision.

4—DOSAGE & USAGE INFORMATION: HOW TO TAKE

Drugs are available in tablets, capsules, liquids, suppositories, injections, aerosol inhalers and topical forms such as drops, sprays, creams, ointments and lotions. This section gives general instructions for taking each form.

This information supplements drug-label information. If your doctor's instructions differ from the suggestions, follow your *doctor's* instructions.

Instructions are left out for how *much* to take. Dose amounts can't be generalized. They must be individualized for you by your doctor, or you must read the drug label.

5—WHEN TO TAKE

Dose schedules vary for medicines and for patients.

Drugs prescribed on a schedule should usually be taken at approximately the same times each day. Some *must* be taken at regular intervals to maintain a steady level of the drug in the body. If the schedule interferes with your sleep, consult with your doctor.

Instructions to take on an empty stomach mean the drug is absorbed best in your body this way. Many drugs must be taken with liquid or food because they irritate the stomach.

Instructions for other dose schedules are usually on the label. Variations in standard dose schedules may apply because some medicines interact with others if you take them at the same time.

6—IF YOU FORGET A DOSE

Suggestions in this section vary from drug to drug. Most tell you when to resume taking the medicine if you forget a scheduled dose.

Establish habits so you won't forget doses. Forgotten doses decrease a drug's therapeutic effect.

7—WHAT DRUG DOES

This is a simple description of the drug's action in the body. The wording is generalized and may not be a complete explanation of the complex chemical process that takes place.

8—TIME LAPSE BEFORE DRUG WORKS

The times given are approximations. Times vary a great deal from person to person, and from time to time in the same person. The figures give you some idea of when to expect improvement.

9—DON'T TAKE WITH

Some drugs create problems when taken in combination with other substances. Most problems are detailed in the Interaction column of each chart. This section mentions substances that don't appear in the Interaction column.

Occasionally, an interaction is singled out if the combination is particularly harmful.

10—OVERDOSE: SYMPTOMS

The symptoms listed are most likely to develop with accidental or purposeful overdose. An overdose patient may not show all symptoms listed. Sometimes symptoms are identical to ones listed as side effects. The difference is intensity and severity. You will have to judge. Consult a doctor or poison-control center if you have any doubt.

11—WHAT TO DO

If you suspect an overdose, whether symptoms are apparent or not, follow instructions in this section. Expanded instructions for emergency treatment for overdose are on page 886.

12—HABIT FORMING

A drug habit can be physical or psychological. A drug that produces physical dependence leads to addiction. It causes painful and sometimes dangerous effects when withdrawn.

Psychological dependence does not cause dangerous withdrawal effects. It may cause stress and unwanted behavior changes until the habit is broken.

13—PRESCRIPTION NEEDED?

"Yes" means a doctor must prescribe the drug for you. "No" means you can buy this drug without prescription. Sometimes low strengths of a drug are available without prescription, while high strengths require prescription.

The information about the generic drug applies whether it requires prescription or not. If the generic ingredients are the same, non-prescription drugs have the same dangers, warnings, precautions and interactions as prescribed drugs.

14—AVAILABLE AS GENERIC?

Some generic drugs have copyright restrictions that protect the manufacturer or distributor of that drug. These drugs may be purchased only by brand name.

In recent years, drug manufacturers have marketed more drugs under generic names. Drugs purchased by generic name sometimes are less expensive than brand names.

Some states allow pharmacists to fill prescriptions by brand names or generic names. This allows patients to buy the least-expensive form of a drug.

A doctor may specify a brand name because he or she trusts a known source more than an unknown manufacturer of generic drugs. You and your doctor should decide whether you should buy a medicine by generic or brand name.

Generic drugs manufactured in other countries are not subject to regulation by the U.S. Food and Drug

Administration. Drugs manufactured in the United States are subject to regulation.

15—DRUG CLASS

Drugs that possess similar chemical structure and similar therapeutic effects are grouped into classes. Most drugs within a class produce similar benefits, side effects, adverse reactions and interactions with other drugs and substances. For example, there are 15 generic drugs in the narcotic drug class. All have similar effects on the body.

Some information on the charts applies to all drugs in a class. For example, a reference may be made to narcotics. The index lists the class—narcotics—and lists drugs in that class.

Drug classes are not standardized, so classes listed in other references may vary from the classes in this book.

16—POSSIBLE ADVERSE REACTIONS OR SIDE EFFECTS

Adverse reactions or side effects are symptoms that may occur when you take a drug. They are effects on the body other than the desired therapeutic effect.

The term *side effect* implies expected and usually unavoidable effects of a drug. Side effects have nothing to do with the drug's intended use.

For example, the generic drug paregoric reduces intestinal cramps and vomiting. It also often causes a flushed face. The flushing is a side effect that is harmless and does not affect the drug's therapeutic potential.

The term *adverse reaction* is more significant. For example, paregoric can cause serious adverse allergic reaction in some people. This reaction can for valid reasons offer benefits that outweigh potential hazards.

17—SYMPTOMS

Symptoms are grouped by various body systems. Symptoms that don't naturally apply to these body systems or which overlap systems are listed under "Others."

18—FREQUENCY

This is an estimation of how often symptoms occur in persons who take the drug. "Common" means these symptoms are expected and sometimes inevitable. "Infrequent" means the symptoms occur in approximately 1% to 10% of patients. "Rare" means symptoms occur in less than 1%.

19—WHAT TO DO

The numbers refer to the key at the bottom of the column. For example, paregoric produces the rare symptoms of slow heartbeat and irregular breathing—listed under "Heart & lungs." The chart suggests you discontinue the medicine and call your doctor right away.

20—WARNINGS AND PRECAUTIONS

Read these entries to determine special information that applies to you.

21—DON'T TAKE IF

This section lists circumstances that indicate the use of a drug may not be safe. On some drug labels and in formal medical literature, these circumstances are called *contraindications.*

22—BEFORE YOU START, CONSULT YOUR DOCTOR

This section lists conditions under which a drug should be used with caution.

23—OVER AGE 60

As a person ages, physical changes occur that require special consideration in drug use. Liver and kidney functions decrease, metabolism slows and the prostate gland enlarges in men.

Most drugs are metabolized or excreted at a rate dependent on kidney and liver functions. Small doses or longer intervals between doses may be necessary to prevent unhealthy concentration of a drug. Toxic effects and adverse reactions occur more frequently and cause more serious problems in this age group.

24—PREGNANCY

The best rule to follow during pregnancy is to avoid all drugs, including tobacco and alcohol. Any medicine—prescription or non-prescription—requires medical advice and supervision.

This section will alert you if there is evidence that a drug harms the unborn child. Lack of evidence does not guarantee a drug's safety. If safety is undetermined, and reasonable doubt exists, "No proven problems" is indicated.

25—BREAST-FEEDING

Many drugs filter into a mother's milk. Some drugs have dangerous or unwanted effects on the nursing infant. This section suggests ways to minimize harm to the child.

26—INFANTS & CHILDREN

Many drugs carry special warnings and precautions for children because of a child's size and immaturity. In medical terminology, *newborns* are babies up to 2 weeks old, *infants* are 2 weeks to 1 year, and *children* are 1 to 12 years.

27—PROLONGED USE

Most drugs produce no ill effects during short periods of treatment. However, relatively safe drugs taken for long periods may produce unwanted effects. These are listed. Drugs should be taken in the smallest dose and for the shortest time possible. Nevertheless, some diseases and conditions require an indefinite period of treatment. Your doctor may want to change drugs occasionally or alter your treatment regimen to minimize problems.

The words "functional dependence" sometimes appear in this section. This does not mean *physical* or *psychological addiction.* Sometimes a body function ceases to work naturally because it has been replaced or interfered with by the drug. The body then becomes dependent on the drug to continue the function.

28—SKIN & SUNLIGHT

Many drugs cause *photosensitivity,* which means increased skin sensitivity to ultraviolet rays from sunlight or artificial rays from a sunlamp. This section will alert you to this potential problem.

29—DRIVING, PILOTING OR HAZARDOUS WORK

Any drug that decreases alertness, muscular coordination or reflexes may make these activities hazardous. The effects may not appear in all people, or they may disappear after a short exposure to the drug. If this section contains a warning, use caution until you determine how a new drug affects you.

30—AIRPLANE PASSENGERS

Before you fly, check this section to determine how altitude can affect you when taking a drug.

31—DISCONTINUING

Some patients stop taking a drug when symptoms begin to go away, although complete recovery may require longer treatment.

Other patients continue taking a drug when it is no longer needed. This section will tell you when you may safely discontinue a drug.

Some drugs cause symptoms days or weeks after discontinuing. This section warns you so the symptoms won't puzzle you if they occur.

32—OTHERS

Warnings and precautions appear here if they don't fit into the other categories. This section includes storage instructions, how to dispose of outdated drugs, weather influences on drug effect, changes in blood and urine tests, warnings to persons with chronic illness and other information.

33—INTERACTION WITH OTHER DRUGS

Drugs interact in your body with other drugs, whether prescription or non-prescription. Interactions affect absorption, elimination or distribution of either drug. The chart lists interactions by generic name or drug class.

If a drug class appears, the generic drug interacts with any drug in that class. Drugs in each class that are included in the book are listed in the index.

Interactions are sometimes beneficial. You may not be able to determine from the chart which interactions are good and which are bad. Don't guess! Consult your doctor if you take drugs that interact. Some combinations are fatal!

Occasionally, drugs appear in the Interaction column that are not included in this book. These drugs are listed under Interactions for your safety.

Some drugs have too many interactions to list on one chart. The additional interactions appear on the page indicated at the bottom of the list.

34—INTERACTION WITH OTHER SUBSTANCES

The substances listed here are repeated on every drug chart. All people eat food and drink beverages. Many adults consume alcohol. Many people use cocaine and smoke tobacco or marijuana. This section shows possible interactions between these substances and each drug.

Drugs of Abuse

Each of the drug charts beginning on page 18 contains a section listing the interactions of alcohol, marijuana and cocaine with the therapeutic drug in the bloodstream. These three drugs are singled out because of their widespread use and abuse. The information is factual, not judgmental.

The long-term effects of alcohol and tobacco abuse are numerous. They have been well-publicized.

Drugs of potential abuse include those that are addictive and harmful. They usually produce a temporary, false sense of well-being. The long-term effects, however, are harmful and can be devastating to the body and psyche of the addict.

Refresh your memory frequently about the potential harm from prolonged use of *any* drugs or substances you take. Avoid unwise use of habit-forming drugs.

These are the most common drugs of abuse:

MARIJUANA (CANNABIS, HASHISH)

What they do: Heighten perception, cause mood swings, relax mind and body.
Signs of use: Red eyes, lethargy, uncoordinated body movements.
Long-term effects: Decreased motivation. Possible brain, heart, lung and reproductive-system damage.

AMPHETAMINES

What they do: Speed up physical and mental processes to cause a false sense of energy and excitement. The moods are temporary and unreal.
Signs of use: Dilated pupils, insomnia, trembling.
Long-term effects: Violent behavior, paranoia, possible death from overdose.

BARBITURATES

What they do: Produce drowsiness and lethargy.
Signs of use: Confused speech, lack of coordination and balance.
Long-term effects: Disrupts normal sleep pattern. Possible death from overdose, especially in combination with alcohol.

COCAINE

What it does: Stimulates the nervous system, heightens sensations and may produce hallucinations.
Signs of use: Trembling, intoxication, dilated pupils, constant sniffling.
Long-term effects: Ulceration of nasal passages where sniffed. Itching all over body, sometimes with open sores. Possible brain damage. Possible death from overdose.

OPIATES (CODEINE, HEROIN, METHADONE MORPHINE, OPIUM)

What they do: Relieve pain, create temporary and false sense of well-being.
Signs of use: Constricted pupils, mood swings, slurred speech, sore eyes, lethargy, weight loss, sweating.
Long-term effects: Malnutrition, extreme susceptibility to infection, the need to increase drug amount to produce the same effects. Possible death from overdose.

PSYCHEDELIC DRUGS (LSD, MESCALINE)

What they do: Produce hallucinations, either pleasant or frightening.
Signs of use: Dilated pupils, sweating, trembling, fever, chills.
Long-term effects: Lack of motivation, unpredictable behavior, narcissism, recurrent hallucinations without drug use ("flashbacks"). Possible death from overdose.

VOLATILE SUBSTANCES (GLUE, SOLVENTS)

What they do: Produce hallucinations, temporary, false sense of well-being and possible unconsciousness.
Signs of use: Dilated pupils, flushed face, confusion.
Long-term effects: Permanent brain, liver, kidney damage. Possible death from overdose.

Checklist for Safer Drug Use

- Learn all you can about drugs you may take *before* you take them. Information sources are your doctor, your nurse, your pharmacist, this book and other books in your public library.

- Don't take drugs prescribed for someone else—even if your symptoms are the same.

- Keep your prescription drugs to yourself. Your drugs may be harmful to someone else.

- Tell your doctor about any symptoms you believe are caused by a drug—prescription or non-prescription—that you take.

- Take only medicines that are *necessary.* Avoid taking non-prescription drugs while taking prescription drugs for a medical problem.

- Before your doctor prescribes for you, tell him about your previous experiences with any drug—beneficial results, adverse reactions or allergies.

- Take medicine in good light after you have identified it. If you wear glasses to read, put them on to check drug labels. It is easy to take the wrong drug at the wrong time.

- Don't keep by your bedside any drugs that change mood, alertness or judgment such as sedatives, narcotics or tranquilizers. These cause many accidental overdose deaths. You may unknowingly repeat a dose when you are half asleep or confused.

- Know the names of your medicines. These include the generic name, the brand name and the generic names of all ingredients in a drug mixture. Your doctor, nurse or pharmacist can give you this information.

- Study the labels on all non-prescription drugs. If the information is incomplete or if you have questions, ask the pharmacist for more details.

- If you must deviate from your prescribed dose schedule, tell your doctor.

- Shake liquid medicines before taking.

- Store all medicines away from moisture and heat. Bathroom medicine cabinets are usually unsuitable.

- If a drug needs refrigeration, don't freeze.

- Obtain a standard measuring spoon from your pharmacy for liquid medicines. Kitchen teaspoons and tablespoons are not accurate enough.

- Follow diet instructions when you take medicines. Some work better on a full stomach, others on an empty stomach. Some drugs are more useful with special diets. For example, medicine for high blood pressure is more effective if accompanied by a sodium-restricted diet.

- Tell your doctor about any allergies you have. A previous allergy to a drug may make it dangerous to prescribe again. People with other allergies, such as eczema, hay fever, asthma, bronchitis and food allergies, are more likely to be allergic to drugs.

- Prior to surgery, tell your doctor, anesthesiologist or dentist about any drug you have taken in the past few weeks. Advise them of any cortisone drugs you have taken within two years.

- If you become pregnant while taking any medicine, including birth-control pills, tell your doctor immediately.

- Avoid *all* drugs while you are pregnant, if possible. If you must take drugs during pregnancy, record names, amounts, dates and reasons.

- If you see more than one doctor, tell each one about drugs others have prescribed.

- When you use non-prescription drugs, report it so the information is on your medical record.

- Store all drugs away from the reach of children.

- Note the expiration date on each drug label. Discard outdated ones safely.

- Pay attention to the information in the charts about safety while driving, piloting or working in dangerous places.

- Alcohol, cocaine, marijuana, other mood-altering drugs and tobacco—mixed with some drugs—can cause a life-threatening interaction, prevent your medicine from being effective or delay your return to health. Common sense dictates that you avoid them during illness.

ACETAMINOPHEN

BRAND NAMES

Campain
Comtrex
Co-Tylenol
Datril
Dristan
Excedrin
Liquiprin
Midol PMS
Sinarest
Sine-Aid
Tylenol
Vanquish

See complete brand names list, page 820.

GENERAL INFORMATION

Habit forming? No
Prescription needed? No
Available as generic? Yes
Drug class: Analgesic, fever-reducer

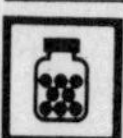

USES

Treatment of mild to moderate pain and fever. Acetaminophen does not relieve redness, stiffness or swelling of joints or tissue inflammation. Use aspirin or other drugs for inflammation.

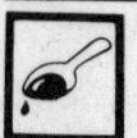

DOSAGE & USAGE INFORMATION

How to take:

- Tablet or capsule—Swallow with liquid.
- Effervescent granules—Dissolve granules in 4 oz. of cool water. Drink all the water.
- Suppositories—Remove wrapper and moisten suppository with water. Gently insert larger end into rectum. Push well into rectum with finger.

When to take:
As needed, no more often than every 3 hours.

If you forget a dose:
Take as soon as you remember. Wait 3 hours for next dose.

What drug does:
May affect hypothalamus—part of brain that helps regulate body heat and receives body's pain messages.

Time lapse before drug works:
15 to 30 minutes. May last 4 hours.

Don't take with:

- Other drugs with acetaminophen. Too much acetaminophen can damage liver and kidneys.
- See Interaction column and consult doctor.

OVERDOSE

Symptoms:
Stomach upset, irritability, convulsions, coma.

What to do:

- Call your doctor or poison-control center for advice if you suspect overdose, even if not sure. Symptoms may not appear until damage has occurred.
- Additional emergency information on page 886.

POSSIBLE ADVERSE REACTIONS OR SIDE EFFECTS

SYMPTOMS	FREQUENCY	WHAT TO DO
Brain & nervous system: Extreme fatigue.	Rare	3
Skin: Rash, itch, hives.	Rare	3
Eyes:	None expected.	
Ears, nose, throat: Sore throat and fever after a few days.	Rare	3
Digestive:	None expected.	
Heart & lungs:	None expected.	
Blood vessels: Unexplained bleeding or bruising.	Rare	3
Muscles, bones, joints:	None expected.	
Genital, urinary: Blood in urine, painful urination or frequent urge to urinate.	Rare	3
Kidneys: Less urine.	Rare	4
Liver: Jaundice (yellow skin and eyes).	Rare	3
Allergic:	None expected.	
Blood: Anemia	Rare	3
Others:	None expected.	

1- Life-threatening. Seek emergency treatment immediately.
2- Discontinue. Seek emergency treatment.
3- Discontinue. Call doctor right away.
4- Continue. Call doctor when convenient.
5- Continue. Tell doctor at next visit.
6- No action necessary.

ACETAMINOPHEN

WARNINGS & PRECAUTIONS

Don't take if:
- You are allergic to acetaminophen.
- Your symptoms don't improve after 2 days use. Call your doctor.

Before you start, consult your doctor:
If you have bronchial asthma, kidney disease or liver damage.

Over age 60:
Don't exceed recommended dose. You can't eliminate drug as efficiently as younger persons.

Pregnancy:
No proven harm to unborn child. Avoid if possible.

Breast-feeding:
No proven harm to nursing infant.

Infants & children:
Use only under medical supervision.

Prolonged use:
May affect blood system and cause anemia. Limit use to 5 days for children 12 and under, and 10 days for adults.

Skin & sunlight:
No problems expected.

Driving, piloting or hazardous work:
Avoid if you feel drowsy. Otherwise, no restrictions.

Airplane passengers:
No problems expected.

Discontinuing:
Discontinue in 2 days if symptoms don't improve.

Others:
No problems expected.

INTERACTION WITH OTHER DRUGS

GENERIC NAME OR DRUG CLASS	COMBINED EFFECT
Anticoagulants (oral)	Danger of hidden bleeding.
Phenobarbital	Quicker elimination of and decreased effect of acetaminophen.
Tetracyclines (effervescent granules or tablets)	May slow tetracycline absorption. Space doses 2 hours apart.

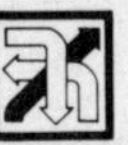

INTERACTION WITH OTHER SUBSTANCES

INTERACTS WITH	COMBINED EFFECT
Alcohol:	Drowsiness
Beverages:	None expected.
Cocaine:	None expected. However, cocaine may slow body's recovery. Avoid.
Foods:	None expected.
Marijuana:	Increased pain relief. However, marijuana may slow body's recovery. Avoid.
Tobacco:	None expected.

ACETOHEXAMIDE

BRAND NAMES

Dymelor
Dimelor

GENERAL INFORMATION

Habit forming? No
Prescription needed? Yes
Available as generic? No
Drug class: Antidiabetic (oral), sulfonurea

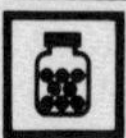

USES

Treatment for diabetes in adults who can't control blood sugar by diet, weight loss and exercise.

DOSAGE & USAGE INFORMATION

How to take:
Tablet—Swallow with liquid or food to lessen stomach irritation. If you can't swallow whole, crumble tablet and take with liquid or food.

When to take:
At the same times each day.

If you forget a dose:
Take as soon as you remember up to 2 hours late. If more than 2 hours, wait for next scheduled dose (don't double this dose).

What drug does:
Stimulates pancreas to produce more insulin. Insulin in blood forces cells to use sugar in blood.

Time lapse before drug works:
3 to 4 hours. May require 2 weeks for maximum benefit.

Don't take with:
See Interaction column and consult doctor.

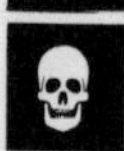

OVERDOSE

Symptoms:
Excessive hunger, nausea, anxiety, cool skin, cold sweats, drowsiness, rapid heartbeat, weakness, unconsciousness, coma.

What to do:
- Dial 0 (operator) or 911 (emergency) for an ambulance or medical help. Then give first aid immediately.
- Additional emergency information on page 886.

POSSIBLE ADVERSE REACTIONS OR SIDE EFFECTS

SYMPTOMS	FREQUENCY	WHAT TO DO
Brain & nervous system:		
• Dizziness	Common	3
• Fatigue	Rare	3
Skin:		
Itching or rash.	Rare	3
Eyes:	None expected.	
Ears, nose, throat:		
• Sore throat, fever.	Rare	3
• Ringing in ears.	Rare	3
Digestive:		
Diarrhea, loss of appetite, nausea, stomach pain, heartburn.	Common	4
Heart & lungs, muscles, bones, joints, genital, urinary, kidneys, allergic, blood:	None expected.	
Blood vessels:		
Unusual bleeding or bruising.	Rare	3
Liver:		
Jaundice (yellow skin and eyes).	Rare	3
Others:		
Low blood sugar (ravenous hunger, nausea, anxiety, cold sweats, cool skin, chills, drowsiness, nervousness, headache, rapid heartbeat, weakness).	Infrequent	2

1- Life-threatening. Seek emergency treatment immediately.
2- Discontinue. Seek emergency treatment.
3- Discontinue. Call doctor right away.
4- Continue. Call doctor when convenient.

WARNINGS & PRECAUTIONS

Don't take if:
- You are allergic to any sulfonurea.
- You have impaired kidney or liver function.

Before you start, consult your doctor:
- If you have a severe infection.
- If you have thyroid disease.
- If you take insulin.
- If you have heart disease.

Over age 60:
Dose usually smaller than for younger adults. Avoid "low-blood-sugar" episodes because repeated ones can damage brain permanently.

Pregnancy:
No proven harm to unborn child. Avoid if possible.

Breast-feeding:
Drug filters into milk. May lower baby's blood sugar. Avoid.

Infants & children:
Don't give to infants or children.

Prolonged use:
None expected.

Skin & sunlight:
May cause rash or intensify sunburn in areas exposed to sun or sunlamp.

Driving, piloting or hazardous work:
No problems expected unless you develop hypoglycemia (low blood sugar). If so, avoid driving or hazardous activity.

Airplane passengers:
No problems expected.

Discontinuing:
Don't discontinue without consulting doctor. Dose may require gradual reduction if you have taken drug for a long time. Doses of other drugs may also require adjustment.

Others:
- Don't exceed 1500 mg. in 1 day.
- Hypoglycemia (low blood sugar) may occur, even with proper dose schedule. You must balance medicine, diet and exercise.

INTERACTION WITH OTHER DRUGS

GENERIC NAME OR DRUG CLASS	COMBINED EFFECT
Androgens	Increased acetohexamide effect.
Anticoagulants (oral)	Unpredictable prothrombin times (see page 848).
Anticonvulsants (hydantoin)	Decreased acetohexamide effect.
Antiinflammatory drugs (non-steroidal)	Increased acetohexamide effect.
Aspirin	Increased acetohexamide effect.
Beta-adrenergic blockers	Increased acetohexamide effect.
Chloramphenicol	Increased acetohexamide effect.
Clofibrate	Increased acetohexamide effect.
Contraceptives (oral)	Decreased acetohexamide effect.
Cortisone drugs	Decreased acetohexamide effect.
Diuretics (thiazide)	Decreased acetohexamide effect.
Epinephrine	Decreased acetohexamide effect.
Estrogens	Increased acetohexamide effect.
Guanethidine	Unpredictable acetohexamide effect.

Additional interactions on page 834.

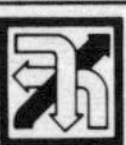

INTERACTION WITH OTHER SUBSTANCES

INTERACTS WITH	COMBINED EFFECT
Alcohol:	Disulfiram reaction (see page 846). Avoid.
Beverages:	None expected.
Cocaine:	No proven problems.
Foods:	None expected.
Marijuana:	Decreased acetohexamide effect. Avoid.
Tobacco:	None expected.

ACETOPHENAZINE

BRAND NAMES

Tindal

GENERAL INFORMATION

Habit forming? No
Prescription needed? Yes
Available as generic? Yes
Drug class: Tranquilizer, antiemetic (phenothiazine)

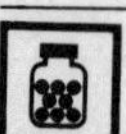

USES

- Stops nausea, vomiting.
- Reduces anxiety, agitation.

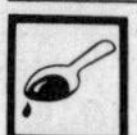

DOSAGE & USAGE INFORMATION

How to take:

- Tablet or capsule—Swallow with liquid or food to lessen stomach irritation.
- Suppositories—Remove wrapper and moisten suppository with water. Gently insert into rectum, large end first.
- Drops or liquid—Dilute dose in beverage.

When to take:

- Nervous and mental disorders—Take at the same times each day.
- Nausea and vomiting—Take as needed, no more often than every 4 hours.

If you forget a dose:

- Nervous and mental disorders—Take up to 2 hours late. If more than 2 hours, wait for next scheduled dose (don't double this).
- Nausea and vomiting—Take as soon as you remember. Wait 4 hours for next dose.

What drug does:

- Suppresses brain's vomiting center.
- Suppresses brain centers that control abnormal emotions and behavior.

Time lapse before drug works:

- Nausea and vomiting—1 hour or less.
- Nervous and mental disorders—4-6 weeks.

Don't take with:

- Antacid or medicine for diarrhea.
- Non-prescription drug for cough, cold or allergy.
- See Interaction column and consult doctor.

OVERDOSE

Symptoms:
Stupor, convulsions, coma.

What to do:

- Dial 0 (operator) or 911 (emergency) for an ambulance or medical help. Then give first aid immediately.
- Additional emergency information on page 886.

POSSIBLE ADVERSE REACTIONS OR SIDE EFFECTS

SYMPTOMS	FREQUENCY	WHAT TO DO
Brain & nervous system:		
• Restlessness, tremor.	Common	3
• Fainting	Infrequent	2
• Drowsiness	Common	3
Skin:		
• Rash	Infrequent	3
• Less perspiration.	Common	4
Eyes:		
Vision changes.	Rare	3
Ears, nose, throat:		
• Sore throat, fever.	Rare	3
• Dry mouth, nasal congestion.	Common	4
Digestive:		
Constipation	Common	4
Heart & lungs, blood vessels, kidneys, allergic, blood:	None expected.	
Muscles, bones, joints:		
Muscle spasms of face and neck, unsteady gait.	Common	2
Genital, urinary:		
Urination difficulty.	Infrequent	4
Liver:		
Jaundice (yellow eyes and skin).	Rare	3
Others:		
Less interest in sex, breast swelling, change in menstrual pattern.	Infrequent	4

1- Life-threatening. Seek emergency treatment immediately.
2- Discontinue. Seek emergency treatment.
3- Discontinue. Call doctor right away.
4- Continue. Call doctor when convenient.
5- Continue. Tell doctor at next visit.
6- No action necessary.

WARNINGS & PRECAUTIONS

Don't take if:
- You are allergic to any phenothiazine.
- You have a blood or bone-marrow disease.

Before you start, consult your doctor:
- If you will have surgery within 2 months, including dental surgery, requiring general or spinal anesthesia.
- If you have asthma, emphysema or other lung disorder.
- If you take non-prescription ulcer medicine, asthma medicine or amphetamines.

Over age 60:
Adverse reactions and side effects may be more frequent and severe than in younger persons. More likely to develop involuntary movement of jaws, lips, tongue, chewing. Report this to your doctor immediately. Early treatment can help.

Pregnancy:
Risk to unborn child outweighs drug benefits. Don't use.

Breast-feeding:
Drug passes into milk. Avoid drug or discontinue nursing until you finish medicine. Consult doctor for advice on maintaining milk supply.

Infants & children:
Don't give to children younger than 2.

Prolonged use:
May lead to tardive dyskinesia (involuntary movement of jaws, lips, tongue, chewing).

Skin & sunlight:
May cause rash or intensify sunburn in areas exposed to sun or sunlamp. Skin may remain sensitive for 3 months after discontinuing.

Driving, piloting or hazardous work:
Don't drive or pilot aircraft until you learn how medicine affects you. Don't work around dangerous machinery. Don't climb ladders or work in high places. Danger increases if you drink alcohol or take medicine affecting alertness and reflexes.

Airplane passengers:
No problems expected.

Discontinuing:
- Nervous and mental disorders—Don't discontinue without doctor's advice until you complete prescribed dose, even though symptoms diminish or disappear.
- Nausea and vomiting—May be unnecessary to finish medicine. Follow doctor's instructions.

INTERACTION WITH OTHER DRUGS

GENERIC NAME OR DRUG CLASS	COMBINED EFFECT
Anticholinergics	Increased anticholinergic effect.
Antidepressants (tricyclic)	Increased acetophenazine effect.
Antihistamines	Increased antihistamine effect.
Appetite suppressants	Decreased suppressant effect.
Levodopa	Decreased levodopa effect.
Mind-altering drugs	Increased effect of mind-altering drugs.
Narcotics	Increased narcotic effect.
Phenytoin	Increased phenytoin effect.
Quinidine	Impaired heart function. Dangerous mixture.
Sedatives	Increased sedative effect.
Tranquilizers (other)	Increased tranquilizer effect.

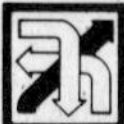

INTERACTION WITH OTHER SUBSTANCES

INTERACTS WITH	COMBINED EFFECT
Alcohol:	Dangerous oversedation.
Beverages:	None expected.
Cocaine:	Decreased acetophenazine effect. Avoid.
Foods:	None expected.
Marijuana:	Drowsiness. May increase antinausea effect.
Tobacco:	None expected.

ACYCLOVIR

BRAND NAMES

Zovirax
Zovirax Ointment

GENERAL INFORMATION

Habit forming? No
Prescription needed? Yes
Available as generic? No
Drug class: Antiviral

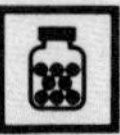

USES

- Treatment of severe herpes infections of genitals occurring for first time in special cases.
- Treatment of severe herpes infections on mucous membrane of mouth and lips in special cases.
- Used (although not yet approved by FDA) for shingles (herpes zoster) and chicken pox (varicella) in special cases.

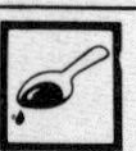

DOSAGE & USAGE INFORMATION

How to take:
- Tablet or capsule—Swallow with liquid.
- Ointment—Apply to skin and mucous membranes every 3 hours (6 times a day) for 7 days. Use rubber glove when applying. Apply 1/2-inch strip to each sore or blister.

When to use:
As directed on label.

If you forget a dose:
Take as soon as you remember up to 2 hours late. If more than 2 hours, wait for next scheduled dose (don't double this dose).

What drug does:
- Inhibits reproduction of virus in cells without killing normal cells.
- Does not cure. Herpes may recur.

Time lapse before drug works:
2 hours.

Don't take with:
See Interaction column and consult doctor.

OVERDOSE

Symptoms:
Hallucinations, seizures, kidney shutdown.

What to do:
- Dial 0 (operator) or 911 (emergency) for an ambulance or medical help. Then give first aid immediately.
- Additional emergency information on page 886.

POSSIBLE ADVERSE REACTIONS OR SIDE EFFECTS

SYMPTOMS	FREQUENCY	WHAT TO DO
Brain & nervous system:		
• Confusion	Infrequent	3
• Hallucinations	Infrequent	3
• Trembling	Infrequent	3
• Lightheadedness, headache.	Common	4
Skin:		
• Rash, hives, itch.	Common	4
• Mild pain, burning, stinging.	Common	4
Eyes:	None expected.	
Ears, nose, throat:	None expected.	
Digestive:		
• Abdominal pain.	Rare	3
• Decreased appetite.	Rare	3
• Nausea, vomiting.	Rare	3
Heart & lungs:		
Breathing difficulty.	Rare	3
Blood vessels:	None expected.	
Muscles, bones, joints:	None expected.	
Genital, urinary:		
Bloody urine, decreased urine volume.	Rare	3
Kidneys, allergic, blood, liver:	None expected.	

1 - Life-threatening. Seek emergency treatment immediately.
2 - Discontinue. Seek emergency treatment.
3 - Discontinue. Call doctor right away.
4 - Continue. Call doctor when convenient.
5 - Continue. Tell doctor at next visit.
6 - No action necessary.

WARNINGS & PRECAUTIONS

Don't take if:
You are allergic to acyclovir.

Before you start, consult your doctor:
- If pregnant or plan pregnancy.
- If breast-feeding.
- If you have kidney disease.
- If you have any nerve disorder.

Over age 60:
Adverse reactions and side effects may be more frequent and severe than in younger persons.

Pregnancy:
Risk to unborn child outweighs drug benefits. Don't use.

Breast-feeding:
Drug passes into milk. Avoid drug or discontinue nursing until you finish medicine. Consult doctor for advice on maintaining milk supply.

Infants & children:
Use only under special medical supervision by experienced clinician.

Prolonged use:
Don't use longer than prescribed time.

Skin & sunlight:
No problems expected.

Driving, piloting or hazardous work:
No problems expected.

Airplane passengers:
No problems expected.

Discontinuing:
May be unnecessary to finish medicine. Follow doctor's instructions.

Others:
Women: Get Pap smear every 6 months because those with herpes infections are more likely to develop cancer of cervix. Avoid sexual activity until all blisters or sores heal. Don't get medicine in eyes.

INTERACTION WITH OTHER DRUGS

GENERIC NAME OR DRUG CLASS	COMBINED EFFECT
Interferon	Neurological abnormalities. Avoid.
Methotrexate	Neurological abnormalities. Avoid.
Other medications that can cause toxic effects on kidneys: **Amikacin** **Amphotericin B** **Capreomycin** **Colistimethate** **Colistin** **Gentamycin** **Kanamycin** **Neomycin** **Netilmicin** **Polymixin B** **Probenecid** **Streptomycin** **Tobramycin** **Vancomycin**	Increase kidney toxicity.

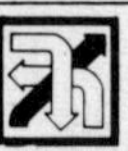

INTERACTION WITH OTHER SUBSTANCES

INTERACTS WITH	COMBINED EFFECT
Alcohol:	Increased chance of brain and nervous system adverse reaction. Avoid.
Beverages:	No problems expected.
Cocaine:	Increased chance of brain and nervous system adverse reaction. Avoid.
Foods:	No problems expected.
Marijuana:	Increased chance of brain and nervous system adverse reaction. Avoid.
Tobacco:	No problems expected.

ADRENOCORTICOIDS (TOPICAL)

BRAND NAMES

Aristocort	Decadron	Medrol	Vioform
Celestone	Decaspray	Neo-Cortef	
Cordran	Hydrocortone	Neo-Decadron	
Cort-Dome	Kenalog	Synalar	
Cortef	Lidex	Topicort	
Cortril	Locorten	Valisone	

See complete brand names list, page 820.

GENERAL INFORMATION

Habit forming? No
Prescription needed? Yes
Available as generic? Yes
Drug class: Adrenocorticoid (topical)

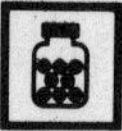

USES

Relieves redness, swelling, itching, skin discomfort of hemorrhoids, insect bites, poison ivy, oak, sumac, soaps, cosmetics and jewelry.

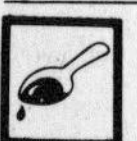

DOSAGE & USAGE INFORMATION

How to use:
- Cream, lotion, ointment—Apply small amount and rub in gently.
- Topical aerosol—Follow directions on container. Don't breathe vapors.

When to use:
When needed or as directed. Don't use more often than directions allow.

If you forget an application:
Use as soon as you remember.

What drug does:
Reduces inflammation by affecting enzymes that produce inflammation.

Time lapse before drug works:
15 to 20 minutes.

Don't use with:
See Interaction column and consult doctor.

OVERDOSE

Symptoms:
None expected.

What to do:
If person swallows or inhales drug, call doctor, poison-control center or hospital emergency room for instructions.

POSSIBLE ADVERSE REACTIONS OR SIDE EFFECTS

SYMPTOMS	FREQUENCY	WHAT TO DO
Brain & nervous system:	None expected.	
Skin:		
• Infection with pain, redness, blisters, pus.	Infrequent	4
• Skin irritation with burning, itching, blistering or peeling.	Infrequent	4
• Acne-like eruptions.	Infrequent	4
Eyes:	None expected.	
Ears, nose, throat:	None expected.	
Digestive:	None expected.	
Heart & lungs:	None expected.	
Blood vessels:	None expected.	
Muscles, bones, joints:	None expected.	
Genital, urinary:	None expected.	
Kidneys:	None expected.	
Liver:	None expected.	
Allergic:	None expected.	
Blood:	None expected.	
Others:	None expected.	

1- Life-threatening. Seek emergency treatment immediately.
2- Discontinue. Seek emergency treatment.
3- Discontinue. Call doctor right away.
4- Continue. Call doctor when convenient.
5- Continue. Tell doctor at next visit.
6- No action necessary.

ADRENOCORTICOIDS (TOPICAL)

WARNINGS & PRECAUTIONS

Don't take if:
You are allergic to any topical adrenocorticoid (cortisone) preparation.

Before you start, consult your doctor:
- If you plan pregnancy within medication period.
- If you have diabetes.
- If you have infection at treatment site.
- If you have stomach ulcer.
- If you have tuberculosis.

Over age 60:
Adverse reactions and side effects may be more frequent and severe than in younger persons, especially thinning of the skin.

Pregnancy:
Risk to unborn child outweighs drug benefits. Don't use.

Breast-feeding:
No problems expected.

Infants & children:
- Use only under medical supervision. Too much for too long can be absorbed into bloodstream through skin and retard growth.
- For infants in diapers, avoid plastic pants or tight diapers.

Prolonged use:
- Increases chance of absorption into bloodstream to cause side effects of oral cortisone drugs (see page 202).
- May thin skin where used.

Skin & sunlight:
No problems expected.

Driving, piloting or hazardous work:
No problems expected.

Airplane passengers:
No problems expected.

Discontinuing:
May be unnecessary to finish medicine. Follow doctor's instructions.

Others:
- Don't use a plastic dressing longer than 2 weeks.
- Aerosol spray—Store in cool place. Don't use near heat or open flame or while smoking. Don't puncture, break or burn container.

INTERACTION WITH OTHER DRUGS

GENERIC NAME OR DRUG CLASS	COMBINED EFFECT
Antibiotics (topical)	Decreased antibiotic effects.
Antifungals (topical)	Decreased antifungal effect.

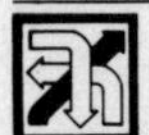

INTERACTION WITH OTHER SUBSTANCES

INTERACTS WITH	COMBINED EFFECT
Alcohol:	None expected.
Beverages:	None expected.
Cocaine:	None expected.
Foods:	None expected.
Marijuana:	None expected.
Tobacco:	None expected.

ALLOPURINOL

BRAND NAMES

Alloprin
Apo-Allopurinol
Lopurin
Novopurol
Purinol
Roucol
Zyloprim

GENERAL INFORMATION

Habit forming? No
Prescription needed? Yes
Available as generic? Yes
Drug class: Antigout

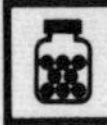

USES

- Treatment for chronic gout.
- Prevention of kidney stones caused by uric acid.

DOSAGE & USAGE INFORMATION

How to take:
Tablet—Swallow with liquid or food to lessen stomach irritation.

When to take:
At the same times each day.

If you forget a dose:
- 1 dose per day—Take as soon as you remember up to 6 hours late. If more than 6 hours, wait for next scheduled dose (don't double this dose).
- More than 1 dose per day—Take as soon as you remember up to 3 hours late. If more than 3 hours, wait for next scheduled dose (don't double this dose).

What drug does:
Slows formation of uric acid by inhibiting enzyme (xanthine oxidase) activity.

Time lapse before drug works:
Reduces blood uric acid in 1 to 3 weeks. May require 6 months to prevent acute gout attacks.

Don't take with:
- Vitamin C.
- See Interaction column and consult doctor.

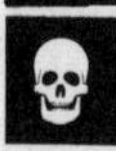

OVERDOSE

Symptoms:
None expected.

What to do:
Overdose unlikely to threaten life. If person takes much larger amount than prescribed, call doctor, poison-control center or hospital emergency room for instructions.

POSSIBLE ADVERSE REACTIONS OR SIDE EFFECTS

SYMPTOMS	FREQUENCY	WHAT TO DO
Brain & nervous system: Drowsiness	Infrequent	4
Skin: Rash, hives, itch.	Common	3
Eyes:	None expected.	
Ears, nose, throat: Sore throat, fever.	Rare	3
Digestive: Diarrhea, stomach pain, nausea, vomiting.	Infrequent	4
Heart & lungs:	None expected.	
Blood vessels: Unusual bleeding or bruising.	Rare	3
Muscles, bones, joints: Numbness, tingling, pain in hands or feet.	Rare	4
Genital, urinary:	None expected.	
Kidneys:	None expected.	
Liver: Jaundice (yellow skin and eyes).	Infrequent	3
Allergic:	None expected.	
Blood:	None expected.	
Others:	None expected.	

1-Life-threatening. Seek emergency treatment immediately.
2-Discontinue. Seek emergency treatment.
3-Discontinue. Call doctor right away.
4-Continue. Call doctor when convenient.
5-Continue. Tell doctor at next visit.
6-No action necessary.

WARNINGS & PRECAUTIONS

Don't take if:
You are allergic to allopurinol.

Before you start, consult your doctor:
If you have had liver or kidney problems.

Over age 60:
Adverse reactions and side effects may be more frequent and severe than in younger persons.

Pregnancy:
Studies inconclusive on harm to unborn child. Animal studies show fetal abnormalities. Decide with your doctor whether drug benefits justify risk to unborn child.

Breast-feeding:
Drug passes into milk. Avoid drug or discontinue nursing.

Infants & children:
Not recommended.

Prolonged use:
No problems expected.

Skin & sunlight:
No problems expected.

Driving, piloting or hazardous work:
Avoid if you feel drowsy. Use may disqualify you for piloting aircraft.

Airplane passengers:
No problems expected.

Discontinuing:
Don't discontinue without doctor's advice until you complete prescribed dose, even though symptoms diminish or disappear.

Others:
Acute gout attacks may increase during first weeks of use. If so, consult doctor about additional medicine.

INTERACTION WITH OTHER DRUGS

GENERIC NAME OR DRUG CLASS	COMBINED EFFECT
Ampicillin	Likely skin rash.
Anticoagulants (oral)	Increased anticoagulant effect.
Antidiabetics (oral)	Increased uric-acid elimination.
Azathioprine	Increased azathioprine effect.
Chlorthalidone	Decreased allopurinol effect.
Cyclophosphamide	Increased cyclophosphamide toxicity.
Diuretics (thiazide)	Decreased allopurinol effect.
Ethacrynic acid	Decreased allopurinol effect.
Furosemide	Decreased allopurinol effect.
Iron supplements	Excessive accumulation of iron in tissues.
Mercaptopurine	Increased mercaptopurine effect.

Additional interactions on page 834.

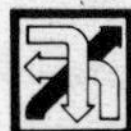

INTERACTION WITH OTHER SUBSTANCES

INTERACTS WITH	COMBINED EFFECT
Alcohol:	None expected, but may impair management of gout.
Beverages: Caffeine drinks	Decreased allopurinol effect.
Cocaine:	Decreased allopurinol effect. Avoid.
Foods:	None expected. Low-purine diet recommended (see page 849).
Marijuana:	Occasional use—None expected. Daily use—Possible increase in uric-acid level.
Tobacco:	None expected.

ALPRAZOLAM

BRAND NAMES

Xanax

GENERAL INFORMATION

Habit forming? Yes
Prescription needed? Yes
Available as generic? No
Drug class: Tranquilizer (benzodiazepine)

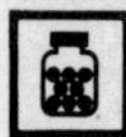

USES

Treatment for nervousness or tension.

DOSAGE & USAGE INFORMATION

How to take:
Tablet or capsule—Swallow with liquid. If you can't swallow whole, crumble tablet or open capsule and take with liquid or food.

When to take:
At the same time each day, according to instructions on prescription label.

If you forget a dose:
Take as soon as you remember up to 2 hours late. If more than 2 hours, wait for next scheduled dose (don't double this dose).

What drug does:
Affects limbic system of brain—part that controls emotions.

Time lapse before drug works:
2 hours. May take 6 weeks for full benefit.

Don't take with:
See Interaction column and consult doctor.

OVERDOSE

Symptoms:
Drowsiness, weakness, tremor, stupor, coma.

What to do:
- Dial 0 (operator) or 911 (emergency) for an ambulance or medical help. Then give first aid immediately.
- If patient is unconscious and not breathing, give mouth-to-mouth breathing. If there is no heartbeat, use cardiac massage and mouth-to-mouth breathing (CPR). Don't try to make patient vomit. If you can't get help quickly, take patient to nearest emergency facility.
- Additional emergency information on page 886.

POSSIBLE ADVERSE REACTIONS OR SIDE EFFECTS

SYMPTOMS	FREQUENCY	WHAT TO DO
Brain & nervous system:		
• Clumsiness, drowsiness, dizziness.	Common	4
• Hallucinations, confusion, depression, irritability.	Infrequent	3
Skin:		
Rash, itch.	Infrequent	3
Eyes:		
Vision changes.	Infrequent	3
Ears, nose, throat:		
Mouth, throat ulcers.	Rare	3
Digestive:		
Constipation or diarrhea, nausea, vomiting.	Infrequent	4
Heart & lungs:		
Slow heartbeat, breathing difficulty.	Rare	2
Blood vessels:	None expected.	
Muscles, bones, joints:	None expected.	
Genital, urinary:		
Urination difficulty.	Infrequent	4
Kidneys:	None expected.	
Liver:		
Jaundice (yellow eyes and skin).	Rare	3
Allergic:	None expected.	
Blood:	None expected.	
Others:	None expected.	

1- Life-threatening. Seek emergency treatment immediately.
2- Discontinue. Seek emergency treatment.
3- Discontinue. Call doctor right away.
4- Continue. Call doctor when convenient.
5- Continue. Tell doctor at next visit.
6- No action necessary.

WARNINGS & PRECAUTIONS

Don't take if:
- You are allergic to any benzodiazepine.
- You have myasthenia gravis.
- You are active or recovering alcoholic.
- Patient is younger than 6 months.

Before you start, consult your doctor:
- If you have liver, kidney or lung disease.
- If you have diabetes, epilepsy or porphyria.

Over age 60:
Adverse reactions and side effects may be more frequent and severe than in younger persons. You need smaller doses for shorter periods of time. May develop agitation, rage or "hangover effect."

Pregnancy:
Risk to unborn child outweighs drug benefits. Don't use.

Breast-feeding:
Drug passes into milk. Avoid drug or discontinue nursing until you finish medicine. Consult doctor for advice on maintaining milk supply.

Infants & children:
Use only under medical supervision for children older than 6 months.

Prolonged use:
May impair liver function.

Skin & sunlight:
No problems expected.

Driving, piloting or hazardous work:
Don't drive or pilot aircraft until you learn how medicine affects you. Don't work around dangerous machinery. Don't climb ladders or work in high places. Danger increases if you drink alcohol or take medicine affecting alertness and reflexes.

Airplane passengers:
No problems expected.

Discontinuing:
Don't discontinue without consulting doctor. Dose may require gradual reduction if you have taken drug for a long time. Doses of other drugs may also require adjustment.

Others:
- Hot weather, heavy exercise and profuse sweat may reduce excretion and cause overdose.
- Blood sugar may rise in diabetics, requiring insulin adjustment.

INTERACTION WITH OTHER DRUGS

GENERIC NAME OR DRUG CLASS	COMBINED EFFECT
Anticonvulsants	Change in seizure frequency or severity.
Antidepressants	Increased sedative effect of both drugs.
Antihistamines	Increased sedative effect of both drugs.
Antihypertensives	Excessively low blood pressure.
Cimetidine	Excess sedation.
Disulfiram	Increased alprazolam effect.
MAO inhibitors	Convulsions, deep sedation, rage.
Narcotics	Increased sedative effect of both drugs.
Sedatives	Increased sedative effect of both drugs.
Sleep inducers	Increased sedative effect of both drugs.
Tranquilizers	Increased sedative effect of both drugs.

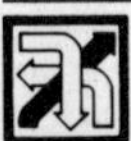

INTERACTION WITH OTHER SUBSTANCES

INTERACTS WITH	COMBINED EFFECT
Alcohol:	Heavy sedation. Avoid.
Beverages:	None expected.
Cocaine:	Decreased alprazolam effect.
Foods:	None expected.
Marijuana:	Heavy sedation. Avoid.
Tobacco:	Decreased alprazolam effect.

ALUMINUM HYDROXIDE

BRAND NAMES

Camalox	Ducon	Mylanta
Chemgel	Kolantyl Wafers	Mucotin
Creamalin	Maalox	Pepsogel
Delcid	Magnatril	Robalate
Di-Gel	Maxamag	Rolaids

See complete brand names list, page 821.

GENERAL INFORMATION

Habit forming? No
Prescription needed? No
Available as generic? Yes
Drug class: Antacid, antidiarrheal

USES

- Binds excess phosphate in intestine.
- Treatment for hyperacidity in upper gastrointestinal tract, including stomach and esophagus. Symptoms may be heartburn or acid indigestion. Diseases include peptic ulcer, gastritis, esophagitis, hiatal hernia.
- Treatment for diarrhea.

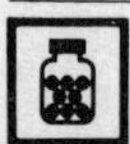

DOSAGE & USAGE INFORMATION

How to take:
- Tablet or capsule—Swallow with liquid.
- Chewable tablets or wafers—Chew well before swallowing.
- Liquid—Shake well and take undiluted.

When to take:
1 to 3 hours after meals unless directed otherwise by your doctor.

If you forget a dose:
Take as soon as you remember, but not simultaneously with any other medicine.

What drug does:
- Neutralizes some of the hydrochloric acid in the stomach.
- Reduces action of pepsin, a digestive enzyme.

Time lapse before drug works:
15 minutes.

Don't take with:
Other medicines at the same time. Decreases absorption of other drugs. Wait 2 hours between doses.

OVERDOSE

Symptoms:
Weakness, fatigue, dizziness.

What to do:
Overdose unlikely to threaten life. If person takes much larger amount than prescribed, call doctor, poison-control center or hospital emergency room for instructions.

POSSIBLE ADVERSE REACTIONS OR SIDE EFFECTS

SYMPTOMS	FREQUENCY	WHAT TO DO
Brain & nervous system:		
Mood changes.	Infrequent	4
Skin:	None expected.	
Eyes:	None expected.	
Ears, nose, throat:	None expected.	
Digestive:		
• Constipation, appetite loss.	Common	4
• Nausea, vomiting.	Infrequent	4
• Lower abdominal pain and swelling.	Infrequent	3
Heart & lungs:	None expected.	
Blood vessels:	None expected.	
Muscles, bones, joints:		
Bone pain, muscle weakness.	Infrequent	3
Genital, urinary:	None expected.	
Kidneys:	None expected.	
Liver:	None expected.	
Allergic:	None expected.	
Blood:	None expected.	
Others:		
• Swelling of wrists or ankles.	Infrequent	3
• Weight loss.	Infrequent	4

1-Life-threatening. Seek emergency treatment immediately.
2-Discontinue. Seek emergency treatment.
3-Discontinue. Call doctor right away.
4-Continue. Call doctor when convenient.
5-Continue. Tell doctor at next visit.
6-No action necessary.

ALUMINUM HYDROXIDE

WARNINGS & PRECAUTIONS

Don't take if:
You are allergic to any antacid.

Before you start, consult your doctor:
- If you have kidney disease.
- If you have chronic constipation, colitis or diarrhea.
- If you have symptoms of appendicitis.
- If you have have stomach or intestinal bleeding.

Over age 60:
Adverse reactions and side effects may be more frequent and severe than in younger persons. Diarrhea or constipation particularly likely.

Pregnancy:
Risk to unborn child outweighs drug benefits. Don't use.

Breast-feeding:
Drug passes into milk. Avoid drug or discontinue nursing until you finish medicine. Consult doctor for advice on maintaining milk supply.

Infants & children:
Use only under medical supervision.

Prolonged use:
Decreased phosphate level in blood weakens bones.

Skin & sunlight:
No problems expected.

Driving, piloting or hazardous work:
No problems expected.

Airplane passengers:
No problems expected.

Discontinuing:
May be unnecessary to finish medicine. Follow doctor's instructions.

Others:
Don't take longer than 2 weeks unless under medical supervision.

INTERACTION WITH OTHER DRUGS

GENERIC NAME OR DRUG CLASS	COMBINED EFFECT
Anticoagulants	Decreased anticoagulant effect.
Chlorpromazine	Decreased chlorpromazine effect.
Digitalis preparations	Decreased digitalis effect.
Iron supplements	Decreased iron effect.
Meperidine	Increased meperidine effect.
Nalidixic acid	Decreased effect of nalidixic acid.
Oxyphenbutazone	Decreased oxyphenbutazone effect.
Para-aminosalicylic acid (PAS)	Decreased PAS effect.
Penicillins	Decreased penicillin effect.
Pentobarbital	Decreased pentobarbital effect.
Phenylbutazone	Decreased phenylbutazone effect.
Pseudoephedrine	Increased pseudoephedrine effect.
Sulfa drugs	Decreased sulfa effect.
Tetracyclines	Decreased tetracycline effect.
Vitamins A and C	Decreased vitamin effect.

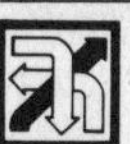

INTERACTION WITH OTHER SUBSTANCES

INTERACTS WITH	COMBINED EFFECT
Alcohol:	Decreased antacid effect.
Beverages:	No proven problems.
Cocaine:	No proven problems.
Foods:	Decreased antacid effect. Wait 1 hour after eating.
Marijuana:	No proven problems.
Tobacco:	Decreased antacid effect.

AMANTADINE

BRAND NAMES

Symmetrel

GENERAL INFORMATION

Habit forming? No
Prescription needed? Yes
Available as generic? No
Drug class: Antiviral, antiparkinsonism

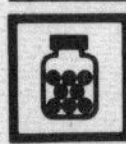

USES

- Treatment for Type-A flu infections.
- Relief for symptoms of Parkinson's disease.

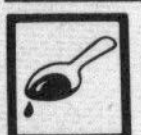

DOSAGE & USAGE INFORMATION

How to take:

- Tablet or capsule—Swallow with liquid or food to lessen stomach irritation.
- Syrup—Dilute dose in beverage before swallowing.

When to take:
At the same times each day. For Type-A flu it is especially important to take regular doses as prescribed.

If you forget a dose:
Take as soon as you remember. Wait 4 hours for next dose. Return to schedule.

What drug does:

- Type-A flu—May block penetration of tissue cells by infectious material from virus cells.
- Parkinson's disease—Improves muscular condition and coordination.

Time lapse before drug works:

- Type-A flu—48 hours.
- Parkinson's disease—2 days to 2 weeks.

Don't take with:

- Alcohol
- See Interaction column and consult doctor.

OVERDOSE

Symptoms:
Heart-rhythm disturbances, blood-pressure drop, convulsions, toxic psychosis.

What to do:

- Dial 0 (operator) or 911 (emergency) for an ambulance or medical help. Then give first aid immediately.
- Additional emergency information on page 886.

POSSIBLE ADVERSE REACTIONS OR SIDE EFFECTS

SYMPTOMS	FREQUENCY	WHAT TO DO
Brain & nervous system:		
• Hallucinations, confusion, mood changes.	Common	4
• Fainting, slurred speech.	Infrequent	3
• Dizziness, headache.	Common	5
Skin:		
• Purple blotches.	Common	5
• Rash	Rare	3
Eyes:		
Uncontrolled rolling of eyes, blurred vision.	Rare	3
Ears, nose, throat:		
• Dry mouth.	Common	6
• Sore throat, fever.	Rare	3
Digestive:		
• Constipation	Rare	5
• Appetite loss, nausea.	Common	5
• Vomiting	Rare	4
Heart & lungs, blood vessels, muscles, bones, joints, liver, allergic, blood:	None expected.	
Genital, urinary:		
Difficult urination.	Infrequent	4
Others:		
Faintness on standing.	Common	4

1- Life-threatening. Seek emergency treatment immediately.
2- Discontinue. Seek emergency treatment.
3- Discontinue. Call doctor right away.
4- Continue. Call doctor when convenient.
5- Continue. Tell doctor at next visit.
6- No action necessary.

WARNINGS & PRECAUTIONS

Don't take if:
You are allergic to amantadine.

Before you start, consult your doctor:
- If you have had epilepsy or other seizures.
- If you have had heart disease or heart failure.
- If you have had liver or kidney disease.
- If you have had peptic ulcers.
- If you have had eczema or skin rashes.
- If you have had emotional or mental disorders or taken drugs for them.

Over age 60:
Adverse reactions and side effects may be more frequent and severe than in younger persons.

Pregnancy:
Studies inconclusive on harm to unborn child. Animal studies show fetal abnormalities. Decide with your doctor whether benefits justify risk to unborn child.

Breast-feeding:
Drug passes into milk. Avoid drug or discontinue nursing until you finish medicine. Consult doctor for advice on maintaining milk supply.

Infants & children:
Use only under medical supervision.

Prolonged use:
Skin splotches, feet swelling, rapid weight gain, shortness of breath. Consult doctor.

Skin & sunlight:
No problems expected.

Driving, piloting or hazardous work:
Don't drive or pilot aircraft until you learn how medicine affects you. Don't work around dangerous machinery. Don't climb ladders or work in high places. Danger increases if you drink alcohol or take medicine affecting alertness and reflexes.

Airplane passengers:
No problems expected.

Discontinuing:
- Parkinson's disease—Don't discontinue without doctor's advice until you complete prescribed dose, even though symptoms diminish or disappear.
- Type-A flu—Discontinue 48 hours after symptoms disappear.

Others:
- Parkinson's disease—May lose effectiveness in 3 to 6 months. Consult doctor.
- Amantadine may increase susceptibility to German measles.

INTERACTION WITH OTHER DRUGS

GENERIC NAME OR DRUG CLASS	COMBINED EFFECT
Amphetamines	Increased amantadine effect. Possible excessive stimulation and agitation.
Anticholinergics	Increased benefit, but excessive anticholinergic dose produces mental confusion, hallucinations, delirium.
Appetite suppressants	Increased amantadine effect. Possible excessive stimulation and agitation.
Levodopa	Increased benefit of levodopa. Can cause agitation.
Sympathomimetics	Increased amantadine effect. Possible excessive stimulation and agitation.

INTERACTION WITH OTHER SUBSTANCES

INTERACTS WITH	COMBINED EFFECT
Alcohol:	Increased alcohol effect. Possible fainting.
Beverages:	None expected.
Cocaine:	Dangerous overstimulation.
Foods:	None expected.
Marijuana:	None expected.
Tobacco:	None expected.

AMBENONIUM

BRAND NAMES

Mytelase

GENERAL INFORMATION

Habit forming? No
Prescription needed? Yes
Available as generic? No
Drug class: Cholinergic (anticholinesterase)

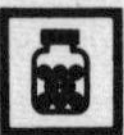

USES

- Treatment of myasthenia gravis.
- Treatment of urinary retention and abdominal distention.

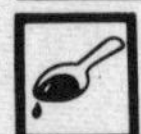

DOSAGE & USAGE INFORMATION

How to take:
Capsule—Swallow with liquid or food to lessen stomach irritation.

When to take:
As directed, usually 3 or 4 times a day.

If you forget a dose:
Take as soon as you remember up to 2 hours late. If more than 2 hours, wait for next scheduled dose (don't double this dose).

What drug does:
Inhibits the chemical activity of an enzyme (cholinesterase) so nerve impulses can cross the junction of nerves and muscles.

Time lapse before drug works:
3 hours.

Don't take with:
See Interaction column and consult doctor.

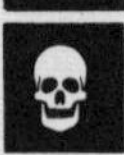

OVERDOSE

Symptoms:
Muscle weakness, cramps, twitching or clumsiness; severe diarrhea, nausea, vomiting, stomach cramps or pain; breathing difficulty; confusion, irritability, nervousness, restlessness, fear; unusually slow heartbeat; seizures.

What to do:
- Dial 0 (operator) or 911 (emergency) for an ambulance or medical help. Then give first aid immediately.
- Additional emergency information on page 886.

POSSIBLE ADVERSE REACTIONS OR SIDE EFFECTS

SYMPTOMS	FREQUENCY	WHAT TO DO
Brain & nervous system:		
Confusion, irritability.	Infrequent	2
Skin:	None expected.	
Eyes:		
Constricted pupils, watery eyes.	Infrequent	4
Ears, nose, throat:		
Excess saliva.	Common	4
Digestive:		
Mild diarrhea, nausea, vomiting, stomach cramps or pain.	Common	3
Heart & lungs:		
Lung congestion.	Infrequent	4
Blood vessels:	None expected.	
Muscles, bones, joints:	None expected.	
Genital, urinary:		
Frequent urge to urinate.	Infrequent	4
Kidneys:	None expected.	
Liver:	None expected.	
Allergic:	None expected.	
Blood:	None expected.	
Others:		
Unusual sweating.	Common	4

1-Life-threatening. Seek emergency treatment immediately.
2-Discontinue. Seek emergency treatment.
3-Discontinue. Call doctor right away.
4-Continue. Call doctor when convenient.
5-Continue. Tell doctor at next visit.
6-No action necessary.

WARNINGS & PRECAUTIONS

Don't take if:
- You are allergic to any cholinergic or bromide.
- You take mecamylamine.

Before you start, consult your doctor:
- If you plan to become pregnant within medication period.
- If you have bronchial asthma.
- If you have heartbeat irregularities.
- If you have urinary obstruction or urinary-tract infection.

Over age 60:
Adverse reactions and side effects may be more frequent and severe than in younger persons.

Pregnancy:
No proven harm to unborn child. Avoid if possible. May increase uterus contractions close to delivery.

Breast-feeding:
No problems expected, but consult doctor.

Infants & children:
Not recommended.

Prolonged use:
Medication may lose effectiveness. Discontinuing for a few days may restore effect.

Skin & sunlight:
No problems expected.

Driving, piloting or hazardous work:
Don't drive or pilot aircraft until you learn how medicine affects you. Don't work around dangerous machinery. Don't climb ladders or work in high places. Danger increases if you drink alcohol or take medicine affecting alertness and reflexes, such as antihistamines, tranquilizers, sedatives, pain medicine, narcotics and mind-altering drugs.

Airplane passengers:
No problems expected.

Discontinuing:
Don't discontinue without doctor's advice until you complete prescribed dose, even though symptoms diminish or disappear.

Others:
No problems expected.

INTERACTION WITH OTHER DRUGS

GENERIC NAME OR DRUG CLASS	COMBINED EFFECT
Anesthetics (local or general)	Decreased ambenonium effect.
Antiarrhythmics	Decreased ambenonium effect.
Antibiotics	Decreased ambenonium effect.
Anticholinergics	Decreased ambenonium effect. May mask severe side effects.
Cholinergics (other)	Reduced intestinal-tract function. Possible brain and nervous-system toxicity.
Mecamylamine	Decreased ambenonium effect.
Quinidine	Decreased ambenonium effect.

INTERACTION WITH OTHER SUBSTANCES

INTERACTS WITH	COMBINED EFFECT
Alcohol:	No proven problems with small doses.
Beverages:	None expected.
Cocaine:	Decreased ambenonium effect. Avoid.
Foods:	None expected.
Marijuana:	No proven problems.
Tobacco:	No proven problems.

AMILORIDE

BRAND NAMES

Midamor
Moduretic

GENERAL INFORMATION

Habit forming? No
Prescription needed? Yes
Available as generic? No
Drug class: Diuretic

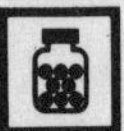

USES

Treatment for high blood pressure and congestive heart failure. Decreases fluid retention and prevents potassium loss.

DOSAGE & USAGE INFORMATION

How to take:
Tablet—Swallow with liquid.

When to take:
At the same time each day, preferably in the morning. May interfere with sleep if taken after 6 p.m.

If you forget a dose:
Take as soon as you remember up to 8 hours late. If more than 8 hours, wait for next scheduled dose (don't double this dose).

What drug does:
Blocks exchange of certain chemicals in the kidney so sodium is excreted. Conserves potassium.

Time lapse before drug works:
2 hours.

Don't take with:
See Interaction column and consult doctor.

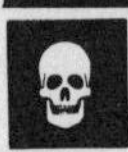

OVERDOSE

Symptoms:
Rapid, irregular heartbeat; confusion; shortness of breath; nervousness; extreme weakness.

What to do:

- Dial 0 (operator) or 911 (emergency) for an ambulance or medical help. Then give first aid immediately.
- If patient is unconscious and not breathing, give mouth-to-mouth breathing. If there is no heartbeat, use cardiac massage and mouth-to-mouth breathing (CPR). Don't try to make patient vomit. If you can't get help quickly, take patient to nearest emergency facility.
- Additional emergency information on page 886.

POSSIBLE ADVERSE REACTIONS OR SIDE EFFECTS

SYMPTOMS	FREQUENCY	WHAT TO DO
Brain & nervous system:		
• Headache	Common	4
• Dizziness	Infrequent	4
Skin:	None expected.	
Eyes:	None expected.	
Ears, nose, throat:	None expected.	
Digestive:		
• Nausea, appetite loss, vomiting, diarrhea.	Common	4
• Constipation, pain, bloating.	Infrequent	4
Heart & lungs:		
Cough, shortness of breath.	Infrequent	3
Blood vessels:	None expected.	
Muscles, bones, joints:		
Muscle cramps.	Infrequent	4
Genital, urinary:	None expected.	
Kidneys:	None expected.	
Liver:	None expected.	
Allergic:	None expected.	
Blood:	None expected.	
Others:	None expected.	

1- Life-threatening. Seek emergency treatment immediately.
2- Discontinue. Seek emergency treatment.
3- Discontinue. Call doctor right away.
4- Continue. Call doctor when convenient.
5- Continue. Tell doctor at next visit.
6- No action necessary.

WARNINGS & PRECAUTIONS

Don't take if:
- You are allergic to amiloride.
- Your serum potassium level is high.

Before you start, consult your doctor:
- If you plan to become pregnant within medication period.
- If you have diabetes.
- If you have heart disease.
- If you have kidney or liver disease.

Over age 60:
Adverse reactions and side effects may be more frequent and severe than in younger persons. More likely to exceed safe potassium blood levels.

Pregnancy:
No proven harm to unborn child. Avoid if possible.

Breast-feeding:
No problems expected, but consult doctor.

Infants & children:
Not recommended.

Prolonged use:
No problems expected.

Skin & sunlight:
No problems expected.

Driving, piloting or hazardous work:
Don't drive or pilot aircraft until you learn how medicine affects you. Don't work around dangerous machinery. Don't climb ladders or work in high places. Danger increases if you drink alcohol or take medicine affecting alertness and reflexes, such as antihistamines, tranquilizers, sedatives, pain medicine, narcotics and mind-altering drugs.

Airplane passengers:
No problems expected.

Discontinuing:
Don't discontinue without doctor's advice until you complete prescribed dose, even though symptoms diminish or disappear.

Others:
Periodic physical checkups and potassium-level tests recommended.

INTERACTION WITH OTHER DRUGS

GENERIC NAME OR DRUG CLASS	COMBINED EFFECT
Antihypertensives	Increased effect of both drugs.
Blood-bank blood	Increased potassium levels.
Diuretics (other)	Increased effect of both drugs.
Lithium	Possible lithium toxicity.
Potassium supplements	Increased potassium levels.
Sodium bicarbonate	Decreased potassium levels.

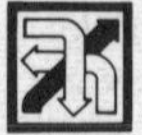

INTERACTION WITH OTHER SUBSTANCES

INTERACTS WITH	COMBINED EFFECT
Alcohol:	Increased blood-pressure drop. Avoid.
Beverages:	
Low-salt milk	Possible excess potassium levels. Low-salt milk has extra potassium.
Cocaine:	Blood-pressure rise. Avoid.
Foods:	
Salt substitutes	Possible excess potassium levels.
Marijuana:	None expected.
Tobacco:	None expected.

AMINOPHYLLINE

BRAND NAMES

Aminodur
Aminodur Dura-tabs
Aminophyl
Amphylline
Corophyllin
Lixaminol
Mini-Lix
Mudrane
Palaron
Phyllocontin
Somophyllin
Somophyllin-DF

GENERAL INFORMATION

Habit forming? No
Prescription needed? Canada—No
U.S: High strength— Yes
Low strength— No
Available as generic? Yes
Drug class: Bronchodilator (xanthine)

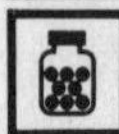

USES

Treatment for bronchial asthma symptoms.

DOSAGE & USAGE INFORMATION

How to take:

- Tablet or capsule—Swallow with liquid.
- Extended-release tablets or capsules—Swallow each dose whole. If you take regular tablets, you may chew or crush them.
- Suppositories—Remove wrapper and moisten suppository with water. Gently insert larger end into rectum. Push well into rectum with finger.
- Syrup—Take as directed on bottle.
- Enema—Use as directed on label.

When to take:
Most effective taken on empty stomach 1 hour before or 2 hours after eating. However, may take with food to lessen stomach upset.

If you forget a dose:
Take as soon as you remember up to 2 hours late. If more than 2 hours, wait for next scheduled dose (don't double this dose).

What drug does:
Relaxes and expands bronchial tubes.

Time lapse before drug works:
15 to 30 minutes.

Don't take with:
See Interaction column and consult doctor.

OVERDOSE

Symptoms:
Restlessness, irritability, confusion, delirium, convulsions, rapid pulse, coma.

What to do:

- Dial 0 (operator) or 911 (emergency) for an ambulance or medical help. Then give first aid immediately.
- Additional emergency information on page 886.

POSSIBLE ADVERSE REACTIONS OR SIDE EFFECTS

SYMPTOMS	FREQUENCY	WHAT TO DO
Brain & nervous system:		
• Headache, irritability, nervousness, restlessness, insomnia.	Common	4
• Dizziness or lightheadedness.	Infrequent	4
Skin:		
• Rash or hives.	Infrequent	3
• Flushed face.	Infrequent	4
Eyes:	None expected.	
Ears, nose, throat:	None expected.	
Digestive:		
• Nausea, vomiting, stomach pain.	Common	4
• Diarrhea, appetite loss.	Infrequent	3
Heart & lungs:		
• Rapid breathing.	Infrequent	3
• Irregular heartbeat.	Infrequent	3
Blood vessels:	None expected.	
Muscles, bones, joints:	None expected.	
Genital, urinary:	None expected.	
Kidneys:	None expected.	
Liver:	None expected.	
Allergic:	None expected.	
Blood:	None expected.	
Others:	None expected.	

1- Life-threatening. Seek emergency treatment immediately.
2- Discontinue. Seek emergency treatment.
3- Discontinue. Call doctor right away.
4- Continue. Call doctor when convenient.
5- Continue. Tell doctor at next visit.
6- No action necessary.

WARNINGS & PRECAUTIONS

Don't take if:
- You are allergic to any bronchodilator.
- You have an active peptic ulcer.

Before you start, consult your doctor:
- If you have had impaired kidney or liver function.
- If you have gastritis.
- If you have a peptic ulcer.
- If you have high blood pressure or heart disease.
- If you take medication for gout.

Over age 60:
Adverse reactions and side effects may be more frequent and severe than in younger persons.

Pregnancy:
Risk to unborn child outweighs drug benefits. Don't use.

Breast-feeding:
Drug passes into milk. Avoid drug or discontinue nursing until you finish medicine. Consult doctor for advice on maintaining milk supply.

Infants & children:
Use only under medical supervision.

Prolonged use:
Stomach irritation.

Skin & sunlight:
No problems expected.

Driving, piloting or hazardous work:
Avoid if lightheaded or dizzy. Otherwise, no problems expected.

Airplane passengers:
No problems expected.

Discontinuing:
May be unnecessary to finish medicine. Follow doctor's instructions.

Others:
No problems expected.

INTERACTION WITH OTHER DRUGS

GENERIC NAME OR DRUG CLASS	COMBINED EFFECT
Allopurinol	Decreased allopurinol effect.
Ephedrine	Increased effect of both drugs.
Epinephrine	Increased effect of both drugs.
Erythromycin	Increased aminophylline effect.
Furosemide	Increased furosemide effect.
Lincomycins	Increased aminophylline effect.
Lithium	Decreased lithium effect.
Probenecid	Decreased effect of both drugs.
Propranolol	Decreased aminophylline effect.
Rauwolfia alkaloids	Rapid heartbeat.
Sulfinpyrazone	Decreased sulfinpyrazone effect.
Troleandomycin	Increased aminophylline effect.

INTERACTION WITH OTHER SUBSTANCES

INTERACTS WITH	COMBINED EFFECT
Alcohol:	None expected.
Beverages: Caffeine drinks	Nervousness and insomnia.
Cocaine:	Excess stimulation. Avoid.
Foods:	None expected.
Marijuana:	Slightly increased antiasthmatic effect of aminophylline.
Tobacco:	Decreased aminophylline effect.

AMITRIPTYLINE

BRAND NAMES

Amitid
Amitril
Apo-Amitriptyline
Elavil
Endep
Etrafon
Levate
Meravil
Novotriptyn
SK-Amitriptyline
Triavil

GENERAL INFORMATION

Habit forming? No
Prescription needed? Yes
Available as generic? Yes
Drug class: Antidepressant (tricyclic)

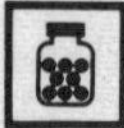

USES

- Gradually relieves, but doesn't cure, symptoms of depression.
- Decreases bed-wetting.

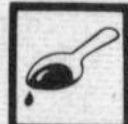

DOSAGE & USAGE INFORMATION

How to take:
Tablet or capsule—Swallow with liquid.

When to take:
At the same time each day, usually bedtime.

If you forget a dose:
Bedtime dose—If you forget your once-a-day bedtime dose, don't take it more than 3 hours late. If more than 3 hours, wait for next scheduled dose. Don't double this dose.

What drug does:
Probably affects part of brain that controls messages between nerve cells.

Time lapse before drug works:
Begins in 1 to 2 weeks. May require 4 to 6 weeks for maximum benefit.

Don't take with:
- Non-prescription drugs without consulting doctor.
- See Interaction column and consult doctor.

OVERDOSE

Symptoms:
Hallucinations, convulsions, coma.

What to do:
- Dial 0 (operator) or 911 (emergency) for an ambulance or medical help. Then give first aid immediately.
- If patient is unconscious and not breathing, give mouth-to-mouth breathing. If there is no heartbeat, use cardiac massage and mouth-to-mouth breathing (CPR). Don't try to make patient vomit. If you can't get help quickly, take patient to nearest emergency facility.
- Additional emergency information on page 886.

POSSIBLE ADVERSE REACTIONS OR SIDE EFFECTS

SYMPTOMS	FREQUENCY	WHAT TO DO
Brain & nervous system:		
• Hallucinations, shakiness, dizziness, fainting.	Infrequent	3
• Headache	Common	4
• Seizures	Rare	1
• Insomnia	Common	5
Skin:		
Rash, itch.	Rare	3
Eyes:		
Blurred vision, pain.	Infrequent	3
Ears, nose, throat:		
• Sore throat.	Rare	3
• Dry mouth or unpleasant taste.	Common	4
Digestive:		
• Constipation or diarrhea, nausea, indigestion.	Common	4
• Vomiting	Infrequent	3
• "Sweet tooth"	Common	5
Heart & lungs:		
Irregular heartbeat or slow pulse.	Infrequent	3
Blood vessels, muscles, bones, joints, kidneys, allergic, blood:	None expected.	
Genital, urinary:		
Difficulty urinating.	Infrequent	4
Liver:		
Jaundice (yellow skin and eyes).	Rare	3
Others:		
• Fever	Rare	3
• Fatigue, weakness.	Common	4

1 - Life-threatening. Seek emergency treatment immediately.
2 - Discontinue. Seek emergency treatment.
3 - Discontinue. Call doctor right away.
4 - Continue. Call doctor when convenient.
5 - Continue. Tell doctor at next visit.

WARNINGS & PRECAUTIONS

Don't take if:
- You are allergic to any tricyclic antidepressant.
- You drink alcohol.
- You have had a heart attack within 6 weeks.
- You have glaucoma.
- You have taken MAO inhibitors within 2 weeks.
- Patient is younger than 12.

Before you start, consult your doctor:
- If you will have surgery within 2 months, including dental surgery, requiring general or spinal anesthesia.
- If you have an enlarged prostate.
- If you have heart disease or high blood pressure.
- If you have stomach or intestinal problems.
- If you have an overactive thyroid.
- If you have asthma.
- If you have liver disease.

Over age 60:
More likely to develop urination difficulty and side effects under Brain & nervous system.

Pregnancy:
Studies inconclusive on harm to unborn child. Animal studies show fetal abnormalities. Decide with your doctor whether drug benefits justify risk to unborn child.

Breast-feeding:
Drug passes into milk. Avoid drug or discontinue nursing until you finish medicine. Consult doctor for advice on maintaining milk supply.

Infants & children:
Don't give to children younger than 12.

Prolonged use:
No problems expected.

Skin & sunlight:
May cause rash or intensify sunburn in areas exposed to sun or sunlamp.

Driving, piloting or hazardous work:
Don't drive or pilot aircraft until you learn how medicine affects you. Don't work around dangerous machinery. Don't climb ladders or work in high places. Danger increases if you drink alcohol or take medicine affecting alertness and reflexes.

Airplane passengers:
No problems expected.

Discontinuing:
Don't discontinue without consulting doctor. Dose may require gradual reduction if you have taken drug for a long time. Doses of other drugs may also require adjustment.

INTERACTION WITH OTHER DRUGS

GENERIC NAME OR DRUG CLASS	COMBINED EFFECT
Anticoagulants (oral)	Increased anticoagulant effect.
Anticholinergics	Increased sedation.
Antihistamines	Increased antihistamine effect.
Barbiturates	Decreased antidepressant effect.
Clonidine	Decreased clonidine effect.
Ethchlorvynol	Delirium
Guanethidine	Decreased guanethidine effect.
MAO inhibitors	Fever, delirium, convulsions.
Methyldopa	Decreased methyldopa effect.
Narcotics	Dangerous oversedation.
Phenytoin	Decreased phenytoin effect.
Quinidine	Irregular heartbeat.
Sedatives	Dangerous oversedation.
Sympathomimetics	Increased sympathomimetic effect.
Thiazide diuretics	Increased amitriptyline effect.
Thyroid hormones	Irregular heartbeat.

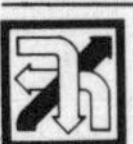

INTERACTION WITH OTHER SUBSTANCES

INTERACTS WITH	COMBINED EFFECT
Alcohol: Beverages or medicines with alcohol.	Excessive intoxication. Avoid.
Beverages:	None expected.
Cocaine:	Excessive intoxication. Avoid.
Foods:	None expected.
Marijuana:	Excessive drowsiness. Avoid.
Tobacco:	None expected.

AMOBARBITAL

BRAND NAMES

Amytal
Dexamyl
Isobec
Novamobarb
Tuinal

GENERAL INFORMATION

Habit forming? Yes
Prescription needed? Yes
Available as generic? Yes
Drug class: Sedative, hypnotic (barbiturate)

USES

- Reduces anxiety or nervous tension (low dose).
- Relieves insomnia (higher bedtime dose).

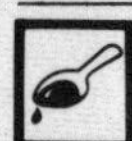

DOSAGE & USAGE INFORMATION

How to take:
Tablet, capsule or liquid—Swallow with food or liquid to lessen stomach irritation. If you can't swallow whole, crumble tablet or open capsule and take with liquid or food.

When to take:
At the same times each day.

If you forget a dose:
Take as soon as you remember up to 2 hours late. If more than 2 hours, wait for next scheduled dose (don't double this dose).

What drug does:
May partially block nerve impulses at nerve-cell connections.

Time lapse before drug works:
60 minutes.

Don't take with:
- Non-prescription drugs without consulting doctor.
- See Interaction column and consult doctor.

OVERDOSE

Symptoms:
Deep sleep, weak pulse, coma.

What to do:
- Dial 0 (operator) or 911 (emergency) for an ambulance or medical help. Then give first aid immediately.
- If patient is unconscious and not breathing, give mouth-to-mouth breathing. If there is no heartbeat use cardiac massage and mouth-to-mouth breathing (CPR). Don't try to make patient vomit. If you can't help quickly, take patient to nearest emergency facility.
- Additional emergency information on page 886.

POSSIBLE ADVERSE REACTIONS OR SIDE EFFECTS

SYMPTOMS	FREQUENCY	WHAT TO DO
Brain & nervous system:		
• Dizziness, drowsiness, "hangover effect."	Common	4
• Depression, confusion, slurred speech.	Infrequent	4
• Agitation	Rare	3
Skin:		
• Rash or hives.	Infrequent	3
• Face, lip swelling.	Infrequent	3
Eyes:		
Eyelid swelling.	Infrequent	3
Ears, nose, throat:		
Sore throat, fever.	Infrequent	3
Digestive:		
Diarrhea, nausea, vomiting.	Infrequent	4
Heart & lungs:		
• Slow heartbeat.	Rare	3
• Breathing difficulty.	Rare	3
Blood vessels:		
Unexplained bleeding or bruising.	Rare	4
Muscles, bones, joints:		
Joint or muscle pain.	Infrequent	4
Genital, urinary:	None expected.	
Kidneys:	None expected.	
Liver:		
Jaundice (yellow skin and eyes).	Rare	3
Allergic:	None expected.	
Blood:	None expected.	
Others:	None expected.	

1-Life-threatening. Seek emergency treatment immediately.
2-Discontinue. Seek emergency treatment.
3-Discontinue. Call doctor right away.
4-Continue. Call doctor when convenient.

WARNINGS & PRECAUTIONS

Don't take if:
- You are allergic to any barbiturate.
- You have porphyria.

Before you start, consult your doctor:
- If you have epilepsy.
- If you have kidney or liver damage.
- If you have asthma.
- If you have anemia.
- If you have chronic pain.
- If you will have surgery within 2 months, including dental surgery, requiring general or spinal anesthesia.

Over age 60:
Adverse reactions and side effects may be more frequent and severe than in younger persons. Use small doses.

Pregnancy:
Risk to unborn child outweighs drug benefits. Don't use.

Breast-feeding:
Drug passes into milk. Avoid drug or discontinue nursing until you finish medicine. Consult doctor for advice on maintaining milk supply.

Infants & children:
Use only under doctor's supervision.

Prolonged use:
- May cause addiction, anemia, chronic intoxication.
- May lower body temperature, making exposure to cold temperatures hazardous.

Skin & sunlight:
May cause rash or intensify sunburn in areas exposed to sun or sunlamp.

Driving, piloting or hazardous work:
Don't drive or pilot aircraft until you learn how medicine affects you. Don't work around dangerous machinery. Don't climb ladders or work in high places. Danger increases if you drink alcohol or take medicine affecting alertness and reflexes.

Airplane passengers:
No problems expected.

Discontinuing:
May be unnecessary to finish medicine. Follow doctor's instructions. If you develop withdrawal symptoms of hallucinations, agitation or sleeplessness after discontinuing, call doctor right away.

Others:
Great potential for abuse.

INTERACTION WITH OTHER DRUGS

GENERIC NAME OR DRUG CLASS	COMBINED EFFECT
Anticoagulants (oral)	Decreased anticoagulant effect.
Anticonvulsants	Changed seizure patterns.
Antidepressants (tricyclic)	Decreased antidepressant effect.
Antidiabetics (oral)	Increased amobarbital effect.
Antihistamines	Dangerous sedation. Avoid.
Antiinflammatory drugs (non-steroidal)	Decreased antiinflammatory effect.
Aspirin	Decreased aspirin effect.
Beta-adrenergic blockers	Decreased effect of beta-adrenergic blocker.
Contraceptives (oral)	Decreased contraceptive effect.
Cortisone drugs	Decreased cortisone effect.
Digitoxin	Decreased digitoxin effect.
Doxycycline	Decreased doxycycline effect.
Griseofulvin	Decreased griseofulvin effect.

Additional interactions on page 834.

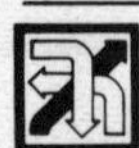

INTERACTION WITH OTHER SUBSTANCES

INTERACTS WITH	COMBINED EFFECT
Alcohol:	Possible fatal oversedation. Avoid.
Beverages:	None expected.
Cocaine:	Decreased amobarbital effect.
Foods:	None expected.
Marijuana:	Excessive sedation. Avoid.
Tobacco:	None expected.

AMOXICILLIN

BRAND NAMES

Amoxil
Augmentin
Larotid
Moxilean
Novamoxin
Penamox
Polymox
Robamox
Sumox
Trimox
Utimox
Wymox

GENERAL INFORMATION

Habit forming? No
Prescription needed? Yes
Available as generic? Yes
Drug class: Antibiotic (penicillin)

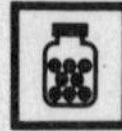

USES

Treatment of bacterial infections that are susceptible to amoxicillin.

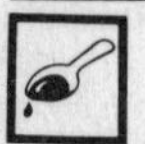

DOSAGE & USAGE INFORMATION

How to take:

- Tablet or capsule—Swallow with liquid on an empty stomach 1 hour before or 2 hours after eating.
- Liquid—Take with cold beverage. Liquid form is perishable and effective for only 7 days at room temperature. Effective for 14 days if stored in refrigerator. Don't freeze.

When to take:
Follow instructions on prescription label or side of package. Doses should be evenly spaced. For example, 4 times a day means every 6 hours.

If you forget a dose:
Take as soon as you remember. Continue regular schedule.

What drug does:
Destroys susceptible bacteria. Does not kill viruses.

Time lapse before drug works:
May be several days before medicine affects infection.

Don't take with:
See Interaction column and consult doctor.

OVERDOSE

Symptoms:
Severe diarrhea, nausea or vomiting.

What to do:
Overdose unlikely to threaten life. If person takes much larger amount than prescribed, call doctor, poison-control center or hospital emergency room for instructions.

POSSIBLE ADVERSE REACTIONS OR SIDE EFFECTS

SYMPTOMS	FREQUENCY	WHAT TO DO
Brain & nervous system:	None expected.	
Skin: Hives, rash, intense itch soon after a dose.	Rare	1
Eyes:	None expected.	
Ears, nose, throat: Dark or discolored tongue.	Common	5
Digestive: Mild nausea, vomiting, diarrhea.	Infrequent	4
Heart & lungs:	None expected.	
Blood vessels: Unexplained bleeding.	Rare	3
Muscles, bones, joints:	None expected.	
Genital, urinary:	None expected.	
Kidneys:	None expected.	
Liver:	None expected.	
Allergic: Life-threatening anaphylaxis may occur!	Rare	1 See Page 888.
Blood:	None expected.	
Others:	None expected.	

1 - Life-threatening. Seek emergency treatment immediately.
2 - Discontinue. Seek emergency treatment.
3 - Discontinue. Call doctor right away.
4 - Continue. Call doctor when convenient.
5 - Continue. Tell doctor at next visit.
6 - No action necessary.

WARNINGS & PRECAUTIONS

Don't take if:
You are allergic to amoxicillin, cephalosporin antibiotics, other penicillins or penicillamine. Life-threatening reaction may occur.

Before you start, consult your doctor:
If you are allergic to any substance or drug.

Over age 60:
You may have skin reactions, particularly around genitals and anus.

Pregnancy:
Studies inconclusive on harm to unborn child. Animal studies show fetal abnormalities. Decide with your doctor whether drug benefits justify risk to unborn child.

Breast-feeding:
Drug passes into milk. Child may become sensitive to penicillins and have allergic reactions to penicillin drugs. Avoid amoxicillin or discontinue nursing until you finish medicine. Consult doctor for advice on maintaining milk supply.

Infants & children:
No problems expected.

Prolonged use:
You may become more susceptible to infections caused by germs not responsive to amoxicillin.

Skin & sunlight:
No problems expected.

Driving, piloting or hazardous work:
Usually not dangerous. Most hazardous reactions likely to occur a few minutes after taking amoxicillin.

Airplane passengers:
No problems expected.

Discontinuing:
Don't discontinue without doctor's advice until you complete prescribed dose, even though symptoms diminish or disappear.

Others:
No problems expected.

INTERACTION WITH OTHER DRUGS

GENERIC NAME OR DRUG CLASS	COMBINED EFFECT
Chloramphenicol	Decreased effect of both drugs.
Erythromycins	Decreased effect of both drugs.
Paromomycin	Decreased effect of both drugs.
Tetracyclines	Decreased effect of both drugs.
Troleandomycin	Decreased effect of both drugs.

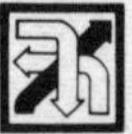

INTERACTION WITH OTHER SUBSTANCES

INTERACTS WITH	COMBINED EFFECT
Alcohol:	Occasional stomach irritation.
Beverages:	None expected.
Cocaine:	No proven problems.
Foods:	None expected.
Marijuana:	No proven problems.
Tobacco:	None expected.

AMPHETAMINE

BRAND NAMES

Amphaplex 10 & 20
Benzedrine
Bexedrine
Biphetamine
Declobese
Obetrol 10 & 20

GENERAL INFORMATION

Habit forming? Yes
Prescription needed? Yes
Available as generic? Yes
Drug class: Central-nervous-system stimulant (amphetamine)

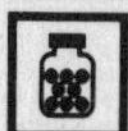

USES

- Prevents narcolepsy (attacks of uncontrollable sleepiness).
- Controls hyperactivity in children.

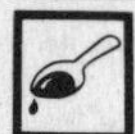

DOSAGE & USAGE INFORMATION

How to take:
- Tablet—Swallow with liquid.
- Extended-release capsules—Swallow each dose whole with liquid.

When to take:
- At the same times each day.
- Short-acting form—Don't take later than 6 hours before bedtime.
- Long-acting form—Take on awakening.

If you forget a dose:
- Short-acting form—Take up to 2 hours late. If more than 2 hours, wait for next dose (don't double this).
- Long-acting form—Take as soon as you remember. Wait 20 hours for next dose.

What drug does:
- Narcolepsy—Apparently affects brain centers to decrease fatigue or sleepiness and increase alertness and motor activity.
- Hyperactive children—Calms children, opposite to effect on narcoleptic adults.

Time lapse before drug works:
15 to 30 minutes.

Don't take with:
See Interaction column and consult doctor.

OVERDOSE

Symptoms:
Rapid heartbeat, hyperactivity, high fever, hallucinations, suicidal or homicidal feelings, convulsions, coma.

What to do:
- Dial 0 (operator) or 911 (emergency) for an ambulance or medical help. Then give first aid immediately.
- Additional emergency information on page 886.

POSSIBLE ADVERSE REACTIONS OR SIDE EFFECTS

SYMPTOMS	FREQUENCY	WHAT TO DO
Brain & nervous system:		
• Headache	Infrequent	4
• Dizziness, lack of alertness.	Infrequent	3
• Mood changes.	Rare	4
• Irritability, nervousness, insomnia.	Common	4
Skin:		
Rash, hives.	Rare	3
Eyes:		
Blurred vision.	Infrequent	3
Ears, nose, throat:		
Dry mouth.	Common	5
Digestive:		
Diarrhea or constipation, appetite loss, stomach pain, nausea, vomiting, weight loss.	Infrequent	5
Heart & lungs:		
• Fast, pounding heartbeat.	Infrequent	3
• Chest pain or irregular heartbeat.	Rare	3
Blood vessels, kidneys, liver, allergic, blood:	None expected.	
Muscles, bones, joints:		
Uncontrolled movements of head, neck, arms, legs.	Rare	3
Genital, urinary:		
Decreased sex drive, impotence.	Infrequent	5
Others:		
• Enlarged breasts.	Rare	4
• Unusual sweating.	Infrequent	3

1- Life-threatening. Seek emergency treatment immediately.
2- Discontinue. Seek emergency treatment.
3- Discontinue. Call doctor right away.
4- Continue. Call doctor when convenient.
5- Continue. Tell doctor at next visit.

WARNINGS & PRECAUTIONS

Don't take if:
- You are allergic to any amphetamine.
- You will have surgery within 2 months, including dental surgery, requiring general or spinal anesthesia.

Before you start, consult your doctor:
- If you plan to become pregnant within medication period.
- If you have glaucoma.
- If you have heart or blood-vessel disease, or high blood pressure.
- If you have overactive thyroid, anxiety or tension.
- If you have a severe mental illness (especially children).

Over age 60:
Adverse reactions and side effects may be more frequent and severe than in younger persons.

Pregnancy:
Risk to unborn child outweighs drug benefits. Don't use.

Breast-feeding:
Drug passes into milk. Avoid drug or discontinue nursing.

Infants & children:
Not recommended for children under 12.

Prolonged use:
Habit forming.

Skin & sunlight:
No problems expected.

Driving, piloting or hazardous work:
Don't drive or pilot aircraft until you learn how medicine affects you. Don't work around dangerous machinery. Don't climb ladders or work in high places. Danger increases if you drink alcohol or take medicine affecting alertness and reflexes.

Airplane passengers:
No problems expected.

Discontinuing:
May be unnecessary to finish medicine. Follow doctor's instructions.

Others:
- This is a dangerous drug and must be closely supervised. Don't use for appetite control or depression. Potential for damage and abuse.
- During withdrawal phase, may cause prolonged sleep of several days.

INTERACTION WITH OTHER DRUGS

GENERIC NAME OR DRUG CLASS	COMBINED EFFECT
Anesthesias (general)	Irregular heartbeat.
Antidepressants (tricyclic)	Decreased amphetamine effect.
Antihypertensives	Decreased antihypertensive effect.
Carbonic anhydrase inhibitors	Increased amphetamine effect.
Guanethidine	Decreased guanethidine effect.
Haloperidol	Decreased amphetamine effect.
MAO inhibitors	May severely increase blood pressure.
Phenothiazines	Decreased amphetamine effect.
Sodium bicarbonate	Increased amphetamine effect.

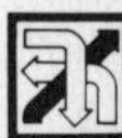

INTERACTION WITH OTHER SUBSTANCES

INTERACTS WITH	COMBINED EFFECT
Alcohol:	Decreased amphetamine effect. Avoid.
Beverages: Caffeine drinks	Overstimulation. Avoid.
Cocaine:	Dangerous stimulation of nervous system. Avoid.
Foods:	None expected.
Marijuana:	Frequent use—Severely impaired mental function.
Tobacco:	None expected.

AMPICILLIN

BRAND NAMES

Alpen
Amcill
Ampicin
Ampilean
Novo-Ampicillin
Omnipen
Penbritin
Polycillin
Principen
SK-Ampicillin
Supen
Totacillin

GENERAL INFORMATION

Habit forming? No
Prescription needed? Yes
Available as generic? Yes
Drug class: Antibiotic (penicillin)

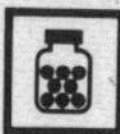

USES

Treatment of bacterial infections that are susceptible to ampicillin.

DOSAGE & USAGE INFORMATION

How to take:

- Tablets or capsules—Swallow with liquid on an empty stomach 1 hour before or 2 hours after eating.
- Liquid—Take with cold beverage. Liquid form is perishable and effective for only 7 days at room temperature. Effective for 14 days if stored in refrigerator. Don't freeze.

When to take:
Follow instructions on prescription label or side of package. Doses should be evenly spaced. For example, 4 times a day means every 6 hours.

If you forget a dose:
Take as soon as you remember. Continue regular schedule.

What drug does:
Destroys susceptible bacteria. Does not kill viruses.

Time lapse before drug works:
May be several days before medicine affects infection.

Don't take with:
See Interaction column and consult doctor.

OVERDOSE

Symptoms:
Severe diarrhea, nausea or vomiting.

What to do:
Overdose unlikely to threaten life. If person takes much larger amount than prescribed, call doctor, poison-control center or hospital emergency room for instructions.

POSSIBLE ADVERSE REACTIONS OR SIDE EFFECTS

SYMPTOMS	FREQUENCY	WHAT TO DO
Brain & nervous system:	None expected.	
Skin: Hives, rash, intense itch soon after a dose.	Rare	1
Eyes:	None expected.	
Ears, nose, throat: Dark or discolored tongue.	Common	5
Digestive: Mild nausea, vomiting, diarrhea.	Infrequent	4
Heart & lungs:	None expected.	
Blood vessels: Unexplained bleeding.	Rare	3
Muscles, bones, joints:	None expected.	
Genital, urinary:	None expected.	
Kidneys:	None expected.	
Liver:	None expected.	
Allergic: Life-threatening anaphylaxis may occur!	Rare	1 See page 888.
Blood:	None expected.	
Others:	None expected.	

1- Life-threatening. Seek emergency treatment immediately.
2- Discontinue. Seek emergency treatment.
3- Discontinue. Call doctor right away.
4- Continue. Call doctor when convenient.
5- Continue. Tell doctor at next visit.
6- No action necessary.

WARNINGS & PRECAUTIONS

Don't take if:
You are allergic to ampicillin, cephalosporin antibiotics, other penicillins or penicillamine. Life-threatening reaction may occur.

Before you start, consult your doctor:
If you are allergic to any substance or drug.

Over age 60:
You may have skin reactions, particularly around genitals and anus.

Pregnancy:
Studies inconclusive on harm to unborn child. Animal studies show fetal abnormalities. Decide with your doctor whether drug benefits justify risk to unborn child.

Breast-feeding:
Drug passes into milk. Child may become sensitive to penicillins and have allergic reactions to penicillin drugs. Avoid ampicillin or discontinue nursing until you finish medicine. Consult doctor for advice on maintaining milk supply.

Infants & children:
No problems expected.

Prolonged use:
You may become more susceptible to infections caused by germs not responsive to ampicillin.

Skin & sunlight:
No problems expected.

Driving, piloting or hazardous work:
Usually not dangerous. Most hazardous reactions likely to occur a few minutes after taking ampicillin.

Airplane passengers:
No problems expected.

Discontinuing:
Don't discontinue without doctor's advice until you complete prescribed dose, even though symptoms diminish or disappear.

Others:
Urine sugar test for diabetes may show false positive result.

INTERACTION WITH OTHER DRUGS

GENERIC NAME OR DRUG CLASS	COMBINED EFFECT
Chloramphenicol	Decreased effect of both drugs.
Erythromycins	Decreased effect of both drugs.
Paromomycin	Decreased effect of both drugs.
Tetracyclines	Decreased effect of both drugs.
Troleandomycin	Decreased effect of both drugs.

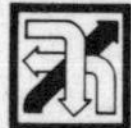

INTERACTION WITH OTHER SUBSTANCES

INTERACTS WITH	COMBINED EFFECT
Alcohol:	Occasional stomach irritation.
Beverages:	None expected.
Cocaine:	No proven problems.
Foods:	None expected.
Marijuana:	No proven problems.
Tobacco:	None expected.

ANDROGENS

BRAND AND GENERIC NAMES

Anabolin | Android
Anabolin LA 100 | Androlone

See complete brand and generic names list, page 821.

GENERAL INFORMATION

Habit forming? No
Prescription needed? Yes
Available as generic? Yes
Drug class: Androgens

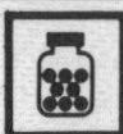

USES

- Corrects male hormone deficiency.
- Reduces "male menopause" symptoms (loss of sex drive, depression, anxiety).
- Decreases calcium loss of osteoporosis (softened bones).
- Blocks growth of breast-cancer cells in females.
- Corrects undescended testicles in male children.
- Reduces breast pain and fullness following childbirth.
- Augments treatment of aplastic anemia.
- Stimulates weight gain after illness, injury or for chronically underweight persons.
- Stimulates growth in treatment of dwarfism.

DOSAGE & USAGE INFORMATION

How to take:
- Tablets—With food to lessen stomach irritation.
- Injection—Once or twice a month.

When to take:
At the same time each day.

If you forget a dose:
Take as soon as you remember up to 2 hours late. If more than 2 hours, wait for next scheduled dose (don't double this dose).

What drug does:
- Stimulates cells that produce male sex characteristics.
- Replaces hormone deficiencies.
- Stimulates red-blood-cell production.
- Suppresses production of estrogen (female sex hormone).

Time lapse before drug works:
Varies with problems treated. May require 2 or 3 months of regular use for desired effects.

Don't take with:
See Interaction column and consult doctor.

OVERDOSE

Overdose unlikely to threaten life. If person takes much larger amount than prescribed, call doctor, poison-control center or hospital emergency room for instructions.

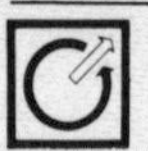

POSSIBLE ADVERSE REACTIONS OR SIDE EFFECTS

SYMPTOMS	FREQUENCY	WHAT TO DO
Brain & nervous system:		
Depression or confusion.	Infrequent	3
Skin:		
• Flushed face.	Infrequent	3
• Rash or itch.	Infrequent	3
• Hives	Rare	2
• Acne or oily skin in females.	Common	4
Eyes, heart & lungs, blood vessels, kidneys, blood:	None expected.	
Ears, nose, throat:		
• Deep voice.	Common	4
• Sore mouth.	Common	5
• Sore throat, fever.	Rare	3
Digestive:		
• Nausea, vomiting, diarrhea.	Infrequent	3
• Abdominal pain.	Rare	3
• Black stool.	Rare	2
Muscles, bones, joints:		
Swollen feet or legs.	Infrequent	3
Genital, urinary:		
• Enlarged clitoris or frequent erections.	Common	4
• Vaginal bleeding.	Infrequent	3
Liver:		
Jaundice (yellow skin and eyes).	Infrequent	2
Allergic:		
Intense itching, weakness, loss of consciousness.	Rare	1
Others:		
• Higher sex drive.	Common	5
• Swollen breasts in men.	Common	4

1- Life-threatening. Seek emergency treatment immediately.
2- Discontinue. Seek emergency treatment.
3- Discontinue. Call doctor right away.
4- Continue. Call doctor when convenient.
5- Continue. Tell doctor at next visit.

WARNINGS & PRECAUTIONS

Don't take if:
You are allergic to any male hormone.

Before you start, consult your doctor:
- If you might be pregnant.
- If you have cancer of prostate.
- If you have heart disease or arteriosclerosis.
- If you have kidney or liver disease.
- If you have breast cancer (males).
- If you have high blood pressure.
- If you have migraine attacks.
- If you have high level of blood calcium.
- If you have epilepsy.

Over age 60:
- May stimulate sexual activity.
- Can make high blood pressure or heart disease worse.
- Can enlarge prostate and cause urinary retention.

Pregnancy:
Risk to unborn child outweighs drug benefits. Don't use.

Breast-feeding:
Drug passes into milk. Avoid drug or discontinue nursing until you finish medicine. Consult doctor for advice on maintaining milk supply.

Infants & children:
Don't give to children younger than 2. Use with older children only under medical supervision.

Prolonged use:
- Reduces sperm count and volume of semen.
- Possible kidney stones.
- Unnatural hair growth and deep voice in women.

Skin & sunlight:
No problems expected.

Driving, piloting or hazardous work:
No problems expected.

Airplane passengers:
No problems expected.

Discontinuing:
No problems expected.

Others:
- May cause atrophy of testicles.
- Will not increase strength in athletes.

INTERACTION WITH OTHER DRUGS

GENERIC NAME OR DRUG CLASS	COMBINED EFFECT
Anticoagulants	Increased anticoagulant effect.
Antidiabetics (oral)	Increased antidiabetic effect.
Chlorzoxazone	Decreased androgen effect.
Oxyphenbutazone	Decreased androgen effect.
Phenobarbital	Decreased androgen effect.
Phenylbutazone	Decreased androgen effect.

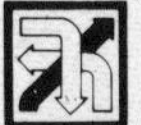

INTERACTION WITH OTHER SUBSTANCES

INTERACTS WITH	COMBINED EFFECT
Alcohol:	None expected.
Beverages:	None expected.
Cocaine:	No proven problems.
Foods:	
Salt	Excessive fluid retention (edema). Decrease salt intake while taking male hormones.
Marijuana:	Decreased blood levels of androgens.
Tobacco:	No proven problems.

ANESTHETICS (TOPICAL)

BRAND AND GENERIC NAMES

Aero Caine Aerosol	**Lidocaine Ointment**
Americaine Aerosol	**Nupercainal Cream**
Americaine Ointment	**Nupercainal Ointment**
Benzocaine Topical	**Nupercainal Spray**
Cyclaine Solution	**Xylocaine Ointment**

See complete brand and generic names list, page 821.

GENERAL INFORMATION

Habit forming? No
Prescription needed? High strength: Yes
Low strength: No
Available as generic? Yes
Drug class: Anesthetic (topical)

USES

- Relieves pain and itch of sunburn, insect bites, scratches and other minor skin irritations.
- Relieves discomfort and itch of hemorrhoids and other disorders of anus and rectum.

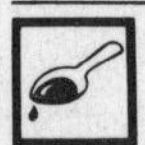

DOSAGE & USAGE INFORMATION

How to use:
- Suppositories—Remove wrapper and moisten suppository with water. Gently insert larger end into rectum. Push well into rectum with finger.
- All other forms—Use only enough to cover irritated area. Follow instructions on label.

When to use:
When needed for discomfort, no more often than every hour.

If you forget an application:
Use as needed.

What drug does:
Blocks pain impulses from skin to brain.

Time lapse before drug works:
3 to 15 minutes.

Don't take with:
See Interaction column and consult doctor.

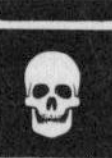

OVERDOSE

Symptoms:
If swallowed or inhaled—Dizziness, nervousness, trembling, seizures.

What to do:
- Dial 0 (operator) or 911 (emergency) for an ambulance or medical help. Then give first aid immediately.
- Additional emergency information on page 886.

POSSIBLE ADVERSE REACTIONS OR SIDE EFFECTS

SYMPTOMS	FREQUENCY	WHAT TO DO
Brain & nervous system:		
• Dizziness	Infrequent	4
• Nervousness, trembling.	Infrequent	3
Skin:		
Hives, rash, itch, inflammation or tenderness not present before application.	Infrequent	3
Eyes:		
Blurred vision.	Infrequent	4
Ears, nose, throat:	None expected.	
Digestive:	None expected.	
Heart & lungs:		
Slow heartbeat.	Infrequent	3
Blood vessels:	None expected.	
Muscles, bones, joints:		
Swelling of feet.	Infrequent	4
Genital, urinary:		
• Bloody urine.	Rare	3
• Increased or painful urination.	Rare	4
Kidneys:	None expected.	
Liver:	None expected.	
Allergic:	None expected.	
Blood:	None expected.	
Others:	None expected.	

1-Life-threatening. Seek emergency treatment immediately.
2-Discontinue. Seek emergency treatment.
3-Discontinue. Call doctor right away.
4-Continue. Call doctor when convenient.

WARNINGS & PRECAUTIONS

Don't use if:
You are allergic to any topical anesthetic.

Before you start, consult your doctor:
- If you have skin infection at site of treatment.
- If you have had severe or extensive skin disorders such as eczema or psoriasis.
- If you have bleeding hemorrhoids.

Over age 60:
Adverse reactions and side effects may be more frequent and severe than in younger persons.

Pregnancy:
No proven harm to unborn child. Avoid if possible.

Breast-feeding:
No problems expected.

Infants & children:
Use caution. More likely to be absorbed through skin and cause adverse reactions.

Prolonged use:
Possible excess absorption. Don't use longer than 3 days for any one problem.

Skin & sunlight:
No problems expected.

Driving, piloting or hazardous work:
No problems expected.

Airplane passengers:
No problems expected.

Discontinuing:
May be unnecessary to finish medicine. Follow doctor's instructions.

Others:
No problems expected.

INTERACTION WITH OTHER DRUGS

GENERIC NAME OR DRUG CLASS	COMBINED EFFECT
Sulfa drugs	Decreased antiinfective effect of sulfa drugs.

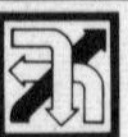

INTERACTION WITH OTHER SUBSTANCES

INTERACTS WITH	COMBINED EFFECT
Alcohol:	None expected.
Beverages:	None expected.
Cocaine:	Possible nervous-system toxicity. Avoid.
Foods:	None expected.
Marijuana:	None expected.
Tobacco:	None expected.

ANTICOAGULANTS (ORAL)

BRAND AND GENERIC NAMES

ANISINDIONE
Anthrombin-K
Coumadin
Danilone
DICUMAROL
Dufalone
Hedulin
Liquamar
Marcumar
Melitoxin
Miradon
Panwarfin
PHENINDIONE
PHENPROCOUMON
WARFARIN POTASSIUM
WARFARIN SODIUM
Warfilone
Warnerin

GENERAL INFORMATION

Habit forming? No
Prescription needed? Yes
Available as generic? Yes
Drug class: Anticoagulant

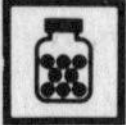

USES

Reduces blood clots. Used for abnormal clotting inside blood vessels.

DOSAGE & USAGE INFORMATION

How to take:
Tablet—Swallow with liquid. If you can't swallow whole, crumble tablet and take with liquid or food.

When to take:
At the same time each day.

If you forget a dose:
Take as soon as you remember up to 12 hours late. If more than 12 hours, wait for next scheduled dose (don't double this dose). Inform your doctor of any missed doses.

What drug does:
Blocks action of vitamin K necessary for blood clotting.

Time lapse before drug works:
36 to 48 hours.

Don't take with:
See Interaction column and consult doctor.

OVERDOSE

Symptoms:
Bloody vomit and bloody or black stools, red urine.

What to do:
- Dial 0 (operator) or 911 (emergency) for an ambulance or medical help. Then give first aid immediately.
- Additional emergency information on page 886.

POSSIBLE ADVERSE REACTIONS OR SIDE EFFECTS

SYMPTOMS	FREQUENCY	WHAT TO DO
Brain & nervous system:		
Dizziness, headache.	Rare	3
Skin:		
Rash, hives, itch.	Infrequent	3
Eyes:		
Blurred vision.	Infrequent	3
Ears, nose, throat:		
• Sore throat.	Infrequent	3
• Mouth sores.	Rare	3
Digestive:		
• Black stools or bloody vomit.	Infrequent	2
• Diarrhea, cramps, nausea, vomiting.	Infrequent	4
• Bloating, gas.	Common	5
Heart & lungs:		
Coughing up blood.	Infrequent	2
Blood vessels:		
Easy bruising, bleeding.	Infrequent	3
Muscles, bones, joints:		
Swollen feet, legs.	Infrequent	4
Genital, urinary:		
Cloudy or red urine.	Infrequent	3
Kidneys:		
Back pain.	Infrequent	3
Liver:		
Jaundice (yellow skin and eyes).	Infrequent	3
Allergic, blood:	None expected.	
Others:		
• Fever, chills.	Infrequent	3
• Hair loss.	Infrequent	4
• Fatigue, weakness.	Infrequent	3

1- Life-threatening. Seek emergency treatment immediately.
2- Discontinue. Seek emergency treatment.
3- Discontinue. Call doctor right away.
4- Continue. Call doctor when convenient.
5- Continue. Tell doctor at next visit.

ANTICOAGULANTS (ORAL)

WARNINGS & PRECAUTIONS

Don't take if:
- You have been allergic to any oral anticoagulant.
- You have a bleeding disorder.
- You have an active peptic ulcer.
- You have ulcerative colitis.

Before you start, consult your doctor:
- If you take any other drugs, including non-prescription drugs.
- If you have high blood pressure.
- If you have heavy or prolonged menstrual periods.
- If you have diabetes.
- If you have a bladder catheter.
- If you have serious liver or kidney disease.
- If you will have surgery within 2 months, including dental surgery, requiring general or spinal anesthesia.

Over age 60:
Adverse reactions and side effects may be more frequent and severe than in younger persons.

Pregnancy:
Risk to unborn child outweighs drug benefits. Don't use.

Breast-feeding:
Drug filters into milk. May harm child. Avoid.

Infants & children:
Use only under doctor's supervision.

Prolonged use:
No problems expected.

Skin & sunlight:
No problems expected.

Driving, piloting or hazardous work:
- Avoid hazardous activities that could cause injury.
- Don't drive if you feel dizzy or have blurred vision.

Airplane passengers:
No problems expected.

Discontinuing:
Don't discontinue without consulting doctor. Dose may require gradual reduction if you have taken drug for a long time. Doses of other drugs may also require adjustment.

Others:
Carry identification to state you take anticoagulants.

INTERACTION WITH OTHER DRUGS

GENERIC NAME OR DRUG CLASS	COMBINED EFFECT
Acetaminophen	Increased anticoagulant effect.
Allopurinol	Increased anticoagulant effect.
Androgens	Increased anticoagulant effect.
Antacids (large doses)	Decreased anticoagulant effect.
Antibiotics	Increased anticoagulant effect.
Anticonvulsants (hydantoin)	Increased effect of both drugs.
Antidepressants (tricyclic)	Increased anticoagulant effect.
Antidiabetics (oral)	Increased anticoagulant effect.
Antihistamines	Unpredictable increased or decreased anticoagulant effect.

Additional interactions on page 834.

INTERACTION WITH OTHER SUBSTANCES

INTERACTS WITH	COMBINED EFFECT
Alcohol:	Can increase or decrease effect of anticoagulant. Use with caution.
Beverages:	None expected.
Cocaine:	None expected.
Foods: High in vitamin K such as fish, liver, spinach, cabbage.	May decrease anticoagulant effect.
Marijuana:	None expected.
Tobacco:	None expected.

ANTICONVULSANTS (DIONE-TYPE)

BRAND AND GENERIC NAMES

PARAMETHADIONE
Paradione
TRIMETHADIONE
Tridione

GENERAL INFORMATION

Habit forming? No
Prescription needed? Yes
Available as generic? No
Drug class: Anticonvulsant (Dione-type)

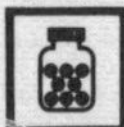

USES

Controls but does not cure petit mal seizures (absence seizures).

DOSAGE & USAGE INFORMATION

How to take:
Tablets, capsules or liquid: Take with food or milk to lessen stomach irritation.

When to take:
At the same time each day.

If you forget a dose:
Take as soon as you remember up to 2 hours late. If more than 2 hours, wait for next scheduled dose (don't double this dose).

What drug does:
Raises threshold of seizures in cerebral cortex. Does not alter seizure pattern.

Time lapse before drug works:
1 to 3 hours.

Don't take with:
See Interaction column and consult doctor.

OVERDOSE

Symptoms:
Bleeding, coma.

What to do:
- Dial 0 (operator) or 911 (emergency) for an ambulance or medical help. Then give first aid immediately.
- If patient is unconscious and not breathing, give mouth-to-mouth breathing. If there is no heartbeat, use cardiac massage and mouth-to-mouth breathing (CPR). Don't try to make patient vomit. If you can't get help quickly, take patient to nearest emergency facility.
- Additional emergency information on page 886.

POSSIBLE ADVERSE REACTIONS OR SIDE EFFECTS

SYMPTOMS	FREQUENCY	WHAT TO DO
Brain & nervous system:		
• Dizziness	Common	4
• Drowsiness	Common	4
• Headache	Common	4
Skin:		
• Rash	Common	4
• Itching	Infrequent	4
Eyes:		
• Changes in vision.	Rare	3
• Sensitivity to light.	Rare	4
Ears, nose, throat:		
• Sore throat with fever and mouth sores.	Rare	3
• Bleeding gums.	Rare	3
Digestive:		
Nausea, vomiting.	Infrequent	4
Heart & lungs:	None expected.	
Blood vessels:		
Easy bleeding.	Rare	3
Muscles, bones, joints:		
Easy bruising.	Rare	3
Genital, urinary:		
Smoky or bloody urine.	Rare	3
Kidneys, allergic, blood, liver:		
Jaundice (yellow skin and eyes).	Rare	3
Others:		
• Puffy hands, face, feet, legs.	Rare	3
• Swollen lymph glands.	Rare	3
• Unusual weakness and fatigue.	Rare	3

1- Life-threatening. Seek emergency treatment immediately.
2- Discontinue. Seek emergency treatment.
3- Discontinue. Call doctor right away.
4- Continue. Call doctor when convenient.
5- Continue. Tell doctor at next visit.

ANTICONVULSANTS (DIONE-TYPE)

WARNINGS & PRECAUTIONS

Don't take if:
You are allergic to this drug or any anticonvulsant.

Before you start, consult your doctor:
- If you are pregnant or plan pregnancy.
- If you have blood disease.
- If you have liver or kidney disease.
- If you have disease of optic nerve or eye.
- If you will have surgery within 2 months, including dental surgery, requiring general or spinal anesthesia.

Over age 60:
Adverse reactions and side effects may be more frequent and severe than in younger persons.

Pregnancy:
Risk to unborn child outweighs drug benefits. Don't use.

Breast-feeding:
No problems proven. Avoid if possible. Consult doctor.

Infants & children:
Use only under close medical supervision of clinician experienced in convulsive disorders.

Prolonged use:
Have regular checkups, especially during early months of treatment.

Skin & sunlight:
Increased sensitivity to sunlight or sun lamp. Avoid overexposure.

Driving, piloting or hazardous work:
Don't drive or pilot aircraft until you learn how medicine affects you. Don't work around dangerous machinery. Don't climb ladders or work in high places. Danger increases if you drink alcohol or take medicine affecting alertness and reflexes, such as antihistamines, tranquilizers, sedatives, pain medicine, narcotics and mind-altering drugs. Be especially careful driving at night because medicine can affect vision.

Airplane passengers:
No problems expected.

Discontinuing:
Don't discontinue without consulting doctor. Dose may require gradual reduction if you have taken drug for a long time. Doses of other drugs may also require adjustment.

Others:
Arrange for eye exams every 6 months as well as blood counts and kidney-function studies.

INTERACTION WITH OTHER DRUGS

GENERIC NAME OR DRUG CLASS	COMBINED EFFECT
Antidepressants (tricyclic)	Greater likelihood of seizures.
Antipsychotic medicines	Greater likelihood of seizures.
Anticonvulsants	Increased chance of blood toxicity.
Sedatives, sleeping pills, antihistamines, pain medicine, alchohol, tranquilizers, narcotics, mind-altering drugs.	Extreme drowsiness. Avoid.

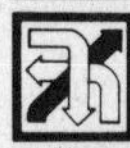

INTERACTION WITH OTHER SUBSTANCES

INTERACTS WITH	COMBINED EFFECT
Alcohol:	Increased chance of seizures and liver damage. Avoid.
Beverages:	No problems expected.
Cocaine:	Increased chance of seizures. Avoid.
Foods:	No problems expected.
Marijuana:	Increased chance of seizures. Avoid.
Tobacco:	Decreased absorption of medicine leading to uneven control of disease.

ANTITHYROID MEDICINES

BRAND AND GENERIC NAMES

METHIMAZOLE
PROPYLTHIOURACIL
Propyl-Thyracil
Tapazole
Thiamazole

GENERAL INFORMATION

Habit forming? No
Prescription needed? Yes
Available as generic? Yes
Drug class: Antihyperthyroid

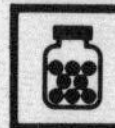

USES

- Treatment of overactive thyroid (hyperthyroidism).
- Treatment of angina in patients who have overactive thyroid.

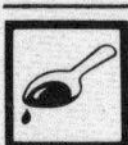

DOSAGE & USAGE INFORMATION

How to take:
- Tablet or capsule—Swallow with liquid or food to lessen stomach irritation. If you can't swallow whole, crumble tablet or open capsule and take with liquid or food.

When to take:
At the same times each day.

If you forget a dose:
Take as soon as you remember up to 2 hours late. If more than 2 hours, wait for next scheduled dose (don't double this dose).

What drug does:
- Prevents thyroid gland from producing excess thyroid hormone.

Time lapse before drug works:
10 to 20 days.

Don't take with:
- Anticoagulants
- See Interaction column and consult doctor.

OVERDOSE

Symptoms:
Bleeding, spots on skin, jaundice (yellow eyes and skin), loss of consciousness.

What to do:
Overdose unlikely to threaten life. If person takes much larger amount than prescribed, call doctor, poison-control center or hospital emergency room for instructions.

POSSIBLE ADVERSE REACTIONS OR SIDE EFFECTS

SYMPTOMS	FREQUENCY	WHAT TO DO
Brain & nervous system:		
• Dizziness	Infrequent	3
• Taste loss.	Infrequent	3
• Headache	Rare	3
Skin:		
• Enlarged lymph glands.	Rare	3
• Skin rash, itching, dryness.	Common	3
Eyes:	None expected.	
Ears, nose, throat:		
• Sore throat with chills and fever.	Infrequent	3
• Taste loss.	Infrequent	3
Digestive:		
• Abdominal pain.	Infrequent	3
• Constipation, diarrhea.	Infrequent	3
Heart & lungs:		
Irregular or rapid heartbeat.	Rare	3
Blood vessels:		
Unusual bruising or or bleeding.	Rare	3
Muscles, bones, joints:		
• Backache	Rare	3
• Numbness/tingling toes, fingers, face.	Rare	3
• Joint pain.	Rare	3
• Muscle aches.	Rare	3
Genital, urinary:		
Menstrual cycle changes.	Rare	3
Kidneys, allergic, blood, liver:		
Jaundice (yellow skin and eyes).	Rare	3
Others:		
Tired, weak, sleepy, listless; swelling around eyes or feet.	Rare	3

3- Discontinue. Call doctor right away.

ANTITHYROID MEDICINES

WARNINGS & PRECAUTIONS

Don't take if:
You are allergic to antithyroid medicines.

Before you start, consult your doctor:
- If you have liver disease.
- If you have blood disease.
- If you have an infection.
- If you take anticoagulants.

Over age 60:
Adverse reactions and side effects may be more frequent and severe than in younger persons.

Pregnancy:
Risk to unborn child outweighs drug benefits. Don't use.

Breast-feeding:
Drug filters into milk. May harm child. Avoid.

Infants & children:
Use only under special medical supervision by experienced clinician.

Prolonged use:
Adverse reactions and side effects more common.

Skin & sunlight:
No problems expected.

Driving, piloting or hazardous work:
Don't drive or pilot aircraft until you learn how medicine affects you. Don't work around dangerous machinery. Don't climb ladders or work in high places. Danger increases if you drink alcohol or take medicine affecting alertness and reflexes, such as antihistamines, tranquilizers, sedatives, pain medicine, narcotics and mind-altering drugs.

Airplane passengers:
No problems expected.

Discontinuing:
Don't discontinue without consulting doctor. Dose may require gradual reduction if you have taken drug for a long time. Doses of other drugs may also require adjustment.

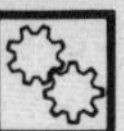

INTERACTION WITH OTHER DRUGS

GENERIC NAME OR DRUG CLASS	COMBINED EFFECT
Anticoagulants	Increased effect of anticoagulants.
Chloramphenicol	Increased chance to suppress bone marrow.
Antineoplastic drugs	Increased chance to suppress bone marrow.

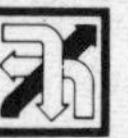

INTERACTION WITH OTHER SUBSTANCES

INTERACTS WITH	COMBINED EFFECT
Alcohol:	Increased possibility of liver toxicity. Avoid.
Beverages:	No problems expected.
Cocaine:	Increased toxicity potential of medicines. Avoid.
Foods:	No problems expected.
Marijuana:	Increased rapid or irregular heartbeat. Avoid.
Tobacco:	Increased chance of rapid heartbeat. Avoid.

APPETITE SUPPRESSANTS

BRAND AND GENERIC NAMES

Adipex-D	Obephen	Parmine
Fastin	Obermine	Phentrol
Ionamin	Obestrin-30	Wilpowr

See complete brand and generic names list, page 821.

GENERAL INFORMATION

Habit forming? Yes
Prescription needed? Yes
Available as generic? Yes
Drug class: Appetite suppressant

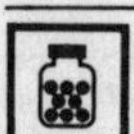

USES

Suppresses appetite.

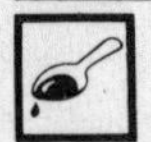

DOSAGE & USAGE INFORMATION

How to take:
- Tablet or capsule—Swallow with liquid. You may chew or crush tablet.
- Extended-release tablets or capsules—Swallow each dose whole with liquid.

When to take:
- Long-acting forms—10 to 14 hours before bedtime.
- Short-acting forms—1 hour before meals. Last dose no later than 4 to 6 hours before bedtime.

If you forget a dose:
- Long-acting form—Take as soon as you remember up to 2 hours late. If more than 2 hours, wait for next scheduled dose (don't double this dose).
- Short-acting form—Wait for next scheduled dose. Don't double this dose.

What drug does:
Apparently stimulates brain's appetite-control center.

Time lapse before drug works:
Begins in 1 hour. Short-acting form lasts 4 hours. Long-acting form lasts 14 hours.

Don't take with:
- Non-prescription drugs without consulting doctor.
- See Interaction column and consult doctor.

OVERDOSE

Symptoms:
Irritability, overactivity, trembling, insomnia, mood changes, rapid heartbeat, confusion, disorientation, hallucinations, convulsions, coma.

What to do:
- Dial 0 (operator) or 911 (emergency) for an ambulance or medical help. Then give first aid immediately.
- Additional emergency information on page 886.

POSSIBLE ADVERSE REACTIONS OR SIDE EFFECTS

SYMPTOMS	FREQUENCY	WHAT TO DO
Brain & nervous system:		
• Irritability, nervousness, insomnia.	Common	4
• Mood changes.	Rare	3
Skin:		
• Hair loss.	Rare	4
• Rash or hives.	Rare	3
Eyes:		
Blurred vision.	Infrequent	4
Ears, nose, throat:		
Unpleasant taste or dry mouth.	Infrequent	4
Digestive:		
Constipation or diarrhea, nausea, vomiting, cramps.	Infrequent	4
Heart & lungs:		
• Irregular or pounding heartbeat.	Infrequent	3
• Breathing difficulty.	Rare	3
Blood vessels, muscles, bones, joints, kidneys, liver, allergic, blood:	None expected.	
Genital, urinary:		
Urinary urgency and difficulty.	Infrequent	3
Others:		
• False sense of well-being.	Common	4
• Changes in sex drive.	Infrequent	4
• Sweat increase.	Infrequent	4

1- Life-threatening. Seek emergency treatment immediately.
2- Discontinue. Seek emergency treatment.
3- Discontinue. Call doctor right away.
4- Continue. Call doctor when convenient.

APPETITE SUPPRESSANTS

WARNINGS & PRECAUTIONS

Don't take if:
- You are allergic to any sympathomimetic or phenylpropanolamine.
- You have glaucoma.
- You have taken MAO inhibitors within 2 weeks.
- You plan to become pregnant within medication period.
- You have a history of drug abuse.
- You have irregular or rapid heartbeat.

Before you start, consult your doctor:
- If you have high blood pressure or heart disease.
- If you have an overactive thyroid, nervous tension or "anxiety."
- If you have epilepsy.
- If you will have surgery within 2 months, including dental surgery, requiring general or spinal anesthesia.

Over age 60:
Adverse reactions and side effects may be more frequent and severe than in younger persons.

Pregnancy:
Safety not established. Avoid.

Breast-feeding:
No proven problems. Consult doctor.

Infants & children:
Don't give to children younger than 12.

Prolonged use:
Loses effectiveness. Avoid.

Skin & sunlight:
No problems expected.

Driving, piloting or hazardous work:
Don't drive or pilot aircraft until you learn how medicine affects you. Don't work around dangerous machinery. Don't climb ladders or work in high places. Danger increases if you drink alcohol or take medicine affecting alertness and reflexes, such as antihistamines, tranquilizers, sedatives, pain medicine, narcotics and mind-altering drugs.

Airplane passengers:
No problems expected.

Discontinuing:
Don't discontinue without consulting doctor. Dose may require gradual reduction if you have taken drug for a long time. Doses of other drugs may also require adjustment.

Others:
Don't increase dose.

INTERACTION WITH OTHER DRUGS

GENERIC NAME OR DRUG CLASS	COMBINED EFFECT
Appetite suppressants (other)	Dangerous overstimulation.
Caffeine	Increased stimulant effect of phentermine.
Guanethidine	Decreased guanethidine effect.
Hydralazine	Decreased hydralazine effect.
MAO inhibitors	Dangerous blood-pressure rise.
Methyldopa	Decreased methyldopa effect.
Phenothiazines	Decreased appetite suppressant effect.
Rauwolfia alkaloids	Decreased effect of rauwolfia alkaloids.

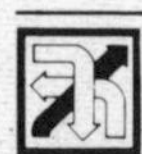

INTERACTION WITH OTHER SUBSTANCES

INTERACTS WITH	COMBINED EFFECT
Alcohol: Beer, chianti wines, vermouth.	Dangerous blood-pressure rise.
Beverages: • Caffeine drinks	Excessive stimulation.
• Drinks containing tyramine (see page 849).	Blood-pressure rise.
Cocaine:	Excessive stimulation.
Foods: Foods containing tyramine (see page 849).	Blood-pressure rise.
Marijuana:	Frequent use—Irregular heartbeat.
Tobacco:	None expected.

ASPIRIN

BRAND NAMES

Alka-Seltzer **Bayer** **Empirin** **Vanquish**
Anacin **Bufferin** **St. Joseph**

See complete brand names list on page 822.

GENERAL INFORMATION

Habit forming? No
Prescription needed? No
Available as generic? Yes
Drug class: Analgesic, antinflammatory (salicylate)

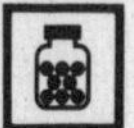

USES

- Reduces pain, fever, inflammation.
- Relieves swelling, stiffness, joint pain of arthritis or rheumatism.

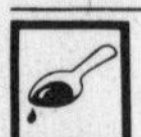

DOSAGE & USAGE INFORMATION

How to take:
- Tablet or capsule—Swallow with liquid.
- Extended-release tablets or capsules—Swallow each dose whole.
- Suppositories—Remove wrapper and moisten suppository with water. Gently insert into rectum, large end first.

When to take:
Pain, fever, inflammation—As needed, no more often than every 4 hours.

If you forget a dose:
- Pain, fever—Take as soon as you remember. Wait 4 hours for next dose.
- Arthritis—Take as soon as you remember up to 2 hours late. Return to regular schedule.

What drug does:
- Affects hypothalamus, part of brain which regulates temperature by dilating small blood vessels in skin.
- Prevents clumping of platelets (small blood cells) so blood vessels remain open.
- Decreases prostaglandin effect.
- Suppresses body's pain messages.

Time lapse before drug works:
30 minutes for pain, fever, arthritis.

Don't take with:
- Tetracyclines. Space doses 1 hour apart.
- See Interaction column and consult doctor.

OVERDOSE

Symptoms:
Ringing in ears; nausea; vomiting; dizziness; fever; deep, rapid breathing; hallucinations; convulsions; coma.

What to do:
- Dial 0 (operator) or 911 (emergency) for an ambulance or medical help. Then give first aid immediately.
- Additional emergency information on page 886.

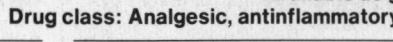

POSSIBLE ADVERSE REACTIONS OR SIDE EFFECTS

SYMPTOMS	FREQUENCY	WHAT TO DO
Brain & nervous system:		
Drowsiness	Rare	4
Skin:		
Rash, hives, itch.	Rare	3
Eyes:		
Diminished vision.	Rare	3
Ears, nose, throat:		
Ringing in ears.	Common	5
Digestive:		
• Nausea, vomiting, abdominal pain.	Common	2
• Black stools.	Rare	2
• Black or bloody vomit.	Rare	1
• Heartburn, indigestion.	Common	4
Heart & lungs:		
Shortness of breath, wheezing.	Rare	3
Blood vessels, muscles, bones, joints, kidneys, blood:	None expected.	
Genital, urinary:		
Blood in urine.	Rare	1
Liver:		
Jaundice (yellow eyes and skin).	Rare	3
Allergic:		
Life-threatening anaphylaxis may occur!	Rare	1 See page 888.
Others:		
Unexplained fever.	Rare	2

1- Life-threatening. Seek emergency treatment immediately.
2- Discontinue. Seek emergency treatment.
3- Discontinue. Call doctor right away.
4- Continue. Call doctor when convenient.
5- Continue. Tell doctor at next visit.
6- No action necessary.

WARNINGS & PRECAUTIONS

Don't take if:
- You need to restrict sodium in your diet. Buffered effervescent tablets and sodium salicylate are high in sodium.
- Aspirin has a strong vinegar-like odor, which means it has decomposed.
- You have a peptic ulcer of stomach or duodenum.
- You have a bleeding disorder.

Before you start, consult your doctor:
- If you have had stomach or duodenal ulcers.
- If you have had gout.
- If you have asthma or nasal polyps.

Over age 60:
More likely to cause hidden bleeding in stomach or intestines. Watch for dark stools.

Pregnancy:
Risk to unborn child outweighs drug benefits. Don't use.

Breast-feeding:
Drug passes into milk. Avoid drug or discontinue nursing until you finish medicine. Consult doctor for advice on maintaining milk supply.

Infants & children:
Overdose frequent and severe. Keep bottles out of children's reach.

Prolonged use:
Kidney damage. Periodic kidney-function test recommended.

Skin & sunlight:
Aspirin combined with sunscreen may decrease sunburn.

Driving, piloting or hazardous work:
No restrictions unless you feel drowsy.

Airplane passengers:
No problems expected.

Discontinuing:
For chronic illness—Don't discontinue without doctor's advice until you complete prescribed dose, even though symptoms diminish or disappear.

Others:
- Aspirin can complicate surgery, pregnancy, labor and delivery, and illness.
- For arthritis—Don't change dose without consulting doctor.
- Urine tests for blood sugar may be inaccurate.

INTERACTION WITH OTHER DRUGS

GENERIC NAME OR DRUG CLASS	COMBINED EFFECT
Allopurinol	Decreased allopurinol effect.
Antacids	Decreased aspirin effect.
Anticoagulants	Increased anticoagulant effect. Abnormal bleeding.
Antidiabetics (oral)	Low blood sugar.
Antiinflammatory drugs (non-steroid)	Risk of stomach bleeding and ulcers.
Aspirin (other)	Likely aspirin toxicity.
Cortisone drugs	Increased cortisone effect. Risk of ulcers and stomach bleeding.
Furosemide	Possible aspirin toxicity.
Indomethacin	Risk of stomach bleeding and ulcers.
Methotrexate	Increased methotrexate effect.
Para-aminosalicylic acid (PAS)	Possible aspirin toxicity.
Penicillins	Increased effect of both drugs.
Phenobarbital	Decreased aspirin effect.
Phenytoin	Increased phenytoin effect.

Additional interactions on page 834.

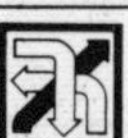

INTERACTION WITH OTHER SUBSTANCES

INTERACTS WITH	COMBINED EFFECT
Alcohol:	Possible stomach irritation and bleeding. Avoid.
Beverages:	None expected.
Cocaine:	None expected.
Foods:	None expected.
Marijuana:	Possible increased pain relief, but marijuana may slow body's recovery. Avoid.
Tobacco:	None expected.

ATENOLOL

BRAND NAMES

Tenormin

GENERAL INFORMATION

Habit forming? No
Prescription needed? Yes
Available as generic? No
Drug class: Beta-adrenergic blocker

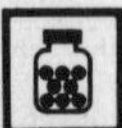

USES

- Reduces angina attacks.
- Stabilizes irregular heartbeat.
- Lowers blood pressure.
- Reduces frequency of migraine headaches. (Does not relieve headache pain.)
- Other uses prescribed by your doctor.

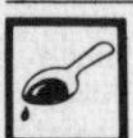

DOSAGE & USAGE INFORMATION

How to take:
Tablet or capsule—Swallow with liquid. If you can't swallow whole, crumble tablet or open capsule and take with liquid or food.

When to take:
With meals or immediately after.

If you forget a dose:
Take as soon as you remember. Return to regular schedule, but allow 3 hours between doses.

What drug does:
- Blocks certain actions of sympathetic nervous system.
- Lowers heart's oxygen requirements.
- Slows nerve impulses through heart.
- Reduces blood vessel contraction in heart, scalp and other body parts.

Time lapse before drug works:
1 to 4 hours.

Don't take with:
Non-prescription drugs or drugs in Interaction column without consulting doctor.

OVERDOSE

Symptoms:
Weakness, slow or weak pulse, blood pressure drop, fainting, convulsions, cold and sweaty skin.

What to do:
- Dial O (operator) or 911 (emergency) for an ambulance or medical help. Then give first aid immediately.
- Additional emergency information on page 886.

POSSIBLE ADVERSE REACTIONS OR SIDE EFFECTS

SYMPTOMS	FREQUENCY	WHAT TO DO
Brain & nervous system:		
• Hallucinations, nightmares, insomnia, headache.	Infrequent	3
• Confusion, depression, reduced alertness.	Infrequent	4
• Drowsiness, numbness or tingling of fingers or toes, dizziness.	Common	4
Skin:		
Rash	Rare	3
Eyes:	None expected.	
Ears, nose, throat:		
Sore throat, fever.	Rare	3
Digestive:		
• Diarrhea, nausea.	Common	4
• Constipation	Infrequent	5
Heart & lungs:		
• Pulse slower than 50 beats per minute.	Common	3
• Breathing difficulty.	Infrequent	3
Blood vessels:		
Cold hands, feet.	Common	5
Muscles, bones, joints, genital, urinary, kidneys, liver, allergic:	None expected.	
Blood:		
Unusual bleeding and bruising.	Rare	4
Others:		
• Fatigue, weakness.	Common	4
• Dry mouth, eyes, skin.	Common	5

1-Life-threatening. Seek emergency treatment immediately.
2-Discontinue. Seek emergency treatment.
3-Discontinue. Call doctor right away.
4-Continue. Call doctor when convenient.
5-Continue. Tell doctor at next visit.

WARNINGS & PRECAUTIONS

Don't take if:

- You are allergic to any beta-adrenergic blocker.
- You have asthma.
- You have hay fever symptoms.
- You have taken MAO inhibitors in past 2 weeks.

Before you start, consult your doctor:

- If you have heart disease or poor circulation to the extremities.
- If you have hay fever, asthma, chronic bronchitis, emphysema.
- If you have overactive thyroid function.
- If you have impaired liver or kidney function.
- If you will have surgery within 2 months, including dental surgery, requiring general or spinal anesthesia.
- If you have diabetes or hypoglycemia.

Over age 60:
Adverse reactions and side effects may be more frequent and severe than in younger persons.

Pregnancy:
Risk to unborn child outweighs drug benefits. Don't use.

Breast-feeding:
Drug passes into milk. Avoid drug or discontinue nursing until you finish medicine. Consult doctor for advice on maintaining milk supply.

Infants & children:
Not recommended.

Prolonged use:
Weakens heart muscle contractions.

Skin & sunlight:
No problems expected.

Driving, piloting or hazardous work:
Don't drive or pilot aircraft until you learn how medicine affects you. Don't work around dangerous machinery. Don't climb ladders or work in high places. Danger increases if you drink alcohol or take medicine affecting alertness and reflexes.

Airplane passengers:
No problems expected.

Discontinuing:
Don't discontinue without consulting doctor. Dose may require gradual reduction if you have taken drug for a long time. Doses of other drugs may also require adjustment.

Others:
May mask hypoglycemia.

INTERACTION WITH OTHER DRUGS

GENERIC NAME OR DRUG CLASS	COMBINED EFFECT
Antidiabetics	Increased antidiabetic effect.
Antihistamines	Decreased antihistamine effect.
Antihypertensives	Increased antihypertensive effect.
Antiinflammatory drugs	Decreased antiinflammatory effect.
Barbiturates	Increased barbiturate effect. Dangerous sedation.
Digitalis preparations	Can either increase or decrease heart rate. Improves irregular heartbeat.
Narcotics	Increased narcotic effect. Dangerous sedation.
Phenytoin	Increased atenolol effect.
Quinidine	Slows heart excessively.
Reserpine	Increased reserpine effect. Excessive sedation and depression.

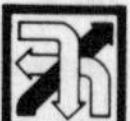

INTERACTION WITH OTHER SUBSTANCES

INTERACTS WITH	COMBINED EFFECT
Alcohol:	Excessive blood pressure drop. Avoid.
Beverages:	None expected.
Cocaine:	Irregular heartbeat. Avoid.
Foods:	None expected.
Marijuana:	Daily use—Impaired circulation to hands and feet.
Tobacco:	Possible irregular heartbeat.

ATROPINE

BRAND NAMES

Atrobarbital
Atrosed
Barbidonna
Belladenal
Bellergal
Bellergal-S
Butibel
Chardonna
Contac
Donnagel
Donnamine
Donnatal
Isopto Atropine
Kinesed
Prydon

See complete brand names list, page 822.

GENERAL INFORMATION

Habit forming? No
Prescription needed? Low strength: No
High strength: Yes
Available as generic? Yes
Drug class: Antispasmodic, anticholinergic

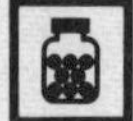

USES

Reduces spasms of digestive system, bladder and urethra.

DOSAGE & USAGE INFORMATION

How to take:
Tablet—Swallow with liquid or food to lessen stomach irritation.

When to take:
30 minutes before meals (unless directed otherwise by doctor).

If you forget a dose:
Take as soon as you remember up to 2 hours late. If more than 2 hours, wait for next scheduled dose (don't double this dose).

What drug does:
Blocks nerve impulses at parasympathetic nerve endings, preventing muscle contractions and gland secretions of organs involved.

Time lapse before drug works:
15 to 30 minutes.

Don't take with:
See Interaction column and consult doctor.

OVERDOSE

Symptoms:
Dilated pupils; rapid pulse and breathing; dizziness; fever; hallucinations; confusion; slurred speech; agitation; flushed face; convulsions; coma.

What to do:
- Dial 0 (operator) or 911 (emergency) for an ambulance or medical help. Then give first aid immediately.
- Additional emergency information on page 886.

POSSIBLE ADVERSE REACTIONS OR SIDE EFFECTS

SYMPTOMS	FREQUENCY	WHAT TO DO
Brain & nervous system:		
• Headache	Infrequent	4
• Confusion, delirium.	Common	3
Skin:		
Rash or hives.	Rare	3
Eyes:		
Pain, blurred vision.	Rare	3
Ears, nose, throat:		
Dryness	Common	6
Digestive:		
• Constipation	Common	5
• Nausea, vomiting.	Common	4
Heart & lungs:		
Rapid heartbeat.	Common	3
Blood vessels:	None expected.	
Muscles, bones, joints:	None expected.	
Genital, urinary:		
Difficult urination.	Infrequent	4
Kidneys:	None expected.	
Liver:	None expected.	
Allergic:	None expected.	
Blood:	None expected.	
Others:		
Less perspiration.	Common	4

1- Life-threatening. Seek emergency treatment immediately.
2- Discontinue. Seek emergency treatment.
3- Discontinue. Call doctor right away.
4- Continue. Call doctor when convenient.
5- Continue. Tell doctor at next visit.
6- No action necessary.

WARNINGS & PRECAUTIONS

Don't take if:
- You are allergic to any anticholinergic.
- You have trouble with stomach bloating.
- You have difficulty emptying your bladder completely.
- You have narrow-angle glaucoma.
- You have severe ulcerative colitis.

Before you start, consult your doctor:
- If you have open-angle glaucoma.
- If you have angina.
- If you have chronic bronchitis or asthma.
- If you have liver disease.
- If you have hiatal hernia.
- If you have enlarged prostate.
- If you have myasthenia gravis.
- If you have peptic ulcer.
- If you will have surgery within 2 months, including dental surgery, requiring general or spinal anesthesia.

Over age 60:
Adverse reactions and side effects may be more frequent and severe than in younger persons.

Pregnancy:
Studies inconclusive on harm to unborn child. Animal studies show fetal abnormalities. Decide with your doctor whether drug benefits justify risk to unborn child.

Breast-feeding:
Drug passes into milk and decreases milk flow. Avoid drug or discontinue nursing until you finish medicine. Consult doctor for advice on maintaining milk supply.

Infants & children:
Use only under medical supervision.

Prolonged use:
Chronic constipation, possible fecal impaction. Consult doctor immediately.

Skin & sunlight:
No problems expected.

Driving, piloting or hazardous work:
Use disqualifies you for piloting aircraft. Otherwise, no problems expected.

Airplane passengers:
No problems expected.

Discontinuing:
May be unnecessary to finish medicine. Follow doctor's instructions.

Others:
No problems expected.

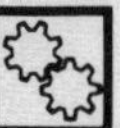

INTERACTION WITH OTHER DRUGS

GENERIC NAME OR DRUG CLASS	COMBINED EFFECT
Amantadine	Increased atropine effect.
Anticholinergics (other)	Increased atropine effect.
Antidepressants (tricyclic)	Increased atropine effect.
Antihistamines	Increased atropine effect.
Cortisone drugs	Increased internal-eye pressure.
Haloperidol	Increased internal-eye pressure.
MAO inhibitors	Increased atropine effect.
Meperidine	Increased atropine effect.
Methylphenidate	Increased atropine effect.
Orphenadrine	Increased atropine effect.
Phenothiazines	Increased atropine effect.
Pilocarpine	Loss of pilocarpine effect in glaucoma treatment.
Vitamin C	Decreased atropine effect. Avoid large doses of vitamin C.

INTERACTION WITH OTHER SUBSTANCES

INTERACTS WITH	COMBINED EFFECT
Alcohol:	None expected.
Beverages:	None expected.
Cocaine:	Excessively rapid heartbeat. Avoid.
Foods:	None expected.
Marijuana:	Drowsiness and dry mouth.
Tobacco:	None expected.

AZATADINE

BRAND NAMES

Optimine
Trinalin Repetabs

GENERAL INFORMATION

Habit forming? No
Prescription needed? Yes
Available as generic? No
Drug class: Antihistamine

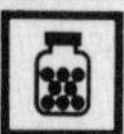

USES

- Reduces allergic symptoms such as hay fever, hives, rash or itching.
- Induces sleep.

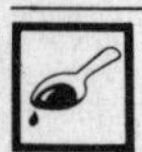

DOSAGE & USAGE INFORMATION

How to take:
Tablet—Swallow with liquid or food to lessen stomach irritation.

When to take:
Varies with form. Follow label directions.

If you forget a dose:
Take as soon as you remember up to 2 hours late. If more than 2 hours, wait for next scheduled dose (don't double this dose).

What drug does:
Blocks action of histamine after an allergic response triggers histamine release in sensitive cells.

Time lapse before drug works:
30 minutes.

Don't take with:
See Interaction column and consult doctor.

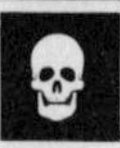

OVERDOSE

Symptoms:
Convulsions, red face, hallucinations, coma.

What to do:
- Dial 0 (operator) or 911 (emergency) for an ambulance or medical help. Then give first aid immediately.
- If patient is unconscious and not breathing, give mouth-to-mouth breathing. If there is no heartbeat, use cardiac massage and mouth-to-mouth breathing (CPR). Don't try to make patient vomit. If you can't get help quickly, take patient to nearest emergency facility.
- Additional emergency information on page 886.

POSSIBLE ADVERSE REACTIONS OR SIDE EFFECTS

SYMPTOMS	FREQUENCY	WHAT TO DO
Brain & nervous system:		
• Nightmares, agitation, irritability.	Rare	3
• Drowsiness, dizziness.	Common	5
Skin:	None expected.	
Eyes:		
• Vision changes.	Infrequent	3
• Less tolerance for contact lenses.	Infrequent	4
Ears, nose, throat:		
• Sore throat, fever.	Rare	3
• Dry mouth, nose, throat.	Common	5
Digestive:		
• Nausea	Common	5
• Appetite loss.	Infrequent	5
Heart & lungs:		
Rapid heartbeat.	Rare	3
Blood vessels:		
Unusual bleeding or bruising.	Rare	3
Muscles, bones, joints, kidneys, liver, allergic, blood:	None expected.	
Genital, urinary:		
Urination difficulty.	Infrequent	4
Others:		
Fatigue, weakness.	Rare	3

1 - Life-threatening. Seek emergency treatment immediately.
2 - Discontinue. Seek emergency treatment.
3 - Discontinue. Call doctor right away.
4 - Continue. Call doctor when convenient.
5 - Continue. Tell doctor at next visit.
6 - No action necessary.

WARNINGS & PRECAUTIONS

Don't take if:
You are allergic to any antihistamine.

Before you start, consult your doctor:
- If you have glaucoma.
- If you have enlarged prostate.
- If you have asthma.
- If you have kidney disease.
- If you have peptic ulcer.
- If you will have surgery within 2 months, including dental surgery, requiring general or spinal anesthesia.

Over age 60:
Don't exceed recommended dose. Adverse reactions and side effects may be more frequent and severe than in younger persons, especially urination difficulty, diminished alertness and other brain and nervous-system symptoms.

Pregnancy:
No proven harm to unborn child. Avoid if possible.

Breast-feeding:
Drug passes into milk. Avoid drug or discontinue nursing until you finish medicine. Consult doctor for advice on maintaining milk supply.

Infants & children:
Not recommended for premature or newborn infants. Otherwise, no problems expected.

Prolonged use:
Avoid. May damage bone-marrow and nerve cells.

Skin & sunlight:
May cause rash or intensify sunburn in areas exposed to sun or sunlamp.

Driving, piloting or hazardous work:
Don't drive or pilot aircraft until you learn how medicine affects you. Don't work around dangerous machinery. Don't climb ladders or work in high places. Danger increases if you drink alcohol or take medicine affecting alertness and reflexes, such as antihistamines, tranquilizers, sedatives, pain medicine, narcotics and mind-altering drugs.

Airplane passengers:
No problems expected.

Discontinuing:
No problems expected.

Others:
May mask symptoms of hearing damage from aspirin, other salicylates, cisplatin, paromomycin, vancomycin or anticonvulsants. Consult doctor if you use these.

INTERACTION WITH OTHER DRUGS

GENERIC NAME OR DRUG CLASS	COMBINED EFFECT
Anticholinergics	Increased anticholinergic effect.
Antidepressants	Excess sedation. Avoid.
Antihistamines (other)	Excess sedation. Avoid.
Hypnotics	Excess sedation. Avoid.
MAO inhibitors	Increased azatadine effect.
Mind-altering drugs	Excess sedation. Avoid.
Narcotics	Excess sedation. Avoid.
Sedatives	Excess sedation. Avoid.
Sleep inducers	Excess sedation. Avoid.
Tranquilizers	Excess sedation. Avoid.

INTERACTION WITH OTHER SUBSTANCES

INTERACTS WITH	COMBINED EFFECT
Alcohol:	Excess sedation. Avoid.
Beverages:	
Caffeine drinks	Less azatadine sedation.
Cocaine:	Decreased azatadine effect. Avoid.
Foods:	None expected.
Marijuana:	Excess sedation. Avoid.
Tobacco:	None expected.

BACAMPICILLIN

BRAND NAMES

Spectrobid

GENERAL INFORMATION

Habit forming? No
Prescription needed? Yes
Available as generic? No
Drug class: Antibiotic (penicillin)

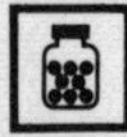

USES

Treatment of bacterial infections that are susceptible to bacampicillin.

DOSAGE & USAGE INFORMATION

How to take:

- Tablets or capsules—Swallow with liquid on an empty stomach 1 hour before meals or 2 hours after eating.
- Liquid—Take with cold beverage. Liquid form is perishable and effective for only 7 days at room temperature. Effective for 14 days if stored in refrigerator. Don't freeze.

When to take:
Follow instructions on prescription label or side of package. Doses should be evenly spaced. For example, 4 times a day means every 6 hours.

If you forget a dose:
Take as soon as you remember. Continue regular schedule.

What drug does:
Destroys susceptible bacteria. Does not kill viruses.

Time lapse before drug works:
May be several days before medicine affects infection.

Don't take with:
See Interaction column and consult doctor.

OVERDOSE

Symptoms:
Severe diarrhea, nausea or vomiting.

What to do:
Overdose unlikely to threaten life. If person takes much larger amount than prescribed, call doctor, poison-control center or hospital emergency room for specific instructions.

POSSIBLE ADVERSE REACTIONS OR SIDE EFFECTS

SYMPTOMS	FREQUENCY	WHAT TO DO
Brain & nervous system:	None expected.	
Skin: Hives, rash, intense itch soon after a dose.	Rare	1
Eyes:	None expected.	
Ears, nose, throat: Dark or discolored tongue.	Common	5
Digestive: Mild nausea, vomiting, diarrhea.	Infrequent	4
Heart & lungs:	None expected.	
Blood vessels: Unexplained bleeding.	Rare	3
Muscles, bones, joints:	None expected.	
Genital, urinary:	None expected.	
Kidneys:	None expected.	
Liver:	None expected.	
Allergic: Life-threatening anaphylaxis may occur!	Rare	1 See Page 888.
Blood:	None expected.	

1-Life-threatening. Seek emergency treatment immediately.
2-Discontinue. Seek emergency treatment.
3-Discontinue. Call doctor right away.
4-Continue. Call doctor when convenient.
5-Continue. Tell doctor at next visit.
6-No action necessary.

WARNINGS & PRECAUTIONS

Don't take if:
You are allergic to bacampicillin, cephalosporin antibiotics, other penicillins or penicillamine. Life-threatening reaction may occur.

Before you start, consult your doctor:
If you are allergic to any substance or drug.

Over age 60:
You may have skin reactions, particularly around genitals and anus.

Pregnancy:
Studies inconclusive on harm to unborn child. Animal studies show fetal abnormalities. Decide with your doctor whether drug benefits justify risk to unborn child.

Breast-feeding:
Drug passes into milk. Child may become sensitive to this and all penicillins. Avoid bacampicillin or discontinue nursing until you finish medicine. Consult doctor for advice on maintaining milk supply.

Infants & children:
No problems expected.

Prolonged use:
You may become more susceptible to infections caused by germs not responsive to bacampicillin.

Skin & sunlight:
No problems expected.

Driving, piloting, or hazardous work:
Usually not dangerous. Most hazardous reactions likely to occur a few minutes after taking bacampicillin.

Airplane passengers:
No problems expected.

Discontinuing:
Don't discontinue without doctor's advice until you complete prescribed dose, even though symptoms diminish or disappear.

Others:
Urine sugar test for diabetes may show false positive result.

INTERACTION WITH OTHER DRUGS

GENERIC NAME OR DRUG CLASS	COMBINED EFFECT
Chloramphenicol	Decreased effect of both drugs.
Erythromycins	Decreased effect of both drugs.
Paromomycin	Decreased effect of both drugs.
Tetracyclines	Decreased effect of both drugs.
Troleandomycin	Decreased effect of both drugs.

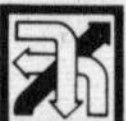

INTERACTION WITH OTHER SUBSTANCES

INTERACTS WITH	COMBINED EFFECT
Alcohol:	Occasional stomach irritation.
Beverages:	None expected.
Cocaine:	No proven problems.
Foods:	None expected.
Marijuana:	No proven problems.
Tobacco:	None expected.

BACLOFEN

BRAND NAMES

Lioresal

GENERAL INFORMATION

Habit forming? No
Prescription needed? Yes
Available as generic? No
Drug class: Muscle relaxant (analgesic)

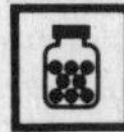

USES

- Relieves spasms, cramps and spasticity of muscles caused by medical problems, including multiple sclerosis and spine injuries.
- Reduces number and severity of trigeminal neuralgia attacks.

DOSAGE & USAGE INFORMATION

How to take:
Tablet or capsule—Swallow with liquid or food to lessen stomach irritation.

When to take:
3 or 4 times daily as directed.

If you forget a dose:
Take as soon as you remember up to 2 hours late. If more than 2 hours, wait for next scheduled dose (don't double this dose).

What drug does:
Blocks body's pain and reflex messages to brain.

Time lapse before drug works:
Variable. Few hours to weeks.

Don't take with:
See Interaction column and consult doctor.

OVERDOSE

Symptoms:
Blurred vision, blindness, difficult breathing, muscle weakness, convulsive seizures.

What to do:
- Dial 0 (operator) or 911 (emergency) for an ambulance or medical help. Then give first aid immediately.
- If patient is unconscious and not breathing, give mouth-to-mouth breathing. If there is no heartbeat, use cardiac massage and mouth-to-mouth breathing (CPR). Don't try to make patient vomit. If you can't get help quickly, take patient to nearest emergency facility.
- Additional emergency information on page 886.

POSSIBLE ADVERSE REACTIONS OR SIDE EFFECTS

SYMPTOMS	FREQUENCY	WHAT TO DO
Brain & nervous system:		
• Dizziness, lightheadedness, confusion, drowsiness.	Common	4
• Fainting, hallucinations, depression, weakness.	Rare	3
• Headache	Infrequent	4
Skin:		
Rash with itching.	Infrequent	3
Eyes:	None expected.	
Ears, nose, throat:		
Ringing in ears.	Rare	4
Digestive:		
• Nausea	Common	4
• Abdominal pain, diarrhea or constipation.	Infrequent	4
• Appetite loss.	Infrequent	4
Heart & lungs:		
• Chest pain.	Rare	3
• Lowered blood pressure.	Rare	4
• Pounding heartbeat.	Rare	4
Blood vessels:	None expected.	
Muscles, bones, joints:		
Muscle weakness.	Infrequent	4
Genital, urinary:		
• Difficult urination.	Infrequent	4
• Male sex problems.	Infrequent	4
Kidneys, allergic, blood, liver:	None expected.	
Others:		
Numbness, tingling in hands or feet.	Infrequent	3

2- Discontinue. Seek emergency treatment.
3- Discontinue. Call doctor right away.
4- Continue. Call doctor when convenient.
5- Continue. Tell doctor at next visit.
6- No action necessary.

WARNINGS & PRECAUTIONS

Don't take if:
You are allergic to any muscle relaxant.

Before you start, consult your doctor:
- If you have Parkinson's disease.
- If you have cerebral palsy.
- If you have had a recent stroke.
- If you have had a recent head injury.
- If you have arthritis.
- If you have diabetes.
- If you have epilepsy.
- If you have psychosis.
- If you have kidney disease.
- If you will have surgery within 2 months, including dental surgery, requiring general or spinal anesthesia.

Over age 60:
Adverse reactions and side effects may be more frequent and severe than in younger persons.

Pregnancy:
Risk to unborn child outweighs drug benefits. Don't use.

Breast-feeding:
Avoid nursing or discontinue until you finish medicine.

Infants & children:
Not recommended.

Prolonged use:
Epileptic patients should be monitored with EEGs. Diabetics should more closely monitor blood sugar levels. Obtain periodic liver function tests.

Skin & sunlight:
No problems expected.

Driving, piloting or hazardous work:
Don't drive or pilot aircraft until you learn how medicine affects you. Don't work around dangerous machinery. Don't climb ladders or work in high places. Danger increases if you drink alcohol or take medicine affecting alertness and reflexes, such as antihistamines, tranquilizers, sedatives, pain medicine, narcotics and mind-altering drugs.

Airplane passengers:
No problems expected.

Discontinuing:
Don't discontinue without consulting doctor. Dose may require gradual reduction if you have taken drug for a long time. Doses of other drugs may also require adjustment.

INTERACTION WITH OTHER DRUGS

GENERIC NAME OR DRUG CLASS	COMBINED EFFECT
General anesthetics	Increased sedation. Low blood pressure. Avoid.
CNS depressants: **Sedatives** **Sleeping pills** **Tranquilizers** **Antidepressants** **Antihistamines** **Narcotics** **Other muscle relaxants**	Increased sedation. Low blood pressure. Avoid.
Insulin and oral medications for diabetes.	Need to adjust diabetes medicine dosage.

INTERACTION WITH OTHER SUBSTANCES

INTERACTS WITH	COMBINED EFFECT
Alcohol:	Increased sedation. Low blood pressure. Avoid.
Beverages:	No problems expected.
Cocaine:	Increased spasticity. Avoid.
Foods:	No problems expected.
Marijuana:	Increased spasticity. Avoid.
Tobacco:	May interfere with absorption of medicine.

BECLOMETHASONE

BRAND NAMES

Beclovent Inhaler
Beconase Inhaler
Propaderm
Vancenase Inhaler
Vanceril Inhaler

GENERAL INFORMATION

Habit forming? No
Prescription needed? Yes
Available as generic? No
Drug class: Cortisone drug (adrenal corticosteroid), antiasthmatic

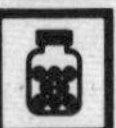

USES

Prevents attacks of bronchial asthma and allergic hay fever. Does not stop an active asthma attack.

DOSAGE & USAGE INFORMATION

How to take:
Follow package instructions. Don't inhale more than twice per dose. Rinse mouth after use to prevent hoarseness, throat irritation and mouth infection.

When to take:
Regularly at the same times each day.

If you forget a dose:
Take as soon as you remember up to 2 hours late. If more than 2 hours, wait for next scheduled dose (don't double this dose).

What drug does:
Reduces inflammation in bronchial tubes.

Time lapse before drug works:
1 to 4 weeks.

Don't take with:
See Interaction column and consult doctor.

OVERDOSE

Symptoms:
Fluid retention, flushed face, nervousness, stomach irritation.

What to do:
Overdose unlikely to threaten life. If person inhales much larger amount than prescribed, call doctor, poison-control center or hospital emergency room for instructions.

POSSIBLE ADVERSE REACTIONS OR SIDE EFFECTS

SYMPTOMS	FREQUENCY	WHAT TO DO
Brain & nervous system:	None expected.	
Skin:		
Rash	Infrequent	3
Eyes:	None expected.	
Ears, nose, throat:		
Fungus infection with white patches in mouth, dryness, sore throat.	Common	4
Digestive:	None expected.	
Heart & lungs:		
Lung inflammation, spasm of bronchial tubes.	Infrequent	4
Blood vessels:	None expected.	
Muscles, bones, joints:	None expected.	
Genital, urinary:	None expected.	
Kidneys:	None expected.	
Liver:	None expected.	
Allergic:	None expected.	
Blood:	None expected.	
Others:	None expected.	

1- Life-threatening. Seek emergency treatment immediately.
2- Discontinue. Seek emergency treatment.
3- Discontinue. Call doctor right away.
4- Continue. Call doctor when convenient.
5- Continue. Tell doctor at next visit.
6- No action necessary.

WARNINGS & PRECAUTIONS

Don't take if:
- You are allergic to beclomethasone.
- You have had tuberculosis.
- You are having an asthma attack.

Before you start, consult your doctor:
- If you take other cortisone drugs.
- If you have an infection.

Over age 60:
More likely to develop lung infections.

Pregnancy:
Risk to unborn child outweighs drug benefits. Don't use.

Breast-feeding:
Drug passes into milk. Avoid drug or discontinue nursing.

Infants & children:
Use only under medical supervision.

Prolonged use:
No problems expected.

Skin & sunlight:
No problems expected.

Driving, piloting or hazardous work:
No problems expected.

Airplane passengers:
No problems expected.

Discontinuing:
Don't discontinue without doctor's advice until you complete prescribed dose, even though symptoms diminish or disappear.

Others:
- Unrelated illness or injury may require cortisone drugs by mouth or injection. Notify your doctor.
- Consult doctor as soon as possible if your asthma returns while using beclamethasone as a preventive.
- Drug can reactivate tuberculosis.

INTERACTION WITH OTHER DRUGS

GENERIC NAME OR DRUG CLASS	COMBINED EFFECT
Antiasthmatics (other)	Increased antiasthmatic effect.
Ephedrine	Increased beclomethasone effect.
Epinephrine	Increased beclomethasone effect.
Isoetharine	Increased beclomethasone effect.
Isoproterenol	Increased beclomethasone effect.
Terbutaline	Increased beclomethasone effect.
Theophylline	Increased beclomethasone effect.

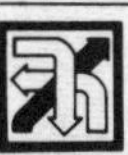

INTERACTION WITH OTHER SUBSTANCES

INTERACTS WITH	COMBINED EFFECT
Alcohol:	None expected.
Beverages:	None expected.
Cocaine:	None expected.
Foods:	None expected.
Marijuana:	Decreased beclomethasone effect.
Tobacco:	Decreased beclomethasone effect.

BELLADONNA

BRAND NAMES

Atrosed
Barbidonna
Butabar Elixir
Butibel Elixir
Chardonna
Spasnil
Wigraine

See complete brand names list, page 823.

GENERAL INFORMATION

Habit forming? No
Prescription needed? Low strength: No
High strength: Yes
Available as generic? Yes
Drug class: Antispasmodic, anticholinergic

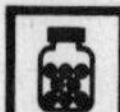

USES

Reduces spasms of digestive system, bladder and urethra.

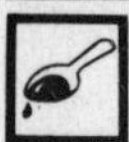

DOSAGE & USAGE INFORMATION

How to take:

- Tablet, elixir or capsule—Swallow with liquid or food to lessen stomach irritation.
- Drops—Dilute dose in beverage before swallowing.

When to take:
30 minutes before meals (unless directed otherwise by doctor).

If you forget a dose:
Take as soon as you remember up to 2 hours late. If more than 2 hours, wait for next scheduled dose (don't double this dose).

What drug does:
Blocks nerve impulses at parasympathetic nerve endings, preventing muscle contractions and gland secretions of organs involved.

Time lapse before drug works:
15 to 30 minutes.

Don't take with:
See Interaction column and consult doctor.

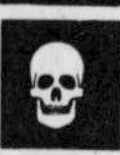

OVERDOSE

Symptoms:
Dilated pupils; rapid pulse and breathing; dizziness; fever; hallucinations; confusion; slurred speech; agitation; flushed face; convulsions; coma.

What to do:

- Dial 0 (operator) or 911 (emergency) for an ambulance or medical help. Then give first aid immediately.
- Additional emergency information on page 886.

POSSIBLE ADVERSE REACTIONS OR SIDE EFFECTS

SYMPTOMS	FREQUENCY	WHAT TO DO
Brain & nervous system:		
• Headache	Infrequent	4
• Confusion, delirium.	Common	3
Skin:		
Rash or hives.	Rare	3
Eyes:		
Pain, blurred vision.	Rare	3
Ears, nose, throat:		
Dryness	Common	6
Digestive:		
• Constipation	Common	5
• Nausea, vomiting.	Common	4
Heart & lungs:		
Rapid heartbeat.	Common	3
Blood vessels:	None expected.	
Muscles, bones, joints:	None expected.	
Genital, urinary:		
Difficult urination.	Infrequent	4
Kidneys:	None expected.	
Liver:	None expected.	
Allergic:	None expected.	
Blood:	None expected.	
Others:		
Less perspiration.	Common	4

1- Life-threatening. Seek emergency treatment immediately.
2- Discontinue. Seek emergency treatment.
3- Discontinue. Call doctor right away.
4- Continue. Call doctor when convenient.
5- Continue. Tell doctor at next visit.
6- No action necessary.

WARNINGS & PRECAUTIONS

Don't take if:

- You are allergic to any anticholinergic.
- You have trouble with stomach bloating.
- You have difficulty emptying your bladder completely.
- You have narrow-angle glaucoma.
- You have severe ulcerative colitis.

Before you start, consult your doctor:

- If you have open-angle glaucoma.
- If you have angina.
- If you have chronic bronchitis or asthma.
- If you have hiatal hernia.
- If you have liver disease.
- If you have enlarged prostate.
- If you have myasthenia gravis.
- If you have peptic ulcer.
- If you will have surgery within 2 months, including dental surgery, requiring general or spinal anesthesia.

Over age 60:
Adverse reactions and side effects may be more frequent and severe than in younger persons.

Pregnancy:
Studies inconclusive on harm to unborn child. Animal studies show fetal abnormalities. Decide with your doctor whether drug benefits justify risk to unborn child.

Breast-feeding:
Drug passes into milk and decreases milk flow. Avoid drug or discontinue nursing until you finish medicine. Consult doctor for advice on maintaining milk supply.

Infants & children:
Use only under medical supervision.

Prolonged use:
Chronic constipation, possible fecal impaction. Consult doctor immediately.

Skin & sunlight:
No problems expected.

Driving, piloting or hazardous work:
Use disqualifies you for piloting aircraft. Otherwise, no problems expected.

Airplane passengers:
No problems expected.

Discontinuing:
May be unnecessary to finish medicine. Follow doctor's instructions.

Others:
No problems expected.

INTERACTION WITH OTHER DRUGS

GENERIC NAME OR DRUG CLASS	COMBINED EFFECT
Amantadine	Increased belladonna effect.
Anticholinergics (other)	Increased belladonna effect.
Antidepressants (tricyclic)	Increased belladonna effect.
Antihistamines	Increased belladonna effect.
Cortisone drugs	Increased internal-eye pressure.
Haloperidol	Increased internal-eye pressure.
MAO inhibitors	Increased belladonna effect.
Meperidine	Increased belladonna effect.
Methylphenidate	Increased belladonna effect.
Orphenadrine	Increased belladonna effect.
Phenothiazines	Increased belladonna effect.
Pilocarpine	Loss of pilocarpine effect in glaucoma treatment.
Vitamin C	Decreased belladonna effect. Avoid large doses of vitamin C.

INTERACTION WITH OTHER SUBSTANCES

INTERACTS WITH	COMBINED EFFECT
Alcohol:	None expected.
Beverages:	None expected.
Cocaine:	Excessively rapid heartbeat. Avoid.
Foods:	None expected.
Marijuana:	Drowsiness and dry mouth.
Tobacco:	None expected.

BENDROFLUMETHIAZIDE

BRAND NAMES

Corzide
Naturetin
Rauzide

GENERAL INFORMATION

Habit forming? No
Prescription needed? Yes
Available as generic? Yes
Drug class: Antihypertensive, diuretic (thiazide)

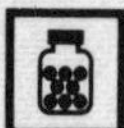

USES

- Controls, but doesn't cure, high blood pressure.
- Reduces fluid retention (edema) caused by conditions such as heart disorders and liver disease.

DOSAGE & USAGE INFORMATION

How to take:
Tablet or capsule—Swallow with liquid. If you can't swallow whole, crumble tablet or open capsule and take with liquid or food. Don't exceed dose.

When to take:
At the same time each day.

If you forget a dose:
Take as soon as you remember up to 2 hours late. If more than 2 hours, wait for next scheduled dose (don't double this dose).

What drug does:
- Forces sodium and water excretion, reducing body fluid.
- Relaxes muscle cells of small arteries.
- Reduced body fluid and relaxed arteries lower blood pressure.

Time lapse before drug works:
4 to 6 hours. May require several weeks to lower blood pressure.

Don't take with:
- See Interaction column and consult doctor.
- Non-prescription drugs without consulting doctor.

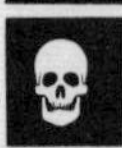

OVERDOSE

Symptoms:
Cramps, weakness, drowsiness, weak pulse, coma.

What to do:
- Dial O (operator) or 911 (emergency) for an ambulance or medical help. Then give first aid immediately.
- Additional emergency information on page 886.

POSSIBLE ADVERSE REACTIONS OR SIDE EFFECTS

SYMPTOMS	FREQUENCY	WHAT TO DO
Brain & nervous system:		
• Dizziness	Infrequent	4
• Mood changes.	Infrequent	4
• Headaches	Infrequent	4
Skin:		
Rash or hives.	Rare	2
Eyes:		
Blurred vision.	Infrequent	3
Ears, nose, throat:		
• Sore throat, fever.	Rare	3
• Dry mouth, thirst.	Infrequent	5
Digestive:		
Severe abdominal pain, nausea, vomiting.	Infrequent	3
Heart & lungs:		
Irregular heartbeat, weak pulse.	Infrequent	3
Blood vessels:	None expected.	
Muscles, bones, joints:		
Weakness, tiredness.	Infrequent	4
Genital, urinary:	None expected.	
Kidneys:	None expected.	
Liver:		
Jaundice (yellow skin and eyes).	Rare	3
Blood:	None expected.	
Allergic:	None expected.	
Others:		
Weight changes.	Infrequent	4

1- Life-threatening. Seek emergency treatment immediately.
2- Discontinue. Seek emergency treatment.
3- Discontinue. Call doctor right away.
4- Continue. Call doctor when convenient.
5- Continue. Call doctor at next visit.
6- No action necessary.

BENDROFLUMETHIAZIDE

WARNINGS & PRECAUTIONS

Don't take if:
You are allergic to any thiazide diuretic drug.

Before you start, consult your doctor:
- If you are allergic to any sulfa drug.
- If you have gout.
- If you have liver, pancreas or kidney disorder.

Over age 60:
Adverse reactions and side effects may be more frequent and severe than in younger persons, especially dizziness and excessive potassium loss.

Pregnancy:
Risk to unborn child outweighs drug benefits. Don't use.

Breast-feeding:
Drug passes into milk. Avoid this medicine or discontinue nursing.

Infants & children:
No problems expected.

Prolonged use:
You may need medicine to treat high blood pressure for the rest of your life.

Skin & sunlight:
May cause rash or intensify sunburn in areas exposed to sun or sunlamp.

Driving, piloting or hazardous work:
Don't drive or pilot aircraft until you learn how medicine affects you. Don't work around dangerous machinery. Don't climb ladders or work in high places. Danger increases if you drink alcohol or take medicine affecting alertness and reflexes, such as antihistamines, tranquilizers, sedatives, pain medicine, narcotics and mind-altering drugs.

Airplane passengers:
No problems expected.

Discontinuing:
Don't discontinue without medical advice.

Others:
- Hot weather and fever may cause dehydration and drop in blood pressure. Dose may require temporary adjustment. Weigh daily and report any unexpected weight decreases to your doctor.
- May cause rise in uric acid, leading to gout.
- May cause blood-sugar rise in diabetics.

INTERACTION WITH OTHER DRUGS

GENERIC NAME OR DRUG CLASS	COMBINED EFFECT
Allopurinol	Decreased allopurinol effect.
Antidepressants (tricyclic)	Dangerous drop in blood pressure. Avoid combination unless under medical supervision.
Barbiturates	Increased bendroflumethiazide effect.
Cholestyramine	Decreased bendroflumethiazide effect.
Cortisone drugs	Excessive potassium loss that causes dangerous heart rhythms.
Digitalis preparations	Excessive potassium loss that causes dangerous heart rhythms.
Diuretics (thiazide)	Increased effect of other thiazide diuretics.
Lithium	Increased effect of lithium.
MAO inhibitors	Increased bendroflumethiazide effect.
Probenecid	Decreased probenecid effect.

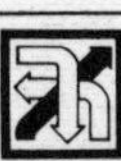

INTERACTIONS WITH OTHER SUBSTANCES

INTERACTS WITH	COMBINED EFFECT
Alcohol:	Dangerous blood-pressure drop.
Beverages:	None expected.
Cocaine:	None expected.
Foods:	
Licorice	Excessive potassium loss that causes dangerous heart rhythms.
Marijuana:	May increase blood pressure.
Tobacco:	None expected.

BENZOYL PEROXIDE

BRAND NAMES

Benoxyl
Benzac
Benzagel
Clearasil BP
Clear By Design
Dermodex
Desquam-X
Dry and Clean
Epi-Clear
Fostex BPO
Oxy-5
Oxy-10
Panoxyl
Persadox
Persa-Gel

See complete brand names list, page 823.

GENERAL INFORMATION

Habit forming? No
Prescription needed? No
Available as generic? Yes
Drug class: Antiacne (topical)

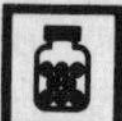

USES

Treatment for acne.

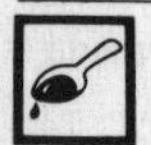

DOSAGE & USAGE INFORMATION

How to use:
Cream, gel, pads, sticks or lotion—Wash affected area with plain soap and water. Dry gently with towel. Rub medicine into affected areas. Keep away from eyes, nose, mouth.

When to use:
Apply 1 or more times daily. If you have a fair complexion, start with single application at bedtime.

If you forget an application:
Use as soon as you remember.

What drug does:
Slowly releases oxygen from skin, which controls some skin bacteria. Also causes peeling and drying, helping control blackheads and whiteheads.

Time lapse before drug works:
1 to 2 weeks.

Don't use with:
See Interaction column and consult doctor.

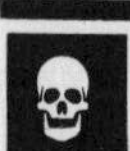

OVERDOSE

Symptoms:
None expected.

What to do:
If person swallows drug, call doctor, poison-control center or hospital emergency room for instructions.

POSSIBLE ADVERSE REACTIONS OR SIDE EFFECTS

SYMPTOMS	FREQUENCY	WHAT TO DO
Brain & nervous system:	None expected.	
Skin:		
• Painful skin irritation.	Infrequent	4
• Rash	Infrequent	3
• Excessive dryness.	Infrequent	3
Eyes:	None expected.	
Ears, nose, throat:	None expected.	
Digestive:	None expected.	
Heart & lungs:	None expected.	
Blood vessels:	None expected.	
Muscles, bones, joints:	None expected.	
Genital, urinary:	None expected.	
Kidneys:	None expected.	
Liver:	None expected.	
Allergic:	None expected.	
Blood:	None expected.	
Others:	None expected.	

1-Life-threatening. Seek emergency treatment immediately.
2-Discontinue. Seek emergency treatment.
3-Discontinue. Call doctor right away.
4-Continue. Call doctor when convenient.
5-Continue. Tell doctor at next visit.
6-No action necessary.

WARNINGS & PRECAUTIONS

Don't take if:
You are allergic to benzoyl peroxide.

Before you start, consult your doctor:
- If you plan to become pregnant within medication period.
- If you take oral contraceptives.

Over age 60:
No problems expected.

Pregnancy:
No proven problems. Consult doctor.

Breast-feeding:
No proven problems. Consult doctor.

Infants & children:
Not recommended.

Prolonged use:
Permanent rash or scarring.

Skin & sunlight:
No problems expected.

Driving, piloting or hazardous work:
No problems expected.

Airplane passengers:
No problems expected.

Discontinuing:
- May be unnecessary to finish medicine. Discontinue when acne improves.
- If acne doesn't improve in 2 weeks, call doctor.

Others:
- Keep away from hair and clothing. May bleach.
- Store away from heat in cool, dry place.
- Avoid contact with eyes, lips, nose and sensitive areas of the neck.

INTERACTION WITH OTHER DRUGS

GENERIC NAME OR DRUG CLASS	COMBINED EFFECT
Antiacne topical preparations (other)	Excessive skin irritation.
Skin-peeling agents (salicylic acid, sulfur, resorcinol, tretinoin)	Excessive skin irritation.

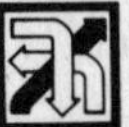

INTERACTION WITH OTHER SUBSTANCES

INTERACTS WITH	COMBINED EFFECT
Alcohol:	None expected.
Beverages:	None expected.
Cocaine:	None expected.
Foods: Cinnamon, foods with benzoic acid.	Skin rash.
Marijuana:	None expected.
Tobacco:	None expected.

BENZTHIAZIDE

BRAND NAMES

Aquastat
Aquatag
Exna
Hydrex

GENERAL INFORMATION

Habit forming? No
Prescription needed? Yes
Available as generic? Yes
Drug class: Antihypertensive, diuretic (thiazide)

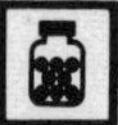

USES

- Controls, but doesn't cure, high blood pressure.
- Reduces fluid retention (edema) caused by conditions such as heart disorders and liver disease.

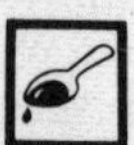

DOSAGE & USAGE INFORMATION

How to take:
Tablet or capsule—Swallow with liquid. If you can't swallow whole, crumble tablet or open capsule and take with liquid or food. Don't exceed dose.

When to take:
At the same time each day.

If you forget a dose:
Take as soon as you remember up to 2 hours late. If more than 2 hours, wait for next scheduled dose (don't double this dose).

What drug does:
- Forces sodium and water excretion, reducing body fluid.
- Relaxes muscle cells of small arteries.
- Reduced body fluid and relaxed arteries lower blood pressure.

Time lapse before drug works:
4 to 6 hours. May require several weeks to lower blood pressure.

Don't take with:
- See Interaction column and consult doctor.
- Non-prescription drugs without consulting doctor.

OVERDOSE

Symptoms:
Cramps, weakness, drowsiness, weak pulse, coma.

What to do:
- Dial 0 (operator) or 911 (emergency) for an ambulance or medical help. Then give first aid immediately.
- Additional emergency information on page 886.

POSSIBLE ADVERSE REACTIONS OR SIDE EFFECTS

SYMPTOMS	FREQUENCY	WHAT TO DO
Brain & nervous system:		
• Dizziness	Infrequent	4
• Mood changes.	Infrequent	4
• Headaches	Infrequent	4
Skin:		
Rash or hives.	Rare	2
Eyes:		
Blurred vision.	Infrequent	3
Ears, nose, throat:		
• Sore throat, fever.	Rare	3
• Dry mouth, thirst.	Infrequent	5
Digestive:		
Severe abdominal pain, nausea, vomiting.	Infrequent	3
Heart & lungs:		
Irregular heartbeat, weak pulse.	Infrequent	3
Blood vessels:	None expected.	
Muscles, bones, joints:		
Weakness, tiredness.	Infrequent	4
Genital, urinary:	None expected.	
Kidneys:	None expected.	
Liver:		
Jaundice (yellow skin and eyes).	Rare	3
Allergic:	None expected.	
Blood:	None expected.	
Others:		
Weight changes.	Infrequent	4

1- Life-threatening. Seek emergency treatment immediately.
2- Discontinue. Seek emergency treatment.
3- Discontinue. Call doctor right away.
4- Continue. Call doctor when convenient.
5- Continue. Tell doctor at next visit.
6- No action necessary.

WARNINGS & PRECAUTIONS

Don't take if:
You are allergic to any thiazide diuretic drug.

Before you start, consult your doctor:
- If you are allergic to any sulfa drug.
- If you have gout.
- If you have liver, pancreas or kidney disorder.

Over age 60:
Adverse reactions and side effects may be more frequent and severe than in younger persons, especially dizziness and excessive potassium loss.

Pregnancy:
Risk to unborn child outweighs drug benefits. Don't use.

Breast-feeding:
Drug passes into milk. Avoid drug or discontinue nursing.

Infants & children:
No problems expected.

Prolonged use:
You may need medicine to treat high blood pressure for the rest of your life.

Skin & sunlight:
May cause rash or intensify sunburn in areas exposed to sun or sunlamp.

Driving, piloting or hazardous work:
Don't drive or pilot aircraft until you learn how medicine affects you. Don't work around dangerous machinery. Don't climb ladders or work in high places. Danger increases if you drink alcohol or take medicine affecting alertness and reflexes, such as antihistamines, tranquilizers, sedatives, pain medicine, narcotics and mind-altering drugs.

Airplane passengers:
No problems expected.

Discontinuing:
Don't discontinue without medical advice.

Others:
- Hot weather and fever may cause dehydration and drop in blood pressure. Dose may require temporary adjustment. Weigh daily and report any unexpected weight decreases to your doctor.
- May cause rise in uric acid, leading to gout.
- May cause blood-sugar rise in diabetics.

INTERACTION WITH OTHER DRUGS

GENERIC NAME OR DRUG CLASS	COMBINED EFFECT
Allopurinol	Decreased allopurinol effect.
Antidepressants (tricyclic)	Dangerous drop in blood pressure. Avoid combination unless under medical supervision.
Barbiturates	Increased benzthiazide effect.
Cholestyramine	Decreased benzthiazide effect.
Cortisone drugs	Excessive potassium loss that causes dangerous heart rhythms.
Digitalis preparations	Excessive potassium loss that causes dangerous heart rhythms.
Diuretics (thiazide)	Increased effect of other thiazide diuretics.
Lithium	Increased effect of lithium.
MAO inhibitors	Increased benzthiazide effect.
Probenecid	Decreased probenecid effect.

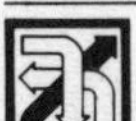

INTERACTION WITH OTHER SUBSTANCES

INTERACTS WITH	COMBINED EFFECT
Alcohol:	Dangerous blood-pressure drop.
Beverages:	None expected.
Cocaine:	None expected.
Foods:	
Licorice	Excessive potassium loss that causes dangerous heart rhythms.
Marijuana:	May increase blood pressure.
Tobacco:	None expected.

BENZTROPINE

BRAND NAMES

Apo-Benztropine
Bensylate
Cogentin

GENERAL INFORMATION

Habit forming? No
Prescription needed? Yes
Available as generic? No
Drug class: Antidyskinetic, antiparkinsonism

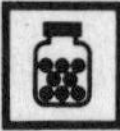

USES

- Treatment of Parkinson's disease.
- Treatment of adverse effects of phenothiazines.

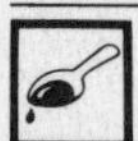

DOSAGE & USAGE INFORMATION

How to take:
Tablets or capsules—Take with food to lessen stomach irritation.

When to take:
At the same times each day.

If you forget a dose:
Take as soon as you remember up to 2 hours late. If more than 2 hours, wait for next scheduled dose (don't double this dose).

What drug does:
- Balances chemical reactions necessary to send nerve impulses within base of brain.
- Improves muscle control and reduces stiffness.

Time lapse before drug works:
1 to 2 hours.

Don't take with:
- Non-prescription drugs for colds, cough or allergy.
- See Interaction column and consult doctor.

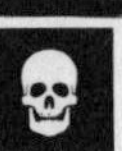

OVERDOSE

Symptoms:
Agitation, dilated pupils, hallucinations, dry mouth, rapid heartbeat, sleepiness.

What to do:
- Dial 0 (operator) or 911 (emergency) for an ambulance or medical help. Then give first aid immediately.
- If patient is unconscious and not breathing, give mouth-to-mouth breathing. If there is no heartbeat, use cardiac massage and mouth-to-mouth breathing (CPR). Don't try to make patient vomit. If you can't get help quickly, take patient to nearest emergency facility.
- Additional emergency information on page 886.

POSSIBLE ADVERSE REACTIONS OR SIDE EFFECTS

SYMPTOMS	FREQUENCY	WHAT TO DO
Brain & nervous system:		
Confusion, dizziness.	Rare	4
Skin:		
Rash	Rare	3
Eyes:		
• Pain	Rare	3
• Blurred vision, light sensitivity.	Common	4
Ears, nose, throat:		
Sore mouth or tongue.	Rare	4
Digestive:		
• Constipation	Common	4
• Nausea, vomiting.	Common	4
Heart & lungs:	None expected.	
Blood vessels:	None expected.	
Muscles, bones, joints:		
• Muscle cramps.	Rare	4
• Numbness, weakness in hands or feet.	Rare	4
Genital, urinary:		
Difficult or painful urination.	Common	5
Kidneys:	None expected.	
Liver:	None expected.	
Allergic:	None expected.	
Blood:	None expected.	
Others:	None expected.	

1- Life-threatening. Seek emergency treatment immediately.
2- Discontinue. Seek emergency treatment.
3- Discontinue. Call doctor right away.
4- Continue. Call doctor when convenient.
5- Continue. Tell doctor at next visit.
6- No action necessary.

WARNINGS & PRECAUTIONS

Don't take if:
You are allergic to any antidyskinetic.

Before you start, consult your doctor:
- If you have had glaucoma.
- If you have had high blood pressure or heart disease.
- If you have had impaired liver function.
- If you have had kidney disease or urination difficulty.

Over age 60:
More sensitive to drug. Aggravates symptoms of enlarged prostate. Causes impaired thinking, hallucinations, nightmares. Consult doctor about any of these.

Pregnancy:
Studies inconclusive on harm to unborn child. Animal studies show fetal abnormalities. Decide with your doctor whether drug benefits justify risk to unborn child.

Breast-feeding:
No problems expected.

Infants & children:
Not recommended for children 3 and younger. Use for older children only under doctor's supervision.

Prolonged use:
Possible glaucoma.

Skin & sunlight:
No problems expected.

Driving, piloting or hazardous work:
Don't drive or pilot aircraft until you learn how medicine affects you. Don't work around dangerous machinery. Don't climb ladders or work in high places. Danger increases if you drink alcohol or take medicine affecting alertness and reflexes, such as antihistamines, tranquilizers, sedatives, pain medicine, narcotics and mind-altering drugs.

Airplane passengers:
No problems expected.

Discontinuing:
Don't discontinue without consulting doctor. Dose may require gradual reduction if you have taken drug for a long time. Doses of other drugs may also require adjustment.

Others:
- Internal eye pressure should be measured regularly.
- Avoid becoming overheated.

INTERACTION WITH OTHER DRUGS

GENERIC NAME OR DRUG CLASS	COMBINED EFFECT
Amantadine	Increased amantadine effect.
Antidepressants (tricyclic)	Increased benztropine effect. May cause glaucoma.
Antihistamines	Increased benztropine effect.
Levodopa	Increased levodopa effect. Improved results in treating Parkinson's disease.
Meperidine	Increased benztropine effect.
MAO inhibitors	Increased benztropine effect.
Orphenadrine	Increased benztropine effect.
Phenothiazines	Behavior changes.
Primidone	Excessive sedation.
Procainamide	Increased procainamide effect.
Quinidine	Increased benztropine effect.
Tranquilizers	Excessive sedation.

INTERACTION WITH OTHER SUBSTANCES

INTERACTS WITH	COMBINED EFFECT
Alcohol:	None expected.
Beverages:	None expected.
Cocaine:	Decreased benztropine effect. Avoid.
Foods:	None expected.
Marijuana:	None expected.
Tobacco:	None expected.

BETAMETHASONE

BRAND NAMES

Beconase
Betnelan
Betnesol
Celestoject
Celestone
Cel-U-Sec
Vancerace

See complete brand names list, page 823.

GENERAL INFORMATION

Habit forming? No
Prescription needed? Yes
Available as generic? Yes
Drug class: Cortisone drug (adrenal corticosteroid)

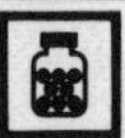

USES

- Reduces inflammation caused by many different medical problems.
- Treatment for some allergic diseases, blood disorders, kidney diseases, asthma and emphysema.
- Replaces corticosteroid deficiencies.

DOSAGE & USAGE INFORMATION

How to take:

- Tablet or liquid—Swallow with liquid or food to lessen stomach irritation. If you can't swallow whole, crumble tablet and take with liquid or food.
- Inhaler—Follow label instructions.

When to take:
At the same times each day. Take once-a-day or once-every-other-day doses in mornings.

If you forget a dose:

- Several-doses-per-day prescription—Take as soon as you remember up to 2 hours late. If more than 2 hours, wait for next scheduled dose (don't double this dose).
- Once-a-day dose or less—Wait for next dose. Double this dose.

What drug does:
Decreases inflammatory responses.

Time lapse before drug works:
2 to 4 days.

Don't take with:
See Interaction column and consult doctor.

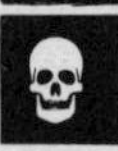

OVERDOSE

Symptoms:
Headache, convulsions, heart failure.

What to do:

- Dial 0 (operator) or 911 (emergency) for an ambulance or medical help. Then give first aid immediately.
- Additional emergency information on page 886.

POSSIBLE ADVERSE REACTIONS OR SIDE EFFECTS

SYMPTOMS	FREQUENCY	WHAT TO DO
Brain & nervous system:		
Mood changes, insomnia, restlessness.	Infrequent	4
Skin:		
• Acne	Common	4
• Rash	Rare	3
• Poor wound healing.	Common	4
Eyes:		
Blurred vision, halos around lights.	Infrequent	3
Ears, nose, throat:		
• Sore throat, fever.	Infrequent	3
• Thirst	Common	4
Digestive:		
• Indigestion, nausea, vomiting.	Common	4
• Bloody or black, tarry stool.	Infrequent	2
Heart & lungs:		
Irregular heartbeat.	Rare	2
Blood vessels, kidneys, liver, allergic, blood:	None expected.	
Muscles, bones, joints:		
Muscle cramps, swollen legs, feet.	Infrequent	3
Genital, urinary:		
Frequent urination.	Infrequent	4
Others:		
• Weight gain, round face.	Infrequent	4
• Fatigue, weakness.	Infrequent	4
• TB recurrence.	Infrequent	4
• Irregular menstrual periods.	Infrequent	4

1- Life-threatening. Seek emergency treatment immediately.
2- Discontinue. Seek emergency treatment.
3- Discontinue. Call doctor right away.
4- Continue. Call doctor when convenient.

BETAMETHASONE

WARNINGS & PRECAUTIONS

Don't take if:
- You are allergic to any cortisone drug.
- You have tuberculosis or fungus infection.
- You have herpes infection of eyes, lips or genitals.

Before you start, consult your doctor:
- If you have had tuberculosis.
- If you have congestive heart failure.
- If you have diabetes.
- If you have peptic ulcer.
- If you have glaucoma.
- If you have underactive thyroid.
- If you have high blood pressure.
- If you have myasthenia gravis.
- If you have blood clots in legs or lungs.

Over age 60:
Adverse reactions and side effects may be more frequent and severe than in younger persons. Likely to aggravate edema, diabetes or ulcers. Likely to cause cataracts and osteoporosis (softening of the bones).

Pregnancy:
Risk to unborn child outweighs drug benefits. Don't use.

Breast-feeding:
Drug passes into milk. Avoid drug or discontinue nursing until you finish medicine. Consult doctor for advice on maintaining milk supply.

Infants & children:
Use only under medical supervision.

Prolonged use:
- Retards growth in children.
- Possible glaucoma, cataracts, diabetes, fragile bones and thin skin.
- Functional dependence.

Skin & sunlight:
No problems expected.

Driving, piloting or hazardous work:
No problems expected.

Airplane passengers:
No problems expected.

Discontinuing:
- Don't discontinue without doctor's advice until you complete prescribed dose, even though symptoms diminish or disappear.
- Drug affects your response to surgery, illness, injury or stress for 2 years after discontinuing. Tell about drug to anyone who takes medical care of you within 2 years.

Others:
Avoid immunizations if possible.

INTERACTION WITH OTHER DRUGS

GENERIC NAME OR DRUG CLASS	COMBINED EFFECT
Amphoterecin B	Potassium depletion.
Anticholinergics	Possible glaucoma.
Anticoagulants (oral)	Decreased anticoagulant effect.
Anticonvulsants (hydantoin)	Decreased betamethasone effect.
Antidiabetics (oral)	Decreased antidiabetic effect.
Antihistamines	Decreased betamethasone effect.
Aspirin	Increased betamethasone effect.
Barbiturates	Decreased betamethasone effect. Oversedation.
Beta-adrenergic blockers	Decreased betamethasone effect.
Chloral hydrate	Decreased betamethasone effect.
Chlorthalidone	Potassium depletion.
Cholinergics	Decreased cholinergic effect.
Contraceptives (oral)	Increased betamethasone effect.
Digitalis preparations	Dangerous potassium depletion. Possible digitalis toxicity.
Diuretics (thiazide)	Potassium depletion.

Additional interactions on page 835.

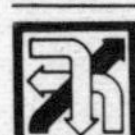

INTERACTION WITH OTHER SUBSTANCES

INTERACTS WITH	COMBINED EFFECT
Alcohol:	Risk of stomach ulcers.
Beverages:	No proven problems.
Cocaine:	Overstimulation. Avoid.
Foods:	No proven problems.
Marijuana:	Decreased immunity.
Tobacco:	Increased betamethasone effect. Possible toxicity.

BETHANECHOL

BRAND NAMES

Duvoid
Myotonachol
Urecholine

GENERAL INFORMATION

Habit forming? No
Prescription needed? Yes
Available as generic? Yes
Drug class: Cholinergic

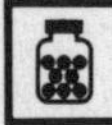

USES

Helps initiate urination following surgery, or for persons with urinary infections or enlarged prostate.

DOSAGE & USAGE INFORMATION

How to take:
Tablet or capsule—Swallow with liquid, 1 hour before or 2 hours after eating.

When to take:
At the same times each day.

If you forget a dose:
Take as soon as you remember up to 2 hours late. If more than 2 hours, wait for next scheduled dose (don't double this dose).

What drug does:
Affects chemical reactions in the body that strengthen bladder muscles.

Time lapse before drug works:
30 to 90 minutes.

Don't take with:
See Interaction column and consult doctor.

OVERDOSE

Symptoms:
Shortness of breath, wheezing or chest tightness, unconsciousness, coma.

What to do:
- Dial 0 (operator) or 911 (emergency) for an ambulance or medical help. Then give first aid immediately.
- If patient is unconscious and not breathing, give mouth-to-mouth breathing. If there is no heartbeat, use cardiac massage and mouth-to-mouth breathing (CPR). Don't try to make patient vomit. If you can't get help quickly, take patient to nearest emergency facility.
- Additional emergency information on page 886.

POSSIBLE ADVERSE REACTIONS OR SIDE EFFECTS

SYMPTOMS	FREQUENCY	WHAT TO DO
Brain & nervous system: Dizziness, headache, faintness.	Infrequent	4
Skin:	None expected.	
Eyes: Blurred or changed vision.	Infrequent	4
Ears, nose, throat:	None expected.	
Digestive: Diarrhea, nausea, vomiting, stomach discomfort, belching.	Infrequent	4
Heart & lungs: Shortness of breath, wheezing, tightness in chest.	Rare	3
Blood vessels:	None expected.	
Muscles, bones, joints:	None expected.	
Genital, urinary: Excessive urge to urinate.	Infrequent	4
Kidneys:	None expected.	
Liver:	None expected.	
Allergic:	None expected.	
Blood:	None expected.	
Others:	None expected.	

1- Life-threatening. Seek emergency treatment immediately.
2- Discontinue. Seek emergency treatment.
3- Discontinue. Call doctor right away.
4- Continue. Call doctor when convenient.
5- Continue. Tell doctor at next visit.
6- No action necessary.

WARNINGS & PRECAUTIONS

Don't take if:
You are allergic to any cholinergic.

Before you start, consult your doctor:
- If you plan to become pregnant within medication period.
- If you have asthma.
- If you have epilepsy.
- If you have heart or blood-vessel disease.
- If you have high or low blood pressure.
- If you have overactive thyroid.
- If you have intestinal blockage.
- If you have Parkinson's disease.
- If you have stomach problems (including ulcer).
- If you have had bladder or intestinal surgery within 1 month.

Over age 60:
Adverse reactions and side effects may be more frequent and severe than in younger persons.

Pregnancy:
Risk to unborn child outweighs drug benefits. Don't use.

Breast-feeding:
Drug filters into milk. May harm child. Avoid.

Infants & children:
Use only under medical supervision.

Prolonged use:
No problems expected.

Skin & sunlight:
No problems expected.

Driving, piloting or hazardous work:
Don't drive or pilot aircraft until you learn how medicine affects you. Don't work around dangerous machinery. Don't climb ladders or work in high places. Danger increases if you drink alcohol or take medicine affecting alertness and reflexes, such as antihistamines, tranquilizers, sedatives, pain medicine, narcotics and mind-altering drugs.

Airplane passengers:
No problems expected.

Discontinuing:
May be unnecessary to finish medicine. Follow doctor's instructions.

Others:
- Be cautious about standing up suddenly.
- Interferes with laboratory studies of liver and pancreas function.
- Side effects more likely with injections.

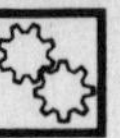

INTERACTION WITH OTHER DRUGS

GENERIC NAME OR DRUG CLASS	COMBINED EFFECT
Cholinergics (other)	Increased effect of both drugs. Possible toxicity.
Procainamide	Decreased bethanechol effect.
Quinidine	Decreased bethanechol effect.

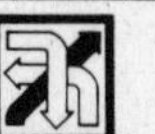

INTERACTION WITH OTHER SUBSTANCES

INTERACTS WITH	COMBINED EFFECT
Alcohol:	None expected.
Beverages:	None expected.
Cocaine:	None expected.
Foods:	None expected.
Marijuana:	None expected.
Tobacco:	None expected.

BIPERIDEN

BRAND NAMES

Akineton

GENERAL INFORMATION

Habit forming? No
Prescription needed? Yes
Available as generic? No
Drug class: Antidyskinetic, antiparkinsonism

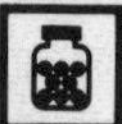

USES

- Treatment of Parkinson's disease.
- Treatment of adverse effects of phenothiazines.

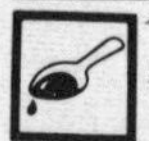

DOSAGE & USAGE INFORMATION

How to take:
Tablets or capsules—Take with food to lessen stomach irritation.

When to take:
At the same times each day.

If you forget a dose:
Take as soon as you remember up to 2 hours late. If more than 2 hours, wait for next scheduled dose (don't double this dose).

What drug does:
- Balances chemical reactions necessary to send nerve impulses within base of brain.
- Improves muscle control and reduces stiffness.

Time lapse before drug works:
1 to 2 hours.

Don't take with:
- Non-prescription drugs for colds, cough or allergy.
- See Interaction column and consult doctor.

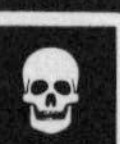

OVERDOSE

Symptoms:
Agitation, dilated pupils, hallucinations, dry mouth, rapid heartbeat, sleepiness.

What to do:
- Dial 0 (operator) or 911 (emergency) for an ambulance or medical help. Then give first aid immediately.
- If patient is unconscious and not breathing, give mouth-to-mouth breathing. If there is no heartbeat, use cardiac massage and mouth-to-mouth breathing (CPR). Don't try to make patient vomit. If you can't get help quickly, take patient to nearest emergency facility.
- Additional emergency information on page 886.

POSSIBLE ADVERSE REACTIONS OR SIDE EFFECTS

SYMPTOMS	FREQUENCY	WHAT TO DO
Brain & nervous system:		
Confusion, dizziness.	Rare	4
Skin:		
Rash	Rare	3
Eyes:		
• Pain	Rare	3
• Blurred vision, light sensitivity.	Common	4
Ears, nose, throat:		
Sore mouth or tongue.	Rare	4
Digestive:		
• Constipation	Common	4
• Nausea, vomiting.	Common	4
Heart & lungs:	None expected.	
Blood vessels:	None expected.	
Muscles, bones, joints:		
• Muscle cramps.	Rare	4
• Numbness, weakness in hands or feet.	Rare	4
Genital, urinary:		
Difficult or painful urination.	Common	5
Kidneys:	None expected.	
Liver:	None expected.	
Allergic:	None expected.	
Blood:	None expected.	
Others:	None expected.	

1- Life-threatening. Seek emergency treatment immediately.
2- Discontinue. Seek emergency treatment.
3- Discontinue. Call doctor right away.
4- Continue. Call doctor when convenient.
5- Continue. Tell doctor at next visit.
6- No action necessary.

WARNINGS & PRECAUTIONS

Don't take if:
You are allergic to any antidyskinetic.

Before you start, consult your doctor:
- If you have had glaucoma.
- If you have had high blood pressure or heart disease.
- If you have had impaired liver function.
- If you have had kidney disease or urination difficulty.

Over age 60:
More sensitive to drug. Aggravates symptoms of enlarged prostate. Causes impaired thinking, hallucinations, nightmares. Consult doctor about any of these.

Pregnancy:
Studies inconclusive on harm to unborn child. Animal studies show fetal abnormalities. Decide with your doctor whether drug benefits justify risk to unborn child.

Breast-feeding:
May inhibit milk secretion. Consult doctor.

Infants & children:
Not recommended for children 3 and younger. Use for older children only under doctor's supervision.

Prolonged use:
Possible glaucoma.

Skin & sunlight:
No problems expected.

Driving, piloting or hazardous work:
Don't drive or pilot aircraft until you learn how medicine affects you. Don't work around dangerous machinery. Don't climb ladders or work in high places. Danger increases if you drink alcohol or take medicine affecting alertness and reflexes, such as antihistamines, tranquilizers, sedatives, pain medicine, narcotics and mind-altering drugs.

Airplane passengers:
No problems expected.

Discontinuing:
Don't discontinue without consulting doctor. Dose may require gradual reduction if you have taken drug for a long time. Doses of other drugs may also require adjustment.

Others:
- Internal eye pressure should be measured regularly.
- Avoid becoming overheated.

INTERACTION WITH OTHER DRUGS

GENERIC NAME OR DRUG CLASS	COMBINED EFFECT
Amantadine	Increased amantadine effect.
Antidepressants (tricyclic)	Increased biperiden effect. May cause glaucoma.
Antihistamines	Increased biperiden effect.
Levodopa	Increased levodopa effect. Improved results in treating Parkinson's disease.
Meperidine	Increased biperiden effect.
MAO inhibitors	Increased biperiden effect.
Orphenadrine	Increased biperiden effect.
Phenothiazines	Behavior changes.
Primidone	Excessive sedation.
Procainamide	Increased procainamide effect.
Quinidine	Increased biperiden effect.
Tranquilizers	Excessive sedation.

INTERACTION WITH OTHER SUBSTANCES

INTERACTS WITH	COMBINED EFFECT
Alcohol:	None expected.
Beverages:	None expected.
Cocaine:	Decreased biperiden effect. Avoid.
Foods:	None expected.
Marijuana:	None expected.
Tobacco:	None expected.

BISACODYL

BRAND NAMES

Apo-Bisacodyl
Bisco-Lax
Cenalax
Clysodrast
Codylax
Deficol
Dulcolax
Evac-Q-Kwik
Fleet Enema
Nulac
Theralax

GENERAL INFORMATION

Habit forming? No
Prescription needed? No
Available as generic? Yes
Drug class: Laxative (stimulant)

USES

Constipation relief.

DOSAGE & USAGE INFORMATION

How to take:
- Tablet—Swallow with liquid.
- Suppository—Remove wrapper and moisten suppository with water. Gently insert larger end into rectum. Push well into rectum with finger.

When to take:
Usually at bedtime with a snack, unless directed otherwise.

If you forget a dose:
Take as soon as you remember.

What drug does:
Acts on smooth muscles of intestine wall to cause vigorous bowel movement.

Time lapse before drug works:
6 to 10 hours.

Don't take with:
- See Interaction column and consult doctor.
- Don't take within 2 hours of taking another medicine. Laxative interferes with medicine absorption.

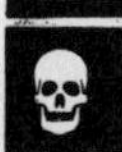

OVERDOSE

Symptoms:
Vomiting, electrolyte depletion.

What to do:
Overdose unlikely to threaten life. If person takes much larger amount than prescribed, call doctor, poison-control center or hospital emergency room for instructions.

POSSIBLE ADVERSE REACTIONS OR SIDE EFFECTS

SYMPTOMS	FREQUENCY	WHAT TO DO
Brain & nervous system:		
Irritability, confusion, headache.	Rare	3
Skin:		
Rash	Rare	3
Eyes:	None expected.	
Ears, nose, throat:	None expected.	
Digestive:		
Belching, cramps, nausea.	Infrequent	4
Heart & lungs:		
Breathing difficulty, irregular heartbeat.	Rare	3
Blood vessels:	None expected.	
Muscles, bones, joints:		
Muscle cramps.	Rare	3
Genital, urinary:	None expected.	
Kidneys:		
Burning on urination.	Rare	4
Liver:	None expected.	
Allergic:	None expected.	
Blood:	None expected.	
Others:		
• Rectal irritation.	Common	4
• Dangerous potassium loss.	Infrequent	3
• Unusual tiredness or weakness.	Rare	3

1- Life-threatening. Seek emergency treatment immediately.
2- Discontinue. Seek emergency treatment.
3- Discontinue. Call doctor right away.
4- Continue. Call doctor when convenient.
5- Continue. Tell doctor at next visit.
6- No action necessary.

WARNINGS & PRECAUTIONS

Don't take if:
- You have symptoms of appendicitis, inflamed bowel or intestinal blockage.
- You are allergic to a stimulant laxative.
- You have missed a bowel movement for only 1 or 2 days.

Before you start, consult your doctor:
- If you have a colostomy or ileostomy.
- If you have congestive heart disease.
- If you have diabetes.
- If you have high blood pressure.
- If you have a laxative habit.
- If you have rectal bleeding.
- If you take other laxatives.

Over age 60:
Adverse reactions and side effects may be more frequent and severe than in younger persons.

Pregnancy:
Risk to mother and unborn child outweighs drug benefits. Don't use.

Breast-feeding:
Drug passes into milk. Avoid drug or discontinue nursing until you finish medicine. Consult doctor for advice on maintaining milk supply.

Infants & children:
Use only under medical supervision.

Prolonged use:
Don't take for more than 1 week unless under doctor's supervision. May cause laxative dependence.

Skin & sunlight:
No problems expected.

Driving, piloting or hazardous work:
No problems expected.

Airplane passengers:
No problems expected.

Discontinuing:
May be unnecessary to finish medicine. Follow doctor's instructions.

Others:
Don't take to "flush out" your system or as a "tonic."

INTERACTION WITH OTHER DRUGS

GENERIC NAME OR DRUG CLASS	COMBINED EFFECT
Antacids	Tablet coating may dissolve too rapidly, irritating stomach or bowel.
Antihypertensives	May cause dangerous low potassium level.
Cimetidine	Stomach or bowel irritation.
Diuretics	May cause dangerous low potassium level.
Ranitidine	Stomach or bowel irritation.

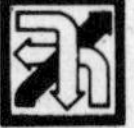

INTERACTION WITH OTHER SUBSTANCES

INTERACTS WITH	COMBINED EFFECT
Alcohol:	None expected.
Beverages:	None expected.
Cocaine:	None expected.
Foods:	None expected.
Marijuana:	None expected.
Tobacco:	None expected.

BROMOCRIPTINE

BRAND NAMES

Parlodel

GENERAL INFORMATION

Available as generic? Yes
Drug class: Antiparkinsonism
Habit forming? No
Prescription needed? Yes

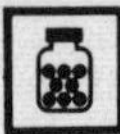

USES

- Controls Parkinson's disease symptoms such as rigidity, tremors and unsteady gait.
- Treats female infertility.
- Prevents lactation.

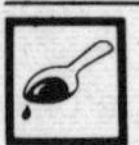

DOSAGE & USAGE INFORMATION

How to take:
Tablet or capsule—Swallow with liquid or food to lessen stomach irritation. If you can't swallow whole, crumble tablet or open capsule and take with liquid or food.

When to take:
At the same times each day.

If you forget a dose:
Take as soon as you remember up to 2 hours late. If more than 2 hours, wait for next scheduled dose (don't double this dose).

What drug does:
Restores chemical balance necessary for normal nerve impulses.

Time lapse before drug works:
2 to 3 weeks to improve; 6 weeks or longer for maximum benefit.

Don't take with:
See Interaction column and consult doctor.

OVERDOSE

Symptoms:
Muscle twitch, spastic eyelid closure, nausea, vomiting, diarrhea, irregular and rapid pulse, weakness, fainting, confusion, agitation, hallucination, coma.

What to do:
- Dial 0 (operator) or 911 (emergency) for an ambulance or medical help. Then give first aid immediately.
- If patient is unconscious and not breathing, give mouth-to-mouth breathing. If there is no heartbeat, use cardiac massage and mouth-to-mouth breathing (CPR). Don't try to make patient vomit. If you can't get help quickly, take patient to nearest emergency facility.
- Additional emergency information on page 886.

POSSIBLE ADVERSE REACTIONS OR SIDE EFFECTS

SYMPTOMS	FREQUENCY	WHAT TO DO
Brain & nervous system:		
• Fainting, severe dizziness, headache, insomnia, nightmares.	Infrequent	3
• Mood changes, uncontrolled body movements.	Common	4
Skin:		
• Flushed face.	Infrequent	4
• Rash, itch.	Infrequent	3
Eyes:		
Blurred vision.	Infrequent	4
Ears, nose, throat:		
Dry mouth.	Common	6
Digestive:		
• Duodenal ulcer.	Rare	4
• Diarrhea	Common	4
• Constipation	Infrequent	5
• Nausea, vomiting.	Infrequent	3
Heart & lungs:		
Irregular heartbeat.	Infrequent	3
Blood vessels:		
High blood pressure.	Rare	3
Muscles, bones, joints:		
Muscle twitching.	Infrequent	4
Genital, urinary:		
• Discolored or dark urine.	Infrequent	4
• Difficult urination.	Infrequent	4
Kidneys, liver, allergic:	None expected.	
Blood:		
Anemia	Rare	4
Others:		
• Tiredness	Infrequent	5
• Body odor.	Common	6

1- Life-threatening. Seek emergency treatment immediately.
2- Discontinue. Seek emergency treatment.
3- Discontinue. Call doctor right away.
4- Continue. Call doctor when convenient.
5- Continue. Tell doctor at next visit.
6- No action necessary.

WARNINGS & PRECAUTIONS

Don't take if:

- You are allergic to bromocriptine.
- You have taken MAO inhibitors in past 2 weeks.
- You have glaucoma (narrow-angle type).

Before you start, consult your doctor:

- If you have diabetes or epilepsy.
- If you have had high blood pressure, heart or lung disease.
- If you have had liver or kidney disease.
- If you have a peptic ulcer.
- If you have malignant melanoma.
- If you will have surgery within 2 months, including dental surgery, requiring general or spinal anesthesia.

Over age 60:
Adverse reactions and side effects may be more frequent and severe than in younger persons.

Pregnancy:
Risk to unborn child outweighs drug benefits. Don't use.

Breast-feeding:
Drug filters into milk. May harm child. Avoid.

Infants & children:
Not recommended.

Prolonged use:
May lead to uncontrolled movements of head, face, mouth, tongue, arms or legs.

Skin & sunlight:
No problems expected.

Driving, piloting or hazardous work:
Don't drive or pilot aircraft until you learn how medicine affects you. Don't work around dangerous machinery. Don't climb ladders or work in high places. Danger increases if you drink alcohol or take medicine affecting alertness and reflexes, such as antihistamines, tranquilizers, sedatives, pain medicine, narcotics and mind-altering drugs.

Airplane passengers:
No problems expected.

Discontinuing:
Don't discontinue without doctor's advice until you complete prescribed dose, even though symptoms diminish or disappear.

Others:
Expect to start with small doses and increase gradually to lessen frequency and severity of adverse reactions.

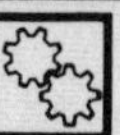

INTERACTION WITH OTHER DRUGS

GENERIC NAME OR DRUG CLASS	COMBINED EFFECT
Antiparkinsonism drugs (other)	Increased bromocriptine effect.
Haloperidol	Decreased bromocriptine effect.
MAO inhibitors	Dangerous rise in blood pressure.
Methyldopa	Decreased bromocriptine effect.
Papaverine	Decreased bromocriptine effect.
Phenothiazines	Decreased bromocriptine effect.
Pyridoxine (Vitamin B-6)	Decreased bromocriptine effect.
Rauwolfia alkaloids	Decreased bromocriptine effect.

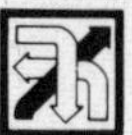

INTERACTION WITH OTHER SUBSTANCES

INTERACTS WITH	COMBINED EFFECT
Alcohol:	None expected.
Beverages:	None expected.
Cocaine:	Decreased bromocriptine effect. Avoid.
Foods:	None expected.
Marijuana:	Increased fatigue, lethargy, fainting. Avoid.
Tobacco:	Interferes with absorption. Avoid.

BROMODIPHENHYDRAMINE

BRAND NAMES

Ambenyl Expectorant
Ambodryl

GENERAL INFORMATION

Habit forming? No
Prescription needed? Yes
Available as generic? No
Drug class: Antihistamine

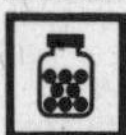

USES

- Reduces allergic symptoms such as hay fever, hives, rash or itching.
- Induces sleep.

DOSAGE & USAGE INFORMATION

How to take:
Capsule or liquid—Swallow with liquid or food to lessen stomach irritation.

When to take:
Varies with form. Follow label directions.

If you forget a dose:
Take as soon as you remember up to 2 hours late. If more than 2 hours, wait for next scheduled dose (don't double this dose).

What drug does:
Blocks action of histamine after an allergic response triggers histamine release in sensitive cells.

Time lapse before drug works:
30 minutes.

Don't take with:
See Interaction column and consult doctor.

OVERDOSE

Symptoms:
Convulsions, red face, hallucinations, coma.

What to do:
- Dial 0 (operator) or 911 (emergency) for an ambulance or medical help. Then give first aid immediately.
- If patient is unconscious and not breathing, give mouth-to-mouth breathing. If there is no heartbeat, use cardiac massage and mouth-to-mouth breathing (CPR). Don't try to make patient vomit. If you can't get help quickly, take patient to nearest emergency facility.
- Additional emergency information on page 886.

POSSIBLE ADVERSE REACTIONS OR SIDE EFFECTS

SYMPTOMS	FREQUENCY	WHAT TO DO
Brain & nervous system:		
• Nightmares, agitation, irritability.	Rare	3
• Drowsiness, dizziness.	Common	5
Skin:	None expected.	
Eyes:		
• Vision changes.	Infrequent	3
• Less tolerance for contact lenses.	Infrequent	4
Ears, nose, throat:		
• Sore throat, fever.	Rare	3
• Dry mouth, nose, throat.	Common	5
Digestive:		
• Nausea	Common	5
• Appetite loss.	Infrequent	5
Heart & lungs:		
Rapid heartbeat.	Rare	3
Blood vessels:		
Unusual bleeding or bruising.	Rare	3
Muscles, bones, joints, kidneys, liver, allergic, blood:	None expected.	
Genital, urinary:		
Urination difficulty.	Infrequent	4
Others:		
Fatigue, weakness.	Rare	3

1-Life-threatening. Seek emergency treatment immediately.
2-Discontinue. Seek emergency treatment.
3-Discontinue. Call doctor right away.
4-Continue. Call doctor when convenient.
5-Continue. Tell doctor at next visit.
6-No action necessary.

BROMODIPHENHYDRAMINE

WARNINGS & PRECAUTIONS

Don't take if:
You are allergic to any antihistamine.

Before you start, consult your doctor:
- If you have glaucoma.
- If you have enlarged prostate.
- If you have asthma.
- If you have kidney disease.
- If you have peptic ulcer.
- If you will have surgery within 2 months, including dental surgery, requiring general or spinal anesthesia.

Over age 60:
Don't exceed recommended dose. Adverse reactions and side effects may be more frequent and severe than in younger persons, especially urination difficulty, diminished alertness and other brain and nervous-system symptoms.

Pregnancy:
No proven harm to unborn child. Avoid if possible.

Breast-feeding:
Drug passes into milk. Avoid drug or discontinue nursing until you finish medicine. Consult doctor for advice on maintaining milk supply.

Infants & children:
Not recommended for premature or newborn infants. Otherwise, no problems expected.

Prolonged use:
Avoid. May damage bone-marrow and nerve cells.

Skin & sunlight:
May cause rash or intensify sunburn in areas exposed to sun or sunlamp.

Driving, piloting or hazardous work:
Don't drive or pilot aircraft until you learn how medicine affects you. Don't work around dangerous machinery. Don't climb ladders or work in high places. Danger increases if you drink alcohol or take medicine affecting alertness and reflexes, such as antihistamines, tranquilizers, sedatives, pain medicine, narcotics and mind-altering drugs.

Airplane passengers:
No problems expected.

Discontinuing:
No problems expected.

Others:
May mask symptoms of hearing damage from aspirin, other salicylates, cisplatin, paromomycin, vancomycin or anticonvulsants. Consult doctor if you use these.

INTERACTION WITH OTHER DRUGS

GENERIC NAME OR DRUG CLASS	COMBINED EFFECT
Anticholinergics	Increased anticholinergic effect.
Antidepressants	Excess sedation. Avoid.
Antihistamines (other)	Excess sedation. Avoid.
Hypnotics	Excess sedation. Avoid.
MAO inhibitors	Increased bromodiphenhydramine effect.
Mind-altering drugs	Excess sedation. Avoid.
Narcotics	Excess sedation. Avoid.
Sedatives	Excess sedation. Avoid.
Sleep inducers	Excess sedation. Avoid.
Tranquilizers	Excess sedation. Avoid.

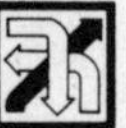

INTERACTION WITH OTHER SUBSTANCES

INTERACTS WITH	COMBINED EFFECT
Alcohol:	Excess sedation. Avoid.
Beverages: Caffeine drinks	Less bromodiphenhydramine sedation.
Cocaine:	Decreased bromodiphenhydramine effect. Avoid.
Foods:	None expected.
Marijuana:	Excess sedation. Avoid.
Tobacco:	None expected.

BROMPHENIRAMINE

BRAND NAMES

Brocon	Drixoral	Rynatapp
Bromepath	Eldatapp	Symptom 3
Bromphen	Histatapp	Taltapp
Dimetane	Poly-Histine	Tapp
Dimetapp	Ralabromophen	Veltap

See complete brand names list, page 823.

GENERAL INFORMATION

Habit forming? No
Prescription needed? Yes
Available as generic? Yes
Drug class: Antihistamine

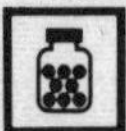

USES

- Reduces allergic symptoms such as hay fever, hives, rash or itching.
- Induces sleep.

DOSAGE & USAGE INFORMATION

How to take:
- Tablet, capsule or syrup—Swallow with liquid or food to lessen stomach irritation.
- Extended-release tablets or capsules—Swallow each dose whole.

When to take:
Varies with form. Follow label directions.

If you forget a dose:
Take as soon as you remember up to 2 hours late. If more than 2 hours, wait for next scheduled dose (don't double this dose).

What drug does:
Blocks action of histamine after an allergic response triggers histamine release in sensitive cells.

Time lapse before drug works:
30 minutes.

Don't take with:
See Interaction column and consult doctor.

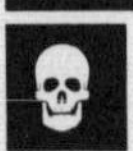

OVERDOSE

Symptoms:
Convulsions, red face, hallucinations, coma.

What to do:
- Dial 0 (operator) or 911 (emergency) for an ambulance or medical help. Then give first aid immediately.
- Additional emergency information on page 886.

POSSIBLE ADVERSE REACTIONS OR SIDE EFFECTS

SYMPTOMS	FREQUENCY	WHAT TO DO
Brain & nervous system:		
• Nightmares, agitation, irritability.	Rare	3
• Drowsiness, dizziness.	Common	5
Skin:	None expected.	
Eyes:		
• Vision changes.	Infrequent	3
• Less tolerance for contact lenses.	Infrequent	4
Ears, nose, throat:		
• Sore throat, fever.	Rare	3
• Dry mouth, nose, throat.	Common	5
Digestive:		
• Nausea	Common	5
• Appetite loss.	Infrequent	5
Heart & lungs:		
Rapid heartbeat.	Rare	3
Blood vessels:		
Unusual bleeding or bruising.	Rare	3
Muscles, bones, joints, kidneys, liver, allergic, blood:	None expected.	
Genital, urinary:		
Urination difficulty.	Infrequent	4
Others:		
Fatigue, weakness.	Rare	3

1- Life-threatening. Seek emergency treatment immediately.
2- Discontinue. Seek emergency treatment.
3- Discontinue. Call doctor right away.
4- Continue. Call doctor when convenient.
5- Continue. Tell doctor at next visit.
6- No action necessary.

WARNINGS & PRECAUTIONS

Don't take if:
You are allergic to any antihistamine.

Before you start, consult your doctor:
- If you have glaucoma.
- If you have enlarged prostate.
- If you have asthma.
- If you have kidney disease.
- If you have peptic ulcer.
- If you will have surgery within 2 months, including dental surgery, requiring general or spinal anesthesia.

Over age 60:
Don't exceed recommended dose. Adverse reactions and side effects may be more frequent and severe than in younger persons, especially urination difficulty, diminished alertness and other brain and nervous-system symptoms.

Pregnancy:
No proven harm to unborn child. Avoid if possible.

Breast-feeding:
Drug passes into milk. Avoid drug or discontinue nursing until you finish medicine. Consult doctor for advice on maintaining milk supply.

Infants & children:
Not recommended for premature or newborn infants. Otherwise, no problems expected.

Prolonged use:
Avoid. May damage bone marrow and nerve cells.

Skin & sunlight:
May cause rash or intensify sunburn in areas exposed to sun or sunlamp.

Driving, piloting or hazardous work:
Don't drive or pilot aircraft until you learn how medicine affects you. Don't work around dangerous machinery. Don't climb ladders or work in high places. Danger increases if you drink alcohol or take medicine affecting alertness and reflexes, such as antihistamines, tranquilizers, sedatives, pain medicine, narcotics and mind-altering drugs.

Airplane passengers:
No problems expected.

Discontinuing:
No problems expected.

Others:
May mask symptoms of hearing damage from aspirin, other salicylates, cisplatin, paromomycin, vancomycin or anticonvulsants. Consult doctor if you use these.

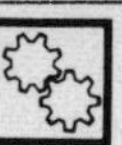

INTERACTION WITH OTHER DRUGS

GENERIC NAME OR DRUG CLASS	COMBINED EFFECT
Anticholinergics	Increased anticholinergic effect.
Antidepressants	Excess sedation. Avoid.
Antihistamines (other)	Excess sedation. Avoid.
Hypnotics	Excess sedation. Avoid.
MAO inhibitors	Increased brompheniramine effect.
Mind-altering drugs	Excess sedation. Avoid.
Narcotics	Excess sedation. Avoid.
Sedatives	Excess sedation. Avoid.
Sleep inducers	Excess sedation. Avoid.
Tranquilizers	Excess sedation. Avoid.

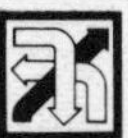

INTERACTION WITH OTHER SUBSTANCES

INTERACTS WITH	COMBINED EFFECT
Alcohol:	Excess sedation. Avoid.
Beverages: Caffeine drinks	Less brompheniramine sedation.
Cocaine:	Decreased brompheniramine effect. Avoid.
Foods:	None expected.
Marijuana:	Excess sedation. Avoid.
Tobacco:	None expected.

BUCLIZINE

BRAND NAMES

Bucladin-S

GENERAL INFORMATION

Habit forming? No
Prescription needed? U.S.: No
Canada: Yes
Available as generic? No
Drug class: Antihistamine, antiemetic

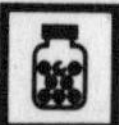

USES

Prevents motion sickness.

DOSAGE & USAGE INFORMATION

How to take:
Tablet—Swallow with liquid or food to lessen stomach irritation. If you can't swallow whole, crumble tablet and chew or take with liquid or food.

When to take:
30 minutes to 1 hour before traveling.

If you forget a dose:
Take as soon as you remember. Wait 4 hours for next dose.

What drug does:
Reduces sensitivity of nerve endings in inner ear, blocking messages to brain's vomiting center.

Time lapse before drug works:
30 to 60 minutes.

Don't take with:
See Interaction column and consult doctor.

OVERDOSE

Symptoms:
Drowsiness, confusion, incoordination, stupor, coma, weak pulse, shallow breathing.

What to do:
- Dial 0 (operator) or 911 (emergency) for an ambulance or medical help. Then give first aid immediately.
- Additional emergency information on page 886.

POSSIBLE ADVERSE REACTIONS OR SIDE EFFECTS

SYMPTOMS	FREQUENCY	WHAT TO DO
Brain & nervous system:		
• Drowsiness	Common	5
• Headache	Infrequent	4
• Restlessness, excitement, insomnia.	Rare	4
Skin:		
Rash or hives.	Rare	3
Eyes:		
Blurred vision.	Rare	4
Ears, nose, throat:		
Dry mouth, nose, throat.	Infrequent	5
Digestive:		
• Appetite loss, nausea.	Rare	5
• Diarrhea or constipation.	Infrequent	4
Heart & lungs:		
Fast heartbeat.	Infrequent	4
Blood vessels:	None expected.	
Muscles, bones, joints:	None expected.	
Genital, urinary:		
Urinary frequency, difficult urination.	Rare	4
Kidneys:	None expected.	
Liver:	None expected.	
Allergic:	None expected.	
Blood:	None expected.	
Others:	None expected.	

1- Life-threatening. Seek emergency treatment immediately.
2- Discontinue. Seek emergency treatment.
3- Discontinue. Call doctor right away.
4- Continue. Call doctor when convenient.
5- Continue. Tell doctor at next visit.

WARNINGS & PRECAUTIONS

Don't take if:
- You are allergic to meclizine, buclizine or cyclizine.
- You have taken MAO inhibitors in the past 2 weeks.

Before you start, consult your doctor:
- If you have glaucoma.
- If you have prostate enlargement.
- If you have reacted badly to any antihistamine.

Over age 60:
Adverse reactions and side effects may be more frequent and severe than in younger persons, especially impaired urination from enlarged prostate gland.

Pregnancy:
Studies inconclusive on harm to unborn child. Animal studies show fetal abnormalities. Decide with your doctor whether drug benefits justify risk to unborn child.

Breast-feeding:
Drug passes into milk. Avoid drug or discontinue nursing until you finish medicine. Consult doctor for advice on maintaining milk supply.

Infants & children:
No problems expected.

Prolonged use:
No problems expected.

Skin & sunlight:
No problems expected.

Driving, piloting or hazardous work:
Don't fly aircraft. Don't drive until you learn how medicine affects you. Don't work around dangerous machinery. Don't climb ladders or work in high places. Danger increases if you drink alcohol or take medicine affecting alertness and reflexes, such as antihistamines, tranquilizers, sedatives, pain medicine, narcotics and mind-altering drugs.

Airplane passengers:
Take 30 minutes before takeoff and every 4 hours while in the air.

Discontinuing:
No problems expected.

Others:
No problems expected.

INTERACTION WITH OTHER DRUGS

GENERIC NAME OR DRUG CLASS	COMBINED EFFECT
Amphetamines	May decrease drowsiness caused by buclizine.
Anticholinergics	Increased effect of both drugs.
Antidepressants (tricyclic)	Increased effect of both drugs.
MAO inhibitors	Increased buclizine effect.
Narcotics	Increased effect of both drugs.
Pain relievers	Increased effect of both drugs.
Sedatives	Increased effect of both drugs.
Sleep inducers	Increased effect of both drugs.
Tranquilizers	Increased effect of both drugs.

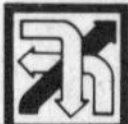

INTERACTION WITH OTHER SUBSTANCES

INTERACTS WITH	COMBINED EFFECT
Alcohol:	Increased sedation. Avoid.
Beverages: Caffeine drinks	May decrease drowsiness.
Cocaine:	None expected.
Foods:	None expected.
Marijuana:	Increased drowsiness, dry mouth.
Tobacco:	None expected.

BUMETANIDE

BRAND NAMES

Bumex

GENERAL INFORMATION

Habit forming? No
Prescription needed? Yes
Available as generic? No
Drug class: Diuretic

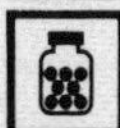

USES

Decreases fluid retention.

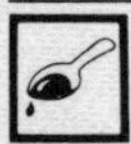

DOSAGE & USAGE INFORMATION

How to take:
Tablet or capsule—Swallow with liquid or food to lessen stomach irritation. If you can't swallow whole, crumble tablet or open capsule and take with liquid or food.

When to take:
- 1 dose a day—Take after breakfast.
- More than 1 dose a day—Take last dose no later than 6 p.m. unless otherwise directed.

If you forget a dose:
- 1 dose a day—Take as soon as you remember up to 12 hours late. If more than 12 hours, wait for next scheduled dose (don't double this dose).
- More than 1 dose a day—Take as soon as you remember up to 2 hours late. If more than 2 hours, wait for next scheduled dose (don't double this dose).

What drug does:
Increases elimination of sodium and water from body. Decreased body fluid reduces blood pressure.

Time lapse before drug works:
1 hour to increase water loss.

Don't take with:
See Interaction column and consult doctor.

OVERDOSE

Symptoms:
Weakness, lethargy, dizziness, confusion, nausea, vomiting, leg-muscle cramps, thirst, stupor, deep sleep, weak and rapid pulse, cardiac arrest.

What to do:
- Dial 0 (operator) or 911 (emergency) for an ambulance or medical help. Then give first aid immediately.
- Additional emergency information on page 886.

POSSIBLE ADVERSE REACTIONS OR SIDE EFFECTS

SYMPTOMS	FREQUENCY	WHAT TO DO
Brain & nervous system:		
• Dizziness	Common	4
• Mood changes.	Infrequent	3
Skin:		
Rash or hives.	Rare	3
Eyes:		
Yellow vision.	Rare	3
Ears, nose, throat:		
• Ringing in ears, hearing loss.	Rare	3
• Sore throat, fever.	Rare	3
• Dry mouth, thirst.	Rare	3
Digestive:		
• Side or stomach pain, nausea, vomiting.	Rare	3
• Appetite loss, diarrhea.	Infrequent	3
Heart & lungs:		
Irregular heartbeat.	Infrequent	3
Blood vessels:		
Unusual bleeding or bruising.	Rare	3
Muscles, bones, joints:		
• Joint pain.	Rare	3
• Muscle cramps.	Infrequent	3
Genital, urinary, kidneys, allergic blood:	None expected.	
Liver:		
Jaundice (yellow skin and eyes).	Rare	3
Others:		
Fatigue, weakness.	Infrequent	3

1- Life-threatening. Seek emergency treatment immediately.
2- Discontinue. Seek emergency treatment.
3- Discontinue. Call doctor right away.
4- Continue. Call doctor when convenient.
5- Continue. Tell doctor at next visit.
6- No action necessary.

WARNINGS & PRECAUTIONS

Don't take if:
You are allergic to bumetanide.

Before you start, consult your doctor:
- If you have liver or kidney disease.
- If you have gout.
- If you have diabetes.
- If you have impaired hearing.
- If you will have surgery within 2 months, including dental surgery, requiring general or spinal anesthesia.

Over age 60:
Adverse reactions and side effects may be more frequent and severe than in younger persons.

Pregnancy:
Risk to unborn child outweighs drug benefits. Don't use.

Breast-feeding:
Drug filters into milk. May harm child. Avoid.

Infants & children:
Use only under medical supervision.

Prolonged use:
- Impaired balance of water, salt and potassium in blood and body tissues. Request periodic laboratory studies of electrolytes in blood.
- Possible diabetes.

Skin & sunlight:
May cause rash or intensify sunburn in areas exposed to sun or sunlamp.

Driving, piloting or hazardous work:
No problems expected.

Airplane passengers:
No problems expected.

Discontinuing:
Don't discontinue without doctor's advice until you complete prescribed dose, even though symptoms diminish or disappear.

Others:
Frequent laboratory studies to monitor potassium level in blood recommended. Eat foods rich in potassium (see page 848) or take potassium supplements. Consult doctor.

INTERACTION WITH OTHER DRUGS

GENERIC NAME OR DRUG CLASS	COMBINED EFFECT
Cephalosporin antibiotics	Increased possibility of hearing loss.
Amitracin, gentamycin, kanamycin, streptomycin, tobramycin, cisplatin, ethacrynic acid, furosemide, mercaptopurine, polymixins.	Increased possibility of hearing loss.
Antihypertensives	Increased blood-pressure drop.
Indomethicin	Decreased effect of bumetanide.
Probenecid	Decreased effect of bumetanide.
Lithium	Increased possibility of lithium toxicity.

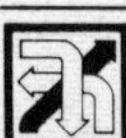

INTERACTION WITH OTHER SUBSTANCES

INTERACTS WITH	COMBINED EFFECT
Alcohol:	Blood-pressure drop. Avoid.
Beverages:	
Caffeine	Decreased bumetanide effect.
Cocaine:	Dangerous blood-pressure drop. Avoid.
Foods:	None expected.
Marijuana:	Increased thirst and urinary frequency, fainting.
Tobacco:	Decreased bumetanide effect.

BUSULFAN

BRAND NAMES

Myleran

GENERAL INFORMATION

Habit forming? No
Prescription needed? Yes
Available as generic? No
Drug class: Antineoplastic, immunosuppressant

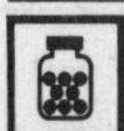

USES

- Treatment for some kinds of cancer.
- Suppresses immune response after transplant and in immune disorders.

DOSAGE & USAGE INFORMATION

How to take:
Tablet or capsule—Swallow with liquid after light meal. Don't drink fluids with meals. Drink extra fluids between meals. Avoid sweet or fatty foods.

When to take:
At the same time each day.

If you forget a dose:
Take as soon as you remember. Don't ever double dose.

What drug does:
Inhibits abnormal cell reproduction. May suppress immune system.

Time lapse before drug works:
Up to 6 weeks for full effect.

Don't take with:
See Interaction column and consult doctor.

OVERDOSE

Symptoms:
Bleeding, chills, fever, collapse, stupor, seizure.

What to do:
- Dial 0 (operator) or 911 (emergency) for an ambulance or medical help. Then give first aid immediately.
- If patient is unconscious and not breathing, give mouth-to-mouth breathing. If there is no heartbeat, use cardiac massage and mouth-to-mouth breathing (CPR). Don't try to make patient vomit. If you can't get help quickly, take patient to nearest emergency facility.
- Additional emergency information on page 886.

POSSIBLE ADVERSE REACTIONS OR SIDE EFFECTS

SYMPTOMS	FREQUENCY	WHAT TO DO
Brain & nervous system:		
Mental confusion.	Infrequent	4
Skin:		
• Unusual bleeding or bruising.	Common	3
• Hair loss.	Common	4
Eyes:	None expected.	
Ears, nose, throat:		
Mouth sores with sore throat, chills and fever.	Common	3
Digestive:		
• Black stools.	Common	3
• Sores in mouth and lips.	Common	3
• Nausea, vomiting, diarrhea (unavoidable).	Common	5
Heart & lungs:		
• Shortness of breath.	Infrequent	4
• Cough	Infrequent	5
Blood vessels:	None expected.	
Muscles, bones, joints:		
Joint pain.	Common	4
Genital, urinary:		
Menstrual changes.	Common	3
Kidneys, allergic, blood, liver:		
• Jaundice (yellow skin and eyes).	Rare	3
• May increase chance of developing leukemia.	Infrequent	4
Others:		
Tiredness, weakness.	Common	5

1- Life-threatening. Seek emergency treatment immediately.
2- Discontinue. Seek emergency treatment.
3- Discontinue. Call doctor right away.
4- Continue. Call doctor when convenient.
5- Continue. Tell doctor at next visit.

WARNINGS & PRECAUTIONS

Don't take if:
- You have had hypersensitivity to alkylating antineoplastic drugs.
- Your physician has not explained serious nature of your medical problem and risks of taking this medicine.

Before you start, consult your doctor:
- If you have gout.
- If you have had kidney stones.
- If you have active infection.
- If you have impaired kidney or liver function.
- If you have taken other antineoplastic drugs or had radiation treatment in last 3 weeks.

Over age 60:
Adverse reactions and side effects may be more frequent and severe than in younger persons.

Pregnancy:
Consult doctor. Risk to child is significant.

Breast-feeding:
Drug passes into milk. Don't nurse.

Infants & children:
Use only under care of medical supervisors who are experienced in anticancer drugs.

Prolonged use:
Adverse reactions more likely the longer drug is required.

Skin & sunlight:
No problems expected.

Driving, piloting or hazardous work:
No problems expected.

Airplane passengers:
No problems expected.

Discontinuing:
Don't discontinue without doctor's advice until you complete prescribed dose, even though symptoms diminish or disappear. Some side effects may follow discontinuing. Report to doctor blurred vision, convulsions, confusion, persistent headache.

Others:
May cause sterility.

INTERACTION WITH OTHER DRUGS

GENERIC NAME OR DRUG CLASS	COMBINED EFFECT
Antigout drugs	Decreased antigout effect.
Antineoplastic drugs (other)	Increased effect of all drugs, (may be beneficial).
Chloramphenicol	Increased likelihood of toxic effects of both drugs.

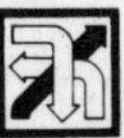

INTERACTION WITH OTHER SUBSTANCES

INTERACTS WITH	COMBINED EFFECT
Alcohol:	May increase chance of intestinal bleeding.
Beverages:	No problems expected.
Cocaine:	Increases chance of toxicity.
Foods:	Reduces irritation in stomach.
Marijuana:	No problems expected.
Tobacco:	Increases lung toxicity.

BUTABARBITAL

BRAND NAMES

Butalan	Cytospaz SR
Butatran	Levamine
Buticaps	Quibron Plus
Butisol	Sarisol No. 2

See complete brand names list, page 823.

GENERAL INFORMATION

Habit forming? Yes
Prescription needed? Yes
Available as generic? Yes
Drug class: Sedative, hypnotic (barbiturate)

USES

- Reduces anxiety or nervous tension (low dose).
- Relieves insomnia (higher bedtime dose).

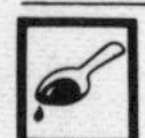

DOSAGE & USAGE INFORMATION

How to take:
Tablet, capsule or liquid—Swallow with food or liquid to lessen stomach irritation. If you can't swallow whole, crumble tablet or open capsule and take with liquid or food.

When to take:
At the same times each day.

If you forget a dose:
Take as soon as you remember up to 2 hours late. If more than 2 hours, wait for next scheduled dose (don't double this dose).

What drug does:
May partially block nerve impulses at nerve-cell connections.

Time lapse before drug works:
60 minutes.

Don't take with:
- Non-prescription drugs without consulting doctor.
- See Interaction column and consult doctor.

OVERDOSE

Symptoms:
Deep sleep, weak pulse, coma.

What to do:
- Dial 0 (operator) or 911 (emergency) for an ambulance or medical help. Then give first aid immediately.
- Additional emergency information on page 886.

POSSIBLE ADVERSE REACTIONS OR SIDE EFFECTS

SYMPTOMS	FREQUENCY	WHAT TO DO
Brain & nervous system:		
• Dizziness, drowsiness, "hangover effect."	Common	4
• Depression, confusion, slurred speech.	Infrequent	4
• Agitation	Rare	3
Skin:		
• Rash or hives.	Infrequent	3
• Face, lip swelling.	Infrequent	3
Eyes:		
Eyelid swelling.	Infrequent	3
Ears, nose, throat:		
Sore throat, fever.	Infrequent	3
Digestive:		
Diarrhea, nausea, vomiting.	Infrequent	4
Heart & lungs:		
• Slow heartbeat.	Rare	3
• Breathing difficulty.	Rare	3
Blood vessels:		
Unexplained bleeding or bruising.	Rare	4
Muscles, bones, joints:		
Joint or muscle pain.	Infrequent	4
Genital, urinary:	None expected.	
Kidneys:	None expected.	
Liver:		
Jaundice (yellow skin and eyes).	Rare	3
Allergic:	None expected.	
Blood:	None expected.	
Others:	None expected.	

1- Life-threatening. Seek emergency treatment immediately.
2- Discontinue. Seek emergency treatment.
3- Discontinue. Call doctor right away.
4- Continue. Call doctor when convenient.

WARNINGS & PRECAUTIONS

Don't take if:
- You are allergic to any barbiturate.
- You have porphyria.

Before you start, consult your doctor:
- If you have epilepsy.
- If you have kidney or liver damage.
- If you have asthma.
- If you have anemia.
- If you have chronic pain.
- If you will have surgery within 2 months, including dental surgery, requiring general or spinal anesthesia.

Over age 60:
Adverse reactions and side effects may be more frequent and severe than in younger persons. Use small doses.

Pregnancy:
Risk to unborn child outweighs drug benefits. Don't use.

Breast-feeding:
Drug passes into milk. Avoid drug or discontinue nursing until you finish medicine. Consult doctor for advice on maintaining milk supply.

Infants & children:
Use only under doctor's supervision.

Prolonged use:
- May cause addiction, anemia, chronic intoxication.
- May lower body temperature, making exposure to cold temperatures hazardous.

Skin & sunlight:
May cause rash or intensify sunburn in areas exposed to sun or sunlamp.

Driving, piloting or hazardous work:
Don't drive or pilot aircraft until you learn how medicine affects you. Don't work around dangerous machinery. Don't climb ladders or work in high places. Danger increases if you drink alcohol or take medicine affecting alertness and reflexes.

Airplane passengers:
No problems expected.

Discontinuing:
May be unnecessary to finish medicine. Follow doctor's instructions. If you develop withdrawal symptoms of hallucinations, agitation or sleeplessness after discontinuing, call doctor right away.

Others:
High potential for abuse.

INTERACTION WITH OTHER DRUGS

GENERIC NAME OR DRUG CLASS	COMBINED EFFECT
Anticoagulants (oral)	Decreased anticoagulant effect.
Anticonvulsants	Changed seizure patterns.
Antidepressants (tricyclic)	Decreased antidepressant effect.
Antidiabetics (oral)	Increased butabarbital effect.
Antihistamines	Dangerous sedation. Avoid.
Antiinflammatory drugs (non-steroidal)	Decreased antiinflammatory effect.
Aspirin	Decreased aspirin effect.
Beta-adrenergic blockers	Decreased effect of beta-adrenergic blocker.
Contraceptives (oral)	Decreased contraceptive effect.
Cortisone drugs	Decreased cortisone effect.
Digitoxin	Decreased digitoxin effect.
Doxycycline	Decreased doxycycline effect.
Griseofulvin	Decreased griseofulvin effect.

Additional interactions on page 835.

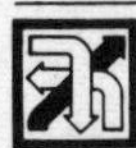

INTERACTION WITH OTHER SUBSTANCES

INTERACTS WITH	COMBINED EFFECT
Alcohol:	Possible fatal oversedation. Avoid.
Beverages:	None expected.
Cocaine:	Decreased butabarbital effect.
Foods:	None expected.
Marijuana:	Excessive sedation. Avoid.
Tobacco:	None expected.

BUTAPERAZINE

BRAND NAMES

Repoise

GENERAL INFORMATION

Habit forming? No
Prescription needed? Yes
Available as generic? Yes
Drug class: Tranquilizer, antiemetic (phenothiazine)

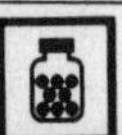

USES

- Stops nausea, vomiting.
- Reduces anxiety, agitation.

DOSAGE & USAGE INFORMATION

How to take:
- Tablet or capsule—Swallow with liquid or food to lessen stomach irritation.
- Suppositories—Remove wrapper and moisten suppository with water. Gently insert into rectum, large end first.
- Drops or liquid—Dilute dose in beverage.

When to take:
- Nervous and mental disorders—Take at the same times each day.
- Nausea and vomiting—Take as needed, no more often than every 4 hours.

If you forget a dose:
- Nervous and mental disorders—Take up to 2 hours late. If more than 2 hours, wait for next scheduled dose (don't double this).
- Nausea and vomiting—Take as soon as you remember. Wait 4 hours for next dose.

What drug does:
- Suppresses brain's vomiting center.
- Suppresses brain centers that control abnormal emotions and behavior.

Time lapse before drug works:
- Nausea and vomiting—1 hour or less.
- Nervous and mental disorders—4-6 weeks.

Don't take with:
- Antacid or medicine for diarrhea.
- Non-prescription drug for cough, cold or allergy.
- See Interaction column and consult doctor.

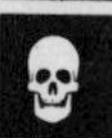

OVERDOSE

Symptoms:
Stupor, convulsions, coma.

What to do:
- Dial 0 (operator) or 911 (emergency) for an ambulance or medical help. Then give first aid immediately.
- Additional emergency information on page 886.

POSSIBLE ADVERSE REACTIONS OR SIDE EFFECTS

SYMPTOMS	FREQUENCY	WHAT TO DO
Brain & nervous system:		
• Restlessness, tremor.	Common	3
• Fainting	Infrequent	2
• Drowsiness	Common	3
Skin:		
• Rash	Infrequent	3
• Less perspiration.	Common	4
Eyes:		
Vision changes.	Rare	3
Ears, nose, throat:		
• Sore throat, fever.	Rare	3
• Dry mouth, nasal congestion.	Common	4
Digestive:		
Constipation	Common	4
Heart & lungs, blood vessels, kidneys, allergic, blood:	None expected.	
Muscles, bones, joints:		
Muscle spasms of face and neck, unsteady gait.	Common	2
Genital, urinary:		
Urination difficulty.	Infrequent	4
Liver:		
Jaundice (yellow eyes and skin).	Rare	3
Others:		
Less interest in sex, breast swelling, change in menstrual pattern.	Infrequent	4

1 - Life-threatening. Seek emergency treatment immediately.
2 - Discontinue. Seek emergency treatment.
3 - Discontinue. Call doctor right away.
4 - Continue. Call doctor when convenient.
5 - Continue. Tell doctor at next visit.
6 - No action necessary.

WARNINGS & PRECAUTIONS

Don't take if:
- You are allergic to any phenothiazine.
- You have a blood or bone-marrow disease.

Before you start, consult your doctor:
- If you will have surgery within 2 months, including dental surgery, requiring general or spinal anesthesia.
- If you have asthma, emphysema or other lung disorder.
- If you take non-prescription ulcer medicine, asthma medicine or amphetamines.

Over age 60:
Adverse reactions and side effects may be more frequent and severe than in younger persons. More likely to develop involuntary movement of jaws, lips, tongue, chewing. Report this to your doctor immediately. Early treatment can help.

Pregnancy:
Risk to unborn child outweighs drug benefits. Don't use.

Breast-feeding:
Drug passes into milk. Avoid drug or discontinue nursing until you finish medicine. Consult doctor for advice on maintaining milk supply.

Infants & children:
Don't give to children younger than 2.

Prolonged use:
May lead to tardive dyskinesia (involuntary movement of jaws, lips, tongue, chewing).

Skin & sunlight:
May cause rash or intensify sunburn in areas exposed to sun or sunlamp. Skin may remain sensitive for 3 months after discontinuing.

Driving, piloting or hazardous work:
Don't drive or pilot aircraft until you learn how medicine affects you. Don't work around dangerous machinery. Don't climb ladders or work in high places. Danger increases if you drink alcohol or take medicine affecting alertness and reflexes.

Airplane passengers:
No problems expected.

Discontinuing:
- Nervous and mental disorders—Don't discontinue without doctor's advice until you complete prescribed dose, even though symptoms diminish or disappear.
- Nausea and vomiting—May be unnecessary to finish medicine. Follow doctor's instructions.

INTERACTION WITH OTHER DRUGS

GENERIC NAME OR DRUG CLASS	COMBINED EFFECT
Anticholinergics	Increased anticholinergic effect.
Antidepressants (tricyclic)	Increased butaperazine effect.
Antihistamines	Increased antihistamine effect.
Appetite suppressants	Decreased suppressant effect.
Levodopa	Decreased levodopa effect.
Mind-altering drugs	Increased effect of mind-altering drugs.
Narcotics	Increased narcotic effect.
Phenytoin	Increased phenytoin effect.
Quinidine	Impaired heart function. Dangerous mixture.
Sedatives	Increased sedative effect.
Tranquilizers (other)	Increased tranquilizer effect.

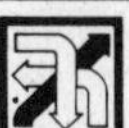

INTERACTION WITH OTHER SUBSTANCES

INTERACTS WITH	COMBINED EFFECT
Alcohol:	Dangerous oversedation.
Beverages:	None expected.
Cocaine:	Decreased butaperazine effect. Avoid.
Foods:	None expected.
Marijuana:	Drowsiness. May increase antinausea effect.
Tobacco:	None expected.

CAFFEINE

BRAND NAMES

Anacin
Ban-Drow 2
Cafacetin
Cafecon
Cafergot
Cafermine
Cafetrate
Excedrin Extra Strength
Midol
Nodoz
Percodan
Tirend
Vanquish
Vivarin

See complete brand names list, page 824.

GENERAL INFORMATION

Habit forming? Yes
Prescription needed? No
Available as generic? Yes
Drug class: Stimulant (xanthine), vasoconstrictor

USES

- Treatment for drowsiness and fatigue.
- Treatment for migraine and other vascular headaches in combination with ergot.

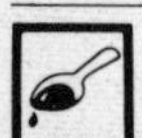

DOSAGE & USAGE INFORMATION

How to take:
- Tablet—Swallow with liquid or food to lessen stomach irritation. If you can't swallow whole, crumble tablet or open capsule and take with liquid or food.
- Extended-release capsules—Swallow whole with liquid.

When to take:
At the same times each day.

If you forget a dose:
Take as soon as you remember up to 2 hours late. If more than 2 hours, wait for next scheduled dose (don't double this dose).

What drug does:
- Constricts blood-vessel walls.
- Stimulates central nervous system.

Time lapse before drug works:
30 minutes.

Don't take with:
- Non-prescription drugs without consulting doctor.
- See Interaction column and consult doctor.

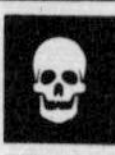

OVERDOSE

Symptoms:
Excitement, rapid heartbeat, hallucinations, convulsions, coma.

What to do:
- Dial 0 (operator) or 911 (emergency) for an ambulance or medical help. Then give first aid immediately.
- Additional emergency information on page 886.

POSSIBLE ADVERSE REACTIONS OR SIDE EFFECTS

SYMPTOMS	FREQUENCY	WHAT TO DO
Brain & nervous system:		
• Nervousness, insomnia.	Common	5
• Confusion, irritability.	Infrequent	3
Skin:	None expected.	
Eyes:	None expected.	
Ears, nose, throat:	None expected.	
Digestive:		
Nausea, indigestion, burning feeling in stomach.	Infrequent	4
Heart & lungs:		
Rapid heartbeat.	Common	4
Blood vessels:	None expected.	
Muscles, bones, joints:	None expected.	
Genital, urinary:		
Increased urination.	Common	6
Kidneys:	None expected.	
Liver:	None expected.	
Allergic:	None expected.	
Blood:	None expected.	
Others:		
Low blood sugar with tremor, irritability, weakness, sweating.	Common	4

1- Life-threatening. Seek emergency treatment immediately.
2- Discontinue. Seek emergency treatment.
3- Discontinue. Call doctor right away.
4- Continue. Call doctor when convenient.
5- Continue. Tell doctor at next visit.
6- No action necessary.

WARNINGS & PRECAUTIONS

Don't take if:
- You are allergic to any stimulant.
- You have heart disease.
- You have active peptic ulcer of stomach or duodenum.

Before you start, consult your doctor:
- If you have irregular heartbeat.
- If you have hypoglycemia (low blood sugar).
- If you have epilepsy.

Over age 60:
Adverse reactions and side effects may be more frequent and severe than in younger persons.

Pregnancy:
Risk to unborn child outweighs drug benefits. Don't use.

Breast-feeding:
Drug passes into milk. Avoid drug or discontinue nursing until you finish medicine. Consult doctor for advice on maintaining milk supply.

Infants & children:
Not recommended.

Prolonged use:
Stomach ulcers.

Skin & sunlight:
No problems expected.

Driving, piloting or hazardous work:
No problems expected.

Airplane passengers:
No problems expected.

Discontinuing:
Will cause withdrawal symptoms of headache, irritability, drowsiness. Discontinue gradually if you use caffeine for a month or more.

Others:
May produce or aggravate fibrocystic disease of the breast in women.

INTERACTION WITH OTHER DRUGS

GENERIC NAME OR DRUG CLASS	COMBINED EFFECT
Contraceptives (oral)	Increased caffeine effect.
Isoniazid	Increased caffeine effect.
MAO inhibitors	Dangerous blood-pressure rise.
Sedatives	Decreased sedative effect.
Sleep inducers	Decreased sedative effect.
Sympathomimetics	Overstimulation.
Thyroid hormones	Increased thyroid effect.
Tranquilizers	Decreased tranquilizer effect.

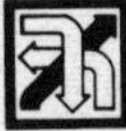

INTERACTION WITH OTHER SUBSTANCES

INTERACTS WITH	COMBINED EFFECT
Alcohol:	Decreased alcohol effect.
Beverages: Caffeine drinks	Increased caffeine effect.
Cocaine:	Overstimulation. Avoid.
Foods:	No proven problems.
Marijuana:	Increased effect of both drugs. May lead to dangerous, rapid heartbeat. Avoid.
Tobacco:	Increased heartbeat. Avoid.

CALCIUM CARBONATE

BRAND NAMES

Alka-2
Alkets
Amitone
Bio Cal
Calcilac
Calglycine
Camalox
Chooz
Dicarbosil
Ducon
El-Da-Mint
Equilet
Gustalac
Mallamint
Os-Cal
Pama No. 1.
Pepto-Bismol
Ratio
Titracid
Titralac
Trialka
Tums

See complete brand names list, page 824.

GENERAL INFORMATION

Habit forming? No
Prescription needed? No
Available as generic? Yes
Drug class: Antacid

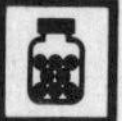

USES

Treatment for hyperacidity in upper gastrointestinal tract, including stomach and esophagus. Symptoms may be heartburn or acid indigestion. Diseases include peptic ulcer, gastritis, esophagitis, hiatal hernia.

DOSAGE & USAGE INFORMATION

How to take:

- Tablet—Swallow with liquid.
- Chewable tablets or wafers—Chew well before swallowing.

When to take:
1 to 3 hours after meals unless directed otherwise by your doctor.

If you forget a dose:
Take as soon as you remember.

What drug does:

- Neutralizes some of the hydrochloric acid in the stomach.
- Reduces action of pepsin, a digestive enzyme.

Time lapse before drug works:
15 minutes.

Don't take with:
Other medicines at the same time. Decreases absorption of other drugs.

OVERDOSE

Symptoms:
Weakness, fatigue, dizziness.

What to do:
Overdose unlikely to threaten life. If person takes much larger amount than prescribed, call doctor, poison-control center or hospital emergency room for instructions.

POSSIBLE ADVERSE REACTIONS OR SIDE EFFECTS

SYMPTOMS	FREQUENCY	WHAT TO DO
Brain & nervous system: Mood changes.	Infrequent	4
Skin:	None expected.	
Eyes:	None expected.	
Ears, nose, throat:	None expected.	
Digestive:		
• Constipation, appetite loss.	Common	4
• Nausea, vomiting.	Infrequent	4
• Lower abdominal pain and swelling.	Infrequent	3
Heart & lungs: Difficult or painful urination.	Rare	3
Blood vessels:	None expected.	
Muscles, bones, joints: Bone pain, muscle weakness.	Infrequent	3
Genital, urinary:	None expected.	
Kidneys:	None expected.	
Liver:	None expected.	
Allergic:	None expected.	
Blood:	None expected.	
Others:		
• Swelling of wrists or ankles.	Infrequent	3
• Unusual tiredness or weakness.	Rare	3
• Weight loss.	Infrequent	4

1 - Life-threatening. Seek emergency treatment immediately.
2 - Discontinue. Seek emergency treatment.
3 - Discontinue. Call doctor right away.
4 - Continue. Call doctor when convenient.
5 - Continue. Tell doctor at next visit.
6 - No action necessary.

CALCIUM CARBONATE

WARNINGS & PRECAUTIONS

Don't take if:
- You are allergic to any antacid.
- You have a high blood-calcium level.

Before you start, consult your doctor:
- If you have kidney disease.
- If you have chronic constipation, colitis or diarrhea.
- If you have symptoms of appendicitis.
- If you have stomach or intestinal bleeding.
- If you have irregular heartbeat.

Over age 60:
Adverse reactions and side effects may be more frequent and severe than in younger persons. Diarrhea or constipation particularly likely.

Pregnancy:
Risk to unborn child outweighs drug benefits. Don't use.

Breast-feeding:
Drug passes into milk. Avoid drug or discontinue nursing until you finish medicine. Consult doctor for advice on maintaining milk supply.

Infants & children:
Use only under medical supervision.

Prolonged use:
- High blood level of calcium which disturbs electrolyte balance.
- Kidney stones, impaired kidney function.

Skin & sunlight:
No problems expected.

Driving, piloting or hazardous work:
No problems expected.

Airplane passengers:
No problems expected.

Discontinuing:
May be unnecessary to finish medicine. Follow doctor's instructions.

Others:
Don't take longer than 2 weeks unless under medical supervision.

INTERACTION WITH OTHER DRUGS

GENERIC NAME OR DRUG CLASS	COMBINED EFFECT
Anticoagulants	Decreased anticoagulant effect.
Calcitonin	Decreased calcitonin effect.
Chlorpromazine	Decreased chlorpromazine effect.
Digitalis preparations	Decreased digitalis effect.
Diuretics	Increased calcium in blood.
Iron supplements	Decreased iron effect.
Meperidine	Increased meperidine effect.
Nalidixic acid	Decreased effect of nalidixic acid.
Oxyphenbutazone	Decreased oxyphenbutazone effect.
Para-aminosalicylic acid (PAS)	Decreased PAS effect.
Penicillins	Decreased penicillin effect.
Pentobarbital	Decreased pentobarbital effect.
Phenylbutazone	Decreased phenylbutazone effect.
Pseudoephedrine	Increased pseudoephedrine effect.

Additional interactions on page 835.

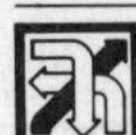

INTERACTION WITH OTHER SUBSTANCES

INTERACTS WITH	COMBINED EFFECT
Alcohol:	Decreased antacid effect.
Beverages:	No proven problems.
Cocaine:	No proven problems.
Foods:	Decreased antacid effect if taken with food. Wait 1 hour after eating.
Marijuana:	No proven problems.
Tobacco:	Decreased antacid effect.

CAPTOPRIL

BRAND NAMES

Capoten

GENERAL INFORMATION

Habit forming? No
Prescription needed? Yes
Available as generic? No
Drug class: Antihypertensive

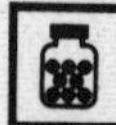

USES

Treatment for high blood pressure and congestive heart failure.

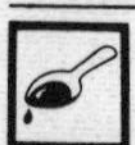

DOSAGE & USAGE INFORMATION

How to take:
Tablets—Swallow with liquid. Instructions to take on empty stomach mean 1 hour before or 2 hours after eating.

When to take:
At the same times each day, usually 3 times daily. Take first dose at bedtime and lie down immediately.

If you forget a dose:
Take as soon as you remember up to 2 hours late. If more than 2 hours, wait for next scheduled dose (don't double this dose).

What drug does:
- Reduces resistance in arteries.
- Strengthens heartbeat.

Time lapse before drug works:
60 to 90 minutes.

Don't take with:
See Interaction column and consult doctor.

OVERDOSE

Symptoms:
Fever, chills, sore throat, fainting, convulsions, coma.

What to do:
- Dial 0 (operator) or 911 (emergency) for an ambulance or medical help. Then give first aid immediately.
- Additional emergency information on page 886.

POSSIBLE ADVERSE REACTIONS OR SIDE EFFECTS

SYMPTOMS	FREQUENCY	WHAT TO DO
Brain & nervous system:		
Dizziness, fainting.	Infrequent	3
Skin:		
Rash	Common	3
Eyes:	None expected.	
Ears, nose, throat:		
• Sore throat.	Rare	3
• Loss of taste.	Common	3
Digestive:		
Nausea, vomiting, indigestion, abdominal pain.	Rare	4
Heart & lungs:		
Chest pain, fast or irregular heartbeat.	Infrequent	3
Blood vessels:	None expected.	
Muscles, bones, joints:	None expected.	
Genital, urinary:		
Cloudy urine.	Rare	3
Kidneys:	None expected.	
Liver:	None expected.	
Allergic:		
Swelling of face, hands, mouth or feet.	Infrequent	2
Blood:	None expected.	
Others:		
Fever, chills.	Rare	3

1-Life-threatening. Seek emergency treatment immediately.
2-Discontinue. Seek emergency treatment.
3-Discontinue. Call doctor right away.
4-Continue. Call doctor when convenient.
5-Continue. Tell doctor at next visit.
6-No action necessary.

WARNINGS & PRECAUTIONS

Don't take if:

- You are allergic to captopril.
- You have any autoimmune disease, including AIDS or lupus.
- You are receiving blood from a blood bank.
- You take drugs for cancer.
- You will have surgery within 2 months, including dental surgery, requiring general or spinal anesthesia.

Before you start, consult your doctor:

- If you have had a stroke.
- If you have angina or heart or blood-vessel disease.
- If you have high level of potassium in blood.
- If you have kidney disease.
- If you are on severe salt-restricted diet.
- If you have lupus.

Over age 60:
Adverse reactions and side effects may be more frequent and severe than in younger persons.

Pregnancy:
Risk to unborn child outweighs drug benefits. Don't use.

Breast-feeding:
Drug passes into milk. Avoid drug or discontinue nursing.

Infants & children:
Not recommended.

Prolonged use:
May decrease white cells in blood or cause protein loss in urine. Request periodic laboratory blood counts and urine tests.

Skin & sunlight:
No problems expected.

Driving, piloting or hazardous work:
Avoid if you become dizzy or faint. Otherwise, no problems expected.

Airplane passengers:
No problems expected.

Discontinuing:
Don't discontinue without consulting doctor. Dose may require gradual reduction if you have taken drug for a long time. Doses of other drugs may also require adjustment.

Others:

- Stop taking diuretics or increase salt intake 1 week before starting captopril.
- Avoid exercising in hot weather.

INTERACTION WITH OTHER DRUGS

GENERIC NAME OR DRUG CLASS	COMBINED EFFECT
Amiloride	Possible excessive potassium in blood.
Antihypertensives (other)	Possible excessive blood-pressure drop.
Chloramphenicol	Possible blood disorders.
Diuretics	Severe blood-pressure drop with first dose.
Potassium supplements	Excessive potassium in blood.
Spironolactone	Possible excessive potassium in blood.
Triamterene	Possible excessive potassium in blood.

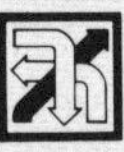

INTERACTION WITH OTHER SUBSTANCES

INTERACTS WITH	COMBINED EFFECT
Alcohol:	Possible excessive blood-pressure drop.
Beverages: Low-salt milk	Possible excessive potassium in blood.
Cocaine:	Increased dizziness and chest pain.
Foods: Salt substitutes	Possible excessive potassium.
Marijuana:	Increased dizziness.
Tobacco:	May decrease captopril effect.

CARBAMAZEPINE

BRAND NAMES

Apo-Carbamazepine
Mazepine
Tegretol

GENERAL INFORMATION

Habit forming? No
Prescription needed? Yes
Available as generic? No
Drug class: Analgesic, anticonvulsant

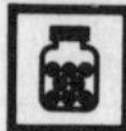

USES

- Decreased frequency, severity and duration of attacks of tic douloureux.
- Prevents seizures.

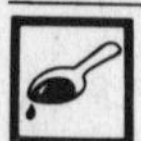

DOSAGE & USAGE INFORMATION

How to take:
Regular or chewable tablet—Swallow with liquid or food to lessen stomach irritation.

When to take:
At the same times each day.

If you forget a dose:
Take as soon as you remember up to 2 hours late. If more than 2 hours, wait for next scheduled dose (don't double this dose).

What drug does:
- Reduces transmission of pain messages at certain nerve terminals.
- Reduces excitability of nerve fibers in brain, thus inhibiting repetitive spread of nerve impulses.

Time lapse before drug works:
- Tic douloureaux—24 to 72 hours.
- Seizures—1 to 2 weeks.

Don't take with:
See Interaction column and consult doctor.

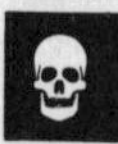

OVERDOSE

Symptoms:
Involuntary movements, dilated pupils, flushed skin, stupor, coma.

What to do:
- Dial 0 (operator) or 911 (emergency) for an ambulance or medical help. Then give first aid immediately.
- If patient is unconscious and not breathing, give mouth-to-mouth breathing. If there is no heartbeat, use cardiac massage and mouth-to-mouth breathing (CPR). Don't try to make patient vomit. If you can't get help quickly, take patient to nearest emergency facility.
- Additional emergency information on page 886.

POSSIBLE ADVERSE REACTIONS OR SIDE EFFECTS

SYMPTOMS	FREQUENCY	WHAT TO DO
Brain & nervous system:		
Confusion, slurred speech, fainting, depression, headache, hallucinations.	Infrequent	3
Skin:		
Hives, rash.	Infrequent	3
Eyes:		
• Blurred vision.	Common	4
• Back-and-forth eye movements.	Rare	3
Ears, nose, throat:		
Sores in mouth, sore throat, fever.	Infrequent	3
Digestive:		
Diarrhea	Infrequent	4
Heart & lungs:		
Breathing difficulty; irregular, pounding or slow heartbeat; pain in chest.	Rare	3
Blood vessels:		
Unusual bleeding or bruising.	Infrequent	3
Muscles, bones, joints:		
Uncontrolled body jerks; numbness, weakness, tingling in hands and feet; tender, bluish legs or feet.	Rare	3
Genital, urinary:		
Frequent urination.	Rare	4
Kidneys:		
Less urine.	Rare	3
Liver, allergic, blood:	None expected.	
Others:		
• Unusual fatigue.	Infrequent	3
• Swollen lymph glands.	Rare	3

3- Discontinue. Call doctor right away.
4- Continue. Call doctor when convenient.

WARNINGS & PRECAUTIONS

Don't take if:
- You are allergic to carbamazepine.
- You have had liver or bone-marrow disease.
- You have taken MAO inhibitors in the past 2 weeks.

Before you start, consult your doctor:
- If you have high blood pressure, thrombophlebitis or heart disease.
- If you have glaucoma.
- If you have emotional or mental problems.
- If you have liver or kidney disease.
- If you drink more than 2 alcoholic drinks per day.

Over age 60:
Adverse reactions and side effects may be more frequent and severe than in younger persons.

Pregnancy:
Studies inconclusive on harm to unborn child. Animal studies show fetal abnormalities. Decide with your doctor whether drug benefits justify risk to unborn child.

Breast-feeding:
Drug passes into milk. Avoid drug or discontinue nursing until you finish medicine. Consult doctor for advice on maintaining milk supply.

Infants & children:
Not recommended.

Prolonged use:
- Jaundice and liver damage.
- Hair loss.
- Ringing in ears.
- Lower sex drive.

Skin & sunlight:
May cause rash or intensify sunburn in areas exposed to sun or sunlamp.

Driving, piloting or hazardous work:
Don't drive or pilot aircraft until you learn how medicine affects you. Don't work around dangerous machinery. Don't climb ladders or work in high places. Danger increases if you drink alcohol or take medicine affecting alertness and reflexes.

Airplane passengers:
No problems expected.

Discontinuing:
Don't discontinue without doctor's advice until you complete prescribed dose, even though symptoms diminish or disappear.

Others:
Use only if less-hazardous drugs are not effective. Stay under medical supervision.

INTERACTION WITH OTHER DRUGS

GENERIC NAME OR DRUG CLASS	COMBINED EFFECT
Anticoagulants (oral)	Decreased anticoagulant effect.
Anticonvulsants (hydantoin)	Decreased effect of both drugs.
Antidepressants (tricyclic)	Confusion. Possible psychosis.
Contraceptives (oral)	Reduced contraceptive protection. Use another birth-control method.
Digitalis preparations	Excess slowing of heart.
Doxycycline	Decreased doxycycline effect.
MAO inhibitors	Dangerous overstimulation. Avoid.
Tranquilizers (benzodiazepine)	Increased carbamazepine effect.

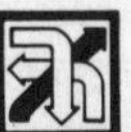

INTERACTION WITH OTHER SUBSTANCES

INTERACTS WITH	COMBINED EFFECT
Alcohol:	Increased sedative effect of alcohol. Avoid.
Beverages:	None expected.
Cocaine:	Increased adverse effect of carbamazepine. Avoid.
Foods:	None expected.
Marijuana:	Increased adverse effects of carbamazepine. Avoid.
Tobacco:	None expected.

CARBENICILLIN

BRAND NAMES

Geocillin
Geopen
Pyopen

GENERAL INFORMATION

Habit forming? No
Prescription needed? Yes
Available as generic? Yes
Drug class: Antibiotic (penicillin)

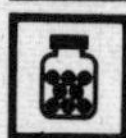

USES

Treatment of bacterial infections that are susceptible to carbenicillin.

DOSAGE & USAGE INFORMATION

How to take:

- Tablets or capsules—Swallow with liquid on an empty stomach 1 hour before or 2 hours after eating.
- Liquid—Take with cold beverage. Liquid form is perishable and effective for only 7 days at room temperature. Effective for 14 days if stored in refrigerator. Don't freeze.

When to take:
Follow instructions on prescription label or side of package. Doses should be evenly spaced. For example, 4 times a day means every 6 hours.

If you forget a dose:
Take as soon as you remember. Continue regular schedule.

What drug does:
Destroys susceptible bacteria. Does not kill viruses.

Time lapse before drug works:
May be several days before medicine affects infection.

Don't take with:
See Interaction column and consult doctor.

OVERDOSE

Symptoms:
Severe diarrhea, nausea or vomiting.

What to do:
Overdose unlikely to threaten life. If person takes much larger amount than prescribed, call doctor, poison-control center or hospital emergency room for instructions.

POSSIBLE ADVERSE REACTIONS OR SIDE EFFECTS

SYMPTOMS	FREQUENCY	WHAT TO DO
Brain & nervous system:	None expected.	
Skin: Hives, rash, intense itch soon after a dose.	Rare	1
Eyes:	None expected.	
Ears, nose, throat: Dark or discolored tongue.	Common	5
Digestive: Mild nausea, vomiting, diarrhea.	Infrequent	4
Heart & lungs:	None expected.	
Blood vessels: Unexplained bleeding.	Rare	3
Muscles, bones, joints:	None expected.	
Genital, urinary:	None expected.	
Kidneys:	None expected.	
Liver:	None expected.	
Allergic: Life-threatening anaphylaxis may occur!	Rare	1 See Page 888.
Blood:	None expected.	
Others:	None expected.	

1- Life-threatening. Seek emergency treatment immediately.
2- Discontinue. Seek emergency treatment.
3- Discontinue. Call doctor right away.
4- Continue. Call doctor when convenient.
5- Continue. Tell doctor at next visit.
6- No action necessary.

WARNINGS & PRECAUTIONS

Don't take if:
You are allergic to carbenicillin, cephalosporin antibiotics, other penicillins or penicillamine. Life-threatening reaction may occur.

Before you start, consult your doctor:
If you are allergic to any substance or drug.

Over age 60:
You may have skin reactions, particularly around genitals and anus.

Pregnancy:
Studies inconclusive on harm to unborn child. Animal studies show fetal abnormalities. Decide with your doctor whether drug benefits justify risk to unborn child.

Breast-feeding:
Drug passes into milk. Child may become sensitive to penicillins and have allergic reactions to penicillin drugs. Avoid carbenicillin or discontinue nursing until you finish medicine. Consult doctor for advice on maintaining milk supply.

Infants & children:
No problems expected.

Prolonged use:
You may become more susceptible to infections caused by germs not responsive to carbenicillin.

Skin & sunlight:
No problems expected.

Driving, piloting or hazardous work:
Usually not dangerous. Most hazardous reactions likely to occur a few minutes after taking carbenicillin.

Airplane passengers:
No problems expected.

Discontinuing:
Don't discontinue without doctor's advice until you complete prescribed dose, even though symptoms diminish or disappear.

Others:
Injection forms may cause fluid retention (edema) with weakness and low potassium in the blood.

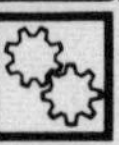

INTERACTION WITH OTHER DRUGS

GENERIC NAME OR DRUG CLASS	COMBINED EFFECT
Chloramphenicol	Decreased effect of both drugs.
Erythromycins	Decreased effect of both drugs.
Paromomycin	Decreased effect of both drugs.
Tetracyclines	Decreased effect of both drugs.
Troleandomycin	Decreased effect of both drugs.

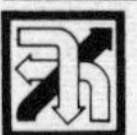

INTERACTION WITH OTHER SUBSTANCES

INTERACTS WITH	COMBINED EFFECT
Alcohol:	Occasional stomach irritation.
Beverages:	None expected.
Cocaine:	No proven problems.
Foods:	Decreased effect of oral carbenicillin.
Marijuana:	No proven problems.
Tobacco:	None expected.

CARBIDOPA & LEVODOPA

BRAND NAMES

Larodopa
Sinemet

GENERAL INFORMATION

Habit forming? No
Prescription needed? Yes
Available as generic? Yes
Drug class: Antiparkinsonism

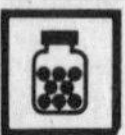

USES

Controls Parkinson's disease symptoms such as rigidity, tremor and unsteady gait.

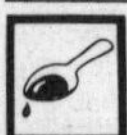

DOSAGE & USAGE INFORMATION

How to take:
Tablet or capsule—Swallow with liquid or food to lessen stomach irritation. If you can't swallow whole, crumble tablet or open capsule and take with liquid or food.

When to take:
At the same times each day.

If you forget a dose:
Take as soon as you remember up to 2 hours late. If more than 2 hours, wait for next scheduled dose (don't double this dose).

What drug does:
Restores chemical balance necessary for normal nerve impulses.

Time lapse before drug works:
2 to 3 weeks to improve; 6 weeks or longer for maximum benefit.

Don't take with:
See Interaction column and consult doctor.

OVERDOSE

Symptoms:
Muscle twitch, spastic eyelid closure, nausea, vomiting, diarrhea, irregular and rapid pulse, weakness, fainting, confusion, agitation, hallucination, coma.

What to do:
- Dial 0 (operator) or 911 (emergency) for an ambulance or medical help. Then give first aid immediately.
- If patient is unconscious and not breathing, give mouth-to-mouth breathing. If there is no heartbeat, use cardiac massage and mouth-to-mouth breathing (CPR). Don't try to make patient vomit. If you can't get help quickly, take patient to nearest emergency facility.
- Additional emergency information on page 886.

POSSIBLE ADVERSE REACTIONS OR SIDE EFFECTS

SYMPTOMS	FREQUENCY	WHAT TO DO
Brain & nervous system:		
• Fainting, severe dizziness, headache, insomnia, nightmares.	Infrequent	3
• Mood changes, uncontrolled body movements.	Common	4
Skin:		
• Flushed face.	Infrequent	4
• Rash, itch.	Infrequent	3
Eyes:		
Blurred vision.	Infrequent	4
Ears, nose, throat:		
Dry mouth.	Common	6
Digestive:		
• Duodenal ulcer.	Rare	4
• Diarrhea	Common	4
• Constipation	Infrequent	5
• Nausea, vomiting.	Infrequent	3
Heart & lungs:		
Irregular heartbeat.	Infrequent	3
Blood vessels:		
High blood pressure.	Rare	3
Muscles, bones, joints:		
Muscle twitching.	Infrequent	4
Genital, urinary:		
• Discolored or dark urine.	Infrequent	4
• Difficult urination.	Infrequent	4
Kidneys, liver, allergic:	None expected.	
Blood:		
Anemia	Rare	4
Others:		
• Tiredness	Infrequent	5
• Body odor.	Common	6

1-Life-threatening. Seek emergency treatment immediately.
2-Discontinue. Seek emergency treatment.
3-Discontinue. Call doctor right away.
4-Continue. Call doctor when convenient.
5-Continue. Tell doctor at next visit.
6-No action necessary.

CARBIDOPA & LEVODOPA

WARNINGS & PRECAUTIONS

Don't take if:
- You are allergic to levodopa or carbidopa.
- You have taken MAO inhibitors in past 2 weeks.
- You have glaucoma (narrow-angle type).

Before you start, consult your doctor:
- If you have diabetes or epilepsy.
- If you have had high blood pressure, heart or lung disease.
- If you have had liver or kidney disease.
- If you have a peptic ulcer.
- If you have malignant melanoma.
- If you will have surgery within 2 months, including dental surgery, requiring general or spinal anesthesia.

Over age 60:
Adverse reactions and side effects may be more frequent and severe than in younger persons.

Pregnancy:
Risk to unborn child outweighs drug benefits. Don't use.

Breast-feeding:
Drug filters into milk. May harm child. Avoid.

Infants & children:
Not recommended.

Prolonged use:
May lead to uncontrolled movements of head, face, mouth, tongue, arms or legs.

Skin & sunlight:
No problems expected.

Driving, piloting or hazardous work:
Don't drive or pilot aircraft until you learn how medicine affects you. Don't work around dangerous machinery. Don't climb ladders or work in high places. Danger increases if you drink alcohol or take medicine affecting alertness and reflexes, such as antihistamines, tranquilizers, sedatives, pain medicine, narcotics and mind-altering drugs.

Airplane passengers:
No problems expected.

Discontinuing:
Don't discontinue without doctor's advice until you complete prescribed dose, even though symptoms diminish or disappear.

Others:
Expect to start with small dose and increase gradually to lessen frequency and severity of adverse reactions.

INTERACTION WITH OTHER DRUGS

GENERIC NAME OR DRUG CLASS	COMBINED EFFECT
Antiparkinsonism drugs (other)	Increased effect of carbidopa and levodopa.
Haloperidol	Decreased effect of carbidopa and levodopa.
MAO inhibitors	Dangerous rise in blood pressure.
Methyldopa	Decreased effect of carbidopa and levodopa.
Papaverine	Decreased effect of carbidopa and levodopa.
Phenothiazines	Decreased effect of carbidopa and levodopa.
Pyridoxine (Vitamin B-6)	Decreased effect carbidopa and levodopa.
Rauwolfia alkaloids	Decreased effect carbidopa and levodopa.

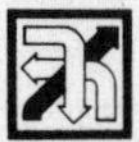

INTERACTION WITH OTHER SUBSTANCES

INTERACTS WITH	COMBINED EFFECT
Alcohol:	None expected.
Beverages:	None expected.
Cocaine:	Decreased carbidopa and levodopa effect.
Foods:	None expected.
Marijuana:	Increased fatigue, lethargy, fainting.
Tobacco:	None expected.

CARBINOXAMINE

BRAND NAMES

Clistin
Clistin R-A

GENERAL INFORMATION

Habit forming? No
Prescription needed? Yes
Available as generic? No
Drug class: Antihistamine

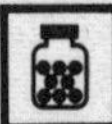

USES

Reduces allergic symptoms such as hay fever, hives, rash or itching.

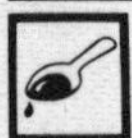

DOSAGE & USAGE INFORMATION

How to take:
- Tablet—Swallow with liquid or food to lessen stomach irritation.
- Extended-release tablets—Swallow each dose whole. If you take regular tablets, you may chew or crush them.

When to take:
Varies with form. Follow label directions.

If you forget a dose:
Take as soon as you remember up to 2 hours late. If more than 2 hours, wait for next scheduled dose (don't double this dose).

What drug does:
Blocks action of histamine after an allergic response triggers histamine release in sensitive cells.

Time lapse before drug works:
30 minutes.

Don't take with:
See Interaction column and consult doctor.

OVERDOSE

Symptoms:
Convulsions, red face, hallucinations, coma.

What to do:
- Dial 0 (operator) or 911 (emergency) for an ambulance or medical help. Then give first aid immediately.
- If patient is unconscious and not breathing, give mouth-to-mouth breathing. If there is no heartbeat, use cardiac massage and mouth-to-mouth breathing (CPR). Don't try to make patient vomit. If you can't get help quickly, take patient to nearest emergency facility.
- Additional emergency information on page 886.

POSSIBLE ADVERSE REACTIONS OR SIDE EFFECTS

SYMPTOMS	FREQUENCY	WHAT TO DO
Brain & nervous system:		
• Nightmares, agitation, irritability.	Rare	3
• Drowsiness, dizziness.	Common	5
Skin:	None expected.	
Eyes:		
• Vision changes.	Infrequent	3
• Less tolerance for contact lenses.	Infrequent	4
Ears, nose, throat:		
• Sore throat, fever.	Rare	3
• Dry mouth, nose, throat.	Common	5
Digestive:		
• Nausea	Common	5
• Appetite loss.	Infrequent	5
Heart & lungs:		
Rapid heartbeat.	Rare	3
Blood vessels:		
Unusual bleeding or bruising.	Rare	3
Muscles, bones, joints, kidneys, liver, allergic, blood:	None expected.	
Genital, urinary:		
Urination difficulty.	Infrequent	4
Others:		
Fatigue, weakness.	Rare	3

1- Life-threatening. Seek emergency treatment immediately.
2- Discontinue. Seek emergency treatment.
3- Discontinue. Call doctor right away.
4- Continue. Call doctor when convenient.
5- Continue. Tell doctor at next visit.
6- No action necessary.

WARNINGS & PRECAUTIONS

Don't take if:
You are allergic to any antihistamine.

Before you start, consult your doctor:
- If you have glaucoma.
- If you have enlarged prostate.
- If you have asthma.
- If you have kidney disease.
- If you have peptic ulcer.
- If you will have surgery within 2 months, including dental surgery, requiring general or spinal anesthesia.

Over age 60:
Don't exceed recommended dose. Adverse reactions and side effects may be more frequent and severe than in younger persons, especially urination difficulty, diminished alertness and other brain and nervous-system symptoms.

Pregnancy:
No proven harm to unborn child. Avoid if possible.

Breast-feeding:
Drug passes into milk. Avoid drug or discontinue nursing until you finish medicine. Consult doctor for advice on maintaining milk supply.

Infants & children:
Not recommended for premature or newborn infants. Otherwise, no problems expected.

Prolonged use:
Avoid. May damage bone marrow and nerve cells.

Skin & sunlight:
May cause rash or intensify sunburn in areas exposed to sun or sunlamp.

Driving, piloting or hazardous work:
Don't drive or pilot aircraft until you learn how medicine affects you. Don't work around dangerous machinery. Don't climb ladders or work in high places. Danger increases if you drink alcohol or take medicine affecting alertness and reflexes, such as antihistamines, tranquilizers, sedatives, pain medicine, narcotics and mind-altering drugs.

Airplane passengers:
No problems expected.

Discontinuing:
No problems expected.

Others:
May mask symptoms of hearing damage from aspirin, other salicylates, cisplatin, paromomycin, vancomycin or anticonvulsants. Consult doctor if you use these.

INTERACTION WITH OTHER DRUGS

GENERIC NAME OR DRUG CLASS	COMBINED EFFECT
Anticholinergics	Increased anticholinergic effect.
Antidepressants	Excess sedation. Avoid.
Antihistamines (other)	Excess sedation. Avoid.
Hypnotics	Excess sedation. Avoid.
MAO inhibitors	Increased carbinoxamine effect.
Mind-altering drugs	Excess sedation. Avoid.
Narcotics	Excess sedation. Avoid.
Sedatives	Excess sedation. Avoid.
Sleep inducers	Excess sedation. Avoid.
Tranquilizers	Excess sedation. Avoid.

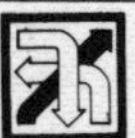

INTERACTION WITH OTHER SUBSTANCES

INTERACTS WITH	COMBINED EFFECT
Alcohol:	Excess sedation. Avoid.
Beverages:	
Caffeine drinks	Less carbinoxamine sedation.
Cocaine:	Decreased carbinoxamine effect. Avoid.
Foods:	None expected.
Marijuana:	Excess sedation. Avoid.
Tobacco:	None expected.

CARBONIC ANHYDRASE INHIBITORS

BRAND AND GENERIC NAMES

Acetazolam
ACETAZOLAMIDE
Ak-Zol
Apo-Acetazolamide
Cetazol
Daranide
Diamox
DICHLORPHENAMIDE
METHAZOLAMIDE
Neptazane
Oratrol

GENERAL INFORMATION

Habit forming? No
Prescription needed? Yes
Available as generic? No
Drug class: Carbonic anhydrase inhibitor

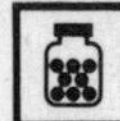

USES

- Treatment of glaucoma.
- Treatment of epileptic seizures.
- Treatment of body-fluid retention.
- Treatment for shortness of breath, insomnia and fatigue in high altitudes.

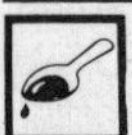

DOSAGE & USAGE INFORMATION

How to take:
Tablets—Swallow whole with liquid or food to lessen stomach irritation.

When to take:
- 1 dose per day—At the same time each morning.
- More than 1 dose per day—Take last dose several hours before bedtime.

If you forget a dose:
Take as soon as you remember. Continue regular schedule.

What drug does:
- Inhibits action of carbonic anhydrase, an enzyme. This lowers the internal eye pressure by decreasing fluid formation in the eye.
- Forces sodium and water excretion, reducing body fluid.

Time lapse before drug works:
2 hours.

Don't take with:
- Non-prescription drugs without consulting doctor.
- See Interaction column and consult doctor.

OVERDOSE

Symptoms:
Drowsiness, confusion, excitement, nausea, vomiting, numbness in hands and feet, coma.

What to do:
- Call your doctor or poison-control center for advice if you suspect overdose, even if not sure. Symptoms may not appear until damage has occurred.
- Additional emergency information on page 886.

POSSIBLE ADVERSE REACTIONS OR SIDE EFFECTS

SYMPTOMS	FREQUENCY	WHAT TO DO
Brain & nervous system:		
• Headache, mood changes, nervousness, clumsiness, trembling, confusion.	Rare	3
• Convulsions	Rare	1
Skin:		
Hives, itch, rash, or sores.	Rare	3
Ears, nose, throat:		
• Ringing in ears, hoarseness, dry mouth, thirst.	Rare	3
• Sore throat, fever.	Rare	3
Digestive:		
• Appetite change, nausea, vomiting.	Rare	3
• Black, tarry stool.	Rare	3
Heart & lungs:		
Breathing difficulty, irregular or weak heartbeat.	Rare	3
Blood vessels:		
Easy bleeding or bruising.	Rare	3
Muscles, bones, joints:		
Muscle cramps.	Rare	3
Genital, urinary:		
Painful or frequent urination, bloody urine.	Rare	3
Kidneys:		
Back pain.	Infrequent	3
Allergic, blood, liver, eyes:	None expected.	
Others:		
• Fatigue, weakness.	Infrequent	4
• Tingling or burning in feet or hands.	Infrequent	4

1- Life-threatening. Seek emergency treatment immediately.
2- Discontinue. Seek emergency treatment.
3- Discontinue. Call doctor right away.
4- Continue. Call doctor when convenient.

CARBONIC ANHYDRASE INHIBITORS

WARNINGS & PRECAUTIONS

Don't take if:
- You are allergic to any carbonic anhydrase inhibitor.
- You have liver or kidney disease.
- You have Addison's disease (adrenal gland failure).
- You have diabetes.

Before you start, consult your doctor:
- If you have gout or lupus.
- If you are allergic to any sulfa drug.
- If you will have surgery within 2 months, including dental surgery, requiring general or spinal anesthesia.

Over age 60:
- Don't exceed recommended dose.
- If you take a digitalis preparation, eat foods high in potassium content or take a potassium supplement.

Pregnancy:
No proven harm to unborn child. Avoid if possible, especially first 3 months.

Breast-feeding:
Avoid drug or don't nurse your infant.

Infants & children:
Not recommended for children younger than 12.

Prolonged use:
May cause kidney stones, vision change, loss of taste and smell, jaundice (yellow skin and eyes) or weight loss.

Skin & sunlight:
No problems expected.

Driving, piloting or hazardous work:
Avoid if you feel drowsy or dizzy. Otherwise, no problems expected.

Airplane passengers:
No problems expected.

Discontinuing:
Don't discontinue without medical advice.

Others:
Medicine may increase sugar levels in blood and urine. Diabetics may need insulin adjustment.

INTERACTION WITH OTHER DRUGS

GENERIC NAME OR DRUG CLASS	COMBINED EFFECT
Amphetamines	Increased amphetamine effect.
Anticonvulsants	Increased loss of bone minerals.
Antidepressants (tricyclic)	Increased antidepressant effect.
Antidiabetics (oral)	Increased potassium loss.
Aspirin	Decreased aspirin effect.
Cortisone drugs	Increased potassium loss.
Digitalis preparations	Possible digitalis toxicity.
Diuretics	Increased potassium loss.
Lithium	Decreased lithium effect.
Methenamine	Decreased methenamine effect.
Quinidine	Increased quinidine effect.
Salicylates	Salicylate toxicity.
Sympathomimetics	Increased sympathomimetic effect.

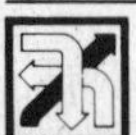

INTERACTION WITH OTHER SUBSTANCES

INTERACTS WITH	COMBINED EFFECT
Alcohol:	None expected.
Beverages:	None expected.
Cocaine:	Avoid. Decreased carbonic anhydrase inhibitor effect.
Foods: Potassium-rich foods.	Eat these to decrease potassium loss. See page 848.
Marijuana:	Avoid. Increased carbonic anhydrase inhibitor effect.
Tobacco:	May decrease absorption of carbonic anhydrase inhibitors.

CARISOPRODOL

BRAND NAMES

Rela
Soma
Soma Compound
Soprodol

GENERAL INFORMATION

Habit forming? No
Prescription needed? Yes
Available as generic? Yes
Drug class: Muscle relaxant (skeletal)

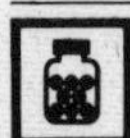

USES

Treatment for sprains, strains and muscle spasms.

DOSAGE & USAGE INFORMATION

How to take:
Tablet or capsule—Swallow with liquid.

When to take:
As needed, no more often than every 4 hours.

If you forget a dose:
Take as soon as you remember. Wait 4 hours for next dose.

What drug does:
Blocks body's pain messages to brain. May also sedate.

Time lapse before drug works:
60 minutes.

Don't take with:
See Interaction column and consult doctor.

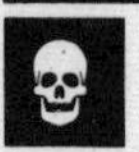

OVERDOSE

Symptoms:
Nausea, vomiting, diarrhea, headache. May progress to severe weakness, difficult breathing, sensation of paralysis, coma.

What to do:
- Dial 0 (operator) or 911 (emergency) for an ambulance or medical help. Then give first aid immediately.
- Additional emergency information on page 886.

POSSIBLE ADVERSE REACTIONS OR SIDE EFFECTS

SYMPTOMS	FREQUENCY	WHAT TO DO
Brain & nervous system:		
• Drowsiness, fainting, dizziness.	Common	4
• Agitation	Infrequent	3
Skin:		
Rash, hives or itch.	Rare	3
Eyes:	None expected.	
Ears, nose, throat:		
Sore throat, fever.	Rare	3
Digestive:		
• Constipation or diarrhea; nausea, cramps, vomiting.	Infrequent	3
• Bloody or tarry, black stool.	Rare	2
Heart & lungs:		
Wheezing, shortness of breath.	Infrequent	3
Blood vessels:	None expected.	
Muscles, bones, joints:	None expected.	
Genital, urinary:		
Orange or red-purple urine.	Common	6
Kidneys:	None expected.	
Liver:		
Jaundice (yellow eyes and skin).	Rare	3
Allergic:	None expected.	
Blood:	None expected.	
Others:		
Tiredness, weakness.	Rare	3

1- Life-threatening. Seek emergency treatment immediately.
2- Discontinue. Seek emergency treatment.
3- Discontinue. Call doctor right away.
4- Continue. Call doctor when convenient.
5- Continue. Tell doctor at next visit.
6- No action necessary.

WARNINGS & PRECAUTIONS

Don't take if:
- You are allergic to any skeletal-muscle relaxant.
- You have porphyria.

Before you start, consult your doctor:
- If you have had liver or kidney disease.
- If you plan pregnancy within medication period.

Over age 60:
Adverse reactions and side effects may be more frequent and severe than in younger persons.

Pregnancy:
No proven harm to unborn child. Avoid if possible.

Breast-feeding:
Drug passes into milk. Avoid drug or discontinue nursing until you finish medicine. Consult doctor for advice on maintaining milk supply.

Infants & children:
Not recommended.

Prolonged use:
Periodic liver-function tests recommended if you use this drug for a long time.

Skin & sunlight:
No problems expected.

Driving, piloting or hazardous work:
Don't drive or pilot aircraft until you learn how medicine affects you. Don't work around dangerous machinery. Don't climb ladders or work in high places. Danger increases if you drink alcohol or take medicine affecting alertness and reflexes, such as antihistamines, tranquilizers, sedatives, pain medicine, narcotics and mind-altering drugs.

Airplane passengers:
No problems expected.

Discontinuing:
Don't discontinue without doctor's advice until you complete prescribed dose, even though symptoms diminish or disappear.

Others:
No problems expected.

INTERACTION WITH OTHER DRUGS

GENERIC NAME OR DRUG CLASS	COMBINED EFFECT
Antidepressants	Increased sedation.
Antihistamines	Increased sedation.
Mind-altering drugs	Increased sedation.
Muscle relaxants (others)	Increased sedation.
Narcotics	Increased sedation.
Sedatives	Increased sedation.
Sleep inducers	Increased sedation.
Testosterone	Decreased carisoprodol effect.
Tranquilizers	Increased sedation.

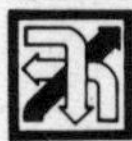

INTERACTION WITH OTHER SUBSTANCES

INTERACTS WITH	COMBINED EFFECT
Alcohol:	Increased sedation.
Beverages:	None expected.
Cocaine:	Lack of coordination, increased sedation.
Foods:	None expected.
Marijuana:	Lack of coordination, drowsiness, fainting.
Tobacco:	None expected.

CARPHENAZINE

BRAND NAMES

Proketazine

GENERAL INFORMATION

Habit forming? No
Prescription needed? Yes
Available as generic? Yes
Drug class: Tranquilizer, antiemetic (phenothiazine)

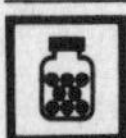

USES

- Stops nausea, vomiting.
- Reduces anxiety, agitation.

DOSAGE & USAGE INFORMATION

How to take:

- Tablet or capsule—Swallow with liquid or food to lessen stomach irritation.
- Suppositories—Remove wrapper and moisten suppository with water. Gently insert into rectum, large end first.
- Drops or liquid—Dilute dose in beverage.

When to take:

- Nervous and mental disorders—Take at the same times each day.
- Nausea and vomiting—Take as needed, no more often than every 4 hours.

If you forget a dose:

- Nervous and mental disorders—Take up to 2 hours late. If more than 2 hours, wait for next scheduled dose (don't double this).
- Nausea and vomiting—Take as soon as you remember. Wait 4 hours for next dose.

What drug does:

- Suppresses brain's vomiting center.
- Suppresses brain centers that control abnormal emotions and behavior.

Time lapse before drug works:

- Nausea and vomiting—1 hour or less.
- Nervous and mental disorders—4-6 weeks.

Don't take with:

- Antacid or medicine for diarrhea.
- Non-prescription drug for cough, cold or allergy.
- See Interaction column and consult doctor.

OVERDOSE

Symptoms:
Stupor, convulsions, coma.

What to do:

- Dial 0 (operator) or 911 (emergency) for an ambulance or medical help. Then give first aid immediately.
- Additional emergency information on page 886.

POSSIBLE ADVERSE REACTIONS OR SIDE EFFECTS

SYMPTOMS	FREQUENCY	WHAT TO DO
Brain & nervous system:		
• Restlessness, tremor.	Common	3
• Fainting	Infrequent	2
• Drowsiness	Common	3
Skin:		
• Rash	Infrequent	3
• Less perspiration.	Common	4
Eyes:		
Vision changes.	Rare	3
Ears, nose, throat:		
• Sore throat, fever.	Rare	3
• Dry mouth, nasal congestion.	Common	4
Digestive:		
Constipation	Common	4
Heart & lungs, blood vessels, kidneys, allergic, blood:	None expected.	
Muscles, bones, joints:		
Muscle spasms of face and neck, unsteady gait.	Common	2
Genital, urinary:		
Urination difficulty.	Infrequent	4
Liver:		
Jaundice (yellow eyes and skin).	Rare	3
Others:		
Less interest in sex, breast swelling, change in menstrual pattern.	Infrequent	4

1- Life-threatening. Seek emergency treatment immediately.
2- Discontinue. Seek emergency treatment.
3- Discontinue. Call doctor right away.
4- Continue. Call doctor when convenient.
5- Continue. Tell doctor at next visit.
6- No action necessary.

WARNINGS & PRECAUTIONS

Don't take if:
- You are allergic to any phenothiazine.
- You have a blood or bone-marrow disease.

Before you start, consult your doctor:
- If you will have surgery within 2 months, including dental surgery, requiring general or spinal anesthesia.
- If you have asthma, emphysema or other lung disorder.
- If you take non-prescription ulcer medicine, asthma medicine or amphetamines.

Over age 60:
Adverse reactions and side effects may be more frequent and severe than in younger persons. More likely to develop involuntary movement of jaws, lips, tongue, chewing. Report this to your doctor immediately. Early treatment can help.

Pregnancy:
Risk to unborn child outweighs drug benefits. Don't use.

Breast-feeding:
Drug passes into milk. Avoid drug or discontinue nursing until you finish medicine. Consult doctor for advice on maintaining milk supply.

Infants & children:
Don't give to children younger than 2.

Prolonged use:
May lead to tardive dyskinesia (involuntary movement of jaws, lips, tongue, chewing).

Skin & sunlight:
May cause rash or intensify sunburn in areas exposed to sun or sunlamp. Skin may remain sensitive for 3 months after discontinuing.

Driving, piloting or hazardous work:
Don't drive or pilot aircraft until you learn how medicine affects you. Don't work around dangerous machinery. Don't climb ladders or work in high places. Danger increases if you drink alcohol or take medicine affecting alertness and reflexes.

Airplane passengers:
No problems expected.

Discontinuing:
- Nervous and mental disorders—Don't discontinue without doctor's advice until you complete prescribed dose, even though symptoms diminish or disappear.
- Nausea and vomiting—May be unnecessary to finish medicine. Follow doctor's instructions.

INTERACTION WITH OTHER DRUGS

GENERIC NAME OR DRUG CLASS	COMBINED EFFECT
Anticholinergics	Increased anticholinergic effect.
Antidepressants (tricyclic)	Increased carphenazine effect.
Antihistamines	Increased antihistamine effect.
Appetite suppressants	Decreased suppressant effect.
Levodopa	Decreased levodopa effect.
Mind-altering drugs	Increased effect of mind-altering drugs.
Narcotics	Increased narcotic effect.
Phenytoin	Increased phenytoin effect.
Quinidine	Impaired heart function. Dangerous mixture.
Sedatives	Increased sedative effect.
Tranquilizers (other)	Increased tranquilizer effect.

INTERACTION WITH OTHER SUBSTANCES

INTERACTS WITH	COMBINED EFFECT
Alcohol:	Dangerous oversedation.
Beverages:	None expected.
Cocaine:	Decreased carphenazine effect. Avoid.
Foods:	None expected.
Marijuana:	Drowsiness. May increase antinausea effect.
Tobacco:	None expected.

CASCARA

BRAND NAMES

Aromatic Cascara Fluidextract
Cascara Sagrada
Cas-Evac
Milk of Magnesia-Cascara
Peri-Colace

GENERAL INFORMATION

Habit forming? No
Prescription needed? No
Available as generic? Yes
Drug class: Laxative (stimulant)

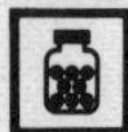

USES

Constipation relief.

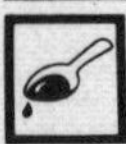

DOSAGE & USAGE INFORMATION

How to take:
- Tablet—Swallow with liquid. If you can't swallow whole, chew or crumble tablet and take with liquid or food.
- Liquid—Drink 6 to 8 glasses of water each day, in addition to one taken with each dose.

When to take:
Usually at bedtime with a snack, unless directed otherwise.

If you forget a dose:
Take as soon as you remember.

What drug does:
Acts on smooth muscles of intestine wall to cause vigorous bowel movement.

Time lapse before drug works:
6 to 10 hours.

Don't take with:
- See Interaction column and consult doctor.
- Don't take within 2 hours of taking another medicine. Laxative interferes with medicine absorption.

OVERDOSE

Symptoms:
Vomiting, electrolyte depletion.

What to do:
Overdose unlikely to threaten life. If person takes much larger amount than prescribed, call doctor, poison-control center or hospital emergency room for instructions.

POSSIBLE ADVERSE REACTIONS OR SIDE EFFECTS

SYMPTOMS	FREQUENCY	WHAT TO DO
Brain & nervous system: Irritability, confusion, headache.	Rare	3
Skin: Rash	Rare	3
Eyes:	None expected.	
Ears, nose, throat:	None expected.	
Digestive: Belching, cramps, nausea.	Infrequent	4
Heart & lungs: Breathing difficulty, irregular heartbeat.	Rare	3
Blood vessels:	None expected.	
Muscles, bones, joints: Muscle cramps.	Rare	3
Genital, urinary:	None expected.	
Kidneys: Burning on urination.	Rare	4
Liver:	None expected.	
Allergic:	None expected.	
Blood:	None expected.	
Others:		
• Rectal irritation.	Common	4
• Dangerous potassium loss.	Infrequent	3
• Unusual tiredness or weakness.	Rare	3

1- Life-threatening. Seek emergency treatment immediately.
2- Discontinue. Seek emergency treatment.
3- Discontinue. Call doctor right away.
4- Continue. Call doctor when convenient.
5- Continue. Tell doctor at next visit.
6- No action necessary.

WARNINGS & PRECAUTIONS

Don't take if:
- You have symptoms of appendicitis, inflamed bowel or intestinal blockage.
- You are allergic to a stimulant laxative.
- You have missed a bowel movement for only 1 or 2 days.

Before you start, consult your doctor:
- If you have a colostomy or ileostomy.
- If you have congestive heart disease.
- If you have diabetes.
- If you have high blood pressure.
- If you have a laxative habit.
- If you have rectal bleeding.
- If you take other laxatives.

Over age 60:
Adverse reactions and side effects may be more frequent and severe than in younger persons.

Pregnancy:
Risk to mother and unborn child outweighs drug benefits. Don't use.

Breast-feeding:
Drug passes into milk. Avoid drug or discontinue nursing until you finish medicine. Consult doctor for advice on maintaining milk supply.

Infants & children:
Use only under medical supervision.

Prolonged use:
Don't take for more than 1 week unless under a doctor's supervision. May cause laxative dependence.

Skin & sunlight:
No problems expected.

Driving, piloting or hazardous work:
No problems expected.

Airplane passengers:
No problems expected.

Discontinuing:
May be unnecessary to finish medicine. Follow doctor's instructions.

Others:
Don't take to "flush out" your system or as a "tonic."

INTERACTION WITH OTHER DRUGS

GENERIC NAME OR DRUG CLASS	COMBINED EFFECT
Antihypertensives	May cause dangerous low potassium level.
Diuretics	May cause dangerous low potassium level.

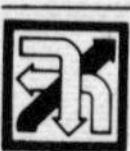

INTERACTION WITH OTHER SUBSTANCES

INTERACTS WITH	COMBINED EFFECT
Alcohol:	None expected.
Beverages:	None expected.
Cocaine:	None expected.
Foods:	None expected.
Marijuana:	None expected.
Tobacco:	None expected.

CASTOR OIL

BRAND NAMES

Alphamul
Emulsoil
Fleet Prep Kit
Granulex
Hydrisinol
Neoloid
Purge
Stimuzyme Plus
Unisoil

GENERAL INFORMATION

Habit forming? No
Prescription needed? No
Available as generic? Yes
Drug class: Laxative (stimulant)

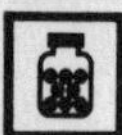

USES

Constipation relief.

DOSAGE & USAGE INFORMATION

How to take:
Liquid—Drink 6 to 8 glasses of water each day, in addition to one taken with each dose.

When to take:
Usually at bedtime with a snack, unless directed otherwise.

If you forget a dose:
Take as soon as you remember.

What drug does:
Acts on smooth muscles of intestine wall to cause vigorous bowel movement.

Time lapse before drug works:
2 to 6 hours.

Don't take with:
- See Interaction column and consult doctor.
- Don't take within 2 hours of taking another medicine. Laxative interferes with medicine absorption.

OVERDOSE

Symptoms:
Vomiting, electrolyte depletion.

What to do:
Overdose unlikely to threaten life. If person takes much larger amount than prescribed, call doctor, poison-control center or hospital emergency room for instructions.

POSSIBLE ADVERSE REACTIONS OR SIDE EFFECTS

SYMPTOMS	FREQUENCY	WHAT TO DO
Brain & nervous system:		
Irritability, confusion, headache.	Rare	3
Skin:		
Rash	Rare	3
Eyes:	None expected.	
Ears, nose, throat:	None expected.	
Digestive:		
Belching, cramps, nausea.	Infrequent	4
Heart & lungs:		
Breathing difficulty, irregular heartbeat.	Rare	3
Blood vessels:	None expected.	
Muscles, bones, joints:		
Muscle cramps.	Rare	3
Genital, urinary:	None expected.	
Kidneys:		
Burning on urination.	Rare	4
Liver:	None expected.	
Allergic:	None expected.	
Blood:	None expected.	
Others:		
• Rectal irritation.	Common	4
• Dangerous potassium loss.	Infrequent	3
• Unusual tiredness or weakness.	Rare	3

1- Life-threatening. Seek emergency treatment immediately.
2- Discontinue. Seek emergency treatment.
3- Discontinue. Call doctor right away.
4- Continue. Call doctor when convenient.
5- Continue. Tell doctor at next visit.
6- No action necessary.

WARNINGS & PRECAUTIONS

Don't take if:
- You have symptoms of appendicitis, inflamed bowel or intestinal blockage.
- You are allergic to a stimulant laxative.
- You have missed a bowel movement for only 1 or 2 days.

Before you start, consult your doctor:
- If you have a colostomy or ileostomy.
- If you have congestive heart disease.
- If you have diabetes.
- If you have high blood pressure.
- If you have a laxative habit.
- If you have rectal bleeding.
- If you take other laxatives.

Over age 60:
Adverse reactions and side effects may be more frequent and severe than in younger persons.

Pregnancy:
Risk to mother and unborn child outweighs drug benefits. Don't use.

Breast-feeding:
Drug passes into milk. Avoid drug or discontinue nursing until you finish medicine. Consult doctor for advice on maintaining milk supply.

Infants & children:
Use only under medical supervision.

Prolonged use:
Don't take for more than 1 week unless under doctor's supervision. May cause laxative dependence.

Skin & sunlight:
No problems expected.

Driving, piloting or hazardous work:
No problems expected.

Airplane passengers:
No problems expected.

Discontinuing:
May be unnecessary to finish medicine. Follow doctor's instructions.

Others:
Don't take to "flush out" your system or as a "tonic."

INTERACTION WITH OTHER DRUGS

GENERIC NAME OR DRUG CLASS	COMBINED EFFECT
Antihypertensives	May cause dangerous low potassium level.
Diuretics	May cause dangerous low potassium level.

INTERACTION WITH OTHER SUBSTANCES

INTERACTS WITH	COMBINED EFFECT
Alcohol:	None expected.
Beverages:	None expected.
Cocaine:	None expected.
Foods:	None expected.
Marijuana:	None expected.
Tobacco:	None expected.

CEFACLOR

BRAND NAMES

Ceclor

GENERAL INFORMATION

Habit forming? No
Prescription needed? Yes
Available as generic? Yes
Drug class: Antibiotic (cephalosporin)

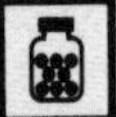

USES

Treatment of bacterial infections. Will not cure viral infections such as cold and flu.

DOSAGE & USAGE INFORMATION

How to take:
- Tablet or capsule—Swallow with liquid. If you can't swallow whole, crumble tablet or open capsule and take with liquid or food.
- Liquid—Use measuring spoon.

When to take:
At same times each day, 1 hour before or 2 hours after eating.

If you forget a dose:
Take as soon as you remember or double next dose. Return to regular schedule.

What drug does:
Kills susceptible bacteria.

Time lapse before drug works:
May require several days to affect infection.

Don't take with:
See Interaction column and consult doctor.

OVERDOSE

Symptoms:
Abdominal cramps, nausea, vomiting, severe diarrhea with mucus or blood in stool.

What to do:
Overdose unlikely to threaten life. If person takes much larger amount than prescribed, call doctor, poison-control center or hospital emergency room for instructions.

POSSIBLE ADVERSE REACTIONS OR SIDE EFFECTS

SYMPTOMS	FREQUENCY	WHAT TO DO
Brain & nervous system:	None expected.	
Skin:		
• Rash, redness, itching.	Common	3
• Rectal itching.	Infrequent	4
Eyes:	None expected.	
Ears, nose, throat:	None expected.	
Digestive:		
Mild, nausea, vomiting, cramps, severe diarrhea with mucus or blood in stool.	Rare	3
Heart & lungs:	None expected.	
Blood vessels:	None expected.	
Muscles, bones, joints:	None expected.	
Genital, urinary:	None expected.	
Kidneys:	None expected.	
Liver:	None expected.	
Allergic:		
Life-threatening anaphylaxis may occur!	Rare	1 See page 888.
Blood:	None expected.	
Others:		
Unusual weakness, tiredness, weight loss or fever.	Rare	3

1-Life-threatening. Seek emergency treatment immediately.
2-Discontinue. Seek emergency treatment.
3-Discontinue. Call doctor right away.
4-Continue. Call doctor when convenient.
5-Continue. Tell doctor at next visit.
6-No action necessary.

WARNINGS & PRECAUTIONS

Don't take if:
You are allergic to any cephalosporin antibiotic.

Before you start, consult your doctor:
- If you are allergic to any penicillin antibiotic.
- If you have a kidney disorder.
- If you have colitis or enteritis.

Over age 60:
Adverse reactions and side effects may be more frequent and severe than in younger persons. More likely to itch around rectum and genitals.

Pregnancy:
No proven harm to unborn child. Avoid if possible.

Breast-feeding:
Drug passes into milk. Avoid drug or discontinue nursing until you finish medicine. Consult doctor for advice on maintaining milk supply.

Infants & children:
No special warnings.

Prolonged use:
Kills beneficial bacteria that protect body against other germs. Unchecked germs may cause secondary infections.

Skin & sunlight:
No problems expected.

Driving, piloting or hazardous work:
No problems expected.

Airplane passengers:
No problems expected.

Discontinuing:
Don't discontinue without doctor's advice until you complete prescribed dose, even though symptoms diminish or disappear.

Others:
No problems expected.

INTERACTION WITH OTHER DRUGS

GENERIC NAME OR DRUG CLASS	COMBINED EFFECT
Anticoagulants	Increased anticoagulant effect.
Probenecid	Increased cefaclor effect.

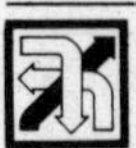

INTERACTION WITH OTHER SUBSTANCES

INTERACTS WITH	COMBINED EFFECT
Alcohol:	None expected.
Beverages:	None expected.
Cocaine:	None expected, but cocaine may slow body's recovery. Avoid.
Foods:	Slow absorption. Take with liquid 1 hour before or 2 hours after eating.
Marijuana:	None expected, but marijuana may slow body's recovery. Avoid.
Tobacco:	None expected.

CEFADROXIL

BRAND NAMES

Duricef
Ultracef

GENERAL INFORMATION

Habit forming? No
Prescription needed? Yes
Available as generic? Yes
Drug class: Antibiotic (cephalosporin)

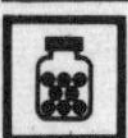

USES

Treatment of bacterial infections. Will not cure viral infections such as cold and flu.

DOSAGE & USAGE INFORMATION

How to take:
- Tablet or capsule—Swallow with liquid. If you can't swallow whole, crumble tablet or open capsule and take with liquid or food.
- Liquid—Use measuring spoon.

When to take:
At same times each day, 1 hour before or 2 hours after eating.

If you forget a dose:
Take as soon as you remember or double next dose. Return to regular schedule.

What drug does:
Kills susceptible bacteria.

Time lapse before drug works:
May require several days to affect infection.

Don't take with:
See Interaction column and consult doctor.

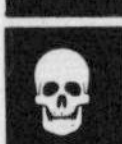

OVERDOSE

Symptoms:
Abdominal cramps, nausea, vomiting, severe diarrhea with mucus or blood in stool.

What to do:
Overdose unlikely to threaten life. If person takes much larger amount than prescribed, call doctor, poison-control center or hospital emergency room for instructions.

POSSIBLE ADVERSE REACTIONS OR SIDE EFFECTS

SYMPTOMS	FREQUENCY	WHAT TO DO
Brain & nervous system:	None expected.	
Skin:		
• Rash, redness, itching.	Common	3
• Rectal itching.	Infrequent	4
Eyes:	None expected.	
Ears, nose, throat:	None expected.	
Digestive:		
Mild nausea, vomiting, cramps, severe diarrhea with mucus or blood in stool.	Rare	3
Heart & lungs:	None expected.	
Blood vessels:	None expected.	
Muscles, bones, joints:	None expected.	
Genital, urinary:	None expected.	
Kidneys:	None expected.	
Liver:	None expected.	
Allergic:		
Life-threatening anaphylaxis may occur!	Rare	1 See page 888.
Blood:	None expected.	
Others:		
Unusual weakness, tiredness, weight loss or fever.	Rare	3

1- Life-threatening. Seek emergency treatment immediately.
2- Discontinue. Seek emergency treatment.
3- Discontinue. Call doctor right away.
4- Continue. Call doctor when convenient.
5- Continue. Tell doctor at next visit.
6- No action necessary.

WARNINGS & PRECAUTIONS

Don't take if:
You are allergic to any cephalosporin antibiotic.

Before you start, consult your doctor:
- If you are allergic to any penicillin antibiotic.
- If you have a kidney disorder.
- If you have colitis or enteritis.

Over age 60:
Adverse reactions and side effects may be more frequent and severe than in younger persons. More likely to itch around rectum and genitals.

Pregnancy:
No proven harm to unborn child. Avoid if possible.

Breast-feeding:
Drug passes into milk. Avoid drug or discontinue nursing until you finish medicine. Consult doctor for advice on maintaining milk supply.

Infants & children:
No special warnings.

Prolonged use:
Kills beneficial bacteria that protect body against other germs. Unchecked germs may cause secondary infections.

Skin & sunlight:
No problems expected.

Driving, piloting or hazardous work:
No problems expected.

Airplane passengers:
No problems expected.

Discontinuing:
Don't discontinue without doctor's advice until you complete prescribed dose, even though symptoms diminish or disappear.

Others:
No problems expected.

INTERACTION WITH OTHER DRUGS

GENERIC NAME OR DRUG CLASS	COMBINED EFFECT
Anticoagulants	Increased anticoagulant effect.
Probenecid	Increased cefadroxil effect.

INTERACTION WITH OTHER SUBSTANCES

INTERACTS WITH	COMBINED EFFECT
Alcohol:	None expected.
Beverages:	None expected.
Cocaine:	None expected, but cocaine may slow body's recovery. Avoid.
Foods:	Slow absorption. Take with liquid 1 hour before or 2 hours after eating.
Marijuana:	None expected, but marijuana may slow body's recovery. Avoid.
Tobacco:	None expected.

CEPHALEXIN

BRAND NAMES

Ceporex
Keflex
Novolexin

GENERAL INFORMATION

Habit forming? No
Prescription needed? Yes
Available as generic? Yes
Drug class: Antibiotic (cephalosporin)

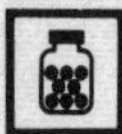

USES

Treatment of bacterial infections. Will not cure viral infections such as cold and flu.

DOSAGE & USAGE INFORMATION

How to take:

- Tablet or capsule—Swallow with liquid. If you can't swallow whole, crumble tablet or open capsule and take with liquid or food.
- Liquid—Use measuring spoon.

When to take:
At same times each day, 1 hour before or 2 hours after eating.

If you forget a dose:
Take as soon as you remember or double next dose. Return to regular schedule.

What drug does:
Kills susceptible bacteria.

Time lapse before drug works:
May require several days to affect infection.

Don't take with:
See Interaction column and consult doctor.

OVERDOSE

Symptoms:
Abdominal cramps, nausea, vomiting, severe diarrhea with mucus or blood in stool.

What to do:
Overdose unlikely to threaten life. If person takes much larger amount than prescribed, call doctor, poison-control center or hospital emergency room for instructions.

POSSIBLE ADVERSE REACTIONS OR SIDE EFFECTS

SYMPTOMS	FREQUENCY	WHAT TO DO
Brain & nervous system:	None expected.	
Skin:		
• Rash, redness, itching.	Common	3
• Rectal itching.	Infrequent	4
Eyes:	None expected.	
Ears, nose, throat:	None expected.	
Digestive:		
Mild nausea, vomiting, cramps, severe diarrhea with mucus or blood in stool.	Rare	3
Heart & lungs:	None expected.	
Blood vessels:	None expected.	
Muscles, bones, joints:	None expected.	
Genital, urinary:	None expected.	
Kidneys:	None expected.	
Liver:	None expected.	
Allergic:		
Life-threatening anaphylaxis may occur!	Rare	1 See page 888.
Blood:	None expected.	
Others:		
Unusual weakness, tiredness, weight loss or fever.	Rare	3

1- Life-threatening. Seek emergency treatment immediately.
2- Discontinue. Seek emergency treatment.
3- Discontinue. Call doctor right away.
4- Continue. Call doctor when convenient.
5- Continue. Tell doctor at next visit.
6- No action necessary.

WARNINGS & PRECAUTIONS

Don't take if:
You are allergic to any cephalosporin antibiotic.

Before you start, consult your doctor:
- If you are allergic to any penicillin antibiotic.
- If you have a kidney disorder.
- If you have colitis or enteritis.

Over age 60:
Adverse reactions and side effects may be more frequent and severe than in younger persons. More likely to itch around rectum and genitals.

Pregnancy:
No proven harm to unborn child. Avoid if possible.

Breast-feeding:
Drug passes into milk. Avoid drug or discontinue nursing until you finish medicine. Consult doctor for advice on maintaining milk supply.

Infants & children:
No special warnings.

Prolonged use:
Kills beneficial bacteria that protect body against other germs. Unchecked germs may cause secondary infections.

Skin & sunlight:
No problems expected.

Driving, piloting or hazardous work:
No problems expected.

Airplane passengers:
No problems expected.

Discontinuing:
Don't discontinue without doctor's advice until you complete prescribed dose, even though symptoms diminish or disappear.

Others:
No problems expected.

INTERACTION WITH OTHER DRUGS

GENERIC NAME OR DRUG CLASS	COMBINED EFFECT
Anticoagulants	Increased anticoagulant effect.
Probenecid	Increased cephalexin effect.

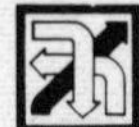

INTERACTION WITH OTHER SUBSTANCES

INTERACTS WITH	COMBINED EFFECT
Alcohol:	None expected.
Beverages:	None expected.
Cocaine:	None expected, but cocaine may slow body's recovery. Avoid.
Foods:	Slow absorption. Take with liquid 1 hour before or 2 hours after eating.
Marijuana:	None expected, but marijuana may slow body's recovery. Avoid.
Tobacco:	None expected.

CEPHRADINE

BRAND NAMES

Anspor
Velosef

GENERAL INFORMATION

Habit forming? No
Prescription needed? Yes
Available as generic? Yes
Drug class: Antibiotic (cephalosporin)

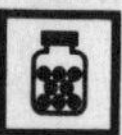

USES

Treatment of bacterial infections. Will not cure viral infections such as cold and flu.

DOSAGE & USAGE INFORMATION

How to take:

- Tablet or capsule—Swallow with liquid. If you can't swallow whole, crumble tablet or open capsule and take with liquid or food.
- Liquid—Use measuring spoon.

When to take:
At same times each day, 1 hour before or 2 hours after eating.

If you forget a dose:
Take as soon as you remember or double next dose. Return to regular schedule.

What drug does:
Kills susceptible bacteria.

Time lapse before drug works:
May require several days to affect infection.

Don't take with:
See Interaction column and consult doctor.

OVERDOSE

Symptoms:
Abdominal cramps, nausea, vomiting, severe diarrhea with mucus or blood in stool.

What to do:
Overdose unlikely to threaten life. If person takes much larger amount than prescribed, call doctor, poison-control center or hospital emergency room for instructions.

POSSIBLE ADVERSE REACTIONS OR SIDE EFFECTS

SYMPTOMS	FREQUENCY	WHAT TO DO
Brain & nervous system:	None expected.	
Skin:		
• Rash, redness, itching.	Common	3
• Rectal itching.	Infrequent	4
Eyes:	None expected.	
Ears, nose, throat:	None expected.	
Digestive:		
Mild nausea, vomiting, cramps, severe diarrhea with mucus or blood in stool.	Rare	3
Heart & lungs:	None expected.	
Blood vessels:	None expected.	
Muscles, bones, joints:	None expected.	
Genital, urinary:	None expected.	
Kidneys:	None expected.	
Liver:	None expected.	
Allergic:		
Life-threatening anaphylaxis may occur!	Rare	1 See page 888.
Blood:	None expected.	
Others:		
Unusual weakness, tiredness, weight loss or fever.	Rare	3

1- Life-threatening. Seek emergency treatment immediately.
2- Discontinue. Seek emergency treatment.
3- Discontinue. Call doctor right away.
4- Continue. Call doctor when convenient.
5- Continue. Tell doctor at next visit.
6- No action necessary.

WARNINGS & PRECAUTIONS

Don't take if:
You are allergic to any cephalosporin antibiotic.

Before you start, consult your doctor:
- If you are allergic to any penicillin antibiotic.
- If you have a kidney disorder.
- If you have colitis or enteritis.

Over age 60:
Adverse reactions and side effects may be more frequent and severe than in younger persons. More likely to itch around rectum and genitals.

Pregnancy:
No proven harm to unborn child. Avoid if possible.

Breast-feeding:
Drug passes into milk. Avoid drug or discontinue nursing until you finish medicine. Consult doctor for advice on maintaining milk supply.

Infants & children:
No special warnings.

Prolonged use:
Kills beneficial bacteria that protect body against other germs. Unchecked germs may cause secondary infections.

Skin & sunlight:
No problems expected.

Driving, piloting or hazardous work:
No problems expected.

Airplane passengers:
No problems expected.

Discontinuing:
Don't discontinue without doctor's advice until you complete prescribed dose, even though symptoms diminish or disappear.

Others:
No problems expected.

INTERACTION WITH OTHER DRUGS

GENERIC NAME OR DRUG CLASS	COMBINED EFFECT
Anticoagulants	Increased anticoagulant effect.
Probenecid	Increased cephradine effect.

INTERACTION WITH OTHER SUBSTANCES

INTERACTS WITH	COMBINED EFFECT
Alcohol:	None expected.
Beverages:	None expected.
Cocaine:	None expected, but cocaine may slow body's recovery. Avoid.
Foods:	Slow absorption. Take with liquid 1 hour before or 2 hours after eating.
Marijuana:	None expected, but marijuana may slow body's recovery. Avoid.
Tobacco:	None expected.

CHLOPHEDIANOL

BRAND NAMES

Ulo
Ulone

GENERAL INFORMATION

Habit forming? No
Prescription needed? Yes
Available as generic? No
Drug class: Cough suppressant

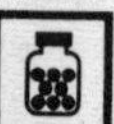

USES

Reduces non-productive cough due to bronchial irritation.

DOSAGE & USAGE INFORMATION

How to take:
Take syrup without diluting. Don't drink fluids immediately after medicine.

When to take:
3 or 4 times a day when needed. No more often than every 3 hours.

If you forget a dose:
Take as soon as you remember up to 2 hours late. If more than 2 hours, wait for next scheduled dose (don't double this dose).

What drug does:
Reduces cough reflex by direct effect on cough center in brain, and by local anesthetic action.

Time lapse before drug works:
30 minutes to 1 hour.

Don't take with:
- Alcohol or brain depressant or stimulant drugs.
- See Interaction column and consult doctor.

OVERDOSE

Symptoms:
Blurred vision, hallucinations, coma.

What to do:
- Dial 0 (operator) or 911 (emergency) for an ambulance or medical help. Then give first aid immediately.
- If patient is unconscious and not breathing, give mouth-to-mouth breathing. If there is no heartbeat, use cardiac massage and mouth-to-mouth breathing (CPR). Don't try to make patient vomit. If you can't get help quickly, take patient to nearest emergency facility.
- Additional emergency information on page 886.

POSSIBLE ADVERSE REACTIONS OR SIDE EFFECTS

SYMPTOMS	FREQUENCY	WHAT TO DO
Brain & nervous system:		
• Hallucinations	Rare	3
• Nightmares	Rare	4
• Excitement or irritability.	Rare	4
• Drowsiness	Rare	3
Skin:		
Rash or hives.	Rare	3
Eyes:		
Blurred vision.	Rare	4
Ears, nose, throat:		
Dry mouth.	Rare	4
Digestive:		
• Nausea, vomiting.	Rare	3
• Dry mouth.	Rare	4
Heart & lungs:		
Irregular heartbeat.	Rare	3
Blood vessels:	None expected.	
Muscles, bones, joints:	None expected.	
Genital, urinary:		
Difficult urination in older men with enlarged prostate.	Common	4
Kidneys, allergic, blood, liver:	None expected.	

1 - Life-threatening. Seek emergency treatment immediately.
2 - Discontinue. Seek emergency treatment.
3 - Discontinue. Call doctor right away.
4 - Continue. Call doctor when convenient.
5 - Continue. Tell doctor at next visit.
6 - No action necessary.

WARNINGS & PRECAUTIONS

Don't take if:
You are allergic to chlophedianol.

Before you start, consult your doctor:
- If medicine is for hyperactive child who takes medicine for treatment.
- If your cough brings up sputum (phlegm).
- If you have heart disease.
- If you will have surgery within 2 months, including dental surgery, requiring general or spinal anesthesia.

Over age 60:
Adverse reactions and side effects may be more frequent and severe than in younger persons.

Pregnancy:
Risk to unborn child outweighs drug benefits. Don't use.

Breast-feeding:
Unknown whether medicine filters into milk. Consult doctor.

Infants & children:
Not recommended for children under age 2.

Prolonged use:
Not recommended. If cough persists despite medicine, consult doctor.

Skin & sunlight:
No problems expected.

Driving, piloting or hazardous work:
Don't drive or pilot aircraft until you learn how medicine affects you. Don't work around dangerous machinery. Don't climb ladders or work in high places. Danger increases if you drink alcohol or take medicine affecting alertness and reflexes, such as antihistamines, tranquilizers, sedatives, pain medicine, narcotics and mind-altering drugs.

Airplane passengers:
No problems expected.

Discontinuing:
May be unnecessary to finish medicine. Follow doctor's instructions.

Others:
Consult doctor if cough persists despite medication for 7 days or if fever, skin rash or headache accompany cough.

INTERACTION WITH OTHER DRUGS

GENERIC NAME OR DRUG CLASS	COMBINED EFFECT
Appetite suppressants	Excess stimulation.
Sympathomimetics	Excess stimulation.
Other medicine for hyperactivity in children.	Excess stimulation.
Anticonvulsants	Interferes with actions of both.
Brain depressing medicines: antihistamines, sedatives, sleeping pills, tranquilizers, pain pills, antidepressants, narcotics, muscle relaxants.	Excess sedation.
Antidepressants (tricyclic)	Excess sedation.
MAO inhibitors	Excess sedation.

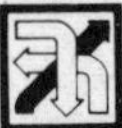

INTERACTION WITH OTHER SUBSTANCES

INTERACTS WITH	COMBINED EFFECT
Alcohol:	Excess sedation. Avoid.
Beverages: Coffee, tea, cocoa, cola.	Excess stimulation. Avoid.
Cocaine:	Increased chance of toxic stimulation. Avoid.
Foods:	None expected.
Marijuana:	Increased chance of toxic stimulation. Avoid.
Tobacco:	Decreased effect of chlophedianol.

CHLORAL HYDRATE

BRAND NAMES

Aquachloral
Colidrate
Noctec
Novochlorhydrate
Oradrate
SK-Chloral Hydrate

GENERAL INFORMATION

Habit forming? Yes
Prescription needed? Yes
Available as generic? Yes
Drug class: Hypnotic

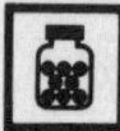

USES

- Reduces anxiety.
- Relieves insomnia.

DOSAGE & USAGE INFORMATION

How to take:

- Tablet or capsule—Swallow with milk or food to lessen stomach irritation.
- Drops—Dilute dose in beverage before swallowing.
- Suppositories—Remove wrapper and moisten suppository with water. Gently insert larger end into rectum. Push well into rectum with finger.

When to take:
At the same time each day.

If you forget a dose:
Take as soon as you remember up to 2 hours late. If more than 2 hours, wait for next scheduled dose (don't double this dose).

What drug does:
Affects brain centers that control wakefulness and alertness.

Time lapse before drug works:
30 to 60 minutes.

Don't take with:
See Interaction column and consult doctor.

OVERDOSE

Symptoms:
Confusion, weakness, breathing difficulty, stagger, slow or irregular heartbeat.

What to do:

- Dial 0 (operator) or 911 (emergency) for an ambulance or medical help. Then give first aid immediately.
- If patient is unconscious and not breathing, give mouth-to-mouth breathing. If there is no heartbeat, use cardiac massage and mouth-to-mouth breathing (CPR). Don't try to make patient vomit. If you can't get help quickly, take patient to nearest emergency facility.
- Additional emergency information on page 886.

POSSIBLE ADVERSE REACTIONS OR SIDE EFFECTS

SYMPTOMS	FREQUENCY	WHAT TO DO
Brain & nervous system:		
• Hallucinations, agitation, confusion.	Rare	3
• "Hangover" effect, clumsiness or unsteadiness, drowsiness, dizziness or lightheadedness.	Infrequent	4
Skin:		
Hives, rash.	Rare	4
Eyes:	None expected.	
Ears, nose, throat:	None expected.	
Digestive:		
Nausea, stomach pain, vomiting.	Common	3
Heart & lungs:	None expected.	
Blood vessels:	None expected.	
Muscles, bones, joints:	None expected.	
Genital, urinary:	None expected.	
Kidneys:	None expected.	
Liver:	None expected.	
Allergic:	None expected.	
Blood:	None expected.	
Others:	None expected.	

1- Life-threatening. Seek emergency treatment immediately.
2- Discontinue. Seek emergency treatment.
3- Discontinue. Call doctor right away.
4- Continue. Call doctor when convenient.
5- Continue. Tell doctor at next visit.
6- No action necessary.

CHLORAL HYDRATE

WARNINGS & PRECAUTIONS

Don't take if:
You are allergic to chloral hydrate.

Before you start, consult your doctor:
- If you have had liver, kidney or heart trouble.
- If you are prone to stomach upsets (if medicine is in oral form).
- If you have colitis or a rectal inflammation (if medicine is in suppository form).

Over age 60:
Adverse reactions and side effects may be more frequent and severe than in younger persons. More likely to have "hangover" effect.

Pregnancy:
Risk to unborn child outweighs drug benefits. Unborn child may become addicted to drug. Don't use.

Breast-feeding:
Drug filters into milk. May harm child. Avoid.

Infants & children:
Use only under medical supervision.

Prolonged use:
Addiction and possible kidney damage.

Skin & sunlight:
No problems expected.

Driving, piloting or hazardous work:
Don't drive or pilot aircraft until you learn how medicine affects you. Don't work around dangerous machinery. Don't climb ladders or work in high places. Danger increases if you drink alcohol or take medicine affecting alertness and reflexes, such as antihistamines, tranquilizers, sedatives, pain medicine, narcotics and mind-altering drugs.

Airplane passengers:
No problems expected.

Discontinuing:
Don't discontinue without consulting doctor. Dose may require gradual reduction if you have taken drug for a long time. Doses of other drugs may also require adjustment.

Others:
Frequent kidney-function tests recommended when drug is used for long time.

INTERACTION WITH OTHER DRUGS

GENERIC NAME OR DRUG CLASS	COMBINED EFFECT
Anticoagulants	Possible hemorrhaging.
Antidepressants	Increased chloral hydrate effect.
Antihistamines	Increased chloral hydrate effect.
Cortisone drugs	Decreased cortisone effect.
MAO inhibitors	Increased chloral hydrate effect.
Mind-altering drugs	Increased chloral hydrate effect.
Narcotics	Increased chloral hydrate effect.
Pain relievers	Increased chloral hydrate effect.
Phenothiazines	Increased chloral hydrate effect.
Sedatives	Increased chloral hydrate effect.
Sleep inducers	Increased chloral hydrate effect.
Tranquilizers	Increased chloral hydrate effect.

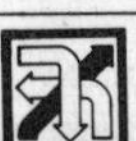

INTERACTION WITH OTHER SUBSTANCES

INTERACTS WITH	COMBINED EFFECT
Alcohol:	Increased sedative effect of both. Avoid.
Beverages:	None expected.
Cocaine:	Decreased chloral hydrate effect. Avoid.
Foods:	None expected.
Marijuana:	May severely impair mental and physical functioning. Avoid.
Tobacco:	None expected.

CHLORAMBUCIL

BRAND NAMES

Leukeran

GENERAL INFORMATION

Habit forming? No
Prescription needed? Yes
Available as generic? No
Drug class: Antineoplastic, immunosuppressant

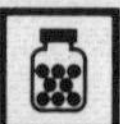

USES

- Treatment for some kinds of cancer.
- Suppresses immune response after transplant and in immune disorders.

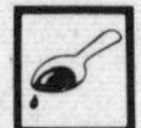

DOSAGE & USAGE INFORMATION

How to take:
Tablet or capsule—Swallow with liquid after light meal. Don't drink fluids with meals. Drink extra fluids between meals. Avoid sweet or fatty foods.

When to take:
At the same time each day.

If you forget a dose:
Take as soon as you remember. Don't ever double dose.

What drug does:
Inhibits abnormal cell reproduction. May suppress immune system.

Time lapse before drug works:
Up to 6 weeks for full effect.

Don't take with:
See Interaction column and consult doctor.

OVERDOSE

Symptoms:
Bleeding, chills, fever, collapse, stupor, seizure.

What to do:
- Dial 0 (operator) or 911 (emergency) for an ambulance or medical help. Then give first aid immediately.
- If patient is unconscious and not breathing, give mouth-to-mouth breathing. If there is no heartbeat, use cardiac massage and mouth-to-mouth breathing (CPR). Don't try to make patient vomit. If you can't get help quickly, take patient to nearest emergency facility.
- Additional emergency information on page 886.

POSSIBLE ADVERSE REACTIONS OR SIDE EFFECTS

SYMPTOMS	FREQUENCY	WHAT TO DO
Brain & nervous system:		
Mental confusion.	Infrequent	4
Skin:		
• Unusual bleeding or bruising.	Common	3
• Hair loss.	Common	4
Eyes:		
Ears, nose, throat:		
Mouth sores with sore throat, chills and fever.	Common	3
Digestive:		
• Black stools.	Common	3
• Sores in mouth and lips.	Common	3
• Nausea, vomiting, diarrhea (unavoidable).	Common	5
Heart & lungs:		
• Shortness of breath.	Infrequent	4
• Cough	Infrequent	5
Blood vessels:	None expected.	
Muscles, bones, joints:		
Joint pain.	Common	4
Genital, urinary:		
Menstrual changes.	Common	3
Kidneys, allergic, blood, liver:		
• Jaundice (yellow skin and eyes).	Rare	3
• May increase chance of developing leukemia.	Infrequent	4
Others:		
Tiredness, weakness.	Common	5

1- Life-threatening. Seek emergency treatment immediately.
2- Discontinue. Seek emergency treatment.
3- Discontinue. Call doctor right away.
4- Continue. Call doctor when convenient.
5- Continue. Tell doctor at next visit.

WARNINGS & PRECAUTIONS

Don't take if:
- You have had hypersensitivity to alkylating antineoplastic drugs.
- Your physician has not explained serious nature of your medical problem and risks of taking this medicine.

Before you start, consult your doctor:
- If you have gout.
- If you have had kidney stones.
- If you have active infection.
- If you have impaired kidney or liver function.
- If you have taken other antineoplastic drugs or had radiation treatment in last 3 weeks.

Over age 60:
Adverse reactions and side effects may be more frequent and severe than in younger persons.

Pregnancy:
Consult doctor. Risk to child is significant.

Breast-feeding:
Drug passes into milk. Don't nurse.

Infants & children:
Use only under care of medical supervisors who are experienced in anticancer drugs.

Prolonged use:
Adverse reactions more likely the longer drug is required.

Skin & sunlight:
No problems expected.

Driving, piloting or hazardous work:
No problems expected.

Airplane passengers:
No problems expected.

Discontinuing:
Don't discontinue without doctor's advice until you complete prescribed dose, even though symptoms diminish or disappear. Some side effects may follow discontinuing. Report to doctor blurred vision, convulsions, confusion, persistent headache.

Others:
May cause sterility.

INTERACTION WITH OTHER DRUGS

GENERIC NAME OR DRUG CLASS	COMBINED EFFECT
Antigout drugs	Decreased antigout effect.
Antineoplastic drugs (other)	Increased effect of all drugs, (may be beneficial).
Chloramphenicol	Increased likelihood of toxic effects of both drugs.

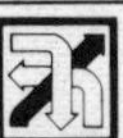

INTERACTION WITH OTHER SUBSTANCES

INTERACTS WITH	COMBINED EFFECT
Alcohol:	May increase chance of intestinal bleeding.
Beverages:	No problems expected.
Cocaine:	Increases chance of toxicity.
Foods:	Reduces irritation in stomach.
Marijuana:	No problems expected.
Tobacco:	Increases lung toxicity.

CHLORAMPHENICOL

BRAND NAMES

Amphicol
Antibiopto
Chloromycetin
Chloroptic
Econochlor
Fenicol
Isopto Fenicol
Minims
Mychel
Nova-Phenicol
Novochlorocap
Ophthochlor
Ophthocort
Pentamycetin
Sopamycetin

GENERAL INFORMATION

Habit forming? No
Prescription needed? Yes
Available as generic? Yes
Drug class: Antibiotic

USES

Treatment of infections susceptible to chloramphenicol.

DOSAGE & USAGE INFORMATION

How to take:

- Tablet or capsule—Swallow with liquid.
- Eye solution or ointment, ear solution or cream—Follow label instructions.

When to take:
Tablet or capsule—1 hour before or 2 hours after eating.

If you forget a dose:
Take as soon as you remember up to 2 hours late. If more than 2 hours, wait for next scheduled dose (don't double this dose).

What drug does:
Prevents bacteria from growing and reproducing. Will not kill viruses.

Time lapse before drug works:
2 to 5 days, depending on type and severity of infection.

Don't take with:
See Interaction column and consult doctor.

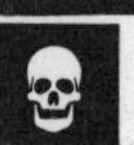

OVERDOSE

Symptoms:
Nausea, vomiting, diarrhea.

What to do:
Overdose unlikely to threaten life. If person takes much larger amount than prescribed, call doctor, poison-control center or hospital emergency room for instructions.

POSSIBLE ADVERSE REACTIONS OR SIDE EFFECTS

SYMPTOMS	FREQUENCY	WHAT TO DO
Brain & nervous system: Headache, confusion.	Infrequent	4
Skin: Rash, hives, swelling of face or extremities.	Infrequent	3
Eyes: Pain, blurred vision, possible vision loss.	Rare	3
Ears, nose, throat: Sore throat, fever.	Rare	3
Digestive: Diarrhea, nausea, vomiting.	Infrequent	3
Heart & lungs, blood vessels, genital, urinary, kidneys:	None expected.	
Muscles, bones, joints: Numbness, tingling, burning pain or weakness in hands and feet.	Infrequent	3
Liver: Jaundice (yellow eyes and skin).	Rare	3
Allergic: Life-threatening anaphylaxis!	Rare	1 See page 888.
Blood: Anemia	Rare	3

1 - Life-threatening. Seek emergency treatment immediately.
2 - Discontinue. Seek emergency treatment.
3 - Discontinue. Call doctor right away.
4 - Continue. Call doctor when convenient.

CHLORAMPHENICOL

WARNINGS & PRECAUTIONS

Don't take if:
- You are allergic to chloramphenicol.
- It is prescribed for a minor disorder such as flu, cold or mild sore throat.

Before you start, consult your doctor:
- If you have had a blood disorder or bone-marrow disease.
- If you have had kidney or liver disease.
- If you have diabetes.

Over age 60:
Adverse reactions and side effects may be more frequent and severe than in younger persons, particularly skin irritation around rectum.

Pregnancy:
Risk to unborn child outweighs drug benefits. Don't use.

Breast-feeding:
Drug passes into milk. Avoid drug or discontinue nursing until you finish medicine. Consult doctor for advice on maintaining milk supply.

Infants & children:
Don't give to infants younger than 2.

Prolonged use:
You may become more susceptible to infections caused by germs not responsive to chloramphenicol.

Skin & sunlight:
No problems expected.

Driving, piloting or hazardous work:
Don't drive or pilot aircraft until you learn how medicine affects you. Don't work around dangerous machinery. Don't climb ladders or work in high places. Danger increases if you drink alcohol or take medicine affecting alertness and reflexes.

Airplane passengers:
No problems expected.

Discontinuing:
Don't discontinue without doctor's advice until you complete prescribed dose, even though symptoms diminish or disappear.

Others:
- Chloramphenicol can cause serious anemia. Frequent laboratory blood studies, liver and kidney tests recommended.
- Second medical opinion recommended before starting.

INTERACTION WITH OTHER DRUGS

GENERIC NAME OR DRUG CLASS	COMBINED EFFECT
Anticoagulants	Increased anticoagulant effect.
Antidiabetics (oral)	Increased antidiabetic effect.
Cyclophosphamide	Decreased cyclophosphamide effect.
Penicillins	Decreased penicillin effect.
Phenytoin	Increased phenytoin effect.

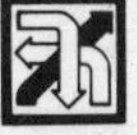

INTERACTION WITH OTHER SUBSTANCES

INTERACTS WITH	COMBINED EFFECT
Alcohol:	Possible liver problems. May cause disulfiram reaction (see page 846).
Beverages:	None expected.
Cocaine:	No proven problems.
Foods:	None expected.
Marijuana:	None expected.
Tobacco:	None expected.

CHLORDIAZEPOXIDE

BRAND NAMES

A-poxide
Apo-Chlordiazepoxide
C-Tran
Chlordiazachel
Corax
Libritabs
Librium
Limbitrol
Medilium
Menrium
Murcil
Novopoxide
Relaxil
Relium
Reposans
SK-Lygen
Sereen
Solium
Tenax
Trilium
Zetran

GENERAL INFORMATION

Habit forming? Yes
Prescription needed? Yes
Available as generic? No
Drug class: Tranquilizer (benzodiazepine)

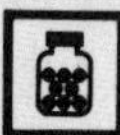

USES

- Treatment for nervousness or tension.
- Treatment for muscle spasm.
- Treatment for convulsive disorders.

DOSAGE & USAGE INFORMATION

How to take:
Tablet or capsule—Swallow with liquid. If you can't swallow whole, crumble tablet or open capsule and take with liquid or food.

When to take:
At the same time each day, according to instructions on prescription label.

If you forget a dose:
Take as soon as you remember up to 2 hours late. If more than 2 hours, wait for next scheduled dose (don't double this dose).

What drug does:
Affects limbic system of brain—part that controls emotions.

Time lapse before drug works:
2 hours. May take 6 weeks for full benefit.

Don't take with:
See Interaction column and consult doctor.

OVERDOSE

Symptoms:
Drowsiness, weakness, tremor, stupor, coma.

What to do:
- Dial 0 (operator) or 911 (emergency) for an ambulance or medical help. Then give first aid immediately.
- If patient is unconscious and not breathing, give mouth-to-mouth breathing. If there is no heartbeat, use cardiac massage and mouth-to-mouth breathing (CPR). Don't try to make patient vomit. If you can't get help quickly, take patient to nearest emergency facility.
- Additional emergency information on page 886.

POSSIBLE ADVERSE REACTIONS OR SIDE EFFECTS

SYMPTOMS	FREQUENCY	WHAT TO DO
Brain & nervous system:		
• Clumsiness, drowsiness, dizziness.	Common	4
• Hallucinations, confusion, depression, irritability.	Infrequent	3
Skin: Rash, itch.	Infrequent	3
Eyes: Vision changes.	Infrequent	3
Ears, nose, throat: Mouth, throat ulcers.	Rare	3
Digestive: Constipation or diarrhea, nausea, vomiting.	Infrequent	4
Heart & lungs: Slow heartbeat, breathing difficulty.	Rare	2
Blood vessels:	None expected.	
Muscles, bones, joints:	None expected.	
Genital, urinary: Urination difficulty.	Infrequent	4
Kidneys:	None expected.	
Liver: Jaundice (yellow eyes and skin).	Rare	3
Allergic:	None expected.	
Blood:	None expected.	
Others:	None expected.	

1- Life-threatening. Seek emergency treatment immediately.
2- Discontinue. Seek emergency treatment.
3- Discontinue. Call doctor right away.
4- Continue. Call doctor when convenient.
5- Continue. Tell doctor at next visit.
6- No action necessary.

CHLORDIAZEPOXIDE

WARNINGS & PRECAUTIONS

Don't take if:
- You are allergic to any benzodiazepine.
- You have myasthenia gravis.
- You are active or recovering alcoholic.
- Patient is younger than 6 months.

Before you start, consult your doctor:
- If you have liver, kidney or lung disease.
- If you have diabetes, epilepsy or porphyria.

Over age 60:
Adverse reactions and side effects may be more frequent and severe than in younger persons. You need smaller doses for shorter periods of time. May develop agitation, rage or "hangover effect."

Pregnancy:
Risk to unborn child outweighs drug benefits. Don't use.

Breast-feeding:
Drug passes into milk. Avoid drug or discontinue nursing until you finish medicine. Consult doctor for advice on maintaining milk supply.

Infants & children:
Use only under medical supervision for children older than 6 months.

Prolonged use:
May impair liver function.

Skin & sunlight:
No problems expected.

Driving, piloting or hazardous work:
Don't drive or pilot aircraft until you learn how medicine affects you. Don't work around dangerous machinery. Don't climb ladders or work in high places. Danger increases if you drink alcohol or take medicine affecting alertness and reflexes.

Airplane passengers:
No problems expected.

Discontinuing:
Don't discontinue without consulting doctor. Dose may require gradual reduction if you have taken drug for a long time. Doses of other drugs may also require adjustment.

Others:
- Hot weather, heavy exercise and profuse sweat may reduce excretion and cause overdose.
- Blood sugar may rise in diabetics, requiring insulin adjustment.

INTERACTION WITH OTHER DRUGS

GENERIC NAME OR DRUG CLASS	COMBINED EFFECT
Anticonvulsants	Change in seizure frequency or severity.
Antidepressants	Increased sedative effect of both drugs.
Antihistamines	Increased sedative effect of both drugs.
Antihypertensives	Excessively low blood pressure.
Cimetidine	Excess sedation.
Disulfiram	Increased chlordiazepoxide effect.
MAO inhibitors	Convulsions, deep sedation, rage.
Narcotics	Increased sedative effect of both drugs.
Sedatives	Increased sedative effect of both drugs.
Sleep inducers	Increased sedative effect of both drugs.
Tranquilizers	Increased sedative effect of both drugs.

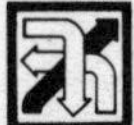

INTERACTION WITH OTHER SUBSTANCES

INTERACTS WITH	COMBINED EFFECT
Alcohol:	Heavy sedation. Avoid.
Beverages:	None expected.
Cocaine:	Decreased chlordiazepoxide effect.
Foods:	None expected.
Marijuana:	Heavy sedation. Avoid.
Tobacco:	Decreased chlordiazepoxide effect.

CHLOROQUINE

BRAND NAMES

Aralen

GENERAL INFORMATION

Habit forming? No
Prescription needed? Yes
Available as generic? Yes
Drug class: Antiprotozoal, antirheumatic

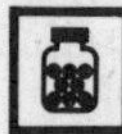

USES

- Treatment for protozoal infections, such as malaria and amebiasis.
- Treatment for some forms of arthritis and lupus.

DOSAGE & USAGE INFORMATION

How to take:
Tablet—Swallow with food or milk to lessen stomach irritation.

When to take:
- Depends on condition. Is adjusted during treatment.
- Malaria prevention—Begin taking medicine 2 weeks before entering areas with malaria.

If you forget a dose:
- 1 or more doses a day—Take as soon as you remember up to 2 hours late. If more than 2 hours, wait for next scheduled dose (don't double this dose).
- 1 dose weekly—Take as soon as possible, then return to regular dosing schedule.

What drug does:
- Inhibits parasite multiplication.
- Decreases inflammatory response in diseased joint.

Time lapse before drug works:
1 to 2 hours.

Don't take with:
See Interaction column and consult doctor.

OVERDOSE

Symptoms:
Severe breathing difficulty, drowsiness, faintness.

What to do:
- Dial 0 (operator) or 911 (emergency) for an ambulance or medical help. Then give first aid immediately.
- Additional emergency information on page 886.

POSSIBLE ADVERSE REACTIONS OR SIDE EFFECTS

SYMPTOMS	FREQUENCY	WHAT TO DO
Brain & nervous system:		
• Mood or mental changes, seizures.	Rare	3
• Headache	Common	5
Skin:		
Rash or itch.	Infrequent	4
Eyes:		
Blurred or changed vision.	Infrequent	3
Ears, nose, throat:		
• Ringing or buzzing in ears, hearing loss.	Rare	4
• Sore throat, fever.	Rare	3
Digestive:		
Diarrhea, nausea, vomiting.	Infrequent	4
Heart & lungs:	None expected.	
Blood vessels:		
Unusual bleeding or bruising.	Rare	3
Muscles, bones, joints:		
Muscle weakness.	Rare	3
Genital, urinary:	None expected.	
Kidneys:	None expected.	
Liver:	None expected.	
Allergic:	None expected.	
Blood:	None expected.	
Others:	None expected.	

1- Life threatening. Seek emergency treatment immediately.
2- Discontinue. Seek emergency treatment.
3- Discontinue. Call doctor right away.
4- Continue. Call doctor when convenient.
5- Continue. Tell doctor at next visit.
6- No action necessary.

WARNINGS & PRECAUTIONS

Don't take if:
You are allergic to chloroquine or hydroxychloroquine.

Before you start, consult your doctor:
- If you plan to become pregnant within the medication period.
- If you have blood disease.
- If you have eye or vision problems.
- If you have a G6PD deficiency.
- If you have liver disease.
- If you have nerve or brain disease (including seizure disorders).
- If you have porphyria.
- If you have psoriasis.
- If you have stomach or intestinal disease.
- If you drink more than 3 oz. of alcohol daily.

Over age 60:
Adverse reactions and side effects may be more frequent and severe than in younger persons.

Pregnancy:
Risk to unborn child outweighs drug benefits. Don't use.

Breast-feeding:
Drug passes into milk. Avoid drug or discontinue nursing.

Infants & children:
Not recommended. Dangerous.

Prolonged use:
Permanent damage to the retina (back part of the eye) or nerve deafness.

Skin & sunlight:
May cause rash or intensify sunburn in areas exposed to sun or sunlamp.

Driving, piloting or hazardous work:
Don't drive or pilot aircraft until you learn how medicine affects you. Don't work around dangerous machinery. Don't climb ladders or work in high places. Danger increases if you drink alcohol or take medicine affecting alertness and reflexes.

Airplane passengers:
No problems expected.

Discontinuing:
Don't discontinue without doctor's advice until you complete prescribed dose, even though symptoms diminish or disappear.

Others:
- Periodic physical and blood examinations recommended.
- If you are in a malaria area for a long time, you may need to change to another preventive drug every 2 years.

INTERACTION WITH OTHER DRUGS

GENERIC NAME OR DRUG CLASS	COMBINED EFFECT
Estrogens	Possible liver toxicity.
Gold compounds	Risk of severe rash and itch.
Oxyphenbutazone	Risk of severe rash and itch.
Penicillamine	Possible blood or kidney toxicity.
Phenylbutazone	Risk of severe rash and itch.
Sulfa drugs	Possible liver toxicity.

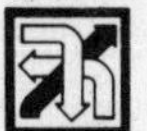

INTERACTION WITH OTHER SUBSTANCES

INTERACTS WITH	COMBINED EFFECT
Alcohol:	Possible liver toxicity. Avoid.
Beverages:	None expected.
Cocaine:	None expected.
Foods:	None expected.
Marijuana:	None expected.
Tobacco:	None expected.

CHLOROTHIAZIDE

BRAND NAMES

Aldoclor
Chloroserpine
Diupres
Diuril
SK-Chlorothiazide

GENERAL INFORMATION

Habit forming? No
Prescription needed? Yes
Available as generic? Yes
Drug class: Antihypertensive, diuretic (thiazide)

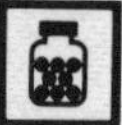

USES

- Controls, but doesn't cure, high blood pressure.
- Reduces fluid retention (edema) caused by conditions such as heart disorders and liver disease.

DOSAGE & USAGE INFORMATION

How to take:
Tablet or capsule—Swallow with liquid. If you can't swallow whole, crumble tablet or open capsule and take with liquid or food. Don't exceed dose.

When to take:
At the same time each day.

If you forget a dose:
Take as soon as you remember up to 2 hours late. If more than 2 hours, wait for next scheduled dose (don't double this dose).

What drug does:
- Forces sodium and water excretion, reducing body fluid.
- Relaxes muscle cells of small arteries.
- Reduced body fluid and relaxed arteries lower blood pressure.

Time lapse before drug works:
4 to 6 hours. May require several weeks to lower blood pressure.

Don't take with:
- See Interaction column and consult doctor.
- Non-prescription drugs without consulting doctor.

OVERDOSE

Symptoms:
Cramps, weakness, drowsiness, weak pulse, coma.

What to do:
- Dial 0 (operator) or 911 (emergency) for an ambulance or medical help. Then give first aid immediately.
- Additional emergency information on page 886.

POSSIBLE ADVERSE REACTIONS OR SIDE EFFECTS

SYMPTOMS	FREQUENCY	WHAT TO DO
Brain & nervous system:		
• Dizziness	Infrequent	4
• Mood changes.	Infrequent	4
• Headaches	Infrequent	4
Skin:		
Rash or hives.	Rare	2
Eyes:		
Blurred vision.	Infrequent	3
Ears, nose, throat:		
• Sore throat, fever.	Rare	5
• Dry mouth, thirst.	Infrequent	5
Digestive:		
Severe abdominal pain, nausea, vomiting.	Infrequent	3
Heart & lungs:		
Irregular heartbeat, weak pulse.	Infrequent	3
Blood vessels:	None expected.	
Muscles, bones, joints:		
Weakness, tiredness.	Infrequent	4
Genital, urinary:	None expected.	
Kidneys:	None expected.	
Liver:		
Jaundice (yellow skin and eyes).	Rare	3
Allergic:	None expected.	
Blood:	None expected.	
Others:		
Weight changes.	Infrequent	4

1- Life-threatening. Seek emergency treatment immediately.
2- Discontinue. Seek emergency treatment.
3- Discontinue. Call doctor right away.
4- Continue. Call doctor when convenient.
5- Continue. Tell doctor at next visit.
6- No action necessary.

WARNINGS & PRECAUTIONS

Don't take if:
You are allergic to any thiazide diuretic drug.

Before you start, consult your doctor:
- If you are allergic to any sulfa drug.
- If you have gout.
- If you have liver, pancreas or kidney disorder.

Over age 60:
Adverse reactions and side effects may be more frequent and severe than in younger persons, especially dizziness and excessive potassium loss.

Pregnancy:
Risk to unborn child outweighs drug benefits. Don't use.

Breast-feeding:
Drug passes into milk. Avoid drug or discontinue nursing.

Infants & children:
No problems expected.

Prolonged use:
You may need medicine to treat high blood pressure for the rest of your life.

Skin & sunlight:
May cause rash or intensify sunburn in areas exposed to sun or sunlamp.

Driving, piloting or hazardous work:
Don't drive or pilot aircraft until you learn how medicine affects you. Don't work around dangerous machinery. Don't climb ladders or work in high places. Danger increases if you drink alcohol or take medicine affecting alertness and reflexes, such as antihistamines, tranquilizers, sedatives, pain medicine, narcotics and mind-altering drugs.

Airplane passengers:
No problems expected.

Discontinuing:
Don't discontinue without medical advice.

Others:
- Hot weather and fever may cause dehydration and drop in blood pressure. Dose may require temporary adjustment. Weigh daily and report any unexpected weight decreases to your doctor.
- May cause rise in uric acid, leading to gout.
- May cause blood-sugar rise in diabetics.

INTERACTION WITH OTHER DRUGS

GENERIC NAME OR DRUG CLASS	COMBINED EFFECT
Allopurinol	Decreased allopurinol effect.
Antidepressants (tricyclic)	Dangerous drop in blood pressure. Avoid combination unless under medical supervision.
Barbiturates	Increased chlorothiazide effect.
Cholestyramine	Decreased chlorothiazide effect.
Cortisone drugs	Excessive potassium loss that causes dangerous heart rhythms.
Digitalis preparations	Excessive potassium loss that causes dangerous heart rhythms.
Diuretics (thiazide)	Increased effect of other thiazide diuretics.
Lithium	Increased effect of lithium.
MAO inhibitors	Increased chlorothiazide effect.
Probenecid	Decreased probenecid effect.

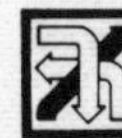

INTERACTION WITH OTHER SUBSTANCES

INTERACTS WITH	COMBINED EFFECT
Alcohol:	Dangerous blood-pressure drop.
Beverages:	None expected.
Cocaine:	None expected.
Foods:	
Licorice	Excessive potassium loss that causes dangerous heart rhythms.
Marijuana:	May increase blood pressure.
Tobacco:	None expected.

CHLOROTRIANISENE

BRAND NAMES

TACE

GENERAL INFORMATION

Habit forming? No
Prescription needed? Yes
Available as generic? Yes
Drug class: Female sex hormone (estrogen)

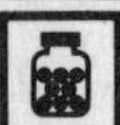

USES

- Treatment for symptoms of menopause and menstrual-cycle irregularity.
- Replacement for female hormone deficiency.
- Treatment for cancer of prostate.

DOSAGE & USAGE INFORMATION

How to take:
Capsule—Swallow with liquid. If you can't swallow whole, open capsule and take with liquid or food.

When to take:
At the same time each day.

If you forget a dose:
Take as soon as you remember up to 12 hours late. If more than 12 hours, wait for next scheduled dose (don't double this dose).

What drug does:
Restores normal estrogen level in tissues.

Time lapse before drug works:
10 to 20 days.

Don't take with:
See Interaction column and consult doctor.

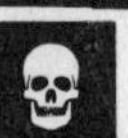

OVERDOSE

Symptoms:
Nausea, vomiting, fluid retention, breast enlargement and discomfort, abnormal vaginal bleeding.

What to do:
Overdose unlikely to threaten life. If person takes much larger amount than prescribed, call doctor, poison-control center or hospital emergency room for instructions.

POSSIBLE ADVERSE REACTIONS OR SIDE EFFECTS

SYMPTOMS	FREQUENCY	WHAT TO DO
Brain & nervous system:		
Depression, dizziness, irritability.	Infrequent	4
Skin:		
• Rash	Infrequent	3
• Brown blotches.	Infrequent	5
• Hair loss.	Infrequent	5
Eyes, ears, nose, throat, heart & lungs, muscles, bones, joints, kidneys, allergic, blood:	None expected.	
Digestive:		
• Stomach or side pain.	Infrequent	3
• Stomach cramps.	Common	3
• Appetite loss.	Common	4
• Nausea, diarrhea.	Common	5
• Vomiting	Infrequent	4
Blood vessels:		
Swollen ankles, feet.	Common	5
Genital, urinary:		
Vaginal discharge or bleeding.	Infrequent	5
Liver:		
Jaundice (yellow skin and eyes).	Rare	3
Others:		
• Breast lumps.	Infrequent	4
• Swollen, tender breasts.	Common	5
• Changes in sex drive.	Infrequent	5

1- Life-threatening. Seek emergency treatment immediately.
2- Discontinue. Seek emergency treatment.
3- Discontinue. Call doctor right away.
4- Continue. Call doctor when convenient.
5- Continue. Tell doctor at next visit.

WARNINGS & PRECAUTIONS

Don't take if:
- You are allergic to any estrogen-containing drugs.
- You have impaired liver function.
- You have had blood clots, stroke or heart attack.
- You have unexplained vaginal bleeding.

Before you start, consult your doctor:
- If you have had cancer of breast or reproductive organs, fibrocystic breast disease, fibroid tumors of the uterus or endometriosis.
- If you have had migraine headaches, epilepsy or porphyria.
- If you have diabetes, high blood pressure, asthma, congestive heart failure, kidney disease or gallstones.
- If you plan to become pregnant within 3 months.

Over age 60:
Controversial. You and your doctor must decide if drug risks outweigh benefits.

Pregnancy:
Risk to unborn child outweighs drug benefits. Don't use.

Breast-feeding:
Drug filters into milk. May harm child. Avoid.

Infants & children:
Not recommended.

Prolonged use:
Increased growth of fibroid tumors of uterus. Possible association with cancer of uterus.

Skin & sunlight:
May cause rash or intensify sunburn in areas exposed to sun or sunlamp.

Driving, piloting or hazardous work:
No problems expected.

Airplane passengers:
No problems expected.

Discontinuing:
You may need to discontinue chlorotrianisene periodically. Consult your doctor.

Others:
In rare instances, may cause blood clot in lung, brain or leg. Symptoms are *sudden* severe headache, coordination loss, vision change, chest pain, breathing difficulty, slurred speech, pain in legs or groin. Seek emergency treatment immediately.

INTERACTION WITH OTHER DRUGS

GENERIC NAME OR DRUG CLASS	COMBINED EFFECT
Anticoagulants (oral)	Decreased anticoagulant effect.
Anticonvulsants (hydantoin)	Increased seizures.
Antidiabetics (oral)	Unpredictable increase or decrease in blood sugar.
Clofibrate	Decreased clofibrate effect.
Carbamazepine	Increased seizures.
Meprobamate	Increased chlorotrianisene effect.
Phenobarbital	Decreased chlorotrianisene effect.
Primidone	Decreased chlorotrianisene effect.
Rifampin	Decreased chlorotrianisene effect.
Thyroid hormones	Decreased thyroid effect.

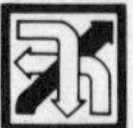

INTERACTION WITH OTHER SUBSTANCES

INTERACTS WITH	COMBINED EFFECT
Alcohol:	None expected.
Beverages:	None expected.
Cocaine:	No proven problems.
Foods:	None expected.
Marijuana:	Possible menstrual irregularities and bleeding between periods.
Tobacco:	Increased risk of blood clots leading to stroke or heart attack.

CHLORPHENESIN

BRAND NAMES

Maolate
Mycil

GENERAL INFORMATION

Habit forming? No
Prescription needed? Yes
Available as generic? Yes
Drug class: Muscle relaxant (skeletal)

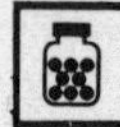

USES

Treatment for sprains, strains and muscle spasms.

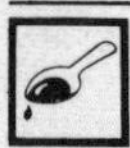

DOSAGE & USAGE INFORMATION

How to take:
Tablet or capsule—Swallow with liquid.

When to take:
As needed, no more often than every 4 hours.

If you forget a dose:
Take as soon as you remember. Wait 4 hours for next dose.

What drug does:
Blocks body's pain messages to brain. May also sedate.

Time lapse before drug works:
60 minutes.

Don't take with:
See Interaction column and consult doctor.

OVERDOSE

Symptoms:
Nausea, vomiting, diarrhea, headache. May progress to severe weakness, difficult breathing, sensation of paralysis, coma.

What to do:
- Dial 0 (operator) or 911 (emergency) for an ambulance or medical help. Then give first aid immediately.
- Additional emergency information on page 886.

POSSIBLE ADVERSE REACTIONS OR SIDE EFFECTS

SYMPTOMS	FREQUENCY	WHAT TO DO
Brain & nervous system:		
• Drowsiness, fainting, dizziness.	Common	4
• Agitation	Infrequent	3
Skin:		
Rash, hives or itch.	Rare	3
Eyes:	None expected.	
Ears, nose, throat:		
Sore throat, fever.	Rare	3
Digestive:		
• Constipation or diarrhea, nausea, cramps, vomiting.	Infrequent	3
• Bloody or tarry, black stool.	Rare	2
Heart & lungs:		
Wheezing, shortness of breath.	Infrequent	3
Allergic:	None expected.	
Blood vessels:	None expected.	
Muscles, bones, joints:	None expected.	
Genital, urinary:		
Orange or red-purple urine.	Common	6
Kidneys:	None expected.	
Liver:		
Jaundice (yellow eyes and skin).	Rare	3
Blood:	None expected.	
Others:		
Tiredness, weakness.	Rare	3

1- Life-threatening. Seek emergency treatment immediately.
2- Discontinue. Seek emergency treatment.
3- Discontinue. Call doctor right away.
4- Continue. Call doctor when convenient.
5- Continue. Tell doctor at next visit.
6- No action necessary.

WARNINGS & PRECAUTIONS

Don't take if:

- You are allergic to any skeletal-muscle relaxant.
- You have porphyria.

Before you start, consult your doctor:

- If you have had liver or kidney disease.
- If you plan pregnancy within medication period.
- If you will have surgery within 2 months, including dental surgery, requiring general or spinal anesthesia.

Over age 60:
Adverse reactions and side effects may be more frequent and severe than in younger persons.

Pregnancy:
No proven harm to unborn child. Avoid if possible.

Breast-feeding:
Drug passes into milk. Avoid drug or discontinue nursing until you finish medicine. Consult doctor for advice on maintaining milk supply.

Infants & children:
Not recommended.

Prolonged use:
Periodic liver-function tests recommended if you use this drug for a long time.

Skin & sunlight:
No problems expected.

Driving, piloting or hazardous work:
Don't drive or pilot aircraft until you learn how medicine affects you. Don't work around dangerous machinery. Don't climb ladders or work in high places. Danger increases if you drink alcohol or take medicine affecting alertness and reflexes, such as antihistamines, tranquilizers, sedatives, pain medicine, narcotics and mind-altering drugs.

Airplane passengers:
No problems expected.

Discontinuing:
Don't discontinue without doctor's advice until you complete prescribed dose, even though symptoms diminish or disappear.

Others:
No problems expected.

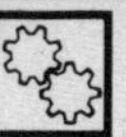

INTERACTION WITH OTHER DRUGS

GENERIC NAME OR DRUG CLASS	COMBINED EFFECT
Antidepressants	Increased sedation.
Antihistamines	Increased sedation.
Mind-altering drugs	Increased sedation.
Muscle relaxants (other)	Increased sedation.
Narcotics	Increased sedation.
Sedatives	Increased sedation.
Sleep inducers	Increased sedation.
Testosterone	Decreased metaxalone effect.
Tranquilizers	Increased sedation.

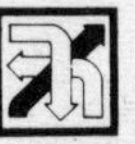

INTERACTION WITH OTHER SUBSTANCES

INTERACTS WITH	COMBINED EFFECT
Alcohol:	Increased sedation. Avoid.
Beverages:	None expected.
Cocaine:	Lack of coordination, increased sedation. Avoid.
Foods:	None expected.
Marijuana:	Lack of coordination, drowsiness, fainting. Avoid.
Tobacco:	None expected.

CHLORPHENIRAMINE

BRAND NAMES

Acutuss	Chlor-Span	Naldecon
Alermine	Chlor-Trimeton	Novahistine
Aller-chlor	Coricidin	Novopheniram
Allerest	Co-Tylenol	Phenetron
Allergesic	Histalon	Sinarest
Anamine	Hycoff	Teldrin

See complete brand names list, page 824.

GENERAL INFORMATION

Habit forming? No
Prescription needed? No
Available as generic? Yes
Drug class: Antihistamine

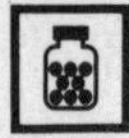

USES

- Reduces allergic symptoms such as hay fever, hives, rash or itching.
- Prevents motion sickness, nausea, vomiting.
- Induces sleep.

DOSAGE & USAGE INFORMATION

How to take:
- Tablet or syrup—Swallow with liquid or food to lessen stomach irritation.
- Extended-release tablets or capsules—Swallow each dose whole.

When to take:
Varies with form. Follow label directions.

If you forget a dose:
Take as soon as you remember up to 2 hours late. If more than 2 hours, wait for next scheduled dose (don't double this dose).

What drug does:
Blocks action of histamine after an allergic response triggers histamine release in sensitive cells.

Time lapse before drug works:
30 minutes.

Don't take with:
See Interaction column and consult doctor.

OVERDOSE

Symptoms:
Convulsions, red face, hallucinations, coma.

What to do:
- Dial 0 (operator) or 911 (emergency) for an ambulance or medical help. Then give first aid immediately.
- Additional emergency information on page 886.

POSSIBLE ADVERSE REACTIONS OR SIDE EFFECTS

SYMPTOMS	FREQUENCY	WHAT TO DO
Brain & nervous system:		
• Nightmares, agitation, irritability.	Rare	3
• Drowsiness, dizziness.	Common	5
Skin:	None expected.	
Eyes:		
• Vision changes.	Infrequent	3
• Less tolerance for contact lenses.	Infrequent	4
Ears, nose, throat:		
• Sore throat, fever.	Rare	3
• Dry mouth, nose, throat.	Common	5
Digestive:		
• Nausea	Common	5
• Appetite loss.	Infrequent	5
Heart & lungs:		
Rapid heartbeat.	Rare	3
Blood vessels:		
Unusual bleeding or bruising.	Rare	3
Muscles, bones, joints, kidneys, liver, allergic, blood:	None expected.	
Genital, urinary:		
Urination difficulty.	Infrequent	4
Others:		
Fatigue, weakness.	Rare	3

1-Life-threatening. Seek emergency treatment immediately.
2-Discontinue. Seek emergency treatment.
3-Discontinue. Call doctor right away.
4-Continue. Call doctor when convenient.
5-Continue. Tell doctor at next visit.
6-No action necessary.

WARNINGS & PRECAUTIONS

Don't take if:
You are allergic to any antihistamine.

Before you start, consult your doctor:
- If you have glaucoma.
- If you have enlarged prostate.
- If you have asthma.
- If you have kidney disease.
- If you have peptic ulcer.
- If you will have surgery within 2 months, including dental surgery, requiring general or spinal anesthesia.

Over age 60:
Don't exceed recommended dose. Adverse reactions and side effects may be more frequent and severe than in younger persons, especially urination difficulty, diminished alertness and other brain and nervous-system symptoms.

Pregnancy:
No proven harm to unborn child. Avoid if possible.

Breast-feeding:
Drug passes into milk. Avoid drug or discontinue nursing until you finish medicine. Consult doctor for advice on maintaining milk supply.

Infants & children:
Not recommended for premature or newborn infants. Otherwise, no problems expected.

Prolonged use:
Avoid. May damage bone marrow and nerve cells.

Skin & sunlight:
May cause rash or intensify sunburn in areas exposed to sun or sunlamp.

Driving, piloting or hazardous work:
Don't drive or pilot aircraft until you learn how medicine affects you. Don't work around dangerous machinery. Don't climb ladders or work in high places. Danger increases if you drink alcohol or take medicine affecting alertness and reflexes, such as antihistamines, tranquilizers, sedatives, pain medicine, narcotics and mind-altering drugs.

Airplane passengers:
No problems expected.

Discontinuing:
No problems expected.

Others:
May mask symptoms of hearing damage from aspirin, other salicylates, cisplatin, paromomycin, vancomycin or anticonvulsants. Consult doctor if you use these.

INTERACTION WITH OTHER DRUGS

GENERIC NAME OR DRUG CLASS	COMBINED EFFECT
Anticholinergics	Increased anticholinergic effect.
Antidepressants	Excess sedation. Avoid.
Antihistamines (other)	Excess sedation. Avoid.
Hypnotics	Excess sedation. Avoid.
MAO inhibitors	Increased chlorpheniramine effect.
Mind-altering drugs	Excess sedation. Avoid.
Narcotics	Excess sedation. Avoid.
Sedatives	Excess sedation. Avoid.
Sleep inducers	Excess sedation. Avoid.
Tranquilizers	Excess sedation. Avoid.

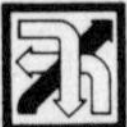

INTERACTION WITH OTHER SUBSTANCES

INTERACTS WITH	COMBINED EFFECT
Alcohol:	Excess sedation. Avoid.
Beverages: Caffeine drinks	Less chlorpheniramine sedation.
Cocaine:	Decreased chlorpheniramine effect. Avoid.
Foods:	None expected.
Marijuana:	Excess sedation. Avoid.
Tobacco:	None expected.

CHLORPROMAZINE

BRAND NAMES

Apo-Chlorpromazine
Chloramead
Chlor-Promanyl
Chlorprom
Largactil
Novochlorpromazine
Promapar
Promosol
Thorazine

GENERAL INFORMATION

Habit forming? No
Prescription needed? Yes
Available as generic? Yes
Drug class: Tranquilizer, antiemetic (phenothiazine)

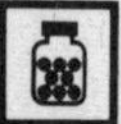

USES

- Stops nausea, vomiting.
- Reduces anxiety, agitation.

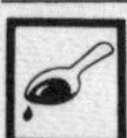

DOSAGE & USAGE INFORMATION

How to take:
- Tablet or capsule—Swallow with liquid or food to lessen stomach irritation.
- Suppositories—Remove wrapper and moisten suppository with water. Gently insert into rectum, large end first.
- Drops or liquid—Dilute dose in beverage.

When to take:
- Nervous and mental disorders—Take at the same times each day.
- Nausea and vomiting—Take as needed, no more often than every 4 hours.

If you forget a dose:
- Nervous and mental disorders—Take up to 2 hours late. If more than 2 hours, wait for next scheduled dose (don't double this).
- Nausea and vomiting—Take as soon as you remember. Wait 4 hours for next dose.

What drug does:
- Suppresses brain's vomiting center.
- Suppresses brain centers that control abnormal emotions and behavior.

Time lapse before drug works:
- Nausea and vomiting—1 hour or less.
- Nervous and mental disorders—4-6 weeks.

Don't take with:
- Antacid or medicine for diarrhea.
- Non-prescription drug for cough, cold or allergy.
- See Interaction column and consult doctor.

OVERDOSE

Symptoms:
Stupor, convulsions, coma.

What to do:
- Dial 0 (operator) or 911 (emergency) for an ambulance or medical help. Then give first aid immediately.
- Additional emergency information on page 886.

POSSIBLE ADVERSE REACTIONS OR SIDE EFFECTS

SYMPTOMS	FREQUENCY	WHAT TO DO
Brain & nervous system:		
• Restlessness, tremor.	Common	3
• Fainting	Infrequent	2
• Drowsiness	Common	3
Skin:		
• Rash	Infrequent	3
• Less perspiration.	Common	4
Eyes:		
Vision changes.	Rare	3
Ears, nose, throat:		
• Sore throat, fever.	Rare	3
• Dry mouth, nasal congestion.	Common	4
Digestive:		
Constipation	Common	4
Heart & lungs, blood vessels, kidneys, allergic, blood:	None expected.	
Muscles, bones, joints:		
Muscle spasms of face and neck, unsteady gait.	Common	2
Genital, urinary:		
Urination difficulty.	Infrequent	4
Liver:		
Jaundice (yellow eyes and skin).	Rare	3
Others:		
Less interest in sex, breast swelling, change in menstrual pattern.	Infrequent	4

1- Life-threatening. Seek emergency treatment immediately.
2- Discontinue. Seek emergency treatment.
3- Discontinue. Call doctor right away.
4- Continue. Call doctor when convenient.
5- Continue. Tell doctor at next visit.
6- No action necessary.

WARNINGS & PRECAUTIONS

Don't take if:
- You are allergic to any phenothiazine.
- You have a blood or bone-marrow disease.

Before you start, consult your doctor:
- If you will have surgery within 2 months, including dental surgery, requiring general or spinal anesthesia.
- If you have asthma, emphysema or other lung disorder.
- If you take non-prescription ulcer medicine, asthma medicine or amphetamines.

Over age 60:
Adverse reactions and side effects may be more frequent and severe than in younger persons. More likely to develop involuntary movement of jaws, lips, tongue, chewing. Report this to your doctor immediately. Early treatment can help.

Pregnancy:
Risk to unborn child outweighs drug benefits. Don't use.

Breast-feeding:
Drug passes into milk. Avoid drug or discontinue nursing until you finish medicine. Consult doctor for advice on maintaining milk supply.

Infants & children:
Don't give to children younger than 2.

Prolonged use:
May lead to tardive dyskinesia (involuntary movement of jaws, lips, tongue, chewing).

Skin & sunlight:
May cause rash or intensify sunburn in areas exposed to sun or sunlamp. Skin may remain sensitive for 3 months after discontinuing.

Driving, piloting or hazardous work:
Don't drive or pilot aircraft until you learn how medicine affects you. Don't work around dangerous machinery. Don't climb ladders or work in high places. Danger increases if you drink alcohol or take medicine affecting alertness and reflexes.

Airplane passengers:
No problems expected.

Discontinuing:
- Nervous and mental disorders—Don't discontinue without doctor's advice until you complete prescribed dose, even though symptoms diminish or disappear.
- Nausea and vomiting—May be unnecessary to finish medicine. Follow doctor's instructions.

INTERACTION WITH OTHER DRUGS

GENERIC NAME OR DRUG CLASS	COMBINED EFFECT
Anticholinergics	Increased anticholinergic effect.
Antidepressants (tricyclic)	Increased chlorpromazine effect.
Antihistamines	Increased antihistamine effect.
Appetite suppressants	Decreased suppressant effect.
Levodopa	Decreased levodopa effect.
Mind-altering drugs	Increased effect of mind-altering drugs.
Narcotics	Increased narcotic effect.
Phenytoin	Increased phenytoin effect.
Quinidine	Impaired heart function. Dangerous mixture.
Sedatives	Increased sedative effect.
Tranquilizers (other)	Increased tranquilizer effect.

INTERACTION WITH OTHER SUBSTANCES

INTERACTS WITH	COMBINED EFFECT
Alcohol:	Dangerous oversedation.
Beverages:	None expected.
Cocaine:	Decreased chlorpromazine effect. Avoid.
Foods:	None expected.
Marijuana:	Drowsiness. May increase antinausea effect.
Tobacco:	None expected.

CHLORPROPAMIDE

BRAND NAMES

Apo-Chlorpropamide
Chloromide
Chloronase
Diabinese
Novopropamide
Stabinol

GENERAL INFORMATION

Habit forming? No
Prescription needed? Yes
Available as generic? No
Drug class: Antidiabetic (oral), sulfonurea

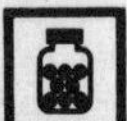

USES

Treatment for diabetes in adults who can't control blood sugar by diet, weight loss and exercise.

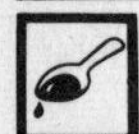

DOSAGE & USAGE INFORMATION

How to take:
Tablet—Swallow with liquid or food to lessen stomach irritation. If you can't swallow whole, crumble tablet and take with liquid or food.

When to take:
At the same times each day.

If you forget a dose:
Take as soon as you remember up to 2 hours late. If more than 2 hours, wait for next scheduled dose (don't double this dose).

What drug does:
Stimulates pancreas to produce more insulin. Insulin in blood forces cells to use sugar in blood.

Time lapse before drug works:
3 to 4 hours. May require 2 weeks for maximum benefit.

Don't take with:
See Interaction column and consult doctor.

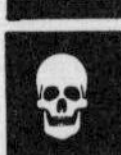

OVERDOSE

Symptoms:
Excessive hunger, nausea, anxiety, cool skin, cold sweats, drowsiness, rapid heartbeat, weakness, unconsciousness, coma.

What to do:
- Dial 0 (operator) or 911 (emergency) for an ambulance or medical help. Then give first aid immediately.
- Additional emergency information on page 886.

POSSIBLE ADVERSE REACTIONS OR SIDE EFFECTS

SYMPTOMS	FREQUENCY	WHAT TO DO
Brain & nervous system:		
• Dizziness	Common	3
• Fatigue	Rare	3
Skin:		
Itching or rash.	Rare	3
Eyes:	None expected.	
Ears, nose, throat:		
• Sore throat, fever.	Rare	3
• Ringing in ears.	Rare	3
Digestive:		
Diarrhea, loss of appetite, nausea, stomach pain, heartburn.	Common	4
Heart & lungs, muscles, bones, joints, genital, urinary, kidneys, allergic, blood:	None expected.	
Blood vessels:		
Unusual bleeding or bruising.	Rare	3
Liver:		
Jaundice (yellow skin, eyes).	Rare	3
Others:		
Low blood sugar (ravenous hunger, nausea, anxiety, cold sweats, cool skin, chills, drowsiness, nervousness, headache, rapid heartbeat, weakness).	Infrequent	2

1- Life-threatening. Seek emergency treatment immediately.
2- Discontinue. Seek emergency treatment.
3- Discontinue. Call doctor right away.
4- Continue. Call doctor when convenient.

WARNINGS & PRECAUTIONS

Don't take if:
- You are allergic to any sulfonurea.
- You have impaired kidney or liver function.

Before you start, consult your doctor:
- If you have a severe infection.
- If you have thyroid disease.
- If you take insulin.
- If you have heart disease.

Over age 60:
Dose usually smaller than for younger adults. Avoid "low-blood-sugar" episodes because repeated ones can damage brain permanently.

Pregnancy:
No proven harm to unborn child. Avoid if possible.

Breast-feeding:
Drug filters into milk. May lower baby's blood sugar. Avoid.

Infants & children:
Don't give to infants or children.

Prolonged use:
None expected.

Skin & sunlight:
May cause rash or intensify sunburn in areas exposed to sun or sunlamp.

Driving, piloting or hazardous work:
No problems expected unless you develop hypoglycemia (low blood sugar). If so, avoid driving or hazardous activity.

Airplane passengers:
No problems expected.

Discontinuing:
Don't discontinue without consulting doctor. Dose may require gradual reduction if you have taken drug for a long time. Doses of other drugs may also require adjustment.

Others:
- Don't exceed 1500 mg. in 1 day.
- Hypoglycemia (low blood sugar) may occur, even with proper dose schedule. You must balance medicine, diet and exercise.

INTERACTION WITH OTHER DRUGS

GENERIC NAME OR DRUG CLASS	COMBINED EFFECT
Androgens	Increased chlorpropamide effect.
Anticoagulants (oral)	Unpredictable prothrombin times (see page 848).
Anticonvulsants (hydantoin)	Decreased chlorpropamide effect.
Antiinflammatory drugs (non-steroidal)	Increased chlorpropamide effect.
Aspirin	Increased chlorpropamide effect.
Beta-adrenergic blockers	Increased chlorpropamide effect.
Chloramphenicol	Increased chlorpropamide effect.
Clofibrate	Increased chlorpropamide effect.
Contraceptives (oral)	Decreased chlorpropamide effect.
Cortisone drugs	Decreased chlorpropamide effect.
Diuretics (thiazide)	Decreased chlorpropamide effect.
Epinephrine	Decreased chlorpropamide effect.
Estrogens	Increased chlorpropamide effect.
Guanethidine	Unpredictable chlorpropamide effect.

Additional interactions on page 835.

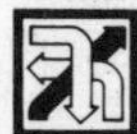

INTERACTION WITH OTHER SUBSTANCES

INTERACTS WITH	COMBINED EFFECT
Alcohol:	Disulfiram reaction (see page 846). Avoid.
Beverages:	None expected.
Cocaine:	No proven problems.
Foods:	None expected.
Marijuana:	Decreased chlorpropamide effect. Avoid.
Tobacco:	None expected.

CHLORPROTHIXENE

BRAND NAMES

Taractan
Tarasan

GENERAL INFORMATION

Habit forming? No
Prescription needed? Yes
Available as generic? No
Drug class: Tranquilizer (thioxanthine), antiemetic

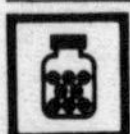

USES

- Reduces anxiety, agitation, psychosis.
- Stops vomiting.

DOSAGE & USAGE INFORMATION

How to take:

- Tablet—Swallow with liquid. If you can't swallow whole, crumble tablet and take with liquid or food.
- Syrup—Dilute dose in beverage before swallowing.

When to take:
At the same time each day.

If you forget a dose:
Take as soon as you remember up to 2 hours late. If more than 2 hours, wait for next scheduled dose (don't double this dose).

What drug does:
Corrects imbalance of nerve impulses.

Time lapse before drug works:
3 weeks.

Don't take with:
See Interaction column and consult doctor.

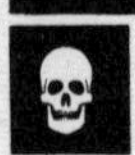

OVERDOSE

Symptoms:
Drowsiness, dizziness, weakness, muscle rigidity, twitching, tremors, confusion, dry mouth, blurred vision, rapid pulse, shallow breathing, low blood pressure, convulsions, coma.

What to do:

- Dial 0 (operator) or 911 (emergency) for an ambulance or medical help. Then give first aid immediately.
- If patient is unconscious and not breathing, give mouth-to-mouth breathing. If there is no heartbeat, use cardiac massage and mouth-to-mouth breathing (CPR). Don't try to make patient vomit. If you can't get help quickly, take patient to nearest emergency facility.
- Additional emergency information on page 886.

POSSIBLE ADVERSE REACTIONS OR SIDE EFFECTS

SYMPTOMS	FREQUENCY	WHAT TO DO
Brain & nervous system:		
• Fainting; restlessness; jerky, involuntary movements.	Common	3
• Dizziness, drowsiness.	Common	4
Skin:		
Rash	Infrequent	3
Eyes:		
Blurred vision.	Common	3
Ears, nose, throat:		
• Sore throat, fever.	Rare	3
• Dry mouth, nasal congestion.	Common	5
Digestive:		
Constipation	Common	4
Heart & lungs:		
Rapid heartbeat.	Common	3
Blood vessels, kidneys, allergic, blood:	None expected.	
Muscles, bones, joints:		
• Muscle spasms.	Common	4
• Shuffling walk.	Common	4
Genital, urinary:		
• Less sexual ability.	Infrequent	4
• Difficult urination.	Infrequent	4
Liver:		
Jaundice (yellow skin and eyes).	Rare	3
Others:		
• Less perspiration.	Common	4
• Menstrual changes.	Infrequent	5
• Breast swelling.	Infrequent	5

1-Life-threatening. Seek emergency treatment immediately.
2-Discontinue. Seek emergency treatment.
3-Discontinue. Call doctor right away.
4-Continue. Call doctor when convenient.
5-Continue. Tell doctor at next visit.

CHLORPROTHIXENE

WARNINGS & PRECAUTIONS

Don't take if:
- You are allergic to any thioxanthine or phenothiazine tranquilizer.
- You have serious blood disorder.
- You have Parkinson's disease.
- Patient is younger than 12.

Before you start, consult your doctor:
- If you have had liver or kidney disease.
- If you have epilepsy or glaucoma.
- If you have high blood pressure or heart disease (especially angina).
- If you use alcohol daily.
- If you will have surgery within 2 months, including dental surgery, requiring general or spinal anesthesia.

Over age 60:
Adverse reactions and side effects may be more frequent and severe than in younger persons.

Pregnancy:
No proven harm to unborn child. Avoid if possible.

Breast-feeding:
Studies inconclusive. Consult your doctor.

Infants & children:
Not recommended.

Prolonged use:
- Pigment deposits in lens and retina of eye.
- Involuntary movements of jaws, lips, tongue (tardive dyskinesia).

Skin & sunlight:
May cause rash or intensify sunburn in areas exposed to sun or sunlamp.

Driving, piloting or hazardous work:
Don't drive or pilot aircraft until you learn how medicine affects you. Don't work around dangerous machinery. Don't climb ladders or work in high places. Danger increases if you drink alcohol or take medicine affecting alertness and reflexes.

Airplane passengers:
No problems expected.

Discontinuing:
Don't discontinue without consulting doctor. Dose may require gradual reduction if you have taken drug for a long time. Doses of other drugs may also require adjustment.

Others:
Hot temperatures increase chance of heat stroke.

INTERACTION WITH OTHER DRUGS

GENERIC NAME OR DRUG CLASS	COMBINED EFFECT
Anticholinergics	Increased anticholinergic effect.
Anticonvulsants	Change in seizure pattern.
Antidepressants (tricyclic)	Increased chlorprothixene effect. Excessive sedation.
Antihistamines	Increased chlorprothixene effect. Excessive sedation.
Antihypertensives	Excessively low blood pressure.
Barbiturates	Increased chlorprothixene effect. Excessive sedation.
Bethanechol	Decreased bethanechol effect.
Guanethidine	Decreased guanethidine effect.
Levodopa	Decreased levodopa effect.
MAO inhibitors	Excessive sedation.
Mind-altering drugs	Increased chlorprothixene effect. Excessive sedation.

Additional interactions on page 835.

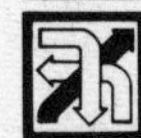

INTERACTION WITH OTHER SUBSTANCES

INTERACTS WITH	COMBINED EFFECT
Alcohol:	Excessive brain depression. Avoid.
Beverages:	None expected.
Cocaine:	Decreased chlorprothixene effect. Avoid.
Foods:	None expected.
Marijuana:	Daily use—Fainting likely, possible psychosis.
Tobacco:	None expected.

CHLORTHALIDONE

BRAND NAMES

Apo-Chlorthalide
Combipres
Demi-Regroton
Hygroton
Novothalidone
Regroton
Tenoretic
Thalitone
Uridon

GENERAL INFORMATION

Habit forming? No
Prescription needed? Yes
Available as generic? Yes
Drug class: Antihypertensive, diuretic (thiazide)

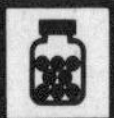

USES

- Controls, but doesn't cure, high blood pressure.
- Reduces fluid retention (edema) caused by conditions such as heart disorders and liver disease.

DOSAGE & USAGE INFORMATION

How to take:
Tablet or capsule—Swallow with liquid. If you can't swallow whole, crumble tablet or open capsule and take with liquid or food. Don't exceed dose.

When to take:
At the same time each day.

If you forget a dose:
Take as soon as you remember up to 2 hours late. If more than 2 hours, wait for next scheduled dose (don't double this dose).

What drug does:
- Forces sodium and water excretion, reducing body fluid.
- Relaxes muscle cells of small arteries.
- Reduced body fluid and relaxed arteries lower blood pressure.

Time lapse before drug works:
4 to 6 hours. May require several weeks to lower blood pressure.

Don't take with:
- See Interaction column and consult doctor.
- Non-prescription drugs without consulting doctor.

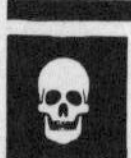

OVERDOSE

Symptoms:
Cramps, weakness, drowsiness, weak pulse, coma.

What to do:
- Dial 0 (operator) or 911 (emergency) for an ambulance or medical help. Then give first aid immediately.
- Additional emergency information on page 886.

POSSIBLE ADVERSE REACTIONS OR SIDE EFFECTS

SYMPTOMS	FREQUENCY	WHAT TO DO
Brain & nervous system:		
• Dizziness	Infrequent	4
• Mood changes.	Infrequent	4
• Headaches	Infrequent	4
Skin:		
Rash or hives.	Rare	2
Eyes:		
Blurred vision.	Infrequent	3
Ears, nose, throat:		
• Sore throat, fever.	Rare	3
• Dry mouth, thirst.	Infrequent	5
Digestive:		
Severe abdominal pain, nausea, vomiting.	Infrequent	3
Heart & lungs:		
Irregular heartbeat, weak pulse.	Infrequent	3
Blood vessels:	None expected.	
Muscles, bones, joints:		
Weakness, tiredness.	Infrequent	4
Genital, urinary:	None expected.	
Kidneys:	None expected.	
Liver:		
Jaundice (yellow skin and eyes).	Rare	3
Allergic:	None expected.	
Blood:	None expected.	
Others:		
Weight changes.	Infrequent	4

1- Life-threatening. Seek emergency treatment immediately.
2- Discontinue. Seek emergency treatment.
3- Discontinue. Call doctor right away.
4- Continue. Call doctor when convenient.
5- Continue. Tell doctor at next visit.
6- No action necessary.

WARNINGS & PRECAUTIONS

Don't take if:
You are allergic to any thiazide diuretic drug.

Before you start, consult your doctor:
- If you are allergic to any sulfa drug.
- If you have gout.
- If you have liver, pancreas or kidney disorder.

Over age 60:
Adverse reactions and side effects may be more frequent and severe than in younger persons, especially dizziness and excessive potassium loss.

Pregnancy:
Risk to unborn child outweighs drug benefits. Don't use.

Breast-feeding:
Drug passes into milk. Avoid this medicine or discontinue nursing.

Infants & children:
No problems expected.

Prolonged use:
You may need medicine to treat high blood pressure for the rest of your life.

Skin & sunlight:
May cause rash or intensify sunburn in areas exposed to sun or sunlamp.

Driving, piloting or hazardous work:
Don't drive or pilot aircraft until you learn how medicine affects you. Don't work around dangerous machinery. Don't climb ladders or work in high places. Danger increases if you drink alcohol or take medicine affecting alertness and reflexes, such as antihistamines, tranquilizers, sedatives, pain medicine, narcotics and mind-altering drugs.

Airplane passengers:
No problems expected.

Discontinuing:
Don't discontinue without medical advice.

Others:
- Hot weather and fever may cause dehydration and drop in blood pressure. Dose may require temporary adjustment. Weigh daily and report any unexpected weight decreases to your doctor.
- May cause rise in uric acid, leading to gout.
- May cause blood-sugar rise in diabetics.

INTERACTION WITH OTHER DRUGS

GENERIC NAME OR DRUG CLASS	COMBINED EFFECT
Allopurinol	Decreased allopurinol effect.
Antidepressants (tricyclic)	Dangerous drop in blood pressure. Avoid combination unless under medical supervision.
Barbiturates	Increased chlorthalidone effect.
Cholestyramine	Decreased chlorthalidone effect.
Cortisone drugs	Excessive potassium loss that causes dangerous heart rhythms.
Digitalis preparations	Excessive potassium loss that causes dangerous heart rhythms.
Diuretics (thiazide)	Increased effect of other thiazide diuretics.
Lithium	Increased effect of lithium.
MAO inhibitors	Increased chlorthalidone effect.
Probenecid	Decreased probenecid effect.

INTERACTION WITH OTHER SUBSTANCES

INTERACTS WITH	COMBINED EFFECT
Alcohol:	Dangerous blood-pressure drop.
Beverages:	None expected.
Cocaine:	None expected.
Foods:	
Licorice	Excessive potassium loss that causes dangerous heart rhythms.
Marijuana:	May increase blood pressure.
Tobacco:	None expected.

CHLORZOXAZONE

BRAND NAMES

Algisin
Chlorzone Forte
Paraflex
Parafon Forte

GENERAL INFORMATION

Habit forming? No
Prescription needed? Yes
Available as generic? No
Drug class: Muscle relaxant (skeletal)

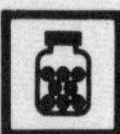

USES

Treatment for sprains, strains and muscle spasms.

DOSAGE & USAGE INFORMATION

How to take:
Tablet or capsule—Swallow with liquid.

When to take:
As needed, no more often than every 4 hours.

If you forget a dose:
Take as soon as you remember. Wait 4 hours for next dose.

What drug does:
Blocks body's pain messages to brain. May also sedate.

Time lapse before drug works:
60 minutes.

Don't take with:
See Interaction column and consult doctor.

OVERDOSE

Symptoms:
Nausea, vomiting, diarrhea, headache, severe weakness, breathing difficulty, sensation of paralysis.

What to do:

- Overdose unlikely to threaten life. Depending on severity of symptoms and amount taken, call doctor, poison-control center or hospital emergency room for instructions.
- Additional emergency information on page 886.

POSSIBLE ADVERSE REACTIONS OR SIDE EFFECTS

SYMPTOMS	FREQUENCY	WHAT TO DO
Brain & nervous system:		
• Drowsiness, dizziness.	Common	4
• Agitation	Infrequent	3
Skin:		
Rash or itch.	Rare	3
Eyes:	None expected.	
Ears, nose, throat:		
Sore throat, fever.	Rare	3
Digestive:		
• Constipation or diarrhea, nausea, cramps, vomiting.	Infrequent	3
• Bloody or tarry, black stool.	Rare	2
Heart & lungs:	None expected.	
Blood vessels:	None expected.	
Muscles, bones, joints:	None expected.	
Genital, urinary:		
Orange or red-purple urine.	Common	6
Kidneys:	None expected.	
Liver:		
Jaundice (yellow eyes and skin).	Rare	3
Allergic:	None expected.	
Blood:	None expected.	
Others:		
Tiredness, weakness.	Rare	3

1- Life-threatening. Seek emergency treatment immediately.
2- Discontinue. Seek emergency treatment.
3- Discontinue. Call doctor right away.
4- Continue. Call doctor when convenient.
5- Continue. Tell doctor at next visit.
6- No action necessary.

WARNINGS & PRECAUTIONS

Don't take if:
You are allergic to any skeletal-muscle relaxant.

Before you start, consult your doctor:
- If you have had liver disease.
- If you plan pregnancy within medication period.

Over age 60:
Adverse reactions and side effects may be more frequent and severe than in younger persons.

Pregnancy:
No proven harm to unborn child. Avoid if possible.

Breast-feeding:
Drug passes into milk. Avoid drug or discontinue nursing until you finish medicine. Consult doctor for advice on maintaining milk supply.

Infants & children:
Not recommended.

Prolonged use:
No problems expected.

Skin & sunlight:
No problems expected.

Driving, piloting or hazardous work:
Don't drive or pilot aircraft until you learn how medicine affects you. Don't work around dangerous machinery. Don't climb ladders or work in high places. Danger increases if you drink alcohol or take medicine affecting alertness and reflexes, such as antihistamines, tranquilizers, sedatives, pain medicine, narcotics and mind-altering drugs.

Airplane passengers:
No problems expected.

Discontinuing:
Don't discontinue without doctor's advice until you complete prescribed dose, even though symptoms diminish or disappear.

Others:
Periodic liver-function tests recommended if you use this drug for a long time.

INTERACTION WI
OTHER DRUGS

GENERIC NAME OR DRUG CLASS	COMBINED EF
Antidepressants	Increased sedatio
Antihistamines	Increased sedation.
MAO inhibitors	Increased effect of both drugs.
Mind-altering drugs	Increased sedation.
Muscle relaxants (others)	Increased sedation.
Narcotics	Increased sedation.
Sedatives	Increased sedation.
Sleep inducers	Increased sedation.
Testosterone	Decreased chlorzoxazone effect.
Tranquilizers	Increased sedation.

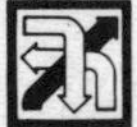

INTERACTION WITH OTHER SUBSTANCES

INTERACTS WITH	COMBINED EFFECT
Alcohol:	Increased sedation.
Beverages:	No problems expected.
Cocaine:	Lack of coordination.
Foods:	No problems expected.
Marijuana:	Lack of coordination, drowsiness, fainting.
Tobacco:	No problems expected.

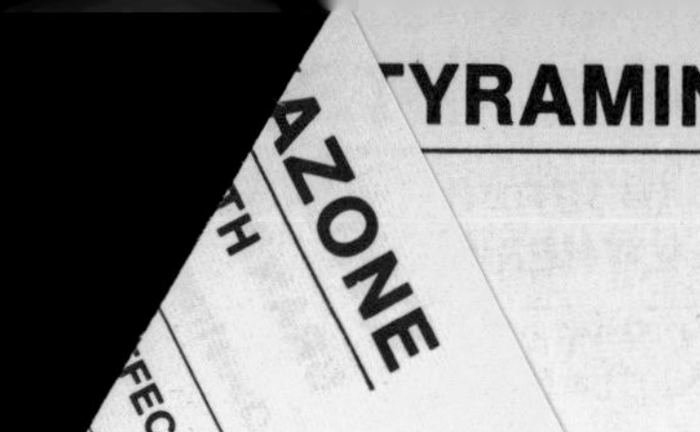

TYRAMINE

GENERAL INFORMATION

Habit forming? No
Prescription needed? Yes
Available as generic? No
Drug class: Antihyperlipidemic, antipruritic

ES

emoves excess bile acids that occur with some liver problems. Reduces persistent itch caused by bile acids.
- Lowers cholesterol level.

DOSAGE & USAGE INFORMATION

How to take:
Powder, granules—Sprinkle into 8 oz. liquid. Let stand for 2 minutes, then mix with liquid before swallowing. Or mix with cereal, soup or pulpy fruit. Don't swallow dry.

When to take:
3 or 4 times a day on an empty stomach, 1 hour before or 2 hours after eating.

If you forget a dose:
Take as soon as you remember up to 2 hours late. If more than 2 hours, wait for next scheduled dose (don't double this dose).

What drug does:
Binds with bile acids to prevent their absorption.

Time lapse before drug works:
- Cholesterol reduction—1 day.
- Bile-acid reduction—3 to 4 weeks.

Don't take with:
- Any drug or vitamin simultaneously. Space doses 2 hours apart.
- See Interaction column and consult doctor.

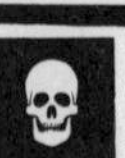

OVERDOSE

Symptoms:
Increased side effects and adverse reactions.

What to do:
Overdose unlikely to threaten life. If person takes much larger amount than prescribed, call doctor, poison-control center or hospital emergency room for instructions.

POSSIBLE ADVERSE REACTIONS OR SIDE EFFECTS

SYMPTOMS	FREQUENCY	WHAT TO DO
Brain & nervous system:	None expected.	
Skin:		
Rash	Rare	3
Eyes:	None expected.	
Ears, nose, throat:		
Sore tongue.	Rare	4
Digestive:		
• Constipation	Common	4
• Belching, bloating, diarrhea, mild nausea, vomiting, stomach pain.	Infrequent	3
• Severe stomach pain; nausea, vomiting; black, tarry stool.	Rare	2
Heart & lungs:	None expected.	
Blood vessels:	None expected.	
Muscles, bones, joints:	None expected.	
Genital, urinary:	None expected.	
Kidneys:	None expected.	
Liver:	None expected.	
Allergic:	None expected.	
Blood:	None expected.	
Others:	None expected.	

1-Life-threatening. Seek emergency treatment immediately.
2-Discontinue. Seek emergency treatment.
3-Discontinue. Call doctor right away.
4-Continue. Call doctor when convenient.
5-Continue. Tell doctor at next visit.
6-No action necessary.

WARNINGS & PRECAUTIONS

Don't take if:
You are allergic to cholestyramine.

Before you start, consult your doctor:
- If you plan to become pregnant within medication period.
- If you have angina, heart or blood-vessel disease.
- If you have stomach problems (including ulcer).
- If you have constipation or hemorrhoids.
- If you have kidney disease.

Over age 60:
Adverse reactions and side effects may be more frequent and severe than in younger persons.

Pregnancy:
No proven harm to unborn child. Avoid if possible.

Breast-feeding:
No problems expected, but consult doctor.

Infants & children:
Not recommended.

Prolonged use:
No problems expected.

Skin & sunlight:
No problems expected.

Driving, piloting or hazardous work:
No problems expected.

Airplane passengers:
No problems expected.

Discontinuing:
Don't discontinue without doctor's advice until you complete prescribed dose, even though symptoms diminish or disappear.

Others:
No problems expected.

INTERACTION WITH OTHER DRUGS

GENERIC NAME OR DRUG CLASS	COMBINED EFFECT
Anticoagulants	Increased anticoagulant effect.
Digitalis preparations	Decreased digitalis effect.
Thyroid hormones	Decreased thyroid effect.
All other medicines	Decreases absorption, so may need dosages or dosage interval adjusted

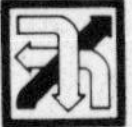

INTERACTION WITH OTHER SUBSTANCES

INTERACTS WITH	COMBINED EFFECT
Alcohol:	None expected.
Beverages:	None expected.
Cocaine:	None expected.
Foods:	Absorption of vitamins in foods decreased. Take vitamin supplements particularly A, D, E & K
Marijuana:	None expected.
Tobacco:	None expected.

CIMETIDINE

BRAND NAMES

Apo-Cimetidine
Novo-Cimetine
Peptol
Tagamet

GENERAL INFORMATION

Habit forming? No
Prescription needed? Yes
Available as generic? No
Drug class: Histamine H-2 antagonist

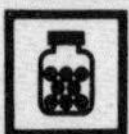

USES

Treatment for duodenal ulcers and other conditions in which stomach produces excess hydrochloric acid.

DOSAGE & USAGE INFORMATION

How to take:
Tablet or capsule—Swallow with liquid.

When to take:
- 1 dose per day—Take at bedtime.
- 2 or more doses per day—Take at the same times each day.

If you forget a dose:
Take as soon as you remember up to 2 hours late. If more than 2 hours, wait for next scheduled dose (don't double this dose).

What drug does:
Blocks histamine release so stomach secretes less acid.

Time lapse before drug works:
Begins in 30 minutes. May require several days to relieve pain.

Don't take with:
See Interaction column and consult doctor.

OVERDOSE

Symptoms:
Confusion, slurred speech, breathing difficulty, rapid heartbeat, delirium.

What to do:
Overdose unlikely to threaten life. If person takes much larger amount than prescribed, call doctor, poison-control center or hospital emergency room for instructions.

POSSIBLE ADVERSE REACTIONS OR SIDE EFFECTS

SYMPTOMS	FREQUENCY	WHAT TO DO
Brain & nervous system:		
• Confusion	Rare	3
• Dizziness or headache.	Infrequent	4
Skin:		
Rash, hives.	Rare	3
Eyes, kidneys, liver, allergic, blood:	None expected.	
Ears, nose, throat:		
Sore throat, fever.	Rare	3
Digestive:		
Diarrhea	Infrequent	4
Heart & lungs:		
Slow, fast or irregular heartbeat.	Rare	3
Blood vessels:		
Unusual bleeding or bruising.	Rare	3
Muscles, bones, joints:		
Muscle cramps or pain.	Rare	3
Genital, urinary:		
Decreased sperm production.	Infrequent	4
Others:		
• Decreased sex drive, breast swelling and soreness in males; unusual milk flow in females; hair loss.	Infrequent	5
• Fatigue, weakness.	Rare	3

1-Life-threatening. Seek emergency treatment immediately.
2-Discontinue. Seek emergency treatment.
3-Discontinue. Call doctor right away.
4-Continue. Call doctor when convenient.
5-Continue. Tell doctor at next visit.

WARNINGS & PRECAUTIONS

Don't take if:
You are allergic to cimetidine or other histamine H-2 antagonist.

Before you start, consult your doctor:
- If you plan to become pregnant during medication period.
- If you take aspirin. Aspirin may irritate stomach.

Over age 60:
Adverse reactions and side effects may be more frequent and severe than in younger persons.

Pregnancy:
No proven harm to unborn child. Avoid if possible.

Breast-feeding:
No problems expected.

Infants & children:
Not recommended.

Prolonged use:
Possible liver damage.

Skin & sunlight:
No problems expected.

Driving, piloting or hazardous work:
Don't drive or pilot aircraft until you learn how medicine affects you. Don't work around dangerous machinery. Don't climb ladders or work in high places. Danger increases if you drink alcohol or take medicine affecting alertness and reflexes, such as antihistamines, tranquilizers, sedatives, pain medicine, narcotics and mind-altering drugs.

Airplane passengers:
No problems expected.

Discontinuing:
Don't discontinue without consulting doctor. Dose may require gradual reduction if you have taken drug for a long time. Doses of other drugs may also require adjustment.

Others:
Patients on kidney dialysis—Take at end of dialysis treatment.

INTERACTION WITH OTHER DRUGS

GENERIC NAME OR DRUG CLASS	COMBINED EFFECT
Anticoagulants (oral)	Increased anticoagulant effect.
Anticholinergics	Decreased cimetidine effect.
Bethanechol	Increased cimetidine effect.
Carmustine (BCNU)	Severe impairment of red-blood-cell production; some interference with white-blood-cell formation.

Additional interactions on page 836.

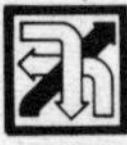

INTERACTION WITH OTHER SUBSTANCES

INTERACTS WITH	COMBINED EFFECT
Alcohol:	No interactions expected, but alcohol may slow body's recovery. Avoid.
Beverages:	
Milk	Enhanced effectiveness. Small amounts useful for taking medication.
Caffeine drinks	May increase acid secretion and delay healing.
Cocaine:	Decreased cimetidine effect.
Foods:	Enhanced effectiveness. Protein-rich foods should be eaten in moderation to minimize secretion of stomach acid.
Marijuana:	Increased chance of low sperm count. Marijuana may slow body's recovery. Avoid.
Tobacco:	No interactions expected, but tobacco may slow body's recovery. Avoid.

CLEMASTINE

BRAND NAMES

Tavist

GENERAL INFORMATION

Habit forming? No
Prescription needed? No
Available as generic? No
Drug class: Antihistamine

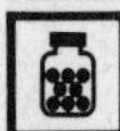

USES

Reduces allergic symptoms such as hay fever, hives, rash or itching.

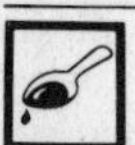

DOSAGE & USAGE INFORMATION

How to take:
Tablet—Swallow with liquid or food to lessen stomach irritation.

When to take:
Varies with form. Follow label directions.

If you forget a dose:
Take as soon as you remember up to 2 hours late. If more than 2 hours, wait for next scheduled dose (don't double this dose).

What drug does:
Blocks action of histamine after an allergic response triggers histamine release in sensitive cells.

Time lapse before drug works:
30 minutes.

Don't take with:
See Interaction column and consult doctor.

OVERDOSE

Symptoms:
Convulsions, red face, hallucinations, coma.

What to do:
- Dial 0 (operator) or 911 (emergency) for an ambulance or medical help. Then give first aid immediately.
- If patient is unconscious and not breathing, give mouth-to-mouth breathing. If there is no heartbeat, use cardiac massage and mouth-to-mouth breathing (CPR). Don't try to make patient vomit. If you can't get help quickly, take patient to nearest emergency facility.
- Additional emergency information on page 886.

POSSIBLE ADVERSE REACTIONS OR SIDE EFFECTS

SYMPTOMS	FREQUENCY	WHAT TO DO
Brain & nervous system:		
• Nightmares, agitation, irritability.	Rare	3
• Drowsiness, dizziness.	Common	5
Skin:	None expected.	
Eyes:		
• Vision changes.	Infrequent	3
• Less tolerance for contact lenses.	Infrequent	4
Ears, nose, throat:		
• Sore throat, fever.	Rare	3
• Dry mouth, nose, throat.	Common	5
Digestive:		
• Nausea	Common	5
• Appetite loss.	Infrequent	5
Heart & lungs:		
Rapid heartbeat.	Rare	3
Blood vessels:		
Unusual bleeding or bruising.	Rare	3
Muscles, bones, joints, kidneys, liver, allergic, blood:	None expected.	
Genital, urinary:		
Urination difficulty.	Infrequent	4
Others:		
Fatigue, weakness.	Rare	3

1- Life-threatening. Seek emergency treatment immediately.
2- Discontinue. Seek emergency treatment.
3- Discontinue. Call doctor right away.
4- Continue. Call doctor when convenient.
5- Continue. Tell doctor at next visit.
6- No action necessary.

WARNINGS & PRECAUTIONS

Don't take if:
You are allergic to any antihistamine.

Before you start, consult your doctor:
- If you have glaucoma.
- If you have enlarged prostate.
- If you have asthma.
- If you have kidney disease.
- If you have peptic ulcer.
- If you will have surgery within 2 months, including dental surgery, requiring general or spinal anesthesia.

Over age 60:
Don't exceed recommended dose. Adverse reactions and side effects may be more frequent and severe than in younger persons, especially urination difficulty, diminished alertness and other brain and nervous-system symptoms.

Pregnancy:
No proven harm to unborn child. Avoid if possible.

Breast-feeding:
Drug passes into milk. Avoid drug or discontinue nursing until you finish medicine. Consult doctor for advice on maintaining milk supply.

Infants & children:
Not recommended for premature or newborn infants. Otherwise, no problems expected.

Prolonged use:
Avoid. May damage bone marrow and nerve cells.

Skin & sunlight:
May cause rash or intensify sunburn in areas exposed to sun or sunlamp.

Driving, piloting or hazardous work:
Don't drive or pilot aircraft until you learn how medicine affects you. Don't work around dangerous machinery. Don't climb ladders or work in high places. Danger increases if you drink alcohol or take medicine affecting alertness and reflexes, such as antihistamines, tranquilizers, sedatives, pain medicine, narcotics and mind-altering drugs.

Airplane passengers:
No problems expected.

Discontinuing:
No problems expected.

Others:
May mask symptoms of hearing damage from aspirin, other salicylates, cisplatin, paromomycin, vancomycin or anticonvulsants. Consult doctor if you use these.

INTERACTION WITH OTHER DRUGS

GENERIC NAME OR DRUG CLASS	COMBINED EFFECT
Anticholinergics	Increased anticholinergic effect.
Antidepressants	Excess sedation. Avoid.
Antihistamines (other)	Excess sedation. Avoid.
Hypnotics	Excess sedation. Avoid.
MAO inhibitors	Increased clemastine effect.
Mind-altering drugs	Excess sedation. Avoid.
Narcotics	Excess sedation. Avoid.
Sedatives	Excess sedation. Avoid.
Sleep inducers	Excess sedation. Avoid.
Tranquilizers	Excess sedation. Avoid.

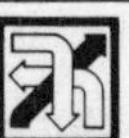

INTERACTION WITH OTHER SUBSTANCES

INTERACTS WITH	COMBINED EFFECT
Alcohol:	Excess sedation. Avoid.
Beverages:	
Caffeine drinks	Less clemastine sedation.
Cocaine:	Decreased clemastine effect. Avoid.
Foods:	None expected.
Marijuana:	Excess sedation. Avoid.
Tobacco:	None expected.

CLIDINIUM

BRAND NAMES

Clipoxide
Librax
Quarzan

GENERAL INFORMATION

Habit forming? No
Prescription needed? Low strength: No
High strength: Yes
Available as generic? Yes
Drug class: Antispasmodic, anticholinergic

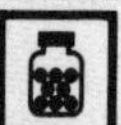

USES

Reduces spasms of digestive system, bladder and urethra.

DOSAGE & USAGE INFORMATION

How to take:
Capsule—Swallow with liquid or food to lessen stomach irritation.

When to take:
30 minutes before meals (unless directed otherwise by doctor).

If you forget a dose:
Take as soon as you remember up to 2 hours late. If more than 2 hours, wait for next scheduled dose (don't double this dose).

What drug does:
Blocks nerve impulses at parasympathetic nerve endings, preventing muscle contractions and gland secretions of organs involved.

Time lapse before drug works:
15 to 30 minutes.

Don't take with:
See Interaction column and consult doctor.

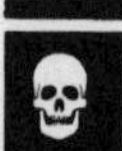

OVERDOSE

Symptoms:
Dilated pupils; rapid pulse and breathing; dizziness; fever; hallucinations; confusion; slurred speech; agitation; flushed face; convulsions; coma.

What to do:
- Dial 0 (operator) or 911 (emergency) for an ambulance or medical help. Then give first aid immediately.
- Additional emergency information on page 886.

POSSIBLE ADVERSE REACTIONS OR SIDE EFFECTS

SYMPTOMS	FREQUENCY	WHAT TO DO
Brain & nervous system:		
• Headache	Infrequent	4
• Confusion, delirium.	Common	3
Skin:		
Rash or hives.	Rare	3
Eyes:		
Pain, blurred vision.	Rare	3
Ears, nose, throat:		
• Dryness	Common	6
• Nasal congestion, altered taste.	Infrequent	3
Digestive:		
• Constipation	Common	5
• Nausea, vomiting.	Common	4
Heart & lungs:		
Rapid heartbeat.	Common	3
Blood vessels:	None expected.	
Muscles, bones, joints:	None expected.	
Genital, urinary:		
Difficult urination.	Infrequent	4
Kidneys:	None expected.	
Liver:	None expected.	
Allergic:	None expected.	
Blood:	None expected.	
Others:		
Less perspiration.	Common	4

1- Life-threatening. Seek emergency treatment immediately.
2- Discontinue. Seek emergency treatment.
3- Discontinue. Call doctor right away.
4- Continue. Call doctor when convenient.
5- Continue. Tell doctor at next visit.
6- No action necessary.

WARNINGS & PRECAUTIONS

Don't take if:

- You are allergic to any anticholinergic.
- You have trouble with stomach bloating.
- You have difficulty emptying your bladder completely.
- You have narrow-angle glaucoma.
- You have severe ulcerative colitis.

Before you start, consult your doctor:

- If you have open-angle glaucoma.
- If you have angina.
- If you have chronic bronchitis or asthma.
- If you have hiatal hernia.
- If you have liver disease.
- If you have enlarged prostate.
- If you have myasthenia gravis.
- If you have peptic ulcer.
- If you will have surgery within 2 months, including dental surgery, requiring general or spinal anesthesia.

Over age 60:
Adverse reactions and side effects may be more frequent and severe than in younger persons.

Pregnancy:
Studies inconclusive on harm to unborn child. Animal studies show fetal abnormalities. Decide with your doctor whether drug benefits justify risk to unborn child.

Breast-feeding:
Drug passes into milk and decreases milk flow. Avoid drug or discontinue nursing until you finish medicine. Consult doctor for advice on maintaining milk supply.

Infants & children:
Use only under medical supervision.

Prolonged use:
Chronic constipation, possible fecal impaction. Consult doctor immediately.

Skin & sunlight:
No problems expected.

Driving, piloting or hazardous work:
Don't drive or pilot aircraft until you learn how medicine affects you. Don't work around dangerous machinery. Don't climb ladders or work in high places. Danger increases if you drink alcohol or take medicine affecting alertness and reflexes, such as antihistamines, tranquilizers, sedatives, pain medicine, narcotics, or mind-altering drugs.

Airplane passengers:
No problems expected.

Discontinuing:
May be unnecessary to finish medicine. Follow doctor's instructions.

INTERACTION WITH OTHER DRUGS

GENERIC NAME OR DRUG CLASS	COMBINED EFFECT
Amantadine	Increased clidinium effect.
Antacids	Decreased clidinium effect.
Anticholinergics (other)	Increased clidinium effect.
Antidepressants (tricyclic)	Increased clidinium effect.
Antihistamines	Increased clidinium effect.
Haloperidol	Increased internal-eye pressure.
MAO inhibitors	Increased clidinium effect.
Meperidine	Increased clidinium effect.
Methylphenidate	Increased clidinium effect.
Orphenadrine	Increased clidinium effect.
Phenothiazines	Increased clidinium effect.
Pilocarpine	Loss of pilocarpine effect in glaucoma treatment.
Tranquilizers	Decreased clidinium effect.
Vitamin C	Decreased clidinium effect. Avoid large doses of vitamin C.

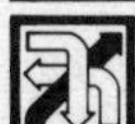

INTERACTION WITH OTHER SUBSTANCES

INTERACTS WITH	COMBINED EFFECT
Alcohol:	None expected.
Beverages:	None expected.
Cocaine:	Excessively rapid heartbeat. Avoid.
Foods:	None expected.
Marijuana:	Drowsiness and dry mouth.
Tobacco:	None expected.

CLINDAMYCIN

BRAND NAMES

Cleocin
Cleocin-T
Dalacin C

GENERAL INFORMATION

Habit forming? No
Prescription needed? Yes
Available as generic? No
Drug class: Antibiotic (lincomycin)

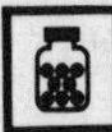

USES

Treatment of bacterial infections that are susceptible to clindamycin.

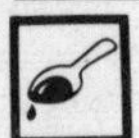

DOSAGE & USAGE INFORMATION

How to take:
Capsule or liquid—Swallow with liquid 1 hour before or 2 hours after eating.

When to take:
At the same times each day.

If you forget a dose:
Take as soon as you remember up to 2 hours late. If more than 2 hours, wait for next scheduled dose (don't double this dose).

What drug does:
Destroys susceptible bacteria. Does not kill viruses.

Time lapse before drug works:
3 to 5 days.

Don't take with:
See Interaction column and consult doctor.

OVERDOSE

Symptoms:
Severe nausea, vomiting, diarrhea.

What to do:
Overdose unlikely to threaten life. If person takes much larger amount than prescribed, call doctor, poison-control center or hospital emergency room for instructions.

POSSIBLE ADVERSE REACTIONS OR SIDE EFFECTS

SYMPTOMS	FREQUENCY	WHAT TO DO
Brain & nervous system:	None expected.	
Skin:		
Rash, itch around groin, rectum or armpits.	Infrequent	4
Eyes:	None expected.	
Ears, nose, throat:		
• Unusual thirst.	Infrequent	3
• White patches in mouth.	Infrequent	4
Digestive:		
Vomiting, stomach cramps, severe and watery diarrhea with blood or mucus.	Infrequent	3
Heart & lungs:	None expected.	
Blood vessels:	None expected.	
Muscles, bones, joints:		
Painful, swollen joints.	Infrequent	3
Genital, urinary:		
Vaginal discharge, itching.	Infrequent	4
Kidneys:	None expected.	
Liver:		
Jaundice (yellow skin and eyes).	Infrequent	3
Allergic:	None expected.	
Blood:	None expected.	
Others:		
• Fever	Infrequent	3
• Tiredness, weakness, weight loss.	Infrequent	3

1- Life-threatening. Seek emergency treatment immediately.
2- Discontinue. Seek emergency treatment.
3- Discontinue. Call doctor right away.
4- Continue. Call doctor when convenient.

WARNINGS & PRECAUTIONS

Don't take if:
- You are allergic to lincomycins.
- You have had ulcerative colitis.
- Prescribed for infant under 1 month old.

Before you start, consult your doctor:
- If you have had yeast infections of mouth, skin or vagina.
- If you will have surgery within 2 months, including dental surgery, requiring general or spinal anesthesia.
- If you have kidney or liver disease.
- If you have allergies of any kind.

Over age 60:
Adverse reactions and side effects may be more frequent and severe than in younger persons.

Pregnancy:
Risk to unborn child outweighs drug benefits. Don't use.

Breast-feeding:
Drug passes into milk. Avoid drug or discontinue nursing until you finish medicine. Consult doctor for advice on maintaining milk supply.

Infants & children:
Don't give to infants younger than 1 month. Use for children only under medical supervision.

Prolonged use:
- Severe colitis with diarrhea and bleeding.
- You may become more susceptible to infections caused by germs not responsive to clindamycin.

Skin & sunlight:
No problems expected.

Driving, piloting or hazardous work:
No problems expected.

Airplane passengers:
No problems expected.

Discontinuing:
Don't discontinue without doctor's advice until you complete prescribed dose, even though symptoms diminish or disappear.

Others:
No problems expected.

INTERACTION WITH OTHER DRUGS

GENERIC NAME OR DRUG CLASS	COMBINED EFFECT
Antidiarrheal preparations	Decreased clindamycin effect.
Chloramphenicol	Decreased clindamycin effect.
Erythromycin	Decreased clindamycin effect.

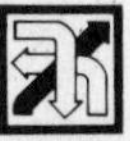

INTERACTION WITH OTHER SUBSTANCES

INTERACTS WITH	COMBINED EFFECT
Alcohol:	None expected.
Beverages:	None expected.
Cocaine:	None expected.
Foods:	None expected.
Marijuana:	None expected.
Tobacco:	None expected.

CLOFIBRATE

BRAND NAMES

Atromid-S
Claripex
Liprinal
Novofibrate

GENERAL INFORMATION

Habit forming? No
Prescription needed? Yes
Available as generic? No
Drug class: Antihyperlipidemic

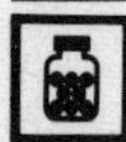

USES

Reduces fatty substances in the blood (cholesterol and triglycerides).

DOSAGE & USAGE INFORMATION

How to take:
Capsule—Swallow with liquid or food to lessen stomach irritation.

When to take:
At the same times each day.

If you forget a dose:
Take as soon as you remember up to 2 hours late. If more than 2 hours, wait for next scheduled dose (don't double this dose).

What drug does:
Inhibits formation of fatty substances.

Time lapse before drug works:
3 months or more.

Don't take with:
See Interaction column and consult doctor.

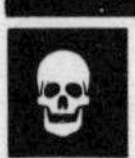

OVERDOSE

Symptoms:
Diarrhea, headache, muscle pain.

What to do:
Overdose unlikely to threaten life. If person takes much larger amount than prescribed, call doctor, poison-control center or hospital emergency room for instructions.

POSSIBLE ADVERSE REACTIONS OR SIDE EFFECTS

SYMPTOMS	FREQUENCY	WHAT TO DO
Brain & nervous system:		
Dizziness, drowsiness, headache.	Rare	4
Skin:		
• Dryness, hair loss.	Rare	4
• Rash, itch.	Rare	3
Eyes, blood vessels, allergic, blood:	None expected.	
Ears, nose, throat:		
• Sores in mouth, on lips.	Rare	3
• Sore throat.	Rare	3
Digestive:		
Nausea, vomiting, diarrhea, stomach pain.	Infrequent	4
Heart & lungs:		
Chest pain, shortness of breath, irregular heartbeat.	Infrequent	3
Muscles, bones, joints:		
• Muscle cramps.	Rare	4
• Swollen feet, legs.	Rare	3
Genital, urinary:		
Bloody urine, painful urination.	Rare	3
Kidneys:		
Backache	Rare	4
Liver:		
Gallstones	Infrequent	3
Others:		
• Decreased sex drive.	Rare	4
• Fever, chills.	Rare	3

1 - Life-threatening. Seek emergency treatment immediately.
2 - Discontinue. Seek emergency treatment.
3 - Discontinue. Call doctor right away.
4 - Continue. Call doctor when convenient.

WARNINGS & PRECAUTIONS

Don't take if:
You are allergic to any antihyperlipidemic.

Before you start, consult your doctor:
- If you have had liver or kidney disease.
- If you have had peptic-ulcer disease.
- If you have diabetes.

Over age 60:
Adverse reactions and side effects may be more frequent and severe than in younger persons. May develop flu-like symptoms.

Pregnancy:
Risk to unborn child outweighs drug benefits. Don't use.

Breast-feeding:
May harm child. Avoid.

Infants & children:
Not recommended.

Prolonged use:
No problems expected.

Skin & sunlight:
No problems expected.

Driving, piloting or hazardous work:
Avoid if you feel drowsy or dizzy. Otherwise, no problems expected.

Airplane passengers:
No problems expected.

Discontinuing:
Don't discontinue without doctor's advice until you complete prescribed dose, even though symptoms diminish or disappear.

Others:
- Periodic blood-cell counts and liver-function studies recommended if you take clofibrate for a long time.
- Some studies question effectiveness. Many studies warn against toxicity.

INTERACTION WITH OTHER DRUGS

GENERIC NAME OR DRUG CLASS	COMBINED EFFECT
Anticoagulants (oral)	Increased anticoagulant effect. Dose reduction of anticoagulant necessary.
Antidiabetics (oral)	Increased antidiabetic effect.
Contraceptives (oral)	Decreased clofibrate effect.
Estrogens	Decreased clofibrate effect.
Furosemide	Possible toxicity of both drugs.
Insulin	Increased insulin effect.
Thyroid hormones	Increased clofibrate effect.

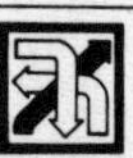

INTERACTION WITH OTHER SUBSTANCES

INTERACTS WITH	COMBINED EFFECT
Alcohol:	None expected.
Beverages:	None expected.
Cocaine:	None expected.
Foods:	
Fatty foods	Decreased clofibrate effect.
Marijuana:	None expected.
Tobacco:	None expected.

CLOMIPHENE

BRAND NAMES

Clomid
Serophene

GENERAL INFORMATION

Habit forming? No
Prescription needed? Yes
Available as generic? No
Drug class: Gonad stimulant

USES

- Treatment for men with low sperm counts.
- Treatment for ovulatory failure in women who wish to become pregnant.

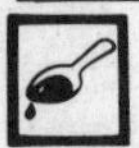

DOSAGE & USAGE INFORMATION

How to take:
Tablet—Swallow with liquid.

When to take:
- Men—Take at the same time each day.
- Women—If you are to begin treatment on "Day 5," count your first menstrual day as "Day 1." Take a tablet each day for 5 days.

If you forget a dose:
Take as soon as you remember. If you forget a day, double next dose. If you miss 2 or more doses, consult doctor.

What drug does:
Antiestrogen effect stimulates ovulation and sperm production.

Time lapse before drug works:
Usually 3 to 6 months. Ovulation may occur 6 to 10 days after last day of treatment in any cycle.

Don't take with:
No restrictions.

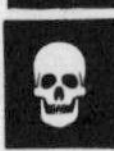

OVERDOSE

Symptoms:
Increased severity of adverse reactions and side effects.

What to do:
Overdose unlikely to threaten life. If person takes much larger amount than prescribed, call doctor, poison-control center or hospital emergency room for instructions.

POSSIBLE ADVERSE REACTIONS OR SIDE EFFECTS

SYMPTOMS	FREQUENCY	WHAT TO DO
Brain & nervous system:		
Dizziness, headache, tiredness, depression, nervousness.	Rare	4
Skin:		
Rash, itch.	Infrequent	3
Eyes:		
Vision changes.	Rare	3
Ears, nose, throat:	None expected.	
Digestive:		
• Bloating, stomach pain.	Common	3
• Constipation, diarrhea, increased appetite.	Infrequent	4
Heart & lungs:	None expected.	
Blood vessels:		
Hot flashes.	Common	5
Muscles, bones, joints:	None expected.	
Genital, urinary:		
• Pelvic pain.	Common	3
• Heavy menstrual flow.	Infrequent	4
Kidneys:		
Frequent urination.	Infrequent	4
Liver:		
Jaundice (yellow skin and eyes).	Infrequent	3
Allergic:	None expected.	
Blood:	None expected.	
Others:		
Breast discomfort, weight change, hair loss.	Infrequent	4

1-Life-threatening. Seek emergency treatment immediately.
2-Discontinue. Seek emergency treatment.
3-Discontinue. Call doctor right away.
4-Continue. Call doctor when convenient.
5-Continue. Tell doctor at next visit.

WARNINGS & PRECAUTIONS

Don't take if:
You are allergic to clomiphene.

Before you start, consult your doctor:
- If you have an ovarian cyst, fibroid uterine tumors or unusual vaginal bleeding.
- If you have inflamed veins caused by blood clots.
- If you have liver disease.
- If you are depressed.

Over age 60:
Not recommended.

Pregnancy:
Stop taking at first sign of pregnancy.

Breast-feeding:
Not used.

Infants & children:
Not used.

Prolonged use:
Not recommended.

Skin & sunlight:
No problems expected.

Driving, piloting or hazardous work:
Avoid if you feel dizzy. Otherwise, no problems expected.

Airplane passengers:
No problems expected.

Discontinuing:
May be unnecessary to finish medicine. Follow doctor's instructions.

Others:
- Have a complete pelvic examination before treatment.
- If you become pregnant, twins or triplets are possible.

INTERACTION WITH OTHER DRUGS

GENERIC NAME OR DRUG CLASS	COMBINED EFFECT
None	

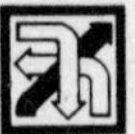

INTERACTION WITH OTHER SUBSTANCES

INTERACTS WITH	COMBINED EFFECT
Alcohol:	None expected.
Beverages:	None expected.
Cocaine:	None expected.
Foods:	None expected.
Marijuana:	None expected.
Tobacco:	None expected.

CLONIDINE

BRAND NAMES

Catapres
Combipres

GENERAL INFORMATION

Habit forming? No
Prescription needed? Yes
Available as generic? No
Drug class: Antihypertensive

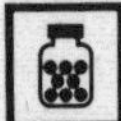

USES

- Treatment of high blood pressure.
- Prevention of vascular headaches.
- Treatment of dysmenorrhea.
- Treatment of narcotic withdrawal syndrome.
- Treatment of congestive heart failure.

DOSAGE & USAGE INFORMATION

How to take:
Tablet or capsule—Swallow with liquid.

When to take:
Daily dose at bedtime.

If you forget a dose:
Bedtime dose—If you forget your once-a-day bedtime dose, don't take it more than 3 hours late.

What drug does:
Relaxes and allows expansion of blood vessel walls.

Time lapse before drug works:
1 to 3 hours.

Don't take with:
- Non-prescription medicines containing alcohol.
- See Interaction column and consult doctor.

OVERDOSE

Symptoms:
Difficult breathing, vomiting, fainting, slow heartbeat, coma, diminished reflexes.

What to do:
- Dial 0 (operator) or 911 (emergency) for an ambulance or medical help. Then give first aid immediately.
- If patient is unconscious and not breathing, give mouth-to-mouth breathing. If there is no heartbeat, use cardiac massage and mouth-to-mouth breathing (CPR). Don't try to make patient vomit. If you can't get help quickly, take patient to nearest emergency facility.
- Additional emergency information on page 886.

POSSIBLE ADVERSE REACTIONS OR SIDE EFFECTS

SYMPTOMS	FREQUENCY	WHAT TO DO
Brain & nervous system:		
• Dizziness	Common	4
• Drowsiness	Common	4
• Insomnia	Infrequent	5
• Headache	Infrequent	4
• Depression	Rare	4
• Nightmares	Infrequent	4
Skin:		
Rash, itch.	Rare	3
Eyes:		
Dryness, burning.	Infrequent	4
Ears, nose, throat:		
• Dry mouth.	Common	5
• Painful glands in neck.	Infrequent	4
Digestive:		
• Constipation	Infrequent	5
• Appetite loss.	Infrequent	5
• Nausea, vomiting.	Infrequent	4
Heart & lungs:		
Abnormal heart rhythm.	Infrequent	3
Blood vessels:		
Cold fingers & toes.	Infrequent	4
Muscles, bones, joints:	None expected.	
Genital, urinary:		
• Decreased sex drive.	Infrequent	5
• Urinary retention.	Infrequent	3
Kidneys, allergic, blood, liver:	None expected.	
Others:		
• Weight gain		
• Lightheadedness upon rising from sitting or lying.	Common	4
• Enlarged breasts.	Common	4

1- Life-threatening. Seek emergency treatment immediately.
2- Discontinue. Seek emergency treatment.
3- Discontinue. Call doctor right away.
4- Continue. Call doctor when convenient.
5- Continue. Tell doctor at next visit.
6- No action necessary.

WARNINGS & PRECAUTIONS

Don't take if:

- You are allergic to any alpha adrenergic blocker.
- Under age 12.

Before you start, consult your doctor:

- If you will have surgery within 2 months, including dental surgery, requiring general or spinal anesthesia.
- If you have heart disease.
- If you have circulation disorder (intermittent claudication, Buerger's disease).

Over age 60:
Adverse reactions and side effects may be more frequent and severe than in younger persons.

Pregnancy:
Studies inconclusive on harm to unborn child. Animal studies show fetal abnormalities. Decide with your doctor whether drug benefits justify risk to unborn child.

Breast-feeding:
Unknown whether safe or not. Consult doctor.

Infants & children:
Use only under careful medical supervision after age 12. Avoid before age 12.

Prolonged use:
Don't discontinue without consulting doctor. Dose may require gradual reduction if you have taken drug for a long time. Doses of other drugs may also require adjustment.

Skin & sunlight:
No problems expected.

Driving, piloting or hazardous work:
Don't drive or pilot aircraft until you learn how medicine affects you. Don't work around dangerous machinery. Don't climb ladders or work in high places. Danger increases if you drink alcohol or take medicine affecting alertness and reflexes, such as antihistamines, tranquilizers, sedatives, pain medicine, narcotics and mind-altering drugs.

Airplane passengers:
No problems expected.

Discontinuing:
Don't discontinue abruptly. May cause anxiety, chest pain, insomnia, headache, nausea, irregular heartbeat, flushed face, sweating.

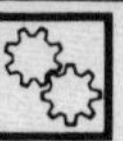

INTERACTION WITH OTHER DRUGS

GENERIC NAME OR DRUG CLASS	COMBINED EFFECT
Antidepressants (tricyclic)	Decreased effect of clonidine.
Antihypertensives (other)	Excessive blood-pressure drop.
Beta-blockers	Blood-pressure control impaired.
Diuretics	Excessive blood-pressure drop.

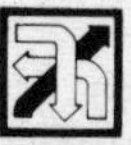

INTERACTION WITH OTHER SUBSTANCES

INTERACTS WITH	COMBINED EFFECT
Alcohol:	Increased sensitivity to sedative effect of alcohol and very low blood pressure. Avoid.
Beverages: Caffeine containing drinks.	Decreased clonidine effect.
Cocaine:	Blood pressure rise. Avoid.
Foods:	No problems expected.
Marijuana:	Weakness on standing.
Tobacco:	No problems expected.

CLORAZEPATE

BRAND NAMES

Tranxene
Tranxene-SD

GENERAL INFORMATION

Habit forming? Yes
Prescription needed? Yes
Available as generic? No
Drug class: Tranquilizer (benzodiazepine)

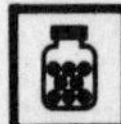

USES

- Treatment for nervousness or tension.
- Treatment for convulsive disorders.

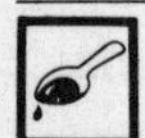

DOSAGE & USAGE INFORMATION

How to take:
Tablet or capsule—Swallow with liquid. If you can't swallow whole, crumble tablet or open capsule and take with liquid or food.

When to take:
At the same time each day, according to instructions on prescription label.

If you forget a dose:
Take as soon as you remember up to 2 hours late. If more than 2 hours, wait for next scheduled dose (don't double this dose).

What drug does:
Affects limbic system of brain—part that controls emotions.

Time lapse before drug works:
2 hours. May take 6 weeks for full benefit.

Don't take with:
See Interaction column and consult doctor.

OVERDOSE

Symptoms:
Drowsiness, weakness, tremor, stupor, coma.

What to do:
- Dial 0 (operator) or 911 (emergency) for an ambulance or medical help. Then give first aid immediately.
- If patient is unconscious and not breathing, give mouth-to-mouth breathing. If there is no heartbeat, use cardiac massage and mouth-to-mouth breathing (CPR). Don't try to make patient vomit. If you can't get help quickly, take patient to nearest emergency facility.
- Additional emergency information on page 886.

POSSIBLE ADVERSE REACTIONS OR SIDE EFFECTS

SYMPTOMS	FREQUENCY	WHAT TO DO
Brain & nervous system:		
• Clumsiness, drowsiness, dizziness.	Common	4
• Hallucinations, confusion, depression, irritability.	Infrequent	3
Skin:		
Rash, itch.	Infrequent	3
Eyes:		
Vision changes.	Infrequent	3
Ears, nose, throat:		
Mouth, throat ulcers.	Rare	3
Digestive:		
Constipation or diarrhea, nausea, vomiting.	Infrequent	4
Heart & lungs:		
Slow heartbeat, breathing difficulty.	Rare	2
Blood vessels:	None expected.	
Muscles, bones, joints:	None expected.	
Genital, urinary:		
Urination difficulty.	Infrequent	4
Kidneys:	None expected.	
Liver:		
Jaundice (yellow eyes and skin).	Rare	3
Allergic:	None expected.	
Blood:	None expected.	
Others:	None expected.	

1- Life-threatening. Seek emergency treatment immediately.
2- Discontinue. Seek emergency treatment.
3- Discontinue. Call doctor right away.
4- Continue. Call doctor when convenient.
5- Continue. Tell doctor at next visit.
6- No action necessary.

WARNINGS & PRECAUTIONS

Don't take if:
- You are allergic to any benzodiazepine.
- You have myasthenia gravis.
- You are active or recovering alcoholic.
- Patient is younger than 6 months.

Before you start, consult your doctor:
- If you have liver, kidney or lung disease.
- If you have diabetes, epilepsy or porphyria.

Over age 60:
Adverse reactions and side effects may be more frequent and severe than in younger persons. You need smaller doses for shorter periods of time. May develop agitation, rage or "hangover effect."

Pregnancy:
Risk to unborn child outweighs drug benefits. Don't use.

Breast-feeding:
Drug passes into milk. Avoid drug or discontinue nursing until you finish medicine. Consult doctor for advice on maintaining milk supply.

Infants & children:
Use only under medical supervision for children older than 6 months.

Prolonged use:
May impair liver function.

Skin & sunlight:
No problems expected.

Driving, piloting or hazardous work:
Don't drive or pilot aircraft until you learn how medicine affects you. Don't work around dangerous machinery. Don't climb ladders or work in high places. Danger increases if you drink alcohol or take medicine affecting alertness and reflexes.

Airplane passengers:
No problems expected.

Discontinuing:
Don't discontinue without consulting doctor. Dose may require gradual reduction if you have taken drug for a long time. Doses of other drugs may also require adjustment.

Others:
- Hot weather, heavy exercise and profuse sweat may reduce excretion and cause overdose.
- Blood sugar may rise in diabetics, requiring insulin adjustment.

INTERACTION WITH OTHER DRUGS

GENERIC NAME OR DRUG CLASS	COMBINED EFFECT
Anticonvulsants	Change in seizure frequency or severity.
Antidepressants	Increased sedative effect of both drugs.
Antihistamines	Increased sedative effect of both drugs.
Antihypertensives	Excessively low blood pressure.
Cimetidine	Excess sedation.
Disulfiram	Increased clorazepate effect.
MAO inhibitors	Convulsions, deep sedation, rage.
Narcotics	Increased sedative effect of both drugs.
Sedatives	Increased sedative effect of both drugs.
Sleep inducers	Increased sedative effect of both drugs.
Tranquilizers	Increased sedative effect of both drugs.

INTERACTION WITH OTHER SUBSTANCES

INTERACTS WITH	COMBINED EFFECT
Alcohol:	Heavy sedation. Avoid.
Beverages:	None expected.
Cocaine:	Decreased clorazepate effect.
Foods:	None expected.
Marijuana:	Heavy sedation. Avoid.
Tobacco:	Decreased clorazepate effect.

CLOXACILLIN

BRAND NAMES

Bactopen
Cloxapen
Cloxilean
Novocloxin
Orbenin
Tegopen

GENERAL INFORMATION

Habit forming? No
Prescription needed? Yes
Available as generic? Yes
Drug class: Antibiotic (penicillin)

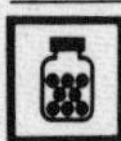

USES

Treatment of bacterial infections that are susceptible to cloxacillin.

DOSAGE & USAGE INFORMATION

How to take:

- Tablets or capsules—Swallow with liquid on an empty stomach 1 hour before or 2 hours after eating.
- Liquid—Take with cold beverage. Liquid form is perishable and effective for only 7 days at room temperature. Effective for 14 days if stored in refrigerator. Don't freeze.

When to take:
Follow instructions on prescription label or side of package. Doses should be evenly spaced. For example, 4 times a day means every 6 hours.

If you forget a dose:
Take as soon as you remember. Continue regular schedule.

What drug does:
Destroys susceptible bacteria. Does not kill viruses.

Time lapse before drug works:
May be several days before medicine affects infection.

Don't take with:
See Interaction column and consult doctor.

OVERDOSE

Symptoms:
Severe diarrhea, nausea or vomiting.

What to do:
Overdose unlikely to threaten life. If person takes much larger amount than prescribed, call doctor, poison-control center or hospital emergency room for instructions.

POSSIBLE ADVERSE REACTIONS OR SIDE EFFECTS

SYMPTOMS	FREQUENCY	WHAT TO DO
Brain & nervous system:	None expected.	
Skin: Hives, rash, intense itch soon after a dose.	Rare	1
Eyes:	None expected.	
Ears, nose, throat: Dark or discolored tongue.	Common	5
Digestive: Mild nausea, vomiting, diarrhea.	Infrequent	4
Heart & lungs:	None expected.	
Blood vessels: Unexplained bleeding.	Rare	3
Muscles, bones, joints:	None expected.	
Genital, urinary:	None expected.	
Kidneys:	None expected.	
Liver:	None expected.	
Allergic: Life-threatening anaphylaxis may occur!	Rare	1 See Page 888.
Blood:	None expected.	
Others:	None expected.	

1- Life-threatening. Seek emergency treatment immediately.
2- Discontinue. Seek emergency treatment.
3- Discontinue. Call doctor right away.
4- Continue. Call doctor when convenient.
5- Continue. Tell doctor at next visit.
6- No action necessary.

WARNINGS & PRECAUTIONS

Don't take if:
You are allergic to cloxacillin, cephalosporin antibiotics, other penicillins or penicillamine. Life-threatening reaction may occur.

Before you start, consult your doctor:
If you are allergic to any substance or drug.

Over age 60:
You may have skin reactions, particularly around genitals and anus.

Pregnancy:
Studies inconclusive on harm to unborn child. Animal studies show fetal abnormalities. Decide with your doctor whether drug benefits justify risk to unborn child.

Breast-feeding:
Drug passes into milk. Child may become sensitive to penicillins and have allergic reactions to penicillin drugs. Avoid cloxacillin or discontinue nursing until you finish medicine. Consult doctor for advice on maintaining milk supply.

Infants & children:
No problems expected.

Prolonged use:
You may become more susceptible to infections caused by germs not responsive to cloxacillin.

Skin & sunlight:
No problems expected.

Driving, piloting or hazardous work:
Usually not dangerous. Most hazardous reactions likely to occur a few minutes after taking cloxacillin.

Airplane passengers:
No problems expected.

Discontinuing:
Don't discontinue without doctor's advice until you complete prescribed dose, even though symptoms diminish or disappear.

Others:
No problems expected.

INTERACTION WITH OTHER DRUGS

GENERIC NAME OR DRUG CLASS	COMBINED EFFECT
Chloramphenicol	Decreased effect of both drugs.
Erythromycins	Decreased effect of both drugs.
Paromomycin	Decreased effect of both drugs.
Tetracyclines	Decreased effect of both drugs.
Troleandomycin	Decreased effect of both drugs.

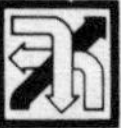

INTERACTION WITH OTHER SUBSTANCES

INTERACTS WITH	COMBINED EFFECT
Alcohol:	Occasional stomach irritation.
Beverages:	None expected.
Cocaine:	No proven problems.
Foods:	None expected.
Marijuana:	No proven problems.
Tobacco:	None expected.

COLCHICINE

BRAND NAMES

ColBenemid
Col-Probenecid
Novocolchine

GENERAL INFORMATION

Habit forming? No
Prescription needed? Yes
Available as generic? Yes
Drug class: Antigout

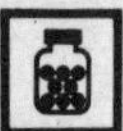

USES

Relieves joint pain, inflammation, swelling of gout.

DOSAGE & USAGE INFORMATION

How to take:

- Tablet—Swallow with liquid or food to lessen stomach irritation.
- Granules—Dissolve in 3 oz. of fluid. Drink all fluid.

When to take:
As prescribed. Stop taking when pain stops or at first sign of digestive upset. Wait at least 3 days between treatments.

If you forget a dose:
Don't double next dose. Consult doctor.

What drug does:
Decreases acidity of joint tissues and prevents deposits of uric-acid crystals.

Time lapse before drug works:
12 to 48 hours.

Don't take with:
See Interaction column and consult doctor.

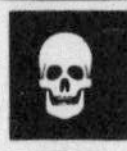

OVERDOSE

Symptoms:
Bloody urine, diarrhea, muscle weakness, fever, shortness of breath, stupor, convulsions, coma.

What to do:

- Dial 0 (operator) or 911 (emergency) for an ambulance or medical help. Then give first aid immediately.
- Additional emergency information on page 886.

POSSIBLE ADVERSE REACTIONS OR SIDE EFFECTS

SYMPTOMS	FREQUENCY	WHAT TO DO
Brain & nervous system:	None expected.	
Skin: Rash, itch.	Infrequent	3
Eyes:	None expected.	
Ears, nose, throat:	None expected.	
Digestive: Diarrhea, nausea, vomiting, abdominal pain.	Common	3
Heart & lungs:	None expected.	
Blood vessels: Unusual bruising.	Infrequent	3
Muscles, bones, joints: Numbness, tingling, pain, weakness in hands or feet.	Infrequent	4
Genital, urinary: Bloody urine.	Infrequent	3
Kidneys:	None expected.	
Liver: Jaundice (yellow eyes and skin).	Rare	3
Allergic: Life-threatening anaphylaxis (with injections).	Rare	1 See page 888.
Blood:	None expected.	
Others: Unusual tiredness or weakness, fever.	Infrequent	4

1- Life-threatening. Seek emergency treatment immediately.
2- Discontinue. Seek emergency treatment.
3- Discontinue. Call doctor right away.
4- Continue. Call doctor when convenient.
5- Continue. Tell doctor at next visit.
6- No action necessary.

WARNINGS & PRECAUTIONS

Don't take if:
You are allergic to colchicine.

Before you start, consult your doctor:
- If you have had peptic ulcers or ulcerative colitis.
- If you have heart, liver or kidney disease.
- If you will have surgery within 2 months, including dental surgery, requiring general or spinal anesthesia.

Over age 60:
Adverse reactions and side effects may be more frequent and severe than in younger persons. Colchicine has a narrow margin of safety for people in this age group.

Pregnancy:
Risk to unborn child outweighs drug benefits. Don't use.

Breast-feeding:
No problems expected, but consult doctor.

Infants & children:
Not recommended.

Prolonged use:
- Permanent hair loss.
- Anemia. Request blood counts.
- Numbness or tingling in hands and feet.

Skin & sunlight:
No problems expected.

Driving, piloting or hazardous work:
Don't drive or pilot aircraft until you learn how medicine affects you. Don't work around dangerous machinery. Don't climb ladders or work in high places. Danger increases if you drink alcohol or take medicine affecting alertness and reflexes, such as antihistamines, tranquilizers, sedatives, pain medicine, narcotics and mind-altering drugs.

Airplane passengers:
Carry drug with you to treat gout attacks while traveling.

Discontinuing:
- May be unnecessary to finish medicine. Follow doctor's instructions.
- Stop taking if digestive upsets occur before symptoms are relieved.

Others:
- Limit each course of treatment to 8 mg. Don't exceed 3 mg. per 24 hours.
- Possible sperm damage. May cause birth defects if child conceived while father taking colchicine.

INTERACTION WITH OTHER DRUGS

GENERIC NAME OR DRUG CLASS	COMBINED EFFECT
Amphetamines	Increased amphetamine effect.
Anticoagulants	Decreased anticoagulant effect.
Antidepressants	Oversedation.
Antihistamines	Oversedation.
Antihypertensives	Decreased antihypertensive effect.
Appetite suppressants	Increased suppressant effect.
Mind-altering drugs	Oversedation.
Narcotics	Oversedation.
Sedatives	Oversedation.
Sleep inducers	Oversedation.
Tranquilizers	Oversedation.

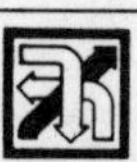

INTERACTION WITH OTHER SUBSTANCES

INTERACTS WITH	COMBINED EFFECT
Alcohol:	No proven problems.
Beverages: Herbal teas	Increased colchicine effect. Avoid.
Cocaine:	Overstimulation. Avoid.
Foods:	No proven problems.
Marijuana:	Decreased colchicine effect.
Tobacco:	No proven problems.

COLESTIPOL

BRAND NAMES

Colestid

GENERAL INFORMATION

Habit forming? No
Prescription needed? Yes
Available as generic? No
Drug class: Antihyperlipidemic

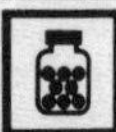

USES

- Reduces cholesterol level in blood in patients with type IIa hyperlipidemia.
- Treats overdose of digitalis.
- Reduces skin itching associated with some forms of liver disease.
- Treats diarrhea after some surgical operations.

DOSAGE & USAGE INFORMATION

How to take:
Mix well with 6 ounces or more or water or liquid, or in soups, pulpy fruits, with milk or in cereals. Will not dissolve.

When to take:
Before meals.

If you forget a dose:
Take as soon as you remember up to 2 hours late. If more than 2 hours, wait for next scheduled dose (don't double this dose).

What drug does:
Binds with bile acids in intestines, preventing reabsorption.

Time lapse before drug works:
3 to 12 months.

Don't take with:
See Interaction column and consult doctor.

OVERDOSE

Symptoms:
Fecal impaction.

What to do:
Overdose unlikely to threaten life. If person takes much larger amount than prescribed, call doctor, poison-control center or hospital emergency room for instructions.

POSSIBLE ADVERSE REACTIONS OR SIDE EFFECTS

SYMPTOMS	FREQUENCY	WHAT TO DO
Brain & nervous system:	None expected.	
Skin:	None expected.	
Eyes:	None expected.	
Ears, nose, throat:	None expected.	
Digestive:		
• Constipation	Infrequent	4
• Black, tarry stools from gastrointestinal bleeding.	Infrequent	2
• Severe abdominal pain.	Infrequent	3
• Belching	Infrequent	4
• Diarrhea	Infrequent	4
• Nausea	Infrequent	4
Heart & lungs:	None expected.	
Blood vessels:	None expected.	
Muscles, bones, joints:	None expected.	
Genital, urinary:	None expected.	
Kidneys, allergic, blood, liver:	None expected.	
Others:		
Unexpected weight loss.	Infrequent	4

1- Life-threatening. Seek emergency treatment immediately.
2- Discontinue. Seek emergency treatment.
3- Discontinue. Call doctor right away.
4- Continue. Call doctor when convenient.
5- Continue. Tell doctor at next visit.
6- No action necessary.

WARNINGS & PRECAUTIONS

Don't take if:
You are allergic to colestipol.

Before you start, consult your doctor:
- If you have liver disease such as cirrhosis.
- If you are jaundiced.
- If you will have surgery within 2 months, including dental surgery, requiring general or spinal anesthesia.
- If you are constipated.
- If you have peptic ulcer.
- If you have coronary artery disease.

Over age 60:
Constipation more likely. Other adverse effects more likely.

Pregnancy:
No proven harm to unborn child. Avoid if possible.

Breast-feeding:
No proven harm to child. Consult doctor.

Infants & children:
Only under expert medical supervision.

Prolonged use:
Request lab studies to determine serum cholesterol and serum triglycerides.

Skin & sunlight:
No problems expected.

Driving, piloting or hazardous work:
No problems expected.

Airplane passengers:
No problems expected.

Discontinuing:
Don't discontinue without consulting doctor. Dose may require gradual reduction if you have taken drug for a long time. Doses of other drugs may also require adjustment, particularly digitalis.

Others:
This medicine does not cure disorders, but helps to control them.

INTERACTION WITH OTHER DRUGS

GENERIC NAME OR DRUG CLASS	COMBINED EFFECT
Anticoagulants	Decreased anticoagulant effect.
Digitalis preparations	Decreased absorption.
Penicillins	Decreased absorption.
Tetracyclines	Decreased absorption.
Diuretics (thiazide)	Decreased absorption.
Vitamins	Decreased absorption of fat-soluble vitamins (A,D,E,K)
Other medicines	May delay or reduce absorption.

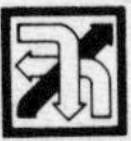

INTERACTION WITH OTHER SUBSTANCES

INTERACTS WITH	COMBINED EFFECT
Alcohol:	None expected.
Beverages:	None expected.
Cocaine:	None expected.
Foods:	Interferes with absorption of vitamins. Take supplements.
Marijuana:	None expected.
Tobacco:	None expected.

CONJUGATED ESTROGENS

BRAND NAMES

Premarin

GENERAL INFORMATION

Habit forming? No
Prescription needed? Yes
Available as generic? Yes
Drug class: Female sex hormone (estrogen)

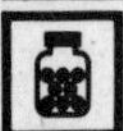

USES

- Treatment for symptoms of menopause and menstrual-cycle irregularity.
- Replacement for female hormone deficiency.
- Treatment for estrogen-deficiency osteoporosis (bone softening from calcium loss).
- Treatment for cancer of prostate and breast.

DOSAGE & USAGE INFORMATION

How to take:
- Tablet—Swallow with liquid. If you can't swallow whole, crumble tablet and take with liquid or food.
- Vaginal cream—Use as directed on label.

When to take:
At the same time each day.

If you forget a dose:
Take as soon as you remember up to 12 hours late. If more than 12 hours, wait for next scheduled dose (don't double this dose).

What drug does:
Restores normal estrogen level in tissues.

Time lapse before drug works:
10 to 20 days.

Don't take with:
See Interaction column and consult doctor.

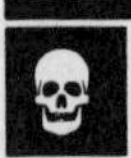

OVERDOSE

Symptoms:
Nausea, vomiting, fluid retention, breast enlargement and discomfort, abnormal vaginal bleeding.

What to do:
Overdose unlikely to threaten life. If person takes much larger amount than prescribed, call doctor, poison-control center or hospital emergency room for instructions.

POSSIBLE ADVERSE REACTIONS OR SIDE EFFECTS

SYMPTOMS	FREQUENCY	WHAT TO DO
Brain & nervous system:		
Depression, dizziness, irritability.	Infrequent	4
Skin:		
• Rash	Infrequent	3
• Brown blotches.	Infrequent	5
• Hair loss.	Infrequent	5
Eyes, ears, nose, throat, heart & lungs, muscles, bones, joints, kidneys, allergic, blood:	None expected.	
Digestive:		
• Stomach or side pain.	Infrequent	3
• Stomach cramps.	Common	3
• Appetite loss.	Common	4
• Nausea, diarrhea.	Common	5
• Vomiting	Infrequent	4
Blood vessels:		
Swollen ankles, feet.	Common	5
Genital, urinary:		
Vaginal discharge or bleeding.	Infrequent	5
Liver:		
Jaundice (yellow skin and eyes).	Rare	3
Others:		
• Breast lumps.	Infrequent	4
• Swollen, tender breasts.	Common	5
• Changes in sex drive.	Infrequent	5

1- Life-threatening. Seek emergency treatment immediately.
2- Discontinue. Seek emergency treatment.
3- Discontinue. Call doctor right away.
4- Continue. Call doctor when convenient.
5- Continue. Tell doctor at next visit.

CONJUGATED ESTROGENS

WARNINGS & PRECAUTIONS

Don't take if:
- You are allergic to any estrogen-containing drugs.
- You have impaired liver function.
- You have had blood clots, stroke or heart attack.
- You have unexplained vaginal bleeding.

Before you start, consult your doctor:
- If you have had cancer of breast or reproductive organs, fibrocystic breast disease, fibroid tumors of the uterus or endometriosis.
- If you have had migraine headaches, epilepsy or porphyria.
- If you have diabetes, high blood pressure, asthma, congestive heart failure, kidney disease or gallstones.
- If you plan to become pregnant within 3 months.

Over age 60:
Controversial. You and your doctor must decide if drug risks outweigh benefits.

Pregnancy:
Risk to unborn child outweighs drug benefits. Don't use.

Breast-feeding:
Drug filters into milk. May harm child. Avoid.

Infants & children:
Not recommended.

Prolonged use:
Increased growth of fibroid tumors of uterus. Possible association with cancer of uterus.

Skin & sunlight:
May cause rash or intensify sunburn in areas exposed to sun or sunlamp.

Driving, piloting or hazardous work:
No problems expected.

Airplane passengers:
No problems expected.

Discontinuing:
You may need to discontinue estrogen periodically. Consult your doctor.

Others:
In rare instances, may cause blood clot in lung, brain or leg. Symptoms are *sudden* severe headache, coordination loss, vision change, chest pain, breathing difficulty, slurred speech, pain in legs or groin. Seek emergency treatment immediately.

INTERACTION WITH OTHER DRUGS

GENERIC NAME OR DRUG CLASS	COMBINED EFFECT
Anticoagulants (oral)	Decreased anticoagulant effect.
Anticonvulsants (hydantoin)	Increased seizures.
Antidiabetics (oral)	Unpredictable increase or decrease in blood sugar.
Clofibrate	Decreased clofibrate effect.
Carbamazepine	Increased seizures.
Meprobamate	Increased effect of conjugated estrogens.
Phenobarbital	Decreased effect of conjugated estrogens.
Primidone	Decreased effect of conjugated estrogens.
Rifampin	Decreased effect of conjugated estrogens.
Thyroid hormones	Decreased thyroid effect.

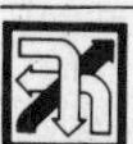

INTERACTION WITH OTHER SUBSTANCES

INTERACTS WITH	COMBINED EFFECT
Alcohol:	None expected.
Beverages:	None expected.
Cocaine:	No proven problems.
Foods:	None expected.
Marijuana:	Possible menstrual irregularities and bleeding between periods.
Tobacco:	Increased risk of blood clots leading to stroke or heart attack.

CONTRACEPTIVES (ORAL)

BRAND NAMES

Anoryol
Brevicon
Demulen
Enovid
Loestrin
Lo-Ovral
Micronor
Min-Ovral
Modacon
Modicon
Norlestrin
Norlinyl
Nor-Q.D.
Ortho-Novum
Ovcon
Ovral
Ovrette
Ovulen

GENERAL INFORMATION

Habit forming? No
Prescription needed? Yes
Available as generic? Yes
Drug class: Female sex hormone, contraceptive

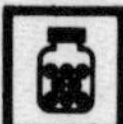

USES

- Prevents pregnancy.
- Regulates menstrual periods.

DOSAGE & USAGE INFORMATION

How to take:
Tablet or capsule—Swallow with liquid or food to lessen stomach irritation.

When to take:
At same time each day according to prescribed instructions, usually for 21 days of 28-day cycle.

If you forget a dose:
Call doctor's office for advice about additional protection against pregnancy.

What drug does:
- Alters mucus at cervix entrance to prevent sperm entry.
- Alters uterus lining to resist implantation of fertilized egg.
- Creates same chemical atmosphere in blood that exists during pregnancy, suppressing pituitary hormones which stimulate ovulation.

Time lapse before drug works:
10 days or more to provide contraception.

Don't take with:
- Tobacco
- See Interaction column and consult doctor.

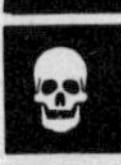

OVERDOSE

Symptoms:
Drowsiness

What to do:
Overdose unlikely to threaten life. If person takes much larger amount than prescribed, call doctor, poison-control center or hospital emergency room for instructions.

POSSIBLE ADVERSE REACTIONS OR SIDE EFFECTS

SYMPTOMS	FREQUENCY	WHAT TO DO
Brain & nervous system:		
• Headache, depression.	Infrequent	3
• Stroke	Rare	1
Skin:		
• Brown blotches.	Common	4
• Rash, hives, itch.	Rare	3
Eyes:		
Blue tinge to objects, lights.	Infrequent	4
Ears, nose, throat, kidneys, allergic:	None expected.	
Digestive:		
Appetite change, nausea, bloating, vomiting, pain.	Infrequent	4
Heart & lungs:		
Chest pain.	Rare	1
Blood vessels:		
Blood clots—Pain, swelling in leg.	Infrequent	3
Muscles, bones, joints:		
Muscle, joint pain.	Infrequent	3
Genital, urinary:		
Vaginal discharge, itch.	Common	4
Liver:		
Jaundice (yellow skin and eyes).	Rare	3
Blood:		
Clotting tendency.	Rare	2
Others:		
• Changed sex drive.	Infrequent	4
• Fluid retention.	Common	4

1- Life-threatening. Seek emergency treatment immediately.
2- Discontinue. Seek emergency treatment.
3- Discontinue. Call doctor right away.
4- Continue. Call doctor when convenient.

WARNINGS & PRECAUTIONS

Don't take if:
- You are allergic to any female hormone.
- You have had heart disease, blood clots or stroke.
- You have liver disease.
- You have cancer of breast, uterus or ovaries.
- You have unexplained vaginal bleeding.

Before you start, consult your doctor:
- If you have fibrocystic disease of breast.
- If you have migraine headaches.
- If you have fibroid tumors of uterus.
- If you have epilepsy.
- If you have asthma.
- If you have high blood pressure.
- If you will have surgery within 2 months, including dental surgery, requiring general or spinal anesthesia.
- If you have endometriosis.
- If you have diabetes.
- If you have sickle-cell anemia.
- If you smoke cigarettes.

Over age 60:
Not used.

Pregnancy:
May harm child. Discontinue at first sign of pregnancy.

Breast-feeding:
Drug passes into milk. Avoid drug or discontinue nursing.

Infants & children:
Not recommended.

Prolonged use:
- Gallstones
- Gradual blood-pressure rise.
- Possible difficulty becoming pregnant after discontinuing.

Skin & sunlight:
May cause rash or intensify sunburn in areas exposed to sun or sunlamp.

Driving, piloting or hazardous work:
No problems expected.

Airplane passengers:
No problems expected.

Discontinuing:
Don't become pregnant for 6 months after discontinuing.

Others:
Failure to take oral contraceptives for 1 day may cancel pregnancy protection. If you forget a dose, use other contraceptive measures and call doctor for instructions on re-starting oral contraceptive.

INTERACTION WITH OTHER DRUGS

GENERIC NAME OR DRUG CLASS	COMBINED EFFECT
Ampicillin	Decreased contraceptive effect.
Anticoagulants	Decreased anticoagulant effect.
Anticonvulsants (hydantoin)	Decreased contraceptive effect.
Antidiabetics	Decreased antidiabetic effect.
Antihistamines	Decreased contraceptive effect.
Antiinflammatory drugs (non-steroid)	Decreased contraceptive effect.
Barbiturates	Decreased contraceptive effect.
Chloramphenicol	Decreased contraceptive effect.
Clofibrate	Decreased clofibrate effect.
Guanethidine	Decreased guanethidine effect.
Meperidine	Increased meperidine effect.
Meprobamate	Decreased contraceptive effect.
Mineral oil	Decreased contraceptive effect.

Additional interactions on page 836.

INTERACTION WITH OTHER SUBSTANCES

INTERACTS WITH	COMBINED EFFECT
Alcohol:	No proven problems.
Beverages:	No proven problems.
Cocaine:	No proven problems.
Foods:	
Salt	Increased edema (fluid retention).
Marijuana:	Increased bleeding between periods. Avoid.
Tobacco:	Possible heart attack, blood clots and stroke.

CORTISONE

BRAND NAMES

Cortone

GENERAL INFORMATION

Habit forming? No
Prescription needed? Yes
Available as generic? Yes
Drug class: Cortisone drug (adrenal corticosteroid)

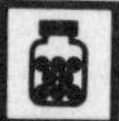

USES

- Reduces inflammation caused by many different medical problems.
- Treatment for some allergic diseases, blood disorders, kidney diseases, asthma and emphysema.
- Replaces corticosteroid deficiencies.

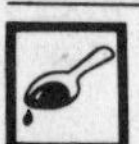

DOSAGE & USAGE INFORMATION

How to take:
Tablet—Swallow with liquid or food to lessen stomach irritation. If you can't swallow whole, crumble tablet and take with liquid or food.

When to take:
At the same times each day. Take once-a-day or once-every-other-day doses in mornings.

If you forget a dose:
- Several-doses-per-day prescription—Take as soon as you remember up to 2 hours late. If more than 2 hours, wait for next scheduled dose (don't double this dose).
- Once-a-day dose or less—Wait for next dose. Double this dose.

What drug does:
Decreases inflammatory responses.

Time lapse before drug works:
2 to 4 days.

Don't take with:
See Interaction column and consult doctor.

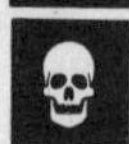

OVERDOSE

Symptoms:
Headache, convulsions, heart failure.

What to do:
- Dial 0 (operator) or 911 (emergency) for an ambulance or medical help. Then give first aid immediately.
- Additional emergency information on page 886.

POSSIBLE ADVERSE REACTIONS OR SIDE EFFECTS

SYMPTOMS	FREQUENCY	WHAT TO DO
Brain & nervous system:		
Mood changes, insomnia, restlessness.	Infrequent	4
Skin:		
• Acne	Common	4
• Rash	Rare	3
• Poor wound healing.	Common	4
Eyes:		
Blurred vision, halos around lights.	Infrequent	3
Ears, nose, throat:		
• Sore throat, fever.	Infrequent	3
• Thirst	Common	4
Digestive:		
• Indigestion, nausea, vomiting.	Common	4
• Bloody or black, tarry stool.	Infrequent	2
Heart & lungs:		
Irregular heartbeat.	Rare	2
Blood vessels, kidneys, liver, allergic, blood:	None expected.	
Muscles, bones, joints:		
Muscle cramps, swollen legs, feet.	Infrequent	3
Genital, urinary:		
Frequent urination.	Infrequent	4
Others:		
• Weight gain, round face.	Infrequent	4
• Fatigue, weakness.	Infrequent	4
• TB recurrence.	Infrequent	4
• Irregular menstrual periods.	Infrequent	4

1- Life-threatening. Seek emergency treatment immediately.
2- Discontinue. Seek emergency treatment.
3- Discontinue. Call doctor right away.
4- Continue. Call doctor when convenient.

WARNINGS & PRECAUTIONS

Don't take if:
- You are allergic to any cortisone drug.
- You have tuberculosis or fungus infection.
- You have herpes infection of eyes, lips or genitals.

Before you start, consult your doctor:
- If you have had tuberculosis.
- If you have congestive heart failure.
- If you have diabetes.
- If you have peptic ulcer.
- If you have glaucoma.
- If you have underactive thyroid.
- If you have high blood pressure.
- If you have myasthenia gravis.
- If you have blood clots in legs or lungs.

Over age 60:
Adverse reactions and side effects may be more frequent and severe than in younger persons. Likely to aggravate edema, diabetes or ulcers. Likely to cause cataracts and osteoporosis (softening of the bones).

Pregnancy:
Risk to unborn child outweighs drug benefits. Don't use.

Breast-feeding:
Drug passes into milk. Avoid drug or discontinue nursing until you finish medicine. Consult doctor for advice on maintaining milk supply.

Infants & children:
Use only under medical supervision.

Prolonged use:
- Retards growth in children.
- Possible glaucoma, cataracts, diabetes, fragile bones and thin skin.
- Functional dependence.

Skin & sunlight:
No problems expected.

Driving, piloting or hazardous work:
No problems expected.

Airplane passengers:
No problems expected.

Discontinuing:
- Don't discontinue without doctor's advice until you complete prescribed dose, even though symptoms diminish or disappear.
- Drug affects your response to surgery, illness, injury or stress for 2 years after discontinuing. Tell about drug to anyone who takes medical care of you within 2 years.

Others:
Avoid immunizations if possible.

INTERACTION WITH OTHER DRUGS

GENERIC NAME OR DRUG CLASS	COMBINED EFFECT
Amphoterecin B	Potassium depletion.
Anticholinergics	Possible glaucoma.
Anticoagulants (oral)	Decreased anticoagulant effect.
Anticonvulsants (hydantoin)	Decreased cortisone effect.
Antidiabetics (oral)	Decreased antidiabetic effect.
Antihistamines	Decreased cortisone effect.
Aspirin	Increased cortisone effect.
Barbiturates	Decreased cortisone effect. Oversedation.
Beta-adrenergic blockers	Decreased cortisone effect.
Chloral hydrate	Decreased cortisone effect.
Chlorthalidone	Potassium depletion.
Cholinergics	Decreased cholinergic effect.
Contraceptives (oral)	Increased cortisone effect.
Digitalis preparations	Dangerous potassium depletion. Possible digitalis toxicity.
Diuretics (thiazide)	Potassium depletion.

Additional interactions on page 836.

INTERACTION WITH OTHER SUBSTANCES

INTERACTS WITH	COMBINED EFFECT
Alcohol:	Risk of stomach ulcers.
Beverages:	No proven problems.
Cocaine:	Overstimulation. Avoid.
Foods:	No proven problems.
Marijuana:	Decreased immunity.
Tobacco:	Increased cortisone effect. Possible toxicity.

CROMOLYN

BRAND NAMES

Fivent
Intal
Nalcrom
Nasalcrom
Opticrom
Rynacrom

GENERAL INFORMATION

Habit forming? No
Prescription needed? Yes
Available as generic? No
Drug class: Antiasthmatic

USES

Prevents asthma attacks. Will not stop an active asthma attack.

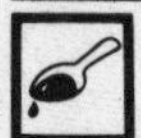

DOSAGE & USAGE INFORMATION

How to take:
Inhaler—Follow instructions enclosed with inhaler. Don't swallow cartridges for inhaler. Gargle and rinse mouth after inhalations.

When to take:
At the same times each day. If you also use a bronchodilator inhaler, use the bronchodilator before the cromolyn.

If you forget a dose:
Take as soon as you remember up to 2 hours late. If more than 2 hours, wait for next scheduled dose (don't double this dose).

What drug does:
Prevents constriction of bronchial tubes by blocking histamine release from mast cells. Has no direct bronchodilator, antihistamine or antiinflammatory action.

Time lapse before drug works:
4 weeks.

Don't take with:
See Interaction column and consult doctor.

OVERDOSE

Symptoms:
Increased side effects and adverse reactions listed.

What to do:
Overdose unlikely to threaten life. If person inhales much larger amount than prescribed, call doctor, poison-control center or hospital emergency room for instructions.

POSSIBLE ADVERSE REACTIONS OR SIDE EFFECTS

SYMPTOMS	FREQUENCY	WHAT TO DO
Brain & nervous system:		
Drowsiness, dizziness, headache.	Infrequent	4
Skin:		
Rash, hives.	Infrequent	3
Eyes:		
Watering	Infrequent	4
Ears, nose, throat:		
• Swallowing difficulty.	Infrequent	3
• Hoarseness	Common	4
• Stuffy nose, throat irritation.	Infrequent	4
• Nosebleed	Rare	4
Digestive:		
Nausea, vomiting.	Infrequent	3
Heart & lungs:		
• Increased wheezing.	Infrequent	3
• Cough	Common	4
Blood vessels, kidneys, liver, blood:	None expected.	
Muscles, bones, joints:		
• Joint pain or swelling.	Infrequent	3
• Muscle pain, weakness.	Infrequent	3
Genital, urinary:		
Difficult or painful urination.	Infrequent	3
Allergic:		
Life-threatening anaphylaxis may occur.	Rare	1 See page 888.

1- Life-threatening. Seek emergency treatment immediately.
2- Discontinue. Seek emergency treatment.
3- Discontinue. Call doctor right away.
4- Continue. Call doctor when convenient.

WARNINGS & PRECAUTIONS

Don't take if:
You are allergic to cromolyn, lactose, milk or milk products.

Before you start, consult your doctor:
- If you plan to become pregnant within medication period.
- If you have kidney or liver disease.

Over age 60:
Adverse reactions and side effects may be more frequent and severe than in younger persons.

Pregnancy:
Risk to unborn child outweighs drug benefits. Don't use.

Breast-feeding:
Drug passes into milk. Avoid drug or discontinue nursing.

Infants & children:
Use only under medical supervision.

Prolonged use:
No problems expected.

Skin & sunlight:
No problems expected.

Driving, piloting or hazardous work:
No problems expected.

Airplane passengers:
No problems expected.

Discontinuing:
No problems expected.

Others:
- Inhaler must be cleaned and work well for drug to be effective.
- This treatment does not stop an acute asthma attack. It may aggravate it.

INTERACTION WITH OTHER DRUGS

GENERIC NAME OR DRUG CLASS	COMBINED EFFECT
Cortisone drugs	Increased cortisone effect in treating asthma. Cortisone dose may be decreased.

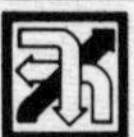

INTERACTION WITH OTHER SUBSTANCES

INTERACTS WITH	COMBINED EFFECT
Alcohol:	None expected.
Beverages:	None expected.
Cocaine:	None expected.
Foods:	None expected.
Marijuana:	None expected.
Tobacco:	None expected, but tobacco smoke aggravates asthma. Avoid.

CYCLACILLIN

BRAND NAMES

Cyclapen-W

GENERAL INFORMATION

Habit forming? No
Prescription needed? Yes
Available as generic? Yes
Drug class: Antibiotic (penicillin)

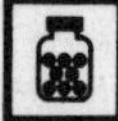

USES

Treatment of bacterial infections that are susceptible to cyclacillin.

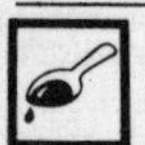

DOSAGE & USAGE INFORMATION

How to take:

- Tablets or capsules—Swallow with liquid on an empty stomach 1 hour before or 2 hours after eating.
- Liquid—Take with cold beverage. Liquid form is perishable and effective for only 7 days at room temperature. Effective for 14 days if stored in refrigerator. Don't freeze.

When to take:
Follow instructions on prescription label or side of package. Doses should be evenly spaced. For example, 4 times a day means every 6 hours.

If you forget a dose:
Take as soon as you remember. Continue regular schedule.

What drug does:
Destroys susceptible bacteria. Does not kill viruses.

Time lapse before drug works:
May be several days before medicine affects infection.

Don't take with:
See Interaction column and consult doctor.

OVERDOSE

Symptoms:
Severe diarrhea, nausea or vomiting.

What to do:
Overdose unlikely to threaten life. If person takes much larger amount than prescribed, call doctor, poison-control center or hospital emergency room for instructions.

POSSIBLE ADVERSE REACTIONS OR SIDE EFFECTS

SYMPTOMS	FREQUENCY	WHAT TO DO
Brain & nervous system:	None expected.	
Skin: Hives, rash, intense itch soon after a dose.	Rare	1
Eyes:	None expected.	
Ears, nose, throat: Dark or discolored tongue.	Common	5
Digestive: Mild nausea, vomiting, diarrhea.	Infrequent	4
Heart & lungs:	None expected.	
Blood vessels: Unexplained bleeding.	Rare	3
Muscles, bones, joints:	None expected.	
Genital, urinary:	None expected.	
Kidneys:	None expected.	
Liver:	None expected.	
Allergic: Life-threatening anaphylaxis may occur!	Rare	1 See page 888.
Blood:	None expected.	
Others:	None expected.	

1- Life-threatening. Seek emergency treatment immediately.
2- Discontinue. Seek emergency treatment.
3- Discontinue. Call doctor right away.
4- Continue. Call doctor when convenient.
5- Continue. Tell doctor at next visit.
6- No action necessary.

WARNINGS & PRECAUTIONS

Don't take if:
Your are allergic to cyclacillin, cephalosporin antibiotics, other penicillins or penicillamine. Life-threatening reaction may occur.

Before you start, consult your doctor:
If you are allergic to any substance or drug.

Over age 60:
You may have skin reactions, particularly around genitals and anus.

Pregnancy:
Studies inconclusive on harm to unborn child. Animal studies show fetal abnormalities. Decide with your doctor whether drug benefits justify risk to unborn child.

Breast-feeding:
Drug passes into milk. Child may become sensitive to penicillins and have allergic reactions to penicillin drugs. Avoid cyclacillin or discontinue nursing until you finish medicine. Consult doctor for advice on maintaining milk supply.

Infants & children:
No problems expected.

Prolonged use:
You may become more susceptible to infections caused by germs not responsive to cyclacillin.

Skin & sunlight:
No problems expected.

Driving, piloting or hazardous work:
Usually not dangerous. Most hazardous reactions likely to occur a few minutes after taking cyclacillin.

Airplane passengers:
No problems expected.

Discontinuing:
Don't discontinue without doctor's advice until you complete prescribed dose, even though symptoms diminish or disappear.

Others:
No problems expected.

INTERACTION WITH OTHER DRUGS

GENERIC NAME OR DRUG CLASS	COMBINED EFFECT
Chloramphenicol	Decreased effect of both drugs.
Erythromycins	Decreased effect of both drugs.
Paromomycin	Decreased effect of both drugs.
Tetracyclines	Decreased effect of both drugs.
Troleandomycin	Decreased effect of both drugs.

INTERACTION WITH OTHER SUBSTANCES

INTERACTS WITH	COMBINED EFFECT
Alcohol:	Occasional stomach irritation.
Beverages:	None expected.
Cocaine:	No proven problems.
Foods:	Decreased effect of cyclacillin.
Marijuana:	No proven problems.
Tobacco:	None expected.

CYCLANDELATE

BRAND NAMES

Cyclospasmol
Cyraso-400

GENERAL INFORMATION

Habit forming? No
Prescription needed? U.S.: Yes
Canada: No
Available as generic? Yes
Drug class: Vasodilator

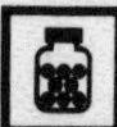

USES

Improves poor blood flow to brain and extremities.

DOSAGE & USAGE INFORMATION

How to take:
Tablet or capsule—Swallow with liquid. If you can't swallow whole, crumble tablet or open capsule and take with liquid or food.

When to take:
At the same time each day.

If you forget a dose:
Take as soon as you remember up to 2 hours late. If more than 2 hours, wait for next scheduled dose (don't double this dose).

What drug does:
Increases blood flow by relaxing and expanding blood-vessel walls.

Time lapse before drug works:
3 weeks.

Don't take with:
See Interaction column and consult doctor.

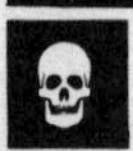

OVERDOSE

Symptoms:
Severe headache, dizziness; nausea, vomiting; flushed, hot face.

What to do:
Overdose unlikely to threaten life. If person takes much larger amount than prescribed, call doctor, poison-control center or hospital emergency room for instructions.

POSSIBLE ADVERSE REACTIONS OR SIDE EFFECTS

SYMPTOMS	FREQUENCY	WHAT TO DO
Brain & nervous system: Dizziness, headache, weakness.	Infrequent	4
Skin: Flushed face.	Infrequent	4
Eyes:	None expected.	
Ears, nose, throat:	None expected.	
Digestive: Belching, heartburn, nausea or stomach pain.	Infrequent	5
Heart & lungs: Rapid heartbeat.	Infrequent	3
Blood vessels:	None expected.	
Muscles, bones, joints: Tingling in face, fingers or toes.	Infrequent	4
Genital, urinary:	None expected.	
Kidneys:	None expected.	
Liver:	None expected.	
Allergic:	None expected.	
Blood:	None expected.	
Others: Unusual sweating.	Infrequent	4

1-Life-threatening. Seek emergency treatment immediately.
2-Discontinue. Seek emergency treatment.
3-Discontinue. Call doctor right away.
4-Continue. Call doctor when convenient.
5-Continue. Tell doctor at next visit.
6-No action necessary.

WARNINGS & PRECAUTIONS

Don't take if:
You have had allergic reaction to cyclandelate.

Before you start, consult your doctor:
- If you have glaucoma.
- If you have had heart attack or stroke.

Over age 60:
Adverse reactions and side effects may be more frequent and severe than in younger persons.

Pregnancy:
No proven harm to unborn child. Avoid if possible.

Breast-feeding:
No proven problems. Consult doctor.

Infants & children:
Not recommended.

Prolonged use:
No problems expected.

Skin & sunlight:
No problems expected.

Driving, piloting or hazardous work:
Avoid if you feel dizzy or weak. Otherwise, no problems expected.

Airplane passengers:
No problems expected.

Discontinuing:
Don't discontinue without doctor's advice until you complete prescribed dose, even though symptoms diminish or disappear.

Others:
Response to drug varies. If your symptoms don't improve after 3 weeks of use, consult doctor.

INTERACTION WITH OTHER DRUGS

GENERIC NAME OR DRUG CLASS	COMBINED EFFECT
None	

INTERACTION WITH OTHER SUBSTANCES

INTERACTS WITH	COMBINED EFFECT
Alcohol:	None expected.
Beverages:	None expected.
Cocaine:	Decreased cyclandelate effect. Avoid.
Foods:	None expected.
Marijuana:	None expected.
Tobacco:	May decrease cyclandelate effect.

CYCLIZINE

BRAND NAMES

Marezine

GENERAL INFORMATION

Habit forming? No
Prescription needed? U.S.: No
Canada: Yes
Available as generic? No
Drug class: Antihistamine, antiemetic

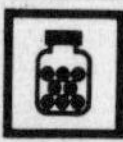

USES

Prevents motion sickness.

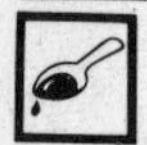

DOSAGE & USAGE INFORMATION

How to take:
Tablet—Swallow with liquid or food to lessen stomach irritation. If you can't swallow whole, crumble tablet and chew or take with liquid or food.

When to take:
30 minutes to 1 hour before traveling.

If you forget a dose:
Take as soon as you remember. Wait 4 hours for next dose.

What drug does:
Reduces sensitivity of nerve endings in inner ear, blocking messages to brain's vomiting center.

Time lapse before drug works:
30 to 60 minutes.

Don't take with:
See Interaction column and consult doctor.

OVERDOSE

Symptoms:
Drowsiness, confusion, incoordination, stupor, coma, weak pulse, shallow breathing.

What to do:
- Dial 0 (operator) or 911 (emergency) for an ambulance or medical help. Then give first aid immediately.
- Additional emergency information on page 886.

POSSIBLE ADVERSE REACTIONS OR SIDE EFFECTS

SYMPTOMS	FREQUENCY	WHAT TO DO
Brain & nervous system:		
• Drowsiness	Common	5
• Headache	Infrequent	4
• Restlessness, excitement, insomnia.	Rare	4
Skin:		
Rash or hives.	Rare	3
Eyes:		
Blurred vision.	Rare	4
Ears, nose, throat:		
Dry mouth, nose, throat.	Infrequent	5
Digestive:		
• Appetite loss, nausea.	Rare	5
• Diarrhea or constipation.	Infrequent	4
Heart & lungs:		
Fast heartbeat.	Infrequent	4
Blood vessels:	None expected.	
Muscles, bones, joints:	None expected.	
Genital, urinary:		
Urinary frequency, difficult urination.	Rare	4
Kidneys:	None expected.	
Liver:		
Jaundice (yellow eyes and skin).	Rare	3
Allergic:	None expected.	
Blood:	None expected.	
Others:	None expected.	

1- Life-threatening. Seek emergency treatment immediately.
2- Discontinue. Seek emergency treatment.
3- Discontinue. Call doctor right away.
4- Continue. Call doctor when convenient.
5- Continue. Tell doctor at next visit.

WARNINGS & PRECAUTIONS

Don't take if:
- You are allergic to meclizine, buclizine or cyclizine.
- You have taken MAO inhibitors in the past 2 weeks.

Before you start, consult your doctor:
- If you have glaucoma.
- If you have prostate enlargement.
- If you have reacted badly to any antihistamine.

Over age 60:
Adverse reactions and side effects may be more frequent and severe than in younger persons, especially impaired urination from enlarged prostate gland.

Pregnancy:
Studies inconclusive on harm to unborn child. Animal studies show fetal abnormalities. Decide with your doctor whether drug benefits justify risk to unborn child.

Breast-feeding:
Drug passes into milk. Avoid drug or discontinue nursing until you finish medicine. Consult doctor for advice on maintaining milk supply.

Infants & children:
No problems expected.

Prolonged use:
No problems expected.

Skin & sunlight:
No problems expected.

Driving, piloting or hazardous work:
Don't fly aircraft. Don't drive until you learn how medicine affects you. Don't work around dangerous machinery. Don't climb ladders or work in high places. Danger increases if you drink alcohol or take medicine affecting alertness and reflexes, such as antihistamines, tranquilizers, sedatives, pain medicine, narcotics and mind-altering drugs.

Airplane passengers:
Take 30 minutes before takeoff and every 4 hours while in the air.

Discontinuing:
No problems expected.

Others:
No problems expected.

INTERACTION WITH OTHER DRUGS

GENERIC NAME OR DRUG CLASS	COMBINED EFFECT
Amphetamines	May decrease drowsiness caused by cyclizine.
Anticholinergics	Increased effect of both drugs.
Antidepressants (tricyclic)	Increased effect of both drugs.
MAO inhibitors	Increased cyclizine effect.
Narcotics	Increased effect of both drugs.
Pain relievers	Increased effect of both drugs.
Sedatives	Increased effect of both drugs.
Sleep inducers	Increased effect of both drugs.
Tranquilizers	Increased effect of both drugs.

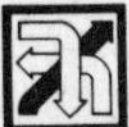

INTERACTION WITH OTHER SUBSTANCES

INTERACTS WITH	COMBINED EFFECT
Alcohol:	Increased sedation. Avoid.
Beverages: Caffeine drinks	May decrease drowsiness.
Cocaine:	None expected.
Foods:	None expected.
Marijuana:	Increased drowsiness, dry mouth.
Tobacco:	None expected.

CYCLOBENZAPRINE

BRAND NAMES

Flexeril

GENERAL INFORMATION

Habit forming? No
Prescription needed? Yes
Available as generic? No
Drug class: Muscle relaxant (skeletal)

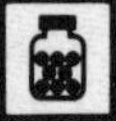

USES

Treatment for pain and limited motion caused by spasms in voluntary muscles.

DOSAGE & USAGE INFORMATION

How to take:
Tablet or capsule—Swallow with liquid.

When to take:
At the same time each day or according to label instructions.

If you forget a dose:
Take as soon as you remember. Wait 4 hours for next dose.

What drug does:
Blocks body's pain messages to brain. May also sedate.

Time lapse before drug works:
30 to 60 minutes.

Don't take with:
- Non-prescription drugs without consulting doctor.
- See Interaction column and consult doctor.

OVERDOSE

Symptoms:
Drowsiness, confusion, difficulty concentrating, visual problems, vomiting, blood-pressure drop, low body temperature, weak and rapid pulse, convulsions, coma.

What to do:
- Dial 0 (operator) or 911 (emergency) for an ambulance or medical help. Then give first aid immediately.
- If patient is unconscious and not breathing, give mouth-to-mouth breathing. If there is no heartbeat, use cardiac massage and mouth-to-mouth breathing (CPR). Don't try to make patient vomit. If you can't get help quickly, take patient to nearest emergency facility.
- Additional emergency information on page 886.

POSSIBLE ADVERSE REACTIONS OR SIDE EFFECTS

SYMPTOMS	FREQUENCY	WHAT TO DO
Brain & nervous system:		
• Drowsiness, dizziness.	Common	4
• Unsteadiness, confusion, depression, hallucinations.	Rare	3
Skin:		
Rash, itch, swelling.	Rare	3
Eyes:		
Blurred vision.	Infrequent	3
Ears, nose, throat:		
• Dry mouth.	Common	4
• Bad taste in mouth.	Infrequent	4
Digestive:	None expected.	
Heart & lungs:		
• Breathing difficulty.	Rare	3
• Fast heartbeat.	Infrequent	3
Blood vessels:	None expected.	
Muscles, bones, joints:	None expected.	
Genital, urinary:		
Difficulty urinating.	Rare	4
Kidneys:	None expected.	
Liver:	None expected.	
Allergic:	None expected.	
Blood:	None expected.	
Others:		
Insomnia, numbness in extremities.	Infrequent	4

1- Life-threatening. Seek emergency treatment immediately.
2- Discontinue. Seek emergency treatment.
3- Discontinue. Call doctor right away.
4- Continue. Call doctor when convenient.
5- Continue. Tell doctor at next visit.
6- No action necessary.

WARNINGS & PRECAUTIONS

Don't take if:
- You are allergic to any skeletal-muscle relaxant.
- You have taken MAO inhibitors in last 2 weeks.
- You have had a heart attack within 6 weeks, or suffer from congestive heart failure.
- You have overactive thyroid.

Before you start, consult your doctor:
- If you have a heart problem.
- If you have reacted to tricyclic antidepressants.
- If you have glaucoma.
- If you have a prostate condition and urination difficulty.
- If you intend to pilot aircraft.

Over age 60:
Adverse reactions and side effects may be more frequent and severe than in younger persons. Avoid extremes of heat and cold.

Pregnancy:
Risk to unborn child outweighs drug benefits. Don't use.

Breast-feeding:
Drug passes into milk. Avoid drug or discontinue nursing until you finish medicine. Consult doctor for advice on maintaining milk supply.

Infants & children:
Don't use for children younger than 15.

Prolonged use:
No problems expected.

Skin & sunlight:
May cause rash or intensify sunburn in areas exposed to sun or sunlamp.

Driving, piloting or hazardous work:
Don't drive or pilot aircraft until you learn how medicine affects you. Don't work around dangerous machinery. Don't climb ladders or work in high places. Danger increases if you drink alcohol or take medicine affecting alertness and reflexes.

Airplane passengers:
Possible side effects may make flying difficult. Consult your doctor.

Discontinuing:
May be unnecessary to finish medicine. Follow doctor's instructions.

Others:
No problems expected.

INTERACTION WITH OTHER DRUGS

GENERIC NAME OR DRUG CLASS	COMBINED EFFECT
Anticholinergics	Increased anticholinergic effect.
Antidepressants	Increased sedation.
Antihistamines	Increased antihistamine effect.
Clonidine	Decreased clonidine effect.
Guanethidine	Decreased guanethidine effect.
MAO inhibitors	High fever, convulsions, possible death.
Mind-altering drugs	Increased mind-altering effect.
Narcotics	Increased sedation.
Pain relievers	Increased pain reliever effect.
Rauwolfia alkaloids	Decreased effect of rauwolfia alkaloids.
Sedatives	Increased sedative effect.
Sleep inducers	Increased sedation.
Tranquilizers	Increased tranquilizer effect.

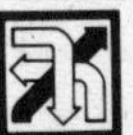

INTERACTION WITH OTHER SUBSTANCES

INTERACTS WITH	COMBINED EFFECT
Alcohol:	Depressed brain function. Avoid.
Beverages:	None expected.
Cocaine:	Decreased cyclobenzaprine effect.
Foods:	None expected.
Marijuana:	Occasional use—Drowsiness. Frequent use—Severe mental and physical impairment.
Tobacco:	None expected.

CYCLOPHOSPHAMIDE

BRAND NAMES

Cytoxan
Neosar
Procytox

GENERAL INFORMATION

Habit forming? No
Prescription needed? Yes
Available as generic? No
Drug class: Immunosuppressant

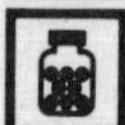

USES

- Treatment for cancer.
- Treatment for severe rheumatoid arthritis.
- Treatment for blood-vessel disease.
- Treatment for skin disease.

DOSAGE & USAGE INFORMATION

How to take:
Tablet—Swallow with liquid. If you can't swallow whole, crumble tablet and take with liquid or food.

When to take:
Works best if taken first thing in morning. However, may take with food to lessen stomach irritation. Don't take at bedtime.

If you forget a dose:
Take as soon as you remember up to 12 hours late. If more than 12 hours, wait for next scheduled dose (don't double this dose).

What drug does:
- Kills cancer cells.
- Suppresses spread of cancer cells.
- Suppresses immune system.

Time lapse before drug works:
7 to 10 days continual use.

Don't take with:
See Interaction column and consult doctor.

OVERDOSE

Symptoms:
Bloody urine, water retention, weight gain, severe infection.

What to do:
Overdose unlikely to threaten life. If person takes much larger amount than prescribed, call doctor, poison-control center or hospital emergency room for instructions.

POSSIBLE ADVERSE REACTIONS OR SIDE EFFECTS

SYMPTOMS	FREQUENCY	WHAT TO DO
Brain & nervous system:		
Confusion, agitation, headache, dizziness.	Infrequent	4
Skin:		
• Rash, hives, itch.	Infrequent	3
• Flushed face.	Infrequent	4
• Dark skin, nails.	Common	4
Eyes:		
Blurred vision.	Rare	4
Ears, nose, throat:		
• Sore throat, fever.	Common	3
• Mouth, lip sores.	Rare	3
Digestive:		
• Black stool.	Rare	3
• Nausea, appetite loss, vomiting.	Common	4
• Stomach pain.	Infrequent	4
Heart & lungs:		
Shortness of breath, rapid heartbeat, cough.	Infrequent	3
Blood vessels, allergic, liver:	None expected.	
Muscles, bones, joints:		
Joint pain.	Infrequent	4
Genital, urinary:		
• Bloody urine, painful urination.	Infrequent	3
• More urination.	Rare	4
Kidneys:		
Pain in side.	Infrequent	3
Blood:		
Bleeding, bruising.	Infrequent	3
Others:		
• Missed period.	Common	4
• Fatigue, weakness.	Infrequent	4
• Unusual thirst.	Rare	3
• More sweating.	Infrequent	3

1- Life-threatening. Seek emergency treatment immediately.
2- Discontinue. Seek emergency treatment.
3- Discontinue. Call doctor right away.
4- Continue. Call doctor when convenient.

CYCLOPHOSPHAMIDE

WARNINGS & PRECAUTIONS

Don't take if:
- You are allergic to any alkylating agent.
- You have an infection.
- You have bloody urine.
- You will have surgery within 2 months, including dental surgery, requiring general or spinal anesthesia.

Before you start, consult your doctor:
- If you have impaired liver or kidney function.
- If you have impaired bone-marrow or blood-cell production.
- If you have had chemotherapy or X-ray therapy.
- If you have taken cortisone drugs in the past year.

Over age 60:
Adverse reactions and side effects may be more frequent and severe than in younger persons. To reduce risk of chemical bladder inflammation, drink 8 to 10 glasses of water daily.

Pregnancy:
Risk to unborn child outweighs drug benefits. Don't use.

Breast-feeding:
Drug passes into milk. Avoid drug or discontinue nursing until you finish medicine. Consult doctor for advice on maintaining milk supply.

Infants & children:
Use only under medical supervision.

Prolonged use:
- Development of fibrous lung tissue.
- Possible jaundice (yellow skin and eyes).
- Swelling of feet, lower legs.

Skin & sunlight:
No problems expected.

Driving, piloting or hazardous work:
Avoid if you feel dizzy or have blurred vision. Otherwise, no problems expected.

Airplane passengers:
No problems expected.

Discontinuing:
Don't discontinue without consulting doctor. Dose may require gradual reduction if you have taken drug for a long time. Doses of other drugs may also require adjustment.

Others:
Frequently causes hair loss. After treatment ends, hair should grow back.

INTERACTION WITH OTHER DRUGS

GENERIC NAME OR DRUG CLASS	COMBINED EFFECT
Allopurinol	Possible anemia.
Antidiabetics (oral)	Increased antidiabetic effect.
Insulin	Increased insulin effect.
Phenobarbital	Increased cyclophosphamide effect.

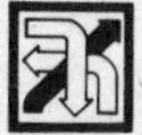

INTERACTION WITH OTHER SUBSTANCES

INTERACTS WITH	COMBINED EFFECT
Alcohol:	No problems expected.
Beverages:	No problems expected. Drink at least 2 quarts fluid every day.
Cocaine:	None expected.
Foods:	None expected.
Marijuana:	Increased impairment of immunity.
Tobacco:	None expected.

CYCLOTHIAZIDE

BRAND NAMES

Anhydron
Fluidil

GENERAL INFORMATION

Habit forming? No
Prescription needed? Yes
Available as generic? Yes
Drug class: Antihypertensive, diuretic (thiazide)

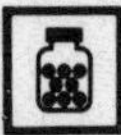

USES

- Controls, but doesn't cure, high blood pressure.
- Reduces fluid retention (edema) caused by conditions such as heart disorders and liver disease.

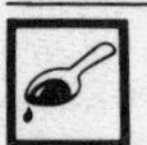

DOSAGE & USAGE INFORMATION

How to take:
Tablet or capsule—Swallow with liquid. If you can't swallow whole, crumble tablet or open capsule and take with liquid or food.

When to take:
At the same time each day.

If you forget a dose:
Take as soon as you remember up to 2 hours late. If more than 2 hours, wait for next scheduled dose (don't double this dose).

What drug does:
- Forces sodium and water excretion, reducing body fluid.
- Relaxes muscle cells of small arteries.
- Reduced body fluid and relaxed arteries lower blood pressure.

Time lapse before drug works:
4 to 6 hours. May require several weeks to lower blood pressure.

Don't take with:
- See Interaction column and consult doctor.
- Non-prescription drugs without consulting doctor.

OVERDOSE

Symptoms:
Cramps, weakness, drowsiness, weak pulse, coma.

What to do:
- Dial 0 (operator) or 911 (emergency) for an ambulance or medical help. Then give first aid immediately.
- Additional emergency information on page 886.

POSSIBLE ADVERSE REACTIONS OR SIDE EFFECTS

SYMPTOMS	FREQUENCY	WHAT TO DO
Brain & nervous system:		
• Dizziness	Infrequent	4
• Mood changes.	Infrequent	4
• Headaches	Infrequent	4
Skin:		
Rash or hives.	Rare	2
Eyes:		
Blurred vision.	Infrequent	3
Ears, nose, throat:		
• Sore throat, fever.	Rare	3
• Dry mouth, thirst.	Infrequent	5
Digestive:		
Severe abdominal pain, nausea, vomiting.	Infrequent	3
Heart & lungs:		
Irregular heartbeat, weak pulse.	Infrequent	3
Blood vessels:	None expected.	
Muscles, bones, joints:		
Weakness, tiredness.	Infrequent	4
Genital, urinary:	None expected.	
Kidneys:	None expected.	
Liver:		
Jaundice (yellow skin and eyes).	Rare	3
Blood:	None expected.	
Others:		
Weight changes.	Infrequent	4

1- Life-threatening. Seek emergency treatment immediately.
2- Discontinue. Seek emergency treatment.
3- Discontinue. Call doctor right away.
4- Continue. Call doctor when convenient.
5- Continue. Tell doctor at next visit.
6- No action necessary.

WARNINGS & PRECAUTIONS

Don't take if:
You are allergic to any thiazide diuretic drugs.

Before you start, consult your doctor:
- If you are allergic to any sulfa drug.
- If you have gout.
- If you have liver, pancreas or kidney disorder.

Over age 60:
Adverse reactions and side effects may be more frequent and severe than in younger persons, especially dizziness and excessive potassium loss.

Pregnancy:
Risk to unborn child outweighs drug benefits. Don't use.

Breast-feeding:
Drug passes into milk. Avoid drug or discontinue nursing.

Infants & children:
No problems expected.

Prolonged use:
You may need medicine to treat high blood pressure for the rest of your life.

Skin & sunlight:
May cause rash or intensify sunburn in areas exposed to sun or sunlamp.

Driving, piloting or hazardous work:
Don't drive or pilot aircraft until you learn how medicine affects you. Don't work around dangerous machinery. Don't climb ladders or work in high places. Danger increases if you drink alcohol or take medicine affecting alertness and reflexes, such as antihistamines, tranquilizers, sedatives, pain medicine, narcotics and mind-altering drugs.

Airplane passengers:
No problems expected.

Discontinuing:
Don't discontinue without medical advice.

Others:
- Hot weather and fever may cause dehydration and drop in blood pressure. Dose may require temporary adjustment. Weigh daily and report any unexpected weight decreases to your doctor.
- May cause rise in uric acid, leading to gout.
- May cause blood-sugar rise in diabetics.

INTERACTION WITH OTHER DRUGS

GENERIC NAME OR DRUG CLASS	COMBINED EFFECT
Allopurinol	Decreased allopurinol effect.
Antidepressants (tricyclic)	Dangerous drop in blood pressure. Avoid combination unless under medical supervision.
Barbiturates	Increased cyclothiazide effect.
Cholestyramine	Decreased cyclothiazide effect.
Cortisone drugs	Excessive potassium loss that causes dangerous heart rhythms.
Digitalis preparations	Excessive potassium loss that causes dangerous heart rhythms.
Diuretics (thiazide)	Increased effect of other thiazide diuretics.
Lithium	Increased effect of lithium.
MAO inhibitors	Increased cyclothiazide effect.
Probenecid	Decreased probenecid effect.

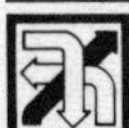

INTERACTION WITH OTHER SUBSTANCES

INTERACTS WITH	COMBINED EFFECT
Alcohol:	Dangerous blood-pressure drop.
Beverages:	None expected.
Cocaine:	None expected.
Foods:	
Licorice	Excessive potassium loss that causes dangerous heart rhythms.
Marijuana:	May increase blood pressure.
Tobacco:	None expected.

CYCRIMINE

BRAND NAMES

Pagitane

GENERAL INFORMATION

Habit forming? No
Prescription needed? Yes
Available as generic? No
Drug class: Antidyskinetic, antiparkinsonism

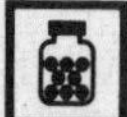

USES

- Treatment of Parkinson's disease.
- Treatment of adverse effects of phenothiazines.

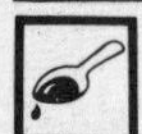

DOSAGE & USAGE INFORMATION

How to take:
Tablets or capsules—Take with food to lessen stomach irritation.

When to take:
At the same times each day.

If you forget a dose:
Take as soon as you remember up to 2 hours late. If more than 2 hours, wait for next scheduled dose (don't double this dose).

What drug does:
- Balances chemical reactions necessary to send nerve impulses within base of brain.
- Improves muscle control and reduces stiffness.

Time lapse before drug works:
1 to 2 hours.

Don't take with:
- Non-prescription drugs for colds, cough or allergy.
- See Interaction column and consult doctor.

OVERDOSE

Symptoms:
Agitation, dilated pupils, hallucinations, dry mouth, rapid heartbeat, sleepiness.

What to do:
- Dial 0 (operator) or 911 (emergency) for an ambulance or medical help. Then give first aid immediately.
- If patient is unconscious and not breathing, give mouth-to-mouth breathing. If there is no heartbeat, use cardiac massage and mouth-to-mouth breathing (CPR). Don't try to make patient vomit. If you can't get help quickly, take patient to nearest emergency facility.
- Additional emergency information on page 886.

POSSIBLE ADVERSE REACTIONS OR SIDE EFFECTS

SYMPTOMS	FREQUENCY	WHAT TO DO
Brain & nervous system:		
Confusion, dizziness.	Rare	4
Skin:		
Rash	Rare	3
Eyes:		
• Pain	Rare	3
• Blurred vision, light sensitivity.	Common	4
Ears, nose, throat:		
Sore mouth or tongue.	Rare	4
Digestive:		
• Constipation	Common	4
• Nausea, vomiting.	Common	4
Heart & lungs:	None expected.	
Blood vessels:	None expected.	
Muscles, bones, joints:		
• Muscle cramps.	Rare	4
• Numbness, weakness in hands or feet.	Rare	4
Genital, urinary:		
Difficult or painful urination.	Common	5
Kidneys:	None expected.	
Liver:	None expected.	
Allergic:	None expected.	
Blood:	None expected.	
Others:	None expected.	

1 - Life-threatening. Seek emergency treatment immediately.
2 - Discontinue. Seek emergency treatment.
3 - Discontinue. Call doctor right away.
4 - Continue. Call doctor when convenient.
5 - Continue. Tell doctor at next visit.
6 - No action necessary.

WARNINGS & PRECAUTIONS

Don't take if:
You are allergic to any antidyskinetic.

Before you start, consult your doctor:
- If you have had glaucoma.
- If you have had high blood pressure or heart disease.
- If you have had impaired liver function.
- If you have had kidney disease or urination difficulty.

Over age 60:
More sensitive to drug. Aggravates symptoms of enlarged prostate. Causes impaired thinking, hallucinations, nightmares. Consult doctor about any of these.

Pregnancy:
Studies inconclusive on harm to unborn child. Animal studies show fetal abnormalities. Decide with your doctor whether drug benefits justify risk to unborn child.

Breast-feeding:
No problems expected.

Infants & children:
Not recommended for children 3 and younger. Use for older children only under doctor's supervision.

Prolonged use:
Possible glaucoma.

Skin & sunlight:
No problems expected.

Driving, piloting or hazardous work:
Don't drive or pilot aircraft until you learn how medicine affects you. Don't work around dangerous machinery. Don't climb ladders or work in high places. Danger increases if you drink alcohol or take medicine affecting alertness and reflexes, such as antihistamines, tranquilizers, sedatives, pain medicine, narcotics and mind-altering drugs.

Airplane passengers:
No problems expected.

Discontinuing:
Don't discontinue without consulting doctor. Dose may require gradual reduction if you have taken drug for a long time. Doses of other drugs may also require adjustment.

Others:
- Internal eye pressure should be measured regularly.
- Avoid becoming overheated.

INTERACTION WITH OTHER DRUGS

GENERIC NAME OR DRUG CLASS	COMBINED EFFECT
Amantadine	Increased amantadine effect.
Antidepressants (tricyclic)	Increased cycrimine effect. May cause glaucoma.
Antihistamines	Increased cycrimine effect.
Levodopa	Increased levodopa effect. Improved results in treating Parkinson's disease.
Meperidine	Increased cycrimine effect.
MAO inhibitors	Increased cycrimine effect.
Orphenadrine	Increased cycrimine effect.
Phenothiazines	Behavior changes.
Primidone	Excessive sedation.
Procainamide	Increased procainamide effect.
Quinidine	Increased cycrimine effect.
Tranquilizers	Excessive sedation.

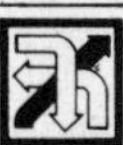

INTERACTION WITH OTHER SUBSTANCES

INTERACTS WITH	COMBINED EFFECT
Alcohol:	None expected.
Beverages:	None expected.
Cocaine:	Decreased cycrimine effect. Avoid.
Foods:	None expected.
Marijuana:	None expected.
Tobacco:	None expected.

CYPROHETPADINE

BRAND NAMES

Cyprodine
Periactin
Vimicon

GENERAL INFORMATION

Habit forming? No
Prescription needed? Yes
Available as generic? Yes
Drug class: Antihistamine

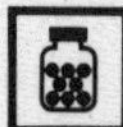

USES

- Reduces allergic symptoms such as hay fever, hives, rash or itching.
- Induces sleep.
- Reduces symptoms of cold urticaria.

DOSAGE & USAGE INFORMATION

How to take:
Tablet or syrup—Swallow with liquid or food to lessen stomach irritation.

When to take:
Varies with form. Follow label directions.

If you forget a dose:
Take as soon as you remember up to 2 hours late. If more than 2 hours, wait for next scheduled dose (don't double this dose).

What drug does:
Blocks action of histamine after an allergic response triggers histamine release in sensitive cells.

Time lapse before drug works:
30 minutes.

Don't take with:
See Interaction column and consult doctor.

OVERDOSE

Symptoms:
Convulsions, red face, hallucinations, coma.

What to do:
- Dial 0 (operator) or 911 (emergency) for an ambulance or medical help. Then give first aid immediately.
- If patient is unconscious and not breathing, give mouth-to-mouth breathing. If there is no heartbeat, use cardiac massage and mouth-to-mouth breathing (CPR). Don't try to make patient vomit. If you can't get help quickly, take patient to nearest emergency facility.
- Additional emergency information on page 886.

POSSIBLE ADVERSE REACTIONS OR SIDE EFFECTS

SYMPTOMS	FREQUENCY	WHAT TO DO
Brain & nervous system:		
• Nightmares, agitation, irritability.	Rare	3
• Drowsiness, dizziness.	Common	5
Skin:	None expected.	
Eyes:		
• Vision changes.	Infrequent	3
• Less tolerance for contact lenses.	Infrequent	4
Ears, nose, throat:		
• Sore throat, fever.	Rare	3
• Dry mouth, nose, throat.	Common	5
Digestive:		
• Nausea	Common	5
• Appetite loss.	Infrequent	5
Heart & lungs:		
Rapid heartbeat.	Rare	3
Blood vessels:		
Unusual bleeding or bruising.	Rare	3
Muscles, bones, joints, kidneys, liver, allergic, blood:	None expected.	
Genital, urinary:		
Urination difficulty.	Infrequent	4
Others:		
Fatigue, weakness.	Rare	3

1 - Life-threatening. Seek emergency treatment immediately.
2 - Discontinue. Seek emergency treatment.
3 - Discontinue. Call doctor right away.
4 - Continue. Call doctor when convenient.
5 - Continue. Tell doctor at next visit.
6 - No action necessary.

WARNINGS & PRECAUTIONS

Don't take if:
You are allergic to any antihistamine.

Before you start, consult your doctor:
- If you have glaucoma.
- If you have enlarged prostate.
- If you have asthma.
- If you have kidney disease.
- If you have peptic ulcer.
- If you will have surgery within 2 months, including dental surgery, requiring general or spinal anesthesia.

Over age 60:
Don't exceed recommended dose. Adverse reactions and side effects may be more frequent and severe than in younger persons, especially urination difficulty, diminished alertness and other brain and nervous-system symptoms.

Pregnancy:
No proven harm to unborn child. Avoid if possible.

Breast-feeding:
Drug passes into milk. Avoid drug or discontinue nursing until you finish medicine. Consult doctor for advice on maintaining milk supply.

Infants & children:
Not recommended for premature or newborn infants. Otherwise, no problems expected.

Prolonged use:
Avoid. May damage bone marrow and nerve cells.

Skin & sunlight:
May cause rash or intensify sunburn in areas exposed to sun or sunlamp.

Driving, piloting or hazardous work:
Don't drive or pilot aircraft until you learn how medicine affects you. Don't work around dangerous machinery. Don't climb ladders or work in high places. Danger increases if you drink alcohol or take medicine affecting alertness and reflexes, such as antihistamines, tranquilizers, sedatives, pain medicine, narcotics and mind-altering drugs.

Airplane passengers:
No problems expected.

Discontinuing:
No problems expected.

Others:
May mask symptoms of hearing damage from aspirin, other salicylates, cisplatin, paromomycin, vancomycin or anticonvulsants. Consult doctor if you use these.

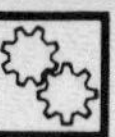

INTERACTION WITH OTHER DRUGS

GENERIC NAME OR DRUG CLASS	COMBINED EFFECT
Anticholinergics	Increased anticholinergic effect.
Antidepressants	Excess sedation. Avoid.
Antihistamines (other)	Excess sedation. Avoid.
Hypnotics	Excess sedation. Avoid.
MAO inhibitors	Increased cyproheptadine effect.
Mind-altering drugs	Excess sedation. Avoid.
Narcotics	Excess sedation. Avoid.
Sedatives	Excess sedation. Avoid.
Sleep inducers	Excess sedation. Avoid.
Tranquilizers	Excess sedation. Avoid.

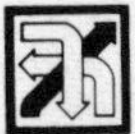

INTERACTION WITH OTHER SUBSTANCES

INTERACTS WITH	COMBINED EFFECT
Alcohol:	Excess sedation. Avoid.
Beverages:	
Caffeine drinks	Less cyproheptadine sedation.
Cocaine:	Decreased cyproheptadine effect. Avoid.
Foods:	None expected.
Marijuana:	Excess sedation. Avoid.
Tobacco:	None expected.

DANAZOL

BRAND NAMES

Cyclomen
Danocrine

GENERAL INFORMATION

Habit forming? No
Prescription needed? Yes
Available as generic? No
Drug class: Gonadotropin inhibitor

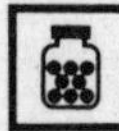

USES

Treatment of endometriosis, fibrocystic breast disease, angioneurotic edema except in pregnant women, gynecomastia, infertility, excessive menstruation, precocious puberty.

DOSAGE & USAGE INFORMATION

How to take:
Tablet or capsule—Swallow with liquid or food to lessen stomach irritation. If you can't swallow whole, crumble tablet or open capsule and take with liquid or food.

When to take:
At the same times each day.

If you forget a dose:
Take as soon as you remember (don't double dose).

What drug does:
Partially prevents output of pituitary follicle-stimulating hormone and lutenizing hormone reducing estrogen production.

Time lapse before drug works:
Takes 3 to 6 months to treat endometriosis.

Don't take with:
- Birth control pills.
- See Interaction column and consult doctor.

OVERDOSE

Symptoms:
Unnatural hair growth in women.

What to do:
Overdose unlikely to threaten life. If person takes much larger amount than prescribed, call doctor, poison-control center or hospital emergency room for instructions.

POSSIBLE ADVERSE REACTIONS OR SIDE EFFECTS

SYMPTOMS	FREQUENCY	WHAT TO DO
Brain & nervous system:		
• Dizziness	Infrequent	4
• Headache	Infrequent	5
Skin:		
• Acne	Infrequent	5
• Unnatural hair growth in women.	Infrequent	3
Eyes:	None expected.	
Ears, nose, throat:		
• Nosebleeds	Infrequent	3
• Hoarseness, voice deepens.	Infrequent	4
Digestive:	None expected.	
Heart & lungs:	None expected.	
Blood vessels:		
Flushed or red skin.	Infrequent	4
Muscles, bones, joints:		
Muscle cramps.	Infrequent	4
Genital, urinary:		
• Enlarged clitoris.	Infrequent	4
• Decreased testicle size.	Infrequent	4
• Vaginal burning, itch.	Infrequent	4
Kidneys, allergic, blood, liver:		
Jaundice (yellow skin and eyes).	Rare	3
Others:		
• Feet swelling.	Infrequent	4
• Weight gain.	Infrequent	5
• Decreased breast size.	Infrequent	4

1- Life-threatening. Seek emergency treatment immediately.
2- Discontinue. Seek emergency treatment.
3- Discontinue. Call doctor right away.
4- Continue. Call doctor when convenient.
5- Continue. Tell doctor at next visit.
6- No action necessary.

WARNINGS & PRECAUTIONS

Don't take if:
You become pregnant.

Before you start, consult your doctor:
- If you take birth control pills.
- If you have diabetes.
- If you have heart disease.
- If you have epilepsy.
- If you have kidney disease.
- If you have liver disease.
- If you have migraine headache.

Over age 60:
Adverse reactions and side effects may be more frequent and severe than in younger persons.

Pregnancy:
Risk to unborn child outweighs drug benefits. Don't use. Stop if you get pregnant.

Breast-feeding:
Unknown whether medicine filters into milk. Consult doctor.

Infants & children:
Not recommended.

Prolonged use:
Required for full effect. Don't discontinue without consulting doctor.

Skin & sunlight:
No problems expected.

Driving, piloting or hazardous work:
No problems expected.

Airplane passengers:
No problems expected.

Discontinuing:
Don't discontinue without consulting doctor. Dose may require gradual reduction if you have taken drug for a long time. Doses of other drugs may also require adjustment. May have no menstrual periods for 2 or 3 months following discontinuation.

INTERACTION WITH OTHER DRUGS

GENERIC NAME OR DRUG CLASS	COMBINED EFFECT
Brain depressing medicines: Antihistamines, sedatives, sleeping pills, tranquilizers, pain medicines.	Excessive nervous system depression; lowered blood pressure.
Estrogens	Increased chance of liver toxicity.

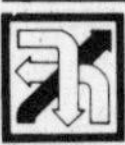

INTERACTION WITH OTHER SUBSTANCES

INTERACTS WITH	COMBINED EFFECT
Alcohol:	Excessive nervous system depression. Avoid.
Beverages:	
Caffeine	Rapid, irregular heartbeat. Avoid.
Cocaine:	May interfere with expected action of danazol. Avoid.
Foods:	No problems expected.
Marijuana:	May interfere with expected action of danazol. Avoid.
Tobacco:	Rapid, irregular heartbeat. Avoid. Increased leg cramps.

DANTHRON

BRAND NAMES

Dorbane
Dorbantyl L
Doxidan
Modane
Roydan

GENERAL INFORMATION

Habit forming? No
Prescription needed? No
Available as generic? Yes
Drug class: Laxative (stimulant)

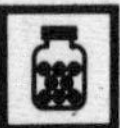

USES

Constipation relief.

DOSAGE & USAGE INFORMATION

How to take:
- Tablet—Swallow with liquid or food.
- Liquid—Drink 6 to 8 glasses of water each day, in addition to one taken with each dose.

When to take:
Usually at bedtime with a snack, unless directed otherwise.

If you forget a dose:
Take as soon as you remember.

What drug does:
Acts on smooth muscles of intestine wall to cause vigorous bowel movement.

Time lapse before drug works:
6 to 10 hours.

Don't take with:
- See Interaction column and consult doctor.
- Don't take within 2 hours of taking another medicine. Laxative interferes with medicine absorption.

OVERDOSE

Symptoms:
Vomiting, electrolyte depletion.

What to do:
Overdose unlikely to threaten life. If person takes much larger amount than prescribed, call doctor, poison-control center or hospital emergency room for instructions.

POSSIBLE ADVERSE REACTIONS OR SIDE EFFECTS

SYMPTOMS	FREQUENCY	WHAT TO DO
Brain & nervous system:		
Irritability, confusion, headache.	Rare	3
Skin:		
Rash	Rare	3
Eyes:	None expected.	
Ears, nose, throat:	None expected.	
Digestive:		
Belching, cramps, nausea.	Infrequent	4
Heart & lungs:		
Breathing difficulty, irregular heartbeat.	Rare	3
Blood vessels:	None expected.	
Muscles, bones, joints:		
Muscle cramps.	Rare	3
Genital, urinary:	None expected.	
Kidneys:		
Burning on urination.	Rare	4
Liver:	None expected.	
Allergic:	None expected.	
Blood:	None expected.	
Others:		
• Rectal irritation.	Common	4
• Dangerous potassium loss.	Infrequent	3
• Unusual tiredness or weakness.	Rare	3

1- Life-threatening. Seek emergency treatment immediately.
2- Discontinue. Seek emergency treatment.
3- Discontinue. Call doctor right away.
4- Continue. Call doctor when convenient.
5- Continue. Tell doctor at next visit.
6- No action necessary.

WARNINGS & PRECAUTIONS

Don't take if:
- You have symptoms of appendicitis, inflamed bowel or intestinal blockage.
- You are allergic to a stimulant laxative.
- You have missed a bowel movement for only 1 or 2 days.

Before you start, consult your doctor:
- If you have a colostomy or ileostomy.
- If you have congestive heart disease.
- If you have diabetes.
- If you have high blood pressure.
- If you have a laxative habit.
- If you have rectal bleeding.
- If you take other laxatives.

Over age 60:
Adverse reactions and side effects may be more frequent and severe than in younger persons.

Pregnancy:
Risk to mother and unborn child outweighs drug benefits. Don't use.

Breast-feeding:
Drug passes into milk. Avoid drug or discontinue nursing until you finish medicine. Consult doctor for advice on maintaining milk supply.

Infants & children:
Use only under medical supervision.

Prolonged use:
Don't take for more than 1 week unless under a doctor's supervision. May cause laxative dependence.

Skin & sunlight:
No problems expected.

Driving, piloting or hazardous work:
No problems expected.

Airplane passengers:
No problems expected.

Discontinuing:
May be unnecessary to finish medicine. Follow doctor's instructions.

Others:
Don't take to "flush out" your system or as a "tonic."

INTERACTION WITH OTHER DRUGS

GENERIC NAME OR DRUG CLASS	COMBINED EFFECT
Antihypertensives	May cause dangerous low potassium level.
Diuretics	May cause dangerous low potassium level.
Docusate calcium	Liver toxicity.
Docusate sodium	Liver toxicity.

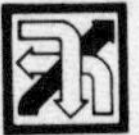

INTERACTION WITH OTHER SUBSTANCES

INTERACTS WITH	COMBINED EFFECT
Alcohol:	None expected.
Beverages:	None expected.
Cocaine:	None expected.
Foods:	None expected.
Marijuana:	None expected.
Tobacco:	None expected.

DANTROLENE

BRAND NAMES

Dantrium

GENERAL INFORMATION

Habit forming? No
Prescription needed? Yes
Available as generic? No
Drug class: Muscle relaxant, antispastic

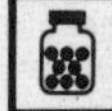

USES

- Relieves muscle spasticity caused by diseases such as multiple sclerosis, cerebral palsy, stroke.
- Relieves muscle spasticity caused by injury to spinal cord.
- Relieves or prevents excess body temperature brought on by some surgical procedures.

DOSAGE & USAGE INFORMATION

How to take:
Capsules—Swallow with liquid.

When to take:
Once a day for muscle spasticity during first 6 days. Later, every 6 hours. For excess temperature, follow label instructions.

If you forget a dose:
Take as soon as you remember up to 2 hours late. If more than 2 hours, wait for next scheduled dose (don't double this dose).

What drug does:
Acts directly on muscles to prevent excess contractions.

Time lapse before drug works:
1 or more weeks.

Don't take with:
See Interaction column and consult doctor.

OVERDOSE

Symptoms:
Bloody stools, chest pain, convulsive seizures.

What to do:
- Dial 0 (operator) or 911 (emergency) for an ambulance or medical help. Then give first aid immediately.
- If patient is unconscious and not breathing, give mouth-to-mouth breathing. If there is no heartbeat, use cardiac massage and mouth-to-mouth breathing (CPR). Don't try to make patient vomit. If you can't get help quickly, take patient to nearest emergency facility.
- Additional emergency information on page 886.

POSSIBLE ADVERSE REACTIONS OR SIDE EFFECTS

SYMPTOMS	FREQUENCY	WHAT TO DO
Brain & nervous system:		
• Seizure	Infrequent	1
• Depression, confusion.	Infrequent	4
• Headache, slurred speech, nervousness, insomnia.	Infrequent	4
Skin:		
Rash, hives.	Infrequent	3
Eyes:		
Blurred vision.	Infrequent	4
Ears, nose, throat:	None expected.	
Digestive:		
• Black or bloody stools.	Infrequent	3
• Diarrhea	Infrequent	4
• Difficult swallowing.	Infrequent	4
• Appetite loss.	Infrequent	4
Heart & lungs:		
• Chest pain.	Infrequent	3
• Fast heartbeat.		
Blood vessels:	None expected.	
Muscles, bones, joints:		
Backache	Infrequent	3
Genital, urinary:		
• Bloody urine.	Infrequent	3
• Difficult urination.	Infrequent	4
Kidneys, allergic blood, liver:		
Jaundice (yellow skin and eyes).	Rare	3
Others:		
• Painful, swollen feet.	Infrequent	3
• Chills, fever.	Infrequent	3
• Decreased sexual function in males.	Infrequent	4

1- Life-threatening. Seek emergency treatment immediately.
2- Discontinue. Seek emergency treatment.
3- Discontinue. Call doctor right away.
4- Continue. Call doctor when convenient.

WARNINGS & PRECAUTIONS

Don't take if:
You are allergic to dantrolene or any muscle relaxant or antispastic medication.

Before you start, consult your doctor:
- If you have liver disease.
- If you have heart disease.
- If you have lung disease (especially emphysema).
- If you are over age 35.
- If you will have surgery within 2 months, including dental surgery, requiring general or spinal anesthesia.

Over age 60:
Adverse reactions and side effects may be more frequent and severe than in younger persons.

Pregnancy:
No proven harm to unborn child. Avoid if possible.

Breast-feeding:
Avoid nursing or discontinue until you finish drug.

Infants & children:
Only under close medical supervision.

Prolonged use:
Blood counts, G6PD tests before treatment begins in Negroes and Caucasians of Mediterranean heritage, liver function studies—all recommended periodically during prolonged use.

Skin & sunlight:
May cause rash or intensify sunburn in areas exposed to sun or sunlamp.

Driving, piloting or hazardous work:
Don't drive or pilot aircraft until you learn how medicine affects you. Don't work around dangerous machinery. Don't climb ladders or work in high places. Danger increases if you drink alcohol or take medicine affecting alertness and reflexes, such as antihistamines, tranquilizers, sedatives, pain medicine, narcotics and mind-altering drugs.

Airplane passengers:
Move cautiously while in flight.

Discontinuing:
Don't discontinue without consulting doctor. Dose may require gradual reduction if you have taken drug for a long time. Doses of other drugs may also require adjustment.

INTERACTION WITH OTHER DRUGS

GENERIC NAME OR DRUG CLASS	COMBINED EFFECT
Central nervous system depressants: Sedatives, sleeping pills, tranquilizers, antidepressants, antihistamines, narcotics, other muscle relaxants	Increased sedation, low blood pressure. Avoid.

INTERACTION WITH OTHER SUBSTANCES

INTERACTS WITH	COMBINED EFFECT
Alcohol:	Increased sedation, low blood pressure. Avoid.
Beverages:	No problems expected.
Cocaine:	Increased spasticity. Avoid.
Foods:	No problems expected.
Marijuana:	Increased spasticity. Avoid.
Tobacco:	May interfere with absorption of medicine.

DAPSONE

BRAND NAMES

Avlosulfon

GENERAL INFORMATION

Habit forming? No
Prescription needed? Yes
Available as generic? No
Drug class: Antibacterial (Antileprosy), Sulfone

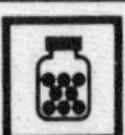

USES

- Treatment of dermatitis herpetiformis.
- Treatment of leprosy.

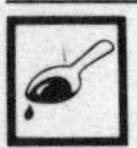

DOSAGE & USAGE INFORMATION

How to take:
Tablet or capsule—Swallow with liquid or food to lessen stomach irritation.

When to take:
Once a day at same time.

If you forget a dose:
Take as soon as you remember up to 2 hours late. If more than 2 hours, wait for next scheduled dose (don't double this dose).

What drug does:
Inhibits enzymes. Kills leprosy germs.

Time lapse before drug works:
- 3 years for leprosy.
- 1 to 2 weeks for dermatitis herpetiformis.

Don't take with:
See Interaction column and consult doctor.

OVERDOSE

Symptoms:
Bleeding, vomiting, coma.

What to do:
- Dial 0 (operator) or 911 (emergency) for an ambulance or medical help. Then give first aid immediately.
- If patient is unconscious and not breathing, give mouth-to-mouth breathing. If there is no heartbeat, use cardiac massage and mouth-to-mouth breathing (CPR). Don't try to make patient vomit. If you can't get help quickly, take patient to nearest emergency facility.
- Additional emergency information on page 886.

POSSIBLE ADVERSE REACTIONS OR SIDE EFFECTS

SYMPTOMS	FREQUENCY	WHAT TO DO
Brain & nervous system:		
• Dizziness	Rare	3
• Headache	Rare	4
• Mental changes.	Rare	3
Skin:		
• Pale	Infrequent	3
• Rash	Common	3
• Itching	Rare	4
Eyes:	None expected.	
Ears, nose, throat:		
Sore throat, fever.	Rare	3
Digestive:		
• Nausea, vomiting.	Rare	4
• Abdominal pain, appetite loss.	Common	4
Heart & lungs:		
Difficult breathing.	Rare	3
Blood vessels:		
Bleeding	Rare	3
Muscles, bones, joints:	None expected.	
Genital, urinary:	None expected.	
Kidneys, allergic, blood, liver:		
Jaundice (yellow skin and eyes).	Rare	3
Others:		
• Blue fingernails, lips.	Rare	4
• Numbness, tingling, pain, burning hands or feet.	Rare	3

1-Life-threatening. Seek emergency treatment immediately.
2-Discontinue. Seek emergency treatment.
3-Discontinue. Call doctor right away.
4-Continue. Call doctor when convenient.
5-Continue. Tell doctor at next visit.
6-No action necessary.

WARNINGS & PRECAUTIONS

Don't take if:

- You have G6PD deficiency.
- You are allergic to furosemide, thiazide diuretics, sulfonureas, carbonic anhydrase inhibitors, sulfonamides.

Before you start, consult your doctor:

- If you are anemic.
- If you have liver or kidney disease.
- If you are Negro or Caucasian with Mediterranean heritage.
- If you will have surgery within 2 months, including dental surgery, requiring general or spinal anesthesia.

Over age 60:
Adverse reactions and side effects may be more frequent and severe than in younger persons.

Pregnancy:
No problems expected.

Breast-feeding:
Consult doctor.

Infants & children:
Under close medical supervision only.

Prolonged use:
Request blood counts, liver function studies.

Skin & sunlight:
No problems expected.

Driving, piloting or hazardous work:
Don't drive or pilot aircraft until you learn how medicine affects you. Don't work around dangerous machinery. Don't climb ladders or work in high places. Danger increases if you drink alcohol or take medicine affecting alertness and reflexes, such as antihistamines, tranquilizers, sedatives, pain medicine, narcotics and mind-altering drugs.

Airplane passengers:
No problems expected.

Discontinuing:
Don't discontinue without consulting doctor. Dose may require gradual reduction if you have taken drug for a long time. Doses of other drugs may also require adjustment.

INTERACTION WITH OTHER DRUGS

GENERIC NAME OR DRUG CLASS	COMBINED EFFECT
Aminobenzoic acid (PABA)	Decreased dapsone effect. Avoid.
Probenecid	Increased toxicity of dapsone.
Rifampin	Decreased effect of dapsone.

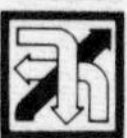

INTERACTION WITH OTHER SUBSTANCES

INTERACTS WITH	COMBINED EFFECT
Alcohol:	Increased chance of toxicity to liver.
Beverages:	No problems expected.
Cocaine:	Increased chance of toxicity. Avoid.
Foods:	No problems expected.
Marijuana:	Increased chance of toxicity. Avoid.
Tobacco:	May interfere with absorption of medicine.

DEHYDROCHOLIC ACID

BRAND NAMES

Bilaz
Cholan-DH
Cholan-HMB
Decholin
Dycholium
G.B.S.
Hepahydrin
Neocholan
Neolax
Trilax

GENERAL INFORMATION

Habit forming? No
Prescription needed? No
Available as generic? Yes
Drug class: Laxative (stimulant)

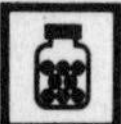

USES

Constipation relief.

DOSAGE & USAGE INFORMATION

How to take:
Tablet—Swallow with liquid.

When to take:
Usually at bedtime with a snack, unless directed otherwise.

If you forget a dose:
Take as soon as you remember.

What drug does:
Acts on smooth muscles of intestine wall to cause vigorous bowel movement.

Time lapse before drug works:
6 to 10 hours.

Don't take with:
- See Interaction column and consult doctor.
- Don't take within 2 hours of taking another medicine. Laxative interferes with medicine absorption.

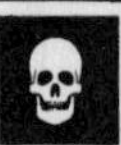

OVERDOSE

Symptoms:
Vomiting, electrolyte depletion.

What to do:
Overdose unlikely to threaten life. If person takes much larger amount than prescribed, call doctor, poison-control center or hospital emergency room for instructions.

POSSIBLE ADVERSE REACTIONS OR SIDE EFFECTS

SYMPTOMS	FREQUENCY	WHAT TO DO
Brain & nervous system: Irritability, confusion, headache.	Rare	3
Skin: Rash	Rare	3
Eyes:	None expected.	
Ears, nose, throat:	None expected.	
Digestive: Belching, cramps, nausea.	Infrequent	4
Heart & lungs: Breathing difficulty, irregular heartbeat.	Rare	3
Blood vessels:	None expected.	
Muscles, bones, joints: Muscle cramps.	Rare	3
Genital, urinary:	None expected.	
Kidneys: Burning on urination.	Rare	4
Liver:	None expected.	
Allergic:	None expected.	
Blood:	None expected.	
Others:		
• Rectal irritation.	Common	4
• Dangerous potassium loss.	Infrequent	3
• Unusual tiredness or weakness.	Rare	3

1- Life-threatening. Seek emergency treatment immediately.
2- Discontinue. Seek emergency treatment.
3- Discontinue. Call doctor right away.
4- Continue. Call doctor when convenient.
5- Continue. Tell doctor at next visit.
6- No action necessary.

DEHYDROCHOLIC ACID

WARNINGS & PRECAUTIONS

Don't take if:
- You have symptoms of appendicitis, inflamed bowel or intestinal blockage.
- You are allergic to a stimulant laxative.
- You have missed a bowel movement for only 1 or 2 days.
- You have liver disease.

Before you start, consult your doctor:
- If you have a colostomy or ileostomy.
- If you have congestive heart disease.
- If you have diabetes.
- If you have enlarged prostate.
- If you have a laxative habit.
- If you have rectal bleeding.
- If you take other laxatives.

Over age 60:
Adverse reactions and side effects may be more frequent and severe than in younger persons.

Pregnancy:
Risk to mother and unborn child outweighs drug benefits. Don't use.

Breast-feeding:
Drug passes into milk. Avoid drug or discontinue nursing until you finish medicine. Consult doctor for advice on maintaining milk supply.

Infants & children:
Use only under medical supervision.

Prolonged use:
Don't take for more than 1 week unless under a doctor's supervision. May cause laxative dependence.

Skin & sunlight:
No problems expected.

Driving, piloting or hazardous work:
No problems expected.

Airplane passengers:
No problems expected.

Discontinuing:
May be unnecessary to finish medicine. Follow doctor's instructions.

Others:
Don't take to "flush out" your system or as a "tonic."

INTERACTION WITH OTHER DRUGS

GENERIC NAME OR DRUG CLASS	COMBINED EFFECT
Antihypertensives	May cause dangerous low potassium level.
Diuretics	May cause dangerous low potassium level.

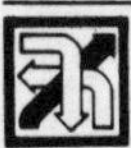

INTERACTION WITH OTHER SUBSTANCES

INTERACTS WITH	COMBINED EFFECT
Alcohol:	None expected.
Beverages:	None expected.
Cocaine:	None expected.
Foods:	None expected.
Marijuana:	None expected.
Tobacco:	None expected.

DESIPRAMINE

BRAND NAMES

Norpramin
Pertofrane

GENERAL INFORMATION

Habit forming? No
Prescription needed? Yes
Available as generic? Yes
Drug class: Antidepressant (tricyclic)

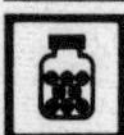

USES

Gradually relieves, but doesn't cure, symptoms of depression.

DOSAGE & USAGE INFORMATION

How to take:
Tablet or capsule—Swallow with liquid.

When to take:
At the same time each day, usually bedtime.

If you forget a dose:
Bedtime dose—If you forget your once-a-day bedtime dose, don't take it more than 3 hours late. If more than 3 hours, wait for next scheduled dose. Don't double this dose.

What drug does:
Probably affects part of brain that controls messages between nerve cells.

Time lapse before drug works:
Begins in 1 to 2 weeks. May require 4 to 6 weeks for maximum benefit.

Don't take with:
- Non-prescription drugs without consulting doctor.
- See Interaction column and consult doctor.

OVERDOSE

Symptoms:
Hallucinations, convulsions, coma.

What to do:
- Dial 0 (operator) or 911 (emergency) for an ambulance or medical help. Then give first aid immediately.
- If patient is unconscious and not breathing, give mouth-to-mouth breathing. If there is no heartbeat, use cardiac massage and mouth-to-mouth breathing (CPR). Don't try to make patient vomit. If you can't get help quickly, take patient to nearest emergency facility.
- Additional emergency information on page 886.

POSSIBLE ADVERSE REACTIONS OR SIDE EFFECTS

SYMPTOMS	FREQUENCY	WHAT TO DO
Brain & nervous system:		
• Hallucinations, shakiness, dizziness, fainting.	Infrequent	3
• Headache	Common	4
• Seizures	Rare	1
• Insomnia	Common	5
Skin:		
Rash, itch.	Rare	3
Eyes:		
Blurred vision, pain.	Infrequent	3
Ears, nose, throat:		
• Sore throat.	Rare	3
• Dry mouth or unpleasant taste.	Common	4
Digestive:		
• Constipation or diarrhea, nausea, indigestion.	Common	4
• Vomiting	Infrequent	3
• "Sweet tooth"	Common	5
Heart & lungs:		
Irregular heartbeat or slow pulse.	Infrequent	3
Blood vessels, muscles, bones, joints, kidneys, allergic, blood:	None expected.	
Genital, urinary:		
Difficulty urinating.	Infrequent	4
Liver:		
Jaundice (yellow skin and eyes).	Rare	3
Others:		
• Fever	Rare	3
• Fatigue, weakness.	Common	4

1- Life-threatening. Seek emergency treatment immediately.
2- Discontinue. Seek emergency treatment.
3- Discontinue. Call doctor right away.
4- Continue. Call doctor when convenient.
5- Continue. Tell doctor at next visit.

WARNINGS & PRECAUTIONS

Don't take if:
- You are allergic to any tricyclic antidepressant.
- You drink alcohol.
- You have had a heart attack within 6 weeks.
- You have glaucoma.
- You have taken MAO inhibitors within 2 weeks.
- Patient is younger than 12.

Before you start, consult your doctor:
- If you will have surgery within 2 months, including dental surgery, requiring general or spinal anesthesia.
- If you have an enlarged prostate.
- If you have heart disease or high blood pressure.
- If you have stomach or intestinal problems.
- If you have an overactive thyroid.
- If you have asthma.
- If you have liver disease.

Over age 60:
More likely to develop urination difficulty and side effects under *Brain & nervous system*, opposite page.

Pregnancy:
Studies inconclusive on harm to unborn child. Animal studies show fetal abnormalities. Decide with your doctor whether drug benefits justify risk to unborn child.

Breast-feeding:
Drug passes into milk. Avoid drug or discontinue nursing until you finish medicine. Consult doctor on maintaining milk supply.

Infants & children:
Don't give to children younger than 12.

Prolonged use:
No problems expected.

Skin & sunlight:
May cause rash or intensify sunburn in areas exposed to sun or sunlamp.

Driving, piloting or hazardous work:
Don't drive or pilot aircraft until you learn how medicine affects you. Don't work around dangerous machinery. Don't climb ladders or work in high places. Danger increases if you drink alcohol or take medicine affecting alertness and reflexes.

Airplane passengers:
No problems expected.

Discontinuing:
Don't discontinue without consulting doctor. Dose may require gradual reduction if you have taken drug for a long time. Doses of other drugs may also require adjustment.

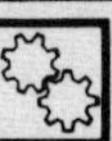

INTERACTION WITH OTHER DRUGS

GENERIC NAME OR DRUG CLASS	COMBINED EFFECT
Anticoagulants (oral)	Increased anticoagulant effect.
Anticholinergics	Increased sedation.
Antihistamines	Increased antihistamine effect.
Barbiturates	Decreased antidepressant effect.
Clonidine	Decreased clonidine effect.
Diuretics (thiazide)	Increased desipramine effect.
Ethchlorvynol	Delirium
Guanethidine	Decreased guanethidine effect.
MAO inhibitors	Fever, delirium, convulsions.
Methyldopa	Decreased methyldopa effect.
Narcotics	Dangerous oversedation.
Phenytoin	Decreased phenytoin effect.
Quinidine	Irregular heartbeat.
Sedatives	Dangerous oversedation.
Sympathomimetics	Increased sympathomimetic effect.
Thyroid hormones	Irregular heartbeat.

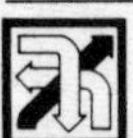

INTERACTION WITH OTHER SUBSTANCES

INTERACTS WITH	COMBINED EFFECT
Alcohol: Beverages or medicines with alcohol.	Excessive intoxication. Avoid.
Beverages:	None expected.
Cocaine:	Excessive intoxication. Avoid.
Foods:	None expected.
Marijuana:	Excessive drowsiness. Avoid.
Tobacco:	None expected.

DEXAMETHASONE

BRAND NAMES

Dalalon L.A.
Decadron
Decadron L.A.
Decadron Respihaler
Decadron with Xylocaine
Dexasone
Dexone
Hexadrol

See complete brand names list, page 825.

GENERAL INFORMATION

Habit forming? No
Prescription needed? Yes
Available as generic? Yes
Drug class: Cortisone drug (adrenal corticosteroid)

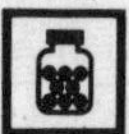

USES

- Reduces inflammation caused by many different medical problems.
- Treatment for some allergic diseases, blood disorders, kidney diseases, asthma and emphysema.
- Replaces corticosteroid deficiencies.

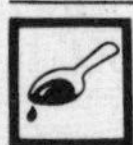

DOSAGE & USAGE INFORMATION

How to take:
- Tablet or liquid—Swallow with liquid or food to lessen stomach irritation. If you can't swallow whole, crumble tablet and take with liquid or food.
- Inhaler—Follow label instructions.

When to take:
At the same times each day. Take once-a-day or once-every-other-day doses in mornings.

If you forget a dose:
- Several-doses-per-day prescription—Take as soon as you remember up to 2 hours late. If more than 2 hours, wait for next scheduled dose (don't double this dose).
- Once-a-day dose or less—Wait for next dose. Double this dose.

What drug does:
Decreases inflammatory responses.

Time lapse before drug works:
2 to 4 days.

Don't take with:
See Interaction column and consult doctor.

OVERDOSE

Symptoms:
Headache, convulsions, heart failure.

What to do:
- Dial 0 (operator) or 911 (emergency) for an ambulance or medical help. Then give first aid immediately.
- Additional emergency information on page 886.

POSSIBLE ADVERSE REACTIONS OR SIDE EFFECTS

SYMPTOMS	FREQUENCY	WHAT TO DO
Brain & nervous system:		
Mood changes, insomnia, restlessness.	Infrequent	4
Skin:		
• Acne	Common	4
• Rash	Rare	3
• Poor wound healing.	Common	4
Eyes:		
Blurred vision, halos around lights.	Infrequent	3
Ears, nose, throat:		
• Sore throat, fever.	Infrequent	3
• Thirst	Common	4
Digestive:		
• Indigestion, nausea, vomiting.	Common	4
• Bloody or black, tarry stool.	Infrequent	2
Heart & lungs:		
Irregular heartbeat.	Rare	2
Blood vessels, kidneys, liver, allergic, blood:	None expected.	
Muscles, bones, joints:		
Muscle cramps, swollen legs, feet.	Infrequent	3
Genital, urinary:		
Frequent urination.	Infrequent	4
Others:		
• Weight gain, round face.	Infrequent	4
• Fatigue, weakness.	Infrequent	4
• TB recurrence.	Infrequent	4
• Irregular menstrual periods.	Infrequent	4

1-Life-threatening. Seek emergency treatment immediately.
2-Discontinue. Seek emergency treatment.
3-Discontinue. Call doctor right away.
4-Continue. Call doctor when convenient.

DEXAMETHASONE

WARNINGS & PRECAUTIONS

Don't take if:
- You are allergic to any cortisone drug.
- You have tuberculosis or fungus infection.
- You have herpes infection of eyes, lips or genitals.

Before you start, consult your doctor:
- If you have had tuberculosis.
- If you have congestive heart failure.
- If you have diabetes.
- If you have peptic ulcer.
- If you have glaucoma.
- If you have underactive thyroid.
- If you have high blood pressure.
- If you have myasthenia gravis.
- If you have blood clots in legs or lungs.

Over age 60:
Adverse reactions and side effects may be more frequent and severe than in younger persons. Likely to aggravate edema, diabetes or ulcers. Likely to cause cataracts and osteoporosis (softening of the bones).

Pregnancy:
Risk to unborn child outweighs drug benefits. Don't use.

Breast-feeding:
Drug passes into milk. Avoid drug or discontinue nursing until you finish medicine. Consult doctor for advice on maintaining milk supply.

Infants & children:
Use only under medical supervision.

Prolonged use:
- Retards growth in children.
- Possible glaucoma, cataracts, diabetes, fragile bones and thin skin.
- Functional dependence.

Skin & sunlight:
No problems expected.

Driving, piloting or hazardous work:
No problems expected.

Airplane passengers:
No problems expected.

Discontinuing:
- Don't discontinue without doctor's advice until you complete prescribed dose, even though symptoms diminish or disappear.
- Drug affects your response to surgery, illness, injury or stress for 2 years after discontinuing. Tell about drug to anyone who takes medical care of you within 2 years.

Others:
Avoid immunizations if possible.

INTERACTION WITH OTHER DRUGS

GENERIC NAME OR DRUG CLASS	COMBINED EFFECT
Amphoterecin B	Potassium depletion.
Anticholinergics	Possible glaucoma.
Anticoagulants (oral)	Decreased anticoagulant effect.
Anticonvulsants (hydantoin)	Decreased dexamethasone effect.
Antidiabetics (oral)	Decreased antidiabetic effect.
Antihistamines	Decreased dexamethasone effect.
Aspirin	Increased dexamethasone effect.
Barbiturates	Decreased dexamethasone effect. Oversedation.
Beta-adrenergic blockers	Decreased dexamethasone effect.
Chloral hydrate	Decreased dexamethasone effect.
Chlorthalidone	Potassium depletion.
Cholinergics	Decreased cholinergic effect.
Contraceptives (oral)	Increased dexamethasone effect.
Digitalis preparations	Dangerous potassium depletion. Possible digitalis toxicity.

Additional interactions on page 836.

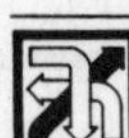

INTERACTION WITH OTHER SUBSTANCES

INTERACTS WITH	COMBINED EFFECT
Alcohol:	Risk of stomach ulcers.
Beverages:	No proven problems.
Cocaine:	Overstimulation. Avoid.
Foods:	No proven problems.
Marijuana:	Decreased immunity.
Tobacco:	Increased dexamethasone effect. Possible toxicity.

DEXCHLORPHENIRAMINE

BRAND NAMES

Dexchlor Repeat Action Tablets
Polaramine
Polaramine Repetabs

GENERAL INFORMATION

Habit forming? No
Prescription needed? Yes
Available as generic? No
Drug class: Antihistamine

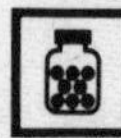

USES

- Reduces allergic symptoms such as hay fever, hives, rash or itching.
- Induces sleep.

DOSAGE & USAGE INFORMATION

How to take:
- Tablet or syrup—Swallow with liquid or food to lessen stomach irritation.
- Extended-release tablets or capsules—Swallow each dose whole. If you take regular tablets, you may chew or crush them.

When to take:
Varies with form. Follow label directions.

If you forget a dose:
Take as soon as you remember up to 2 hours late. If more than 2 hours, wait for next scheduled dose (don't double this dose).

What drug does:
Blocks action of histamine after an allergic response triggers histamine release in sensitive cells.

Time lapse before drug works:
30 minutes.

Don't take with:
See Interaction column and consult doctor.

OVERDOSE

Symptoms:
Convulsions, red face, hallucinations, coma.

What to do:
- Dial 0 (operator) or 911 (emergency) for an ambulance or medical help. Then give first aid immediately.
- If patient is unconscious and not breathing, give mouth-to-mouth breathing. If there is no heartbeat, use cardiac massage and mouth-to-mouth breathing (CPR). Don't try to make patient vomit. If you can't get help quickly, take patient to nearest emergency facility.
- Additional emergency information on page 886.

POSSIBLE ADVERSE REACTIONS OR SIDE EFFECTS

SYMPTOMS	FREQUENCY	WHAT TO DO
Brain & nervous system:		
• Nightmares, agitation, irritability.	Rare	3
• Drowsiness, dizziness.	Common	5
Skin:	None expected.	
Eyes:		
• Vision changes.	Infrequent	3
• Less tolerance for contact lenses.	Infrequent	4
Ears, nose, throat:		
• Sore throat, fever.	Rare	3
• Dry mouth, nose, throat.	Common	5
Digestive:		
• Nausea	Common	5
• Appetite loss.	Infrequent	5
Heart & lungs:		
Rapid heartbeat.	Rare	3
Blood vessels:		
Unusual bleeding or bruising.	Rare	3
Muscles, bones, joints, kidneys, liver, allergic, blood:	None expected.	
Genital, urinary:		
Urination difficulty.	Infrequent	4
Others:		
Fatigue, weakness.	Rare	3

1- Life-threatening. Seek emergency treatment immediately.
2- Discontinue. Seek emergency treatment.
3- Discontinue. Call doctor right away.
4- Continue. Call doctor when convenient.
5- Continue. Tell doctor at next visit.
6- No action necessary.

DEXCHLORPHENIRAMINE

WARNINGS & PRECAUTIONS

Don't take if:
You are allergic to any antihistamine.

Before you start, consult your doctor:
- If you have glaucoma.
- If you have enlarged prostate.
- If you have asthma.
- If you have kidney disease.
- If you have peptic ulcer.
- If you will have surgery within 2 months, including dental surgery, requiring general or spinal anesthesia.

Over age 60:
Don't exceed recommended dose. Adverse reactions and side effects may be more frequent and severe than in younger persons, especially urination difficulty, diminished alertness and other brain and nervous-system symptoms.

Pregnancy:
No proven harm to unborn child. Avoid if possible.

Breast-feeding:
Drug passes into milk. Avoid drug or discontinue nursing until you finish medicine. Consult doctor for advice on maintaining milk supply.

Infants & children:
Not recommended for premature or newborn infants. Otherwise, no problems expected.

Prolonged use:
Avoid. May damage bone marrow and nerve cells.

Skin & sunlight:
May cause rash or intensify sunburn in areas exposed to sun or sunlamp.

Driving, piloting or hazardous work:
Don't drive or pilot aircraft until you learn how medicine affects you. Don't work around dangerous machinery. Don't climb ladders or work in high places. Danger increases if you drink alcohol or take medicine affecting alertness and reflexes, such as antihistamines, tranquilizers, sedatives, pain medicine, narcotics and mind-altering drugs.

Airplane passengers:
No problems expected.

Discontinuing:
No problems expected.

Others:
May mask symptoms of hearing damage from aspirin, other salicylates, cisplatin, paromomycin, vancomycin or anticonvulsants. Consult doctor if you use these.

INTERACTION WITH OTHER DRUGS

GENERIC NAME OR DRUG CLASS	COMBINED EFFECT
Anticholinergics	Increased anticholinergic effect.
Antidepressants	Excess sedation. Avoid.
Antihistamines (other)	Excess sedation. Avoid.
Hypnotics	Excess sedation. Avoid.
MAO inhibitors	Increased dexchlorpheniramine effect.
Mind-altering drugs	Excess sedation. Avoid.
Narcotics	Excess sedation. Avoid.
Sedatives	Excess sedation. Avoid.
Sleep inducers	Excess sedation. Avoid.
Tranquilizers	Excess sedation. Avoid.

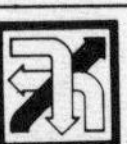

INTERACTION WITH OTHER SUBSTANCES

INTERACTS WITH	COMBINED EFFECT
Alcohol:	Excess sedation. Avoid.
Beverages: Caffeine drinks	Less dexchlorpheniramine sedation.
Cocaine:	Decreased dexchlorpheniramine effect. Avoid.
Foods:	None expected.
Marijuana:	Excess sedation. Avoid.
Tobacco:	None expected.

DEXTROAMPHETAMINE

BRAND NAMES

Amphaplex
Biphetamine
Declobese
Dexampex
Dexedrine
Eskatrol
Ferndex
Obetrol
Obotan
Oxydess II
Spancap No. 1

GENERAL INFORMATION

Habit forming? Yes
Prescription needed? Yes
Available as generic? Yes
Drug class: Central-nervous-system stimulant (amphetamine)

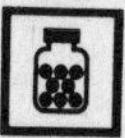

USES

- Prevents narcolepsy (attacks of uncontrollable sleepiness).
- Controls hyperactivity in children.

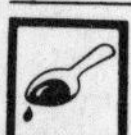

DOSAGE & USAGE INFORMATION

How to take:

- Tablet or liquid—Swallow with water.
- Extended-release capsules—Swallow each dose whole with liquid.

When to take:

- At the same times each day.
- Short-acting form—Don't take later than 6 hours before bedtime.
- Long-acting form—Take on awakening.

If you forget a dose:

- Short-acting form—Take up to 2 hours late. If more than 2 hours, wait for next dose (don't double this).
- Long-acting form—Take as soon as you remember. Wait 20 hours for next dose.

What drug does:

- Narcolepsy—Apparently affects brain centers to decrease fatigue or sleepiness and increase alertness and motor activity.
- Hyperactive children—Calms children, opposite to effect on narcoleptic adults.

Time lapse before drug works:
15 to 30 minutes.

Don't take with:
See Interaction column and consult doctor.

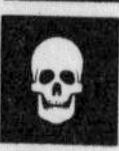

OVERDOSE

Symptoms:
Rapid heartbeat, hyperactivity, high fever, hallucinations, suicidal or homicidal feelings, convulsions, coma.

What to do:

- Dial 0 (operator) or 911 (emergency) for an ambulance or medical help. Then give first aid immediately.
- Additional emergency information on page 886.

POSSIBLE ADVERSE REACTIONS OR SIDE EFFECTS

SYMPTOMS	FREQUENCY	WHAT TO DO
Brain & nervous system:		
• Headache	Infrequent	4
• Dizziness, lack of alertness.	Infrequent	3
• Mood changes.	Rare	4
• Irritability, nervousness, insomnia.	Common	4
Skin:		
Rash, hives.	Rare	3
Eyes:		
Blurred vision.	Infrequent	3
Ears, nose, throat:		
Dry mouth.	Common	5
Digestive:		
Diarrhea or constipation, appetite loss, stomach pain, nausea, vomiting, weight loss.	Infrequent	5
Heart & lungs:		
• Fast, pounding heartbeat.	Infrequent	3
• Chest pain or irregular heartbeat.	Rare	3
Blood vessels, kidneys, liver, allergic, blood:	None expected.	
Muscles, bones, joints:		
Uncontrolled movements of head, neck, arms, legs.	Rare	3
Genital, urinary:		
Decreased sex drive, impotence.	Infrequent	5
Others:		
• Enlarged breasts.	Rare	4
• Unusual sweating.	Infrequent	3

1- Life-threatening. Seek emergency treatment immediately.
2- Discontinue. Seek emergency treatment.
3- Discontinue. Call doctor right away.
4- Continue. Call doctor when convenient.
5- Continue. Tell doctor at next visit.

WARNINGS & PRECAUTIONS

Don't take if:
- You are allergic to any amphetamine or central-nervous-system stimulant.
- You will have surgery within 2 months, including dental surgery, requiring general or spinal anesthesia.

Before you start, consult your doctor:
- If you plan to become pregnant within medication period.
- If you have glaucoma.
- If you have heart or blood-vessel disease, or high blood pressure.
- If you have overactive thyroid, anxiety or tension.
- If you have a severe mental illness (especially children).

Over age 60:
Adverse reactions and side effects may be more frequent and severe than in younger persons.

Pregnancy:
Risk to unborn child outweighs drug benefits. Don't use.

Breast-feeding:
Drug passes into milk. Avoid drug or discontinue nursing.

Infants & children:
Not recommended for children under 12.

Prolonged use:
Habit forming.

Skin & sunlight:
No problems expected.

Driving, piloting or hazardous work:
Don't drive or pilot aircraft until you learn how medicine affects you. Don't work around dangerous machinery. Don't climb ladders or work in high places. Danger increases if you drink alcohol or take medicine affecting alertness and reflexes.

Airplane passengers:
No problems expected.

Discontinuing:
May be unnecessary to finish medicine. Follow doctor's instructions.

Others:
- This is a dangerous drug and must be closely supervised. Don't use for appetite control or depression. Potential for damage and abuse.
- During withdrawal phase, may cause prolonged sleep of several days.

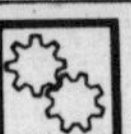

INTERACTION WITH OTHER DRUGS

GENERIC NAME OR DRUG CLASS	COMBINED EFFECT
Anesthesias (general)	Irregular heartbeat.
Antidepressants (tricyclic)	Decreased dextroamphetamine effect.
Antihypertensives	Decreased antihypertensive effect.
Carbonic anhydrase inhibitors	Increased dextroamphetamine effect.
Guanethidine	Decreased guanethidine effect.
Haloperidol	Decreased dextroamphetamine effect.
MAO inhibitors	May severely increase blood pressure.
Phenothiazines	Decreased dextroamphetamine effect.
Sodium bicarbonate	Increased dextroamphetamine effect.

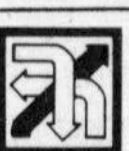

INTERACTION WITH OTHER SUBSTANCES

INTERACTS WITH	COMBINED EFFECT
Alcohol:	Decreased dextroamphetamine effect. Avoid.
Beverages: Caffeine drinks	Overstimulation. Avoid.
Cocaine:	Dangerous stimulation of nervous system. Avoid.
Foods:	None expected.
Marijuana:	Frequent use—Severely impaired mental function.
Tobacco:	None expected.

DEXTROMETHORPHAN

BRAND NAMES

Dristan Cough Formula
Formula 44-D
Hold Cough Suppressant
Nyquil
Robitussin-DM
Romilar
St. Joseph Cough Syrup
Silexin
Trocal
Tussaminic
Vicks Cough Syrup

See complete brand names list, page 825.

GENERAL INFORMATION

Habit forming? No
Prescription needed? No
Available as generic? Yes
Drug class: Cough suppressant

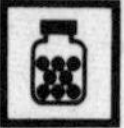

USES

Suppresses cough associated with allergies or infections such as colds, bronchitis, flu and lung disorders.

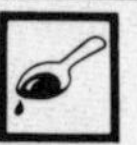

DOSAGE & USAGE INFORMATION

How to take:

- Tablet or capsule—Swallow with liquid. If you can't swallow whole, crumble tablet or open capsule and take with liquid or food.
- Lozenges or syrups—Take as directed on label.

When to take:
As needed, no more often than every 3 hours.

If you forget a dose:
Take as soon as you remember. Wait 3 hours for next dose.

What drug does:
Reduces sensitivity of brain's cough-control center, suppressing urge to cough.

Time lapse before drug works:
15 to 30 minutes.

Don't take with:
See Interaction column and consult doctor.

OVERDOSE

Symptoms:
Euphoria, overactivity, sense of intoxication, visual and auditory hallucinations, lack of coordination, stagger, stupor, shallow breathing.

What to do:

- Dial 0 (operator) or 911 (emergency) for an ambulance or medical help. Then give first aid immediately.
- Additional emergency information on page 886.

POSSIBLE ADVERSE REACTIONS OR SIDE EFFECTS

SYMPTOMS	FREQUENCY	WHAT TO DO
Brain & nervous system: Dizziness, drowsiness.	Rare	3
Skin: Rash	Rare	3
Eyes:	None expected.	
Ears, nose, throat:	None expected.	
Digestive: Diarrhea, nausea or vomiting, stomach pain.	Rare	3
Heart & lungs:	None expected.	
Blood vessels:	None expected.	
Muscles, bones, joints:	None expected.	
Genital, urinary:	None expected.	
Kidneys:	None expected.	
Liver:	None expected.	
Allergic:	None expected.	
Blood:	None expected.	
Others:	None expected.	

1- Life-threatening. Seek emergency treatment immediately.
2- Discontinue. Seek emergency treatment.
3- Discontinue. Call doctor right away.
4- Continue. Call doctor when convenient.
5- Continue. Tell doctor at next visit.
6- No action necessary.

WARNINGS & PRECAUTIONS

Don't take if:
You are allergic to any cough syrup containing dextromethorphan.

Before you start, consult your doctor:
- If you have asthma attacks.
- If you have impaired liver function.

Over age 60:
May become constipated, excessively drowsy or unsteady. If drug is used for cough, other treatment may be necessary to liquefy thick mucus in bronchial tubes.

Pregnancy:
No proven harm to unborn child. Avoid if possible.

Breast-feeding:
No proven problems. Consult doctor.

Infants & children:
Use only as label directs.

Prolonged use:
No problems expected.

Skin & sunlight:
No problems expected.

Driving, piloting or hazardous work:
Don't drive or pilot aircraft until you learn how medicine affects you. Don't work around dangerous machinery. Don't climb ladders or work in high places. Danger increases if you drink alcohol or take medicine affecting alertness and reflexes, such as antihistamines, tranquilizers, sedatives, pain medicine, narcotics and mind-altering drugs.

Airplane passengers:
No problems expected.

Discontinuing:
May be unnecessary to finish medicine. Follow doctor's instructions.

Others:
- If cough persists or if you cough blood or brown-yellow, thick mucus, call your doctor.
- Excessive use may lead to functional dependence.

INTERACTION WITH OTHER DRUGS

GENERIC NAME OR DRUG CLASS	COMBINED EFFECT
MAO inhibitors	Disorientation, high fever, drop in blood pressure and loss of consciousness.

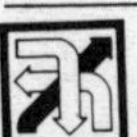

INTERACTION WITH OTHER SUBSTANCES

INTERACTS WITH	COMBINED EFFECT
Alcohol:	None expected.
Beverages:	None expected.
Cocaine:	Decreased dextromethorphan effect. Avoid.
Foods:	None expected.
Marijuana:	None expected.
Tobacco:	None expected.

DIAZEPAM

BRAND NAMES

Apo-Diazepam
D-Tran
E-Pam
Maval
Neo-Calme
Novodipam
Rival
Serenack
Stress-Pam
Valium
Valrelease
Vivol

GENERAL INFORMATION

Habit forming? Yes
Prescription needed? Yes
Available as generic? Yes
Drug class: Tranquilizer (benzodiazepine)

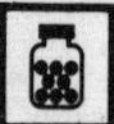

USES

- Treatment for nervousness or tension.
- Treatment for muscle spasm.
- Treatment for convulsive disorders.

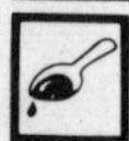

DOSAGE & USAGE INFORMATION

How to take:
Tablet or capsule—Swallow with liquid. If you can't swallow whole, crumble tablet or open capsule and take with liquid or food.

When to take:
At the same time each day, according to instructions on prescription label.

If you forget a dose:
Take as soon as you remember up to 2 hours late. If more than 2 hours, wait for next scheduled dose (don't double this dose).

What drug does:
Affects limbic system of brain—part that controls emotions.

Time lapse before drug works:
2 hours. May take 6 weeks for full benefit.

Don't take with:
See Interaction column and consult doctor.

OVERDOSE

Symptoms:
Drowsiness, weakness, tremor, stupor, coma.

What to do:

- Dial 0 (operator) or 911 (emergency) for an ambulance or medical help. Then give first aid immediately.
- If patient is unconscious and not breathing, give mouth-to-mouth breathing. If there is no heartbeat, use cardiac massage and mouth-to-mouth breathing (CPR). Don't try to make patient vomit. If you can't get help quickly, take patient to nearest emergency facility.
- Additional emergency information on page 886.

POSSIBLE ADVERSE REACTIONS OR SIDE EFFECTS

SYMPTOMS	FREQUENCY	WHAT TO DO
Brain & nervous system:		
• Clumsiness, drowsiness, dizziness.	Common	4
• Hallucinations, confusion, depression, irritability.	Infrequent	3
Skin: Rash, itch.	Infrequent	3
Eyes: Vision changes.	Infrequent	3
Ears, nose, throat: Mouth, throat ulcers.	Rare	3
Digestive: Constipation or diarrhea, nausea, vomiting.	Infrequent	4
Heart & lungs: Slow heartbeat, breathing difficulty.	Rare	2
Blood vessels:	None expected.	
Muscles, bones, joints:	None expected.	
Genital, urinary: Urination difficulty.	Infrequent	4
Kidneys:	None expected.	
Liver: Jaundice (yellow eyes and skin).	Rare	3
Allergic:	None expected.	
Blood:	None expected.	
Others:	None expected.	

1- Life-threatening. Seek emergency treatment immediately.
2- Discontinue. Seek emergency treatment.
3- Discontinue. Call doctor right away.
4- Continue. Call doctor when convenient.
5- Continue. Tell doctor at next visit.
6- No action necessary.

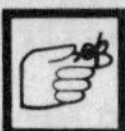

WARNINGS & PRECAUTIONS

Don't take if:

- You are allergic to any benzodiazepine.
- You have myasthenia gravis.
- You are active or recovering alcoholic.
- Patient is younger than 6 months.

Before you start, consult your doctor:

- If you have liver, kidney or lung disease.
- If you have diabetes, epilepsy or porphyria.

Over age 60:
Adverse reactions and side effects may be more frequent and severe than in younger persons. You need smaller doses for shorter periods of time. May develop agitation, rage or "hangover effect."

Pregnancy:
Risk to unborn child outweighs drug benefits. Don't use.

Breast-feeding:
Drug passes into milk. Avoid drug or discontinue nursing until you finish medicine. Consult doctor for advice on maintaining milk supply.

Infants & children:
Use only under medical supervision for children older than 6 months.

Prolonged use:
May impair liver function.

Skin & sunlight:
No problems expected.

Driving, piloting or hazardous work:
Don't drive or pilot aircraft until you learn how medicine affects you. Don't work around dangerous machinery. Don't climb ladders or work in high places. Danger increases if you drink alcohol or take medicine affecting alertness and reflexes.

Airplane passengers:
No problems expected.

Discontinuing:
Don't discontinue without consulting doctor. Dose may require gradual reduction if you have taken drug for a long time. Doses of other drugs may also require adjustment.

Others:

- Hot weather, heavy exercise and profuse sweat may reduce excretion and cause overdose.
- Blood sugar may rise in diabetics, requiring insulin adjustment.

INTERACTION WITH OTHER DRUGS

GENERIC NAME OR DRUG CLASS	COMBINED EFFECT
Anticonvulsants	Change in seizure frequency or severity.
Antidepressants	Increased sedative effect of both drugs.
Antihistamines	Increased sedative effect of both drugs.
Antihypertensives	Excessively low blood pressure.
Cimetidine	Excess sedation.
Disulfiram	Increased diazepam effect.
MAO inhibitors	Convulsions, deep sedation, rage.
Narcotics	Increased sedative effect of both drugs.
Sedatives	Increased sedative effect of both drugs.
Sleep inducers	Increased sedative effect of both drugs.
Tranquilizers	Increased sedative effect of both drugs.

INTERACTION WITH OTHER SUBSTANCES

INTERACTS WITH	COMBINED EFFECT
Alcohol:	Heavy sedation. Avoid.
Beverages:	None expected.
Cocaine:	Decreased diazepam effect.
Foods:	None expected.
Marijuana:	Heavy sedation. Avoid.
Tobacco:	Decreased diazepam effect.

DICLOXACILLIN

BRAND NAMES

Dycill
Dynapen
Pathocil

GENERAL INFORMATION

Habit forming? No
Prescription needed? Yes
Available as generic? Yes
Drug class: Antibiotic (penicillin)

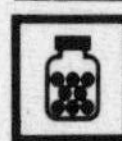

USES

Treatment of bacterial infections that are susceptible to dicloxacillin.

DOSAGE & USAGE INFORMATION

How to take:

- Tablets or capsules—Swallow with liquid on an empty stomach 1 hour before or 2 hours after eating.
- Liquid—Take with cold beverage. Liquid form is perishable and effective for only 7 days at room temperature. Effective for 14 days if stored in refrigerator. Don't freeze.

When to take:
Follow instructions on prescription label or side of package. Doses should be evenly spaced. For example, 4 times a day means every 6 hours.

If you forget a dose:
Take as soon as you remember. Continue regular schedule.

What drug does:
Destroys susceptible bacteria. Does not kill viruses.

Time lapse before drug works:
May be several days before medicine affects infection.

Don't take with:
See Interaction column and consult doctor.

OVERDOSE

Symptoms:
Severe diarrhea, nausea or vomiting.

What to do:
Overdose unlikely to threaten life. If person takes much larger amount than prescribed, call doctor, poison-control center or hospital emergency room for instructions.

POSSIBLE ADVERSE REACTIONS OR SIDE EFFECTS

SYMPTOMS	FREQUENCY	WHAT TO DO
Brain & nervous system:	None expected.	
Skin: Hives, rash, intense itch soon after a dose.	Rare	1
Eyes:	None expected.	
Ears, nose, throat: Dark or discolored tongue.	Common	5
Digestive: Mild nausea, vomiting, diarrhea.	Infrequent	4
Heart & lungs:	None expected.	
Blood vessels: Unexplained bleeding.	Rare	3
Muscles, bones, joints:	None expected.	
Genital, urinary:	None expected.	
Kidneys:	None expected.	
Liver:	None expected.	
Allergic: Life-threatening anaphylaxis may occur!	Rare	1 See page 888.
Blood:	None expected.	
Others:	None expected.	

1- Life-threatening. Seek emergency treatment immediately.
2- Discontinue. Seek emergency treatment.
3- Discontinue. Call doctor right away.
4- Continue. Call doctor when convenient.
5- Continue. Tell doctor at next visit.
6- No action necessary.

WARNINGS & PRECAUTIONS

Don't take if:
You are allergic to dicloxacillin, cephalosporin antibiotics, other penicillins or penicillamine. Life-threatening reaction may occur.

Before you start, consult your doctor:
If you are allergic to any substance or drug.

Over age 60:
You may have skin reactions, particularly around genitals and anus.

Pregnancy:
Studies inconclusive on harm to unborn child. Animal studies show fetal abnormalities. Decide with your doctor whether drug benefits justify risk to unborn child.

Breast-feeding:
Drug passes into milk. Child may become sensitive to penicillins and have allergic reactions to penicillin drugs. Avoid dicloxacillin or discontinue nursing until you finish medicine. Consult doctor for advice on maintaining milk supply.

Infants & children:
No problems expected.

Prolonged use:
You may become more susceptible to infections caused by germs not responsive to dicloxacillin.

Skin & sunlight:
No problems expected.

Driving, piloting or hazardous work:
Usually not dangerous. Most hazardous reactions likely to occur a few minutes after taking dicloxacillin.

Airplane passengers:
No problems expected.

Discontinuing:
Don't discontinue without doctor's advice until you complete prescribed dose, even though symptoms diminish or disappear.

Others:
No problems expected.

INTERACTION WITH OTHER DRUGS

GENERIC NAME OR DRUG CLASS	COMBINED EFFECT
Chloramphenicol	Decreased effect of both drugs.
Erythromycins	Decreased effect of both drugs.
Paromomycin	Decreased effect of both drugs.
Tetracyclines	Decreased effect of both drugs.
Troleandomycin	Decreased effect of both drugs.

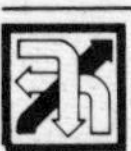

INTERACTION WITH OTHER SUBSTANCES

INTERACTS WITH	COMBINED EFFECT
Alcohol:	Occasional stomach irritation.
Beverages:	None expected.
Cocaine:	No proven problems.
Foods:	None expected.
Marijuana:	No proven problems.
Tobacco:	None expected.

DICYCLOMINE

BRAND NAMES

Antispas
Bentyl
Bentylol
Cyclobec
Dibent
Dicen
Dilomine
Di-Spaz
Dyspas
Formulex
Lomine
Menospasm
Neoquess
Nospaz
Or-Tyl
Protylol
Spasmoban
Spasmoject
Triactin
Viscerol

GENERAL INFORMATION

Habit forming? No
Prescription needed? Low strength: No
High strength: Yes
Available as generic? Yes
Drug class: Antispasmodic, anticholinergic

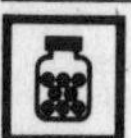

USES

Reduces spasms of digestive system, bladder and urethra.

DOSAGE & USAGE INFORMATION

How to take:

- Tablet, syrup or capsule—Swallow with liquid or food to lessen stomach irritation.
- Drops—Dilute dose in beverage before swallowing.

When to take:
30 minutes before meals (unless directed otherwise by doctor).

If you forget a dose:
Take as soon as you remember up to 2 hours late. If more than 2 hours, wait for next scheduled dose (don't double this dose).

What drug does:
Blocks nerve impulses at parasympathetic nerve endings, preventing muscle contractions and gland secretions of organs involved.

Time lapse before drug works:
15 to 30 minutes.

Don't take with:
See Interaction column and consult doctor.

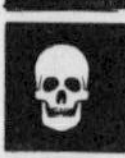

OVERDOSE

Symptoms:
Dilated pupils; rapid pulse and breathing; dizziness; fever; hallucinations; confusion; slurred speech; agitation; flushed face; convulsions; coma.

What to do:

- Dial 0 (operator) or 911 (emergency) for an ambulance or medical help. Then give first aid immediately.
- Additional emergency information on page 886.

POSSIBLE ADVERSE REACTIONS OR SIDE EFFECTS

SYMPTOMS	FREQUENCY	WHAT TO DO
Brain & nervous system:		
• Headache	Infrequent	4
• Confusion, delirium.	Common	3
Skin:		
Rash or hives.	Rare	3
Eyes:		
Pain, blurred vision.	Rare	3
Ears, nose, throat:		
Dryness	Common	6
Digestive:		
• Constipation	Common	5
• Nausea, vomiting.	Common	4
Heart & lungs:		
Rapid heartbeat.	Common	3
Blood vessels:	None expected.	
Muscles, bones, joints:	None expected.	
Genital, urinary:		
Difficult urination.	Infrequent	4
Kidneys:	None expected.	
Liver:	None expected.	
Allergic:	None expected.	
Blood:	None expected.	
Others:		
Less perspiration.	Common	4

1- Life-threatening. Seek emergency treatment immediately.
2- Discontinue. Seek emergency treatment.
3- Discontinue. Call doctor right away.
4- Continue. Call doctor when convenient.
5- Continue. Tell doctor at next visit.
6- No action necessary.

WARNINGS & PRECAUTIONS

Don't take if:
- You are allergic to any anticholinergic.
- You have trouble with stomach bloating.
- You have difficulty emptying your bladder completely.
- You have narrow-angle glaucoma.
- You have severe ulcerative colitis.

Before you start, consult your doctor:
- If you have open-angle glaucoma.
- If you have angina.
- If you have chronic bronchitis or asthma.
- If you have hiatal hernia.
- If you have liver disease.
- If you have enlarged prostate.
- If you have myasthenia gravis.
- If you have peptic ulcer.
- If you will have surgery within 2 months, including dental surgery, requiring general or spinal anesthesia.

Over age 60:
Adverse reactions and side effects may be more frequent and severe than in younger persons.

Pregnancy:
Studies inconclusive on harm to unborn child. Animal studies show fetal abnormalities. Decide with your doctor whether drug benefits justify risk to unborn child.

Breast-feeding:
Drug passes into milk and decreases milk flow. Avoid drug or discontinue nursing until you finish medicine. Consult doctor for advice on maintaining milk supply.

Infants & children:
Use only under medical supervision.

Prolonged use:
Chronic constipation, possible fecal impaction. Consult doctor immediately.

Skin & sunlight:
No problems expected.

Driving, piloting or hazardous work:
Use disqualifies you for piloting aircraft. Otherwise, no problems expected.

Airplane passengers:
No problems expected.

Discontinuing:
May be unnecessary to finish medicine. Follow doctor's instructions.

Others:
No problems expected.

INTERACTION WITH OTHER DRUGS

GENERIC NAME OR DRUG CLASS	COMBINED EFFECT
Amantadine	Increased dicyclomine effect.
Anticholinergics (other)	Increased dicyclomine effect.
Antidepressants (tricyclic)	Increased dicyclomine effect.
Antihistamines	Increased dicyclomine effect.
Cortisone drugs	Increased internal-eye pressure.
Haloperidol	Increased internal-eye pressure.
MAO inhibitors	Increased dicyclomine effect.
Meperidine	Increased dicyclomine effect.
Methylphenidate	Increased dicyclomine effect.
Orphenadrine	Increased dicyclomine effect.
Phenothiazines	Increased dicyclomine effect.
Pilocarpine	Loss of pilocarpine effect in glaucoma treatment.
Vitamin C	Decreased dicyclomine effect. Avoid large doses of vitamin C.

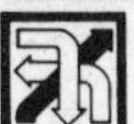

INTERACTION WITH OTHER SUBSTANCES

INTERACTS WITH	COMBINED EFFECT
Alcohol:	None expected.
Beverages:	None expected.
Cocaine:	Excessively rapid heartbeat. Avoid.
Foods:	None expected.
Marijuana:	Drowsiness and dry mouth.
Tobacco:	None expected.

DIETHYLSTILBESTROL

BRAND NAMES

DES
Honvol
Stilbestrol
Stilphostrol

GENERAL INFORMATION

Habit forming? No
Prescription needed? Yes
Available as generic? Yes
Drug class: Female sex hormone (estrogen)

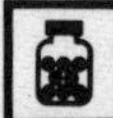

USES

- Treatment for symptoms of menopause and menstrual-cycle irregularity.
- Replacement for female hormone deficiency.
- Treatment for cancer of prostate and breast.

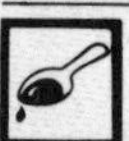

DOSAGE & USAGE INFORMATION

How to take:
- Tablet—Swallow with liquid. If you can't swallow whole, crumble tablet and take with liquid or food.
- Vaginal suppositories—Use as directed on label.

When to take:
At the same time each day.

If you forget a dose:
Take as soon as you remember up to 12 hours late. If more than 12 hours, wait for next scheduled dose (don't double this dose).

What drug does:
Restores normal estrogen level in tissues.

Time lapse before drug works:
10 to 20 days.

Don't take with:
See Interaction column and consult doctor.

OVERDOSE

Symptoms:
Nausea, vomiting, fluid retention, breast enlargement and discomfort, abnormal vaginal bleeding.

What to do:
Overdose unlikely to threaten life. If person takes much larger amount than prescribed, call doctor, poison-control center or hospital emergency room for instructions.

POSSIBLE ADVERSE REACTIONS OR SIDE EFFECTS

SYMPTOMS	FREQUENCY	WHAT TO DO
Brain & nervous system:		
Depression, dizziness, irritability.	Infrequent	4
Skin:		
• Rash	Infrequent	3
• Brown blotches.	Infrequent	5
• Hair loss.	Infrequent	5
Eyes, ears, nose, throat, heart & lungs, muscles, bones, joints, kidneys, allergic, blood:	None expected.	
Digestive:		
• Stomach or side pain.	Infrequent	3
• Stomach cramps.	Common	3
• Appetite loss.	Common	4
• Nausea, diarrhea.	Common	5
• Vomiting	Infrequent	4
Blood vessels:		
Swollen ankles, feet.	Common	5
Genital, urinary:		
Vaginal discharge or bleeding.	Infrequent	5
Liver:		
Jaundice (yellow skin and eyes).	Rare	3
Others:		
• Breast lumps.	Infrequent	4
• Swollen, tender breasts.	Common	5
• Changes in sex drive.	Infrequent	5

1- Life-threatening. Seek emergency treatment immediately.
2- Discontinue. Seek emergency treatment.
3- Discontinue. Call doctor right away.
4- Continue. Call doctor when convenient.
5- Continue. Tell doctor at next visit.

WARNINGS & PRECAUTIONS

Don't take if:
- You are allergic to any estrogen-containing drugs.
- You have impaired liver function.
- You have had blood clots, stroke or heart attack.
- You have unexplained vaginal bleeding.

Before you start, consult your doctor:
- If you have had cancer of breast or reproductive organs, fibrocystic breast disease, fibroid tumors of the uterus or endometriosis.
- If you have had migraine headaches, epilepsy or porphyria.
- If you have diabetes, high blood pressure, asthma, congestive heart failure, kidney disease or gallstones.
- If you plan to become pregnant within 3 months.

Over age 60:
Controversial. You and your doctor must decide if drug risks outweigh benefits.

Pregnancy:
Risk to unborn child outweighs drug benefits. Don't use.

Breast-feeding:
Drug filters into milk. May harm child. Avoid.

Infants & children:
Not recommended.

Prolonged use:
Increased growth of fibroid tumors of uterus. Possible association with cancer of uterus.

Skin & sunlight:
May cause rash or intensify sunburn in areas exposed to sun or sunlamp.

Driving, piloting or hazardous work:
No problems expected.

Airplane passengers:
No problems expected.

Discontinuing:
You may need to discontinue diethylstilbestrol periodically. Consult your doctor.

Others:
In rare instances, may cause blood clot in lung, brain or leg. Symptoms are *sudden* severe headache, coordination loss, vision change, chest pain, breathing difficulty, slurred speech, pain in legs or groin. Seek emergency treatment immediately.

INTERACTION WITH OTHER DRUGS

GENERIC NAME OR DRUG CLASS	COMBINED EFFECT
Anticoagulants (oral)	Decreased anticoagulant effect.
Anticonvulsants (hydantoin)	Increased seizures.
Antidiabetics (oral)	Unpredictable increase or decrease in blood sugar.
Clofibrate	Decreased clofibrate effect.
Carbamazepine	Increased seizures.
Meprobamate	Increased diethylstilbestrol effect.
Phenobarbital	Decreased diethylstilbestrol effect.
Primidone	Decreased diethylstilbestrol effect.
Rifampin	Decreased diethylstilbestrol effect.
Thyroid hormones	Decreased thyroid effect.

INTERACTION WITH OTHER SUBSTANCES

INTERACTS WITH	COMBINED EFFECT
Alcohol:	None expected.
Beverages:	None expected.
Cocaine:	No proven problems.
Foods:	None expected.
Marijuana:	Possible menstrual irregularities and bleeding between periods.
Tobacco:	Increased risk of blood clots leading to stroke or heart attack.

DIFLUNISAL

BRAND NAMES

Dolobid

GENERAL INFORMATION

Habit forming? No
Prescription needed? Yes
Available as generic? Yes
Drug class: Antiinflammatory (non-steroid)

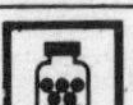

USES

- Treatment for joint pain, stiffness, inflammation and swelling of arthritis and gout.
- Pain reliever.

DOSAGE & USAGE INFORMATION

How to take:
Tablet or capsule—Swallow with liquid or food to lessen stomach irritation. If you can't swallow whole, crumble tablet or open capsule and take with liquid or food.

When to take:
At the same times each day.

If you forget a dose:
Take as soon as you remember up to 2 hours late. If more than 2 hours, wait for next scheduled dose (don't double this dose).

What drug does:
Reduces tissue concentration of prostaglandins (hormones which produce inflammation and pain).

Time lapse before drug works:
Begins in 4 to 24 hours. May require 3 weeks regular use for maximum benefit.

Don't take with:
See Interaction column and consult doctor.

OVERDOSE

Symptoms:
Confusion, agitation, incoherence, convulsions, possible hemorrhage from stomach or intestine, coma.

What to do:
- Dial 0 (operator) or 911 (emergency) for an ambulance or medical help. Then give first aid immediately.
- Additional emergency information on page 886.

POSSIBLE ADVERSE REACTIONS OR SIDE EFFECTS

SYMPTOMS	FREQUENCY	WHAT TO DO
Brain & nervous system:		
• Depression drowsiness.	Infrequent	4
• Convulsions, confusion.	Rare	3
• Dizziness	Common	4
• Headache	Common	5
Skin:		
Rash, hives or itch.	Rare	3
Eyes:		
Blurred vision.	Rare	3
Ears, nose, throat:		
Ringing in ears.	Infrequent	4
Digestive:		
• Bloody or black, tarry stools.	Rare	3
• Nausea, pain.	Common	4
• Constipation or diarrhea, vomiting.	Infrequent	4
Heart & lungs:		
Breathing difficulty, tightness in chest, rapid heartbeat.	Rare	3
Blood vessels:		
Unusual bleeding or bruising.	Rare	3
Muscles, bones, joints:		
Swollen feet, legs.	Infrequent	4
Genital, urinary:		
• Bloody urine.	Rare	3
• Difficult, painful or frequent urination.	Rare	4
Kidneys, allergic, blood:	None expected.	
Liver:		
Jaundice (yellow skin and eyes).	Rare	3
Others:		
Fatigue, weakness.	Rare	4

3- Discontinue. Call doctor right away.
4- Continue. Call doctor when convenient.
5- Continue. Tell doctor at next visit.

WARNINGS & PRECAUTIONS

Don't take if:
- You are allergic to aspirin or any non-steroid, antiinflammatory drug.
- You have gastritis, peptic ulcer, enteritis, ileitis, ulcerative colitis, asthma, heart failure, high blood pressure or bleeding problems.
- Patient is younger than 15.

Before you start, consult your doctor:
- If you have epilepsy.
- If you have Parkinson's disease.
- If you have been mentally ill.
- If you have had kidney disease or impaired kidney function.

Over age 60:
Adverse reactions and side effects may be more frequent and severe than in younger persons.

Pregnancy:
Studies inconclusive on harm to unborn child. Animal studies show fetal abnormalities. Decide with your doctor whether drug benefits justify risk to unborn child.

Breast-feeding:
May harm child. Avoid.

Infants & children:
Not recommended for anyone younger than 15. Use only under medical supervision.

Prolonged use:
- Eye damage.
- Reduced hearing.
- Sore throat, fever.
- Weight gain.

Skin & sunlight:
No problems expected.

Driving, piloting or hazardous work:
Don't drive or pilot aircraft until you learn how medicine affects you. Don't work around dangerous machinery. Don't climb ladders or work in high places. Danger increases if you drink alcohol or take medicine affecting alertness and reflexes, such as antihistamines, tranquilizers, sedatives, pain medicine, narcotics and mind-altering drugs.

Airplane passengers:
No problems expected.

Discontinuing:
Don't discontinue without consulting doctor. Dose may require gradual reduction if you have taken drug for a long time. Doses of other drugs may also require adjustment.

Others:
No problems expected.

INTERACTION WITH OTHER DRUGS

GENERIC NAME OR DRUG CLASS	COMBINED EFFECT
Antacids	Decreased diflunisal effect.
Anticoagulants (oral)	Decreased effect of anticoagulant.
Aspirin, other antiinflammatory drugs	Increased risk of stomach ulcer.
Cortisone drugs	Increased risk of stomach ulcer.
Furosemide	Decreased diuretic effect of furosemide.
Hydrochlorothiazide	Increased risk of severe blood-pressure drop.
Indomethacin	Increased possibility of intestinal hemorrhage.
Oxyphenbutazone	Possible stomach ulcer.
Phenylbutazone	Possible stomach ulcer.
Probenecid	Increased diflunisal effect.
Thyroid hormones	Rapid heartbeat. blood-pressure rise.

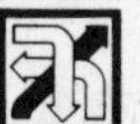

INTERACTION WITH OTHER SUBSTANCES

INTERACTS WITH	COMBINED EFFECT
Alcohol:	Possible stomach ulcer or bleeding.
Beverages:	None expected.
Cocaine:	Increased cocaine toxicity. Avoid.
Foods:	None expected.
Marijuana:	Increased pain relief from diflunisal.
Tobacco:	Decreased absorption of diflunisal. Avoid.

DIGITALIS PREPARATIONS

BRAND AND GENERIC NAMES

Crystodigin
Crystogin
Digifortis
Digiglusin
DIGITALIS
DIGITOXIN
DIGOXIN
Gitaligen
GITALIN
Lanoxicaps
Lanoxin
Natigozine
Novodigoxin
Purodigin

GENERAL INFORMATION

Habit forming? No
prescription needed? Yes
Available as generic? Yes
Drug class: Digitalis preparations

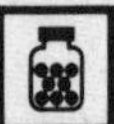

USES

- Strengthens weak heart-muscle contractions to prevent congestive heart failure.
- Corrects irregular heartbeat.

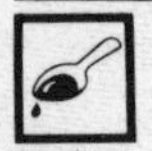

DOSAGE & USAGE INFORMATION

How to take:
- Tablet or capsule—Swallow with liquid. If you can't swallow whole, crumble tablet or open capsule and take with liquid or food.
- Liquid—Dilute dose in beverage before swallowing.

When to take:
At the same time each day.

If you forget a dose:
Take as soon as you remember up to 12 hours late. If more than 12 hours, wait for next scheduled dose (don't double this dose).

What drug does:
- Strengthens heart-muscle contraction.
- Delays nerve impulses to heart.

Time lapse before drug works:
May require regular use for a week or more.

Don't take with:
- Non-prescription drugs without consulting doctor.
- See Interaction column and consult doctor.

OVERDOSE

Symptoms:
Nausea, vomiting, diarrhea, vision disturbances with halos around lights, irregular heartbeat, confusion, hallucinations, convulsions.

What to do:
- Dial 0 (operator) or 911 (emergency) for an ambulance or medical help. Then give first aid immediately.
- Additional emergency information on page 886.

POSSIBLE ADVERSE REACTIONS OR SIDE EFFECTS

SYMPTOMS	FREQUENCY	WHAT TO DO
Brain & nervous system:		
Drowsiness, lethargy, disorientation.	Infrequent	3
Skin:		
Rash, hives.	Rare	3
Eyes:		
Double or yellow-green vision.	Rare	4
Ears, nose, throat:	None expected.	
Digestive:		
Appetite loss, diarrhea.	Common	4
Heart & lungs:	None expected.	
Blood vessels:	None expected.	
Muscles, bones, joints:	None expected.	
Genital, urinary:	None expected.	
Kidneys:	None expected.	
Liver:	None expected.	
Allergic:	None expected.	
Blood:	None expected.	
Others:		
• Enlarged, sensitive male breasts.	Rare	4
• Tiredness, weakness.	Rare	4

1- Life-threatening. Seek emergency treatment immediately.
2- Discontinue. Seek emergency treatment.
3- Discontinue. Call doctor right away.
4- Continue. Call doctor when convenient.
5- Continue. Tell doctor at next visit.
6- No action necessary.

DIGITALIS PREPARATIONS

WARNINGS & PRECAUTIONS

Don't take if:
- You are allergic to any digitalis preparation.
- Your heartbeat is slower than 50 beats per minute.

Before you start, consult your doctor:
- If you have taken another digitalis preparation in past 2 weeks.
- If you have taken a diuretic within 2 weeks.
- If you have liver or kidney disease.
- If you have a thyroid disorder.
- If you will have surgery within 2 months, including dental surgery, requiring general or spinal anesthesia.

Over age 60:
Adverse reactions and side effects may be more frequent and severe than in younger persons.

Pregnancy:
Studies inconclusive on harm to unborn child. Consult your doctor.

Breast-feeding:
Drug filters into milk. May harm child. Avoid.

Infants & children:
Use only under medical supervision.

Prolonged use:
No problems expected.

Skin & sunlight:
No problems expected.

Driving, piloting or hazardous work:
Possible vision disturbances. Otherwise, no problems expected.

Airplane passengers:
Nausea more likely.

Discontinuing:
Don't stop without doctor's advice.

Others:
No problems expected.

INTERACTION WITH OTHER DRUGS

GENERIC NAME OR DRUG CLASS	COMBINED EFFECT
Antacids	Decreased digitalis effect.
Anticonvulsants (hydantoin)	Increased digitalis effect at first, then decreased.
Beta-adrenergic blockers	Increased digitalis effect.
Cortisone drugs	Digitalis toxicity.
Diuretics	Digitalis toxicity.
Ephedrine	Disturbed heart rhythm. Avoid.
Epinephrine	Disturbed heart rhythm. Avoid.
Guanethidine	Increased digitalis effect.
Laxatives	Decreased digitalis effect.
Oxyphenbutazone	Decreased digitalis effect.
Phenobarbital	Decreased digitalis effect.
Phenylbutazone	Decreased digitalis effect.
Quinidine	Increased digitalis effect.
Rauwolfia alkaloids	Increased digitalis effect.
Thyroid hormones	Digitalis toxicity.

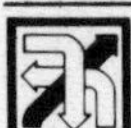

INTERACTION WITH OTHER SUBSTANCES

INTERACTS WITH	COMBINED EFFECT
Alcohol:	None expected.
Beverages: Caffeine drinks	Irregular heartbeat. Avoid.
Cocaine:	Irregular heartbeat. Avoid.
Foods:	None expected.
Marijuana:	Decreased digitalis effect.
Tobacco:	Irregular heartbeat. Avoid.

DILTIAZEM

BRAND NAMES

Cardizem

GENERAL INFORMATION

Habit forming? No
Prescription needed? Yes
Available as generic? No
Drug class: Calcium-channel blocker, antiarrhythmic, antianginal

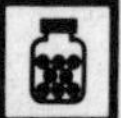

USES

- Prevents angina attacks.
- Stabilizes irregular heartbeat.

DOSAGE & USAGE INFORMATION

How to take:
Tablet or capsule—Swallow with liquid.

When to take:
At the same times each day 1 hour before or 2 hours after eating.

If you forget a dose:
Take as soon as you remember up to 2 hours late. If more than 2 hours, wait for next scheduled dose (don't double this dose).

What drug does:
- Reduces work that heart must perform.
- Reduces normal artery pressure.
- Increases oxygen to heart muscle.

Time lapse before drug works:
1 to 2 hours.

Don't take with:
See Interaction column and consult doctor.

OVERDOSE

Symptoms:
Unusually fast or unusually slow heartbeat; loss of consciousness, cardiac arrest.

What to do:
- Dial 0 (operator) or 911 (emergency) for an ambulance or medical help. Then give first aid immediately.
- Additional emergency information on page 886.

POSSIBLE ADVERSE REACTIONS OR SIDE EFFECTS

SYMPTOMS	FREQUENCY	WHAT TO DO
Brain & nervous system:		
• Dizziness	Infrequent	4
• Headache	Rare	5
• Fainting	Rare	3
Skin:		
Rash	Rare	3
Eyes, ears, nose, throat, kidneys, blood vessels, allergic, blood:	None expected.	
Digestive:		
Nausea, constipation or diarrhea, vomiting, indigestion.	Infrequent	5
Heart & lungs:		
• Unusually fast or slow heartbeat.	Infrequent	3
• Wheezing, cough, shortness of breath.	Infrequent	3
Muscles, bones, joints:		
• Numbness, tingling in hands and feet.	Infrequent	4
• Swelling of ankles, feet, legs.	Infrequent	4
Genital, urinary:		
Difficult urination.	Infrequent	4
Liver:		
Jaundice (yellow eyes and skin).	Rare	3
Others:		
Tiredness	Common	5

1-Life-threatening. Seek emergency treatment immediately.
2-Discontinue. Seek emergency treatment.
3-Discontinue. Call doctor right away.
4-Continue. Call doctor when convenient.
5-Continue. Tell doctor at next visit.

WARNINGS & PRECAUTIONS

Don't take if:
You are allergic to any calcium-channel blocker.

Before you start, consult your doctor:
- If you have kidney or liver disease.
- If you have high or low blood pressure.
- If you have heart disease other than coronary artery disease.

Over age 60:
Adverse reactions and side effects may be more frequent and severe than in younger persons.

Pregnancy:
No proven harm to unborn child. Avoid if possible.

Breast-feeding:
No problems expected.

Infants & children:
Not recommended.

Prolonged use:
No problems expected.

Skin & sunlight:
May cause rash or intensify sunburn in areas exposed to sun or sunlamp.

Driving, piloting or hazardous work:
Avoid if you feel dizzy. Otherwise, no problems expected.

Airplane passengers:
No problems expected.

Discontinuing:
Don't discontinue without consulting doctor.

Others:
Learn to check your own pulse rate. If it drops to 50 beats per minute or lower, don't take diltiazem until your consult your doctor.

INTERACTION WITH OTHER DRUGS

GENERIC NAME OR DRUG CLASS	COMBINED EFFECT
Antihypertensives	Dangerous blood-pressure drop.
Beta-adrenergic blockers	Decreased angina attacks.
Diuretics	Dangerous blood-pressure drop.
Disopyramide	May cause dangerously slow, fast or irregular heartbeat.
Nitrates	Reduced angina attacks.
Quinidine	Increased quinidine effect.

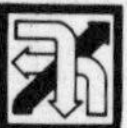

INTERACTION WITH OTHER SUBSTANCES

INTERACTS WITH	COMBINED EFFECT
Alcohol:	Dangerously low blood pressure.
Beverages:	None expected.
Cocaine:	Possible irregular heartbeat. Avoid.
Foods:	None expected.
Marijuana:	Possible irregular heartbeat. Avoid.
Tobacco:	Possible rapaid heartbeat. Avoid.

DIMENHYDRINATE

BRAND NAMES

Apo-Dimenhydrinate
Dimentabs
Dramaban
Dramamine
Dramilin
Dramocen
Dramoject
Dymenate
Eldodram
Gravol
Marine
Marmine
Motion-Aid
Nauseatol
Novodimenate
PMS-Dimenhydrinate
Trav-Arex
Travamine
Vertiban
Wehamine

GENERAL INFORMATION

Habit forming? No
Prescription needed?
High strength: Yes
Low strength: No
Available as generic? Yes
Drug class: Antihistamine

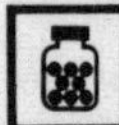

USES

- Reduces allergic symptoms such as hay fever, hives, rash or itching.
- Prevents motion sickness, nausea, vomiting.
- Induces sleep.

DOSAGE & USAGE INFORMATION

How to take:
Tablet or liquid—Swallow with liquid or food to lessen stomach irritation.

When to take:
Varies with form. Follow label directions.

If you forget a dose:
Take as soon as you remember up to 2 hours late. If more than 2 hours, wait for next scheduled dose (don't double this dose).

What drug does:
Blocks action of histamine after an allergic response triggers histamine release in sensitive cells.

Time lapse before drug works:
30 minutes.

Don't take with:
See Interaction column and consult doctor.

OVERDOSE

Symptoms:
Convulsions, red face, hallucinations, coma.

What to do:
- Dial 0 (operator) or 911 (emergency) for an ambulance or medical help. Then give first aid immediately.
- If patient is unconscious and not breathing, give mouth-to-mouth breathing. If there is no heartbeat, use cardiac massage and mouth-to-mouth breathing (CPR). Don't try to make patient vomit. If you can't get help quickly, take patient to nearest emergency facility.
- Additional emergency information on page 886.

POSSIBLE ADVERSE REACTIONS OR SIDE EFFECTS

SYMPTOMS	FREQUENCY	WHAT TO DO
Brain & nervous system:		
• Nightmares, agitation, irritability.	Rare	3
• Drowsiness, dizziness.	Common	5
Skin:	None expected.	
Eyes:		
• Vision changes.	Infrequent	3
• Less tolerance for contact lenses.	Infrequent	4
Ears, nose, throat:		
• Sore throat, fever.	Rare	3
• Dry mouth, nose, throat.	Common	5
Digestive:		
• Nausea	Common	5
• Appetite loss.	Infrequent	5
Heart & lungs:		
Rapid heartbeat.	Rare	3
Blood vessels:		
Unusual bleeding or bruising.	Rare	3
Muscles, bones, joints, kidneys, liver, allergic, blood:	None expected.	
Genital, urinary:		
Urination difficulty.	Infrequent	4
Others:		
Fatigue, weakness.	Rare	3

1 - Life-threatening. Seek emergency treatment immediately.
2 - Discontinue. Seek emergency treatment.
3 - Discontinue. Call doctor right away.
4 - Continue. Call doctor when convenient.
5 - Continue. Tell doctor at next visit.
6 - No action necessary.

WARNINGS & PRECAUTIONS

Don't take if:
You are allergic to any antihistamine.

Before you start, consult your doctor:
- If you have glaucoma.
- If you have enlarged prostate.
- If you have asthma.
- If you have kidney disease.
- If you have peptic ulcer.
- If you will have surgery within 2 months, including dental surgery, requiring general or spinal anesthesia.

Over age 60:
Don't exceed recommended dose. Adverse reactions and side effects may be more frequent and severe than in younger persons, especially urination difficulty, diminished alertness and other brain and nervous-system symptoms.

Pregnancy:
No proven harm to unborn child. Avoid if possible.

Breast-feeding:
Drug passes into milk. Avoid drug or discontinue nursing until you finish medicine. Consult doctor for advice on maintaining milk supply.

Infants & children:
Not recommended for premature or newborn infants. Otherwise, no problems expected.

Prolonged use:
Avoid. May damage bone marrow and nerve cells.

Skin & sunlight:
May cause rash or intensify sunburn in areas exposed to sun or sunlamp.

Driving, piloting or hazardous work:
Don't drive or pilot aircraft until you learn how medicine affects you. Don't work around dangerous machinery. Don't climb ladders or work in high places. Danger increases if you drink alcohol or take medicine affecting alertness and reflexes, such as antihistamines, tranquilizers, sedatives, pain medicine, narcotics and mind-altering drugs.

Airplane passengers:
No problems expected.

Discontinuing:
No problems expected.

Others:
May mask symptoms of hearing damage from aspirin, other salicylates, cisplatin, paromomycin, vancomycin or anticonvulsants. Consult doctor if you use these.

INTERACTION WITH OTHER DRUGS

GENERIC NAME OR DRUG CLASS	COMBINED EFFECT
Anticholinergics	Increased anticholinergic effect.
Antidepressants	Excess sedation. Avoid.
Antihistamines (other)	Excess sedation. Avoid.
Hypnotics	Excess sedation. Avoid.
MAO inhibitors	Increased dimenhydrinate effect.
Mind-altering drugs	Excess sedation. Avoid.
Narcotics	Excess sedation. Avoid.
Sedatives	Excess sedation. Avoid.
Sleep inducers	Excess sedation. Avoid.
Tranquilizers	Excess sedation. Avoid.

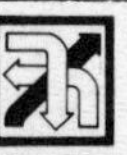

INTERACTION WITH OTHER SUBSTANCES

INTERACTS WITH	COMBINED EFFECT
Alcohol:	Excess sedation. Avoid.
Beverages: Caffeine drinks	Less dimenhydrinate sedation.
Cocaine:	Decreased dimenhydrinate effect. Avoid.
Foods:	None expected.
Marijuana:	Excess sedation. Avoid.
Tobacco:	None expected.

DIMETHINDENE

BRAND NAMES

Forhistal
Triten
Triten Tab-In

GENERAL INFORMATION

Habit forming? No
Prescription needed? Yes
Available as generic? Yes
Drug class: Antihistamine

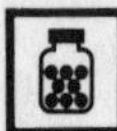

USES

- Reduces allergic symptoms such as hay fever, hives, rash or itching.
- Induces sleep.

DOSAGE & USAGE INFORMATION

How to take:
Extended-release tablets or capsules—Take with liquid or food. Swallow each dose whole.

When to take:
Varies with form. Follow label directions.

If you forget a dose:
Take as soon as you remember up to 2 hours late. If more than 2 hours, wait for next scheduled dose (don't double this dose).

What drug does:
Blocks action of histamine after an allergic response triggers histamine release in sensitive cells.

Time lapse before drug works:
30 minutes.

Don't take with:
See Interaction column and consult doctor.

OVERDOSE

Symptoms:
Convulsions, red face, hallucinations, coma.

What to do:
- Dial 0 (operator) or 911 (emergency) for an ambulance or medical help. Then give first aid immediately.
- If patient is unconscious and not breathing, give mouth-to-mouth breathing. If there is no heartbeat, use cardiac massage and mouth-to-mouth breathing (CPR). Don't try to make patient vomit. If you can't get help quickly, take patient to nearest emergency facility.
- Additional emergency information on page 886.

POSSIBLE ADVERSE REACTIONS OR SIDE EFFECTS

SYMPTOMS	FREQUENCY	WHAT TO DO
Brain & nervous system:		
• Nightmares, agitation, irritability.	Rare	3
• Drowsiness, dizziness.	Common	5
Skin:	None expected.	
Eyes:		
• Vision changes.	Infrequent	3
• Less tolerance for contact lenses.	Infrequent	4
Ears, nose, throat:		
• Sore throat, fever.	Rare	3
• Dry mouth, nose, throat.	Common	5
Digestive:		
• Nausea	Common	5
• Appetite loss.	Infrequent	5
Heart & lungs:		
Rapid heartbeat.	Rare	3
Blood vessels:		
Unusual bleeding or bruising.	Rare	3
Muscles, bones, joints, kidneys, liver, allergic, blood:	None expected.	
Genital, urinary:		
Urination difficulty.	Infrequent	4
Others:		
Fatigue, weakness.	Rare	3

1 - Life-threatening. Seek emergency treatment immediately.
2 - Discontinue. Seek emergency treatment.
3 - Discontinue. Call doctor right away.
4 - Continue. Call doctor when convenient.
5 - Continue. Tell doctor at next visit.
6 - No action necessary.

WARNINGS & PRECAUTIONS

Don't take if:
You are allergic to any antihistamine.

Before you start, consult your doctor:
- If you have glaucoma.
- If you have enlarged prostate.
- If you have asthma.
- If you have kidney disease.
- If you have peptic ulcer.
- If you will have surgery within 2 months, including dental surgery, requiring general or spinal anesthesia.

Over age 60:
Don't exceed recommended dose. Adverse reactions and side effects may be more frequent and severe than in younger persons, especially urination difficulty, diminished alertness and other brain and nervous-system symptoms.

Pregnancy:
No proven harm to unborn child. Avoid if possible.

Breast-feeding:
Drug passes into milk. Avoid drug or discontinue nursing until you finish medicine. Consult doctor for advice on maintaining milk supply.

Infants & children:
Not recommended for premature or newborn infants. Otherwise, no problems expected.

Prolonged use:
Avoid. May damage bone marrow and nerve cells.

Skin & sunlight:
May cause rash or intensify sunburn in areas exposed to sun or sunlamp.

Driving, piloting or hazardous work:
Don't drive or pilot aircraft until you learn how medicine affects you. Don't work around dangerous machinery. Don't climb ladders or work in high places. Danger increases if you drink alcohol or take medicine affecting alertness and reflexes, such as antihistamines, tranquilizers, sedatives, pain medicine, narcotics and mind-altering drugs.

Airplane passengers:
No problems expected.

Discontinuing:
No problems expected.

Others:
May mask symptoms of hearing damage from aspirin, other salicylates, cisplatin, paromomycin, vancomycin or anticonvulsants. Consult doctor if you use these.

INTERACTION WITH OTHER DRUGS

GENERIC NAME OR DRUG CLASS	COMBINED EFFECT
Anticholinergics	Increased anticholinergic effect.
Antidepressants	Excess sedation. Avoid.
Antihistamines (other)	Excess sedation. Avoid.
Hypnotics	Excess sedation. Avoid.
MAO inhibitors	Increased dimethindene effect.
Mind-altering drugs	Excess sedation. Avoid.
Narcotics	Excess sedation. Avoid.
Sedatives	Excess sedation. Avoid.
Sleep inducers	Excess sedation. Avoid.
Tranquilizers	Excess sedation. Avoid.

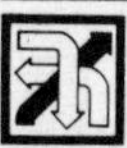

INTERACTION WITH OTHER SUBSTANCES

INTERACTS WITH	COMBINED EFFECT
Alcohol:	Excess sedation. Avoid.
Beverages:	
Caffeine drinks	Less dimethindene sedation.
Cocaine:	Decreased dimethindene effect. Avoid.
Foods:	None expected.
Marijuana:	Excess sedation. Avoid.
Tobacco:	None expected.

DIPHENHYDRAMINE

BRAND NAMES

Ambenyl Expectorant	Eldadryl	SK-Diphenhydramine
Benadryl	Fenylhist	Sominex
Bendylate	Insomnal	Valdrene
Diahist	Nordryl	Wehydryl
	Nytol	

See complete brand names list, page 825.

GENERAL INFORMATION

Habit forming? No
Prescription needed?
High strength: Yes
Low strength: No
Available as generic? Yes
Drug class: Antihistamine

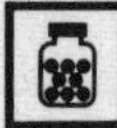

USES

- Reduces allergic symptoms such as hay fever, hives, rash or itching.
- Prevents motion sickness, nausea, vomiting.
- Induces sleep.
- Reduces stiffness and tremors of Parkinson's disease.

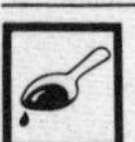

DOSAGE & USAGE INFORMATION

How to take:
- Tablet or capsule—Swallow with liquid or food to lessen stomach irritation.
- Extended-release tablets or capsules—Swallow each dose whole.
- Suppositories—Remove wrapper and moisten suppository with water. Gently insert larger end into rectum. Push well into rectum with finger.

When to take:
Varies with form. Follow label directions.

If you forget a dose:
Take as soon as you remember up to 2 hours late. If more than 2 hours, wait for next scheduled dose (don't double this dose).

What drug does:
Blocks action of histamine after an allergic response triggers histamine release in sensitive cells.

Time lapse before drug works:
30 minutes.

Don't take with:
See Interaction column and consult doctor.

OVERDOSE

Symptoms:
Convulsions, red face, hallucinations, coma.

What to do:
- Dial 0 (operator) or 911 (emergency) for an ambulance or medical help. Then give first aid immediately.
- Additional emergency information on page 886.

POSSIBLE ADVERSE REACTIONS OR SIDE EFFECTS

SYMPTOMS	FREQUENCY	WHAT TO DO
Brain & nervous system:		
• Nightmares, agitation, irritability.	Rare	3
• Drowsiness, dizziness.	Common	5
Skin:	None expected.	
Eyes:		
• Vision changes.	Infrequent	3
• Less tolerance for contact lenses.	Infrequent	4
Ears, nose, throat:		
• Sore throat, fever.	Rare	3
• Dry mouth, nose, throat.	Common	5
Digestive:		
• Nausea	Common	5
• Appetite loss.	Infrequent	5
Heart & lungs:		
Rapid heartbeat.	Rare	3
Blood vessels:		
Unusual bleeding or bruising.	Rare	3
Muscles, bones, joints, kidneys, liver, allergic, blood:	None expected.	
Genital, urinary:		
Urination difficulty.	Infrequent	4
Others:		
Fatigue, weakness.	Rare	3

1-Life-threatening. Seek emergency treatment immediately.
2-Discontinue. Seek emergency treatment.
3-Discontinue. Call doctor right away.
4-Continue. Call doctor when convenient.
5-Continue. Tell doctor at next visit.
6-No action necessary.

WARNINGS & PRECAUTIONS

Don't take if:
You are allergic to any antihistamine.

Before you start, consult your doctor:
- If you have glaucoma.
- If you have enlarged prostate.
- If you have asthma.
- If you have kidney disease.
- If you have peptic ulcer.
- If you will have surgery within 2 months, including dental surgery, requiring general or spinal anesthesia.

Over age 60:
Don't exceed recommended dose. Adverse reactions and side effects may be more frequent and severe than in younger persons, especially urination difficulty, diminished alertness and other brain and nervous-system symptoms.

Pregnancy:
No proven harm to unborn child. Avoid if possible.

Breast-feeding:
Drug passes into milk. Avoid drug or discontinue nursing until you finish medicine. Consult doctor for advice on maintaining milk supply.

Infants & children:
Not recommended for premature or newborn infants. Otherwise, no problems expected.

Prolonged use:
Avoid. May damage bone marrow and nerve cells.

Skin & sunlight:
May cause rash or intensify sunburn in areas exposed to sun or sunlamp.

Driving, piloting or hazardous work:
Don't drive or pilot aircraft until you learn how medicine affects you. Don't work around dangerous machinery. Don't climb ladders or work in high places. Danger increases if you drink alcohol or take medicine affecting alertness and reflexes, such as antihistamines, tranquilizers, sedatives, pain medicine, narcotics and mind-altering drugs.

Airplane passengers:
No problems expected.

Discontinuing:
No problems expected.

Others:
May mask symptoms of hearing damage from aspirin, other salicylates, cisplatin, paromomycin, vancomycin or anticonvulsants. Consult doctor if you use these.

INTERACTION WITH OTHER DRUGS

GENERIC NAME OR DRUG CLASS	COMBINED EFFECT
Anticholinergics	Increased anticholinergic effect.
Antidepressants	Excess sedation. Avoid.
Antihistamines (other)	Excess sedation. Avoid.
Hypnotics	Excess sedation. Avoid.
MAO inhibitors	Increased diphenhydramine effect.
Mind-altering drugs	Excess sedation. Avoid.
Narcotics	Excess sedation. Avoid.
Sedatives	Excess sedation. Avoid.
Sleep inducers	Excess sedation. Avoid.
Tranquilizers	Excess sedation. Avoid.

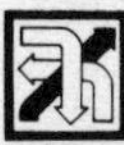

INTERACTION WITH OTHER SUBSTANCES

INTERACTS WITH	COMBINED EFFECT
Alcohol:	Excess sedation. Avoid.
Beverages:	
Caffeine drinks	Less diphenhydramine sedation.
Cocaine:	Decreased diphenhydramine effect. Avoid.
Foods:	None expected.
Marijuana:	Excess sedation. Avoid.
Tobacco:	None expected.

DIPHENIDOL

BRAND NAMES

Vontrol

GENERAL INFORMATION

Habit forming? No
Prescription needed? Yes
Available as generic? No
Drug class: Antiemetic, antivertigo

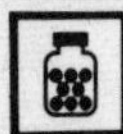

USES

- Prevents motion sickness.
- Controls nausea and vomiting (do not use during pregnancy).

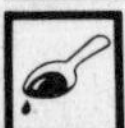

DOSAGE & USAGE INFORMATION

How to take:
Tablet—Swallow with liquid or food to lessen stomach irritation. If you can't swallow whole, crumble tablet and chew or take with liquid or food.

When to take:
30 to 60 minutes before traveling.

If you forget a dose:
Take as soon as you remember. Wait 4 hours for next dose.

What drug does:
Reduces sensitivity of nerve endings in inner ear, blocking messages to brain's vomiting center.

Time lapse before drug works:
30 to 60 minutes.

Don't take with:
See Interaction column and consult doctor.

OVERDOSE

Symptoms:
Drowsiness, confusion, incoordination, weak pulse, shallow breathing, stupor, coma.

What to do:
- Dial 0 (operator) or 911 (emergency) for an ambulance or medical help. Then give first aid immediately.
- Additional emergency information on page 886.

POSSIBLE ADVERSE REACTIONS OR SIDE EFFECTS

SYMPTOMS	FREQUENCY	WHAT TO DO
Brain & nervous system:		
• Drowsiness	Common	5
• Headache	Infrequent	4
• Restlessness, excitement, insomnia.	Rare	4
Skin:		
Rash or hives.	Rare	3
Eyes:		
Blurred vision.	Rare	4
Ears, nose, throat:		
Dry mouth, nose, throat.	Infrequent	5
Digestive:		
• Appetite loss, nausea.	Rare	5
• Diarrhea or constipation.	Infrequent	4
Heart & lungs:		
Fast heartbeat.	Infrequent	4
Blood vessels:	None expected.	
Muscles, bones, joints:	None expected.	
Genital, urinary:		
Urinary frequency, difficult urination.	Rare	4
Kidneys:	None expected.	
Liver:	None expected.	
Allergic:	None expected.	
Blood:	None expected.	
Others:	None expected.	

1- Life-threatening. Seek emergency treatment immediately.
2- Discontinue. Seek emergency treatment.
3- Discontinue. Call doctor right away.
4- Continue. Call doctor when convenient.
5- Continue. Tell doctor at next visit.
6- No action necessary.

WARNINGS & PRECAUTIONS

Don't take if:
- You have severe kidney disease.
- You are allergic to diphenidol or meclizine.

Before you start, consult your doctor:
- If you have prostate enlargement.
- If you have glaucoma.
- If you have heart disease.
- If you have intestinal obstruction or ulcers in the gastrointestinal tract.
- If you have kidney disease.
- If you have low blood pressure.
- If you will have surgery within 2 months, including dental surgery, requiring general or spinal anesthesia.

Over age 60:
Adverse reactions and side effects may be more frequent and severe than in younger persons.

Pregnancy:
Animal studies show fetal abnormalities. Decide with your doctor whether drug benefits justify risk to unborn child.

Breast-feeding:
Drug passes into milk. Avoid drug or discontinue nursing until you finish medicine. Consult doctor for advice on maintaining milk supply.

Infants & children:
No problems expected.

Prolonged use:
No problems expected.

Skin & sunlight:
No problems expected.

Driving, piloting or hazardous work:
Don't fly aircraft. Don't drive until you learn how medicine affects you. Don't work around dangerous machinery. Don't climb ladders or work in high places. Danger increases if you drink alcohol or take medicine affecting alertness and reflexes, such as antihistamines, tranquilizers, sedatives, pain medicine, narcotics and mind-altering drugs.

Airplane passengers:
Take 30 minutes before takeoff and every 4 hours while in the air.

Discontinuing:
No problems expected.

Others:
No problems expected.

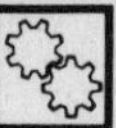

INTERACTION WITH OTHER DRUGS

GENERIC NAME OR DRUG CLASS	COMBINED EFFECT
Anticonvulsants	Increased effect of both drugs.
Antidepressants (tricyclic)	Increased sedative effect of both drugs.
Antihistamines	Increased sedative effect of both drugs.
Atropine	Increased chance of toxic effect of atropine and atropine-like medicines.
Narcotics	Increased sedative effect of both drugs.
Sedatives	Increased sedative effect of both drugs.
Tranquilizers	Increased sedative effect of both drugs.

INTERACTION WITH OTHER SUBSTANCES

INTERACTS WITH	COMBINED EFFECT
Alcohol:	Increased sedation. Avoid.
Beverages: Caffeine	May decrease drowsiness.
Cocaine:	Increased chance of toxic effects of cocaine. Avoid.
Foods:	None expected.
Marijuana:	Increased drowsiness, dry mouth.
Tobacco:	None expected.

DIPHENOXYLATE & ATROPINE

BRAND NAMES

Colonil
Lomotil
SK-Diphenoxylate

GENERAL INFORMATION

Habit forming? Yes
Prescription needed? Yes
Available as generic? Yes
Drug class: Antidiarrheal

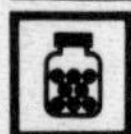

USES

Relieves diarrhea and intestinal cramps.

DOSAGE & USAGE INFORMATION

How to take:

- Tablet or capsule—Swallow with liquid or food to lessen stomach irritation.
- Drops or liquid—Follow label instructions and use marked dropper.

When to take:
No more often than directed on label.

If you forget a dose:
Take as soon as you remember up to 2 hours late. If more than 2 hours, wait for next scheduled dose (don't double this dose).

What drug does:
Blocks digestive tract's nerve supply, which reduces propelling movements.

Time lapse before drug works:
May require 12 to 24 hours of regular doses to control diarrhea.

Don't take with:
See Interaction column and consult doctor.

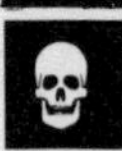

OVERDOSE

Symptoms:
Excitement, constricted pupils, shallow breathing, coma.

What to do:

- Dial 0 (operator) or 911 (emergency) for an ambulance or medical help. Then give first aid immediately.
- If patient is unconscious and not breathing, give mouth-to-mouth breathing. If there is no heartbeat, use cardiac massage and mouth-to-mouth breathing (CPR). Don't try to make patient vomit. If you can't get help quickly, take patient to nearest emergency facility.
- Additional emergency information on page 886.

POSSIBLE ADVERSE REACTIONS OR SIDE EFFECTS

SYMPTOMS	FREQUENCY	WHAT TO DO
Brain & nervous system:		
• Dizziness, depression, drowsiness.	Infrequent	4
• Restlessness, flush, fever, headache.	Rare	3
Skin:		
Rash or itch.	Infrequent	4
Eyes:		
Blurred vision.	Infrequent	4
Ears, nose, throat:		
Dry mouth or swollen gums.	Infrequent	3
Digestive:		
Stomach pain, nausea, vomiting, bloating, constipation.	Rare	3
Heart & lungs:		
Rapid heartbeat.	Infrequent	3
Blood vessels:		
Numbness of hands or feet.	Rare	3
Muscles, bones, joints:	None expected.	
Genital, urinary:		
Decreased urination.	Infrequent	4
Kidneys:	None expected.	
Liver:	None expected.	
Allergic:	None expected.	
Blood:	None expected.	
Others:	None expected.	

1- Life-threatening. Seek emergency treatment immediately.
2- Discontinue. Seek emergency treatment.
3- Discontinue. Call doctor right away.
4- Continue. Call doctor when convenient.
5- Continue. Tell doctor at next visit.
6- No action necessary.

DIPHENOXYLATE & ATROPINE

WARNINGS & PRECAUTIONS

Don't take if:
- You are allergic to diphenoxylate & atropine or any narcotic or anticholinergic.
- You have jaundice (yellow skin and eyes).
- Patient is younger than 2.

Before you start, consult your doctor:
- If you have had liver problems.
- If you have ulcerative colitis.
- If you plan to become pregnant within medication period.
- If you have any medical disorder.
- If you take any medication, including non-prescription drugs.

Over age 60:
Adverse reactions and side effects may be more frequent and severe than in younger persons.

Pregnancy:
No proven harm to unborn child. Avoid because of many side effects.

Breast-feeding:
Drug passes into milk. Avoid drug or discontinue nursing until you finish medicine. Consult doctor for advice on maintaining milk supply.

Infants & children:
Don't give to infants or toddlers. Use only under doctor's supervision for children older than 2.

Prolonged use:
Habit forming.

Skin & sunlight:
No problems expected.

Driving, piloting or hazardous work:
Don't drive or pilot aircraft until you learn how medicine affects you. Don't work around dangerous machinery. Don't climb ladders or work in high places. Danger increases if you drink alcohol or take medicine affecting alertness and reflexes.

Airplane passengers:
No problems expected.

Discontinuing:
- May be unnecessary to finish medicine. Follow doctor's instructions.
- After discontinuing, consult doctor if you experience muscle cramps, nausea, vomiting, trembling, stomach cramps or unusual sweating.

Others:
If diarrhea lasts longer than 4 days, discontinue and call doctor.

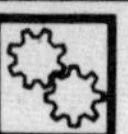

INTERACTION WITH OTHER DRUGS

GENERIC NAME OR DRUG CLASS	COMBINED EFFECT
MAO inhibitors	May increase blood pressure excessively.
Sedatives	Increased effect of both drugs.
Tranquilizers	Increased effect of both drugs.

INTERACTION WITH OTHER SUBSTANCES

INTERACTS WITH	COMBINED EFFECT
Alcohol:	Depressed brain function. Avoid.
Beverages:	None expected.
Cocaine:	Decreased effect of diphenoxylate and atropine.
Foods:	None expected.
Marijuana:	None expected.
Tobacco:	None expected.

DIPHENYLPYRALINE

BRAND NAMES

Diafen
Hispril

GENERAL INFORMATION

Habit forming? No
Prescription needed? High strength: Yes
Low strength: No
Available as generic? No
Drug class: Antihistamine

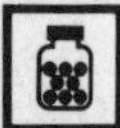

USES

- Reduces allergic symptoms such as hay fever, hives, rash or itching.
- Induces sleep.

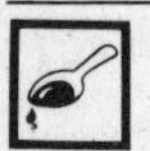

DOSAGE & USAGE INFORMATION

How to take:
Extended-release capsules—Swallow each dose whole with liquid.

When to take:
Varies with form. Follow label directions.

If you forget a dose:
Take as soon as you remember up to 2 hours late. If more than 2 hours, wait for next scheduled dose (don't double this dose).

What drug does:
Blocks action of histamine after an allergic response triggers histamine release in sensitive cells.

Time lapse before drug works:
30 minutes.

Don't take with:
See Interaction column and consult doctor.

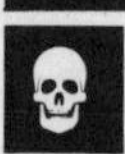

OVERDOSE

Symptoms:
Convulsions, red face, hallucinations, coma.

What to do:
- Dial 0 (operator) or 911 (emergency) for an ambulance or medical help. Then give first aid immediately.
- If patient is unconscious and not breathing, give mouth-to-mouth breathing. If there is no heartbeat, use cardiac massage and mouth-to-mouth breathing (CPR). Don't try to make patient vomit. If you can't get help quickly, take patient to nearest emergency facility.
- Additional emergency information on page 886.

POSSIBLE ADVERSE REACTIONS OR SIDE EFFECTS

SYMPTOMS	FREQUENCY	WHAT TO DO
Brain & nervous system:		
• Nightmares, agitation, irritability.	Rare	3
• Drowsiness, dizziness.	Common	5
Skin:	None expected.	
Eyes:		
• Vision changes.	Infrequent	3
• Less tolerance for contact lenses.	Infrequent	4
Ears, nose, throat:		
• Sore throat, fever.	Rare	3
• Dry mouth, nose, throat.	Common	5
Digestive:		
• Nausea	Common	5
• Appetite loss.	Infrequent	5
Heart & lungs:		
Rapid heartbeat.	Rare	3
Blood vessels:		
Unusual bleeding or bruising.	Rare	3
Muscles, bones, joints, kidneys, liver, allergic, blood:	None expected.	
Genital, urinary:		
Urination difficulty.	Infrequent	4
Others:		
Fatigue, weakness.	Rare	3

1- Life-threatening. Seek emergency treatment immediately.
2- Discontinue. Seek emergency treatment.
3- Discontinue. Call doctor right away.
4- Continue. Call doctor when convenient.
5- Continue. Tell doctor at next visit.
6- No action necessary.

WARNINGS & PRECAUTIONS

Don't take if:
You are allergic to any antihistamine.

Before you start, consult your doctor:
- If you have glaucoma.
- If you have enlarged prostate.
- If you have asthma.
- If you have kidney disease.
- If you have peptic ulcer.
- If you will have surgery within 2 months, including dental surgery, requiring general or spinal anesthesia.

Over age 60:
Don't exceed recommended dose. Adverse reactions and side effects may be more frequent and severe than in younger persons, especially urination difficulty, diminished alertness and other brain and nervous-system symptoms.

Pregnancy:
No proven harm to unborn child. Avoid if possible.

Breast-feeding:
Drug passes into milk. Avoid drug or discontinue nursing until you finish medicine. Consult doctor for advice on maintaining milk supply.

Infants & children:
Not recommended for premature or newborn infants. Otherwise, no problems expected.

Prolonged use:
Avoid. May damage bone marrow and nerve cells.

Skin & sunlight:
May cause rash or intensify sunburn in areas exposed to sun or sunlamp.

Driving, piloting or hazardous work:
Don't drive or pilot aircraft until you learn how medicine affects you. Don't work around dangerous machinery. Don't climb ladders or work in high places. Danger increases if you drink alcohol or take medicine affecting alertness and reflexes, such as antihistamines, tranquilizers, sedatives, pain medicine, narcotics and mind-altering drugs.

Airplane passengers:
No problems expected.

Discontinuing:
No problems expected.

Others:
May mask symptoms of hearing damage from aspirin, other salicylates, cisplatin, paromomycin, vancomycin or anticonvulsants. Consult doctor if you use these.

INTERACTION WITH OTHER DRUGS

GENERIC NAME OR DRUG CLASS	COMBINED EFFECT
Anticholinergics	Increased anticholinergic effect.
Antidepressants	Excess sedation. Avoid.
Antihistamines (other)	Excess sedation. Avoid.
Hypnotics	Excess sedation. Avoid.
MAO inhibitors	Increased diphenylpyraline effect.
Mind-altering drugs	Excess sedation. Avoid.
Narcotics	Excess sedation. Avoid.
Sedatives	Excess sedation. Avoid.
Sleep inducers	Excess sedation. Avoid.
Tranquilizers	Excess sedation. Avoid.

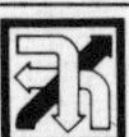

INTERACTION WITH OTHER SUBSTANCES

INTERACTS WITH	COMBINED EFFECT
Alcohol:	Excess sedation. Avoid.
Beverages: Caffeine drinks	Less diphenylpyraline sedation.
Cocaine:	Decreased diphenylpyraline effect. Avoid.
Foods:	None expected.
Marijuana:	Excess sedation. Avoid.
Tobacco:	None expected.

DIPYRIDAMOLE

BRAND NAMES

Apo-Dipyridamole
Persantine
SK-Dipyridamole

GENERAL INFORMATION

Habit forming? No
Prescription needed? U.S.: Yes; Canada: No
Available as generic? No
Drug class: Coronary vasodilator

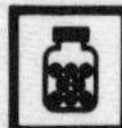

USES

- Reduces frequency and intensity of angina attacks.
- Prevents blood clots after heart surgery.

DOSAGE & USAGE INFORMATION

How to take:
Tablet or capsule—Swallow with liquid. If you can't swallow whole, crumble tablet or open capsule and take with liquid.

When to take:
1 hour before meals.

If you forget a dose:
Take as soon as you remember up to 2 hours late. If more than 2 hours, wait for next scheduled dose (don't double this dose).

What drug does:
- Probably dilates blood vessels to increase oxygen to heart.
- Prevents platelet clumping, which causes blood clots.

Time lapse before drug works:
3 months of continual use.

Don't take with:
See Interaction column and consult doctor.

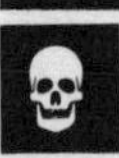

OVERDOSE

Symptoms:
Decreased blood pressure; weak, rapid pulse; cold, clammy skin; collapse.

What to do:
- Dial 0 (operator) or 911 (emergency) for an ambulance or medical help. Then give first aid immediately.
- If patient is unconscious and not breathing, give mouth-to-mouth breathing. If there is no heartbeat, use cardiac massage and mouth-to-mouth breathing (CPR). Don't try to make patient vomit. If you can't get help quickly, take patient to nearest emergency facility.
- Additional emergency information on page 886.

POSSIBLE ADVERSE REACTIONS OR SIDE EFFECTS

SYMPTOMS	FREQUENCY	WHAT TO DO
Brain & nervous system: Dizziness, fainting, headache.	Infrequent	3
Skin: Red flush, rash.	Infrequent	4
Eyes:	None expected.	
Ears, nose, throat:	None expected.	
Digestive: Nausea, vomiting, cramps.	Infrequent	4
Heart & lungs:	None expected.	
Blood vessels:	None expected.	
Muscles, bones, joints:	None expected.	
Genital, urinary:	None expected.	
Kidneys:	None expected.	
Liver:	None expected.	
Allergic:	None expected.	
Blood:	None expected.	
Others: Weakness	Infrequent	4

1- Life-threatening. Seek emergency treatment immediately.
2- Discontinue. Seek emergency treatment.
3- Discontinue. Call doctor right away.
4- Continue. Call doctor when convenient.
5- Continue. Tell doctor at next visit.
6- No action necessary.

WARNINGS & PRECAUTIONS

Don't take if:
- You are allergic to dipyridamole.
- You are recovering from a heart attack.

Before you start, consult your doctor:
- If you have low blood pressure.
- If you have liver disease.

Over age 60:
Begin treatment with small doses.

Pregnancy:
No proven harm to unborn child. Avoid if possible.

Breast-feeding:
No proven problems. Consult doctor.

Infants & children:
Not recommended.

Prolonged use:
No problems expected.

Skin & sunlight:
No problems expected.

Driving, piloting or hazardous work:
Avoid if you feel dizzy. Otherwise, no problems expected.

Airplane passengers:
No problems expected.

Discontinuing:
Don't discontinue without doctor's advice until you complete prescribed dose, even though symptoms diminish or disappear.

Others:
Drug increases your ability to be active without angina pain. Avoid excessive physical exertion that might injure heart.

INTERACTION WITH OTHER DRUGS

GENERIC NAME OR DRUG CLASS	COMBINED EFFECT
Anticoagulants (oral)	Increased anticoagulant effect. Bleeding tendency.
Antihypertensives	Increased antihypertensive effect.
Aspirin	Increased dipyridamole effect. Dose may need adjustment.

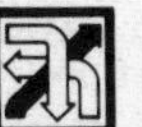

INTERACTION WITH OTHER SUBSTANCES

INTERACTS WITH	COMBINED EFFECT
Alcohol:	May lower blood pressure excessively.
Beverages:	None expected.
Cocaine:	No proven problems.
Foods:	Decreased dipyridamole absorption unless taken 1 hour before eating.
Marijuana:	Daily use—Decreased dipyridamole effect.
Tobacco:	
Nicotine	May decrease dipyridamole effect.

DISOPYRAMIDE

BRAND NAMES

Norpace
Norpace CR
Rythmodan

GENERAL INFORMATION

Habit forming? No
Prescription needed? Yes
Available as generic? No
Drug class: Antiarrhythmic

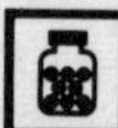

USES

Corrects heart rhythm disorders.

DOSAGE & USAGE INFORMATION

How to take:
Tablet or capsule—Swallow with liquid. If you can't swallow whole, crumble tablet or open capsule and take with liquid or food.

When to take:
At the same times each day.

If you forget a dose:
Take as soon as you remember up to 2 hours late. If more than 2 hours, wait for next scheduled dose (don't double this dose).

What drug does:
Delays nerve impulses to heart to regulate heartbeat.

Time lapse before drug works:
Begins in 30 to 60 minutes. Must use for 5 to 7 days to determine effectiveness.

Don't take with:
See Interaction column and consult doctor.

OVERDOSE

Symptoms:
Blood-pressure drop, irregular heartbeat.

What to do:
- Dial 0 (operator) or 911 (emergency) for an ambulance or medical help. Then give first aid immediately.
- If patient is unconscious and not breathing, give mouth-to-mouth breathing. If there is no heartbeat, use cardiac massage and mouth-to-mouth breathing (CPR). Don't try to make patient vomit. If you can't get help quickly, take patient to nearest emergency facility.
- Additional emergency information on page 886.

POSSIBLE ADVERSE REACTIONS OR SIDE EFFECTS

SYMPTOMS	FREQUENCY	WHAT TO DO
Brain & nervous system:		
Dizziness, fainting, confusion, nervousness, depression.	Infrequent	3
Skin, blood vessels, kidneys, allergic, blood:	None expected.	
Eyes:		
Pain	Rare	4
Ears, nose, throat:		
Sore throat with fever.	Rare	3
Digestive:		
Dry mouth, constipation.	Common	4
Heart & lungs:		
Chest pain, very fast or very slow heartbeat.	Infrequent	3
Muscles, bones, joints:		
Swollen feet.	Infrequent	4
Genital, urinary:		
Difficult urination.	Common	4
Liver:		
Jaundice (yellow skin and eyes).	Rare	3
Others:		
• Hypoglycemia	Common	3
• Lower sex drive.	Rare	4
• Rapid weight gain.	Common	4

1-Life-threatening. Seek emergency treatment immediately.
2-Discontinue. Seek emergency treatment.
3-Discontinue. Call doctor right away.
4-Continue. Call doctor when convenient.

DISOPYRAMIDE

WARNINGS & PRECAUTIONS

Don't take if:
- You are allergic to disopyramide or any antiarrhythmic.
- You have second- or third-degree heart block.

Before you start, consult your doctor:
- If you react unfavorably to other antiarrhythmic drugs.
- If you have had heart disease.
- If you have low blood pressure.
- If you have liver disease.
- If you have glaucoma.
- If you have enlarged prostate.
- If you have myasthenia gravis.
- If you take digitalis preparations or diuretics.

Over age 60:
- May require reduced dose.
- More likely to have difficulty urinating or be constipated.
- More likely to have blood-pressure drop.

Pregnancy:
No proven harm to unborn child. Avoid if possible.

Breast-feeding:
Drug passes into milk. Avoid drug or discontinue nursing until you finish medicine. Consult doctor for advice on maintaining milk supply.

Infants & children:
Safety not established. Don't use.

Prolonged use:
No problems expected.

Skin & sunlight:
No problems expected.

Driving, piloting or hazardous work:
Don't drive or pilot aircraft until you learn how medicine affects you. Don't work around dangerous machinery. Don't climb ladders or work in high places. Danger increases if you drink alcohol or take medicine affecting alertness and reflexes, such as antihistamines, tranquilizers, sedatives, pain medicine, narcotics, or mind-altering drugs.

Airplane passengers:
No problems expected.

Discontinuing:
Don't discontinue without doctor's advice until you complete prescribed dose, even though symptoms diminish or disappear.

Others:
If new illness, injury or surgery occurs, tell doctors of disopyramide use.

INTERACTION WITH OTHER DRUGS

GENERIC NAME OR DRUG CLASS	COMBINED EFFECT
Ambenonium	Decreased ambenonium effect.
Anticholinergics	Increased anticholinergic effect.
Anticoagulants (oral)	Increased anticoagulant effect.
Antihypertensives	Increased antihypertensive effect.
Antimyasthenics	Decreased antimyasthenic effect.

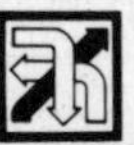

INTERACTION WITH OTHER SUBSTANCES

INTERACTS WITH	COMBINED EFFECT
Alcohol:	Decreased blood pressure and blood sugar. Use caution.
Beverages:	None expected.
Cocaine:	Irregular heartbeat.
Foods:	None expected.
Marijuana:	Unpredictable. May decrease disopyramide effect.
Tobacco:	May decrease disopyramide effect.

DISULFIRAM

BRAND NAMES

Antabuse

GENERAL INFORMATION

Habit forming? No
Prescription needed? Yes
Available as generic? Yes
Drug class: None

USES

Treatment for alcoholism. Will not cure alcoholism, but is a powerful deterrent to drinking.

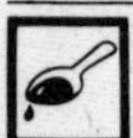

DOSAGE & USAGE INFORMATION

How to take:
Tablet or capsule—Swallow with liquid.

When to take:
Morning or bedtime. Avoid if you have used within 12 hours *any* alcohol, tonics, cough syrups, fermented vinegar, after-shave lotion or backrub solutions.

If you forget a dose:
Take as soon as you remember up to 12 hours late. If more than 12 hours, wait for next scheduled dose (don't double this dose).

What drug does:
In combination with alcohol, produces a metabolic change that causes severe, temporary toxicity.

Time lapse before drug works:
3 weeks or more.

Don't take with:
- See Interaction column and consult doctor.
- Non-prescription drugs that contain *any* alcohol.

OVERDOSE

Symptoms:
Memory loss, behavior disturbances, lethargy, confusion and headaches; nausea, vomiting, stomach pain and diarrhea; weakness and unsteady walk; temporary paralysis.

What to do:
- Dial 0 (operator) or 911 (emergency) for an ambulance or medical help. Then give first aid immediately.
- Additional emergency information on page 886.

POSSIBLE ADVERSE REACTIONS OR SIDE EFFECTS

SYMPTOMS	FREQUENCY	WHAT TO DO
Brain & nervous system:		
• Drowsiness	Common	5
• Mood changes.	Infrequent	5
Skin:		
Rash	Rare	3
Eyes:		
Pain, vision changes.	Infrequent	4
Ears, nose, throat:		
Bad taste in mouth (metal or garlic).	Infrequent	6
Digestive:		
Stomach discomfort.	Infrequent	4
Heart & lungs:	None expected.	
Blood vessels:		
Throbbing headache.	Infrequent	4
Muscles, bones, joints:	None expected.	
Genital, urinary:		
Decreased sexual ability in men.	Infrequent	5
Kidneys:	None expected.	
Liver:		
Jaundice (yellow skin and eyes).	Rare	3
Allergic:	None expected.	
Blood:	None expected.	
Others:		
• Tiredness	Infrequent	5
• Numbness in hands and feet.	Infrequent	4

1 - Life-threatening. Seek emergency treatment immediately.
2 - Discontinue. Seek emergency treatment.
3 - Discontinue. Call doctor right away.
4 - Continue. Call doctor when convenient.
5 - Continue. Tell doctor at next visit.
6 - No action necessary.

WARNINGS & PRECAUTIONS

Don't take if:
- You are allergic to disulfiram. (Alcohol-disulfiram combination is not an allergic reaction).
- You have used alcohol in any form or amount within 12 hours.
- You have taken paraldehyde within 1 week.
- You have heart disease.

Before you start, consult your doctor:
- If you have allergies.
- If you plan to become pregnant within medication period.
- If no one has explained to you how disulfiram reacts.
- If you think you cannot avoid drinking.
- If you have diabetes, epilepsy, liver or kidney disease.
- If you take other drugs.

Over age 60:
Adverse reactions and side effects may be more frequent and severe than in younger persons.

Pregnancy:
Risk to unborn child outweighs drug benefits. Don't use.

Breast-feeding:
Studies inconclusive. Consult your doctor.

Infants & children:
Not recommended.

Prolonged use:
Periodic blood-cell counts and liver-function tests recommended if you take this drug a long time.

Skin & sunlight:
No problems expected.

Driving, piloting or hazardous work:
Avoid if you feel drowsy or have vision side effects. Otherwise, no restrictions.

Airplane passengers:
Avoid if you feel drowsy or dizzy. Otherwise, no restrictions.

Discontinuing:
Don't discontinue without consulting doctor. Dose may require gradual reduction if you have taken drug for a long time. Doses of other drugs may also require adjustment. Avoid alcohol at least 14 days following last dose.

Others:
No problems expected.

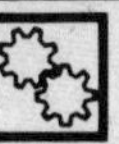

INTERACTION WITH OTHER DRUGS

GENERIC NAME OR DRUG CLASS	COMBINED EFFECT
Anticoagulants	Possible unexplained bleeding.
Anticonvulsants	Excessive sedation.
Barbiturates	Excessive sedation.
Cephalosporins	Disulfiram reaction, see page 846.
Isoniazid	Unsteady walk and disturbed behavior.
Metronidazole	Disulfiram reaction, see page 846.
Sedatives	Excessive sedation.

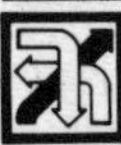

INTERACTION WITH OTHER SUBSTANCES

INTERACTS WITH	COMBINED EFFECT
Alcohol: *Any* form or amount.	Possible life-threatening toxicity. See disulfiram reaction, page 846.
Beverages: Punch or fruit drink that may contain alcohol.	Disulfiram reaction, see page 846.
Cocaine:	Increased disulfiram effect.
Foods: Sauces, fermented vinegar, marinades, desserts or other foods prepared with *any* alcohol.	Disulfiram reaction, see page 846.
Marijuana:	None expected.
Tobacco:	None expected.

DIVALPOREX

BRAND NAMES

Depakote

GENERAL INFORMATION

Habit forming? No
Prescription needed? Yes
Available as generic? No
Drug class: Anticonvulsant

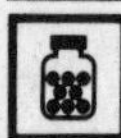

USES

Controls petit mal (absence) seizures in treatment of epilepsy.

DOSAGE & USAGE INFORMATION

How to take:
Tablet or capsule—Swallow with liquid or food to lessen stomach irritation.

When to take:
Once a day.

If you forget a dose:
Take as soon as you remember. Don't ever double dose.

What drug does:
Increases concentration of gamma aminobutyric acid, which inhibits nerve transmission in parts of brain.

Time lapse before drug works:
1 to 4 hours.

Don't take with:
See Interaction column and consult doctor.

OVERDOSE

Symptoms:
Coma.

What to do:

- Dial 0 (operator) or 911 (emergency) for an ambulance or medical help. Then give first aid immediately.
- If patient is unconscious and not breathing, give mouth-to-mouth breathing. If there is no heartbeat, use cardiac massage and mouth-to-mouth breathing (CPR). Don't try to make patient vomit. If you can't get help quickly, take patient to nearest emergency facility.
- Additional emergency information on page 886.

POSSIBLE ADVERSE REACTIONS OR SIDE EFFECTS

SYMPTOMS	FREQUENCY	WHAT TO DO
Brain & nervous system:		
Sleepy, weakness, easily upset emotionally, depression, psychic changes, headache, incoordination.	Infrequent	4
Skin:		
• Rash	Infrequent	3
• Bloody spots under skin.	Infrequent	3
• Hair loss.	Infrequent	3
Eyes:		
Double vision, unusual movements of eyes (nystagmus).	Rare	3
Ears, nose, throat:	None expected.	
Digestive:		
Nausea, vomiting, abdominal cramps, appetite change.	Infrequent	4
Heart & lungs:		
• Bleeding	Infrequent	3
• Easy bruising.	Infrequent	3
Blood vessels:	None expected.	
Muscles, bones, joints:	None expected.	
Genital, urinary:		
Irregular menstruation.	Common	4
Kidneys, allergic, blood, liver:	None expected.	
Others:		
Anemia	Rare	4

1- Life-threatening. Seek emergency treatment immediately.
2- Discontinue. Seek emergency treatment.
3- Discontinue. Call doctor right away.
4- Continue. Call doctor when convenient.
5- Continue. Tell doctor at next visit.
6- No action necessary.

WARNINGS & PRECAUTIONS

Don't take if:
You are allergic to divalporex.

Before you start, consult your doctor:
- If you have blood, kidney or liver disease.
- If you will have surgery within 2 months, including dental surgery, requiring general or spinal anesthesia.

Over age 60:
Adverse reactions and side effects may be more frequent and severe than in younger persons.

Pregnancy:
No proven harm to unborn child. Avoid if possible.

Breast-feeding:
Unknown effect.

Infants & children:
Under close medical supervision only.

Prolonged use:
Request periodic blood tests, liver and kidney function tests.

Skin & sunlight:
No problems expected.

Driving, piloting or hazardous work:
Don't drive or pilot aircraft until you learn how medicine affects you. Don't work around dangerous machinery. Don't climb ladders or work in high places. Danger increases if you drink alcohol or take medicine affecting alertness and reflexes, such as antihistamines, tranquilizers, sedatives, pain medicine, narcotics and mind-altering drugs.

Airplane passengers:
No problems expected.

Discontinuing:
Don't discontinue without consulting doctor. Dose may require gradual reduction if you have taken drug for a long time. Doses of other drugs may also require adjustment.

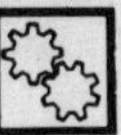

INTERACTION WITH OTHER DRUGS

GENERIC NAME OR DRUG CLASS	COMBINED EFFECT
Central nervous system depressants: Antidepressants, antihistamines, narcotics, sedatives, sleeping pills, tranquilizers.	Increases sedative effect.
Anticoagulants	Increases chance of bleeding.
Aspirin	Increases chance of bleeding.
Dypiradamole	Increases chance of bleeding.
Sulfinpyrazone	Increases chance of bleeding.
Primidone	Increases chance of toxicity.
MAO inhibitors	Increases sedative effect.
Clonazepam	May prolong seizure.
Phenytoin	Unpredictable. May require increased or decreased dosage.

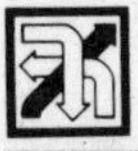

INTERACTION WITH OTHER SUBSTANCES

INTERACTS WITH	COMBINED EFFECT
Alcohol:	Deep sedation. Avoid.
Beverages:	No problems expected.
Cocaine:	Increased brain sensitivity. Avoid.
Foods:	No problems expected.
Marijuana:	Increased brain sensitivity. Avoid.
Tobacco:	Increased brain sensitivity. Avoid.

DOCUSATE CALCIUM

BRAND NAMES

Dioctocal
Doxidan
Surfak

GENERAL INFORMATION

Habit forming? No
Prescription needed? No
Available as generic? Yes
Drug class: Laxative (emollient)

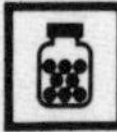

USES

Constipation relief.

DOSAGE & USAGE INFORMATION

How to take:

- Tablet or capsule—Swallow with liquid. Don't open capsules.
- Drops—Dilute dose in beverage before swallowing.
- Syrup—Take as directed on bottle.

When to take:
At the same time each day, preferably bedtime.

If you forget a dose:
Take as soon as you remember. Wait 12 hours for next dose. Return to regular schedule.

What drug does:
Makes stool hold fluid so it is easier to pass.

Time lapse before drug works:
2 to 3 days of continual use.

Don't take with:

- Other medicines at same time. Wait 2 hours.
- See Interaction column and consult doctor.

OVERDOSE

Symptoms:
Appetite loss, nausea, vomiting, diarrhea.

What to do:
Overdose unlikely to threaten life. If person takes much larger amount than prescribed, call doctor, poison-control center or hospital emergency room for instructions.

POSSIBLE ADVERSE REACTIONS OR SIDE EFFECTS

SYMPTOMS	FREQUENCY	WHAT TO DO
Brain & nervous system:	None expected.	
Skin:		
Rash	Rare	3
Eyes:	None expected.	
Ears, nose, throat:		
Throat irritation (liquid only).	Infrequent	4
Digestive:		
Intestinal and stomach cramps.	Infrequent	4
Heart & lungs:	None expected.	
Blood vessels:	None expected.	
Muscles, bones, joints:	None expected.	
Genital, urinary:	None expected.	
Kidneys:	None expected.	
Liver:	None expected.	
Allergic:	None expected.	
Blood:	None expected.	
Others:	None expected.	

1- Life-threatening. Seek emergency treatment immediately.
2- Discontinue. Seek emergency treatment.
3- Discontinue. Call doctor right away.
4- Continue. Call doctor when convenient.
5- Continue. Tell doctor at next visit.
6- No action necessary.

DOCUSATE CALCIUM

WARNINGS & PRECAUTIONS

Don't take if:
- You are allergic to any emollient laxative.
- You have abdominal pain and fever that might be appendicitis.

Before you start, consult your doctor:
- If you are taking other laxatives.
- To be sure constipation isn't a sign of a serious disorder.

Over age 60:
You must drink 6 to 8 glasses of fluid every 24 hours for drug to work.

Pregnancy:
No problems expected. Consult doctor.

Breast-feeding:
No problems expected.

Infants & children:
No problems expected.

Prolonged use:
Avoid. Overuse of laxatives may damage intestine lining.

Skin & sunlight:
No problems expected.

Driving, piloting or hazardous work:
No problems expected.

Airplane passengers:
No problems expected.

Discontinuing:
May be unnecessary to finish medicine. Follow doctor's instructions.

Others:
No problems expected.

INTERACTION WITH OTHER DRUGS

GENERIC NAME OR DRUG CLASS	COMBINED EFFECT
Danthron	Possible liver damage.
Digitalis preparations	Toxic absorption of digitalis.
Mineral oil	Increased mineral oil absorption into bloodstream. Avoid.
Phenolphthalein	Increased phenolphthalein absorption. Possible toxicity.

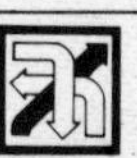

INTERACTION WITH OTHER SUBSTANCES

INTERACTS WITH	COMBINED EFFECT
Alcohol:	None expected.
Beverages:	None expected.
Cocaine:	None expected.
Foods:	None expected.
Marijuana:	None expected.
Tobacco:	None expected.

DOCUSATE POTASSIUM

BRAND NAMES

Dialose
Kasof
Pro-Cal-Sof
Surfac

GENERAL INFORMATION

Habit forming? No
Prescription needed? No
Available as generic? Yes
Drug class: Laxative (emollient)

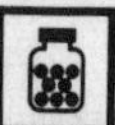

USES

Constipation relief.

DOSAGE & USAGE INFORMATION

How to take:

- Tablet or capsule—Swallow with liquid. Don't open capsules.
- Drops—Dilute dose in beverage before swallowing.
- Syrup—Take as directed on bottle.

When to take:
At the same time each day, preferably bedtime.

If you forget a dose:
Take as soon as you remember. Wait 12 hours for next dose. Return to regular schedule.

What drug does:
Makes stool hold fluid so it is easier to pass.

Time lapse before drug works:
2 to 3 days of continual use.

Don't take with:

- Other medicines at same time. Wait 2 hours.
- See Interaction column and consult doctor.

OVERDOSE

Symptoms:
Appetite loss, nausea, vomiting, diarrhea.

What to do:
Overdose unlikely to threaten life. If person takes much larger amount than prescribed, call doctor, poison-control center or hospital emergency room for instructions.

POSSIBLE ADVERSE REACTIONS OR SIDE EFFECTS

SYMPTOMS	FREQUENCY	WHAT TO DO
Brain & nervous system:	None expected.	
Skin:		
Rash	Rare	3
Eyes:	None expected.	
Ears, nose, throat:		
Throat irritation (liquid only).	Infrequent	4
Digestive:		
Intestinal and stomach cramps.	Infrequent	4
Heart & lungs:	None expected.	
Blood vessels:	None expected.	
Muscles, bones, joints:	None expected.	
Genital, urinary:	None expected.	
Kidneys:	None expected.	
Liver:	None expected.	
Allergic:	None expected.	
Blood:	None expected.	
Others:	None expected.	

1- Life-threatening. Seek emergency treatment immediately.
2- Discontinue. Seek emergency treatment.
3- Discontinue. Call doctor right away.
4- Continue. Call doctor when convenient.
5- Continue. Tell doctor at next visit.
6- No action necessary.

WARNINGS & PRECAUTIONS

Don't take if:
- You are allergic to any emollient laxative.
- You have abdominal pain and fever that might be appendicitis.

Before you start, consult your doctor:
- If you are taking other laxatives.
- To be sure constipation isn't a sign of a serious disorder.

Over age 60:
You must drink 6 to 8 glasses of fluid every 24 hours for drug to work.

Pregnancy:
No problems expected. Consult doctor.

Breast-feeding:
No problems expected.

Infants & children:
No problems expected.

Prolonged use:
Avoid. Overuse of laxatives may damage intestine lining.

Skin & sunlight:
No problems expected.

Driving, piloting or hazardous work:
No problems expected.

Airplane passengers:
No problems expected.

Discontinuing:
May be unnecessary to finish medicine. Follow doctor's instructions.

Others:
No problems expected.

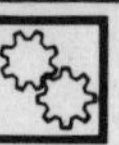

INTERACTION WITH OTHER DRUGS

GENERIC NAME OR DRUG CLASS	COMBINED EFFECT
Danthron	Possible liver damage.
Digitalis preparations	Toxic absorption of digitalis.
Mineral oil	Increased mineral oil absorption into bloodstream. Avoid.
Phenolphthalein	Increased phenolphthalein absorption. Possible toxicity.

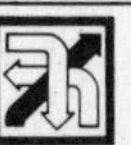

INTERACTION WITH OTHER SUBSTANCES

INTERACTS WITH	COMBINED EFFECT
Alcohol:	None expected.
Beverages:	None expected.
Cocaine:	None expected.
Foods:	None expected.
Marijuana:	None expected.
Tobacco:	None expected.

DOCUSATE SODIUM

BRAND NAMES

Afko-Lube	Dialose
Colace	Doxidan
Colax	Ferro-sequels
Coloctyl	Peri-Colase
Dioctyl Sodium Sulfosuccinate	Regutol
	Stulex

See complete brand names list, page 825.

GENERAL INFORMATION

Habit forming? No
Prescription needed? No
Available as generic? Yes
Drug class: Laxative (emollient)

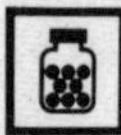

USES

Constipation relief.

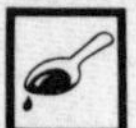

DOSAGE & USAGE INFORMATION

How to take:
- Tablet or capsule—Swallow with liquid. Don't open capsules.
- Drops—Dilute dose in beverage before swallowing.
- Syrup—Take as directed on bottle.

When to take:
At the same time each day, preferably bedtime.

If you forget a dose:
Take as soon as you remember. Wait 12 hours for next dose. Return to regular schedule.

What drug does:
Makes stool hold fluid so it is easier to pass.

Time lapse before drug works:
2 to 3 days of continual use.

Don't take with:
- Other medicines at same time. Wait 2 hours.
- See Interaction column and consult doctor.

OVERDOSE

Symptoms:
Appetite loss, nausea, vomiting, diarrhea.

What to do:
Overdose unlikely to threaten life. If person takes much larger amount than prescribed, call doctor, poison-control center or hospital emergency room for instructions.

POSSIBLE ADVERSE REACTIONS OR SIDE EFFECTS

SYMPTOMS	FREQUENCY	WHAT TO DO
Brain & nervous system:	None expected.	
Skin: Rash	Rare	3
Eyes:	None expected.	
Ears, nose, throat: Throat irritation (liquid only).	Infrequent	4
Digestive: Intestinal and stomach cramps.	Infrequent	4
Heart & lungs:	None expected.	
Blood vessels:	None expected.	
Muscles, bones, joints:	None expected.	
Genital, urinary:	None expected.	
Kidneys:	None expected.	
Liver:	None expected.	
Allergic:	None expected.	
Blood:	None expected.	
Others:	None expected.	

1- Life-threatening. Seek emergency treatment immediately.
2- Discontinue. Seek emergency treatment.
3- Discontinue. Call doctor right away.
4- Continue. Call doctor when convenient.
5- Continue. Tell doctor at next visit.
6- No action necessary.

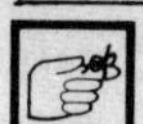

WARNINGS & PRECAUTIONS

Don't take if:
- You are allergic to any emollient laxative.
- You have abdominal pain and fever that might be appendicitis.

Before you start, consult your doctor:
- If you are taking other laxatives.
- To be sure constipation isn't a sign of a serious disorder.

Over age 60:
You must drink 6 to 8 glasses of fluid every 24 hours for drug to work.

Pregnancy:
No problems expected. Consult doctor.

Breast-feeding:
No problems expected.

Infants & children:
No problems expected.

Prolonged use:
Avoid. Overuse of laxatives may damage intestine lining.

Skin & sunlight:
No problems expected.

Driving, piloting or hazardous work:
No problems expected.

Airplane passengers:
No special problems.

Discontinuing:
May be unnecessary to finish medicine. Follow doctor's instructions.

Others:
No problems expected.

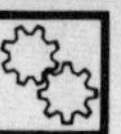

INTERACTION WITH OTHER DRUGS

GENERIC NAME OR DRUG CLASS	COMBINED EFFECT
Danthron	Possible liver damage.
Digitalis preparations	Toxic absorption of digitalis.
Mineral oil	Increased mineral oil absorption into bloodstream. Avoid.
Phenolphthalein	Increased phenolphthalein absorption. Possible toxicity.

INTERACTION WITH OTHER SUBSTANCES

INTERACTS WITH	COMBINED EFFECT
Alcohol:	None expected.
Beverages:	None expected.
Cocaine:	None expected.
Foods:	None expected.
Marijuana:	None expected.
Tobacco:	None expected.

DOXEPIN

BRAND NAMES

Adapin
Sinequan

GENERAL INFORMATION

Habit forming? No
Prescription needed? Yes
Available as generic? Yes
Drug class: Antidepressant (tricyclic)

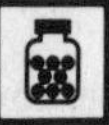

USES

Gradually relieves, but doesn't cure, symptoms of depression.

DOSAGE & USAGE INFORMATION

How to take:

- Tablet or capsule—Swallow with liquid.
- Oral concentrate—Dilute with liquid.

When to take:
At the same time each day, usually bedtime.

If you forget a dose:
Bedtime dose—If you forget your once-a-day bedtime dose, don't take it more than 3 hours late. If more than 3 hours, wait for next scheduled dose. Don't double this dose.

What drug does:
Probably affects part of brain that controls messages between nerve cells.

Time lapse before drug works:
Begins in 1 to 2 weeks. May require 4 to 6 weeks for maximum benefit.

Don't take with:

- Non-prescription drugs without consulting doctor.
- See Interaction column and consult doctor.

OVERDOSE

Symptoms:
Hallucinations, convulsions, coma.

What to do:

- Dial 0 (operator) or 911 (emergency) for an ambulance or medical help. Then give first aid immediately.
- If patient is unconscious and not breathing, give mouth-to-mouth breathing. If there is no heartbeat, use cardiac massage and mouth-to-mouth breathing (CPR). Don't try to make patient vomit. If you can't get help quickly, take patient to nearest emergency facility.
- Additional emergency information on page 886.

POSSIBLE ADVERSE REACTIONS OR SIDE EFFECTS

SYMPTOMS	FREQUENCY	WHAT TO DO
Brain & nervous system:		
• Hallucinations, shakiness, dizziness, fainting.	Infrequent	3
• Headache	Common	4
• Seizures	Rare	1
• Insomnia	Common	5
Skin:		
Rash, itch.	Rare	3
Eyes:		
Blurred vision, pain.	Infrequent	3
Ears, nose, throat:		
• Sore throat.	Rare	3
• Dry mouth or unpleasant taste.	Common	4
Digestive:		
• Constipation or diarrhea, nausea, indigestion.	Common	4
• Vomiting	Infrequent	3
• "Sweet tooth"	Common	5
Heart & lungs:		
Irregular heartbeat or slow pulse.	Infrequent	3
Blood vessels, muscles, bones, joints, kidneys, allergic, blood:	None expected.	
Genital, urinary:		
Difficulty urinating.	Infrequent	4
Liver:		
Jaundice (yellow skin and eyes).	Rare	3
Others:		
• Fever	Rare	3
• Fatigue, weakness.	Common	4

1 - Life-threatening. Seek emergency treatment immediately.
2 - Discontinue. Seek emergency treatment.
3 - Discontinue. Call doctor right away.
4 - Continue. Call doctor when convenient.
5 - Continue. Tell doctor at next visit.

WARNINGS & PRECAUTIONS

Don't take if:
- You are allergic to any tricyclic antidepressant.
- You drink alcohol.
- You have had a heart attack within 6 weeks.
- You have glaucoma.
- You have taken MAO inhibitors within 2 weeks.
- Patient is younger than 12.

Before you start, consult your doctor:
- If you will have surgery within 2 months, including dental surgery, requiring general or spinal anesthesia.
- If you have an enlarged prostate.
- If you have heart disease or high blood pressure.
- If you have stomach or intestinal problems.
- If you have an overactive thyroid.
- If you have asthma.
- If you have liver disease.

Over age 60:
More likely to develop urination difficulty and side effects under *Brain & nervous system*, opposite.

Pregnancy:
Studies inconclusive on harm to unborn child. Animal studies show fetal abnormalities. Decide with your doctor whether drug benefits justify risk to unborn child.

Breast-feeding:
Drug passes into milk. Avoid drug or discontinue nursing until you finish medicine. Consult doctor on maintaining milk supply.

Infants & children:
Don't give to children younger than 12.

Prolonged use:
No problems expected.

Skin & sunlight:
May cause rash or intensify sunburn in areas exposed to sun or sunlamp.

Driving, piloting or hazardous work:
Don't drive or pilot aircraft until you learn how medicine affects you. Don't work around dangerous machinery. Don't climb ladders or work in high places. Danger increases if you drink alcohol or take medicine affecting alertness and reflexes.

Airplane passengers:
No problems expected.

Discontinuing:
Don't discontinue without consulting doctor. Dose may require gradual reduction if you have taken drug for a long time. Doses of other drugs may also require adjustment.

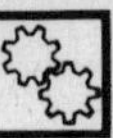

INTERACTION WITH OTHER DRUGS

GENERIC NAME OR DRUG CLASS	COMBINED EFFECT
Anticoagulants (oral)	Increased anticoagulant effect.
Anticholinergics	Increased sedation.
Antihistamines	Increased antihistamine effect.
Barbiturates	Decreased antidepressant effect.
Clonidine	Decreased clonidine effect.
Diuretics (thiazide)	Increased doxepin effect.
Ethchlorvynol	Delirium
Guanethidine	Decreased guanethidine effect.
MAO inhibitors	Fever, delirium, convulsions.
Methyldopa	Decreased methyldopa effect.
Narcotics	Dangerous oversedation.
Phenytoin	Decreased phenytoin effect.
Quinidine	Irregular heartbeat.
Sedatives	Dangerous oversedation.
Sympathomimetics	Increased sympathomimetic effect.
Thyroid hormones	Irregular heartbeat.

INTERACTION WITH OTHER SUBSTANCES

INTERACTS WITH	COMBINED EFFECT
Alcohol: Beverages or medicines with alcohol.	Excessive intoxication. Avoid.
Beverages:	None expected.
Cocaine:	Excessive intoxication. Avoid.
Foods:	None expected.
Marijuana:	Excessive drowsiness. Avoid.
Tobacco:	None expected.

DOXYLAMINE

BRAND NAMES

Bendectin
Cremacoat 4
Decapryn
Unisom Nighttime Sleep Aid

GENERAL INFORMATION

Habit forming? No
Prescription needed? Yes
Available as generic? No
Drug class: Antihistamine

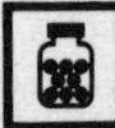

USES

- Reduces allergic symptoms such as hay fever, hives, rash or itching.
- Prevents motion sickness, nausea, vomiting.
- Induces sleep.

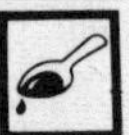

DOSAGE & USAGE INFORMATION

How to take:
- Tablet or syrup—Swallow with liquid or food to lessen stomach irritation.

When to take:
Varies with form. Follow label directions.

If you forget a dose:
Take as soon as you remember up to 2 hours late. If more than 2 hours, wait for next scheduled dose (don't double this dose).

What drug does:
Blocks action of histamine after an allergic response triggers histamine release in sensitive cells.

Time lapse before drug works:
30 minutes.

Don't take with:
See Interaction column and consult doctor.

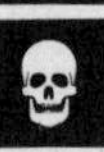

OVERDOSE

Symptoms:
Convulsions, red face, hallucinations, coma.

What to do:
- Dial 0 (operator) or 911 (emergency) for an ambulance or medical help. Then give first aid immediately.
- If patient is unconscious and not breathing, give mouth-to-mouth breathing. If there is no heartbeat, use cardiac massage and mouth-to-mouth breathing (CPR). Don't try to make patient vomit. If you can't get help quickly, take patient to nearest emergency facility.
- Additional emergency information on page 886.

POSSIBLE ADVERSE REACTIONS OR SIDE EFFECTS

SYMPTOMS	FREQUENCY	WHAT TO DO
Brain & nervous system:		
• Nightmares, agitation, irritability.	Rare	3
• Drowsiness, dizziness.	Common	5
Skin:	None expected.	
Eyes:		
• Vision changes.	Infrequent	3
• Less tolerance for contact lenses.	Infrequent	4
Ears, nose, throat:		
• Sore throat, fever.	Rare	3
• Dry mouth, nose, throat.	Common	5
Digestive:		
• Nausea	Common	5
• Appetite loss.	Infrequent	5
Heart & lungs:		
Rapid heartbeat.	Rare	3
Blood vessels:		
Unusual bleeding or bruising.	Rare	3
Muscles, bones, joints, kidneys, liver, allergic, blood:	None expected.	
Genital, urinary:		
Urination difficulty.	Infrequent	4
Others:		
Fatigue, weakness.	Rare	3

1-Life-threatening. Seek emergency treatment immediately.
2-Discontinue. Seek emergency treatment.
3-Discontinue. Call doctor right away.
4-Continue. Call doctor when convenient.
5-Continue. Tell doctor at next visit.
6-No action necessary.

WARNINGS & PRECAUTIONS

Don't take if:
You are allergic to any antihistamine.

Before you start, consult your doctor:
- If you have glaucoma.
- If you have enlarged prostate.
- If you have asthma.
- If you have kidney disease.
- If you have peptic ulcer.
- If you will have surgery within 2 months, including dental surgery, requiring general or spinal anesthesia.

Over age 60:
Don't exceed recommended dose. Adverse reactions and side effects may be more frequent and severe than in younger persons, especially urination difficulty, diminished alertness and other brain and nervous-system symptoms.

Pregnancy:
No proven harm to unborn child. Avoid if possible.

Breast-feeding:
Drug passes into milk. Avoid drug or discontinue nursing until you finish medicine. Consult doctor for advice on maintaining milk supply.

Infants & children:
Not recommended for premature or newborn infants. Otherwise, no problems expected.

Prolonged use:
Avoid. May damage bone marrow and nerve cells.

Skin & sunlight:
May cause rash or intensify sunburn in areas exposed to sun or sunlamp.

Driving, piloting or hazardous work:
Don't drive or pilot aircraft until you learn how medicine affects you. Don't work around dangerous machinery. Don't climb ladders or work in high places. Danger increases if you drink alcohol or take medicine affecting alertness and reflexes, such as antihistamines, tranquilizers, sedatives, pain medicine, narcotics and mind-altering drugs.

Airplane passengers:
No problems expected.

Discontinuing:
No problems expected.

Others:
May mask symptoms of hearing damage from aspirin, other salicylates, cisplatin, paromomycin, vancomycin or anticonvulsants. Consult doctor if you use these.

INTERACTION WITH OTHER DRUGS

GENERIC NAME OR DRUG CLASS	COMBINED EFFECT
Anticholinergics	Increased anticholinergic effect.
Antidepressants	Excess sedation. Avoid.
Antihistamines (other)	Excess sedation. Avoid.
Hypnotics	Excess sedation. Avoid.
MAO inhibitors	Increased doxylamine effect.
Mind-altering drugs	Excess sedation. Avoid.
Narcotics	Excess sedation. Avoid.
Sedatives	Excess sedation. Avoid.
Sleep inducers	Excess sedation. Avoid.
Tranquilizers	Excess sedation. Avoid.

INTERACTION WITH OTHER SUBSTANCES

INTERACTS WITH	COMBINED EFFECT
Alcohol:	Excess sedation. Avoid.
Beverages: Caffeine drinks	Less doxylamine sedation.
Cocaine:	Decreased doxylamine effect. Avoid.
Foods:	None expected.
Marijuana:	Excess sedation. Avoid.
Tobacco:	None expected.

DYPHYLLINE

BRAND NAMES

Aerophylline
Airet
Brosema
Dilin
Dilor
Dilor-G
Droxine
Droxine L.A.
Droxine S.F.
Dyflex
Lufyllin
Neothylline
Protophylline

GENERAL INFORMATION

Habit forming? No
Prescription needed? Canada—No
U.S: High strength—Yes
Low strength—No
Available as generic? Yes
Drug class: Bronchodilator (xanthine)

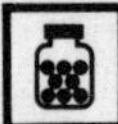

USES

Treatment for bronchial asthma symptoms.

DOSAGE & USAGE INFORMATION

How to take:

- Tablet or capsule—Swallow with liquid.
- Extended-release tablets or capsules—Swallow each dose whole. If you take regular tablets, you may chew or crush them.
- Suppositories—Remove wrapper and moisten suppository with water. Gently insert larger end into rectum. Push well into rectum with finger.
- Syrup—Take as directed on bottle.
- Enema—Use as directed on label.

When to take:
Most effective taken on empty stomach 1 hour before or 2 hours after eating. However, may take with food to lessen stomach upset.

If you forget a dose:
Take as soon as you remember up to 2 hours late. If more than 2 hours, wait for next scheduled dose (don't double this dose).

What drug does:
Relaxes and expands bronchial tubes.

Time lapse before drug works:
15 to 30 minutes.

Don't take with:
See Interaction column and consult doctor.

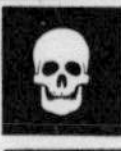

OVERDOSE

Symptoms:
Restlessness, irritability, confusion, delirium, convulsions, rapid pulse, coma.

What to do:

- Dial 0 (operator) or 911 (emergency) for an ambulance or medical help. Then give first aid immediately.
- Additional emergency information on page 886.

POSSIBLE ADVERSE REACTIONS OR SIDE EFFECTS

SYMPTOMS	FREQUENCY	WHAT TO DO
Brain & nervous system:		
• Headache, irritability, nervousness, restlessness, insomnia.	Common	4
• Dizziness or lightheadedness.	Infrequent	4
Skin:		
• Rash or hives.	Infrequent	3
• Flushed face.	Infrequent	4
Eyes:	None expected.	
Ears, nose, throat:	None expected.	
Digestive:		
• Nausea, vomiting, stomach pain.	Common	4
• Diarrhea, appetite loss.	Infrequent	3
Heart & lungs:		
• Rapid breathing.	Infrequent	3
• Irregular heartbeat.	Infrequent	3
Blood vessels:	None expected.	
Muscles, bones, joints:	None expected.	
Genital, urinary:	None expected.	
Kidneys:	None expected.	
Liver:	None expected.	
Allergic:	None expected.	
Blood:	None expected.	
Others:	None expected.	

1- Life-threatening. Seek emergency treatment immediately.
2- Discontinue. Seek emergency treatment.
3- Discontinue. Call doctor right away.
4- Continue. Call doctor when convenient.
5- Continue. Tell doctor at next visit.
6- No action necessary.

WARNINGS & PRECAUTIONS

Don't take if:
- You are allergic to any bronchodilator.
- You have an active peptic ulcer.

Before you start, consult your doctor:
- If you have had impaired kidney or liver function.
- If you have gastritis.
- If you have a peptic ulcer.
- If you have high blood pressure or heart disease.
- If you take medication for gout.

Over age 60:
Adverse reactions and side effects may be more frequent and severe than in younger persons.

Pregnancy:
Risk to unborn child outweighs drug benefits. Don't use.

Breast-feeding:
Drug passes into milk. Avoid drug or discontinue nursing until you finish medicine. Consult doctor for advice on maintaining milk supply.

Infants & children:
Use only under medical supervision.

Prolonged use:
Stomach irritation.

Skin & sunlight:
No problems expected.

Driving, piloting or hazardous work:
Avoid if lightheaded or dizzy. Otherwise, no problems expected.

Airplane passengers:
No problems expected.

Discontinuing:
May be unnecessary to finish medicine. Follow doctor's instructions.

Others:
No problems expected.

INTERACTION WITH OTHER DRUGS

GENERIC NAME OR DRUG CLASS	COMBINED EFFECT
Allopurinol	Decreased allopurinol effect.
Ephedrine	Increased effect of both drugs.
Epinephrine	Increased effect of both drugs.
Erythromycin	Increased dyphylline effect.
Furosemide	Increased furosemide effect.
Lincomycins	Increased dyphylline effect.
Lithium	Decreased lithium effect.
Probenecid	Decreased effect of both drugs.
Propranolol	Decreased dyphylline effect.
Rauwolfia alkaloids	Rapid heartbeat.
Sulfinpyrazone	Decreased sulfinpyrazone effect.
Troleandomycin	Increased dyphylline effect.

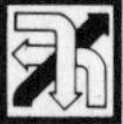

INTERACTION WITH OTHER SUBSTANCES

INTERACTS WITH	COMBINED EFFECT
Alcohol:	None expected.
Beverages: Caffeine drinks	Nervousness and insomnia.
Cocaine:	Excess stimulation. Avoid.
Foods:	None expected.
Marijuana:	Slightly increased antiasthmatic effect of dyphylline.
Tobacco:	Decreased dyphylline effect.

EPHEDRINE

BRAND NAMES

Acet-Am
Amesec
Bronkaid
Bronkotabs
Ectasule Minus
Ephedrol
Marax
Nyquil
Quadrinal
Quelidrine
Quibron Plus
Tedral

See complete brand names list, page 826.

GENERAL INFORMATION

Habit forming? No
Prescription needed? Low strength: No
High strength: Yes
Available as generic? Yes
Drug class: Sympathomimetic

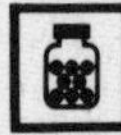

USES

- Relieves bronchial asthma.
- Decreases congestion of breathing passages.
- Suppresses allergic reactions.

DOSAGE & USAGE INFORMATION

How to take:
- Tablet or capsule—Swallow with liquid. You may chew or crush tablet.
- Extended-release tablets or capsules—Swallow each dose whole.
- Syrup—Take as directed on bottle.
- Drops—Dilute dose in beverage.

When to take:
As needed, no more often than every 4 hours.

If you forget a dose:
Take up to 2 hours late. If more than 2 hours, wait for next dose (don't double this).

What drug does:
- Prevents cells from releasing allergy-causing chemicals (histamines).
- Relaxes muscles of bronchial tubes.
- Decreases blood-vessel size and blood flow, thus causing decongestion.

Time lapse before drug works:
30 to 60 minutes.

Don't take with:
- See Interaction column and consult doctor.
- Non-prescription drugs with ephedrine, pseudoephedrine or epinephrine.
- Non-prescription drugs for cough, cold, allergy or asthma without consulting doctor.

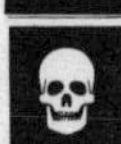

OVERDOSE

Symptoms:
Severe anxiety, confusion, delirium, muscle tremors, rapid and irregular pulse.

What to do:
- Dial 0 (operator) or 911 (emergency) for an ambulance or medical help. Then give first aid immediately.
- Additional emergency information on page 886.

POSSIBLE ADVERSE REACTIONS OR SIDE EFFECTS

SYMPTOMS	FREQUENCY	WHAT TO DO
Brain & nervous system:		
• Nervousness, headache.	Common	4
• Dizziness	Infrequent	4
Skin:		
Paleness	Common	4
Eyes:	None expected.	
Ears, nose, throat:	None expected.	
Digestive:		
Appetite loss, nausea, vomiting.	Infrequent	4
Heart & lungs:		
• Irregular heartbeat.	Infrequent	3
• Rapid heartbeat.	Common	4
Blood vessels:	None expected.	
Muscles, bones, joints:	None expected.	
Genital, urinary:		
Difficult urination.	Infrequent	4
Kidneys:	None expected.	
Liver:	None expected.	
Allergic:	None expected.	
Blood:	None expected.	
Others:		
Insomnia	Common	5

1- Life-threatening. Seek emergency treatment immediately.
2- Discontinue. Seek emergency treatment.
3- Discontinue. Call doctor right away.
4- Continue. Call doctor when convenient.
5- Continue. Tell doctor at next visit.
6- No action necessary.

WARNINGS & PRECAUTIONS

Don't take if:
You are allergic to ephedrine or any sympathomimetic drug.

Before you start, consult your doctor:
- If you have high blood pressure.
- If you have diabetes.
- If you have overactive thyroid gland.
- If you have difficulty urinating.
- If you have taken any MAO inhibitor in past 2 weeks
- If you have taken digitalis preparations in the last 7 days.
- If you will have surgery within 2 months, including dental surgery, requiring general or spinal anesthesia.

Over age 60:
More likely to develop high blood pressure, heart-rhythm disturbances, angina and to feel drug's stimulant effects.

Pregnancy:
No proven harm to unborn child. Avoid if possible.

Breast-feeding:
Drug passes into milk. Avoid drug or discontinue nursing until you finish medicine. Consult doctor for advice on maintaining milk supply.

Infants & children:
No problems expected.

Prolonged use:
- Excessive doses—Rare toxic psychosis.
- Men with enlarged prostate gland may have more urination difficulty.

Skin & sunlight:
No problems expected.

Driving, piloting or hazardous work:
Avoid if you feel dizzy. Otherwise, no problems expected.

Airplane passengers:
No problems expected.

Discontinuing:
May be unnecessary to finish medicine. Follow doctor's instructions.

Others:
No problems expected.

INTERACTION WITH OTHER DRUGS

GENERIC NAME OR DRUG CLASS	COMBINED EFFECT
Antidepressants (tricyclic)	Increased effect of ephedrine. Excessive stimulation of heart and blood pressure.
Antihypertensives	Decreased antihypertensive effect.
Digitalis preparations	Serious heart-rhythm disturbances.
Epinephrine	Increased epinephrine effect.
Ergot preparations	Serious blood-pressure rise.
Guanethidine	Decreased effect of both drugs.
MAO inhibitors	Increased ephedrine effect. Dangerous blood-pressure rise.
Pseudoephedrine	Increased pseudoephedrine effect.

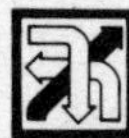

INTERACTION WITH OTHER SUBSTANCES

INTERACTS WITH	COMBINED EFFECT
Alcohol:	None expected.
Beverages: Caffeine drinks.	Nervousness or insomnia.
Cocaine:	Rapid heartbeat. Avoid.
Foods:	None expected.
Marijuana:	Rapid heartbeat, possible heart-rhythm disturbance.
Tobacco:	None expected.

EPINEPHRINE

BRAND NAMES

Adrenalin
Asmolin
Asthma Haler
Asthma Nefrin
Bronitin
Bronkaid Mist
Epifrin
Epitrate
Eppy
Glaucon
microNEFRIN
Primatene Mist
Simplene
Sus-phrine
Vaponefrin

See complete brand names list, page 826.

GENERAL INFORMATION

Habit forming? No
Prescription needed? Yes
Available as generic? Nose drops, aerosol inhaler—No
Eye drops, injection—Yes
Drug class: Sympathomimetic, antiglaucoma

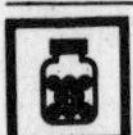

USES

- Relieves allergic symptoms of anaphylaxis.
- Eases symptoms of acute bronchial spasms.
- Relieves congestion of nose, sinuses and throat.
- Reduces internal eye pressure.

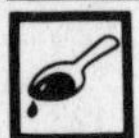

DOSAGE & USAGE INFORMATION

How to take:
Eyedrops, nose drops, aerosol inhaler, injection—Use as directed on labels.

When to take:
As needed, no more often than label directs.

If you forget a dose:
If needed, take when you remember. Wait 3 hours for next dose.

What drug does:
- Contracts blood-vessel walls and raises blood pressure.
- Inhibits release of histamine.
- Dilates constricted bronchial tubes and decreases volume of blood in nasal tissue.
- Reduces fluid formation within the eye.

Time lapse before drug works:
1 to 2 minutes.

Don't take with:
- Non-prescription drugs without consulting doctor.
- See Interaction column and consult doctor.

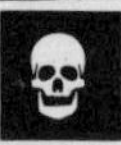

OVERDOSE

Symptoms:
Tremor, rapid breathing, palpitations, extreme rise in blood pressure, irregular heartbeat, breathing difficulty, convulsions, coma.

What to do:
- Dial 0 (operator) or 911 (emergency) for an ambulance or medical help. Then give first aid immediately.
- Additional emergency information on page 886.

POSSIBLE ADVERSE REACTIONS OR SIDE EFFECTS

SYMPTOMS	FREQUENCY	WHAT TO DO
Brain & nervous system:		
• Headache, agitation, dizziness.	Common	4
• Trembling	Infrequent	4
• Insomnia	Common	4
Skin:		
Flushed face or paleness.	Infrequent	4
Eyes, blood vessels, muscles, bones, joints, genital, urinary, kidneys, liver, allergic, blood:	None expected.	
Ears, nose, throat:		
Dry mouth and throat (inhaler only).	Common	5
Digestive:		
Nausea, vomiting.	Infrequent	4
Heart & lungs:		
• Fast or pounding heartbeat.	Common	4
• Chest pain, irregular heartbeat.	Rare	3
• Breathing difficulty.	Infrequent	3
• Cough or bronchial irritation (inhaler only).	Infrequent	4
Others:		
• Sweating	Rare	3
• Weakness	Infrequent	4

1-Life-threatening. Seek emergency treatment immediately.
2-Discontinue. Seek emergency treatment.
3-Discontinue. Call doctor right away.
4-Continue. Call doctor when convenient.
5-Continue. Tell doctor at next visit.

WARNINGS & PRECAUTIONS

Don't take if:

- You are allergic to any sympathomimetic.
- You have narrow-angle glaucoma.
- You have had a stroke or heart attack within 3 weeks.
- You have heart-rhythm disturbance.

Before you start, consult your doctor:

- If you have high blood pressure, heart disease or have had a stroke.
- If you have diabetes.
- If you have overactive thyroid.

Over age 60:

- Use with caution if you have hardening of the arteries.
- If you have enlarged prostate, drug may increase urination difficulty.
- If you have Parkinson's disease, drug may temporarily increase rigidity and tremor.
- If you see "floaters" in field of vision, tell your doctor.

Pregnancy:
No proven harm to unborn child. Avoid if possible.

Breast-feeding:
Drug passes into milk. Avoid drug or discontinue nursing until you finish medicine. Consult doctor for advice on maintaining milk supply.

Infants & children:
Use only under medical supervision.

Prolonged use:

- You may stop responding to drug.
- Drug may reduce blood volume.
- Drug may damage eye retina and impair vision.

Skin & sunlight:
No problems expected.

Driving, piloting or hazardous work:
No problems expected. Use caution if you feel dizzy or nervous.

Airplane passengers:
No problems expected.

Discontinuing:

- May be unnecessary to finish medicine. Follow doctor's instructions.
- If drug fails to provide relief after several doses, discontinue. Don't increase dose or frequency.

Others:

- May temporarily raise blood sugar in diabetics.
- Excessive use can cause sudden death.
- Discard medicine if cloudy or discolored.

INTERACTION WITH OTHER DRUGS

GENERIC NAME OR DRUG CLASS	COMBINED EFFECT
Antidepressants (tricyclic)	Increased epinephrine effect.
Antidiabetics (oral)	Decreased antidiabetic effect.
Antihistamines	Increased epinephrine effect.
Beta-adrenergic blockers	Decreased epinephrine effect.
Carbonic anhydrase inhibitors	Increased epinephrine effect.
Digitalis preparations	Possible irregular heartbeat.
Ephedrine	Increased ephedrine effect.
Guanethidine	Decreased guanethidine effect.
Insulin	Decreased insulin effect.
Isoproterenol	Dangerous to heart.
MAO inhibitors	Dangerous to heart.
Pilocarpine	Increased pilocarpine effect.
Rauwolfia alkaloids	Increased epinephrine effect.
Thyroid preparations	Increased epinephrine effect.

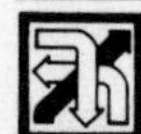

INTERACTION WITH OTHER SUBSTANCES

INTERACTS WITH	COMBINED EFFECT
Alcohol:	May increase urinary excretion of drug and reduce effectiveness.
Beverages:	None expected.
Cocaine:	Dangerous overstimulation. Avoid.
Foods:	None expected.
Marijuana:	Increase in epinephrine's antiasthmatic effect.
Tobacco:	None expected.

ERGOLOID MESYLATES

BRAND NAMES

Circanol
Deapril-ST
Hydergine
Trigot

GENERAL INFORMATION

Habit forming? No
Prescription needed? Yes
Available as generic? No
Drug class: Ergot preparation

USES

Treatment for reduced alertness, poor memory, confusion, depression or lack of motivation in the elderly.

DOSAGE & USAGE INFORMATION

How to take:

- Tablet or capsule—Swallow with liquid. If you can't swallow whole, crumble tablet or open capsule and take with liquid or food.
- Liquid—Take as directed on label.
- Sublingual tablets—Dissolve tablet under tongue.

When to take:
At the same times each day.

If you forget a dose:
Take as soon as you remember up to 2 hours late. If more than 2 hours, wait for next scheduled dose (don't double this dose).

What drug does:
Stimulates brain-cell metabolism to increase use of oxygen and nutrients.

Time lapse before drug works:
Gradual improvement over 3 to 4 months.

Don't take with:

- Non-prescription drugs containing alcohol without consulting doctor.
- See Interaction column and consult doctor.

OVERDOSE

Symptoms:
Headache, flushed face, nasal congestion, nausea, vomiting, blood-pressure drop, weakness, collapse, coma.

What to do:

- Dial 0 (operator) or 911 (emergency) for an ambulance or medical help. Then give first aid immediately.
- Additional emergency information on page 886.

POSSIBLE ADVERSE REACTIONS OR SIDE EFFECTS

SYMPTOMS	FREQUENCY	WHAT TO DO
Brain & nervous system:		
• Dizziness when getting up, drowsiness.	Rare	4
• Nervousness, hostility, confusion, depression.	Infrequent	4
• Fainting	Rare	2
Skin:		
Rash	Rare	3
Eyes:		
Blurred vision.	Infrequent	4
Ears, nose, throat:		
• Soreness under tongue.	Rare	4
• Nasal congestion.	Common	5
Digestive:		
• Appetite loss.	Rare	4
• Nausea, vomiting, stomach cramps.	Rare	3
Heart & lungs:		
Slow heartbeat.	Infrequent	3
Blood vessels:	None expected.	
Muscles, bones, joints:	None expected.	
Genital, urinary:	None expected.	
Kidneys:	None expected.	
Liver:	None expected.	
Allergic:	None expected.	
Blood:	None expected.	
Others:		
• Fever	Rare	4
• Tingling fingers.	Infrequent	3

1-Life-threatening. Seek emergency treatment immediately.
2-Discontinue. Seek emergency treatment.
3-Discontinue. Call doctor right away.
4-Continue. Call doctor when convenient.
5-Continue. Tell doctor at next visit.
6-No action necessary.

WARNINGS & PRECAUTIONS

Don't take if:
- You are allergic to any ergot preparation.
- Your heartbeat is less than 60 beats per minute.
- Your systolic blood pressure is consistently below 100.

Before you start, consult your doctor:
If you have had low blood pressure.

Over age 60:
Primarily used in people older than 60. Results unpredictable, but many patients show improved brain function.

Pregnancy:
Not recommended.

Breast-feeding:
Risk to nursing child outweighs drug benefits. Don't use.

Infants & children:
Not recommended.

Prolonged use:
No problems expected.

Skin & sunlight:
No problems expected.

Driving, piloting or hazardous work:
Avoid if you feel dizzy, faint or have blurred vision. Otherwise, no problems expected.

Airplane passengers:
No problems expected.

Discontinuing:
No problems expected.

Others:
No problems expected.

INTERACTION WITH OTHER DRUGS

GENERIC NAME OR DRUG CLASS	COMBINED EFFECT
Antihypertensives	Increased antihypertensive effect.
Beta-adrenergic blockers	Excessive decrease in heartbeat and/or blood pressure.
Digitalis preparations	Excessively slow heartbeat.

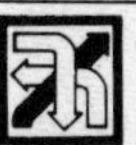

INTERACTION WITH OTHER SUBSTANCES

INTERACTS WITH	COMBINED EFFECT
Alcohol:	Use caution. May drop blood pressure excessively.
Beverages:	None expected.
Cocaine:	Overstimulation. Avoid.
Foods:	None expected.
Marijuana:	Decreased effect of ergot alkaloids.
Tobacco:	None expected.

ERGONOVINE

BRAND NAMES

Ergotrate

GENERAL INFORMATION

Habit forming? No
Prescription needed? Yes
Available as generic? Yes
Drug class: Ergot preparation (uterine stimulant)

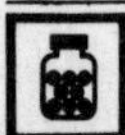

USES

Retards excessive post-delivery bleeding.

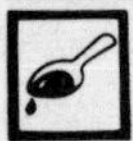

DOSAGE & USAGE INFORMATION

How to take:
Tablet—Swallow with liquid or food to lessen stomach irritation.

When to take:
At the same times each day.

If you forget a dose:
Don't take missed dose and don't double next one. Wait for next scheduled dose.

What drug does:
Causes smooth-muscle cells of uterine wall to contract and surround bleeding blood vessels of relaxed uterus.

Time lapse before drug works:
Tablets—20 to 30 minutes.

Don't take with:
See Interaction column and consult doctor.

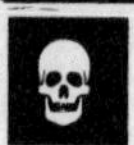

OVERDOSE

Symptoms:
Vomiting, diarrhea, weak pulse, low blood pressure, convulsions.

What to do:
- Dial 0 (operator) or 911 (emergency) for an ambulance or medical help. Then give first aid immediately.
- If patient is unconscious and not breathing, give mouth-to-mouth breathing. If there is no heartbeat, use cardiac massage and mouth-to-mouth breathing (CPR). Don't try to make patient vomit. If you can't get help quickly, take patient to nearest emergency facility.
- Additional emergency information on page 886.

POSSIBLE ADVERSE REACTIONS OR SIDE EFFECTS

SYMPTOMS	FREQUENCY	WHAT TO DO
Brain & nervous system:		
• Sudden, severe headache.	Rare	2
• Confusion	Infrequent	3
Skin:	None expected.	
Eyes:	None expected.	
Ears, nose, throat:		
Ringing in ears.	Infrequent	3
Digestive:		
• Nausea, vomiting.	Common	3
• Diarrhea	Infrequent	3
Heart & lungs:		
Shortness of breath, chest pain.	Rare	2
Blood vessels:	None expected.	
Muscles, bones, joints:		
• Muscle cramps.	Infrequent	3
• Numb, cold hands and feet.	Rare	2
Genital, urinary:	None expected.	
Kidneys:	None expected.	
Liver:	None expected.	
Allergic:	None expected.	
Blood:	None expected.	
Others:		
Unusual sweating.	Infrequent	4

1-Life-threatening. Seek emergency treatment immediately.
2-Discontinue. Seek emergency treatment.
3-Discontinue. Call doctor right away.
4-Continue. Call doctor when convenient.
5-Continue. Tell doctor at next visit.
6-No action necessary.

WARNINGS & PRECAUTIONS

Don't take if:
You are allergic to any ergot preparation.

Before you start, consult your doctor:
- If you have coronary-artery or blood-vessel disease.
- If you have liver or kidney disease.
- If you have high blood pressure.
- If you have postpartum infection.

Over age 60:
Not recommended.

Pregnancy:
Risk to unborn child outweighs drug benefits. Don't use.

Breast-feeding:
Drug passes into milk. Avoid drug or discontinue nursing until you finish medicine. Consult doctor for advice on maintaining milk supply.

Infants & children:
Not recommended.

Prolonged use:
Not recommended.

Skin & sunlight:
No problems expected.

Driving, piloting or hazardous work:
No problems expected.

Airplane passengers:
No problems expected.

Discontinuing:
May be unnecessary to finish medicine. Follow doctor's instructions.

Others:
Drug should be used for short time only following childbirth or miscarriage.

INTERACTION WITH OTHER DRUGS

GENERIC NAME OR DRUG CLASS	COMBINED EFFECT
Ergot preparations (other)	Increased ergonovine effect.

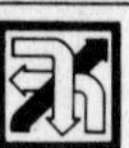

INTERACTION WITH OTHER SUBSTANCES

INTERACTS WITH	COMBINED EFFECT
Alcohol:	None expected.
Beverages:	None expected.
Cocaine:	None expected.
Foods:	None expected.
Marijuana:	None expected.
Tobacco:	None expected.

ERGOTAMINE

BRAND NAMES

Bellergal
Bellergal-S
Cafergot
Cafergot-PB
Cafetrate-PB
Ergomar
Ergostat
Gynergen
Medihaler-Ergotamine
Migraine
Migral
Migrastat
Wigraine
Wigraine-PB
Wigrettes

GENERAL INFORMATION

Habit forming? No
Prescription needed? Yes
Available as generic? Yes
Drug class: Vasoconstrictor, ergot preparation

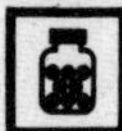

USES

Relieves pain of migraines and other headaches caused by dilated blood vessels. Will not prevent headaches.

DOSAGE & USAGE INFORMATION

How to take:

- Tablet or capsule—Swallow with liquid, or let dissolve under tongue. If you can't swallow whole, crumble tablet or open capsule and take with liquid or food.
- Suppositories—Remove wrapper and moisten suppository with water. Gently insert larger end into rectum. Push well into rectum with finger.
- Aerosol inhaler—Use only as directed on prescription label.
- Lie down in quiet, dark room after taking.

When to take:
At first sign of vascular or migraine headache.

If you forget a dose:
Take as soon as you remember. Wait 4 hours for next dose.

What drug does:
Constricts blood vessels in the head.

Time lapse before drug works:
30 to 60 minutes.

Don't take with:
See Interaction column and consult doctor.

OVERDOSE

Symptoms:
Tingling, cold extremities and muscle pain. Progresses to nausea, vomiting, diarrhea, cold skin, rapid and weak pulse, severe numbness of extremities, confusion, convulsions, coma.

What to do:

- Dial 0 (operator) or 911 (emergency) for an ambulance or medical help. Then give first aid immediately.
- Additional emergency information on page 886.

POSSIBLE ADVERSE REACTIONS OR SIDE EFFECTS

SYMPTOMS	FREQUENCY	WHAT TO DO
Brain & nervous system:		
• Anxiety or confusion.	Rare	3
• Dizziness	Common	4
Skin:		
• Red or purple blisters, especially on hands, feet.	Rare	3
• Itch, swelling.	Infrequent	3
Eyes:		
Vision changes.	Rare	3
Ears, nose, throat:		
Extreme thirst.	Rare	3
Digestive:		
• Stomach pain or bloating.	Rare	3
• Nausea, diarrhea, vomiting.	Common	4
Heart & lungs:		
Unusually fast or slow heartbeat, possible chest pain.	Rare	3
Blood vessels:		
Cold, pale hands or feet.	Infrequent	3
Muscles, bones, joints:		
Pain or weakness in arms, legs, back.	Infrequent	3
Genital, urinary, kidneys, liver, allergic, blood:	None expected.	
Others:		
Numbness or tingling of face, fingers, toes.	Rare	3

1 - Life-threatening. Seek emergency treatment immediately.
2 - Discontinue. Seek emergency treatment.
3 - Discontinue. Call doctor right away.
4 - Continue. Call doctor when convenient.

WARNINGS & PRECAUTIONS

Don't take if:
You are allergic to any ergot preparation.

Before you start, consult your doctor:
- If you plan to become pregnant within medication period.
- If you have an infection.
- If you have angina, heart problems, high blood pressure, hardening of the arteries or vein problems.
- If you have kidney or liver disease.
- If you are allergic to other spray inhalants.

Over age 60:
Adverse reactions and side effects may be more frequent and severe than in younger persons.

Pregnancy:
Risk to unborn child outweighs drug benefits. Don't use.

Breast-feeding:
Drug filters into milk. May harm child. Avoid.

Infants & children:
Studies inconclusive on harm to children. Consult your doctor.

Prolonged use:
Cold skin, muscle pain, gangrene of hands and feet. This medicine not intended for uninterrupted use.

Skin & sunlight:
No problems expected.

Driving, piloting or hazardous work:
Don't drive or pilot aircraft until you learn how medicine affects you. Don't work around dangerous machinery. Don't climb ladders or work in high places. Danger increases if you drink alcohol or take medicine affecting alertness and reflexes, such as antihistamines, tranquilizers, sedatives, pain medicine, narcotics and mind-altering drugs.

Airplane passengers:
No problems expected.

Discontinuing:
May be unnecessary to finish medicine. Follow doctor's instructions.

Others:
Impaired blood circulation can lead to gangrene in intestines or extremities. Never exceed recommended dose.

INTERACTION WITH OTHER DRUGS

GENERIC NAME OR DRUG CLASS	COMBINED EFFECT
Amphetamines	Dangerous blood-pressure rise.
Ephedrine	Dangerous blood-pressure rise.
Epinephrine	Dangerous blood-pressure rise.
Pseudoephedrine	Dangerous blood-pressure rise.
Troleandomycin	Increased adverse reactions of ergotamine.

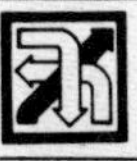

INTERACTION WITH OTHER SUBSTANCES

INTERACTS WITH	COMBINED EFFECT
Alcohol:	Dilates blood vessels. Makes headache worse.
Beverages: Caffeine drinks	May help relieve headache.
Cocaine:	Decreased ergotamine effect.
Foods: Any to which you are allergic.	May make headache worse. Avoid.
Marijuana:	Occasional use—Cool extremities. Regular use—Persistent chill.
Tobacco:	Decreased effect of ergotamine. Makes headache worse.

ERYTHRITYL TETRANITRATE

BRAND NAMES

Cardilate

GENERAL INFORMATION

Habit forming? No
Prescription needed? Yes
Available as generic? No
Drug class: Antianginal (nitrate)

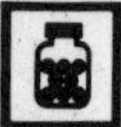

USES

Reduces frequency and severity of angina attacks.

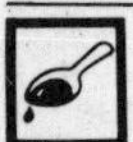

DOSAGE & USAGE INFORMATION

How to take:

- Sublingual tablet—Dissolve under tongue at earliest sign of angina.
- Chewable tablet—Chew tablet at earliest sign of angina, and hold in mouth for 2 minutes.
- Regular tablet—Swallow with liquid. You may chew or crush it.

When to take:
Swallowed tablets—Take at the same times each day, 1 or 2 hours after meals.

If you forget a dose:
Swallowed tablets—Take as soon as you remember up to 2 hours late. If more than 2 hours, wait for next scheduled dose (don't double this dose).

What drug does:
Relaxes blood vessels, increasing blood flow to heart muscle.

Time lapse before drug works:

- Sublingual or chewable tablets—3 to 5 minutes.
- Swallowed tablets—30 minutes.

Don't take with:
See Interaction column and consult doctor.

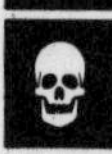

OVERDOSE

Symptoms:
Vomiting, sweating, shortness of breath, loss of consciousness.

What to do:

- Dial 0 (operator) or 911 (emergency) for an ambulance or medical help. Then give first aid immediately.
- Additional emergency information on page 886.

POSSIBLE ADVERSE REACTIONS OR SIDE EFFECTS

SYMPTOMS	FREQUENCY	WHAT TO DO
Brain & nervous system:		
• Headache	Common	5
• Fainting	Infrequent	3
Skin:		
• Rash	Rare	3
• Flushed face and neck.	Common	5
Eyes:	None expected.	
Ears, nose, throat:	None expected.	
Digestive:		
Nausea, vomiting.	Common	5
Heart & lungs:		
Rapid heartbeat.	Common	5
Blood vessels:	None expected.	
Muscles, bones, joints:	None expected.	
Genital, urinary:	None expected.	
Kidneys:	None expected.	
Liver:	None expected.	
Allergic:	None expected.	
Blood:	None expected.	
Others:	None expected.	

1- Life-threatening. Seek emergency treatment immediately.
2- Discontinue. Seek emergency treatment.
3- Discontinue. Call doctor right away.
4- Continue. Call doctor when convenient.
5- Continue. Tell doctor at next visit.
6- No action necessary.

ERYTHRITYL TETRANITRATE

WARNINGS & PRECAUTIONS

Don't take if:
You are allergic to nitrates, including nitroglycerin.

Before you start, consult your doctor:
If you have glaucoma.

Over age 60:
Adverse reactions and side effects may be more frequent and severe than in younger persons.

Pregnancy:
No proven harm to unborn child. Avoid if possible.

Breast-feeding:
No proven problems. Consult your doctor.

Infants & children:
Not recommended.

Prolonged use:
Drug may become less effective and require higher doses.

Skin & sunlight:
No problems expected.

Driving, piloting or hazardous work:
Don't drive or pilot aircraft until you learn how medicine affects you. Don't work around dangerous machinery. Don't climb ladders or work in high places. Danger increases if you drink alcohol or take medicine affecting alertness and reflexes, such as antihistamines, tranquilizers, sedatives, pain medicine, narcotics and mind-altering drugs.

Airplane passengers:
No problems expected.

Discontinuing:
Don't discontinue without doctor's advice until you complete prescribed dose, even though symptoms diminish or disappear.

Others:
Periodic laboratory blood studies recommended if you take erythrityl tetranitrate.

INTERACTION WITH OTHER DRUGS

GENERIC NAME OR DRUG CLASS	COMBINED EFFECT
Anticholinergics	Increased internal eye pressure.
Antidepressants (tricyclic)	Excessive blood-pressure drop.
Antihypertensives	Excessive blood-pressure drop.
Beta-adrenergic blockers	Excessive blood-pressure drop.
Cholinergics	Decreased cholinergic effect.
Ephedrine	Decreased effect of erythrityl tetranitrate.

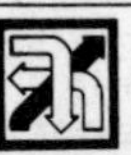

INTERACTION WITH OTHER SUBSTANCES

INTERACTS WITH	COMBINED EFFECT
Alcohol:	Excessive blood-pressure drop.
Beverages:	None expected.
Cocaine:	Flushed face and headache. Avoid.
Foods:	None expected.
Marijuana:	Decreased effect of erythrityl tetranitrate.
Tobacco:	Decreased effect of erythrityl tetranitrate.

ERYTHROMYCINS

BRAND AND GENERIC NAMES

Dowmycin
E-Biotic
E-Mycin
Eryc
Ery-derm
Ery-Tab
Erythromid
Kesso-mycin
Novorythro
Robimycin
RP-Mycin

See complete brand and generic names list, page 826.

GENERAL INFORMATION

Habit forming? No
Prescription needed? Yes
Available as generic? Yes
Drug class: Antibiotic (erythromycin)

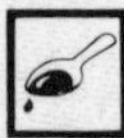

USES

Treatment of infections responsive to erythromycin.

DOSAGE & USAGE INFORMATION

How to take:

- Tablet or capsule—Swallow with liquid.
- Extended-release tablets or capsules—Swallow each dose whole. If you take regular tablets, you may chew or crush them.
- Liquid, drops, granules, skin ointment, eye ointment, skin solution—Follow prescription label directions.

When to take:
At the same times each day, 1 hour before or 2 hours after eating.

If you forget a dose:

- If you take 3 or more doses daily—Take as soon as you remember. Return to regular schedule.
- If you take 2 doses daily—Take as soon as you remember. Wait 5 to 6 hours for next dose. Return to regular schedule.

What drug does:
Prevents growth and reproduction of susceptible bacteria.

Time lapse before drug works:
2 to 5 days.

Don't take with:
See Interaction column and consult doctor.

OVERDOSE

Symptoms:
Nausea, vomiting, abdominal discomfort, diarrhea.

What to do:
Overdose unlikely to threaten life. If person takes much larger amount than prescribed, call doctor, poison-control center or hospital emergency room for instructions.

POSSIBLE ADVERSE REACTIONS OR SIDE EFFECTS

SYMPTOMS	FREQUENCY	WHAT TO DO
Brain & nervous system:	None expected.	
Skin: Dryness, irritation, itch, stinging with use of skin solution.	Infrequent	4
Eyes:	None expected.	
Ears, nose, throat: Sore mouth or tongue.	Infrequent	4
Digestive: Diarrhea, nausea, stomach cramps, discomfort, vomiting.	Infrequent	3
Heart & lungs:	None expected.	
Blood vessels:	None expected.	
Muscles, bones, joints:	None expected.	
Genital, urinary:	None expected.	
Kidneys:	None expected.	
Liver: Jaundice (yellow skin and eyes) in adults.	Rare	3
Allergic:	None expected.	
Blood:	None expected.	
Others: Unusual tiredness or weakness.	Rare	4

1-Life-threatening. Seek emergency treatment immediately.
2-Discontinue. Seek emergency treatment.
3-Discontinue. Call doctor right away.
4-Continue. Call doctor when convenient.
5-Continue. Tell doctor at next visit.
6-No action necessary.

WARNINGS & PRECAUTIONS

Don't take if:
- You are allergic to any erythromycin.
- You have had liver disease or impaired liver function.

Before you start, consult your doctor:
If you have taken erythromycin estolate in the past.

Over age 60:
Adverse reactions and side effects may be more frequent and severe than in younger persons, especially skin reactions around genitals and anus.

Pregnancy:
No proven harm to unborn child. Avoid if possible.

Breast-feeding:
Drug passes into milk. Avoid drug or discontinue nursing until you finish medicine. Consult doctor for advice on maintaining milk supply.

Infants & children:
Use only under medical supervision.

Prolonged use:
You may become more susceptible to infections caused by germs not responsive to erythromycin.

Skin & sunlight:
No problems expected.

Driving, piloting or hazardous work:
No problems expected.

Airplane passengers:
No problems expected.

Discontinuing:
You must take full dose at least 10 consecutive days for streptococcal or staphylococcal infections.

Others:
No problems expected.

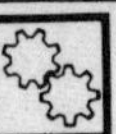

INTERACTION WITH OTHER DRUGS

GENERIC NAME OR DRUG CLASS	COMBINED EFFECT
Aminophylline	Increased effect of aminophylline in blood.
Lincomycins	Decreased lincomycin effect.
Oxtriphylline	Increased level of oxtriphylline in blood.
Penicillins	Decreased penicillin effect.
Theophylline	Increased level of theophylline in blood.

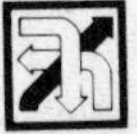

INTERACTION WITH OTHER SUBSTANCES

INTERACTS WITH	COMBINED EFFECT
Alcohol:	Possible liver damage.
Beverages:	None expected.
Cocaine:	None expected.
Foods:	None expected.
Marijuana:	None expected.
Tobacco:	None expected.

ESTERIFIED ESTROGENS

BRAND NAMES

Amnestrogen
Estratab
Estratest
Evex

GENERAL INFORMATION

Habit forming? No
Prescription needed? Yes
Available as generic? Yes
Drug class: Female sex hormone (estrogen)

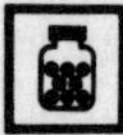

USES

- Treatment for symptoms of menopause and menstrual-cycle irregularity.
- Replacement for female hormone deficiency.
- Treatment for cancer of prostate and breast.

DOSAGE & USAGE INFORMATION

How to take:
Tablet—Swallow with liquid. If you can't swallow whole, crumble tablet and take with liquid or food.

When to take:
At the same time each day.

If you forget a dose:
Take as soon as you remember up to 12 hours late. If more than 12 hours, wait for next scheduled dose (don't double this dose).

What drug does:
Restores normal estrogen level in tissues.

Time lapse before drug works:
10 to 20 days.

Don't take with:
See Interaction column and consult doctor.

OVERDOSE

Symptoms:
Nausea, vomiting, fluid retention, breast enlargement and discomfort, abnormal vaginal bleeding.

What to do:
Overdose unlikely to threaten life. If person takes much larger amount than prescribed, call doctor, poison-control center or hospital emergency room for instructions.

POSSIBLE ADVERSE REACTIONS OR SIDE EFFECTS

SYMPTOMS	FREQUENCY	WHAT TO DO
Brain & nervous system:		
Depression, dizziness, irritability.	Infrequent	4
Skin:		
• Rash	Infrequent	3
• Brown blotches.	Infrequent	5
• Hair loss.	Infrequent	5
Eyes, ears, nose, throat, heart & lungs, muscles, bones, joints, kidneys, allergic, blood:	None expected.	
Digestive:		
• Stomach or side pain.	Infrequent	3
• Stomach cramps.	Common	3
• Appetite loss.	Common	4
• Nausea, diarrhea.	Common	5
• Vomiting	Infrequent	4
Blood vessels:		
Swollen ankles, feet.	Common	5
Genital, urinary:		
Vaginal discharge or bleeding.	Infrequent	5
Liver:		
Jaundice (yellow skin and eyes).	Rare	3
Others:		
• Breast lumps.	Infrequent	4
• Swollen, tender breasts.	Common	5
• Changes in sex drive.	Infrequent	5

1- Life-threatening. Seek emergency treatment immediately.
2- Discontinue. Seek emergency treatment.
3- Discontinue. Call doctor right away.
4- Continue. Call doctor when convenient.
5- Continue. Tell doctor at next visit.

WARNINGS & PRECAUTIONS

Don't take if:
- You are allergic to any estrogen-containing drugs.
- You have impaired liver function.
- You have had blood clots, stroke or heart attack.
- You have unexplained vaginal bleeding.

Before you start, consult your doctor:
- If you have had cancer of breast or reproductive organs, fibrocystic breast disease, fibroid tumors of the uterus or endometriosis.
- If you have had migraine headaches, epilepsy or porphyria.
- If you have diabetes, high blood pressure, asthma, congestive heart failure, kidney disease or gallstones.
- If you plan to become pregnant within 3 months.

Over age 60:
Controversial. You and your doctor must decide if drug risks outweigh benefits.

Pregnancy:
Risk to unborn child outweighs drug benefits. Don't use.

Breast-feeding:
Drug filters into milk. May harm child. Avoid.

Infants & children:
Not recommended.

Prolonged use:
Increased growth of fibroid tumors of uterus. Possible association with cancer of uterus.

Skin & sunlight:
May cause rash or intensify sunburn in areas exposed to sun or sunlamp.

Driving, piloting or hazardous work:
No problems expected.

Airplane passengers:
No problems expected.

Discontinuing:
You may need to discontinue estrogen periodically. Consult your doctor.

Others:
In rare instances, may cause blood clot in lung, brain or leg. Symptoms are *sudden* severe headache, coordination loss, vision change, chest pain, breathing difficulty, slurred speech, pain in legs or groin. Seek emergency treatment immediately.

INTERACTION WITH OTHER DRUGS

GENERIC NAME OR DRUG CLASS	COMBINED EFFECT
Anticoagulants (oral)	Decreased anticoagulant effect.
Anticonvulsants (hydantoin)	Increased seizures.
Antidiabetics (oral)	Unpredictable increase or decrease in blood sugar.
Clofibrate	Decreased clofibrate effect.
Carbamazepine	Increased seizures.
Meprobamate	Increased effect of esterified estrogens.
Phenobarbital	Decreased effect of esterified estrogens.
Primidone	Decreased effect of esterified estrogens.
Rifampin	Decreased effect of esterified estrogens.
Thyroid hormones	Decreased thyroid effect.

INTERACTION WITH OTHER SUBSTANCES

INTERACTS WITH	COMBINED EFFECT
Alcohol:	None expected.
Beverages:	None expected.
Cocaine:	No proven problems.
Foods:	None expected.
Marijuana:	Possible menstrual irregularities and bleeding between periods.
Tobacco:	Increased risk of blood clots leading to stroke or heart attack.

ESTRADIOL

BRAND NAMES

Delestrogen
Estrace

GENERAL INFORMATION

Habit forming? No
Prescription needed? Yes
Available as generic? Yes
Drug class: Female sex hormone (estrogen)

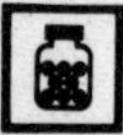

USES

- Treatment for symptoms of menopause and menstrual-cycle irregularity.
- Replacement for female hormone deficiency.
- Treatment for cancer of prostate and breast.

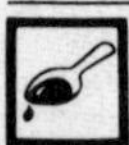

DOSAGE & USAGE INFORMATION

How to take:
Tablet—Swallow with liquid. If you can't swallow whole, crumble tablet and take with liquid or food.

When to take:
At the same time each day.

If you forget a dose:
Take as soon as you remember up to 12 hours late. If more than 12 hours, wait for next scheduled dose (don't double this dose).

What drug does:
Restores normal estrogen level in tissues.

Time lapse before drug works:
10 to 20 days.

Don't take with:
See Interaction column and consult doctor.

OVERDOSE

Symptoms:
Nausea, vomiting, fluid retention, breast enlargement and discomfort, abnormal vaginal bleeding.

What to do:
Overdose unlikely to threaten life. If person takes much larger amount than prescribed, call doctor, poison-control center or hospital emergency room for instructions.

POSSIBLE ADVERSE REACTIONS OR SIDE EFFECTS

SYMPTOMS	FREQUENCY	WHAT TO DO
Brain & nervous system:		
Depression, dizziness, irritability.	Infrequent	4
Skin:		
• Rash	Infrequent	3
• Brown blotches.	Infrequent	5
• Hair loss.	Infrequent	5
Eyes, ears, nose, throat, heart & lungs, muscles, bones, joints, kidneys, allergic, blood:	None expected.	
Digestive:		
• Stomach or side pain.	Infrequent	3
• Stomach cramps.	Common	3
• Appetite loss.	Common	4
• Nausea, diarrhea.	Common	5
• Vomiting	Infrequent	4
Blood vessels:		
Swollen ankles, feet.	Common	5
Genital, urinary:		
Vaginal discharge or bleeding.	Infrequent	5
Liver:		
Jaundice (yellow skin and eyes).	Rare	3
Others:		
• Breast lumps.	Infrequent	4
• Swollen, tender breasts.	Common	5
• Changes in sex drive.	Infrequent	5

1- Life-threatening. Seek emergency treatment immediately.
2- Discontinue. Seek emergency treatment.
3- Discontinue. Call doctor right away.
4- Continue. Call doctor when convenient.
5- Continue. Tell doctor at next visit.

WARNINGS & PRECAUTIONS

Don't take if:

- You are allergic to any estrogen-containing drugs.
- You have impaired liver function.
- You have had blood clots, stroke or heart attack.
- You have unexplained vaginal bleeding.

Before you start, consult your doctor:

- If you have had cancer of breast or reproductive organs, fibrocystic breast disease, fibroid tumors of the uterus or endometriosis.
- If you have had migraine headaches, epilepsy or porphyria.
- If you have diabetes, high blood pressure, asthma, congestive heart failure, kidney disease or gallstones.
- If you plan to become pregnant within 3 months.

Over age 60:
Controversial. You and your doctor must decide if drug risks outweigh benefits.

Pregnancy:
Risk to unborn child outweighs drug benefits. Don't use.

Breast-feeding:
Drug filters into milk. May harm child. Avoid.

Infants & children:
Not recommended.

Prolonged use:
Increased growth of fibroid tumors of uterus. Possible association with cancer of uterus.

Skin & sunlight:
May cause rash or intensify sunburn in areas exposed to sun or sunlamp.

Driving, piloting or hazardous work:
No problems expected.

Airplane passengers:
No problems expected.

Discontinuing:
You may need to discontinue estradiol periodically. Consult your doctor.

Others:
In rare instances, may cause blood clot in lung, brain or leg. Symptoms are *sudden* severe headache, coordination loss, vision change, chest pain, breathing difficulty, slurred speech, pain in legs or groin. Seek emergency treatment immediately.

INTERACTION WITH OTHER DRUGS

GENERIC NAME OR DRUG CLASS	COMBINED EFFECT
Anticoagulants (oral)	Decreased anticoagulant effect.
Anticonvulsants (hydantoin)	Increased seizures.
Antidiabetics (oral)	Unpredictable increase or decrease in blood sugar.
Clofibrate	Decreased clofibrate effect.
Carbamazepine	Increased seizures.
Meprobamate	Increased estradiol effect.
Phenobarbital	Decreased estradiol effect.
Primidone	Decreased estradiol effect.
Rifampin	Decreased estradiol effect.
Thyroid hormones	Decreased thyroid effect.

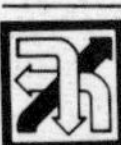

INTERACTION WITH OTHER SUBSTANCES

INTERACTS WITH	COMBINED EFFECT
Alcohol:	None expected.
Beverages:	None expected.
Cocaine:	No proven problems.
Foods:	None expected.
Marijuana:	Possible menstrual irregularities and bleeding between periods.
Tobacco:	Increased risk of blood clots leading to stroke or heart attack.

ESTROGEN

BRAND NAMES

Amnestrogen	Estrocon	Hormonin	Milprem
Clinestrone	Estrovis	Menest	PMB-200
DES	Evex	Menotrol	PMB-400
Delestrogen	Feminone	Menrium	Premarin
Estinyl	Femogen	Oestrilin	Stilphostrol
Estomed	Formatrix	Oagen	Theogen
Estrace			

GENERAL INFORMATION

Habit forming? No
Prescription needed? Yes
Available as generic? Yes
Drug class: Female sex hormone (estrogen)

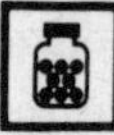

USES

- Treatment for symptoms of menopause and menstrual-cycle irregularity.
- Treatment for estrogen-deficiency osteoporosis (bone softening from calcium loss).
- Treatment for DES-induced cancer.

DOSAGE & USAGE INFORMATION

How to take:

- Tablet or capsule—Swallow with liquid. If you can't swallow whole, crumble tablet or open capsule and take with liquid or food.
- Vaginal cream—Use as directed on label.

When to take:
At the same time each day.

If you forget a dose:
Take as soon as you remember up to 12 hours late. If more than 12 hours, wait for next scheduled dose (don't double this dose).

What drug does:
Restores normal estrogen level in tissues.

Time lapse before drug works:
10 to 20 days.

Don't take with:
See Interaction column and consult doctor.

OVERDOSE

Symptoms:
Nausea, vomiting, fluid retention, breast enlargement and discomfort, abnormal vaginal bleeding.

What to do:
Overdose unlikely to threaten life. If person takes much larger amount than prescribed, call doctor, poison-control center or hospital emergency room for instructions.

POSSIBLE ADVERSE REACTIONS OR SIDE EFFECTS

SYMPTOMS	FREQUENCY	WHAT TO DO
Brain & nervous system:		
Depression, dizziness, irritability.	Infrequent	4
Skin:		
• Rash	Infrequent	3
• Brown blotches.	Infrequent	5
• Hair loss.	Infrequent	5
Eyes, ears, nose, throat, heart & lungs, muscles, bones, joints, kidneys, allergic, blood:	None expected.	
Digestive:		
• Stomach or side pain.	Infrequent	3
• Stomach cramps.	Common	3
• Appetite loss.	Common	4
• Nausea, diarrhea.	Common	5
• Vomiting	Infrequent	4
Blood vessels:		
Swollen ankles, feet.	Common	5
Genital, urinary:		
Vaginal discharge or bleeding.	Infrequent	5
Liver:		
Jaundice (yellow skin and eyes).	Rare	3
Others:		
• Breast lumps.	Infrequent	4
• Swollen, tender breasts.	Common	5
• Changes in sex drive.	Infrequent	5

1- Life-threatening. Seek emergency treatment immediately.
2- Discontinue. Seek emergency treatment.
3- Discontinue. Call doctor right away.
4- Continue. Call doctor when convenient.
5- Continue. Tell doctor at next visit.
6- No action necessary.

WARNINGS & PRECAUTIONS

Don't take if:
- You are allergic to any estrogen-containing drugs.
- You have impaired liver function.
- You have had blood clots, stroke or heart attack.
- You have unexplained vaginal bleeding.

Before you start, consult your doctor:
- If you have had cancer of breast or reproductive organs, fibrocystic breast disease, fibroid tumors of the uterus or endometriosis.
- If you have had migraine headaches, epilepsy or porphyria.
- If you have diabetes, high blood pressure, asthma, congestive heart failure, kidney disease or gallstones.
- If you plan to become pregnant within 3 months.

Over age 60:
Controversial. You and your doctor must decide if drug risks outweigh benefits.

Pregnancy:
Risk to unborn child outweighs drug benefits. Don't use.

Breast-feeding:
Drug filters into milk. May harm child. Avoid.

Infants & children:
Not recommended.

Prolonged use:
Increased growth of fibroid tumors of uterus. Possible association with cancer of utérus.

Skin & sunlight:
May cause rash or intensify sunburn in areas exposed to sun or sunlamp.

Driving, piloting or hazardous work:
No problems expected.

Airplane passengers:
No problems expected.

Discontinuing:
You may need to discontinue estrogens periodically. Consult your doctor.

Others:
In rare instances, may cause blood clot in lung, brain or leg. Symptoms are *sudden* severe headache, coordination loss, vision change, chest pain, breathing difficulty, slurred speech, pain in legs or groin. Seek emergency treatment immediately.

INTERACTION WITH OTHER DRUGS

GENERIC NAME OR DRUG CLASS	COMBINED EFFECT
Anticoagulants (oral)	Decreased anticoagulant effect.
Anticonvulsants (hydantoin)	Increased seizures.
Antidiabetics (oral)	Unpredictable increase or decrease in blood sugar.
Clofibrate	Decreased clofibrate effect.
Carbamazepine	Increased seizures.
Meprobamate	Increased estrogen effect.
Phenobarbital	Decreased estrogen effect.
Primidone	Decreased estrogen effect.
Rifampin	Decreased estrogen effect.
Thyroid hormones	Decreased thyroid effect.

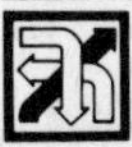

INTERACTION WITH OTHER SUBSTANCES

INTERACTS WITH	COMBINED EFFECT
Alcohol:	None expected.
Beverages:	None expected.
Cocaine:	No proven problems.
Foods:	None expected.
Marijuana:	Possible menstrual irregularities and bleeding between periods.
Tobacco:	Increased risk of blood clots leading to stroke or heart attack.

ESTRONE

BRAND NAMES

Besterone
Femogen
Kestrin
Natural Estrogenic Substance
Ogen
Theelin
Theogen

GENERAL INFORMATION

Habit forming? No
Prescription needed? Yes
Available as generic? Yes
Drug class: Female sex hormone (estrogen)

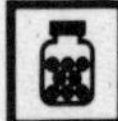

USES

- Treatment for symptoms of menopause and menstrual-cycle irregularity.
- Replacement for female hormone deficiency.
- Treatment for cancer of prostate.

DOSAGE & USAGE INFORMATION

How to take:
By injection under medical supervision.

When to take:
Varies according to doctor's instructions.

If you forget an injection:
Consult doctor.

What drug does:
Restores normal estrogen level in tissues.

Time lapse before drug works:
10 to 20 days.

Don't take with:
See Interaction column and consult doctor.

OVERDOSE

Symptoms:
Nausea, vomiting, fluid retention, breast enlargement and discomfort, abnormal vaginal bleeding.

What to do:
Overdose unlikely to threaten life. If person takes much larger amount than prescribed, call doctor, poison-control center or hospital emergency room for instructions.

POSSIBLE ADVERSE REACTIONS OR SIDE EFFECTS

SYMPTOMS	FREQUENCY	WHAT TO DO
Brain & nervous system:		
Depression, dizziness, irritability.	Infrequent	4
Skin:		
• Rash	Infrequent	3
• Brown blotches.	Infrequent	5
• Hair loss.	Infrequent	5
Eyes, ears, nose, throat, heart & lungs, muscles, bones, joints, kidneys, allergic, blood:	None expected.	
Digestive:		
• Stomach or side pain.	Infrequent	3
• Stomach cramps.	Common	3
• Appetite loss.	Common	4
• Nausea, diarrhea.	Common	5
• Vomiting	Infrequent	4
Blood vessels:		
Swollen ankles, feet.	Common	5
Genital, urinary:		
Vaginal discharge or bleeding.	Infrequent	5
Liver:		
Jaundice (yellow skin and eyes).	Rare	3
Others:		
• Breast lumps.	Infrequent	4
• Swollen, tender breasts.	Common	5
• Changes in sex drive.	Infrequent	5

1 - Life-threatening. Seek emergency treatment immediately.
2 - Discontinue. Seek emergency treatment.
3 - Discontinue. Call doctor right away.
4 - Continue. Call doctor when convenient.
5 - Continue. Tell doctor at next visit.

WARNINGS & PRECAUTIONS

Don't take if:
- You are allergic to any estrogen-containing drugs.
- You have impaired liver function.
- You have had blood clots, stroke or heart attack.
- You have unexplained vaginal bleeding.

Before you start, consult your doctor:
- If you have had cancer of breast or reproductive organs, fibrocystic breast disease, fibroid tumors of the uterus or endometriosis.
- If you have had migraine headaches, epilepsy or porphyria.
- If you have diabetes, high blood pressure, asthma, congestive heart failure, kidney disease or gallstones.
- If you plan to become pregnant within 3 months.

Over age 60:
Controversial. You and your doctor must decide if drug risks outweigh benefits.

Pregnancy:
Risk to unborn child outweighs drug benefits. Don't use.

Breast-feeding:
Drug filters into milk. May harm child. Avoid.

Infants & children:
Not recommended.

Prolonged use:
Increased growth of fibroid tumors of uterus. Possible association with cancer of uterus.

Skin & sunlight:
May cause rash or intensify sunburn in areas exposed to sun or sunlamp.

Driving, piloting or hazardous work:
No problems expected.

Airplane passengers:
No problems expected.

Discontinuing:
You may need to discontinue estrone periodically. Consult your doctor.

Others:
In rare instances, may cause blood clot in lung, brain or leg. Symptoms are *sudden* severe headache, coordination loss, vision change, chest pain, breathing difficulty, slurred speech, pain in legs or groin. Seek emergency treatment immediately.

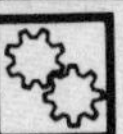

INTERACTION WITH OTHER DRUGS

GENERIC NAME OR DRUG CLASS	COMBINED EFFECT
Anticoagulants (oral)	Decreased anticoagulant effect.
Anticonvulsants (hydantoin)	Increased seizures.
Antidiabetics (oral)	Unpredictable increase or decrease in blood sugar.
Clofibrate	Decreased clofibrate effect.
Carbamazepine	Increased seizures.
Meprobamate	Increased estrone effect.
Phenobarbital	Decreased estrone effect.
Primidone	Decreased estrone effect.
Rifampin	Decreased estrone effect.
Thyroid hormones	Decreased thyroid effect.

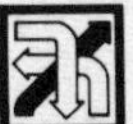

INTERACTION WITH OTHER SUBSTANCES

INTERACTS WITH	COMBINED EFFECT
Alcohol:	None expected.
Beverages:	None expected.
Cocaine:	No proven problems.
Foods:	None expected.
Marijuana:	Possible menstrual irregularities and bleeding between periods.
Tobacco:	Increased risk of blood clots leading to stroke or heart attack.

ESTROPIPATE

BRAND NAMES

Ogen
Piperazine Estrone Sulfate

GENERAL INFORMATION

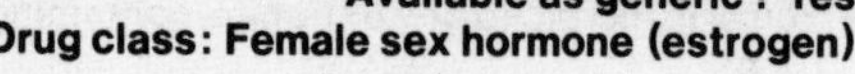

Habit forming? No
Prescription needed? Yes
Available as generic? Yes
Drug class: Female sex hormone (estrogen)

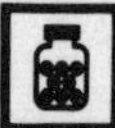

USES

- Treatment for symptoms of menopause and menstrual-cycle irregularity.
- Replacement for female hormone deficiency.

DOSAGE & USAGE INFORMATION

How to take:

- Tablet—Swallow with liquid. If you can't swallow whole, crumble tablet and take with liquid or food.
- Vaginal cream—Use as directed on label.

When to take:
At the same time each day.

If you forget a dose:
Take as soon as you remember up to 12 hours late. If more than 12 hours, wait for next scheduled dose (don't double this dose).

What drug does:
Restores normal estrogen level in tissues.

Time lapse before drug works:
10 to 20 days.

Don't take with:
See Interaction column and consult doctor.

OVERDOSE

Symptoms:
Nausea, vomiting, fluid retention, breast enlargement and discomfort, abnormal vaginal bleeding.

What to do:
Overdose unlikely to threaten life. If person takes much larger amount than prescribed, call doctor, poison-control center or hospital emergency room for instructions.

POSSIBLE ADVERSE REACTIONS OR SIDE EFFECTS

SYMPTOMS	FREQUENCY	WHAT TO DO
Brain & nervous system:		
Depression, dizziness, irritability.	Infrequent	4
Skin:		
• Rash	Infrequent	3
• Brown blotches.	Infrequent	5
• Hair loss.	Infrequent	5
Eyes, ears, nose, throat, heart & lungs, muscles, bones, joints, kidneys, allergic, blood:	None expected.	
Digestive:		
• Stomach or side pain.	Infrequent	3
• Stomach cramps.	Common	3
• Appetite loss.	Common	4
• Nausea, diarrhea.	Common	5
• Vomiting	Infrequent	4
Blood vessels:		
Swollen ankles, feet.	Common	5
Genital, urinary:		
Vaginal discharge or bleeding.	Infrequent	5
Liver:		
Jaundice (yellow skin and eyes).	Rare	3
Others:		
• Breast lumps.	Infrequent	4
• Swollen, tender breasts.	Common	5
• Changes in sex drive.	Infrequent	5

1-Life-threatening. Seek emergency treatment immediately.
2-Discontinue. Seek emergency treatment.
3-Discontinue. Call doctor right away.
4-Continue. Call doctor when convenient.
5-Continue. Tell doctor at next visit.

WARNINGS & PRECAUTIONS

Don't take if:
- You are allergic to any estrogen-containing drugs.
- You have impaired liver function.
- You have had blood clots, stroke or heart attack.
- You have unexplained vaginal bleeding.

Before you start, consult your doctor:
- If you have had cancer of breast or reproductive organs, fibrocystic breast disease, fibroid tumors of the uterus or endometriosis.
- If you have had migraine headaches, epilepsy or porphyria.
- If you have diabetes, high blood pressure, asthma, congestive heart failure, kidney disease or gallstones.
- If you plan to become pregnant within 3 months.

Over age 60:
Controversial. You and your doctor must decide if drug risks outweigh benefits.

Pregnancy:
Risk to unborn child outweighs drug benefits. Don't use.

Breast-feeding:
Drug filters into milk. May harm child. Avoid.

Infants & children:
Not recommended.

Prolonged use:
Increased growth of fibroid tumors of uterus. Possible association with cancer of uterus.

Skin & sunlight:
May cause rash or intensify sunburn in areas exposed to sun or sunlamp.

Driving, piloting or hazardous work:
No problems expected.

Airplane passengers:
No problems expected.

Discontinuing:
You may need to discontinue estropipate periodically. Consult your doctor.

Others:
In rare instances, may cause blood clot in lung, brain or leg. Symptoms are *sudden* severe headache, coordination loss, vision change, chest pain, breathing difficulty, slurred speech, pain in legs or groin. Seek emergency treatment immediately.

INTERACTION WITH OTHER DRUGS

GENERIC NAME OR DRUG CLASS	COMBINED EFFECT
Anticoagulants (oral)	Decreased anticoagulant effect.
Anticonvulsants (hydantoin)	Increased seizures.
Antidiabetics (oral)	Unpredictable increase or decrease in blood sugar.
Clofibrate	Decreased clofibrate effect.
Carbamazepine	Increased seizures.
Meprobamate	Increased estropipate effect.
Phenobarbital	Decreased estropipate effect.
Primidone	Decreased estropipate effect.
Rifampin	Decreased estropipate effect.
Thyroid hormones	Decreased thyroid effect.

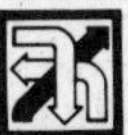

INTERACTION WITH OTHER SUBSTANCES

INTERACTS WITH	COMBINED EFFECT
Alcohol:	None expected.
Beverages:	None expected.
Cocaine:	No proven problems.
Foods:	None expected.
Marijuana:	Possible menstrual irregularities and bleeding between periods.
Tobacco:	Increased risk of blood clots leading to stroke or heart attack.

ETHACRYNIC ACID

BRAND NAMES

Edecrin

GENERAL INFORMATION

Habit forming? No
Prescription needed? Yes
Available as generic? No
Drug class: Diuretic (loop diuretic); antihypertensive

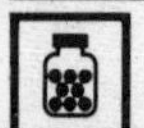

USES

- Lowers blood pressure.
- Decreases fluid retention.

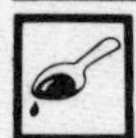

DOSAGE & USAGE INFORMATION

How to take:
Tablet or capsule—Swallow with liquid or food to lessen stomach irritation. If you can't swallow whole, crumble tablet or open capsule and take with liquid or food.

When to take:
- 1 dose a day—Take after breakfast.
- More than 1 dose a day—Take last dose no later than 6 p.m. unless otherwise directed.

If you forget a dose:
- 1 dose a day—Take as soon as you remember up to 12 hours late. If more than 12 hours, wait for next scheduled dose (don't double this dose).
- More than 1 dose a day—Take as soon as you remember up to 2 hours late. If more than 2 hours, wait for next scheduled dose (don't double this dose).

What drug does:
Increases elimination of sodium and water from body. Decreased body fluid reduces blood pressure.

Time lapse before drug works:
1 hour to increase water loss. Requires 2 to 3 weeks to lower blood pressure.

Don't take with:
- Non-prescription drugs with aspirin.
- See Interaction column and consult doctor.

OVERDOSE

Symptoms:
Weakness, lethargy, dizziness, confusion, nausea, vomiting, leg-muscle cramps, thirst, stupor, deep sleep, weak and rapid pulse, cardiac arrest.

What to do:
- Dial 0 (operator) or 911 (emergency) for an ambulance or medical help. Then give first aid immediately.
- Additional emergency information on page 886.

POSSIBLE ADVERSE REACTIONS OR SIDE EFFECTS

SYMPTOMS	FREQUENCY	WHAT TO DO
Brain & nervous system:		
• Dizziness	Common	4
• Mood changes.	Infrequent	3
Skin:		
Rash or hives.	Rare	3
Eyes:		
Yellow vision.	Rare	3
Ears, nose, throat:		
• Ringing in ears, hearing loss.	Rare	3
• Sore throat, fever.	Rare	3
• Dry mouth, thirst.	Rare	3
Digestive:		
• Side or stomach pain, nausea, vomiting.	Rare	3
• Appetite loss, diarrhea.	Infrequent	3
Heart & lungs:		
Irregular heartbeat.	Infrequent	3
Blood vessels:		
Unusual bleeding or bruising.	Rare	3
Muscles, bones, joints:		
• Joint pain.	Rare	3
• Muscle cramps.	Infrequent	3
Genital, urinary, kidneys, allergic, blood:	None expected.	
Liver:		
Jaundice (yellow skin and eyes).	Rare	3
Others:		
Fatigue, weakness.	Infrequent	3

1- Life-threatening. Seek emergency treatment immediately.
2- Discontinue. Seek emergency treatment.
3- Discontinue. Call doctor right away.
4- Continue. Call doctor when convenient.

WARNINGS & PRECAUTIONS

Don't take if:
You are allergic to ethacrynic acid.

Before you start, consult your doctor:
- If you are allergic to any sulfa drug.
- If you have liver or kidney disease.
- If you have gout.
- If you have diabetes.
- If you have impaired hearing.
- If you will have surgery within 2 months, including dental surgery, requiring general or spinal anesthesia.

Over age 60:
Adverse reactions and side effects may be more frequent and severe than in younger persons. Hot weather may cause need to reduce dosage.

Pregnancy:
Risk to unborn child outweighs drug benefits. Don't use.

Breast-feeding:
Drug filters into milk. May harm child. Avoid.

Infants & children:
Use only under medical supervision.

Prolonged use:
- Impaired balance of water, salt and potassium in blood and body tissues.
- Possible diabetes.

Skin & sunlight:
May cause rash or intensify sunburn in areas exposed to sun or sunlamp.

Driving, piloting or hazardous work:
No problems expected.

Airplane passengers:
No problems expected.

Discontinuing:
Don't discontinue without doctor's advice until you complete prescribed dose, even though symptoms diminish or disappear.

Others:
Frequent laboratory studies to monitor potassium level in blood recommended. Eat foods rich in potassium (see page 848) or take potassium supplements. Consult doctor.

INTERACTION WITH OTHER DRUGS

GENERIC NAME OR DRUG CLASS	COMBINED EFFECT
Allopurinol	Decreased allopurinol effect.
Anticoagulants	Abnormal clotting.
Antidepressants (tricyclic)	Excessive blood-pressure drop.
Antidiabetics (oral)	Decreased antidiabetic effect.
Antiinflammatory drugs (non-steroid)	Decreased ethacrynic acid effect.
Antihypertensives	Increased antihypertensive effect.
Barbiturates	Low blood pressure.
Cortisone drugs	Excessive potassium loss.
Digitalis preparations	Serious heart-rhythm disorders.
Insulin	Decreased insulin effect.
Lithium	Increased lithium toxicity.
MAO inhibitors	Increased ethacrynic acid effect.
Narcotics	Dangerous low blood pressure. Avoid.
Phenothiazines	Increased phenothiazine effect.

Additional interactions on page 837.

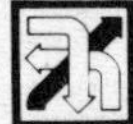

INTERACTION WITH OTHER SUBSTANCES

INTERACTS WITH	COMBINED EFFECT
Alcohol:	Blood-pressure drop. Avoid.
Beverages:	None expected.
Cocaine:	Dangerous blood-pressure drop. Avoid.
Foods:	None expected.
Marijuana:	Increased thirst and urinary frequency, fainting.
Tobacco:	Decreased ethacrynic acid effect.

ETHCHLORVYNOL

BRAND NAMES

Placidyl

GENERAL INFORMATION

Habit forming? Yes
Prescription needed? Yes
Available as generic? No
Drug class: Sleep inducer (hypnotic)

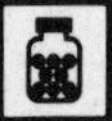

USES

Treatment of insomnia.

DOSAGE & USAGE INFORMATION

How to take:
With food or milk to lessen side effects.

When to take:
At or near bedtime.

If you forget a dose:
Bedtime dose—If you forget your once-a-day bedtime dose, don't take it more than 3 hours late.

What drug does:
Affects brain centers that control waking and sleeping.

Time lapse before drug works:
30 to 60 minutes.

Don't take with:
See Interaction column and consult doctor.

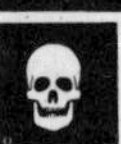

OVERDOSE

Symptoms:
Excitement, delirium, incoordination, excessive drowsiness, deep coma.

What to do:
- Dial 0 (operator) or 911 (emergency) for an ambulance or medical help. Then give first aid immediately.
- If patient is unconscious and not breathing, give mouth-to-mouth breathing. If there is no heartbeat, use cardiac massage and mouth-to-mouth breathing (CPR). Don't try to make patient vomit. If you can't get help quickly, take patient to nearest emergency facility.
- Additional emergency information on page 886.

POSSIBLE ADVERSE REACTIONS OR SIDE EFFECTS

SYMPTOMS	FREQUENCY	WHAT TO DO
Brain & nervous system:		
• Jitters, clumsiness, unsteadiness.	Infrequent	3
• Dizziness	Common	4
• Drowsiness, confusion.	Infrequent	3
Skin:		
Rash, hives.	Infrequent	3
Eyes:		
Blurred vision.	Common	4
Ears, nose, throat:		
Unpleasant taste in mouth.	Common	5
Digestive:		
Indigestion, nausea, vomiting, stomach pain.	Common	3
Heart & lungs:		
Slow heartbeat, breathing difficulty.	Rare	3
Blood vessels:		
Unusual bleeding or bruising.	Infrequent	3
Muscles, bones, joints:	None expected.	
Genital, urinary:	None expected.	
Kidneys:	None expected.	
Liver:		
Jaundice (yellow skin and eyes).	Rare	3
Allergic:	None expected.	
Blood:	None expected.	
Others:		
Fatigue, weakness.	Common	5

1- Life-threatening. Seek emergency treatment immediately.
2- Discontinue. Seek emergency treatment.
3- Discontinue. Call doctor right away.
4- Continue. Call doctor when convenient.
5- Continue. Tell doctor at next visit.

WARNINGS & PRECAUTIONS

Don't take if:
- You are allergic to any hypnotic.
- You have porphyria.
- Patient is younger than 12.

Before you start, consult your doctor:
- If you plan to become pregnant within medication period.
- If you have kidney or liver disease.

Over age 60:
Adverse reactions and side effects, especially a "hangover" effect, may be more frequent and severe than in younger persons.

Pregnancy:
Risk to unborn child outweighs drug benefits. Don't use.

Breast-feeding:
No problems expected, but observe child and ask doctor for guidance.

Infants & children:
Not recommended.

Prolonged use:
Impaired vision.

Skin & sunlight:
No problems expected.

Driving, piloting or hazardous work:
Don't drive or pilot aircraft until you learn how medicine affects you. Don't work around dangerous machinery. Don't climb ladders or work in high places. Danger increases if you drink alcohol or take medicine affecting alertness and reflexes.

Airplane passengers:
No problems expected, except altitude makes "hangover" effect more likely.

Discontinuing:
- Don't discontinue without consulting doctor. Dose may require gradual reduction if you have taken drug for a long time. Doses of other drugs may also require adjustment.
- Many of side effects, plus irritability, muscle twitching, trembling, hallucinations or seizures, may occur when you stop taking this drug. Consult your doctor if so.

Others:
No problems expected.

INTERACTION WITH OTHER DRUGS

GENERIC NAME OR DRUG CLASS	COMBINED EFFECT
Anticoagulants (oral)	Decreased anticoagulant effect.
Antidepressants (tricyclic)	Delirium and deep sedation.
Antihistamines	Increased antihistamine effect.
Narcotics	Increased narcotic effect.
Pain relievers	Increased effect of pain reliever.
Sedatives	Increased sedative effect.
Tranquilizers	Increased tranquilizer effect.

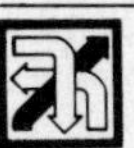

INTERACTION WITH OTHER SUBSTANCES

INTERACTS WITH	COMBINED EFFECT
Alcohol:	Excessive depressant and sedative effect. Avoid.
Beverages:	None expected.
Cocaine:	Decreased ethchlorvynol effect.
Foods:	None expected.
Marijuana:	Occasional use—Drowsiness, unsteadiness, depressed function. Frequent use—Severe drowsiness, impaired physical and mental function.
Tobacco:	None expected.

ETHINYL ESTRADIOL

BRAND NAMES

Brevicon
Demulen
Estinyl
Feminone
Loestrin
Lo-Ovral
Modicon
Norette
Norinyl
Norlestrin
Ortho-Novum
Ovcon
Ovral
Tri-Norinyl

GENERAL INFORMATION

Habit forming? No
Prescription needed? Yes
Available as generic? Yes
Drug class: Female sex hormone (estrogen)

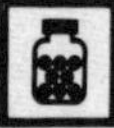

USES

- Treatment for symptoms of menopause and menstrual-cycle irregularity.
- Replacement for female hormone deficiency.
- Prevention of pregnancy.
- Treatment for cancer of breast and prostate.

DOSAGE & USAGE INFORMATION

How to take:

- Tablet—Swallow with liquid. If you can't swallow whole, crumble tablet and take with liquid or food.

When to take:
At the same time each day.

If you forget a dose:
Take as soon as you remember up to 12 hours late. If more than 12 hours, wait for next scheduled dose (don't double this dose).

What drug does:

- Restores normal estrogen level in tissues.
- Prevents pituitary gland from secreting hormone that causes ovary to ripen and release egg.

Time lapse before drug works:
10 to 20 days.

Don't take with:
See Interaction column and consult doctor.

OVERDOSE

Symptoms:
Nausea, vomiting, fluid retention, breast enlargement and discomfort, abnormal vaginal bleeding.

What to do:
Overdose unlikely to threaten life. If person takes much larger amount than prescribed, call doctor, poison-control center or hospital emergency room for instructions.

POSSIBLE ADVERSE REACTIONS OR SIDE EFFECTS

SYMPTOMS	FREQUENCY	WHAT TO DO
Brain & nervous system:		
Depression, dizziness, irritability.	Infrequent	4
Skin:		
• Rash	Infrequent	3
• Brown blotches.	Infrequent	5
• Hair loss.	Infrequent	5
Eyes, ears, nose, throat, heart & lungs, muscles, bones, joints, kidneys, allergic, blood:	None expected.	
Digestive:		
• Stomach or side pain.	Infrequent	3
• Stomach cramps.	Common	3
• Appetite loss.	Common	4
• Nausea, diarrhea.	Common	5
• Vomiting	Infrequent	4
Blood vessels:		
Swollen ankles, feet.	Common	5
Genital, urinary:		
Vaginal discharge or bleeding.	Infrequent	5
Liver:		
Jaundice (yellow skin and eyes).	Rare	3
Others:		
• Breast lumps.	Infrequent	4
• Swollen, tender breasts.	Common	5
• Changes in sex drive.	Infrequent	5

1- Life-threatening. Seek emergency treatment immediately.
2- Discontinue. Seek emergency treatment.
3- Discontinue. Call doctor right away.
4- Continue. Call doctor when convenient.
5- Continue. Tell doctor at next visit.

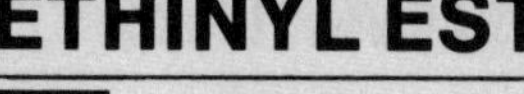

WARNINGS & PRECAUTIONS

Don't take if:
- You are allergic to any estrogen-containing drugs.
- You have impaired liver function.
- You have had blood clots, stroke or heart attack.
- You have unexplained vaginal bleeding.

Before you start, consult your doctor:
- If you have had cancer of breast or reproductive organs, fibrocystic breast disease, fibroid tumors of the uterus or endometriosis.
- If you have had migraine headaches, epilepsy or porphyria.
- If you have diabetes, high blood pressure, asthma, congestive heart failure, kidney disease or gallstones.
- If you plan to become pregnant within 3 months.

Over age 60:
Controversial. You and your doctor must decide if drug risks outweigh benefits.

Pregnancy:
Risk to unborn child outweighs drug benefits. Don't use.

Breast-feeding:
Drug filters into milk. May harm child. Avoid.

Infants & children:
Not recommended.

Prolonged use:
Increased growth of fibroid tumors of uterus. Possible association with cancer of uterus.

Skin & sunlight:
May cause rash or intensify sunburn in areas exposed to sun or sunlamp.

Driving, piloting or hazardous work:
No problems expected.

Airplane passengers:
No problems expected.

Discontinuing:
You may need to discontinue ethinyl estradiol periodically. Consult your doctor.

Others:
In rare instances, may cause blood clot in lung, brain or leg. Symptoms are *sudden* severe headache, coordination loss, vision change, chest pain, breathing difficulty, slurred speech, pain in legs or groin. Seek emergency treatment immediately.

INTERACTION WITH OTHER DRUGS

GENERIC NAME OR DRUG CLASS	COMBINED EFFECT
Anticoagulants (oral)	Decreased anticoagulant effect.
Anticonvulsants (hydantoin)	Increased seizures.
Antidiabetics (oral)	Unpredictable increase or decrease in blood sugar.
Clofibrate	Decreased clofibrate effect.
Carbamazepine	Increased seizures.
Meprobamate	Increased effect of ethinyl estradiol.
Phenobarbital	Decreased effect of ethinyl estradiol.
Primidone	Decreased effect of ethinyl estradiol.
Rifampin	Decreased effect of ethinyl estradiol.
Thyroid hormones	Decreased thyroid effect.

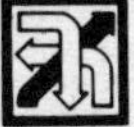

INTERACTION WITH OTHER SUBSTANCES

INTERACTS WITH	COMBINED EFFECT
Alcohol:	None expected.
Beverages:	None expected.
Cocaine:	No proven problems.
Foods:	None expected.
Marijuana:	Possible menstrual irregularities and bleeding between periods.
Tobacco:	Increased risk of blood clots leading to stroke or heart attack.

ETHOPROPAZINE

BRAND NAMES

Parsidol
Parsitan

GENERAL INFORMATION

Habit forming? No
Prescription needed? Yes
Available as generic? No
Drug class: Antidyskinetic, antiparkinsonism

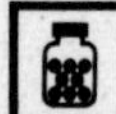

USES

- Treatment of Parkinson's disease.
- Treatment of adverse effects of phenothiazines.

DOSAGE & USAGE INFORMATION

How to take:
Tablets or capsules—Take with food to lessen stomach irritation.

When to take:
At the same times each day.

If you forget a dose:
Take as soon as you remember up to 2 hours late. If more than 2 hours, wait for next scheduled dose (don't double this dose).

What drug does:
- Balances chemical reactions necessary to send nerve impulses within base of brain.
- Improves muscle control and reduces stiffness.

Time lapse before drug works:
1 to 2 hours.

Don't take with:
- Non-prescription drugs for colds, cough or allergy.
- See Interaction column and consult doctor.

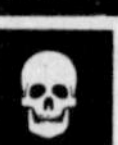

OVERDOSE

Symptoms:
Agitation, dilated pupils, hallucinations, dry mouth, rapid heartbeat, sleepiness.

What to do:
- Dial 0 (operator) or 911 (emergency) for an ambulance or medical help. Then give first aid immediately.
- If patient is unconscious and not breathing, give mouth-to-mouth breathing. If there is no heartbeat, use cardiac massage and mouth-to-mouth breathing (CPR). Don't try to make patient vomit. If you can't get help quickly, take patient to nearest emergency facility.
- Additional emergency information on page 886.

POSSIBLE ADVERSE REACTIONS OR SIDE EFFECTS

SYMPTOMS	FREQUENCY	WHAT TO DO
Brain & nervous system:		
Confusion, dizziness.	Rare	4
Skin:		
Rash	Rare	3
Eyes:		
• Pain	Rare	3
• Blurred vision, light sensitivity.	Common	4
Ears, nose, throat:		
Sore mouth or tongue.	Rare	4
Digestive:		
• Constipation	Common	4
• Nausea, vomiting.	Common	4
Heart & lungs:	None expected.	
Blood vessels:	None expected.	
Muscles, bones, joints:		
• Muscle cramps.	Rare	4
• Numbness, weakness in hands or feet.	Rare	4
Genital, urinary:		
Difficult or painful urination.	Common	5
Kidneys:	None expected.	
Liver:	None expected.	
Allergic:	None expected.	
Blood:	None expected.	
Others:	None expected.	

1 - Life-threatening. Seek emergency treatment immediately.
2 - Discontinue. Seek emergency treatment.
3 - Discontinue. Call doctor right away.
4 - Continue. Call doctor when convenient.
5 - Continue. Tell doctor at next visit.
6 - No action necessary.

WARNINGS & PRECAUTIONS

Don't take if:
You are allergic to any antidyskinetic.

Before you start, consult your doctor:
- If you have had glaucoma.
- If you have had high blood pressure or heart disease.
- If you have had impaired liver function.
- If you have had kidney disease or urination difficulty.

Over age 60:
More sensitive to drug. Aggravates symptoms of enlarged prostate. Causes impaired thinking, hallucinations, nightmares. Consult doctor about any of these.

Pregnancy:
Studies inconclusive on harm to unborn child. Animal studies show fetal abnormalities. Decide with your doctor whether drug benefits justify risk to unborn child.

Breast-feeding:
No problems expected.

Infants & children:
Not recommended for children 3 and younger. Use for older children only under doctor's supervision.

Prolonged use:
Possible glaucoma.

Skin & sunlight:
No problems expected.

Driving, piloting or hazardous work:
Don't drive or pilot aircraft until you learn how medicine affects you. Don't work around dangerous machinery. Don't climb ladders or work in high places. Danger increases if you drink alcohol or take medicine affecting alertness and reflexes, such as antihistamines, tranquilizers, sedatives, pain medicine, narcotics and mind-altering drugs.

Airplane passengers:
No problems expected.

Discontinuing:
Don't discontinue without consulting doctor. Dose may require gradual reduction if you have taken drug for a long time. Doses of other drugs may also require adjustment.

Others:
- Internal eye pressure should be measured regularly.
- Avoid becoming overheated.

INTERACTION WITH OTHER DRUGS

GENERIC NAME OR DRUG CLASS	COMBINED EFFECT
Amantadine	Increased amantadine effect.
Antidepressants (tricyclic)	Increased ethopropazine effect. May cause glaucoma.
Antihistamines	Increased ethopropazine effect.
Levodopa	Increased levodopa effect. Improved results in treating Parkinson's disease.
Meperidine	Increased ethopropazine effect.
MAO inhibitors	Increased ethopropazine effect.
Orphenadrine	Increased ethopropazine effect.
Phenothiazines	Behavior changes.
Primidone	Excessive sedation.
Procainamide	Increased procainamide effect.
Quinidine	Increased ethopropazine effect.
Tranquilizers	Excessive sedation.

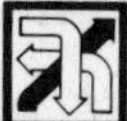

INTERACTION WITH OTHER SUBSTANCES

INTERACTS WITH	COMBINED EFFECT
Alcohol:	None expected.
Beverages:	None expected.
Cocaine:	Decreased ethopropazine effect. Avoid.
Foods:	None expected.
Marijuana:	None expected.
Tobacco:	None expected.

ETHOSUXIMIDE

BRAND NAMES

Zarontin

GENERAL INFORMATION

Habit forming? No
Prescription needed? Yes
Available as generic? No
Drug class: Anticonvulsant (succinimide)

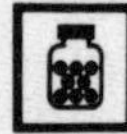

USES

Controls seizures in treatment of epilepsy.

DOSAGE & USAGE INFORMATION

How to take:
Capsule—Swallow with liquid or food to lessen stomach irritation.

When to take:
Every day in regularly-spaced doses, according to prescription.

If you forget a dose:
Take as soon as you remember up to 2 hours late. If more than 2 hours, wait for next scheduled dose (don't double this dose).

What drug does:
Depresses nerve transmissions in part of brain that controls muscles.

Time lapse before drug works:
3 hours.

Don't take with:
See Interaction column and consult doctor.

OVERDOSE

Symptoms:
Coma

What to do:
- Dial 0 (operator) or 911 (emergency) for an ambulance or medical help. Then give first aid immediately.
- If patient is unconscious and not breathing, give mouth-to-mouth breathing. If there is no heartbeat, use cardiac massage and mouth-to-mouth breathing (CPR). Don't try to make patient vomit. If you can't get help quickly, take patient to nearest emergency facility.
- Additional emergency information on page 886.

POSSIBLE ADVERSE REACTIONS OR SIDE EFFECTS

SYMPTOMS	FREQUENCY	WHAT TO DO
Brain & nervous system:		
Dizziness, drowsiness, headache, irritability, mood changes.	Infrequent	4
Skin:		
Rash	Rare	3
Eyes:	None expected.	
Ears, nose, throat:		
Sore throat, fever.	Rare	3
Digestive:		
Nausea, vomiting, stomach cramps, appetite loss.	Common	4
Heart & lungs:	None expected.	
Blood vessels:	None expected.	
Muscles, bones, joints:	None expected.	
Genital, urinary:	None expected.	
Kidneys:	None expected.	
Liver:	None expected.	
Allergic:	None expected.	
Blood:		
Unusual bleeding or bruising.	Rare	3
Others:		
Swollen lymph glands.	Rare	4

1- Life-threatening. Seek emergency treatment immediately.
2- Discontinue. Seek emergency treatment.
3- Discontinue. Call doctor right away.
4- Continue. Call doctor when convenient.
5- Continue. Tell doctor at next visit.
6- No action necessary.

WARNINGS & PRECAUTIONS

Don't take if:
You are allergic to any succinimide anticonvulsant.

Before you start, consult your doctor:
- If you plan to become pregnant within medication period.
- If you take other anticonvulsants.
- If you have blood disease.
- If you have kidney or liver disease.

Over age 60:
Adverse reactions and side effects may be more frequent and severe than in younger persons.

Pregnancy:
Risk to unborn child outweighs drug benefits. Don't use.

Breast-feeding:
Drug passes into milk. Avoid drug or discontinue nursing.

Infants & children:
Use only under medical supervision.

Prolonged use:
No problems expected.

Skin & sunlight:
No problems expected.

Driving, piloting or hazardous work:
Don't drive or pilot aircraft until you learn how medicine affects you. Don't work around dangerous machinery. Don't climb ladders or work in high places. Danger increases if you drink alcohol or take medicine affecting alertness and reflexes, such as antihistamines, tranquilizers, sedatives, pain medicine, narcotics and mind-altering drugs.

Airplane passengers:
No problems expected.

Discontinuing:
Don't discontinue without doctor's advice until you complete prescribed dose, even though symptoms diminish or disappear.

Others:
- Your response to medicine should be checked regularly by your doctor. Dose and schedule may have to be altered frequently to fit individual needs.
- Periodic blood-cell counts, kidney- and liver-function studies recommended.

INTERACTION WITH OTHER DRUGS

GENERIC NAME OR DRUG CLASS	COMBINED EFFECT
Anticonvulsants (other)	Increased effect of both drugs.
Antidepressants (tricyclic)	May provoke seizures.
Antipsychotics	May provoke seizures.

INTERACTION WITH OTHER SUBSTANCES

INTERACTS WITH	COMBINED EFFECT
Alcohol:	May provoke seizures.
Beverages:	None expected.
Cocaine:	May provoke seizures.
Foods:	None expected.
Marijuana:	May provoke seizures.
Tobacco:	None expected.

ETHOTOIN

BRAND NAMES

Peganone

GENERAL INFORMATION

Habit forming? No
Prescription needed? Yes
Available as generic? Yes
Drug class: Anticonvulsant (hydantoin)

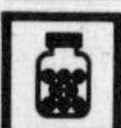

USES

- Prevents epileptic seizures.
- Stabilizes irregular heartbeat.

DOSAGE & USAGE INFORMATION

How to take:
- Tablet or capsule—Swallow with liquid.
- Extended-release tablets or capsules—Swallow each dose whole. If you take regular tablets, you may chew or crush them.

When to take:
At the same time each day.

If you forget a dose:
- If drug taken 1 time per day—Take as soon as you remember up to 12 hours late. If more than 12 hours, wait for next scheduled dose (don't double this dose).
- If taken several times per day—Take as soon as possible, then return to regular schedule.

What drug does:
Promotes sodium loss from nerve fibers. This lessens excitability and inhibits spread of nerve impulses.

Time lapse before drug works:
7 to 10 days continual use.

Don't take with:
See Interaction column and consult doctor.

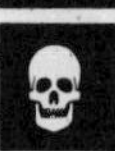

OVERDOSE

Symptoms:
Jerky eye movements; stagger; slurred speech; imbalance; drowsiness; blood-pressure drop; slow, shallow breathing; coma.

What to do:
- Dial 0 (operator) or 911 (emergency) for an ambulance or medical help. Then give first aid immediately.
- Additional emergency information on page 886.

POSSIBLE ADVERSE REACTIONS OR SIDE EFFECTS

SYMPTOMS	FREQUENCY	WHAT TO DO
Brain & nervous system:		
• Mild dizziness, drowsiness.	Common	4
• Headache, sleeplessness.	Infrequent	4
• Hallucinations, confusion, slurred speech, stagger.	Infrequent	3
Skin:		
Rash	Infrequent	3
Eyes:		
Vision changes.	Infrequent	3
Ears, nose, throat:		
Sore throat, fever.	Rare	3
Digestive:		
• Stomach pain.	Rare	3
• Constipation, nausea, vomiting.	Common	4
• Diarrhea	Infrequent	4
Heart & lungs, genital, urinary, kidneys, allergic blood:	None expected.	
Blood vessels:		
Unusual bleeding or bruising.	Rare	3
Muscles, bones, joints:		
Muscle twitching.	Infrequent	4
Liver:		
Jaundice (yellow skin and eyes).	Rare	3
Others:		
Increased body and facial hair.	Infrequent	5

1- Life-threatening. Seek emergency treatment immediately.
2- Discontinue. Seek emergency treatment.
3- Discontinue. Call doctor right away.
4- Continue. Call doctor when convenient.
5- Continue. Tell doctor at next visit.

WARNINGS & PRECAUTIONS

Don't take if:
You are allergic to any hydantoin anticonvulsant.

Before you start, consult your doctor:
- If you have had impaired liver function or disease.
- If you will have surgery within 2 months, including dental surgery, requiring general or spinal anesthesia.

Over age 60:
Adverse reactions and side effects may be more frequent and severe than in younger persons.

Pregnancy:
Risk to unborn child outweighs drug benefits. Don't use.

Breast-feeding:
Drug passes into milk. Avoid drug or discontinue nursing until you finish medicine. Consult doctor for advice on maintaining milk supply.

Infants & children:
Use only under medical supervision.

Prolonged use:
- Weakened bones.
- Lymph gland enlargement.
- Possible liver damage.
- Numbness and tingling of hands and feet.
- Continual back-and-forth eye movements.
- Bleeding, swollen or tender gums.

Skin & sunlight:
May cause rash or intensify sunburn in areas exposed to sun or sunlamp.

Driving, piloting or hazardous work:
Don't drive or pilot aircraft until you learn how medicine affects you. Don't work around dangerous machinery. Don't climb ladders or work in high places. Danger increases if you drink alcohol or take medicine affecting alertness and reflexes.

Airplane passengers:
No problems expected.

Discontinuing:
Don't discontinue without consulting doctor. Dose may require gradual reduction if you have taken drug for a long time. Doses of other drugs may also require adjustment.

INTERACTION WITH OTHER DRUGS

GENERIC NAME OR DRUG CLASS	COMBINED EFFECT
Anticoagulants	Increased effect of both drugs.
Antidepressants (tricyclic)	Need to adjust ethotoin dose.
Antihypertensives	Increased effect of antihypertensive.
Aspirin	Increased ethotoin effect.
Barbiturates	Changed seizure pattern.
Carbonic anhydrase inhibitors	Increased chance of bone disease.
Chloramphenicol	Increased ethotoin effect.
Contraceptives (oral)	Increased seizures.
Cortisone drugs	Decreased cortisone effect.
Digitalis preparations	Decreased digitalis effect.
Disulfiram	Increased ethotoin effect.
Estrogens	Increased ethotoin effect.
Furosemide	Decreased furosemide effect.
Glutethimide	Decreased ethotoin effect.

Additional interactions on page 837.

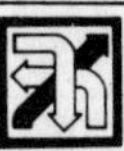

INTERACTION WITH OTHER SUBSTANCES

INTERACTS WITH	COMBINED EFFECT
Alcohol:	Possible decreased anticonvulsant effect. Use with caution.
Beverages:	None expected.
Cocaine:	Possible seizures.
Foods:	None expected.
Marijuana:	Drowsiness, unsteadiness, decreased anti-convulsant effect.
Tobacco:	None expected.

FENOPROFEN

BRAND NAMES

Nalfon

Habit forming? No
Prescription needed? Yes

GENERAL INFORMATION

Available as generic? No
Drug class: Antiinflammatory (non-steroid)

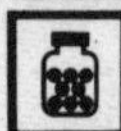

USES

- Treatment for joint pain, stiffness, inflammation and swelling of arthritis and gout.
- Pain reliever.
- Treatment for dysmenorrhea (painful or difficult menstruation).

DOSAGE & USAGE INFORMATION

How to take:
Tablet or capsule—Swallow with liquid or food to lessen stomach irritation. If you can't swallow whole, crumble tablet or open capsule and take with liquid or food.

When to take:
At the same times each day.

If you forget a dose:
Take as soon as you remember up to 2 hours late. If more than 2 hours, wait for next scheduled dose (don't double this dose).

What drug does:
Reduces tissue concentration of prostaglandins (hormones which produce inflammation and pain).

Time lapse before drug works:
Begins in 4 to 24 hours. May require 3 weeks regular use for maximum benefit.

Don't take with:
See Interaction column and consult doctor.

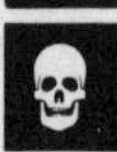

OVERDOSE

Symptoms:
Confusion, agitation, incoherence, convulsions, possible hemorrhage from stomach or intestine, coma.

What to do:
- Dial 0 (operator) or 911 (emergency) for an ambulance or medical help. Then give first aid immediately.
- Additional emergency information on page 886.

POSSIBLE ADVERSE REACTIONS OR SIDE EFFECTS

SYMPTOMS	FREQUENCY	WHAT TO DO
Brain & nervous system:		
• Depression, drowsiness.	Infrequent	4
• Convulsions, confusion.	Rare	3
• Dizziness	Common	4
• Headache	Common	5
Skin:		
Rash, hives or itch.	Rare	3
Eyes:		
Blurred vision.	Rare	3
Ears, nose, throat:		
Ringing in ears.	Infrequent	4
Digestive:		
• Bloody or black, tarry stools.	Rare	3
• Nausea, pain.	Common	4
• Constipation or diarrhea, vomiting.	Infrequent	4
Heart & lungs:		
Breathing difficulty, tightness in chest, rapid heartbeat.	Rare	3
Blood vessels:		
Unusual bleeding or bruising.	Rare	3
Muscles, bones, joints:		
Swollen feet, legs.	Infrequent	4
Genital, urinary:		
• Bloody urine.	Rare	3
• Difficult, painful or frequent urination.	Rare	4
Kidneys, allergic, blood:	None expected.	
Liver:		
Jaundice (yellow skin and eyes).	Rare	3
Others:		
Fatigue, weakness.	Rare	4

1 - Life-threatening. Seek emergency treatment immediately.
2 - Discontinue. Seek emergency treatment.
3 - Discontinue. Call doctor right away.
4 - Continue. Call doctor when convenient.
5 - Continue. Tell doctor at next visit.

WARNINGS & PRECAUTIONS

Don't take if:
- You are allergic to aspirin or any non-steroid, antiinflammatory drug.
- You have gastritis, peptic ulcer, enteritis, ileitis, ulcerative colitis, asthma, heart faiiure, high blood pressure or bleeding problems.
- Patient is younger than 15.

Before you start, consult your doctor:
- If you have epilepsy.
- If you have Parkinson's disease.
- If you have been mentally ill.
- If you have had kidney disease or impaired kidney function.

Over age 60:
Adverse reactions and side effects may be more frequent and severe than in younger persons.

Pregnancy:
Studies inconclusive on harm to unborn child. Decide with your doctor whether drug benefits justify risk to unborn child.

Breast-feeding:
May harm child. Avoid.

Infants & children:
Not recommended for anyone younger than 15. Use only under medical supervision.

Prolonged use:
- Eye damage.
- Reduced hearing.
- Sore throat, fever.
- Weight gain.

Skin & sunlight:
No problems expected.

Driving, piloting or hazardous work:
Don't drive or pilot aircraft until you learn how medicine affects you. Don't work around dangerous machinery. Don't climb ladders or work in high places. Danger increases if you drink alcohol or take medicine affecting alertness and reflexes, such as antihistamines, tranquilizers, sedatives, pain medicine, narcotics and mind-altering drugs.

Airplane passengers:
No problems expected.

Discontinuing:
Don't discontinue without consulting doctor. Dose may require gradual reduction if you have taken drug for a long time. Doses of other drugs may also require adjustment.

Others:
No problems expected.

INTERACTION WITH OTHER DRUGS

GENERIC NAME OR DRUG CLASS	COMBINED EFFECT
Anticoagulants (oral)	Increased risk of bleeding.
Aspirin	Increased risk of stomach ulcer.
Cortisone drugs	Increased risk of stomach ulcer.
Furosemide	Decreased diuretic effect of furosemide.
Oxyphenbutazone	Possible stomach ulcer.
Phenylbutazone	Possible stomach ulcer.
Probenecid	Increased fenoprofen effect.
Thyroid hormones	Rapid heartbeat, blood-pressure rise.

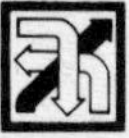

INTERACTION WITH OTHER SUBSTANCES

INTERACTS WITH	COMBINED EFFECT
Alcohol:	Possible stomach ulcer or bleeding.
Beverages:	None expected.
Cocaine:	None expected.
Foods:	None expected.
Marijuana:	Increased pain relief from fenoprofen.
Tobacco:	None expected.

FERROUS FUMARATE

BRAND NAMES

Feco-T	Fumasorb	Toleron
Femiron	Fumerin	Tolfrinic
Feostat	Ircon	Tolifer
Ferrofume	Laud-Iron	Vitron C
Ferro-sequels)	Maniron	
Fersamal	Palafer	

See complete brand names list, page 826.

GENERAL INFORMATION

Habit forming? No
Prescription needed? With folic acid: Yes
Without folic acid: No
Available as generic? Yes
Drug class: Mineral supplement (iron)

USES

Treatment for dietary iron deficiency or iron-deficiency anemia from other causes.

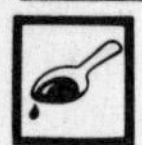

DOSAGE & USAGE INFORMATION

How to take:
- Tablet, capsule or liquid—Swallow with liquid or food to lessen stomach irritation. If you can't swallow whole, crumble tablet or open capsule and take with liquid or food. Place medicine far back on tongue to avoid staining teeth.
- Drops—Dilute dose in beverage before swallowing and drink through a straw.

When to take:
1 hour before or 2 hours after meals.

If you forget a dose:
Take up to 2 hours late. If more than 2 hours, wait for next dose (don't double this).

What drug does:
Stimulates bone-marrow production of hemoglobin (red-blood-cell pigment that carries oxygen to body cells).

Time lapse before drug works:
3 to 7 days. May require 3 weeks for maximum benefit.

Don't take with:
- Multiple vitamin and mineral supplements.
- See Interaction column and consult doctor.

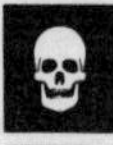

OVERDOSE

Symptoms:
Weakness, collapse; pallor, blue lips, hands and fingernails; weak, rapid heartbeat; shallow breathing; convulsions; coma.

What to do:
- Dial 0 (operator) or 911 (emergency) for an ambulance or medical help. Then give first aid immediately.
- Additional emergency information on page 886.

POSSIBLE ADVERSE REACTIONS OR SIDE EFFECTS

SYMPTOMS	FREQUENCY	WHAT TO DO
Brain & nervous system:		
Drowsiness	Rare	4
Skin, eyes, blood vessels, muscles, bones, joints, kidneys, liver, allergic, blood:	None expected.	
Ears, nose, throat:		
Throat or chest pain on swallowing.	Rare	3
Digestive:		
• Gray or black stool.	Always	6
• Constipation or diarrhea, heartburn, nausea, vomiting.	Infrequent	3
• Pain, cramps, blood in stool.	Rare	3
Heart & lungs:		
Weak, rapid heartbeat.	Rare	1
Genital, urinary:		
Dark urine.	Infrequent	5
Others:		
• Stained teeth with liquid iron.	Common	6
• Fatigue, weakness.	Infrequent	4

1-Life-threatening. Seek emergency treatment immediately.
2-Discontinue. Seek emergency treatment.
3-Discontinue. Call doctor right away.
4-Continue. Call doctor when convenient.
5-Continue. Tell doctor at next visit.
6-No action necessary.

WARNINGS & PRECAUTIONS

Don't take if:
- You are allergic to any iron supplement.
- You take iron injections.
- Your daily iron intake is high.
- You plan to take this supplement for a long time.
- You have acute hepatitis.
- You have hemosiderosis or hemochromatosis (conditions involving excess iron in body).
- You have hemolytic anemia.

Before you start, consult your doctor:
- If you plan to become pregnant within medication period.
- If you have had stomach surgery.
- If you have had peptic ulcer disease, enteritis or colitis.
- If you have had pancreatitis or hepatitis.

Over age 60:
May cause hemochromatosis (iron storage disease) with bronze skin, liver damage, diabetes, heart problems and impotence.

Pregnancy:
No proven harm to unborn child. Avoid if possible. Take only if your doctor prescribes supplement during last half of pregnancy.

Breast-feeding:
No problems expected. Take only if your doctor confirms you have a dietary deficiency or an iron-deficiency anemia.

Infants & children:
Use only under medical supervision. Overdose common and dangerous. Keep out of children's reach.

Prolonged use:
May cause hemochromatosis (iron storage disease) with bronze skin, liver damage, diabetes, heart problems and impotence.

Skin & sunlight:
No problems expected.

Driving, piloting or hazardous work:
No problems expected.

Airplane passengers:
No problems expected.

Discontinuing:
May be unnecessary to finish medicine. Follow doctor's instructions.

Others:
Liquid form stains teeth. Mix with water or juice to lessen the effect. Brush with baking soda or hydrogen peroxide to help remove stain.

INTERACTION WITH OTHER DRUGS

GENERIC NAME OR DRUG CLASS	COMBINED EFFECT
Allopurinol	Possible excess iron storage in liver.
Antacids	Poor iron absorption.
Chloramphenicol	Decreased effect of iron. Interferes with red-blood-cell and hemoglobin formation.
Cholestyramine	Decreased iron effect.
Iron supplements (other)	Possible excess iron storage in liver.
Penicillamine	Decreased penicillamine effect.
Sulfasalazine	Decreased iron effect.
Tetracyclines	Decreased tetracycline effect. Take iron 3 hours before or 2 hours after taking tetracycline.
Vitamin C	Increased iron effect. Contributes to red-blood-cell and hemoglobin formation.
Vitamin E	Decreased iron effect.

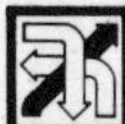

INTERACTION WITH OTHER SUBSTANCES

INTERACTS WITH	COMBINED EFFECT
Alcohol:	Increased iron absorption. May cause organ damage. Avoid or use in moderation.
Beverages: Milk, tea	Decreased iron effect.
Cocaine:	None expected.
Foods: Dairy foods, eggs, whole-grain bread and cereal.	Decreased iron effect.
Marijuana:	None expected.
Tobacco:	None expected.

FERROUS GLUCONATE

BRAND NAMES

Apo-Ferrous Gluconate
Fergon
Ferralet
Ferralet Plus
Ferrous-G
Fertinic
Fosfree
Glytinic
I.L.X. B-12
Iromin-G
Megadose
Mission
Novoferrogluc

GENERAL INFORMATION

Habit forming? No
Prescription needed?
With folic acid—Yes
Without folic acid—No
Available as generic? Yes
Drug class: Mineral supplement (iron)

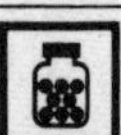

USES

Treatment for dietary iron deficiency or iron-deficiency anemia from other causes.

DOSAGE & USAGE INFORMATION

How to take:
- Tablet or capsule—Swallow with liquid or food to lessen stomach irritation. If you can't swallow whole, crumble tablet or open capsule and take with liquid or food. Place medicine far back on tongue to avoid staining teeth.
- Drops—Dilute dose in beverage before swallowing and drink through a straw.

When to take:
1 hour before or 2 hours after eating.

If you forget a dose:
Take up to 2 hours late. If more than 2 hours, wait for next dose (don't double this).

What drug does:
Stimulates bone-marrow production of hemoglobin (red-blood-cell pigment that carries oxygen to body cells).

Time lapse before drug works:
3 to 7 days. May require 3 weeks for maximum benefit.

Don't take with:
- Multiple vitamin and mineral supplements.
- See Interaction column and consult doctor.

OVERDOSE

Symptoms:
- Moderate overdose—Stomach pain, vomiting, diarrhea, black stools, lethargy.
- Serious overdose—Weakness and collapse; pallor, weak and rapid heartbeat; shallow breathing; convulsions and coma.

What to do:
- Dial 0 (operator) or 911 (emergency) for an ambulance or medical help. Then give first aid immediately.
- Additional emergency information on page 886.

POSSIBLE ADVERSE REACTIONS OR SIDE EFFECTS

SYMPTOMS	FREQUENCY	WHAT TO DO
Brain & nervous system:		
Drowsiness	Rare	4
Skin:		
Blue lips, fingernails, palms of hands; pale, clammy skin.	Rare	2
Ears, nose, throat:		
• Stained teeth with liquid iron.	Common	6
• Throat pain on swallowing.	Rare	3
Digestive:		
• Gray or black stool.	Always	6
• Constipation or diarrhea, heartburn, nausea, vomiting.	Infrequent	3
• Pain, cramps, blood in stool.	Rare	3
Heart & lungs:		
Weak, rapid heartbeat.	Rare	1
Eyes, blood vessels, muscles, bones, joints, genital, urinary, kidneys, liver, allergic, blood:	None expected.	
Others:		
Fatigue, weakness.	Infrequent	4

1- Life-threatening. Seek emergency treatment immediately.
2- Discontinue. Seek emergency treatment.
3- Discontinue. Call doctor right away.
4- Continue. Call doctor when convenient.
5- Continue. Tell doctor at next visit.
6- No action necessary.

WARNINGS & PRECAUTIONS

Don't take if:

- You are allergic to any iron supplement.
- You take iron injections.
- You have acute hepatitis, hemosiderosis or hemochromatosis (conditions involving excess iron in body).
- You have hemolytic anemia.

Before you start, consult your doctor:

- If you plan to become pregnant within medication period.
- If you have had stomach surgery.
- If you have had peptic ulcer, enteritis or colitis.

Over age 60:
May cause hemochromatosis (iron storage disease) with bronze skin, liver damage, diabetes, heart problems and impotence.

Pregnancy:
No proven harm to unborn child. Avoid if possible. Take only if your doctor advises supplement during last half of pregnancy.

Breast-feeding:
No problems expected. Take only if your doctor confirms you have a dietary deficiency or an iron-deficiency anemia.

Infants & children:
Use only under medical supervision. Overdose common and dangerous. Keep out of children's reach.

Prolonged use:
May cause hemochromatosis (iron storage disease) with bronze skin, liver damage, diabetes, heart problems and impotence.

Skin & sunlight:
No problems expected.

Driving, piloting or hazardous work:
No problems expected.

Airplane passengers:
No problems expected.

Discontinuing:
May be unnecessary to finish medicine. Follow doctor's instructions.

Others:
Liquid form stains teeth. Mix with water or juice to lessen the effect. Brush with baking soda or hydrogen peroxide to help remove.

INTERACTION WITH OTHER DRUGS

GENERIC NAME OR DRUG CLASS	COMBINED EFFECT
Allopurinol	Possible excess iron storage in liver.
Antacids	Poor iron absorption.
Chloramphenicol	Decreased effect of iron. Interferes with red-blood-cell and hemoglobin formation.
Cholestyramine	Decreased iron effect.
Iron supplements (other)	Possible excess iron storage in liver.
Sulfasalazine	Decreased iron effect.
Tetracyclines	Decreased tetracycline effect. Take iron 3 hours before or 2 hours after taking tetracycline.
Vitamin C	Increased iron effect. Contributes to red-blood-cell and hemoglobin formation.
Vitamin E	Decreased iron effect.

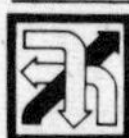

INTERACTION WITH OTHER SUBSTANCES

INTERACTS WITH	COMBINED EFFECT
Alcohol:	Increased iron absorption. May cause organ damage. Avoid or use in moderation.
Beverages: Milk, tea	Decreased iron effect.
Cocaine:	None expected.
Foods: Dairy foods, eggs, whole-grain bread and cereal	Decreased iron effect.
Marijuana:	None expected.
Tobacco:	None expected.

FERROUS SULFATE

BRAND NAMES

Feosol
Fer-In-Sol
Fero-folic-500
Fero-Grad-500
Fero-Gradumet
Ferralyn
Fesofor
Geritol Tablets
Iberet
Iberet-500
Iberet-Folic-500
Mol-Iron
Novoferrosulfa
Slow-Fe

GENERAL INFORMATION

Habit forming? No
Prescription needed?
With folic acid: Yes
Without folic acid: No
Available as generic? Yes
Drug class: Mineral supplement (iron)

USES

Treatment for dietary iron deficiency or iron-deficiency anemia from other causes.

DOSAGE & USAGE INFORMATION

How to take:
- Tablet, capsule, or liquid—Swallow with liquid or food to lessen stomach irritation. Place medicine far back on tongue to avoid staining teeth.
- Drops—Dilute dose in beverage before swallowing and drink through a straw.
- Extended release tablet or capsule—Swallow whole with liquid.

When to take:
1 hour before or 2 hours after meals.

If you forget a dose:
Take up to 2 hours late. If more than 2 hours, wait for next dose (don't double this).

What drug does:
Stimulates bone-marrow production of hemoglobin (red-blood-cell pigment that carries oxygen to body cells).

Time lapse before drug works:
3 to 7 days. May require 3 weeks for maximum benefit.

Don't take with:
- Multiple vitamin and mineral supplements.
- See Interaction column and consult doctor.

OVERDOSE

Symptoms:
Weakness, collapse; pallor, blue lips, hands and fingernails; weak, rapid heartbeat; shallow breathing; convulsions; coma.

What to do:
- Dial 0 (operator) or 911 (emergency) for an ambulance or medical help. Then give first aid immediately.
- Additional information on page 886.

POSSIBLE ADVERSE REACTIONS OR SIDE EFFECTS

SYMPTOMS	FREQUENCY	WHAT TO DO
Brain & nervous system:		
Drowsiness	Rare	4
Skin, eyes, blood vessels, muscles, bones, joints, kidneys, liver, allergic, blood:	None expected.	
Ears, nose, throat:		
Throat or chest pain on swallowing.	Rare	3
Digestive:		
• Gray or black stool.	Always	6
• Constipation or diarrhea, heartburn, nausea, vomiting.	Infrequent	3
• Pain, cramps, blood in stool.	Rare	3
Heart & lungs:		
Weak, rapid heartbeat.	Rare	1
Genital, urinary:		
Dark urine.	Infrequent	5
Others:		
• Stained teeth with liquid iron.	Common	6
• Fatigue, weakness.	Infrequent	4

1-Life-threatening. Seek emergency treatment immediately.
2-Discontinue. Seek emergency treatment.
3-Discontinue. Call doctor right away.
4-Continue. Call doctor when convenient.
5-Continue. Tell doctor at next visit.
6-No action necessary.

WARNINGS & PRECAUTIONS

Don't take if:

- You are allergic to any iron supplement.
- You take iron injections.
- Your daily iron intake is high.
- You plan to take this supplement for a long time.
- You have acute hepatitis.
- You have hemosiderosis or hemochromatosis (conditions involving excess iron in body).
- You have hemolytic anemia.

Before you start, consult your doctor:

- If you plan to become pregnant within medication period.
- If you have had stomach surgery.
- If you have had peptic ulcer disease, enteritis or colitis.
- If you have had pancreatitis or hepatitis.

Over age 60:
May cause hemochromatosis (iron storage disease) with bronze skin, liver damage, diabetes, heart problems and impotence.

Pregnancy:
No proven harm to unborn child. Avoid if possible. Take only if your doctor prescribes supplement during last half of pregnancy.

Breast-feeding:
No problems expected. Take only if your doctor confirms you have a dietary deficiency or an iron-deficiency anemia.

Infants & children:
Use only under medical supervision. Overdose common and dangerous. Keep out of children's reach.

Prolonged use:
May cause hemochromatosis (iron storage disease) with bronze skin, liver damage, diabetes, heart problems and impotence.

Skin & sunlight:
No problems expected.

Driving, piloting or hazardous work:
No problems expected.

Airplane passengers:
No problems expected.

Discontinuing:
May be unnecessary to finish medicine. Follow doctor's instructions.

Others:
Liquid form stains teeth. Mix with water or juice to lessen the effect. Brush with baking soda or hydrogen peroxide to help remove stain.

INTERACTION WITH OTHER DRUGS

GENERIC NAME OR DRUG CLASS	COMBINED EFFECT
Allopurinol	Possible excess iron storage in liver.
Antacids	Poor iron absorption.
Chloramphenicol	Decreased effect of iron. Interferes with red-blood-cell and hemoglobin formation.
Cholestyramine	Decreased iron effect.
Iron supplements (other)	Possible excess iron storage in liver.
Penicillamine	Decreased penicillamine effect.
Sulfasalazine	Decreased iron effect.
Tetracyclines	Decreased tetracycline effect. Take iron 3 hours before or 2 hours after taking tetracycline.
Vitamin C	Increased iron effect. Contributes to red-blood-cell and hemoglobin formation.
Vitamin E	Decreased iron effect.

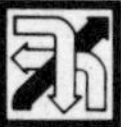

INTERACTION WITH OTHER SUBSTANCES

INTERACTS WITH	COMBINED EFFECT
Alcohol:	Increased iron absorption. May cause organ damage. Avoid or use in moderation.
Beverages: Milk, tea	Decreased iron effect.
Cocaine:	None expected.
Foods: Dairy foods, eggs, whole-grain bread and cereal.	Decreased iron effect.
Marijuana:	None expected.
Tobacco:	None expected.

FLAVOXATE

BRAND NAMES

Urispas

GENERAL INFORMATION

Habit forming? No
Prescription needed? Yes
Available as generic? No
Drug class: Smooth-muscle relaxant, anticholinergic

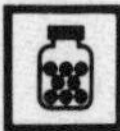

USES

Relieves urinary pain, urgency, nighttime urination, unusual frequency of urination associated with urinary system disorders.

DOSAGE & USAGE INFORMATION

How to take:
Tablet or capsule—Swallow with liquid or food to lessen stomach irritation.

When to take:
30 minutes before meals (unless directed otherwise by doctor).

If you forget a dose:
Take as soon as you remember up to 2 hours late. If more than 2 hours, wait for next scheduled dose (don't double this dose).

What drug does:
Blocks nerve impulses at smooth muscle nerve endings, preventing muscle contractions and gland secretions of organs involved.

Time lapse before drug works:
15 to 30 minutes.

Don't take with:
See Interaction column and consult doctor.

OVERDOSE

Symptoms:
Dilated pupils, rapid pulse and breathing, dizziness, fever, hallucinations, confusion, slurred speech, agitation, flushed face, convulsions, coma.

What to do:
- Dial 0 (operator) or 911 (emergency) for an ambulance or medical help. Then give first aid immediately.
- Additional emergency information on page 886.

POSSIBLE ADVERSE REACTIONS OR SIDE EFFECTS

SYMPTOMS	FREQUENCY	WHAT TO DO
Brain & nervous system:		
• Unusual excitement, irritability, restlessness.	Infrequent	3
• Headache	Infrequent	4
• Confusion, delirium.	Common	3
Skin:		
Rash or hives.	Rare	3
Eyes:		
• Pain, blurred vision.	Rare	3
• Increased sensitivity to light.	Infrequent	4
Ears, nose, throat:		
• Dryness	Common	6
• Sore throat, fever, mouth sores.	Rare	3
Digestive:		
• Constipation	Common	5
• Nausea, vomiting.	Common	4
Heart & lungs:		
• Rapid heartbeat.	Common	3
• Shortness of breath.	Rare	2
Blood vessels:	None expected.	
Muscles, bones, joints:	None expected.	
Genital, urinary:		
Difficult urination.	Infrequent	4
Kidneys:	None expected.	
Liver:	None expected.	
Allergic:	None expected.	
Blood:	None expected.	
Others:		
Less perspiration.	Common	4

2- Discontinue. Seek emergency treatment.
3- Discontinue. Call doctor right away.
4- Continue. Call doctor when convenient.
5- Continue. Tell doctor at next visit.
6- No action necessary.

WARNINGS & PRECAUTIONS

Don't take if:
- You are allergic to any anticholinergic.
- You have trouble with stomach bloating.
- You have difficulty emptying your bladder completely.
- You have narrow-angle glaucoma.
- You have severe ulcerative colitis.

Before you start, consult your doctor:
- If you have open-angle glaucoma.
- If you have angina.
- If you have chronic bronchitis or asthma.
- If you have liver disease.
- If you have hiatal hernia.
- If you have enlarged prostate.
- If you have myasthenia gravis.
- If you have peptic ulcer.
- If you will have surgery within 2 months, including dental surgery, requiring general or spinal anesthesia.

Over age 60:
Adverse reactions and side effects, particularly mental confusion, may be more frequent and severe than in younger persons.

Pregnancy:
Studies inconclusive on harm to unborn child. Animal studies show fetal abnormalities. Decide with your doctor whether drug benefits justify risk to unborn child.

Breast-feeding:
Drug passes into milk. Avoid drug or discontinue nursing until you finish medicine. Consult doctor for advice on maintaining milk supply.

Infants & children:
Use only under medical supervision.

Prolonged use:
Chronic constipation, possible fecal impaction. Consult doctor immediately.

Skin & sunlight:
No problems expected.

Driving, piloting or hazardous work:
Use disqualifies you for piloting aircraft. Otherwise, no problems expected.

Airplane passengers:
No problems expected.

Discontinuing:
May be unnecessary to finish medicine. Follow doctor's instructions.

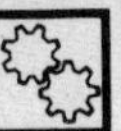

INTERACTION WITH OTHER DRUGS

GENERIC NAME OR DRUG CLASS	COMBINED EFFECT
Amantadine	Increased flavoxate effect.
Anticholinergics (other)	Increased flavoxate effect.
Antidepressants (tricyclic)	Increased flavoxate effect.
Antihistamines	Increased flavoxate effect.
Atropine	Increased effect of both drugs.
Cortisone drugs	Increased internal-eye pressure.
Haloperidol	Increased internal-eye pressure.
MAO inhibitors	Increased flavoxate effect.
Meperidine	Increased flavoxate effect.
Orphenadrine	Increased flavoxate effect.
Phenothiazines	Increased flavoxate effect.
Pilocarpine	Loss of pilocarpine effect in glaucoma treatment.
Vitamin C	Decreased flavoxate effect. Avoid large doses of vitamin C.

INTERACTION WITH OTHER SUBSTANCES

INTERACTS WITH	COMBINED EFFECT
Alcohol:	None expected.
Beverages:	None expected.
Cocaine:	Excessively rapid heartbeat. Avoid.
Foods:	None expected.
Marijuana:	Drowsiness and dry mouth.
Tobacco:	None expected.

FLUPHENAZINE

BRAND NAMES

Apo-Fluphenazine
Modecate
Moditen
Permitil
Prolixin

GENERAL INFORMATION

Habit forming? No
Prescription needed? Yes
Available as generic? Yes
Drug class: Tranquilizer, antiemetic (phenothiazine)

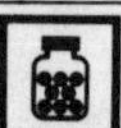

USES

- Stops nausea, vomiting.
- Reduces anxiety, agitation.

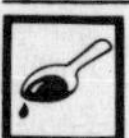

DOSAGE & USAGE INFORMATION

How to take:
- Tablet or capsule—Swallow with liquid or food to lessen stomach irritation.
- Suppositories—Remove wrapper and moisten suppository with water. Gently insert into rectum, large end first.
- Drops or liquid—Dilute dose in beverage.

When to take:
- Nervous and mental disorders—Take at the same times each day.
- Nausea and vomiting—Take as needed, no more often than every 4 hours.

If you forget a dose:
- Nervous and mental disorders—Take up to 2 hours late. If more than 2 hours, wait for next scheduled dose (don't double this).
- Nausea and vomiting—Take as soon as you remember. Wait 4 hours for next dose.

What drug does:
- Suppresses brain's vomiting center.
- Suppresses brain centers that control abnormal emotions and behavior.

Time lapse before drug works:
- Nausea and vomiting—1 hour or less.
- Nervous and mental disorders—4-6 weeks.

Don't take with:
- Antacid or medicine for diarrhea.
- Non-prescription drug for cough, cold or allergy.
- See Interaction column and consult doctor.

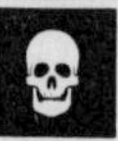

OVERDOSE

Symptoms:
Stupor, convulsions, coma.

What to do:
- Dial 0 (operator) or 911 (emergency) for an ambulance or medical help. Then give first aid immediately.
- Additional emergency information on page 886.

POSSIBLE ADVERSE REACTIONS OR SIDE EFFECTS

SYMPTOMS	FREQUENCY	WHAT TO DO
Brain & nervous system:		
• Restlessness, tremor.	Common	3
• Fainting	Infrequent	2
• Drowsiness	Common	3
Skin:		
• Rash	Infrequent	3
• Less perspiration.	Common	4
Eyes:		
Vision changes.	Rare	3
Ears, nose, throat:		
• Sore throat, fever.	Rare	3
• Dry mouth, nasal congestion.	Common	4
Digestive:		
Constipation	Common	4
Heart & lungs, blood vessels, kidneys, allergic, blood:	None expected.	
Muscles, bones, joints:		
Muscle spasms of face and neck, unsteady gait.	Common	2
Genital, urinary:		
Urination difficulty.	Infrequent	4
Liver:		
Jaundice (yellow eyes and skin).	Rare	3
Others:		
Less interest in sex, breast swelling, change in menstrual pattern.	Infrequent	4

1-Life-threatening. Seek emergency treatment immediately.
2-Discontinue. Seek emergency treatment.
3-Discontinue. Call doctor right away.
4-Continue. Call doctor when convenient.
5-Continue. Tell doctor at next visit.
6-No action necessary.

WARNINGS & PRECAUTIONS

Don't take if:
- You are allergic to any phenothiazine.
- You have a blood or bone-marrow disease.

Before you start, consult your doctor:
- If you will have surgery within 2 months, including dental surgery, requiring general or spinal anesthesia.
- If you have asthma, emphysema or other lung disorder.
- If you take non-prescription ulcer medicine, asthma medicine or amphetamines.

Over age 60:
Adverse reactions and side effects may be more frequent and severe than in younger persons. More likely to develop involuntary movement of jaws, lips, tongue, chewing. Report this to your doctor immediately. Early treatment can help.

Pregnancy:
Risk to unborn child outweighs drug benefits. Don't use.

Breast-feeding:
Drug passes into milk. Avoid drug or discontinue nursing until you finish medicine. Consult doctor for advice on maintaining milk supply.

Infants & children:
Don't give to children younger than 2.

Prolonged use:
May lead to tardive dyskinesia (involuntary movement of jaws, lips, tongue, chewing).

Skin & sunlight:
May cause rash or intensify sunburn in areas exposed to sun or sunlamp. Skin may remain sensitive for 3 months after discontinuing.

Driving, piloting or hazardous work:
Don't drive or pilot aircraft until you learn how medicine affects you. Don't work around dangerous machinery. Don't climb ladders or work in high places. Danger increases if you drink alcohol or take medicine affecting alertness and reflexes.

Airplane passengers:
No problems expected.

Discontinuing:
- Nervous and mental disorders—Don't discontinue without doctor's advice until you complete prescribed dose, even though symptoms diminish or disappear.
- Nausea and vomiting—May be unnecessary to finish medicine. Follow doctor's instructions.

INTERACTION WITH OTHER DRUGS

GENERIC NAME OR DRUG CLASS	COMBINED EFFECT
Anticholinergics	Increased anticholinergic effect.
Antidepressants (tricyclic)	Increased fluphenazine effect.
Antihistamines	Increased antihistamine effect.
Appetite suppressants	Decreased suppressant effect.
Levodopa	Decreased levodopa effect.
Mind-altering drugs	Increased effect of mind-altering drugs.
Narcotics	Increased narcotic effect.
Phenytoin	Increased phenytoin effect.
Quinidine	Impaired heart function. Dangerous mixture.
Sedatives	Increased sedative effect.
Tranquilizers (other)	Increased tranquilizer effect.

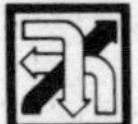

INTERACTION WITH OTHER SUBSTANCES

INTERACTS WITH	COMBINED EFFECT
Alcohol:	Dangerous oversedation.
Beverages:	None expected.
Cocaine:	Decreased fluphenazine effect. Avoid.
Foods:	None expected.
Marijuana:	Drowsiness. May increase antinausea effect.
Tobacco:	None expected.

FLUPREDNISOLONE

BRAND NAMES

Alphadrol

GENERAL INFORMATION

Habit forming? No
Prescription needed? Yes
Available as generic? No
Drug class: Cortisone drug (adrenal corticosteroid)

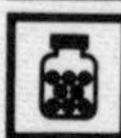

USES

- Reduces inflammation caused by many different medical problems.
- Treatment for some allergic diseases, blood disorders, kidney diseases, asthma and emphysema.
- Replaces corticosteroid deficiencies.

DOSAGE & USAGE INFORMATION

How to take:
Tablet—Swallow with liquid or food to lessen stomach irritation. If you can't swallow whole, crumble tablet.

When to take:
At the same times each day. Take once-a-day or once-every-other-day doses in mornings.

If you forget a dose:
- Several-doses-per-day prescription—Take as soon as you remember up to 2 hours late. If more than 2 hours, wait for next scheduled dose (don't double this dose).
- Once-a-day dose or less—Wait for next dose. Double this dose.

What drug does:
Decreases inflammatory responses.

Time lapse before drug works:
2 to 4 days.

Don't take with:
See Interaction column and consult doctor.

OVERDOSE

Symptoms:
Headache, convulsions, heart failure.

What to do:
- Dial 0 (operator) or 911 (emergency) for an ambulance or medical help. Then give first aid immediately.
- Additional emergency information on page 886.

POSSIBLE ADVERSE REACTIONS OR SIDE EFFECTS

SYMPTOMS	FREQUENCY	WHAT TO DO
Brain & nervous system:		
Mood changes, insomnia, restlessness.	Infrequent	4
Skin:		
• Acne	Common	4
• Rash	Rare	3
• Poor wound healing.	Common	4
Eyes:		
Blurred vision, halos around lights.	Infrequent	3
Ears, nose, throat:		
• Sore throat, fever.	Infrequent	3
• Thirst	Common	4
Digestive:		
• Indigestion, nausea, vomiting.	Common	4
• Bloody or black, tarry stool.	Infrequent	2
Heart & lungs:		
Irregular heartbeat.	Rare	2
Blood vessels, kidneys, liver, allergic, blood:	None expected.	
Muscles, bones, joints:		
Muscle cramps, swollen legs, feet.	Infrequent	3
Genital, urinary:		
Frequent urination.	Infrequent	4
Others:		
• Weight gain, round face.	Infrequent	4
• Fatigue, weakness.	Infrequent	4
• TB recurrence.	Infrequent	4
• Irregular menstrual periods.	Infrequent	4

1-Life-threatening. Seek emergency treatment immediately.
2-Discontinue. Seek emergency treatment.
3-Discontinue. Call doctor right away.
4-Continue. Call doctor when convenient.

WARNINGS & PRECAUTIONS

Don't take if:
- You are allergic to any cortisone drug.
- You have tuberculosis or fungus infection.
- You have herpes infection of eyes, lips or genitals.

Before you start, consult your doctor:
- If you have had tuberculosis.
- If you have congestive heart failure.
- If you have diabetes.
- If you have peptic ulcer.
- If you have glaucoma.
- If you have underactive thyroid.
- If you have high blood pressure.
- If you have myasthenia gravis.
- If you have blood clots in legs or lungs.

Over age 60:
Adverse reactions and side effects may be more frequent and severe than in younger persons. Likely to aggravate edema, diabetes or ulcers. Likely to cause cataracts and osteoporosis (softening of the bones).

Pregnancy:
Risk to unborn child outweighs drug benefits. Don't use.

Breast-feeding:
Drug passes into milk. Avoid drug or discontinue nursing until you finish medicine. Consult doctor for advice on maintaining milk supply.

Infants & children:
Use only under medical supervision.

Prolonged use:
- Retards growth in children.
- Possible glaucoma, cataracts, diabetes, fragile bones and thin skin.
- Functional dependence.

Skin & sunlight:
No problems expected.

Driving, piloting or hazardous work:
No problems expected.

Airplane passengers:
No problems expected.

Discontinuing:
- Don't discontinue without doctor's advice until you complete prescribed dose, even though symptoms diminish or disappear.
- Drug affects your response to surgery, illness, injury or stress for 2 years after discontinuing. Tell about drug to anyone who takes medical care of you within 2 years.

Others:
Avoid immunizations if possible.

INTERACTION WITH OTHER DRUGS

GENERIC NAME OR DRUG CLASS	COMBINED EFFECT
Amphoterecin B	Potassium depletion.
Anticholinergics	Possible glaucoma.
Anticoagulants (oral)	Decreased anticoagulant effect.
Anticonvulsants (hydantoin)	Decreased fluprednisolone effect.
Antidiabetics (oral)	Decreased antidiabetic effect.
Antihistamines	Decreased fluprednisolone effect.
Aspirin	Increased fluprednisolone effect.
Barbiturates	Decreased fluprednisolone effect. Oversedation.
Beta-adrenergic blockers	Decreased fluprednisolone effect.
Chloral hydrate	Decreased fluprednisolone effect.
Chlorthalidone	Potassium depletion.
Cholinergics	Decreased cholinergic effect.
Contraceptives (oral)	Increased fluprednisolone effect.
Digitalis preparations	Dangerous potassium depletion. Possible digitalis toxicity.

Additional interactions on page 837.

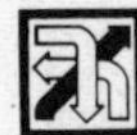

INTERACTION WITH OTHER SUBSTANCES

INTERACTS WITH	COMBINED EFFECT
Alcohol:	Risk of stomach ulcers.
Beverages:	No proven problems.
Cocaine:	Overstimulation. Avoid.
Foods:	No proven problems.
Marijuana:	Decreased immunity.
Tobacco:	Increased fluprednisolone effect. Possible toxicity.

FLURAZEPAM

BRAND NAMES

Apo-Flurazepam
Dalmane
Novoflupam

GENERAL INFORMATION

Habit forming? Yes
Prescription needed? Yes
Available as generic? No
Drug class: Tranquilizer (benzodiazepine)

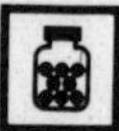

USES

Treatment for insomnia and tension.

DOSAGE & USAGE INFORMATION

How to take:
Tablet or capsule—Swallow with liquid. If you can't swallow whole, crumble tablet or open capsule and take with liquid or food.

When to take:
At the same time each day, according to instructions on prescription label.

If you forget a dose:
Take as soon as you remember up to 2 hours late. If more than 2 hours, wait for next scheduled dose (don't double this dose).

What drug does:
Affects limbic system of brain—part that controls emotions. Induces near-normal sleep pattern.

Time lapse before drug works:
30 minutes.

Don't take with:
See Interaction column and consult doctor.

OVERDOSE

Symptoms:
Drowsiness, weakness, tremor, stupor, coma.

What to do:
- Dial 0 (operator) or 911 (emergency) for an ambulance or medical help. Then give first aid immediately.
- If patient is unconscious and not breathing, give mouth-to-mouth breathing. If there is no heartbeat, use cardiac massage and mouth-to-mouth breathing (CPR). Don't try to make patient vomit. If you can't get help quickly, take patient to nearest emergency facility.
- Additional emergency information on page 886.

POSSIBLE ADVERSE REACTIONS OR SIDE EFFECTS

SYMPTOMS	FREQUENCY	WHAT TO DO
Brain & nervous system:		
• Clumsiness, drowsiness, dizziness.	Common	4
• Hallucinations, confusion, depression, irritability.	Infrequent	3
Skin:		
Rash, itch.	Infrequent	3
Eyes:		
Vision changes.	Infrequent	3
Ears, nose, throat:		
Mouth, throat ulcers.	Rare	3
Digestive:		
Constipation or diarrhea, nausea, vomiting.	Infrequent	4
Heart & lungs:		
Slow heartbeat, breathing difficulty.	Rare	2
Blood vessels:	None expected.	
Muscles, bones, joints:	None expected.	
Genital, urinary:		
Urination difficulty.	Infrequent	4
Kidneys:	None expected.	
Liver:		
Jaundice (yellow eyes and skin).	Rare	3
Allergic:	None expected.	
Blood:	None expected.	
Others:	None expected.	

1 - Life-threatening. Seek emergency treatment immediately.
2 - Discontinue. Seek emergency treatment.
3 - Discontinue. Call doctor right away.
4 - Continue. Call doctor when convenient.
5 - Continue. Tell doctor at next visit.
6 - No action necessary.

WARNINGS & PRECAUTIONS

Don't take if:
- You are allergic to any benzodiazepine.
- You have myasthenia gravis.
- You are active or recovering alcoholic.
- Patient is younger than 6 months.

Before you start, consult your doctor:
- If you have liver, kidney or lung disease.
- If you have diabetes, epilepsy or porphyria.

Over age 60:
Adverse reactions and side effects may be more frequent and severe than in younger persons. May develop agitation, rage or "hangover effect."

Pregnancy:
Risk to unborn child outweighs drug benefits. Don't use.

Breast-feeding:
Drug passes into milk. Avoid drug or discontinue nursing until you finish medicine. Consult doctor for advice on maintaining milk supply.

Infants & children:
Use only under medical supervision for children older than 6 months.

Prolonged use:
May impair liver function.

Skin & sunlight:
No problems expected.

Driving, piloting or hazardous work:
Don't drive or pilot aircraft until you learn how medicine affects you. Don't work around dangerous machinery. Don't climb ladders or work in high places. Danger increases if you drink alcohol or take medicine affecting alertness and reflexes.

Airplane passengers:
No problems expected.

Discontinuing:
Don't discontinue without doctor's advice until you complete prescribed dose, even though symptoms diminish or disappear.

Others:
- Hot weather, heavy exercise and profuse sweat may reduce excretion and cause overdose.
- "Hangover effect" may occur.
- Blood sugar may rise in diabetics, requiring insulin adjustment.

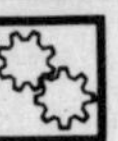

INTERACTION WITH OTHER DRUGS

GENERIC NAME OR DRUG CLASS	COMBINED EFFECT
Anticonvulsants	Change in seizure frequency or severity.
Antidepressants	Increased sedative effect of both drugs.
Antihistamines	Increased sedative effect of both drugs.
Antihypertensives	Excessively low blood pressure.
Cimetidine	Excess sedation.
Disulfiram	Increased flurazepam effect.
MAO inhibitors	Convulsions, deep sedation, rage.
Narcotics	Increased sedative effect of both drugs.
Sedatives	Increased sedative effect of both drugs.
Sleep inducers	Increased sedative effect of both drugs.
Tranquilizers	Increased sedative effect of both drugs.

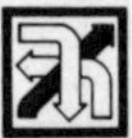

INTERACTION WITH OTHER SUBSTANCES

INTERACTS WITH	COMBINED EFFECT
Alcohol:	Heavy sedation. Avoid.
Beverages:	None expected.
Cocaine:	Decreased flurazepam effect.
Foods:	None expected.
Marijuana:	Heavy sedation. Avoid.
Tobacco:	Decreased flurazepam effect.

FOLIC ACID (VITAMIN B-9)

BRAND NAMES

Apo-Folic
Folvite
Novofolacid
Numerous other multiple vitamin-mineral supplements.

GENERAL INFORMATION

Habit forming? No
Prescription needed? High strength: Yes
Vitamin mixtures: No
Available as generic? Yes
Drug class: Vitamin supplement

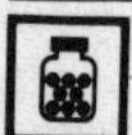

USES

- Dietary supplement to promote normal growth, development and good health.
- Treatment for anemias due to folic-acid deficiency occurring from alcoholism, liver disease, hemolytic anemia, sprue, infants on artificial formula, pregnancy, breast-feeding and oral-contraceptive use.

DOSAGE & USAGE INFORMATION

How to take:
Tablet—Swallow with liquid or food to lessen stomach irritation. If you can't swallow whole, crumble tablet and take with liquid or food.

When to take:
At the same time each day.

If you forget a dose:
Take when you remember. Don't double next dose. Resume regular schedule.

What drug does:
Essential to normal red-blood-cell formation.

Time lapse before drug works:
Not determined.

Don't take with:
See Interaction column and consult doctor.

OVERDOSE

Symptoms:
None expected.

What to do:
Overdose unlikely to threaten life.

POSSIBLE ADVERSE REACTIONS OR SIDE EFFECTS

SYMPTOMS	FREQUENCY	WHAT TO DO
Brain & nervous system:	None expected.	
Skin:	None expected.	
Eyes:	None expected.	
Ears, nose, throat:	None expected.	
Digestive:	None expected.	
Heart & lungs:	None expected.	
Blood vessels:	None expected.	
Muscles, bones, joints:	None expected.	
Genital, urinary:		
Large dose may produce yellow urine.	Common	5
Kidneys:	None expected.	
Liver:	None expected.	
Allergic:	None expected.	
Blood:	None expected.	
Others:	None expected.	

1 - Life-threatening. Seek emergency treatment immediately.
2 - Discontinue. Seek emergency treatment.
3 - Discontinue. Call doctor right away.
4 - Continue. Call doctor when convenient.
5 - Continue. Tell doctor at next visit.
6 - No action necessary.

FOLIC ACID (VITAMIN B-9)

WARNINGS & PRECAUTIONS

Don't take if:
You are allergic to any B vitamin.

Before you start, consult your doctor:
- If you have liver disease.
- If you have pernicious anemia. (Folic acid corrects anemia, but nerve damage of pernicious anemia continues.)

Over age 60:
No problems expected.

Pregnancy:
No problems expected.

Breast-feeding:
No problems expected.

Infants & children:
No problems expected.

Prolonged use:
No problems expected.

Skin & sunlight:
No problems expected.

Driving, piloting or hazardous work:
No problems expected.

Airplane passengers:
No problems expected.

Discontinuing:
Don't discontinue without doctor's advice until you complete prescribed dose, even though symptoms diminish or disappear.

Others:
- Folic acid removed by kidney dialysis. Dialysis patients should increase intake to 300% of RDA.
- A balanced diet should provide all the folic acid a healthy person needs and make supplements unnecessary. Best sources are green, leafy vegetables, fruits, liver and kidney.

INTERACTION WITH OTHER DRUGS

GENERIC NAME OR DRUG CLASS	COMBINED EFFECT
Analgesics	Decreased effect of folic acid.
Anticonvulsants	Decreased effect of folic acid.
Contraceptives (oral)	Decreased effect of folic acid.
Cortisone drugs	Decreased effect of folic acid.
Methotrexate	Decreased effect of folic acid.
Pyrimethamine	Decreased effect of folic acid.
Quinine	Decreased effect of folic acid.
Triamterene	Decreased effect of folic acid.
Trimethoprim	Decreased effect of folic acid.

INTERACTION WITH OTHER SUBSTANCES

INTERACTS WITH	COMBINED EFFECT
Alcohol:	None expected.
Beverages:	None expected.
Cocaine:	None expected.
Foods:	None expected.
Marijuana:	None expected.
Tobacco:	None expected.

FUROSEMIDE

BRAND NAMES

Apo-Furosemide
Furoside
Lasix
Neo-Renal
Novosemide
SK-Furosemide
Uritol

GENERAL INFORMATION

Habit forming? No
Prescription needed? Yes
Available as generic? No
Drug class: Diuretic, antihypertensive

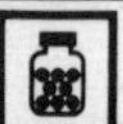

USES

- Lowers high blood pressure.
- Decreases fluid retention.

DOSAGE & USAGE INFORMATION

How to take:
Tablet, liquid or capsule—Swallow with liquid. If you can't swallow whole, crumble tablet or open capsule and take with liquid or food.

When to take:
- 1 dose a day—Take after breakfast.
- More than 1 dose a day—Take last dose no later than 6 p.m. unless otherwise directed.

If you forget a dose:
- 1 dose a day—Take as soon as you remember up to 12 hours late. If more than 12 hours, wait for next scheduled dose (don't double this dose).
- More than 1 dose a day—Take as soon as you remember up to 2 hours late. If more than 2 hours, wait for next scheduled dose (don't double this dose).

What drug does:
Increases elimination of sodium and water from body. Decreased body fluid reduces blood pressure.

Time lapse before drug works:
1 hour to increase water loss. Requires 2 to 3 weeks to lower blood pressure.

Don't take with:
- Non-prescription drugs with aspirin.
- See Interaction column and consult doctor.

OVERDOSE

Symptoms:
Weakness, lethargy, dizziness, confusion, nausea, vomiting, leg-muscle cramps, thirst, stupor, deep sleep, weak and rapid pulse, cardiac arrest.

What to do:
- Dial 0 (operator) or 911 (emergency) for an ambulance or medical help. Then give first aid immediately.
- Additional emergency information on page 886.

POSSIBLE ADVERSE REACTIONS OR SIDE EFFECTS

SYMPTOMS	FREQUENCY	WHAT TO DO
Brain & nervous system:		
• Dizziness	Common	4
• Mood changes.	Infrequent	3
Skin:		
Rash or hives.	Rare	3
Eyes:		
Yellow vision.	Rare	3
Ears, nose, throat:		
• Ringing in ears, hearing loss.	Rare	3
• Sore throat, fever.	Rare	3
• Dry mouth, thirst.	Rare	3
Digestive:		
• Side or stomach pain, nausea, vomiting.	Rare	3
• Appetite loss, diarrhea.	Infrequent	3
Heart & lungs:		
Irregular heartbeat.	Infrequent	3
Blood vessels:		
Unusual bleeding or bruising.	Rare	3
Muscles, bones, joints:		
• Joint pain.	Rare	3
• Muscle cramps.	Infrequent	3
Genital, urinary, kidneys, allergic, blood:	None expected.	
Liver:		
Jaundice (yellow skin and eyes).	Rare	3
Others:		
Fatigue, weakness.	Infrequent	3

1- Life-threatening. Seek emergency treatment immediately.
2- Discontinue. Seek emergency treatment.
3- Discontinue. Call doctor right away.
4- Continue. Call doctor when convenient.

WARNINGS & PRECAUTIONS

Don't take if:
You are allergic to furosemide.

Before you start, consult your doctor:
- If you are allergic to any sulfa drug.
- If you have liver or kidney disease.
- If you have gout.
- If you have diabetes.
- If you have impaired hearing.
- If you will have surgery within 2 months, including dental surgery, requiring general or spinal anesthesia.

Over age 60:
Adverse reactions and side effects may be more frequent and severe than in younger persons.

Pregnancy:
Risk to unborn child outweighs drug benefits. Don't use.

Breast-feeding:
Drug filters into milk. May harm child. Avoid.

Infants & children:
Use only under medical supervision.

Prolonged use:
- Impaired balance of water, salt and potassium in blood and body tissues.
- Possible diabetes.

Skin & sunlight:
May cause rash or intensify sunburn in areas exposed to sun or sunlamp.

Driving, piloting or hazardous work:
No problems expected.

Airplane passengers:
No problems expected.

Discontinuing:
Don't discontinue without doctor's advice until you complete prescribed dose, even though symptoms diminish or disappear.

Others:
Frequent laboratory studies to monitor potassium level in blood recommended. Eat foods rich in potassium (see page 848) or take potassium supplements. Consult doctor.

INTERACTION WITH OTHER DRUGS

GENERIC NAME OR DRUG CLASS	COMBINED EFFECT
Allopurinol	Decreased allopurinol effect.
Anticoagulants	Abnormal clotting.
Antidepressants (tricyclic)	Excessive blood-pressure drop.
Antidiabetics (oral)	Decreased antidiabetic effect.
Antiinflammatory drugs (non-steroid)	Decreased furosemide effect.
Antihypertensives	Increased antihypertensive effect.
Barbiturates	Low blood pressure.
Cortisone drugs	Excessive potassium loss.
Digitalis preparations	Serious heart-rhythm disorders.
Insulin	Decreased insulin effect.
Lithium	Increased lithium toxicity.
MAO inhibitors	Increased furosemide effect.
Narcotics	Dangerous low blood pressure. Avoid.
Phenothiazines	Increased phenothiazine effect.

Additional interactions on page 837.

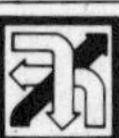

INTERACTION WITH OTHER SUBSTANCES

INTERACTS WITH	COMBINED EFFECT
Alcohol:	Blood-pressure drop. Avoid.
Beverages:	None expected.
Cocaine:	Dangerous blood-pressure drop. Avoid.
Foods:	None expected.
Marijuana:	Increased thirst and urinary frequency, fainting.
Tobacco:	Decreased furosemide effect.

GEMFIBROZIL

BRAND NAMES

Lopid

GENERAL INFORMATION

Habit forming? No
Prescription needed? Yes
Available as generic? No
Drug class: Antihyperlipidemic

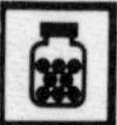

USES

Reduces fatty substances in the blood (cholesterol and triglycerides).

DOSAGE & USAGE INFORMATION

How to take:
Capsule—Swallow with liquid or food to lessen stomach irritation.

When to take:
At the same times each day.

If you forget a dose:
Take as soon as you remember up to 2 hours late. If more than 2 hours, wait for next scheduled dose (don't double this dose).

What drug does:
Inhibits formation of fatty substances.

Time lapse before drug works:
3 months or more.

Don't take with:
See Interaction column and consult doctor.

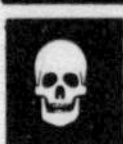

OVERDOSE

Symptoms:
Diarrhea, headache, muscle pain.

What to do:
Overdose unlikely to threaten life. If person takes much larger amount than prescribed, call doctor, poison-control center or hospital emergency room for instructions.

POSSIBLE ADVERSE REACTIONS OR SIDE EFFECTS

SYMPTOMS	FREQUENCY	WHAT TO DO
Brain & nervous system:		
Dizziness, drowsiness, headache.	Rare	4
Skin:		
• Dryness, hair loss.	Rare	4
• Rash, itch.	Rare	3
Eyes, blood vessels, allergic, blood:	None expected.	
Ears, nose, throat:		
• Sores in mouth, on lips.	Rare	3
• Sore throat.	Rare	3
Digestive:		
Nausea, vomiting, diarrhea, stomach pain.	Infrequent	4
Heart & lungs:		
Chest pain, shortness of breath, irregular heartbeat.	Infrequent	3
Muscles, bones, joints:		
• Muscle cramps.	Rare	4
• Swollen feet, legs.	Rare	3
Genital, urinary:		
Bloody urine, painful urination.	Rare	3
Kidneys:		
Backache	Rare	4
Liver:		
Gallstones	Infrequent	3
Others:		
• Decreased sex drive.	Rare	4
• Fever, chills.	Rare	3

1- Life-threatening. Seek emergency treatment immediately.
2- Discontinue. Seek emergency treatment.
3- Discontinue. Call doctor right away.
4- Continue. Call doctor when convenient.

WARNINGS & PRECAUTIONS

Don't take if:
You are allergic to any antihyperlipidemic.

Before you start, consult your doctor:
- If you have had liver or kidney disease.
- If you have had peptic-ulcer disease.
- If you have diabetes.

Over age 60:
Adverse reactions and side effects may be more frequent and severe than in younger persons.

Pregnancy:
Risk to unborn child outweighs drug benefits. Don't use.

Breast-feeding:
May harm child. Avoid.

Infants & children:
Not recommended.

Prolonged use:
Periodic blood-cell counts and liver-function studies recommended if you take gemfibrozil for a long time.

Skin & sunlight:
No problems expected.

Driving, piloting or hazardous work:
Avoid if you feel drowsy or dizzy. Otherwise, no problems expected.

Airplane passengers:
No problems expected.

Discontinuing:
Don't discontinue without doctor's advice until you complete prescribed dose, even though symptoms diminish or disappear.

Others:
Some studies question effectiveness. Many studies warn against toxicity.

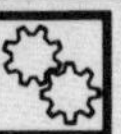

INTERACTION WITH OTHER DRUGS

GENERIC NAME OR DRUG CLASS	COMBINED EFFECT
Anticoagulants (oral)	Increased anticoagulant effect. Dose reduction of anticoagulant necessary.
Antidiabetics (oral)	Increased antidiabetic effect.
Contraceptives (oral)	Decreased gemfibrozil effect.
Estrogens	Decreased gemfibrozil effect.
Furosemide	Possible toxicity of both drugs.
Insulin	Increased insulin effect.
Thyroid hormones	Increased gemfibrozil effect.

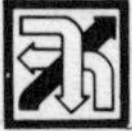

INTERACTION WITH OTHER SUBSTANCES

INTERACTS WITH	COMBINED EFFECT
Alcohol:	None expected.
Beverages:	None expected.
Cocaine:	Decreased effect of gemfibrozil. Avoid cocaine.
Foods:	
Fatty foods	Decreased gemfibrozil effect.
Marijuana:	None expected.
Tobacco:	Decreased gemfibrozil absorption. Avoid.

GLIPIZIDE

BRAND NAMES

Glucatrol

GENERAL INFORMATION

Habit forming? No
Prescription needed? Yes
Available as generic? No
Drug class: Antidiabetic (oral), sulfonurea

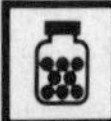

USES

Treatment for diabetes in adults who can't control blood sugar by diet, weight loss and exercise.

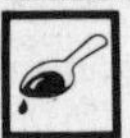

DOSAGE & USAGE INFORMATION

How to take:
Tablet—Swallow with liquid or food to lessen stomach irritation. If you can't swallow whole, crumble tablet and take with liquid or food.

When to take:
At the same times each day.

If you forget a dose:
Take as soon as you remember up to 2 hours late. If more than 2 hours, wait for next scheduled dose (don't double this dose).

What drug does:
Stimulates pancreas to produce more insulin. Insulin in blood forces cells to use sugar in blood.

Time lapse before drug works:
3 to 4 hours. May require 2 weeks for maximum benefit.

Don't take with:
See Interaction column and consult doctor.

OVERDOSE

Symptoms:
Excessive hunger, nausea, anxiety, cool skin, cold sweats, drowsiness, rapid heartbeat, weakness, unconsciousness, coma.

What to do:
- Dial 0 (operator) or 911 (emergency) for an ambulance or medical help. Then give first aid immediately.
- Additional emergency information on page 886.

POSSIBLE ADVERSE REACTIONS OR SIDE EFFECTS

SYMPTOMS	FREQUENCY	WHAT TO DO
Brain & nervous system:		
• Dizziness	Common	3
• Fatigue	Rare	3
Skin:		
Itching or rash.	Rare	3
Eyes:	None expected.	
Ears, nose, throat:		
• Sore throat, fever.	Rare	3
• Ringing in ears.	Rare	3
Digestive:		
Diarrhea, loss of appetite, nausea, stomach pain, heartburn.	Common	4
Heart & lungs, muscles, bones, joints, genital, urinary, kidneys, allergic, blood:	None expected.	
Blood vessels:		
Unusual bleeding or bruising.	Rare	3
Liver:		
Jaundice (yellow skin, eyes).	Rare	3
Others:		
Low blood sugar (ravenous hunger, nausea, anxiety, cold sweats, cool skin, chills, drowsiness, nervousness, headache, rapid heartbeat, weakness).	Infrequent	2

1-Life-threatening. Seek emergency treatment immediately.
2-Discontinue. Seek emergency treatment.
3-Discontinue. Call doctor right away.
4-Continue. Call doctor when convenient.

WARNINGS & PRECAUTIONS

Don't take if:

- You are allergic to any sulfonurea.
- You have impaired kidney or liver function.

Before you start, consult your doctor:

- If you have a severe infection.
- If you have thyroid disease.
- If you take insulin.
- If you have heart disease.

Over age 60:
Dose usually smaller than for younger adults. Avoid "low-blood-sugar" episodes because repeated ones can damage brain permanently.

Pregnancy:
No proven harm to unborn child. Avoid if possible.

Breast-feeding:
Drug filters into milk. May lower baby's blood sugar. Avoid.

Infants & children:
Don't give to infants or children.

Prolonged use:
None expected.

Skin & sunlight:
May cause rash or intensify sunburn in areas exposed to sun or sunlamp.

Driving, piloting or hazardous work:
No problems expected unless you develop hypoglycemia (low blood sugar). If so, avoid driving or hazardous activity.

Airplane passengers:
No problems expected.

Discontinuing:
Don't discontinue without consulting doctor. Dose may require gradual reduction if you have taken drug for a long time. Doses of other drugs may also require adjustment.

Others:

- Don't exceed 1500 mg. in 1 day.
- Hypoglycemia (low blood sugar) may occur, even with proper dose schedule. You must balance medicine, diet and exercise.

INTERACTION WITH OTHER DRUGS

GENERIC NAME OR DRUG CLASS	COMBINED EFFECT
Androgens	Increased glipizide effect.
Anticoagulants (oral)	Unpredictable prothrombin times (see page 848).
Anticonvulsants (hydantoin)	Decreased glipizide effect.
Antiinflammatory drugs (non-steroidal)	Increased glipizide effect.
Aspirin	Increased glipizide effect.
Beta-adrenergic blockers	Increased glipizide effect.
Chloramphenicol	Increased glipizide effect.
Clofibrate	Increased glipizide effect.
Contraceptives (oral)	Decreased glipizide effect.
Cortisone drugs	Decreased glipizide effect.
Diuretics (thiazide)	Decreased glipizide effect.
Epinephrine	Decreased glipizide effect.
Estrogens	Increased glipizide effect.
Guanethidine	Unpredictable glipizide effect.

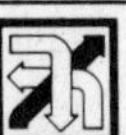

INTERACTION WITH OTHER SUBSTANCES

INTERACTS WITH	COMBINED EFFECT
Alcohol:	Disulfiram reaction (see page 846). Avoid.
Beverages:	None expected.
Cocaine:	No proven problems.
Foods:	None expected.
Marijuana:	Decreased glipizide effect. Avoid.
Tobacco:	None expected.

GLYBURIDE

BRAND NAMES

DiaBeta
Micronase

GENERAL INFORMATION

Habit forming? No
Prescription needed? Yes
Available as generic? No
Drug class: Antidiabetic (oral), sulfonurea

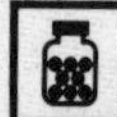

USES

Treatment for diabetes in adults who can't control blood sugar by diet, weight loss and exercise.

DOSAGE & USAGE INFORMATION

How to take:
Tablet—Swallow with liquid or food to lessen stomach irritation. If you can't swallow whole, crumble tablet and take with liquid or food.

When to take:
At the same times each day.

If you forget a dose:
Take as soon as you remember up to 2 hours late. If more than 2 hours, wait for next scheduled dose (don't double this dose).

What drug does:
Stimulates pancreas to produce more insulin. Insulin in blood forces cells to use sugar in blood.

Time lapse before drug works:
3 to 4 hours. May require 2 weeks for maximum benefit.

Don't take with:
See Interaction column and consult doctor.

OVERDOSE

Symptoms:
Excessive hunger, nausea, anxiety, cool skin, cold sweats, drowsiness, rapid heartbeat, weakness, unconsciousness, coma.

What to do:

- Dial 0 (operator) or 911 (emergency) for an ambulance or medical help. Then give first aid immediately.
- Additional emergency information on page 886.

POSSIBLE ADVERSE REACTIONS OR SIDE EFFECTS

SYMPTOMS	FREQUENCY	WHAT TO DO
Brain & nervous system:		
• Dizziness	Common	3
• Fatigue	Rare	3
Skin:		
Itching or rash.	Rare	3
Eyes:	None expected.	
Ears, nose, throat:		
• Sore throat, fever.	Rare	3
• Ringing in ears.	Rare	3
Digestive:		
Diarrhea, loss of appetite, nausea, stomach pain, heartburn.	Common	4
Heart & lungs, muscles, bones, joints, genital, urinary, kidneys, allergic, blood:	None expected.	
Blood vessels:		
Unusual bleeding or bruising.	Rare	3
Liver:		
Jaundice (yellow skin, eyes).	Rare	3
Others:		
Low blood sugar (ravenous hunger, nausea, anxiety, cold sweats, cool skin, chills, drowsiness, nervousness, headache, rapid heartbeat, weakness).	Infrequent	2

1- Life-threatening. Seek emergency treatment immediately.
2- Discontinue. Seek emergency treatment.
3- Discontinue. Call doctor right away.
4- Continue. Call doctor when convenient.

WARNINGS & PRECAUTIONS

Don't take if:
- You are allergic to any sulfonurea.
- You have impaired kidney or liver function.

Before you start, consult your doctor:
- If you have a severe infection.
- If you have thyroid disease.
- If you take insulin.
- If you have heart disease.

Over age 60:
Dose usually smaller than for younger adults. Avoid "low-blood-sugar" episodes because repeated ones can damage brain permanently.

Pregnancy:
No proven harm to unborn child. Avoid if possible.

Breast-feeding:
Drug filters into milk. May lower baby's blood sugar. Avoid.

Infants & children:
Don't give to infants or children.

Prolonged use:
None expected.

Skin & sunlight:
May cause rash or intensify sunburn in areas exposed to sun or sunlamp.

Driving, piloting or hazardous work:
No problems expected unless you develop hypoglycemia (low blood sugar). If so, avoid driving or hazardous activity.

Airplane passengers:
No problems expected.

Discontinuing:
Don't discontinue without consulting doctor. Dose may require gradual reduction if you have taken drug for a long time. Doses of other drugs may also require adjustment.

Others:
- Don't exceed 1500 mg. in 1 day.
- Hypoglycemia (low blood sugar) may occur, even with proper dose schedule. You must balance medicine, diet and exercise.

INTERACTION WITH OTHER DRUGS

GENERIC NAME OR DRUG CLASS	COMBINED EFFECT
Androgens	Increased glyburide effect.
Anticoagulants (oral)	Unpredictable prothrombin times (see page 848).
Anticonvulsants (hydantoin)	Decreased glyburide effect.
Antiinflammatory drugs (non-steroidal)	Increased glyburide effect.
Aspirin	Increased glyburide effect.
Beta-adrenergic blockers	Increased glyburide effect.
Chloramphenicol	Increased glyburide effect.
Clofibrate	Increased glyburide effect.
Contraceptives (oral)	Decreased glyburide effect.
Cortisone drugs	Decreased glyburide effect.
Diuretics (thiazide)	Decreased glyburide effect.
Epinephrine	Decreased glyburide effect.
Estrogens	Increased glyburide effect.
Guanethidine	Unpredictable glyburide effect.

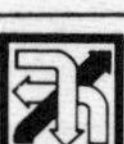

INTERACTION WITH OTHER SUBSTANCES

INTERACTS WITH	COMBINED EFFECT
Alcohol:	Disulfiram reaction (see page 846). Avoid.
Beverages:	None expected.
Cocaine:	No proven problems.
Foods:	None expected.
Marijuana:	Decreased glyburide effect. Avoid.
Tobacco:	None expected.

GRISEOFULVIN

BRAND NAMES

Fulvicin P/G
Fulvicin U/F
Grifulvin V
Grisactin
Grisovin-FP
Gris-PEG
grisOwen

GENERAL INFORMATION

Habit forming? No
Prescription needed? Yes
Available as generic? Yes
Drug class: Antibiotic (antifungal)

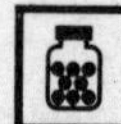

USES

Treatment for fungal infections susceptible to griseofulvin.

DOSAGE & USAGE INFORMATION

How to take:

- Tablet or capsule—Swallow with liquid or food to lessen stomach irritation. If you can't swallow whole, crumble tablet or open capsule and take with liquid or food.
- Liquid—Follow label instructions.

When to take:
With or immediately after meals.

If you forget a dose:
Take as soon as you remember up to 2 hours late. If more than 2 hours, wait for next scheduled dose (don't double this dose).

What drug does:
Prevents fungi from growing and reproducing.

Time lapse before drug works:
2 to 10 days for skin infections. 2 to 4 weeks for infections of fingernails or toenails. Complete cure of either may require several months.

Don't take with:
See Interaction column and consult doctor.

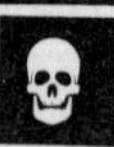

OVERDOSE

Symptoms:
Nausea, vomiting, diarrhea. In sensitive individuals, severe diarrhea may occur without overdosing.

What to do:
Overdose unlikely to threaten life. If person takes much larger amount than prescribed, call doctor, poison-control center or hospital emergency room for instructions.

POSSIBLE ADVERSE REACTIONS OR SIDE EFFECTS

SYMPTOMS	FREQUENCY	WHAT TO DO
Brain & nervous system:		
• Insomnia	Infrequent	4
• Confusion	Infrequent	3
• Headache	Common	5
Skin:		
Rash, hives, itch.	Infrequent	3
Eyes:	None expected.	
Ears, nose, throat:		
• Sore throat, fever.	Rare	3
• Mouth or tongue irritation, soreness.	Infrequent	3
Digestive:		
Nausea, vomiting, diarrhea, stomach pain.	Infrequent	3
Heart & lungs:	None expected.	
Blood vessels:	None expected.	
Muscles, bones, joints:	None expected.	
Genital, urinary:	None expected.	
Kidneys:	None expected.	
Liver:	None expected.	
Allergic:	None expected.	
Blood:	None expected.	
Others:		
• Tiredness	Infrequent	4
• Numbness, tingling, pain or weakness in extremities.	Rare	3

1- Life-threatening. Seek emergency treatment immediately.
2- Discontinue. Seek emergency treatment.
3- Discontinue. Call doctor right away.
4- Continue. Call doctor when convenient.
5- Continue. Tell doctor at next visit.
6- No action necessary.

WARNINGS & PRECAUTIONS

Don't take if:
- You are allergic to any antifungal medicine.
- You have liver disease.
- You have porphyria.
- The infection is minor and will respond to less-potent drugs.

Before you start, consult your doctor:
- If you plan to become pregnant within medication period.
- If you have liver disease.
- If you have lupus.

Over age 60:
Adverse reactions and side effects may be more frequent and severe than in younger persons.

Pregnancy:
Risk to unborn child outweighs drug benefits. Don't use.

Breast-feeding:
No problems expected, but consult your doctor.

Infants & children:
Not recommended for children younger than 2.

Prolonged use:
You may become susceptible to infections caused by germs not responsive to griseofulvin.

Skin & sunlight:
May cause rash or intensify sunburn in areas exposed to sun or sunlamp.

Driving, piloting or hazardous work:
- Don't drive if you feel dizzy or have vision problems.
- Don't pilot aircraft.

Airplane passengers:
No problems expected.

Discontinuing:
Don't discontinue without doctor's advice until you complete prescribed dose, even though symptoms diminish or disappear.

Others:
Periodic laboratory blood studies and liver- and kidney-function tests recommended.

INTERACTION WITH OTHER DRUGS

GENERIC NAME OR DRUG CLASS	COMBINED EFFECT
Anticoagulants (oral)	Decreased anticoagulant effect.
Barbiturates	Decreased griseofulvin effect.

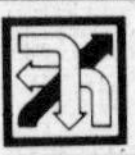

INTERACTION WITH OTHER SUBSTANCES

INTERACTS WITH	COMBINED EFFECT
Alcohol:	Increased intoxication. Possible disulfiram reaction (see page 846).
Beverages:	None expected.
Cocaine:	None expected.
Foods:	None expected, but foods high in fat will improve drug absorption.
Marijuana:	None expected.
Tobacco:	None expected.

GUAIFENESIN

BRAND NAMES

Ambenyl Expectorant
Cheracol Cough Syrup
Chlor-Trimeton Expectorant
Dimetane Expectorant
Dristan Cough Formula
Formula 44-D
Vicks Cough Syrup

See complete brand names list, page 826.

GENERAL INFORMATION

Habit forming? No
Prescription needed? No
Available as generic? Yes
Drug class: Cough/cold preparation

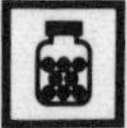

USES

Loosens mucus in respiratory passages from allergies and infections (hay fever, cough, cold).

DOSAGE & USAGE INFORMATION

How to take:

- Tablet or capsule—Swallow with liquid. If you can't swallow whole, crumble tablet or open capsule and take with liquid or food.
- Syrup or lozenge—Take as directed on label. Follow with 8 oz. water.

When to take:
As needed, no more often than every 3 hours.

If you forget a dose:
Take as soon as you remember. Wait 3 hours for next dose.

What drug does:
Increases production of watery fluids to thin mucus so it can be coughed out or absorbed.

Time lapse before drug works:
15 to 30 minutes. Regular use for 5 to 7 days necessary for maximum benefit.

Don't take with:
See Interaction column and consult doctor.

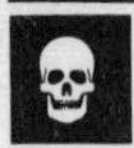

OVERDOSE

Symptoms:
Drowsiness, mild weakness, nausea, vomiting.

What to do:
Overdose unlikely to threaten life. If person takes much larger amount than prescribed, call doctor, poison-control center or hospital emergency room for instructions.

POSSIBLE ADVERSE REACTIONS OR SIDE EFFECTS

SYMPTOMS	FREQUENCY	WHAT TO DO
Brain & nervous system: Drowsiness	Infrequent	4
Skin: Rash	Infrequent	3
Eyes:	None expected.	
Ears, nose, throat:	None expected.	
Digestive:		
• Stomach pain, diarrhea.	Infrequent	3
• Nausea, vomiting.	Infrequent	3
Heart & lungs:	None expected.	
Blood vessels:	None expected.	
Muscles, bones, joints:	None expected.	
Genital, urinary:	None expected.	
Kidneys:	None expected.	
Liver:	None expected.	
Allergic:	None expected.	
Blood:	None expected.	
Others:	None expected.	

1 - Life-threatening. Seek emergency treatment immediately.
2 - Discontinue. Seek emergency treatment.
3 - Discontinue. Call doctor right away.
4 - Continue. Call doctor when convenient.
5 - Continue. Tell doctor at next visit.
6 - No action necessary.

WARNINGS & PRECAUTIONS

Don't take if:
You are allergic to any cough or cold preparation containing guaifenesin.

Before you start, consult your doctor:
See Interaction column and consult doctor.

Over age 60:
Adverse reactions and side effects may be more frequent and severe than in younger persons. For drug to work, you must drink 8 to 10 glasses of fluid per day.

Pregnancy:
No proven harm to unborn child. Avoid if possible.

Breast-feeding:
No proven problems. Consult your doctor.

Infants & children:
No problems expected.

Prolonged use:
No problems expected.

Skin & sunlight:
No problems expected.

Driving, piloting or hazardous work:
Avoid if you feel drowsy. Otherwise, no problems expected.

Airplane passengers:
No problems expected.

Discontinuing:
May be unnecessary to finish medicine. Discontinue when symptoms disappear. If symptoms persist more than 1 week, consult doctor.

Others:
No problems expected.

INTERACTION WITH OTHER DRUGS

GENERIC NAME OR DRUG CLASS	COMBINED EFFECT
Anticoagulants	Risk of bleeding.

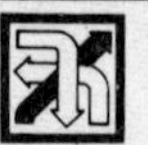

INTERACTION WITH OTHER SUBSTANCES

INTERACTS WITH	COMBINED EFFECT
Alcohol:	No proven problems.
Beverages:	You must drink 8 to 10 glasses of fluid per day for drug to work.
Cocaine:	No proven problems.
Foods:	None expected.
Marijuana:	No proven problems.
Tobacco:	No proven problems.

GUANABENZ

BRAND NAMES

Wytensin

GENERAL INFORMATION

Habit forming? No
Prescription needed? Yes
Available as generic? No
Drug class: Antihypertensive (alpha adrenergic stimulant)

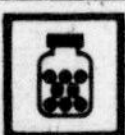

USES

Controls, but doesn't cure, high blood pressure.

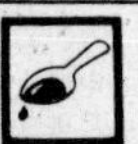

DOSAGE & USAGE INFORMATION

How to take:
Tablet—Swallow with liquid or food to lessen stomach irritation. If you can't swallow whole, crumble tablet and take with liquid or food.

When to take:
At the same times each day.

If you forget a dose:
Take as soon as you remember up to 2 hours late. If more than 2 hours, wait for next scheduled dose (don't double this dose).

What drug does:
- Relaxes muscle cells of small arteries.
- Slows heartbeat.

Time lapse before drug works:
1 hour.

Don't take with:
See Interaction column and consult doctor.

OVERDOSE

Symptoms:
Severe dizziness, slow heartbeat, pinpoint pupils, fainting, coma.

What to do:
- Dial 0 (operator) or 911 (emergency) for an ambulance or medical help. Then give first aid immediately.
- If patient is unconscious and not breathing, give mouth-to-mouth breathing. If there is no heartbeat, use cardiac massage and mouth-to-mouth breathing (CPR). Don't try to make patient vomit. If you can't get help quickly, take patient to nearest emergency facility.
- Additional emergency information on page 886.

POSSIBLE ADVERSE REACTIONS OR SIDE EFFECTS

SYMPTOMS	FREQUENCY	WHAT TO DO
Brain & nervous system:		
• Nervousness, headache.	Common	4
• Dizziness	Infrequent	4
Skin:		
Paleness	Common	4
Eyes:	None expected.	
Ears, nose, throat:		
Dry mouth.	Common	4
Digestive:		
Appetite loss, nausea, vomiting.	Infrequent	4
Heart & lungs:		
• Irregular heartbeat.	Infrequent	3
• Rapid heartbeat.	Common	4
Blood vessels:	None expected.	
Muscles, bones, joints:		
Trembling hands.	Infrequent	3
Genital, urinary:		
Difficult urination.	Infrequent	4
Kidneys:	None expected.	
Liver:	None expected.	
Allergic:	None expected.	
Blood:	None expected.	
Others:		
• Insomnia	Common	5
• Decreased sex drive.	Infrequent	4

1- Life-threatening. Seek emergency treatment immediately.
2- Discontinue. Seek emergency treatment.
3- Discontinue. Call doctor right away.
4- Continue. Call doctor when convenient.
5- Continue. Tell doctor at next visit.
6- No action necessary.

WARNINGS & PRECAUTIONS

Don't take if:
You are allergic to any sympathomimetic drug.

Before you start, consult your doctor:
- If you have blood disease.
- If you have heart disease.
- If you have liver disease.
- If you have diabetes or overactive thyroid.
- If you will have surgery within 2 months, including dental surgery, requiring general or spinal anesthesia.

Over age 60:
Adverse reactions and side effects may be more frequent and severe than in younger persons. Hot weather may cause need to reduce dosage.

Pregnancy:
Risk to unborn child outweighs drug benefits. Don't use.

Breast-feeding:
Avoid nursing.

Infants & children:
Not recommended.

Prolonged use:
Side effects tend to diminish. Request uric-acid and kidney-function studies periodically.

Skin & sunlight:
No problems expected.

Driving, piloting or hazardous work:
Avoid if you feel dizzy; otherwise, no problems expected.

Airplane passengers:
No problems expected.

Discontinuing:
Don't discontinue without consulting doctor. Dose may require gradual reduction if you have taken drug for a long time. Doses of other drugs may also require adjustment. Abrupt discontinuing may cause anxiety, chest pain, salivation, headache, abdominal cramps, fast heartbeat.

Others:
Stay away from high sodium foods. Lose weight if you are overweight.

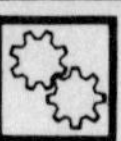

INTERACTION WITH OTHER DRUGS

GENERIC NAME OR DRUG CLASS	COMBINED EFFECT
Brain depressants: Sedatives, Sleeping pills, Tranquilizers, Antidepressants, Narcotics	Increased brain depression. Avoid.
Antihypertensives (other)	Decreases blood pressure more than either alone. May be beneficial, but requires dosage adjustment.
Diuretics	Decreases blood pressure more than either alone. May be beneficial, but requires dosage adjustment.

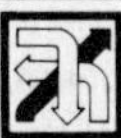

INTERACTION WITH OTHER SUBSTANCES

INTERACTS WITH	COMBINED EFFECT
Alcohol:	Oversedation. Avoid.
Beverages:	
Caffeine	Overstimulation. Avoid.
Cocaine:	Overstimulation. Avoid.
Foods:	
Salt	Decrease salt intake to increase beneficial effects of guanabenz.
Marijuana:	Overstimulation. Avoid.
Tobacco:	Decreased guanabenz effect.

GUANADREL

BRAND NAMES

Hylorel

GENERAL INFORMATION

Habit forming? No
Prescription needed? Yes
Available as generic? No
Drug class: Antihypertensive

USES

Controls, but doesn't cure, high blood pressure.

DOSAGE & USAGE INFORMATION

How to take:
Tablet or capsule—Swallow with liquid or food to lessen stomach irritation. If you can't swallow whole, crumble tablet or open capsule and take with liquid or food.

When to take:
At the same time each day.

If you forget a dose:
Take as soon as you remember up to 2 hours late. If more than 2 hours, wait for next scheduled dose (don't double this dose).

What drug does:
Relaxes muscle cells of small arteries.

Time lapse before drug works:
4 to 6 hours. May need to take for lifetime.

Don't take with:
See Interaction column and consult doctor.

OVERDOSE

Symptoms:
Severe blood-pressure drop; fainting; slow, weak pulse; cold, sweaty skin; loss of consciousness.

What to do:
- Dial 0 (operator) or 911 (emergency) for an ambulance or medical help. Then give first aid immediately.
- Additional emergency information on page 886.

POSSIBLE ADVERSE REACTIONS OR SIDE EFFECTS

SYMPTOMS	FREQUENCY	WHAT TO DO
Brain & nervous system:		
Dizziness, headache.	Common	5
Skin:		
Rash.	Infrequent	3
Eyes:		
Blurred vision, drooping eyelids.	Infrequent	3
Ears, nose, throat:		
Stuffy nose, dry mouth.	Common	6
Digestive:		
• Diarrhea, more bowel movements.	Common	4
• Nausea or vomiting.	Infrequent	4
Heart & lungs:		
Chest pains or shortness of breath.	Infrequent	3
Blood vessels, kidneys, liver, allergic, blood:	None expected.	
Muscles, bones, joints:		
Muscle pain or tremors.	Infrequent	3
Genital, urinary:		
• Impotence	Infrequent	5
• Nighttime urination.	Infrequent	5
Others:		
• Fatigue, weakness.	Common	4
• Lower sex drive.	Common	5

1- Life-threatening. Seek emergency treatment immediately.
2- Discontinue. Seek emergency treatment.
3- Discontinue. Call doctor right away.
4- Continue. Call doctor when convenient.
5- Continue. Tell doctor at next visit.
6- No action necessary.

WARNINGS & PRECAUTIONS

Don't take if:
- You are allergic to guanadrel.
- You have taken MAO inhibitors within 2 weeks.

Before you start, consult your doctor:
- If you have stroke or heart disease.
- If you have asthma.
- If you have had kidney disease.
- If you have peptic ulcer or chronic acid indigestion.
- If you will have surgery within 2 months, including dental surgery, requiring general or spinal anesthesia.

Over age 60:
Adverse reactions and side effects may be more frequent and severe than in younger persons. Start with small doses and monitor blood pressure frequently.

Pregnancy:
No proven harm to unborn child. Avoid if possible.

Breast-feeding:
No proven harm to nursing infant. Avoid if possible.

Infants & children:
Not recommended.

Prolonged use:
Due to drug's cumulative effect, dose will require adjustment to prevent wide fluctuations in blood pressure.

Skin & sunlight:
No problems expected.

Driving, piloting or hazardous work:
Don't drive or pilot aircraft until you learn how medicine affects you. Don't work around dangerous machinery. Don't climb ladders or work in high places. Danger increases if you drink alcohol or take medicine affecting alertness and reflexes, such as antihistamines, tranquilizers, sedatives, pain medicine, narcotics and mind-altering drugs.

Airplane passengers:
No problems expected.

Discontinuing:
Don't discontinue without consulting doctor. Dose may require gradual reduction if you have taken drug for a long time. Doses of other drugs may also require adjustment.

Others:
Hot weather further lowers blood pressure, particularly in patients over 60.

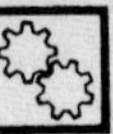

INTERACTION WITH OTHER DRUGS

GENERIC NAME OR DRUG CLASS	COMBINED EFFECT
Beta blockers	Increased likelihood of dizziness and fainting.
Rauwolfia alkaloids	Increased likelihood of dizziness and fainting.
Diuretics	Increased likelihood of dizziness and fainting.
Antihypertensives (other)	Increased effect of guanadrel.
Sympathomimetics	Decreased effect of guanadrel.
Phenothiazines	Decreased effect of guanadrel.
Antidepressants (tricyclic)	Decreased effect of guanadrel.
CNS depressants: Anticonvulsants, antihistamines, muscle relaxants, narcotics, sedatives, tranquilizers.	Decreased effect of guanadrel.
MAO inhibitors	Severe high blood pressure. Avoid.

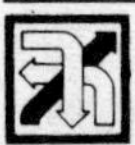

INTERACTION WITH OTHER SUBSTANCES

INTERACTS WITH	COMBINED EFFECT
Alcohol:	Decreased effect of guanadrel. Avoid.
Beverages: Caffeine	Decreased effect of guanadrel.
Cocaine:	Higher blood pressure. Avoid.
Foods:	No problems expected.
Marijuana:	Higher blood pressure. Avoid.
Tobacco:	Higher blood pressure. Avoid.

GUANETHIDINE

BRAND NAMES

Apo-Guanethidine
Esimil
Ismelin
Ismelin-Esidrix

GENERAL INFORMATION

Habit forming? No
Prescription needed? Yes
Available as generic? No
Drug class: Antihypertensive

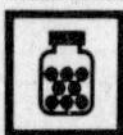

USES

Reduces high blood pressure.

DOSAGE & USAGE INFORMATION

How to take:
Tablet or capsule—Swallow with liquid. If you can't swallow tablet or capsule whole, crumble or open and take with liquid or food.

When to take:
At the same time each day.

If you forget a dose:
Take as soon as you remember up to 2 hours late. If more than 2 hours, wait for next scheduled dose (don't double this dose).

What drug does:
Displaces norepinephrine—hormone necessary to maintain small blood-vessel tone. Blood vessels relax and high blood pressure drops.

Time lapse before drug works:
Regular use for several weeks may be necessary to determine effectiveness.

Don't take with:
- Non-prescription drugs containing alcohol without consulting doctor.
- See Interaction column and consult doctor.

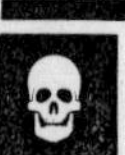

OVERDOSE

Symptoms:
Severe blood-pressure drop; fainting; slow, weak pulse; cold, sweaty skin; loss of consciousness.

What to do:
- Dial 0 (operator) or 911 (emergency) for an ambulance or medical help. Then give first aid immediately.
- Additional emergency information on page 886.

POSSIBLE ADVERSE REACTIONS OR SIDE EFFECTS

SYMPTOMS	FREQUENCY	WHAT TO DO
Brain & nervous system:		
Dizziness, headache.	Common	5
Skin:		
Rash	Infrequent	3
Eyes:		
Blurred vision, drooping eyelids.	Infrequent	3
Ears, nose, throat:		
Stuffy nose, dry mouth.	Common	6
Digestive:		
• Diarrhea, more bowel movements.	Common	4
• Nausea or vomiting.	Infrequent	4
Heart & lungs:		
• Chest pains or shortness of breath.	Infrequent	3
• Unusually slow heartbeat.	Common	3
Blood vessels, kidneys, liver, allergic, blood:	None expected.	
Muscles, bones, joints:		
• Muscle pain or tremors.	Infrequent	3
• Swollen feet, legs.	Common	4
Genital, urinary:		
• Impotence	Infrequent	5
• Nighttime urination.	Infrequent	5
Others:		
• Fatigue, weakness.	Common	4
• Lower sex drive.	Common	5

1- Life-threatening. Seek emergency treatment immediately.
2- Discontinue. Seek emergency treatment.
3- Discontinue. Call doctor right away.
4- Continue. Call doctor when convenient.
5- Continue. Tell doctor at next visit.
6- No action necessary.

WARNINGS & PRECAUTIONS

Don't take if:
- You are allergic to guanethidine.
- You have taken MAO inhibitors within 2 weeks.

Before you start, consult your doctor:
- If you have had stroke or heart disease.
- If you have asthma.
- If you have had kidney disease.
- If you have peptic ulcer or chronic acid indigestion.
- If you will have surgery within 2 months, including dental surgery, requiring general or spinal anesthesia.

Over age 60:
Adverse reactions and side effects may be more frequent and severe than in younger persons. Start with small doses and monitor blood pressure frequently.

Pregnancy:
No proven harm to unborn child. Avoid if possible.

Breast-feeding:
No proven harm to nursing infant. Avoid if possible.

Infants & children:
Not recommended.

Prolonged use:
Due to drug's cumulative effect, dose will require adjustment to prevent wide fluctuations in blood pressure.

Skin & sunlight:
No problems expected.

Driving, piloting or hazardous work:
Don't drive or pilot aircraft until you learn how medicine affects you. Don't work around dangerous machinery. Don't climb ladders or work in high places. Danger increases if you drink alcohol or take medicine affecting alertness and reflexes, such as antihistamines, tranquilizers, sedatives, pain medicine, narcotics and mind-altering drugs.

Airplane passengers:
No problems expected.

Discontinuing:
Don't discontinue without consulting doctor. Dose may require gradual reduction if you have taken drug for a long time. Doses of other drugs may also require adjustment.

Others:
Hot weather further lowers blood pressure.

INTERACTION WITH OTHER DRUGS

GENERIC NAME OR DRUG CLASS	COMBINED EFFECT
Amphetamines	Decreased guanethidine effect.
Antidepressants (tricyclic)	Decreased guanethidine effect.
Antihistamines	Decreased guanethidine effect.
Contraceptives (oral)	Decreased guanethidine effect.
Digitalis preparations	Slower heartbeat.
Diuretics (thiazide)	Increased guanethidine effect.
Rauwolfia alkaloids	Increased guanethidine effect.

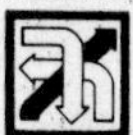

INTERACTION WITH OTHER SUBSTANCES

INTERACTS WITH	COMBINED EFFECT
Alcohol:	Use caution. Decreases blood pressure.
Beverages: Carbonated drinks	Use sparingly. Sodium content increases blood pressure.
Cocaine:	Raises blood pressure. Avoid.
Foods: Spicy or acid foods	Avoid if subject to indigestion or peptic ulcer.
Marijuana:	Excessively low blood pressure. Avoid.
Tobacco:	Possible blood-pressure rise. Avoid.

HALAZEPAM

BRAND NAMES

Paxipam

GENERAL INFORMATION

Habit forming? Yes
Prescription needed? Yes
Available as generic? No
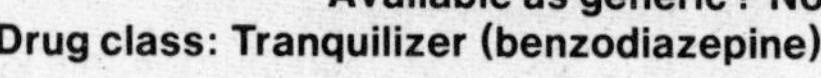
Drug class: Tranquilizer (benzodiazepine)

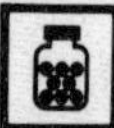

USES

Treatment for nervousness or tension.

DOSAGE & USAGE INFORMATION

How to take:
Tablet or capsule—Swallow with liquid. If you can't swallow whole, crumble tablet or open capsule and take with liquid or food.

When to take:
At the same time each day, according to instructions on prescription label.

If you forget a dose:
Take as soon as you remember up to 2 hours late. If more than 2 hours, wait for next scheduled dose (don't double this dose).

What drug does:
Affects limbic system of brain—part that controls emotions.

Time lapse before drug works:
2 hours. May take 6 weeks for full benefit.

Don't take with:
See Interaction column and consult doctor.

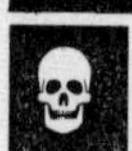

OVERDOSE

Symptoms:
Drowsiness, weakness, tremor, stupor, coma.

What to do:
- Dial 0 (operator) or 911 (emergency) for an ambulance or medical help. Then give first aid immediately.
- If patient is unconscious and not breathing, give mouth-to-mouth breathing. If there is no heartbeat, use cardiac massage and mouth-to-mouth breathing (CPR). Don't try to make patient vomit. If you can't get help quickly, take patient to nearest emergency facility.
- Additional emergency information on page 886.

POSSIBLE ADVERSE REACTIONS OR SIDE EFFECTS

SYMPTOMS	FREQUENCY	WHAT TO DO
Brain & nervous system:		
• Clumsiness, drowsiness, dizziness.	Common	4
• Hallucinations, confusion, depression, irritability.	Infrequent	3
Skin:		
Rash, itch.	Infrequent	3
Eyes:		
Vision changes.	Infrequent	3
Ears, nose, throat:		
Mouth, throat ulcers.	Rare	3
Digestive:		
Constipation or diarrhea, nausea, vomiting.	Infrequent	4
Heart & lungs:		
Slow heartbeat, breathing difficulty.	Rare	2
Blood vessels:	None expected.	
Muscles, bones, joints:	None expected.	
Genital, urinary:		
Urination difficulty.	Infrequent	4
Kidneys:	None expected.	
Liver:		
Jaundice (yellow eyes and skin).	Rare	3
Allergic:	None expected.	
Blood:	None expected.	
Others:	None expected.	

1- Life-threatening. Seek emergency treatment immediately.
2- Discontinue. Seek emergency treatment.
3- Discontinue. Call doctor right away.
4- Continue. Call doctor when convenient.
5- Continue. Tell doctor at next visit.
6- No action necessary.

WARNINGS & PRECAUTIONS

Don't take if:
- You are allergic to any benzodiazepine.
- You have myasthenia gravis.
- You are active or recovering alcoholic.
- Patient is younger than 6 months.

Before you start, consult your doctor:
- If you have liver, kidney or lung disease.
- If you have diabetes, epilepsy or porphyria.

Over age 60:
Adverse reactions and side effects may be more frequent and severe than in younger persons. You need smaller doses for shorter periods of time. May develop agitation, rage or "hangover effect."

Pregnancy:
Risk to unborn child outweighs drug benefits. Don't use.

Breast-feeding:
Drug passes into milk. Avoid drug or discontinue nursing until you finish medicine. Consult doctor for advice on maintaining milk supply.

Infants & children:
Use only under medical supervision for children older than 6 months.

Prolonged use:
May impair liver function.

Skin & sunlight:
No problems expected.

Driving, piloting or hazardous work:
Don't drive or pilot aircraft until you learn how medicine affects you. Don't work around dangerous machinery. Don't climb ladders or work in high places. Danger increases if you drink alcohol or take medicine affecting alertness and reflexes.

Airplane passengers:
No problems expected.

Discontinuing:
Don't discontinue without consulting doctor. Dose may require gradual reduction if you have taken drug for a long time. Doses of other drugs may also require adjustment.

Others:
- Hot weather, heavy exercise and profuse sweat may reduce excretion and cause overdose.
- Blood sugar may rise in diabetics, requiring insulin adjustment.

INTERACTION WITH OTHER DRUGS

GENERIC NAME OR DRUG CLASS	COMBINED EFFECT
Anticonvulsants	Change in seizure frequency or severity.
Antidepressants	Increased sedative effect of both drugs.
Antihistamines	Increased sedative effect of both drugs.
Antihypertensives	Excessively low blood pressure.
Cimetidine	Excess sedation.
Disulfiram	Increased halazepam effect.
MAO inhibitors	Convulsions, deep sedation, rage.
Narcotics	Increased sedative effect of both drugs.
Sedatives	Increased sedative effect of both drugs.
Sleep inducers	Increased sedative effect of both drugs.
Tranquilizers	Increased sedative effect of both drugs.

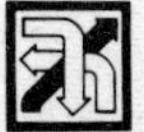

INTERACTION WITH OTHER SUBSTANCES

INTERACTS WITH	COMBINED EFFECT
Alcohol:	Heavy sedation. Avoid.
Beverages:	None expected.
Cocaine:	Decreased halazepam effect.
Foods:	None expected.
Marijuana:	Heavy sedation. Avoid.
Tobacco:	Decreased halazepam effect.

HALOPERIDOL

BRAND NAMES

Apo-Haloperidol
Haldol
Peridol

GENERAL INFORMATION

Habit forming? No
Prescription needed? Yes
Available as generic? No
Drug class: Tranquilizer (antipsychotic)

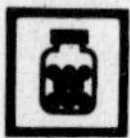

USES

Reduces severe anxiety, agitation and psychotic behavior.

DOSAGE & USAGE INFORMATION

How to take:

- Tablet or capsule—Swallow with liquid. If you can't swallow whole, crumble tablet or open capsule and take with liquid or food.
- Drops—Dilute dose in beverage before swallowing.

When to take:
At the same times each day.

If you forget a dose:
Take as soon as you remember up to 2 hours late. If more than 2 hours, wait for next scheduled dose (don't double this dose).

What drug does:
Corrects an imbalance in nerve impulses from brain.

Time lapse before drug works:
3 weeks to 2 months for maximum benefit.

Don't take with:

- Non-prescription drugs without consulting doctor.
- See Interaction column and consult doctor.

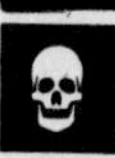

OVERDOSE

Symptoms:
Weak, rapid pulse; shallow, slow breathing; very low blood pressure; convulsions; deep sleep ending in coma.

What to do:

- Dial 0 (operator) or 911 (emergency) for an ambulance or medical help. Then give first aid immediately.
- If patient is unconscious and not breathing, give mouth-to-mouth breathing. If there is no heartbeat, use cardiac massage and mouth-to-mouth breathing (CPR). Don't try to make patient vomit. If you can't get help quickly, take patient to nearest emergency facility.
- Additional emergency information on page 886.

POSSIBLE ADVERSE REACTIONS OR SIDE EFFECTS

SYMPTOMS	FREQUENCY	WHAT TO DO
Brain & nervous system:		
• Shuffling, stiffness, jerkiness, trembling.	Common	4
• Dizziness, faintness, drowsiness.	Infrequent	4
Skin:		
Rash	Infrequent	3
Eyes:		
Blurred vision.	Common	3
Ears, nose, throat:		
• Dry mouth.	Common	6
• Circling motions of tongue.	Infrequent	3
• Sore throat, fever.	Rare	3
Digestive:		
• Constipation	Common	4
• Nausea or vomiting.	Infrequent	4
Heart & lungs, blood vessels, muscles, bones, joints, kidneys, allergic, blood:	None expected.	
Genital, urinary:		
• Urination difficulty.	Infrequent	4
• Decreased sexual ability.	Infrequent	4
Liver:		
Jaundice (yellow skin and eyes).	Rare	3

1-Life-threatening. Seek emergency treatment immediately.
2-Discontinue. Seek emergency treatment.
3-Discontinue. Call doctor right away.
4-Continue. Call doctor when convenient.
5-Continue. Tell doctor at next visit.
6-No action necessary.

WARNINGS & PRECAUTIONS

Don't take if:
- You have ever been allergic to haloperidol.
- You are depressed.
- You have Parkinson's disease.
- Patient is younger than 3 years old.

Before you start, consult your doctor:
- If you take sedatives, sleeping pills, tranquilizers, antidepressants, antihistamines, narcotics or mind-altering drugs.
- If you have a history of mental depression.
- If you have had kidney or liver problems.
- If you have diabetes, epilepsy, glaucoma, high blood pressure or heart disease.
- If you drink alcoholic beverages frequently.

Over age 60:
Adverse reactions and side effects may be more frequent and severe than in younger persons.

Pregnancy:
Risk to unborn child outweighs drug benefits. Don't use.

Breast-feeding:
No proven harm to nursing infant. Avoid if possible.

Infants & children:
Not recommended.

Prolonged use:
May develop tardive dyskinesia (involuntary movements of jaws, lips and tongue).

Skin & sunlight:
May cause rash or intensify sunburn in areas exposed to sun or sunlamp.

Driving, piloting or hazardous work:
Don't drive or pilot aircraft until you learn how medicine affects you. Don't work around dangerous machinery. Don't climb ladders or work in high places. Danger increases if you drink alcohol or take medicine affecting alertness and reflexes.

Airplane passengers:
Don't fly without medical advice.

Discontinuing:
Don't discontinue without consulting doctor. Dose may require gradual reduction if you have taken drug for a long time. Doses of other drugs may also require adjustment.

Others:
No problems expected.

INTERACTION WITH OTHER DRUGS

GENERIC NAME OR DRUG CLASS	COMBINED EFFECT
Anticholinergics	Increased anticholinergic effect. May cause pressure within the eye.
Anticoagulants (oral)	Decreased anticoagulant effect.
Anticonvulsants	Changed seizure pattern.
Antidepressants	Excessive sedation.
Antihistamines	Excessive sedation.
Antihypertensives	May cause severe blood-pressure drop.
Barbiturates	Excessive sedation.
Bethanidine	Decreased bethanidine effect.
Guanethidine	Decreased guanethidine effect.
Levodopa	Decreased levodopa effect.
Methyldopa	Possible psychosis.
Narcotics	Excessive sedation.
Sedatives	Excessive sedation.
Tranquilizers	Excessive sedation.

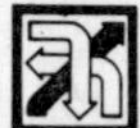

INTERACTION WITH OTHER SUBSTANCES

INTERACTS WITH	COMBINED EFFECT
Alcohol:	Excessive sedation and depressed brain function. Avoid.
Beverages:	None expected.
Cocaine:	Decreased effect of haloperidol. Avoid.
Foods:	None expected.
Marijuana:	Occasional use—Increased sedation. Frequent use—Possible toxic psychosis.
Tobacco:	None expected.

HETACILLIN

BRAND NAMES

Versapen
Versapen-K

GENERAL INFORMATION

Habit forming? No
Prescription needed? Yes
Available as generic? Yes
Drug class: Antibiotic (penicillin)

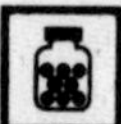

USES

Treatment of bacterial infections that are susceptible to hetacillin.

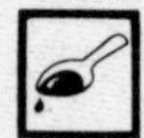

DOSAGE & USAGE INFORMATION

How to take:

- Tablets or capsules—Swallow with liquid on an empty stomach 1 hour before or 2 hours after eating.
- Liquid—Take with cold beverage. Liquid form is perishable and effective for only 7 days at room temperature. Effective for 14 days if stored in refrigerator. Don't freeze.

When to take:
Follow instructions on prescription label or side of package. Doses should be evenly spaced. For example, 4 times a day means every 6 hours.

If you forget a dose:
Take as soon as you remember. Continue regular schedule.

What drug does:
Destroys susceptible bacteria. Does not kill viruses.

Time lapse before drug works:
May be several days before medicine affects infection.

Don't take with:
See Interaction column and consult doctor.

OVERDOSE

Symptoms:
Severe diarrhea, nausea or vomiting.

What to do:
Overdose unlikely to threaten life. If person takes much larger amount than prescribed, call doctor, poison-control center or hospital emergency room for instructions.

POSSIBLE ADVERSE REACTIONS OR SIDE EFFECTS

SYMPTOMS	FREQUENCY	WHAT TO DO
Brain & nervous system:	None expected.	
Skin: Hives, rash, intense itch soon after a dose.	Rare	1
Eyes:	None expected.	
Ears, nose, throat: Dark or discolored tongue.	Common	5
Digestive: Nausea, vomiting, diarrhea.	Infrequent	4
Heart & lungs:	None expected.	
Blood vessels: Unexplained bleeding.	Rare	3
Muscles, bones, joints:	None expected.	
Genital, urinary:	None expected.	
Kidneys:	None expected.	
Liver:	None expected.	
Allergic: Life-threatening anaphylaxis may occur!	Rare	1 See page 888.
Blood:	None expected.	
Others:	None expected.	

1- Life-threatening. Seek emergency treatment immediately.
2- Discontinue. Seek emergency treatment.
3- Discontinue. Call doctor right away.
4- Continue. Call doctor when convenient.
5- Continue. Tell doctor at next visit.
6- No action necessary.

WARNINGS & PRECAUTIONS

Don't take if:
You are allergic to hetacillin, cephalosporin antibiotics, other penicillins or penicillamine. Life-threatening reaction may occur.

Before you start, consult your doctor:
If you are allergic to any substance or drug.

Over age 60:
You may have skin reactions, particularly around genitals and anus.

Pregnancy:
Studies inconclusive on harm to unborn child. Animal studies show fetal abnormalities. Decide with your doctor whether drug benefits justify risk to unborn child.

Breast-feeding:
Drug passes into milk. Child may become sensitive to penicillins and have allergic reactions to penicillin drugs. Avoid hetacillin or discontinue nursing until you finish medicine. Consult doctor for advice on maintaining milk supply.

Infants & children:
No problems expected.

Prolonged use:
You may become more susceptible to infections caused by germs not responsive to hetacillin.

Skin & sunlight:
No problems expected.

Driving, piloting or hazardous work:
Usually not dangerous. Most hazardous reactions likely to occur a few minutes after taking hetacillin.

Airplane passengers:
No problems expected.

Discontinuing:
Don't discontinue without doctor's advice until you complete prescribed dose, even though symptoms diminish or disappear.

Others:
Urine sugar test for diabetes may show false positive result.

INTERACTION WITH OTHER DRUGS

GENERIC NAME OR DRUG CLASS	COMBINED EFFECT
Chloramphenicol	Decreased effect of both drugs.
Erythromycins	Decreased effect of both drugs.
Paromomycin	Decreased effect of both drugs.
Tetracyclines	Decreased effect of both drugs.
Troleandomycin	Decreased effect of both drugs.

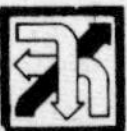

INTERACTION WITH OTHER SUBSTANCES

INTERACTS WITH	COMBINED EFFECT
Alcohol:	Occasional stomach irritation.
Beverages:	None expected.
Cocaine:	No proven problems.
Foods:	None expected.
Marijuana:	No proven problems.
Tobacco:	None expected.

HEXOBARBITAL

BRAND NAMES

Sombulex

GENERAL INFORMATION

Habit forming? Yes
Prescription needed? Yes
Available as generic? Yes
Drug class: Sedative, hypnotic (barbiturate)

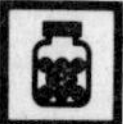

USES

- Reduces anxiety or nervous tension (low dose).
- Relieves insomnia (higher bedtime dose).

DOSAGE & USAGE INFORMATION

How to take:
Tablet—Swallow with liquid or food to lessen stomach irritation. If you can't swallow whole, crumble tablet and take with liquid or food.

When to take:
At the same times each day.

If you forget a dose:
Take as soon as you remember up to 2 hours late. If more than 2 hours, wait for next scheduled dose (don't double this dose).

What drug does:
May partially block nerve impulses at nerve-cell connections.

Time lapse before drug works:
60 minutes.

Don't take with:
- Non-prescription drugs without consulting doctor.
- See Interaction column and consult doctor.

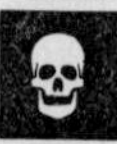

OVERDOSE

Symptoms:
Deep sleep, weak pulse, coma.

What to do:
- Dial 0 (operator) or 911 (emergency) for an ambulance or medical help. Then give first aid immediately.
- If patient is unconscious and not breathing, give mouth-to-mouth breathing. If there is no heartbeat use cardiac massage and mouth-to-mouth breathing (CPR). Don't try to make patient vomit. If you can't help quickly, take patient to nearest emergency facility.
- Additional emergency information on page 886.

POSSIBLE ADVERSE REACTIONS OR SIDE EFFECTS

SYMPTOMS	FREQUENCY	WHAT TO DO
Brain & nervous system:		
• Dizziness, drowsiness, "hangover effect."	Common	4
• Depression, confusion, slurred speech.	Infrequent	4
• Agitation	Rare	3
Skin:		
• Rash or hives.	Infrequent	3
• Face, lip swelling.	Infrequent	3
Eyes:		
Eyelid swelling.	Infrequent	3
Ears, nose, throat:		
Sore throat, fever.	Infrequent	3
Digestive:		
Diarrhea, nausea, vomiting.	Infrequent	4
Heart & lungs:		
• Slow heartbeat.	Rare	3
• Breathing difficulty.	Rare	3
Blood vessels:		
Unexplained bleeding or bruising.	Rare	4
Muscles, bones, joints:		
Joint or muscle pain.	Infrequent	4
Genital, urinary:	None expected.	
Kidneys:	None expected.	
Liver:		
Jaundice (yellow skin and eyes).	Rare	3
Allergic:	None expected.	
Blood:	None expected.	
Others:	None expected.	

1 - Life-threatening. Seek emergency treatment immediately.
2 - Discontinue. Seek emergency treatment.
3 - Discontinue. Call doctor right away.
4 - Continue. Call doctor when convenient.

HEXOBARBITAL

WARNINGS & PRECAUTIONS

Don't take if:
- You are allergic to any barbiturate.
- You have porphyria.

Before you start, consult your doctor:
- If you have epilepsy.
- If you have kidney or liver damage.
- If you have asthma.
- If you have anemia.
- If you have chronic pain.
- If you will have surgery within 2 months, including dental surgery, requiring general or spinal anesthesia.

Over age 60:
Adverse reactions and side effects may be more frequent and severe than in younger persons. Use small doses.

Pregnancy:
Risk to unborn child outweighs drug benefits. Don't use.

Breast-feeding:
Drug passes into milk. Avoid drug or discontinue nursing until you finish medicine. Consult doctor for advice on maintaining milk supply.

Infants & children:
Use only under doctor's supervision.

Prolonged use:
- May cause addiction, anemia, chronic intoxication.
- May lower body temperature, making exposure to cold temperatures hazardous.

Skin & sunlight:
May cause rash or intensify sunburn in areas exposed to sun or sunlamp.

Driving, piloting or hazardous work:
Don't drive or pilot aircraft until you learn how medicine affects you. Don't work around dangerous machinery. Don't climb ladders or work in high places. Danger increases if you drink alcohol or take medicine affecting alertness and reflexes.

Airplane passengers:
No problems expected.

Discontinuing:
May be unnecessary to finish medicine. Follow doctor's instructions. If you develop withdrawal symptoms of hallucinations, agitation or sleeplessness after discontinuing, call doctor right away.

Others:
No problems expected.

INTERACTION WITH OTHER DRUGS

GENERIC NAME OR DRUG CLASS	COMBINED EFFECT
Anticoagulants (oral)	Decreased anticoagulant effect.
Anticonvulsants	Changed seizure patterns.
Antidepressants (tricyclic)	Decreased antidepressant effect.
Antidiabetics (oral)	Increased hexobarbital effect.
Antihistamines	Dangerous sedation. Avoid.
Antiinflammatory drugs (non-steroidal)	Decreased antiinflammatory effect.
Aspirin	Decreased aspirin effect.
Beta-adrenergic blockers	Decreased effect of beta-adrenergic blocker.
Contraceptives (oral)	Decreased contraceptive effect.
Cortisone drugs	Decreased cortisone effect.
Digitoxin	Decreased digitoxin effect.
Doxycycline	Decreased doxycycline effect.
Griseofulvin	Decreased griseofulvin effect.

Additional interactions on page 837.

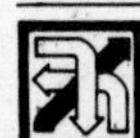

INTERACTION WITH OTHER SUBSTANCES

INTERACTS WITH	COMBINED EFFECT
Alcohol:	Possible fatal oversedation. Avoid.
Beverages:	None expected.
Cocaine:	Decreased hexobarbital effect.
Foods:	None expected.
Marijuana:	Excessive sedation. Avoid.
Tobacco:	None expected.

HYDRALAZINE

BRAND NAMES

Apresazide
Apresoline
H-H-R
Hydralazide
Rolazine
Ser-Ap-Es
Serpasil-Apresoline
Unipes
Uniserp

GENERAL INFORMATION

Habit forming? No
Prescription needed? Yes
Available as generic? Yes
Drug class: Antihypertensive

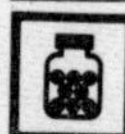

USES

Treatment for high blood pressure and congestive heart failure.

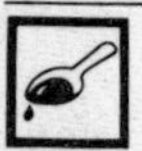

DOSAGE & USAGE INFORMATION

How to take:
Tablet or capsule—Swallow with liquid. If you can't swallow whole, crumble tablet or open capsule and take with liquid or food.

When to take:
At the same time each day.

If you forget a dose:
Take as soon as you remember up to 2 hours late. If more than 2 hours, wait for next scheduled dose (don't double this dose).

What drug does:
Relaxes and expands blood-vessel walls, lowering blood pressure.

Time lapse before drug works:
Regular use for several weeks may be necessary to determine drug's effectiveness.

Don't take with:
- Non-prescription drugs containing alcohol without consulting doctor.
- See Interaction column and consult doctor.

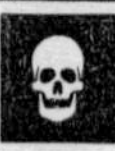

OVERDOSE

Symptoms:
Rapid and weak heartbeat, fainting, extreme weakness, cold and sweaty skin.

What to do:
- Dial 0 (operator) or 911 (emergency) for an ambulance or medical help. Then give first aid immediately.
- If patient is unconscious and not breathing, give mouth-to-mouth breathing. If there is no heartbeat, use cardiac massage and mouth-to-mouth breathing (CPR). Don't try to make patient vomit. If you can't get help quickly, take patient to nearest emergency facility.
- Additional emergency information on page 886.

POSSIBLE ADVERSE REACTIONS OR SIDE EFFECTS

SYMPTOMS	FREQUENCY	WHAT TO DO
Brain & nervous system:		
• Headache	Common	5
• Confusion, dizziness.	Infrequent	4
Skin:		
• Hives or rash.	Infrequent	3
• Flushed face.	Infrequent	3
Eyes:		
Watering, irritation.	Infrequent	5
Ears, nose, throat:		
Sore throat, fever.	Infrequent	3
Digestive:		
• Diarrhea, appetite loss.	Common	5
• Nausea or vomiting.	Common	3
• Constipation	Infrequent	5
Heart & lungs:		
• Chest pain.	Infrequent	3
• Rapid or irregular heartbeat.	Common	3
Blood vessels, kidneys, allergic, blood:	None expected.	
Muscles, bones, joints:		
Joint pain.	Infrequent	4
Genital, urinary:		
Difficult urination.	Common	5
Liver:		
Jaundice (yellow skin and eyes).	Rare	3
Others:		
• Swelling of lymph glands.	Infrequent	3
• General discomfort or weakness.	Infrequent	4

1- Life-threatening. Seek emergency treatment immediately.
2- Discontinue. Seek emergency treatment.
3- Discontinue. Call doctor right away.
4- Continue. Call doctor when convenient.
5- Continue. Tell doctor at next visit.

WARNINGS & PRECAUTIONS

Don't take if:
- You are allergic to hydralazine.
- You have history of coronary-artery disease or rheumatic heart disease.

Before you start, consult your doctor:
- If you feel pain in chest, neck or arms on physical exertion.
- If you have had lupus.
- If you have had a stroke.
- If you have had kidney disease or impaired kidney function.
- If you will have surgery within 2 months, including dental surgery, requiring general or spinal anesthesia.

Over age 60:
Adverse reactions and side effects may be more frequent and severe than in younger persons.

Pregnancy:
Risk to unborn child outweighs drug benefits. Don't use.

Breast-feeding:
Drug filters into milk. May harm child. Avoid.

Infants & children:
Not recommended.

Prolonged use:
- May cause lupus (arthritis-like illness).
- Possible psychosis.
- May cause numbness, tingling in hands or feet.

Skin & sunlight:
No problems expected.

Driving, piloting or hazardous work:
Don't drive or pilot aircraft until you learn how medicine affects you. Don't work around dangerous machinery. Don't climb ladders or work in high places. Danger increases if you drink alcohol or take medicine affecting alertness and reflexes, such as antihistamines, tranquilizers, sedatives, pain medicine, narcotics and mind-altering drugs.

Airplane passengers:
No problems expected.

Discontinuing:
Don't discontinue without doctor's advice until you complete prescribed dose, even though symptoms diminish or disappear.

Others:
Vitamin B-6 diet supplement may be advisable. Consult doctor.

INTERACTION WITH OTHER DRUGS

GENERIC NAME OR DRUG CLASS	COMBINED EFFECT
Amphetamines	Decreased hydralazine effect.
Antidepressants (tricyclic)	Increased hydralazine effect.
Antihypertensives (other)	Increased antihypertensive effect.
Diuretics (oral)	Increased hydralazine effect.
MAO inhibitors	Increased hydralazine effect.

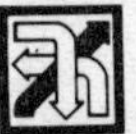

INTERACTION WITH OTHER SUBSTANCES

INTERACTS WITH	COMBINED EFFECT
Alcohol:	May lower blood pressure excessively. Use extreme caution.
Beverages:	None expected.
Cocaine:	Dangerous blood-pressure rise. Avoid.
Foods:	Increased hydralazine absorption.
Marijuana:	Weakness on standing.
Tobacco:	Possible angina attacks.

HYDROCHLOROTHIAZIDE

BRAND NAMES

Aldactazide	Hydrid	Inderide
Apresazide	Hydro-Aquil	Neo-Codema
Diuchlor H	HydroDIURIL	Novohydrazide
Dyazide	Hydrozide-Z-50	Oretic
Esidrix	Hyperetic	Thiuretic

See complete brand names list, page 827.

GENERAL INFORMATION

Habit forming? No
Prescription needed? Yes
Available as generic? Yes
Drug class: Antihypertensive, diuretic (thiazide)

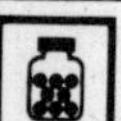

USES

- Controls, but doesn't cure, high blood pressure.
- Reduces fluid retention (edema).

DOSAGE & USAGE INFORMATION

How to take:
Tablet or capsule—Swallow with liquid. If you can't swallow whole, crumble tablet or open capsule and take with liquid or food.

When to take:
At the same time each day.

If you forget a dose:
Take as soon as you remember up to 2 hours late. If more than 2 hours, wait for next scheduled dose (don't double this dose).

What drug does:
- Forces sodium and water excretion, reducing body fluid.
- Relaxes muscle cells of small arteries.
- Reduced body fluid and relaxed arteries lower blood pressure.

Time lapse before drug works:
4 to 6 hours. May require several weeks to lower blood pressure.

Don't take with:
- See Interaction column and consult doctor.
- Non-prescription drugs without consulting doctor.

OVERDOSE

Symptoms:
Cramps, weakness, drowsiness, weak pulse, coma.

What to do:
- Dial 0 (operator) or 911 (emergency) for an ambulance or medical help. Then give first aid immediately.
- Additional emergency information on page 886.

POSSIBLE ADVERSE REACTIONS OR SIDE EFFECTS

SYMPTOMS	FREQUENCY	WHAT TO DO
Brain & nervous system:		
• Dizziness	Infrequent	4
• Mood changes.	Infrequent	4
• Headaches	Infrequent	4
Skin:		
Rash or hives.	Rare	2
Eyes:		
Blurred vision.	Infrequent	3
Ears, nose, throat:		
• Sore throat, fever.	Rare	3
• Dry mouth, thirst.	Infrequent	5
Digestive:		
Severe abdominal pain, nausea, vomiting.	Infrequent	3
Heart & lungs:		
Irregular heartbeat, weak pulse.	Infrequent	3
Blood vessels:	None expected.	
Muscles, bones, joints:		
Weakness, tiredness.	Infrequent	4
Genital, urinary:	None expected.	
Kidneys:	None expected.	
Liver:		
Jaundice (yellow skin and eyes).	Rare	3
Allergic:	None expected.	
Blood:	None expected.	
Others:		
Weight changes.	Infrequent	4

1-Life-threatening. Seek emergency treatment immediately.
2-Discontinue. Seek emergency treatment.
3-Discontinue. Call doctor right away.
4-Continue. Call doctor when convenient.
5-Continue. Tell doctor at next visit.
6-No action necessary.

WARNINGS & PRECAUTIONS

Don't take if:
You are allergic to any thiazide diuretic drug.

Before you start, consult your doctor:
- If you are allergic to any sulfa drug.
- If you have gout.
- If you have liver, pancreas or kidney disorder.

Over age 60:
Adverse reactions and side effects may be more frequent and severe than in younger persons, especially dizziness and excessive potassium loss.

Pregnancy:
Risk to unborn child outweighs drug benefits. Don't use.

Breast-feeding:
Drug passes into milk. Avoid drug or discontinue nursing.

Infants & children:
No problems expected.

Prolonged use:
You may need medicine to treat high blood pressure for the rest of your life.

Skin & sunlight:
May cause rash or intensify sunburn in areas exposed to sun or sunlamp.

Driving, piloting or hazardous work:
Don't drive or pilot aircraft until you learn how medicine affects you. Don't work around dangerous machinery. Don't climb ladders or work in high places. Danger increases if you drink alcohol or take medicine affecting alertness and reflexes, such as antihistamines, tranquilizers, sedatives, pain medicine, narcotics and mind-altering drugs.

Airplane passengers:
No problems expected.

Discontinuing:
Don't discontinue without medical advice.

Others:
- Hot weather and fever may cause dehydration and drop in blood pressure. Dose may require temporary adjustment. Weigh daily and report any unexpected weight decreases to your doctor.
- May cause rise in uric acid, leading to gout.
- May cause blood-sugar rise in diabetics.

INTERACTION WITH OTHER DRUGS

GENERIC NAME OR DRUG CLASS	COMBINED EFFECT
Allopurinol	Decreased allopurinol effect.
Antidepressants (tricyclic)	Dangerous drop in blood pressure. Avoid combination unless under medical supervision.
Barbiturates	Increased hydrochlorothiazide effect.
Cholestyramine	Decreased hydrochlorothiazide effect.
Cortisone drugs	Excessive potassium loss that causes dangerous heart rhythms.
Digitalis preparations	Excessive potassium loss that causes dangerous heart rhythms.
Diuretics (thiazide)	Increased effect of other thiazide diuretics.
Lithium	Increased effect of lithium.
MAO inhibitors	Increased hydrochlorothiazide effect.
Probenecid	Decreased probenecid effect.

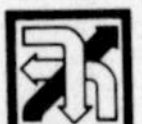

INTERACTION WITH OTHER SUBSTANCES

INTERACTS WITH	COMBINED EFFECT
Alcohol:	Dangerous blood-pressure drop.
Beverages:	None expected.
Cocaine:	None expected.
Foods:	
Licorice	Excessive potassium loss that causes dangerous heart rhythms.
Marijuana:	May increase blood pressure.
Tobacco:	None expected.

HYDROCORTISONE (CORTISOL)

BRAND NAMES

A-hydroCort
Biosone
Cortef
Cortef Fluid
Cortenema
Cortifoam
Fernisone
Hydrocortone
Proctocort
Rectoid
Solu-Cortef
Texacort

See complete brand names list, page 827.

GENERAL INFORMATION

Habit forming? No
Prescription needed? Yes
Available as generic? Yes
Drug class: Cortisone drug (adrenal corticosteroid)

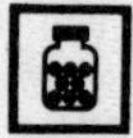

USES

- Reduces inflammation caused by many different medical problems.
- Treatment for some allergic diseases, blood disorders, kidney diseases, asthma and emphysema.
- Replaces corticosteroid deficiencies.

DOSAGE & USAGE INFORMATION

How to take:
- Tablet or liquid—Swallow with liquid or food to lessen stomach irritation. If you can't swallow whole, crumble tablet.
- Other forms—Follow label instructions.

When to take:
At the same times each day. Take once-a-day or once-every-other-day doses in mornings.

If you forget a dose:
- Several-doses-per-day prescription—Take as soon as you remember up to 2 hours late. If more than 2 hours, wait for next scheduled dose (don't double this dose).
- Once-a-day dose or less—Wait for next dose. Double this dose.

What drug does:
Decreases inflammatory responses.

Time lapse before drug works:
2 to 4 days.

Don't take with:
See Interaction column and consult doctor.

OVERDOSE

Symptoms:
Headache, convulsions, heart failure.

What to do:
- Dial 0 (operator) or 911 (emergency) for an ambulance or medical help. Then give first aid immediately.
- Additional emergency information on page 886.

POSSIBLE ADVERSE REACTIONS OR SIDE EFFECTS

SYMPTOMS	FREQUENCY	WHAT TO DO
Brain & nervous system:		
Mood changes, insomnia, restlessness.	Infrequent	4
Skin:		
• Acne	Common	4
• Rash	Rare	3
• Poor wound healing.	Common	4
Eyes:		
Blurred vision, halos around lights.	Infrequent	3
Ears, nose, throat:		
• Sore throat, fever.	Infrequent	3
• Thirst	Common	4
Digestive:		
• Indigestion, nausea, vomiting.	Common	4
• Bloody or black, tarry stool.	Infrequent	2
Heart & lungs:		
Irregular heartbeat.	Rare	2
Blood vessels, kidneys, liver, allergic, blood:	None expected.	
Muscles, bones, joints:		
Muscle cramps, swollen legs, feet.	Infrequent	3
Genital, urinary:		
Frequent urination.	Infrequent	4
Others:		
• Weight gain, round face.	Infrequent	4
• Fatigue, weakness.	Infrequent	4
• TB recurrence.	Infrequent	4
• Irregular menstrual periods.	Infrequent	4

1-Life-threatening. Seek emergency treatment immediately.
2-Discontinue. Seek emergency treatment.
3-Discontinue. Call doctor right away.
4-Continue. Call doctor when convenient.

HYDROCORTISONE (CORTISOL)

WARNINGS & PRECAUTIONS

Don't take if:
- You are allergic to any cortisone drug.
- You have tuberculosis or fungus infection.
- You have herpes infection of eyes, lips or genitals.

Before you start, consult your doctor:
- If you have had tuberculosis.
- If you have congestive heart failure.
- If you have diabetes.
- If you have peptic ulcer.
- If you have glaucoma.
- If you have underactive thyroid.
- If you have high blood pressure.
- If you have myasthenia gravis.
- If you have blood clots in legs or lungs.

Over age 60:
Adverse reactions and side effects may be more frequent and severe than in younger persons. Likely to aggravate edema, diabetes or ulcers. Likely to cause cataracts and osteoporosis (softening of the bones).

Pregnancy:
Risk to unborn child outweighs drug benefits. Don't use.

Breast-feeding:
Drug passes into milk. Avoid drug or discontinue nursing until you finish medicine. Consult doctor for advice on maintaining milk supply.

Infants & children:
Use only under medical supervision.

Prolonged use:
- Retards growth in children.
- Possible glaucoma, cataracts, diabetes, fragile bones and thin skin.
- Functional dependence.

Skin & sunlight:
No problems expected.

Driving, piloting or hazardous work:
No problems expected.

Airplane passengers:
No problems expected.

Discontinuing:
- Don't discontinue without doctor's advice until you complete prescribed dose, even though symptoms diminish or disappear.
- Drug affects your response to surgery, illness, injury or stress for 2 years after discontinuing. Tell about drug to anyone who takes medical care of you within 2 years.

Others:
Avoid immunizations if possible.

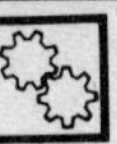

INTERACTION WITH OTHER DRUGS

GENERIC NAME OR DRUG CLASS	COMBINED EFFECT
Amphoterecin B	Potassium depletion.
Anticholinergics	Possible glaucoma.
Anticoagulants (oral)	Decreased anticoagulant effect.
Anticonvulsants (hydantoin)	Decreased hydrocortisone effect.
Antidiabetics (oral)	Decreased antidiabetic effect.
Antihistamines	Decreased hydrocortisone effect.
Aspirin	Increased hydrocortisone effect.
Barbiturates	Decreased hydrocortisone effect. Oversedation.
Beta-adrenergic blockers	Decreased hydrocortisone effect.
Chloral hydrate	Decreased hydrocortisone effect.
Chlorthalidone	Potassium depletion.
Cholinergics	Decreased cholinergic effect.
Contraceptives (oral)	Increased hydrocortisone effect.
Digitalis preparations	Dangerous potassium depletion. Possible digitalis toxicity.
Diuretics (thiazide)	Potassium depletion.

Additional interactions on page 838.

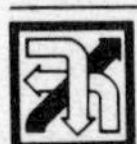

INTERACTION WITH OTHER SUBSTANCES

INTERACTS WITH	COMBINED EFFECT
Alcohol:	Risk of stomach ulcers.
Beverages:	No proven problems.
Cocaine:	Overstimulation. Avoid.
Foods:	No proven problems.
Marijuana:	Decreased immunity.
Tobacco:	Increased hydrocortisone effect. Possible toxicity.

HYDROFLUMETHIAZIDE

BRAND NAMES

Diucardin
Hydro-Fluserpine #1 & #2
Saluron
Salutensin

GENERAL INFORMATION

Habit forming? No
Prescription needed? Yes
Available as generic? Yes
Drug class: Antihypertensive, diuretic (thiazide)

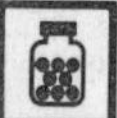

USES

- Controls, but doesn't cure, high blood pressure.
- Reduces fluid retention (edema) caused by conditions such as heart disorders and liver disease.

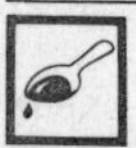

DOSAGE & USAGE INFORMATION

How to take:
Tablet or capsule—Swallow with liquid. If you can't swallow whole, crumble tablet or open capsule and take with liquid or food. Don't exceed dose.

When to take:
At the same time each day.

If you forget a dose:
Take as soon as you remember up to 2 hours late. If more than 2 hours, wait for next scheduled dose (don't double this dose).

What drug does:
- Forces sodium and water excretion, reducing body fluid.
- Relaxes muscle cells of small arteries.
- Reduced body fluid and relaxed arteries lower blood pressure.

Time lapse before drug works:
4 to 6 hours. May require several weeks to lower blood pressure.

Don't take with:
- See Interaction column and consult doctor.
- Non-prescription drugs without consulting doctor.

OVERDOSE

Symptoms:
Cramps, weakness, drowsiness, weak pulse, coma.

What to do:
- Dial 0 (operator) or 911 (emergency) for an ambulance or medical help. Then give first aid immediately.
- Additional emergency information on page 886.

POSSIBLE ADVERSE REACTIONS OR SIDE EFFECTS

SYMPTOMS	FREQUENCY	WHAT TO DO
Brain & nervous system:		
• Dizziness	Infrequent	4
• Mood changes.	Infrequent	4
• Headaches	Infrequent	4
Skin:		
Rash or hives.	Rare	2
Eyes:		
Blurred vision.	Infrequent	3
Ears, nose, throat:		
• Sore throat, fever.	Rare	3
• Dry mouth, thirst.	Infrequent	5
Digestive:		
Severe abdominal pain, nausea, vomiting.	Infrequent	3
Heart & lungs:		
Irregular heartbeat, weak pulse.	Infrequent	3
Blood vessels:	None expected.	
Muscles, bones, joints:		
Weakness, tiredness.	Infrequent	4
Genital, urinary:	None expected.	
Kidneys:	None expected.	
Liver:		
Jaundice (yellow skin and eyes).	Rare	3
Allergic:	None expected.	
Blood:	None expected.	
Others:		
Weight changes.	Infrequent	4

1- Life-threatening. Seek emergency treatment immediately.
2- Discontinue. Seek emergency treatment.
3- Discontinue. Call doctor right away.
4- Continue. Call doctor when convenient.
5- Continue. Tell doctor at next visit.
6- No action necessary.

WARNINGS & PRECAUTIONS

Don't take if:
You are allergic to any thiazide diuretic drug.

Before you start, consult your doctor:
- If you are allergic to any sulfa drug.
- If you have gout.
- If you have liver, pancreas or kidney disorder.

Over age 60:
Adverse reactions and side effects may be more frequent and severe than in younger persons, especially dizziness and excessive potassium loss.

Pregnancy:
Risk to unborn child outweighs drug benefits. Don't use.

Breast-feeding:
Drug passes into milk. Avoid drug or discontinue nursing.

Infants & children:
No problems expected.

Prolonged use:
You may need medicine to treat high blood pressure for the rest of your life.

Skin & sunlight:
May cause rash or intensify sunburn in areas exposed to sun or sunlamp.

Driving, piloting or hazardous work:
Don't drive or pilot aircraft until you learn how medicine affects you. Don't work around dangerous machinery. Don't climb ladders or work in high places. Danger increases if you drink alcohol or take medicine affecting alertness and reflexes, such as antihistamines, tranquilizers, sedatives, pain medicine, narcotics and mind-altering drugs.

Airplane passengers:
No problems expected.

Discontinuing:
Don't discontinue without medical advice.

Others:
- Hot weather and fever may cause dehydration and drop in blood pressure. Dose may require temporary adjustment. Weigh daily and report any unexpected weight decreases to your doctor.
- May cause rise in uric acid, leading to gout.
- May cause blood-sugar rise in diabetics.

INTERACTION WITH OTHER DRUGS

GENERIC NAME OR DRUG CLASS	COMBINED EFFECT
Allopurinol	Decreased allopurinol effect.
Antidepressants (tricyclic)	Dangerous drop in blood pressure. Avoid combination unless under medical supervision.
Barbiturates	Increased hydroflumethiazide effect.
Cholestyramine	Decreased hydroflumethiazide effect.
Cortisone drugs	Excessive potassium loss that causes dangerous heart rhythms.
Digitalis preparations	Excessive potassium loss that causes dangerous heart rhythms.
Diuretics (thiazide)	Increased effect of other thiazide diuretics.
Lithium	Increased effect of lithium.
MAO inhibitors	Increased hydroflumethiazide effect.
Probenecid	Decreased probenecid effect.

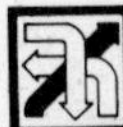

INTERACTION WITH OTHER SUBSTANCES

INTERACTS WITH	COMBINED EFFECT
Alcohol:	Dangerous blood-pressure drop.
Beverages:	None expected.
Cocaine:	None expected.
Foods:	
Licorice	Excessive potassium loss that causes dangerous heart rhythms.
Marijuana:	May increase blood pressure.
Tobacco:	None expected.

HYDROXYCHLOROQUINE

BRAND NAMES

Plaquenil

GENERAL INFORMATION

Habit forming? No
Prescription needed? Yes
Available as generic? Yes
Drug class: Antiprotozoal, antirheumatic

USES

- Treatment for protozoal infections, such as malaria and amebiasis.
- Treatment for some forms of arthritis and lupus.

DOSAGE & USAGE INFORMATION

How to take:
Tablet—Swallow with food or milk to lessen stomach irritation.

When to take:
- Depends on condition. Is adjusted during treatment.
- Malaria prevention—Begin taking medicine 2 weeks before entering areas with malaria.

If you forget a dose:
- 1 or more doses a day—Take as soon as you remember up to 2 hours late. If more than 2 hours, wait for next scheduled dose (don't double this dose).
- 1 dose weekly—Take as soon as possible, then return to regular dosing schedule.

What drug does:
- Inhibits parasite multiplication.
- Decreases inflammatory response in diseased joint.

Time lapse before drug works:
1 to 2 hours.

Don't take with:
See Interaction column and consult doctor.

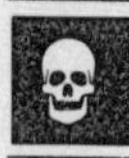

OVERDOSE

Symptoms:
Severe breathing difficulty, drowsiness, faintness.

What to do:
- Dial 0 (operator) or 911 (emergency) for an ambulance or medical help. Then give first aid immediately.
- Additional emergency information on page 886.

POSSIBLE ADVERSE REACTIONS OR SIDE EFFECTS

SYMPTOMS	FREQUENCY	WHAT TO DO
Brain & nervous system:		
• Mood or mental changes, seizures.	Rare	3
• Headache	Common	5
Skin:		
Rash or itch.	Infrequent	4
Eyes:		
Blurred or changed vision.	Infrequent	3
Ears, nose, throat:		
• Ringing or buzzing in ears, hearing loss.	Rare	4
• Sore throat, fever.	Rare	3
Digestive:		
Diarrhea, nausea, vomiting.	Infrequent	4
Heart & lungs:	None expected.	
Blood vessels:		
Unusual bleeding or bruising.	Rare	3
Muscles, bones, joints:		
Muscle weakness.	Rare	3
Genital, urinary:	None expected.	
Kidneys:	None expected.	
Liver:	None expected.	
Allergic:	None expected.	
Blood:	None expected.	
Others:	None expected.	

1-Life threatening. Seek emergency treatment immediately.
2-Discontinue. Seek emergency treatment.
3-Discontinue. Call doctor right away.
4-Continue. Call doctor when convenient.
5-Continue. Tell doctor at next visit.
6-No action necessary.

WARNINGS & PRECAUTIONS

Don't take if:
You are allergic to chloroquine or hydroxychloroquine.

Before you start, consult your doctor:
- If you plan to become pregnant within the medication period.
- If you have blood disease.
- If you have eye or vision problems.
- If you have a G6PD deficiency.
- If you have liver disease.
- If you have nerve or brain disease (including seizure disorders).
- If you have porphyria.
- If you have psoriasis.
- If you have stomach or intestinal disease.
- If you drink more than 3 oz. of alcohol daily.

Over age 60:
Adverse reactions and side effects may be more frequent and severe than in younger persons.

Pregnancy:
Risk to unborn child outweighs drug benefits. Don't use.

Breast-feeding:
Drug passes into milk. Avoid drug or discontinue nursing.

Infants & children:
Not recommended. Dangerous.

Prolonged use:
Permanent damage to the retina (back part of the eye) or nerve deafness.

Skin & sunlight:
May cause rash or intensify sunburn in areas exposed to sun or sunlamp.

Driving, piloting or hazardous work:
Don't drive or pilot aircraft until you learn how medicine affects you. Don't work around dangerous machinery. Don't climb ladders or work in high places. Danger increases if you drink alcohol or take medicine affecting alertness and reflexes.

Airplane passengers:
No problems expected.

Discontinuing:
Don't discontinue without doctor's advice until you complete prescribed dose, even though symptoms diminish or disappear.

Others:
- Periodic physical and blood examinations recommended.
- If you are in a malaria area for a long time, you may need to change to another preventive drug every 2 years.

INTERACTION WITH OTHER DRUGS

GENERIC NAME OR DRUG CLASS	COMBINED EFFECT
Estrogens	Possible liver toxicity.
Gold compounds	Risk of severe rash and itch.
Oxyphenbutazone	Risk of severe rash and itch.
Penicillamine	Possible blood or kidney toxicity.
Phenylbutazone	Risk of severe rash and itch.
Sulfa drugs	Possible liver toxicity.

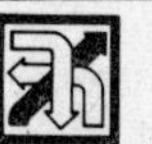

INTERACTION WITH OTHER SUBSTANCES

INTERACTS WITH	COMBINED EFFECT
Alcohol:	Possible liver toxicity. Avoid.
Beverages:	None expected.
Cocaine:	None expected.
Foods:	None expected.
Marijuana:	None expected.
Tobacco:	None expected.

HYDROXYZINE

BRAND NAMES

Atarax
Ataraxoid
Cartrax
Durrax
Enarax
Marax
Multipax
Neucalm 50
Orgatrax
T.E.H. Tablets
Theozine
Vistaril
Vistrax

GENERAL INFORMATION

Habit forming? No
Prescription needed? Yes
Available as generic? No
Drug class: Tranquilizer, antihistamine

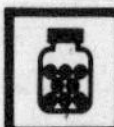

USES

- Treatment for anxiety, tension and agitation.
- Relieves itching from allergic reactions.

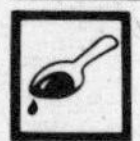

DOSAGE & USAGE INFORMATION

How to take:
- Tablet or capsule—Swallow with liquid. If you can't swallow whole, crumble tablet or open capsule and take with liquid or food.
- Liquid—If desired, dilute dose in beverage before swallowing.

When to take:
At the same times each day.

If you forget a dose:
Take as soon as you remember up to 2 hours late. If more than 2 hours, wait for next scheduled dose (don't double this dose).

What drug does:
May reduce activity in areas of the brain that influence emotional stability.

Time lapse before drug works:
15 to 30 minutes.

Don't take with:
- Non-prescription drugs without consulting doctor.
- See Interaction column and consult doctor.

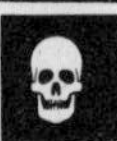

OVERDOSE

Symptoms:
Drowsiness, unsteadiness, agitation, purposeless movements, tremor, convulsions.

What to do:
- Dial 0 (operator) or 911 (emergency) for an ambulance or medical help. Then give first aid immediately.
- Additional emergency information on page 886.

POSSIBLE ADVERSE REACTIONS OR SIDE EFFECTS

SYMPTOMS	FREQUENCY	WHAT TO DO
Brain & nervous system:		
• Headache	Infrequent	5
• Tremor	Rare	3
• Drowsiness	Common	5
Skin:		
Rash	Rare	3
Eyes:	None expected.	
Ears, nose, throat:		
Dry mouth.	Common	5
Digestive:	None expected.	
Heart & lungs:	None expected.	
Blood vessels:	None expected.	
Muscles, bones, joints:	None expected.	
Genital, urinary:		
Difficult urination.	Common	5
Kidneys:	None expected.	
Liver:	None expected.	
Allergic:	None expected.	
Blood:	None expected.	
Others:	None expected.	

1- Life-threatening. Seek emergency treatment immediately.
2- Discontinue. Seek emergency treatment.
3- Discontinue. Call doctor right away.
4- Continue. Call doctor when convenient.
5- Continue. Tell doctor at next visit.
6- No action necessary.

WARNINGS & PRECAUTIONS

Don't take if:
You are allergic to any antihistamine.

Before you start, consult your doctor:
- If you have epilepsy.
- If you will have surgery within 2 months, including dental surgery, requiring general or spinal anesthesia.

Over age 60:
Adverse reactions and side effects may be more frequent and severe than in younger persons. Drug likely to increase urination difficulty caused by enlarged prostate gland.

Pregnancy:
Studies inconclusive on harm to unborn child. Animal studies show fetal abnormalities. Decide with your doctor whether drug benefits justify risk to unborn child.

Breast-feeding:
Drug passes into milk. Avoid drug or discontinue nursing until you finish medicine. Consult doctor for advice on maintaining milk supply.

Infants & children:
Use only under medical supervision.

Prolonged use:
Tolerance develops and reduces effectiveness.

Skin & sunlight:
No problems expected.

Driving, piloting or hazardous work:
Don't drive or pilot aircraft until you learn how medicine affects you. Don't work around dangerous machinery. Don't climb ladders or work in high places. Danger increases if you drink alcohol or take medicine affecting alertness and reflexes, such as antihistamines, tranquilizers, sedatives, pain medicine, narcotics and mind-altering drugs.

Airplane passengers:
No problems expected.

Discontinuing:
Don't discontinue without consulting doctor. Dose may require gradual reduction if you have taken drug for a long time. Doses of other drugs may also require adjustment.

Others:
No problems expected.

INTERACTION WITH OTHER DRUGS

GENERIC NAME OR DRUG CLASS	COMBINED EFFECT
Anticoagulants (oral)	Increased anticoagulant effect.
Anticonvulsants (hydantoin)	Decreased anticonvulsant effect.
Antidepressants (tricyclic)	Increased effect of both drugs.
Antihistamines	Increased hydroxyzine effect.
Narcotics	Increased effect of both drugs.
Pain relievers	Increased effect of both drugs.
Sedatives	Increased effect of both drugs.
Sleep inducers	Increased effect of both drugs.
Tranquilizers	Increased effect of both drugs.

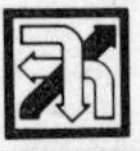

INTERACTION WITH OTHER SUBSTANCES

INTERACTS WITH	COMBINED EFFECT
Alcohol:	Increased sedation and intoxication. Use with caution.
Beverages: Caffeine drinks	Decreased tranquilizer effect of hydroxyzine.
Cocaine:	Decreased hydroxyzine effect. Avoid.
Foods:	None expected.
Marijuana:	None expected.
Tobacco:	None expected.

HYOSCYAMINE

BRAND NAMES

Anaspaz
Barbidonna-CR
Cystospaz
Donnatal
Ergobel
Floramine
Levsin
Omnibel

See complete brand names list, page 827.

GENERAL INFORMATION

Habit forming? No
Prescription needed? Low strength: No
High strength: Yes
Available as generic? Yes
Drug class: Antispasmodic, anticholinergic

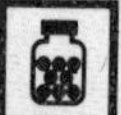

USES

Reduces spasms of digestive system, bladder and urethra.

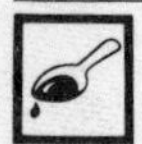

DOSAGE & USAGE INFORMATION

How to take:

- Tablet or liquid—Swallow with liquid or food to lessen stomach irritation.
- Extended-release tablets or capsules—Swallow each dose whole. If you take regular tablets, you may chew or crush them.
- Drops—Dilute dose in beverage before swallowing.

When to take:
30 minutes before meals (unless directed otherwise by doctor).

If you forget a dose:
Take as soon as you remember up to 2 hours late. If more than 2 hours, wait for next scheduled dose (don't double this dose).

What drug does:
Blocks nerve impulses at parasympathetic nerve endings, preventing muscle contractions and gland secretions of organs involved.

Time lapse before drug works:
15 to 30 minutes.

Don't take with:
See Interaction column and consult doctor.

OVERDOSE

Symptoms:
Dilated pupils; rapid pulse and breathing; dizziness; fever; hallucinations; confusion; slurred speech; agitation; flushed face; convulsions; coma.

What to do:

- Dial 0 (operator) or 911 (emergency) for an ambulance or medical help. Then give first aid immediately.
- Additional emergency information on page 886.

POSSIBLE ADVERSE REACTIONS OR SIDE EFFECTS

SYMPTOMS	FREQUENCY	WHAT TO DO
Brain & nervous system:		
• Headache	Infrequent	4
• Confusion, delirium.	Common	3
Skin:		
Rash or hives.	Rare	3
Eyes:		
Pain, blurred vision.	Rare	3
Ears, nose, throat:		
Dryness	Common	6
Digestive:		
• Constipation	Common	5
• Nausea, vomiting.	Common	4
Heart & lungs:		
Rapid heartbeat.	Common	3
Blood vessels:	None expected.	
Muscles, bones, joints:	None expected.	
Genital, urinary:		
Difficult urination.	Infrequent	4
Kidneys:	None expected.	
Liver:	None expected.	
Allergic:	None expected.	
Blood:	None expected.	
Others:		
Less perspiration.	Common	4

1- Life-threatening. Seek emergency treatment immediately.
2- Discontinue. Seek emergency treatment.
3- Discontinue. Call doctor right away.
4- Continue. Call doctor when convenient.
5- Continue. Tell doctor at next visit.
6- No action necessary.

WARNINGS & PRECAUTIONS

Don't take if:
- You are allergic to any anticholinergic.
- You have trouble with stomach bloating.
- You have difficulty emptying your bladder completely.
- You have narrow-angle glaucoma.
- You have severe ulcerative colitis.

Before you start, consult your doctor:
- If you have open-angle glaucoma.
- If you have angina.
- If you have chronic bronchitis or asthma.
- If you have hiatal hernia.
- If you have liver disease.
- If you have enlarged prostate.
- If you have myasthenia gravis.
- If you have peptic ulcer.
- If you will have surgery within 2 months, including dental surgery, requiring general or spinal anesthesia.

Over age 60:
Adverse reactions and side effects may be more frequent and severe than in younger persons.

Pregnancy:
Studies inconclusive on harm to unborn child. Animal studies show fetal abnormalities. Decide with your doctor whether drug benefits justify risk to unborn child.

Breast-feeding:
Drug passes into milk and decreases milk flow. Avoid drug or discontinue nursing until you finish medicine. Consult doctor for advice on maintaining milk supply.

Infants & children:
Use only under medical supervision.

Prolonged use:
Chronic constipation, possible fecal impaction. Consult doctor immediately.

Skin & sunlight:
No problems expected.

Driving, piloting or hazardous work:
Use disqualifies you for piloting aircraft. Otherwise, no problems expected.

Airplane passengers:
No problems expected.

Discontinuing:
May be unnecessary to finish medicine. Follow doctor's instructions.

Others:
No problems expected.

INTERACTION WITH OTHER DRUGS

GENERIC NAME OR DRUG CLASS	COMBINED EFFECT
Amantadine	Increased hyoscyamine effect.
Anticholinergics (other)	Increased hyoscyamine effect.
Antidepressants (tricyclic)	Increased hyoscyamine effect.
Antihistamines	Increased hyoscyamine effect.
Cortisone drugs	Increased internal-eye pressure.
Haloperidol	Increased internal-eye pressure.
MAO inhibitors	Increased hyoscyamine effect.
Meperidine	Increased hyoscyamine effect.
Methylphenidate	Increased hyoscyamine effect.
Orphenadrine	Increased hyoscyamine effect.
Phenothiazines	Increased hyoscyamine effect.
Pilocarpine	Loss of pilocarpine effect in glaucoma treatment.
Vitamin C	Decreased hyoscyamine effect. Avoid large doses of vitamin C.

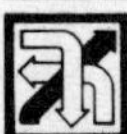

INTERACTION WITH OTHER SUBSTANCES

INTERACTS WITH	COMBINED EFFECT
Alcohol:	None expected.
Beverages:	None expected.
Cocaine:	Excessively rapid heartbeat. Avoid.
Foods:	None expected.
Marijuana:	Drowsiness and dry mouth.
Tobacco:	None expected.

IBUPROFEN

BRAND NAMES

Advil
Motrin
Nuprin
Rufen

Habit forming? No
Prescription needed? No

GENERAL INFORMATION

Available as generic? Yes
Drug class: Antiinflammatory (non-steroid)

USES

- Treatment for joint pain, stiffness, inflammation and swelling of arthritis and gout.
- Pain reliever.
- Treatment for dysmenorrhea (painful or difficult menstruation).

DOSAGE & USAGE INFORMATION

How to take:
Tablet—Swallow with liquid or food to lessen stomach irritation. If you can't swallow whole, crumble tablet and take with liquid or food.

When to take:
At the same times each day.

If you forget a dose:
Take as soon as you remember up to 2 hours late. If more than 2 hours, wait for next scheduled dose (don't double this dose).

What drug does:
Reduces tissue concentration of prostaglandins (hormones which produce inflammation and pain).

Time lapse before drug works:
Begins in 4 to 24 hours. May require 3 weeks regular use for maximum benefit.

Don't take with:
See Interaction column and consult doctor.

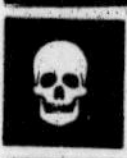

OVERDOSE

Symptoms:
Confusion, agitation, incoherence, convulsions, possible hemorrhage from stomach or intestine, coma.

What to do:
- Dial 0 (operator) or 911 (emergency) for an ambulance or medical help. Then give first aid immediately.
- Additional emergency information on page 886.

POSSIBLE ADVERSE REACTIONS OR SIDE EFFECTS

SYMPTOMS	FREQUENCY	WHAT TO DO
Brain & nervous system:		
• Depression, drowsiness.	Infrequent	4
• Convulsions, confusion.	Rare	3
• Dizziness	Common	4
• Headache	Common	5
Skin:		
Rash, hives or itch.	Rare	3
Eyes:		
Blurred vision.	Rare	3
Ears, nose, throat:		
Ringing in ears.	Infrequent	4
Digestive:		
• Bloody or black, tarry stools.	Rare	3
• Nausea, pain.	Common	4
• Constipation or diarrhea, vomiting.	Infrequent	4
Heart & lungs:		
Breathing difficulty, tightness in chest, rapid heartbeat.	Rare	3
Blood vessels:		
Unusual bleeding or bruising.	Rare	3
Muscles, bones, joints:		
Swollen feet, legs.	Infrequent	4
Genital, urinary:		
• Bloody urine.	Rare	3
• Difficult, painful or frequent urination.	Rare	4
Kidneys, allergic, blood:	None expected.	
Liver:		
Jaundice (yellow skin and eyes).	Rare	3
Others:		
Fatigue, weakness.	Rare	4

2- Discontinue. Seek emergency treatment.
3- Discontinue. Call doctor right away.
4- Continue. Call doctor when convenient.
5- Continue. Tell doctor at next visit.

WARNINGS & PRECAUTIONS

Don't take if:

- You are allergic to aspirin or any non-steroid, antiinflammatory drug.
- You have gastritis, peptic ulcer, enteritis, ileitis, ulcerative colitis, asthma, heart failure, high blood pressure or bleeding problems.
- Patient is younger than 15.

Before you start, consult your doctor:

- If you have epilepsy.
- If you have Parkinson's disease.
- If you have been mentally ill.
- If you have had kidney disease or impaired kidney function.

Over age 60:
Adverse reactions and side effects may be more frequent and severe than in younger persons.

Pregnancy:
Studies inconclusive on harm to unborn child. Decide with your doctor whether drug benefits justify risk to unborn child.

Breast-feeding:
May harm child. Avoid.

Infants & children:
Not recommended for anyone younger than 15. Use only under medical supervision.

Prolonged use:

- Eye damage.
- Reduced hearing.
- Sore throat, fever.
- Weight gain.

Skin & sunlight:
No problems expected.

Driving, piloting or hazardous work:
Don't drive or pilot aircraft until you learn how medicine affects you. Don't work around dangerous machinery. Don't climb ladders or work in high places. Danger increases if you drink alcohol or take medicine affecting alertness and reflexes, such as antihistamines, tranquilizers, sedatives, pain medicine, narcotics and mind-altering drugs.

Airplane passengers:
No problems expected.

Discontinuing:
Don't discontinue without consulting doctor. Dose may require gradual reduction if you have taken drug for a long time. Doses of other drugs may also require adjustment.

Others:
No problems expected.

INTERACTION WITH OTHER DRUGS

GENERIC NAME OR DRUG CLASS	COMBINED EFFECT
Anticoagulants (oral)	Increased risk of bleeding.
Aspirin	Increased risk of stomach ulcer.
Cortisone drugs	Increased risk of stomach ulcer.
Furosemide	Decreased diuretic effect of furosemide.
Oxyphenbutazone	Possible stomach ulcer.
Phenylbutazone	Possible stomach ulcer.
Probenecid	Increased ibuprofen effect.
Thyroid hormones	Rapid heartbeat, blood-pressure rise.

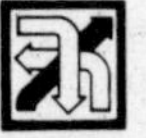

INTERACTION WITH OTHER SUBSTANCES

INTERACTS WITH	COMBINED EFFECT
Alcohol:	Possible stomach ulcer or bleeding.
Beverages:	None expected.
Cocaine:	None expected.
Foods:	None expected.
Marijuana:	Increased pain relief from ibuprofen.
Tobacco:	None expected.

IMIPRAMINE

BRAND NAMES

Apo-Imipramine
Impril
Janimine
Novopramine
Presamine
SK-Pramine
Tofranil
Tofranil-PM

GENERAL INFORMATION

Habit forming? No
Prescription needed? Yes
Available as generic? Yes
Drug class: Antidepressant (tricyclic)

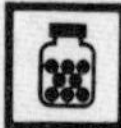

USES

- Gradually relieves, but doesn't cure, symptoms of depression.
- Decreases bed-wetting.

DOSAGE & USAGE INFORMATION

How to take:
Tablet or capsule—Swallow with liquid.

When to take:
At the same time each day, usually bedtime.

If you forget a dose:
Bedtime dose—If you forget your once-a-day bedtime dose, don't take it more than 3 hours late. If more than 3 hours, wait for next scheduled dose. Don't double this dose.

What drug does:
Probably affects part of brain that controls messages between nerve cells.

Time lapse before drug works:
Begins in 1 to 2 weeks. May require 4 to 6 weeks for maximum benefit.

Don't take with:
- Non-prescription drugs without consulting doctor.
- See Interaction column and consult doctor.

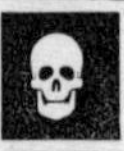

OVERDOSE

Symptoms:
Hallucinations, convulsions, coma.

What to do:
- Dial 0 (operator) or 911 (emergency) for an ambulance or medical help. Then give first aid immediately.
- If patient is unconscious and not breathing, give mouth-to-mouth breathing. If there is no heartbeat, use cardiac massage and mouth-to-mouth breathing (CPR). Don't try to make patient vomit. If you can't get help quickly, take patient to nearest emergency facility.
- Additional emergency information on page 886.

POSSIBLE ADVERSE REACTIONS OR SIDE EFFECTS

SYMPTOMS	FREQUENCY	WHAT TO DO
Brain & nervous system:		
• Hallucinations, shakiness, dizziness, fainting.	Infrequent	3
• Headache	Common	4
• Seizures	Rare	1
• Insomnia	Common	5
Skin:		
Rash, itch.	Rare	3
Eyes:		
Blurred vision, pain.	Infrequent	3
Ears, nose, throat:		
• Sore throat.	Rare	3
• Dry mouth or unpleasant taste.	Common	4
Digestive:		
• Constipation or diarrhea, nausea, indigestion.	Common	4
• Vomiting	Infrequent	3
• "Sweet tooth"	Common	5
Heart & lungs:		
Irregular heartbeat or slow pulse.	Infrequent	3
Blood vessels, muscles, bones, joints, kidneys, allergic, blood:	None expected.	
Genital, urinary:		
Difficulty urinating.	Infrequent	4
Liver:		
Jaundice (yellow skin and eyes).	Rare	3
Others:		
• Fever	Rare	3
• Fatigue, weakness.	Common	4

1 - Life-threatening. Seek emergency treatment immediately.
2 - Discontinue. Seek emergency treatment.
3 - Discontinue. Call doctor right away.
4 - Continue. Call doctor when convenient.
5 - Continue. Tell doctor at next visit.

WARNINGS & PRECAUTIONS

Don't take if:

- You are allergic to any tricyclic antidepressant.
- You drink alcohol.
- You have had a heart attack within 6 weeks.
- You have glaucoma.
- You have taken MAO inhibitors within 2 weeks.
- Patient is younger than 12.

Before you start, consult your doctor:

- If you will have surgery within 2 months, including dental surgery, requiring general or spinal anesthesia.
- If you have an enlarged prostate.
- If you have heart disease or high blood pressure.
- If you have stomach or intestinal problems.
- If you have an overactive thyroid.
- If you have asthma.
- If you have liver disease.

Over age 60:
More likely to develop urination difficulty and side effects under *Brain & nervous system,* opposite.

Pregnancy:
Studies inconclusive on harm to unborn child. Animal studies show fetal abnormalities. Decide with your doctor whether drug benefits justify risk to unborn child.

Breast-feeding:
Drug passes into milk. Avoid drug or discontinue nursing until you finish medicine. Consult doctor on maintaining milk supply.

Infants & children:
Don't give to children younger than 12.

Prolonged use:
No problems expected.

Skin & sunlight:
May cause rash or intensify sunburn in areas exposed to sun or sunlamp.

Driving, piloting or hazardous work:
Don't drive or pilot aircraft until you learn how medicine affects you. Don't work around dangerous machinery. Don't climb ladders or work in high places. Danger increases if you drink alcohol or take medicine affecting alertness and reflexes.

Airplane passengers:
No problems expected.

Discontinuing:
Don't discontinue without consulting doctor. Dose may require gradual reduction if you have taken drug for a long time. Doses of other drugs may also require adjustment.

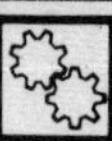

INTERACTION WITH OTHER DRUGS

GENERIC NAME OR DRUG CLASS	COMBINED EFFECT
Anticoagulants (oral)	Increased anticoagulant effect.
Anticholinergics	Increased sedation.
Antihistamines	Increased antihistamine effect.
Barbiturates	Decreased antidepressant effect.
Clonidine	Decreased clonidine effect.
Diuretics (thiazide)	Increased imipramine effect.
Ethchlorvynol	Delirium
Guanethidine	Decreased guanethidine effect.
MAO inhibitors	Fever, delirium, convulsions.
Methyldopa	Decreased methyldopa effect.
Narcotics	Dangerous oversedation.
Phenytoin	Decreased phenytoin effect.
Quinidine	Irregular heartbeat.
Sedatives	Dangerous oversedation.
Sympathomimetics	Increased sympathomimetic effect.
Thyroid hormones	Irregular heartbeat.

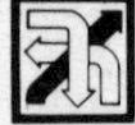

INTERACTION WITH OTHER SUBSTANCES

INTERACTS WITH	COMBINED EFFECT
Alcohol: Beverages or medicines with alcohol.	Excessive intoxication. Avoid.
Beverages:	None expected.
Cocaine:	Excessive intoxication. Avoid.
Foods:	None expected.
Marijuana:	Excessive drowsiness. Avoid.
Tobacco:	None expected.

INDAPAMIDE

BRAND NAMES

Lozol

GENERAL INFORMATION

Habit forming? No
Prescription needed? Yes
Available as generic? No
Drug class: Antihypertensive, diuretic

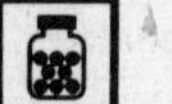

USES

- Controls, but doesn't cure, high blood pressure.
- Reduces fluid retention (edema) caused by conditions such as heart disorders.

DOSAGE & USAGE INFORMATION

How to take:
Tablet or capsule—Swallow with liquid or food to lessen stomach irritation.

When to take:
At the same times each day, usually at bedtime.

If you forget a dose:
Bedtime dose—If you forget your once-a-day bedtime dose, don't take it more than 3 hours late.

What drug does:
Probably reduces constriction of small arteries.

Time lapse before drug works:
8 to 12 weeks before blood pressure effects can be evaluated.

Don't take with:
See Interaction column and consult doctor.

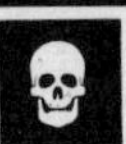

OVERDOSE

Symptoms:
Cramps, weakness, heartbeat irregular, weak pulse, fainting, coma.

What to do:
- Dial 0 (operator) or 911 (emergency) for an ambulance or medical help. Then give first aid immediately.
- If patient is unconscious and not breathing, give mouth-to-mouth breathing. If there is no heartbeat, use cardiac massage and mouth-to-mouth breathing (CPR). Don't try to make patient vomit. If you can't get help quickly, take patient to nearest emergency facility.
- Additional emergency information on page 886.

POSSIBLE ADVERSE REACTIONS OR SIDE EFFECTS

SYMPTOMS	FREQUENCY	WHAT TO DO
Brain & nervous system:		
• Mood changes.	Rare	4
• Headache	Infrequent	4
Skin:	None expected.	
Eyes:	None expected.	
Ears, nose, throat:	None expected.	
Digestive:		
• Dry mouth.	Rare	4
• Nausea/vomiting.	Rare	4
• Appetite loss.	Infrequent	4
Heart & lungs:		
• Irregular heartbeat.	Rare	3
• Weak pulse.	Rare	2
Blood vessels:	None expected.	
Muscles, bones, joints:		
• Muscle cramps.	Rare	4
• Joint pain.	Rare	4
Genital, urinary:		
Frequent urination.	Common	5
Kidneys, allergic, blood, liver:	None expected.	
Others:		
Insomnia	Rare	4

1 - Life-threatening. Seek emergency treatment immediately.
2 - Discontinue. Seek emergency treatment.
3 - Discontinue. Call doctor right away.
4 - Continue. Call doctor when convenient.
5 - Continue. Tell doctor at next visit.

WARNINGS & PRECAUTIONS

Don't take if:
You are allergic to indapamide.

Before you start, consult your doctor:
- If you have severe kidney disease.
- If you have diabetes.
- If you have gout.
- If you have liver disease.
- If you will have surgery within 2 months, including dental surgery, requiring general or spinal anesthesia.

Over age 60:
Adverse reactions and side effects may be more frequent and severe than in younger persons.

Pregnancy:
Risk to unborn child outweighs drug benefits. Don't use.

Breast-feeding:
Unknown effect on child. Consult doctor.

Infants & children:
Use only under close medical supervision.

Prolonged use:
Request laboratory studies for blood sugar, BUN, uric acid and serum electrolytes (potassium and sodium).

Skin & sunlight:
No problems expected.

Driving, piloting or hazardous work:
Don't drive or pilot aircraft until you learn how medicine affects you. Don't work around dangerous machinery. Don't climb ladders or work in high places. Danger increases if you drink alcohol or take medicine affecting alertness and reflexes, such as antihistamines, tranquilizers, sedatives, pain medicine, narcotics and mind-altering drugs.

Airplane passengers:
No problems expected.

Discontinuing:
Don't discontinue without consulting doctor. Dose may require gradual reduction if you have taken drug for a long time. Doses of other drugs may also require adjustment.

INTERACTION WITH OTHER DRUGS

GENERIC NAME OR DRUG CLASS	COMBINED EFFECT
Cortisone drugs	Excess potassium loss that may cause dangerous heart rhythms.
Diuretics (other)	Increased effectiveness of both—sometimes desirable.
Digitalis preparations	Increased chance of digitalis toxicity.
Lithium	Lithium toxicity. Avoid combination.
Sympathomimetics	Decreased sympathomimetic effect.

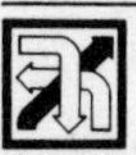

INTERACTION WITH OTHER SUBSTANCES

INTERACTS WITH	COMBINED EFFECT
Alcohol:	Dangerous blood-pressure drop. Avoid.
Beverages:	No problems expected.
Cocaine:	Reduced effectiveness of indapamide. Avoid.
Foods:	None expected.
Marijuana:	Reduced effectiveness of indapamide. Avoid.
Tobacco:	Reduced effectiveness of indapamide. Avoid.

INDOMETHACIN

BRAND NAMES

Indocid
Indocin
Indocin-SR
Indo-Lemmon
Novomethacin

GENERAL INFORMATION

Habit forming? No
Prescription needed? Yes
Available as generic? No
Drug class: Antiinflammatory (non-steroid)

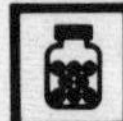

USES

- Treatment for joint pain, stiffness, inflammation and swelling of arthritis and gout.
- Pain reliever.
- Treatment for dysmenorrhea (painful or difficult menstruation).

DOSAGE & USAGE INFORMATION

How to take:

- Tablet or capsule—Swallow with liquid or food to lessen stomach irritation. If you can't swallow whole, crumble tablet or open capsule and take with liquid or food.
- Extended release tablets or capsules—Swallow whole with liquid or food to lessen stomach irritation.

When to take:
At the same times each day.

If you forget a dose:
Take as soon as you remember up to 2 hours late. If more than 2 hours, wait for next scheduled dose (don't double this dose).

What drug does:
Reduces tissue concentration of prostaglandins (hormones which produce inflammation and pain).

Time lapse before drug works:
Begins in 4 to 24 hours. May require 3 weeks regular use for maximum benefit.

Don't take with:
See Interaction column and consult doctor.

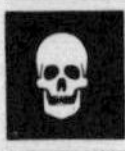

OVERDOSE

Symptoms:
Confusion, agitation, incoherence, convulsions, possible hemorrhage from stomach or intestine, coma.

What to do:

- Dial 0 (operator) or 911 (emergency) for an ambulance or medical help. Then give first aid immediately.
- Additional emergency information on page 886.

POSSIBLE ADVERSE REACTIONS OR SIDE EFFECTS

SYMPTOMS	FREQUENCY	WHAT TO DO
Brain & nervous system:		
• Depression, drowsiness.	Infrequent	4
• Convulsions, confusion.	Rare	3
• Dizziness	Common	4
• Headache	Common	5
Skin:		
Rash, hives or itch.	Rare	3
Eyes:		
Blurred vision.	Rare	3
Ears, nose, throat:		
Ringing in ears.	Infrequent	4
Digestive:		
• Bloody or black, tarry stools.	Rare	3
• Nausea, pain.	Common	4
• Constipation or diarrhea, vomiting.	Infrequent	4
Heart & lungs:		
Breathing difficulty, tightness in chest, rapid heartbeat.	Rare	3
Blood vessels:		
Unusual bleeding or bruising.	Rare	3
Muscles, bones, joints:		
Swollen feet, legs.	Infrequent	4
Genital, urinary:		
• Bloody urine.	Rare	3
• Difficult, painful or frequent urination.	Rare	4
Kidneys, allergic, blood:	None expected.	
Liver:		
Jaundice (yellow skin and eyes).	Rare	3
Others:		
Fatigue, weakness.	Rare	4

1- Life-threatening. Seek emergency treatment immediately.
2- Discontinue. Seek emergency treatment.
3- Discontinue. Call doctor right away.
4- Continue. Call doctor when convenient.
5- Continue. Tell doctor at next visit.

WARNINGS & PRECAUTIONS

Don't take if:
- You are allergic to aspirin or any non-steroid, antiinflammatory drug.
- You have gastritis, peptic ulcer, enteritis, ileitis, ulcerative colitis, asthma, heart failure, high blood pressure or bleeding problems.
- Patient is younger than 15.

Before you start, consult your doctor:
- If you have epilepsy.
- If you have Parkinson's disease.
- If you have been mentally ill.
- If you have had kidney disease or impaired kidney function.

Over age 60:
Adverse reactions and side effects may be more frequent and severe than in younger persons.

Pregnancy:
Studies inconclusive on harm to unborn child. Decide with your doctor whether drug benefits justify risk to unborn child.

Breast-feeding:
May harm child. Avoid.

Infants & children:
Not recommended for anyone younger than 15. Use only under medical supervision.

Prolonged use:
- Eye damage.
- Reduced hearing.
- Sore throat, fever.
- Weight gain.

Skin & sunlight:
No problems expected.

Driving, piloting or hazardous work:
Don't drive or pilot aircraft until you learn how medicine affects you. Don't work around dangerous machinery. Don't climb ladders or work in high places. Danger increases if you drink alcohol or take medicine affecting alertness and reflexes, such as antihistamines, tranquilizers, sedatives, pain medicine, narcotics and mind-altering drugs.

Airplane passengers:
No problems expected.

Discontinuing:
Don't discontinue without consulting doctor. Dose may require gradual reduction if you have taken drug for a long time. Doses of other drugs may also require adjustment.

Others:
No problems expected.

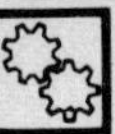

INTERACTION WITH OTHER DRUGS

GENERIC NAME OR DRUG CLASS	COMBINED EFFECT
Anticoagulants (oral)	Increased risk of bleeding.
Aspirin	Increased risk of stomach ulcer.
Cortisone drugs	Increased risk of stomach ulcer.
Furosemide	Decreased diuretic effect of furosemide.
Lithium	Increased lithium effect.
Oxyphenbutazone	Possible stomach ulcer.
Phenylbutazone	Possible stomach ulcer.
Probenecid	Increased indomethacin effect.
Thyroid hormones	Rapid heartbeat, blood-pressure rise.

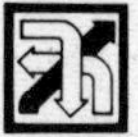

INTERACTION WITH OTHER SUBSTANCES

INTERACTS WITH	COMBINED EFFECT
Alcohol:	Possible stomach ulcer or bleeding.
Beverages:	None expected.
Cocaine:	None expected.
Foods:	None expected.
Marijuana:	Increased pain relief from indomethacin.
Tobacco:	None expected.

INSULIN

BRAND NAMES

Actrapid	Lente Insulin	PZI
Globin Insulin	Mixtard	Protamine Zinc & Iletin II
Insulatard	Monotard	Regular Iletin II
Lentard	NPH	Regular Insulin
Lente Iletin II	NPH Iletin II	

See complete brand names list, page 828.

GENERAL INFORMATION

Habit forming? No
Prescription needed? No
Available as generic? Yes
Drug class: Antidiabetic

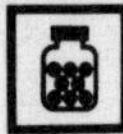

USES

Controls diabetes, a complex metabolic disorder, in which the body does not manufacture insulin.

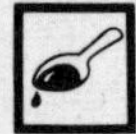

DOSAGE & USAGE INFORMATION

How to take:
Must be taken by injection under the skin. Use disposable, sterile needles. Rotate injection sites.

When to take:
At the same time each day.

If you forget a dose:
Take as soon as you remember. Wait at least 4 hours for next dose. Resume regular schedule.

What drug does:
Facilitates passage of blood sugar through cell membranes so sugar is usable.

Time lapse before drug works:
30 minutes to 8 hours, depending on type of insulin used.

Don't take with:
See Interaction column and consult doctor.

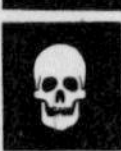

OVERDOSE

Symptoms:
Low blood sugar (hypoglycemia)—Anxiety; chills, cold sweats, pale skin; drowsiness; excess hunger; headache; nausea; nervousness; fast heartbeat; shakiness; unusual tiredness or weakness.

What to do:
- Eat some type of sugar immediately, such as orange juice, honey, sugar cubes, crackers, sandwich.
- If patient loses consciousness, give glucagon if you have it and know how to use it.
- Otherwise, dial 0 (operator) or 911 (emergency) for an ambulance or medical help. Then give first aid immediately.
- Additional emergency information on page 886.

POSSIBLE ADVERSE REACTIONS OR SIDE EFFECTS

SYMPTOMS	FREQUENCY	WHAT TO DO
Brain & nervous system:	None expected.	
Skin:		
• Swelling, redness, itch at injection site.	Infrequent	4
• Hives	Infrequent	3
Eyes:	None expected.	
Ears, nose, throat:	None expected.	
Digestive:	None expected.	
Heart & lungs:	None expected.	
Blood vessels:	None expected.	
Muscles, bones, joints:	None expected.	
Genital, urinary:	None expected.	
Kidneys:	None expected.	
Liver:	None expected.	
Allergic:		
Life-threatening anaphylaxis may occur.	Rare	1 See Page 888.
Blood:	None expected.	
Others:	None expected.	

1- Life-threatening. Seek emergency treatment immediately.
2- Discontinue. Seek emergency treatment.
3- Discontinue. Call doctor right away.
4- Continue. Call doctor when convenient.
5- Continue. Tell doctor at next visit.
6- No action necessary.

WARNINGS & PRECAUTIONS

Don't take if:
- Your diagnosis and dose schedule is not established.
- You don't know how to deal with overdose emergencies.

Before you start, consult your doctor:
- If you are allergic to insulin.
- If you take MAO inhibitors.
- If you have liver or kidney disease or low thyroid function.

Over age 60:
Guard against hypoglycemia. Repeated episodes can cause permanent confusion and abnormal behavior.

Pregnancy:
Possible drug benefits outweigh risk to unborn child. Adhere rigidly to diabetes treatment program.

Breast-feeding:
No problems expected.

Infants & children:
Use only under medical supervision.

Prolonged use:
No problems expected.

Skin & sunlight:
No problems expected.

Driving, piloting or hazardous work:
No problems expected after dose is established.

Airplane passengers:
No problems expected.

Discontinuing:
Don't discontinue without doctor's advice until you complete prescribed dose, even though symptoms diminish or disappear.

Others:
- Diet and exercise affect how much insulin you need. Work with your doctor to determine accurate dose.
- Notify your doctor if you skip a dose, overeat, have fever or infection.
- Notify doctor if you develop symptoms of high blood sugar: drowsiness, dry skin, orange fruit-like odor to breath, increased urination, appetite loss, unusual thirst.

INTERACTION WITH OTHER DRUGS

GENERIC NAME OR DRUG CLASS	COMBINED EFFECT
Anticoagulants (oral)	Increased anticoagulant effect.
Anticonvulsants (hydantoin)	Decreased insulin effect.
Antidiabetics (oral)	Increased antibiabetic effect.
Beta-adrenergic blockers	Can mask symptoms of low blood sugar.
Contraceptives (oral)	Decreased insulin effect.
Cortisone drugs	Decreased insulin effect.
Diuretics	Decreased insulin effect.
Furosemide	Decreased insulin effect.
MAO inhibitors	Increased insulin effect.
Oxyphenbutazone	Increased insulin effect.
Phenylbutazone	Increased insulin effect.
Salicylates	Increased insulin effect.
Sulfa drugs	Increased insulin effect.

Additional interactions on page 838.

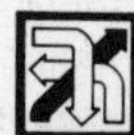

INTERACTION WITH OTHER SUBSTANCES

INTERACTS WITH	COMBINED EFFECT
Alcohol:	Increased insulin effect. May cause hypoglycemia and brain damage.
Beverages:	None expected.
Cocaine:	May cause brain damage.
Foods:	None expected.
Marijuana:	Possible increase in blood sugar.
Tobacco:	None expected.

IRON-POLYSACCHARIDE

BRAND NAMES

Hytinic
Niferex
Nu-Iron

GENERAL INFORMATION

Habit forming? No
Prescription needed? With folic acid: Yes
Without folic acid: No
Available as generic? Yes
Drug class: Mineral supplement (iron)

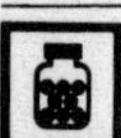

USES

Treatment for dietary iron deficiency or iron-deficiency anemia from other causes.

DOSAGE & USAGE INFORMATION

How to take:
Tablet, capsule or liquid—Swallow with liquid or food to lessen stomach irritation. If you can't swallow whole, crumble tablet or open capsule and take with liquid or food. Place medicine far back on tongue to avoid staining teeth.

When to take:
1 hour before or 2 hours after meals.

If you forget a dose:
Take up to 2 hours late. If more than 2 hours, wait for next dose (don't double this).

What drug does:
Stimulates bone-marrow production of hemoglobin (red-blood-cell pigment that carries oxygen to body cells).

Time lapse before drug works:
3 to 7 days. May require 3 weeks for maximum benefit.

Don't take with:
- Multiple vitamin and mineral supplements.
- See Interaction column and consult doctor.

OVERDOSE

Symptoms:
Weakness, collapse; pallor, blue lips, hands and fingernails; weak, rapid heartbeat; shallow breathing; convulsions; coma.

What to do:
- Dial 0 (operator) or 911 (emergency) for an ambulance or medical help. Then give first aid immediately.
- Additional emergency information on page 886.

POSSIBLE ADVERSE REACTIONS OR SIDE EFFECTS

SYMPTOMS	FREQUENCY	WHAT TO DO
Brain & nervous system:		
Drowsiness	Rare	4
Skin, eyes, blood vessels, muscles, bones, joints, kidneys, liver, allergic, blood:	None expected.	
Ears, nose, throat:		
Throat or chest pain on swallowing.	Rare	3
Digestive:		
• Gray or black stool.	Always	6
• Constipation or diarrhea, heartburn, nausea, vomiting.	Infrequent	3
• Pain, cramps, blood in stool.	Rare	3
Heart & lungs:		
Weak, rapid heartbeat.	Rare	1
Genital, urinary:		
Dark urine.	Infrequent	5
Others:		
• Stained teeth with liquid iron.	Common	6
• Fatigue, weakness.	Infrequent	4

1 - Life-threatening. Seek emergency treatment immediately.
2 - Discontinue. Seek emergency treatment.
3 - Discontinue. Call doctor right away.
4 - Continue. Call doctor when convenient.
5 - Continue. Tell doctor at next visit.
6 - No action necessary.

WARNINGS & PRECAUTIONS

Don't take if:
- You are allergic to any iron supplement.
- You take iron injections.
- Your daily iron intake is high.
- You plan to take this supplement for a long time.
- You have acute hepatitis.
- You have hemosiderosis or hemochromatosis (conditions involving excess iron in body).
- You have hemolytic anemia.

Before you start, consult your doctor:
- If you plan to become pregnant within medication period.
- If you have had stomach surgery.
- If you have had peptic ulcer disease, enteritis or colitis.
- If you have had pancreatitis or hepatitis.

Over age 60:
May cause hemochromatosis (iron storage disease) with bronze skin, liver damage, diabetes, heart problems and impotence.

Pregnancy:
No proven harm to unborn child. Avoid if possible. Take only if your doctor prescribes supplement during last half of pregnancy.

Breast-feeding:
No problems expected. Take only if your doctor confirms you have a dietary deficiency or an iron-deficiency anemia.

Infants & children:
Use only under medical supervision. Overdose common and dangerous. Keep out of children's reach.

Prolonged use:
May cause hemochromatosis (iron storage disease) with bronze skin, liver damage, diabetes, heart problems and impotence.

Skin & sunlight:
No problems expected.

Driving, piloting or hazardous work:
No problems expected.

Airplane passengers:
No problems expected.

Discontinuing:
May be unnecessary to finish medicine. Follow doctor's instructions.

Others:
Liquid form stains teeth. Mix with water or juice to lessen the effect. Brush with baking soda or hydrogen peroxide to help remove stain.

INTERACTION WITH OTHER DRUGS

GENERIC NAME OR DRUG CLASS	COMBINED EFFECT
Allopurinol	Possible excess iron storage in liver.
Antacids	Poor iron absorption.
Chloramphenicol	Decreased effect of iron. Interferes with red-blood-cell and hemoglobin formation.
Cholestyramine	Decreased iron effect.
Iron supplements (other)	Possible excess iron storage in liver.
Penicillamine	Decreased penicillamine effect.
Sulfasalazine	Decreased iron effect.
Tetracyclines	Decreased tetracycline effect. Take iron 3 hours before or 2 hours after taking tetracycline.
Vitamin C	Increased iron effect. Contributes to red-blood-cell and hemoglobin formation.
Vitamin E	Decreased iron effect.

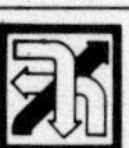

INTERACTION WITH OTHER SUBSTANCES

INTERACTS WITH	COMBINED EFFECT
Alcohol:	Increased iron absorption. May cause organ damage. Avoid or use in moderation.
Beverages: Milk, tea	Decreased iron effect.
Cocaine:	None expected.
Foods: Dairy foods, eggs, whole-grain bread and cereal.	Decreased iron effect.
Marijuana:	None expected.
Tobacco:	None expected.

ISOETHARINE

BRAND NAMES

Beta-2
Bronkometer
Bronkosol
Dilabron

GENERAL INFORMATION

Habit forming? No
Prescription needed? Yes
Available as generic? No
Drug class: Sympathomimetic (bronchodilator)

USES

Eases breathing difficulty from bronchial asthma attacks, bronchitis and emphysema.

DOSAGE & USAGE INFORMATION

How to take:
Aerosol—Use only as directed on label. Don't inhale medicine more than twice per dose unless otherwise directed by doctor.

When to take:
As needed, no more often than every 3 hours.

If you forget a dose:
Take as soon as you remember if you need it. Never double dose.

What drug does:
Dilates constricted bronchial tubes so air can pass.

Time lapse before drug works:
1 to 2 minutes.

Don't take with:
- Non-prescription drugs containing caffeine without consulting doctor.
- See Interaction column and consult doctor.

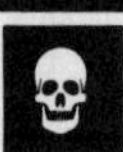

OVERDOSE

Symptoms:
Nervousness, anxiety, dizziness, palpitations, tremor, rapid heartbeat, spasm of bronchial tubes, cardiac arrest.

What to do:
- Dial 0 (operator) or 911 (emergency) for an ambulance or medical help. Then give first aid immediately.
- If patient is unconscious and not breathing, give mouth-to-mouth breathing. If there is no heartbeat, use cardiac massage and mouth-to-mouth breathing (CPR). Don't try to make patient vomit. If you can't get help quickly, take patient to nearest emergency facility.
- Additional emergency information on page 886.

POSSIBLE ADVERSE REACTIONS OR SIDE EFFECTS

SYMPTOMS	FREQUENCY	WHAT TO DO
Brain & nervous system:		
Dizziness, agitation, headache, insomnia.	Common	4
Skin:	None expected.	
Eyes:	None expected.	
Ears, nose, throat:	None expected.	
Digestive:		
Nausea	Common	4
Heart & lungs:		
• Fast or pounding heartbeat.	Common	4
• Constriction of bronchial tubes, particularly after overuse.	Infrequent	3
Blood vessels:	None expected.	
Muscles, bones, joints:	None expected.	
Genital, urinary:	None expected.	
Kidneys:	None expected.	
Liver:	None expected.	
Allergic:	None expected.	
Blood:	None expected.	
Others:		
Weakness	Infrequent	4

1 - Life-threatening. Seek emergency treatment immediately.
2 - Discontinue. Seek emergency treatment.
3 - Discontinue. Call doctor right away.
4 - Continue. Call doctor when convenient.
5 - Continue. Tell doctor at next visit.
6 - No action necessary.

WARNINGS & PRECAUTIONS

Don't take if:
- You are allergic to any sympathomimetic drug.
- You have a heart-rhythm disorder.
- You have taken MAO inhibitors in past 2 weeks.

Before you start, consult your doctor:
- If you use epinephrine for asthma.
- If you have diabetes.
- If you have an overactive thyroid gland.
- If you take a digitalis preparation, have high blood pressure or heart disease.

Over age 60:
- If you have hardening of the arteries, use with caution.
- If you have enlarged prostate gland, drug may increase urination difficulty.
- If you have Parkinson's disease, drug may temporarily increase rigidity and tremor in extremities.

Pregnancy:
No proven harm to unborn child. Avoid if possible.

Breast-feeding:
No problems expected, but consult doctor.

Infants & children:
Don't give to infants younger than 2. For older children, use only under medical supervision.

Prolonged use:
No problems expected.

Skin & sunlight:
No problems expected.

Driving, piloting or hazardous work:
No problems expected. Use caution if you feel nervous or dizzy.

Airplane passengers:
No problems expected.

Discontinuing:
Discontinue if drug fails to provide relief. Don't increase dose or frequency.

Others:
May increase blood- and urine-sugar levels, particularly in diabetics.

INTERACTION WITH OTHER DRUGS

GENERIC NAME OR DRUG CLASS	COMBINED EFFECT
Beta-adrenergic blockers	Decreased isoetharine effect.
Ephedrine	Increased ephedrine effect. Excessive heart stimulation.
Epinephrine	Excessive heart stimulation.
Isoproterenol	Excessive heart stimulation.
MAO inhibitors	Dangerous mixture. Avoid.

INTERACTION WITH OTHER SUBSTANCES

INTERACTS WITH	COMBINED EFFECT
Alcohol:	None expected.
Beverages: Caffeine drinks	May cause irregular or fast heartbeat.
Cocaine:	Excessive stimulation. Avoid.
Foods: Chocolates	May cause irregular or fast heartbeat.
Marijuana:	Improves drug's antiasthmatic effect.
Tobacco:	None expected.

ISONIAZID

BRAND NAMES

Ethionamide
INH
Isotamine
Laniazid C.P.
Nydrazid
Rifamate
Rimifon
Trecator-SC

GENERAL INFORMATION

Habit forming? No
Prescription needed? Yes
Available as generic? Yes
Drug class: Antitubercular (antimicrobial)

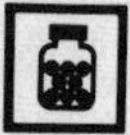

USES

Kills tuberculosis germs.

DOSAGE & USAGE INFORMATION

How to take:
- Tablet or capsule—Swallow with liquid to lessen stomach irritation.
- Syrup—Follow label directions.

When to take:
At the same time each day.

If you forget a dose:
Take as soon as you remember up to 12 hours late. If more than 12 hours, wait for next scheduled dose (don't double this dose).

What drug does:
Interferes with TB germ metabolism. Eventually destroys the germ.

Time lapse before drug works:
3 to 6 months. You may need to take drug as long as 2 years.

Don't take with:
See Interaction column and consult doctor.

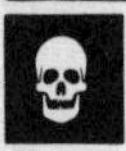

OVERDOSE

Symptoms:
Difficult breathing, convulsions, coma.

What to do:
- Dial 0 (operator) or 911 (emergency) for an ambulance or medical help. Then give first aid immediately.
- If patient is unconscious and not breathing, give mouth-to-mouth breathing. If there is no heartbeat, use cardiac massage and mouth-to-mouth breathing (CPR). Don't try to make patient vomit. If you can't get help quickly, take patient to nearest emergency facility.
- Additional emergency information on page 886.

POSSIBLE ADVERSE REACTIONS OR SIDE EFFECTS

SYMPTOMS	FREQUENCY	WHAT TO DO
Brain & nervous system:		
• Confusion, unsteady walk.	Common	4
• Dizziness	Infrequent	4
Skin:		
Rash, fever.	Rare	3
Eyes:		
Impaired vision.	Rare	3
Ears, nose, throat:		
Swollen glands.	Infrequent	3
Digestive:		
Nausea, indigestion, vomiting, appetite loss.	Infrequent	3
Heart & lungs, blood vessels, genital, urinary, kidneys, allergic:	None expected.	
Muscles, bones, joints:		
Pain in muscles and joints, tingling or numbness in extremities.	Common	3
Liver:		
Jaundice (yellow skin and eyes).	Common	3
Blood:		
• Anemia with fatigue, weakness, fever, sore throat, unusual bruising or bleeding.	Rare	3
• Increase in blood sugar.	Infrequent	4
Others:		
Breast enlargement or discomfort.	Rare	5

1-Life-threatening. Seek emergency treatment immediately.
2-Discontinue. Seek emergency treatment.
3-Discontinue. Call doctor right away.
4-Continue. Call doctor when convenient.
5-Continue. Tell doctor at next visit.

WARNINGS & PRECAUTIONS

Don't take if:
You are allergic to isoniazid.

Before you start, consult your doctor:
- If you plan to become pregnant within medication period.
- If you are allergic to athionamide, pyrazinamide or nicotinic acid.
- If you drink alcohol.
- If you have liver or kidney disease.
- If you have epilepsy, diabetes or lupus.

Over age 60:
Adverse reactions and side effects, especially jaundice, may be more frequent and severe than in younger persons. Kidneys may be less efficient.

Pregnancy:
No proven harm to unborn child. Avoid if possible, especially in the first 6 months of pregnancy. Consult doctor about use in last 3 months.

Breast-feeding:
Drug passes into milk. Avoid drug or discontinue nursing until you finish medicine. Consult doctor for advice on maintaining milk supply.

Infants & children:
Use only under medical supervision.

Prolonged use:
Numbness and tingling of hands and feet.

Skin & sunlight:
No problems expected.

Driving, piloting or hazardous work:
Avoid if you feel dizzy. Otherwise, no problems expected.

Airplane passengers:
Avoid if you feel dizzy. Otherwise, no problems expected.

Discontinuing:
Don't discontinue without doctor's advice until you complete prescribed dose, even though symptoms diminish or disappear.

Others:
- Diabetic patients may have false blood-sugar tests.
- Periodic liver-function tests and laboratory blood studies recommended.
- Prescription for vitamin B-6 (pyridoxine) recommended to prevent nerve damage.

INTERACTION WITH OTHER DRUGS

GENERIC NAME OR DRUG CLASS	COMBINED EFFECT
Antacids	Decreased absorption of isoniazid.
Anticholinergics	May increase pressure within eyeball.
Anticoagulants	Increased anticoagulant effect.
Antidiabetics	Increased antidiabetic effect.
Antihypertensives	Increased antihypertensive effect.
Disulfiram	Increased effect of disulfiram.
Laxatives	Decreased absorption and effect of isoniazid.
Narcotics	Increased narcotic effect.
Phenytoin	Increased phenytoin effect.
Pyridoxine (Vitamin B-6)	Decreased chance of nerve damage in extremities.
Rifampin	Increased isoniazid toxicity to liver.
Sedatives	Increased sedative effect.
Stimulants	Increased stimulant effect.

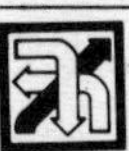

INTERACTION WITH OTHER SUBSTANCES

INTERACTS WITH	COMBINED EFFECT
Alcohol:	Decreased isoniazid effect. Avoid.
Beverages:	None expected.
Cocaine:	None expected.
Foods:	Decreased absorption of isoniazid.
Marijuana:	No interactions expected, but marijuana may slow body's recovery.
Tobacco:	No interactions expected, but tobacco may slow body's recovery.

ISOPROPAMIDE

BRAND NAMES

Allergine
Allernade
Capade
Combid
Darbid
Oraminic
Ornade
Prochlor-Iso
Pro-Iso

GENERAL INFORMATION

Habit forming? No
Prescription needed? Low strength: No
High strength: Yes
Available as generic? Yes
Drug class: Antispasmodic, anticholinergic

USES

Reduces spasms of digestive system, bladder and urethra.

DOSAGE & USAGE INFORMATION

How to take:

- Tablet or capsule—Swallow with liquid or food to lessen stomach irritation.
- Extended-release tablets or capsules—Swallow each dose whole. If you take regular tablets, you may chew or crush them.

When to take:
30 minutes before meals (unless directed otherwise by doctor).

If you forget a dose:
Take as soon as you remember up to 2 hours late. If more than 2 hours, wait for next scheduled dose (don't double this dose).

What drug does:
Blocks nerve impulses at parasympathetic nerve endings, preventing muscle contractions and gland secretions of organs involved.

Time lapse before drug works:
15 to 30 minutes.

Don't take with:
See Interaction column and consult doctor.

OVERDOSE

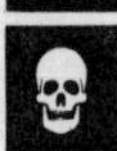

Symptoms:
Dilated pupils; rapid pulse and breathing; dizziness; fever; hallucinations; confusion; slurred speech; agitation; flushed face; convulsions; coma.

What to do:

- Dial 0 (operator) or 911 (emergency) for an ambulance or medical help. Then give first aid immediately.
- Additional emergency information on page 886.

POSSIBLE ADVERSE REACTIONS OR SIDE EFFECTS

SYMPTOMS	FREQUENCY	WHAT TO DO
Brain & nervous system:		
• Headache	Infrequent	4
• Confusion, delirium.	Common	3
Skin:		
Rash or hives.	Rare	3
Eyes:		
Pain, blurred vision.	Rare	3
Ears, nose, throat:		
Dryness	Common	6
Digestive:		
• Constipation	Common	5
• Nausea, vomiting.	Common	4
Heart & lungs:		
Rapid heartbeat.	Common	3
Blood vessels:	None expected.	
Muscles, bones, joints:	None expected.	
Genital, urinary:		
Difficult urination.	Infrequent	4
Kidneys:	None expected.	
Liver:	None expected.	
Allergic:	None expected.	
Blood:	None expected.	
Others:		
Less perspiration.	Common	4

1- Life-threatening. Seek emergency treatment immediately.
2- Discontinue. Seek emergency treatment.
3- Discontinue. Call doctor right away.
4- Continue. Call doctor when convenient.
5- Continue. Tell doctor at next visit.
6- No action necessary.

WARNINGS & PRECAUTIONS

Don't take if:

- You are allergic to any anticholinergic.
- You have trouble with stomach bloating.
- You have difficulty emptying your bladder completely.
- You have narrow-angle glaucoma.
- You have severe ulcerative colitis.

Before you start, consult your doctor:

- If you have open-angle glaucoma.
- If you have angina.
- If you have chronic bronchitis or asthma.
- If you have hiatal hernia.
- If you have liver disease.
- If you have enlarged prostate.
- If you have myasthenia gravis.
- If you have peptic ulcer.
- If you will have surgery within 2 months, including dental surgery, requiring general or spinal anesthesia.

Over age 60:
Adverse reactions and side effects may be more frequent and severe than in younger persons.

Pregnancy:
Studies inconclusive on harm to unborn child. Animal studies show fetal abnormalities. Decide with your doctor whether drug benefits justify risk to unborn child.

Breast-feeding:
Drug passes into milk and decreases milk flow. Avoid drug or discontinue nursing until you finish medicine. Consult doctor for advice on maintaining milk supply.

Infants & children:
Use only under medical supervision.

Prolonged use:
Chronic constipation, possible fecal impaction. Consult doctor immediately.

Skin & sunlight:
No problems expected.

Driving, piloting or hazardous work:
Use disqualifies you for piloting aircraft. Otherwise, no problems expected.

Airplane passengers:
No problems expected.

Discontinuing:
May be unnecessary to finish medicine. Follow doctor's instructions.

Others:
No problems expected.

INTERACTION WITH OTHER DRUGS

GENERIC NAME OR DRUG CLASS	COMBINED EFFECT
Amantadine	Increased isopropamide effect.
Anticholinergics (other)	Increased isopropamide effect
Antidepressants (tricyclic)	Increased isopropamide effect.
Antihistamines	Increased isopropamide effect.
Cortisone drugs	Increased internal-eye pressure.
Haloperidol	Increased internal-eye pressure.
MAO inhibitors	Increased isopropamide effect.
Meperidine	Increased isopropamide effect.
Methylphenidate	Increased isopropamide effect.
Orphenadrine	Increased isopropamide effect.
Phenothiazines	Increased isopropamide effect.
Pilocarpine	Loss of pilocarpine effect in glaucoma treatment.
Vitamin C	Decreased isopropamide effect. Avoid large doses of vitamin C.

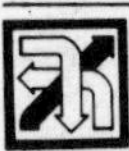

INTERACTION WITH OTHER SUBSTANCES

INTERACTS WITH	COMBINED EFFECT
Alcohol:	None expected.
Beverages:	None expected.
Cocaine:	Excessively rapid heartbeat. Avoid.
Foods:	None expected.
Marijuana:	Drowsiness and dry mouth.
Tobacco:	None expected.

ISOPROTERENOL

BRAND NAMES

Aerolone
Brondilate
Duo-Medihaler
Iprenol
Isuprel
Medihaler-Iso
Norisodrine
Norisodrine Aerotrol
Proternol
Vapo-Iso

GENERAL INFORMATION

Habit forming? No
Prescription needed? Yes
Available as generic? No
Drug class: Sympathomimetic, bronchodilator

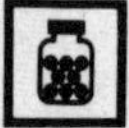

USES

Treatment for breathing difficulty from acute asthma, bronchitis and emphysema.

DOSAGE & USAGE INFORMATION

How to take:
- Tablet—Swallow with liquid or food to lessen stomach irritation.
- Extended-release tablets—Swallow each dose whole.
- Sublingual tablets—Dissolve under tongue.
- Aerosol inhaler—Don't inhale more than twice per dose.

When to take:
As needed, no more often than every 4 hours.

If you forget a dose:
Take as soon as you remember. Wait 4 hours for next dose.

What drug does:
- Dilates constricted bronchial tubes, improving air flow.
- Stimulates heart muscle and dilates blood vessels.

Time lapse before drug works:
2 to 4 minutes.

Don't take with:
See Interaction column and consult doctor.

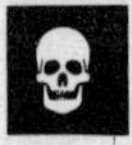

OVERDOSE

Symptoms:
Nervousness, rapid or irregular heartbeat, fainting, sweating, headache, tremor, vomiting, chest pain, blood-pressure drop.

What to do:
- Dial 0 (operator) or 911 (emergency) for an ambulance or medical help. Then give first aid immediately.
- Additional emergency information on page 886.

POSSIBLE ADVERSE REACTIONS OR SIDE EFFECTS

SYMPTOMS	FREQUENCY	WHAT TO DO
Brain & nervous system:		
• Nervousness, insomnia.	Common	4
• Dizziness, headache, trembling, weakness.	Infrequent	4
Skin:		
Flushed face.	Infrequent	4
Eyes:	None expected.	
Ears, nose, throat:		
Dry mouth, throat.	Common	5
Digestive:		
Nausea, vomiting.	Infrequent	4
Heart & lungs:		
Chest pain; irregular, fast or pounding heartbeat.	Infrequent	3
Blood vessels:	None expected.	
Muscles, bones, joints:	None expected.	
Genital, urinary:	None expected.	
Kidneys:	None expected.	
Liver:	None expected.	
Allergic:	None expected.	
Blood:	None expected.	
Others:		
Unusual sweating.	Infrequent	3

1- Life-threatening. Seek emergency treatment immediately.
2- Discontinue. Seek emergency treatment.
3- Discontinue. Call doctor right away.
4- Continue. Call doctor when convenient.
5- Continue. Tell doctor at next visit.
6- No action necessary.

WARNINGS & PRECAUTIONS

Don't take if:
- You are allergic to any sympathomimetic, including some diet pills.
- You have serious heart-rhythm disorder.
- You have taken MAO inhibitors in past 2 weeks.

Before you start, consult your doctor:
- If you are sensitive to sympathomimetics.
- If you use epinephrine.
- If you have high blood pressure, heart disease, or take a digitalis preparation.
- If you have diabetes.
- If you have overactive thyroid.
- If your heartbeat is faster than 100 beats per minute.

Over age 60:
You may be more sensitive to drug's stimulant effects. Use with caution if you have hardening of the arteries.

Pregnancy:
Studies inconclusive on harm to unborn child. Animal studies show fetal abnormalities. Decide with your doctor whether drug benefits justify risk to unborn child.

Breast-feeding:
Drug does not appear in milk. Consult doctor.

Infants & children:
Not recommended.

Prolonged use:
- Salivary glands may swell.
- Mouth ulcers (sublingual tablets).

Skin & sunlight:
No problems expected.

Driving, piloting or hazardous work:
Use caution if you feel dizzy or nervous.

Airplane passengers:
No problems expected.

Discontinuing:
Discontinue if drug fails to provide relief after 2 or 3 days. Consult doctor.

Others:
No problems expected.

INTERACTION WITH OTHER DRUGS

GENERIC NAME OR DRUG CLASS	COMBINED EFFECT
Antidepressants (tricyclic)	Increased effect of both drugs.
Beta-adrenergic blockers	Decreased isoproterenol effect.
Ephedrine	Increased ephedrine effect.
Epinephrine	Increased chance of serious heart disturbances.
Sympathomimetics (other)	Increased effect of both drugs, especially harmful side effects.

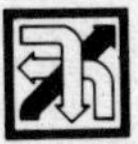

INTERACTION WITH OTHER SUBSTANCES

INTERACTS WITH	COMBINED EFFECT
Alcohol:	Decreased isoproterenol effect.
Beverages:	
Caffeine drinks	Overstimulation. Avoid.
Cocaine:	Overstimulation of brain and heart. Avoid.
Foods:	None expected.
Marijuana:	Increased antiasthmatic effect of isoproterenol.
Tobacco:	None expected.

ISOSORBIDE DINITRATE

BRAND NAMES

Coronex
Dilatrate-SR
Iso-Bid
Isochron
Isogard
Isordil
Isotrate
Novosorbide
Onset
Sorate
Sorbide
Sorbitrate

GENERAL INFORMATION

Habit forming? No
Prescription needed? Yes
Available as generic? Yes
Drug class: Antianginal (nitrate)

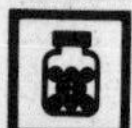

USES

Reduces frequency and severity of angina attacks.

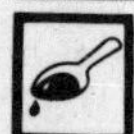

DOSAGE & USAGE INFORMATION

How to take:

- Sublingual tablet—Dissolve under tongue at earliest sign of angina.
- Chewable tablet—Chew tablet at earliest sign of angina, and hold in mouth for 2 minutes.
- Regular tablet—Swallow with liquid. You may chew or crush it.
- Extended-release tablets or capsules—Swallow each dose whole with liquid.

When to take:
Swallowed tablets—Take at the same times each day, 1 or 2 hours after meals.

If you forget a dose:
Swallowed tablets or capsules—Take as soon as you remember up to 2 hours late. If more than 2 hours, wait for next scheduled dose (don't double this dose).

What drug does:
Relaxes blood vessels, increasing blood flow to heart muscle.

Time lapse before drug works:

- Sublingual or chewable tablets—3 to 5 minutes.
- Swallowed tablets or capsules—30 minutes.

Don't take with:
See Interaction column and consult doctor.

OVERDOSE

Symptoms:
Vomiting, sweating, shortness of breath, loss of consciousness.

What to do:

- Dial 0 (operator) or 911 (emergency) for an ambulance or medical help. Then give first aid immediately.
- Additional emergency information on page 886.

POSSIBLE ADVERSE REACTIONS OR SIDE EFFECTS

SYMPTOMS	FREQUENCY	WHAT TO DO
Brain & nervous system:		
• Headache	Common	5
• Fainting	Infrequent	3
Skin:		
• Rash	Rare	3
• Flushed face and neck.	Common	5
Eyes:	None expected.	
Ears, nose, throat:	None expected.	
Digestive:		
Nausea, vomiting.	Common	5
Heart & lungs:		
Rapid heartbeat.	Common	5
Blood vessels:	None expected.	
Muscles, bones, joints:	None expected.	
Genital, urinary:	None expected.	
Kidneys:	None expected.	
Liver:	None expected.	
Allergic:	None expected.	
Blood:	None expected.	
Others:	None expected.	

1-Life-threatening. Seek emergency treatment immediately.
2-Discontinue. Seek emergency treatment.
3-Discontinue. Call doctor right away.
4-Continue. Call doctor when convenient.
5-Continue. Tell doctor at next visit.
6-No action necessary.

WARNINGS & PRECAUTIONS

Don't take if:
You are allergic to nitrates, including nitroglycerin.

Before you start, consult your doctor:
If you have glaucoma.

Over age 60:
Adverse reactions and side effects may be more frequent and severe than in younger persons.

Pregnancy:
No proven harm to unborn child. Avoid if possible.

Breast-feeding:
No proven problems. Consult your doctor.

Infants & children:
Not recommended.

Prolonged use:
Drug may become less effective and require higher doses.

Skin & sunlight:
No problems expected.

Driving, piloting or hazardous work:
Don't drive or pilot aircraft until you learn how medicine affects you. Don't work around dangerous machinery. Don't climb ladders or work in high places. Danger increases if you drink alcohol or take medicine affecting alertness and reflexes, such as antihistamines, tranquilizers, sedatives, pain medicine, narcotics and mind-altering drugs.

Airplane passengers:
No problems expected.

Discontinuing:
Don't discontinue without doctor's advice until you complete prescribed dose, even though symptoms diminish or disappear.

Others:
Periodic laboratory blood studies recommended if you take isosorbide dinitrate.

INTERACTION WITH OTHER DRUGS

GENERIC NAME OR DRUG CLASS	COMBINED EFFECT
Anticholinergics	Increased internal eye pressure.
Antidepressants (tricyclic)	Excessive blood-pressure drop.
Antihypertensives	Excessive blood-pressure drop.
Beta-adrenergic blockers	Excessive blood-pressure drop.
Cholinergics	Decreased cholinergic effect.
Ephedrine	Decreased effect of isosorbide dinitrate.

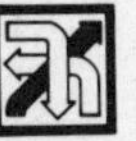

INTERACTION WITH OTHER SUBSTANCES

INTERACTS WITH	COMBINED EFFECT
Alcohol:	Excessive blood-pressure drop.
Beverages:	None expected.
Cocaine:	Flushed face and headache. Avoid.
Foods:	None expected.
Marijuana:	Decreased effect of isosorbide dinitrate.
Tobacco:	Decreased effect of isosorbide dinitrate.

ISOTRETINOIN

BRAND NAMES

Accutane

GENERAL INFORMATION

Habit forming? No
Prescription needed? Yes
Available as generic? No
Drug classification: Antiacne

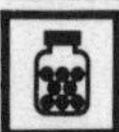

USES

- Decreases cystic acne formation in severe cases.
- Certain other skin disorders involving an overabundance of outer skin layer.

DOSAGE & USAGE INFORMATION

How to take:
Tablet or capsule—Swallow with liquid or food to lessen stomach irritation. If you can't swallow whole, crumble tablet or open capsule and take with liquid or food.

When to take:
Twice a day. Follow prescription directions.

If you forget a dose:
Take as soon as you remember up to 2 hours late. If more than 2 hours, wait for next scheduled dose and double dose.

What drug does:
Reduces sebaceous gland activity and size.

Time lapse before drug works:
May require 15 to 20 weeks to experience full benefit.

Don't take with:
Vitamin A or supplements containing Vitamin A.

OVERDOSE

Symptoms:
None reported.

What to do:
Overdose unlikely to threaten life. If person takes much larger amount than prescribed, call doctor, poison-control center or hospital emergency room for instructions.

POSSIBLE ADVERSE REACTIONS OR SIDE EFFECTS

SYMPTOMS	FREQUENCY	WHAT TO DO
Brain & nervous system:		
Headache	Infrequent	4
Skin:		
Rash, infection.	Infrequent	3
Itching skin.	Common	4
Eyes:		
Burning, redness, itching.	Common	3
Ears, nose, throat:		
Dry mouth.	Frequent	5 (Suck ice or chew gum.)
Digestive:		
Lip scaling, burning pain.	Common	3
Nausea, vomiting.	Infrequent	3
Heart & lungs:	None expected.	
Blood vessels:	None expected.	
Muscles, bones, joints:		
Pain.	Infrequent	4
Genital, urinary:	None expected.	
Kidneys, allergic, blood, liver:	None expected.	
Others:		
Hair thinning.	Infrequent	4
Tiredness.	Infrequent	4

1- Life-threatening. Seek emergency treatment immediately.
2- Discontinue. Seek emergency treatment.
3- Discontinue. Call doctor right away.
4- Continue. Call doctor when convenient.
5- Continue. Tell doctor at next visit.
6- No action necessary.

WARNINGS & PRECAUTIONS

Don't take if:
- You are allergic to isotretinoin.
- You are pregnant or plan pregnancy.

Before you start, consult your doctor:
- If you have diabetes.
- If you or any member of family have high triglyceride levels in blood.

Over age 60:
Adverse reactions and side effects may be more frequent and severe than in younger persons.

Pregnancy:
Risk to unborn child outweighs drug benefits. Don't use.

Breast-feeding:
Drug filters into milk. May harm child. Avoid.

Infants & children:
Not recommended.

Prolonged use:
Possible damage to cornea.

Skin & sunlight:
May cause rash or intensify sunburn in areas exposed to sun or sunlamp.

Driving, piloting or hazardous work:
No problems expected.

Airplane passengers:
No problems expected.

Discontinuing:
Single course of treatment usually all needed. If second course required, wait 8 weeks after completing first course.

Others:
Use only for severe cases of cystic acne that have not responded to less hazardous forms of acne treatment.

INTERACTION WITH OTHER DRUGS

GENERIC NAME OR DRUG CLASS	COMBINED EFFECT
Vitamin A	Additive toxic effect of each. Avoid.

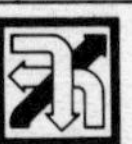

INTERACTION WITH OTHER SUBSTANCES

INTERACTS WITH	COMBINED EFFECT
Alcohol:	Significant increase in triglycerides in blood. Avoid.
Beverages:	No problems expected.
Cocaine:	Increased chance of toxicity of isotretinoin. Avoid.
Foods:	No problems expected.
Marijuana:	Increased chance of toxicity of isotretinoin. Avoid.
Tobacco:	May decrease absorption of medicine. Avoid tobacco while in treatment.

ISOXSUPRINE

BRAND NAMES

Vasodilan
Vasoprine

GENERAL INFORMATION

Habit forming? No
Prescription needed? Yes
Available as generic? Yes
Drug class: Vasodilator

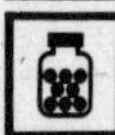

USES

Improves poor blood circulation.

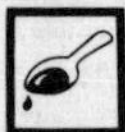

DOSAGE & USAGE INFORMATION

How to take:
Tablet—Swallow with liquid or food to lessen stomach irritation. If you can't swallow whole, crumble tablet and take with liquid or food.

When to take:
At the same times each day.

If you forget a dose:
Take as soon as you remember up to 2 hours late. If more than 2 hours, wait for next scheduled dose (don't double this dose).

What drug does:
Expands blood vessels, increasing flow and permitting distribution of oxygen and nutrients.

Time lapse before drug works:
1 hour.

Don't take with:
See Interaction column and consult doctor.

OVERDOSE

Symptoms:
Headache, dizziness, flush, vomiting, weakness, sweating, fainting, shortness of breath, coma.

What to do:
- Dial 0 (operator) or 911 (emergency) for an ambulance or medical help. Then give first aid immediately.
- If patient is unconscious and not breathing, give mouth-to-mouth breathing. If there is no heartbeat, use cardiac massage and mouth-to-mouth breathing (CPR). Don't try to make patient vomit. If you can't get help quickly, take patient to nearest emergency facility.
- Additional emergency information on page 886.

POSSIBLE ADVERSE REACTIONS OR SIDE EFFECTS

SYMPTOMS	FREQUENCY	WHAT TO DO
Brain & nervous system:		
Dizziness, faintness.	Common	4
Skin:		
Rash	Infrequent	3
Eyes:	None expected.	
Ears, nose, throat:	None expected.	
Digestive:		
Appetite loss, nausea, vomiting.	Common	3
Heart & lungs:		
Rapid or irregular heartbeat.	Rare	3
Blood vessels:	None expected.	
Muscles, bones, joints:	None expected.	
Genital, urinary:	None expected.	
Kidneys:	None expected.	
Liver:	None expected.	
Allergic:	None expected.	
Blood:	None expected.	
Others:		
Weakness, lethargy.	Common	5

1-Life-threatening. Seek emergency treatment immediately.
2-Discontinue. Seek emergency treatment.
3-Discontinue. Call doctor right away.
4-Continue. Call doctor when convenient.
5-Continue. Tell doctor at next visit.
6-No action necessary.

WARNINGS & PRECAUTIONS

Don't take if:
- You are allergic to any vasodilator.
- You have any bleeding disease.

Before you start, consult your doctor:
- If you have high blood pressure, hardening of the arteries or heart disease.
- If you plan to become pregnant within medication period.
- If you have glaucoma.

Over age 60:
Adverse reactions and side effects may be more frequent and severe than in younger persons.

Pregnancy:
Studies inconclusive on harm to unborn child. Decide with your doctor whether drug benefits justify risk to unborn child.

Breast-feeding:
No problems expected, but consult doctor.

Infants & children:
Not recommended.

Prolonged use:
No problems expected.

Skin & sunlight:
No problems expected.

Driving, piloting or hazardous work:
Avoid if you feel dizzy or faint. Otherwise, no problems expected.

Airplane passengers:
No problems expected.

Discontinuing:
Don't discontinue without doctor's advice until you complete prescribed dose, even though symptoms diminish or disappear.

Others:
Be cautious when arising from lying or sitting position, when climbing stairs, or if dizziness occurs.

INTERACTION WITH OTHER DRUGS

GENERIC NAME OR DRUG CLASS	COMBINED EFFECT
None	

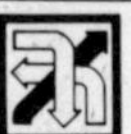

INTERACTION WITH OTHER SUBSTANCES

INTERACTS WITH	COMBINED EFFECT
Alcohol:	None expected.
Beverages:	
Milk	Decreased stomach irritation.
Cocaine:	Decreased blood circulation to extremities. Avoid.
Foods:	None expected.
Marijuana:	Rapid heartbeat.
Tobacco:	Decreased isoxsuprine effect.

KAOLIN AND PECTIN

BRAND NAMES

Kaopectate
K-P
K-Pek
Donnagel-PG
Parepectolin

GENERAL INFORMATION

Habit forming? No
Prescription needed? No
Available as generic? Yes
Drug class: Antidiarrheal

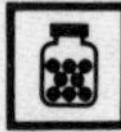

USES

Reduces intestinal cramps and diarrhea.

DOSAGE & USAGE INFORMATION

How to take:
Liquid—Swallow prescribed dosage (without diluting) after each loose bowel movement.

When to take:
After each loose bowel movement.

If you forget a dose:
Take when you remember.

What drug does:
Makes loose stools less watery, but may not prevent loss of fluids.

Time lapse before drug works:
15 to 30 minutes.

Don't take with:
See Interaction column and consult doctor.

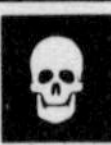

OVERDOSE

Symptoms:
Fecal impaction.

What to do:
Overdose unlikely to threaten life. If person takes much larger amount than prescribed, call doctor, poison-control center or hospital emergency room for instructions.

POSSIBLE ADVERSE REACTIONS OR SIDE EFFECTS

SYMPTOMS	FREQUENCY	WHAT TO DO
Brain & nervous system:	None expected.	
Skin:	None expected.	
Eyes:	None expected.	
Ears, nose, throat:	None expected.	
Digestive: Constipation, mild.	Rare	4
Heart & lungs:	None expected.	
Blood vessels:	None expected.	
Muscles, bones, joints:	None expected.	
Genital, urinary:	None expected.	
Kidneys, allergic, blood, liver:	None expected.	
Others:	None expected.	

1- Life-threatening. Seek emergency treatment immediately.
2- Discontinue. Seek emergency treatment.
3- Discontinue. Call doctor right away.
4- Continue. Call doctor when convenient.
5- Continue. Tell doctor at next visit.
6- No action necessary.

KAOLIN AND PECTIN

WARNINGS & PRECAUTIONS

Don't take if:
You are allergic to kaolin or pectin.

Before you start, consult your doctor:
- If patient is child or infant.
- If you have any chronic medical problem with heart disease, peptic ulcer, asthma or others.
- If you have fever over 101F.

Over age 60:
Fluid loss caused by diarrhea, especially if taking other medicines, may lead to serious disability. Consult doctor.

Pregnancy:
No problems expected.

Breast-feeding:
No problems expected.

Infants & children:
Fluid loss caused by diarrhea in infants and children can cause serious dehydration. Consult doctor before giving any medicine for diarrhea.

Prolonged use:
Not recommended.

Skin & sunlight:
No problems expected.

Driving, piloting or hazardous work:
No problems expected.

Airplane passengers:
No problems expected.

Discontinuing:
May be unnecessary to finish medicine. Follow doctor's instructions.

Others:
Consult doctor about fluids, diet and rest.

INTERACTION WITH OTHER DRUGS

GENERIC NAME OR DRUG CLASS	COMBINED EFFECT
Digoxin	Decreases absorption of digoxin. Separate doses by at least 2 hours.
Lincomycin	Decreases absorption of lincomycin. Separate doses by at least 2 hours.
All other oral medicines.	Decreases absorption of other medicines. Separate doses by at least 2 hours.

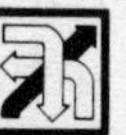

INTERACTION WITH OTHER SUBSTANCES

INTERACTS WITH	COMBINED EFFECT
Alcohol:	Increased diarrhea. Prevents action of kaolin and pectin.
Beverages:	No problems expected.
Cocaine:	Aggravates underlying disease. Avoid.
Foods:	No problems expected.
Marijuana:	Aggravates underlying disease. Avoid.
Tobacco:	Aggravates underlying disease. Avoid.

KETOCONAZOLE

BRAND NAMES

Nizoral

GENERAL INFORMATION

Habit forming? No
Prescription needed? Yes
Available as generic? No
Drug class: Antifungal

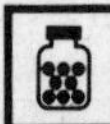

USES

Treatment of fungus infections susceptible to ketoconazole.

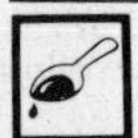

DOSAGE & USAGE INFORMATION

How to take:
Tablet or capsule—Swallow with liquid or food to lessen stomach irritation. If you can't swallow whole, crumble tablet or open capsule and take with liquid or food.

When to take:
At same time once a day.

If you forget a dose:
Take as soon as you remember up to 2 hours late. If more than 2 hours, wait for next scheduled dose (don't double this dose).

What drug does:
Prevents fungi from growing and reproducing.

Time lapse before drug works:
8 to 10 months or longer.

Don't take with:
See Interaction column and consult doctor.

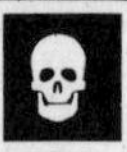

OVERDOSE

Symptoms:
Nausea, vomiting, diarrhea.

What to do:
Overdose unlikely to threaten life. If person takes much larger amount than prescribed, call doctor, poison-control center or hospital emergency room for instructions.

POSSIBLE ADVERSE REACTIONS OR SIDE EFFECTS

SYMPTOMS	FREQUENCY	WHAT TO DO
Brain & nervous system:		
• Drowsiness	Infrequent	4
• Insomnia	Infrequent	4
Skin:		
Rash or itching.	Infrequent	3
Eyes:		
Increased sensitivity to light.	Infrequent	3
Ears, nose, throat:	None expected.	
Digestive:		
• Pale stools.	Rare	3
• Abdominal pain.	Rare	3
• Nausea or vomiting.	Common	3
• Diarrhea	Infrequent	4
Heart & lungs:	None expected.	
Blood vessels:	None expected.	
Muscles, bones, joints:	None expected.	
Genital, urinary:		
Dark or amber urine.	Rare	3
Kidneys, allergic, blood, liver:	None expected.	
Others:		
• Decreased sex drive in males.	Rare	4
• Tiredness, weakness.	Rare	4

1- Life-threatening. Seek emergency treatment immediately.
2- Discontinue. Seek emergency treatment.
3- Discontinue. Call doctor right away.
4- Continue. Call doctor when convenient.
5- Continue. Tell doctor at next visit.
6- No action necessary.

KETOCONAZOLE

WARNINGS & PRECAUTIONS

Don't take if:
You are allergic to ketoconazole.

Before you start, consult your doctor:
- If you have absence of stomach acid (achlorhydria).
- If you have liver disease.

Over age 60:
Adverse reactions and side effects may be more frequent and severe than in younger persons.

Pregnancy:
Risk to unborn child outweighs drug benefits. Don't use.

Breast-feeding:
Drug passes into milk. Avoid drug or discontinue nursing until you finish medicine. Consult doctor for advice on maintaining milk supply.

Infants & children:
Only under close medical supervision.

Prolonged use:
Request liver-function studies.

Skin & sunlight:
No problems expected.

Driving, piloting or hazardous work:
Don't drive or pilot aircraft until you learn how medicine affects you. Don't work around dangerous machinery. Don't climb ladders or work in high places. Danger increases if you drink alcohol or take medicine affecting alertness and reflexes, such as antihistamines, tranquilizers, sedatives, pain medicine, narcotics and mind-altering drugs.

Airplane passengers:
No problems expected.

Discontinuing:
May be unnecessary to finish medicine. Follow doctor's instructions.

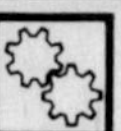

INTERACTION WITH OTHER DRUGS

GENERIC NAME OR DRUG CLASS	COMBINED EFFECT
Antacids	Decreased absorption of ketoconazole.
Anticholinergics	Decreased absorption of ketoconazole.
Atropine	Decreased absorption of ketoconazole.
Belladonna	Decreased absorption of ketoconazole.
Cimetidine	Decreased absorption of ketoconazole.
Clidinium	Decreased absorption of ketoconazole.
Glycopyrrolate	Decreased absorption of ketoconazole.
Hyoscyamine	Decreased absorption of ketoconazole.
Methscopolamine	Decreased absorption of ketoconazole.

Additional interactions on page 838.

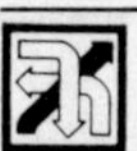

INTERACTION WITH OTHER SUBSTANCES

INTERACTS WITH	COMBINED EFFECT
Alcohol:	Increased chance of liver damage.
Beverages:	No problems expected.
Cocaine:	Decreased ketoconazole effect. Avoid cocaine.
Foods:	No problems expected.
Marijuana:	Decreased ketoconazole effect. Avoid marijuana.
Tobacco:	Decreased ketoconazole effect. Avoid tobacco.

LACTULOSE

BRAND NAMES

Cephalac
Chronulac

GENERAL INFORMATION

Habit forming? No
Prescription needed? No
Available as generic? No
Drug class: Laxative (hyperosmotic)

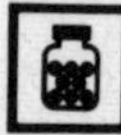

USES

Constipation relief.

DOSAGE & USAGE INFORMATION

How to take:
Liquid—Dilute dose in beverage before swallowing.

When to take:
Usually once a day, preferably in the morning.

If you forget a dose:
Take as soon as you remember up to 8 hours before bedtime. If later, wait for next scheduled dose (don't double this dose). Don't take at bedtime.

What drug does:
Draws water into bowel from other body tissues. Causes distention through fluid accumulation, which promotes soft stool and accelerates bowel motion.

Time lapse before drug works:
30 minutes to 3 hours.

Don't take with:
Another medicine. Space 2 hours apart.

OVERDOSE

Symptoms:
Fluid depletion, weakness, vomiting, fainting.

What to do:
Overdose unlikely to threaten life. If person takes much larger amount than prescribed, call doctor, poison-control center or hospital emergency room for instructions.

POSSIBLE ADVERSE REACTIONS OR SIDE EFFECTS

SYMPTOMS	FREQUENCY	WHAT TO DO
Brain & nervous system: Dizziness, confusion.	Rare	4
Skin:	None expected.	
Eyes:	None expected.	
Ears, nose, throat: Increased thirst.	Infrequent	5
Digestive: Cramps, nausea, diarrhea, gas.	Infrequent	5
Heart & lungs: Irregular heartbeat.	Infrequent	3
Blood vessels:	None expected.	
Muscles, bones, joints:	None expected.	
Genital, urinary:	None expected.	
Kidneys:	None expected.	
Liver:	None expected.	
Allergic:	None expected.	
Blood:	None expected.	
Others: Fatigue, weakness.	Rare	4

1- Life-threatening. Seek emergency treatment immediately.
2- Discontinue. Seek emergency treatment.
3- Discontinue. Call doctor right away.
4- Continue. Call doctor when convenient.
5- Continue. Tell doctor at next visit.
6- No action necessary.

WARNINGS & PRECAUTIONS

Don't take if:
- You are allergic to any hyperosmotic laxative.
- You have symptoms of appendicitis, inflamed bowel or intestinal blockage.
- You have missed a bowel movement for only 1 or 2 days.

Before you start, consult your doctor:
- If you have congestive heart disease.
- If you have diabetes.
- If you have high blood pressure.
- If you have a colostomy or ileostomy.
- If you have kidney disease.
- If you have a laxative habit.
- If you have rectal bleeding.
- If you take another laxative.
- If you require a low-galactose diet.

Over age 60:
Adverse reactions and side effects may be more frequent and severe than in younger persons.

Pregnancy:
No proven problems. Avoid if possible.

Breast-feeding:
No problems expected.

Infants & children:
Use only under medical supervision.

Prolonged use:
Don't take for more than 1 week unless under a doctor's supervision. May cause laxative dependence.

Skin & sunlight:
No problems expected.

Driving, piloting or hazardous work:
No problems expected.

Airplane passengers:
No problems expected.

Discontinuing:
May be unnecessary to finish medicine. Follow doctor's instructions.

Others:
Don't take to "flush out" your system or as a "tonic."

INTERACTION WITH OTHER DRUGS

GENERIC NAME OR DRUG CLASS	COMBINED EFFECT
None	

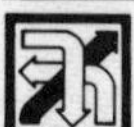

INTERACTION WITH OTHER SUBSTANCES

INTERACTS WITH	COMBINED EFFECT
Alcohol:	None expected.
Beverages:	None expected.
Cocaine:	None expected.
Foods:	None expected.
Marijuana:	None expected.
Tobacco:	None expected.

LEVODOPA

BRAND NAMES

Bendopa
Dopar
Larodopa
Levopa
Sinemet

GENERAL INFORMATION

Habit forming? No
Prescription needed? Yes
Available as generic? Yes
Drug class: Antiparkinsonism

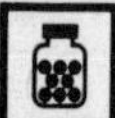

USES

Controls Parkinson's disease symptoms such as rigidity, tremor and unsteady gait.

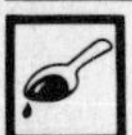

DOSAGE & USAGE INFORMATION

How to take:
Tablet or capsule—Swallow with liquid or food to lessen stomach irritation. If you can't swallow whole, crumble tablet or open capsule and take with liquid or food.

When to take:
At the same times each day.

If you forget a dose:
Take as soon as you remember up to 2 hours late. If more than 2 hours, wait for next scheduled dose (don't double this dose).

What drug does:
Restores chemical balance necessary for normal nerve impulses.

Time lapse before drug works:
2 to 3 weeks to improve; 6 weeks or longer for maximum benefit.

Don't take with:
See Interaction column and consult doctor.

OVERDOSE

Symptoms:
Muscle twitch, spastic eyelid closure, nausea, vomiting, diarrhea, irregular and rapid pulse, weakness, fainting, confusion, agitation, hallucination, coma.

What to do:
- Dial 0 (operator) or 911 (emergency) for an ambulance or medical help. Then give first aid immediately.
- If patient is unconscious and not breathing, give mouth-to-mouth breathing. If there is no heartbeat, use cardiac massage and mouth-to-mouth breathing (CPR). Don't try to make patient vomit. If you can't get help quickly, take patient to nearest emergency facility.
- Additional emergency information on page 886.

POSSIBLE ADVERSE REACTIONS OR SIDE EFFECTS

SYMPTOMS	FREQUENCY	WHAT TO DO
Brain & nervous system:		
• Fainting, severe dizziness, headache, insomnia, nightmares.	Infrequent	3
• Mood changes, uncontrolled body movements.	Common	4
Skin:		
• Flushed face.	Infrequent	4
• Rash, itch.	Infrequent	3
Eyes:		
Blurred vision.	Infrequent	4
Ears, nose, throat:		
Dry mouth.	Common	6
Digestive:		
• Duodenal ulcer.	Rare	4
• Diarrhea	Common	4
• Constipation	Infrequent	5
• Nausea, vomiting.	Infrequent	3
Heart & lungs:		
Irregular heartbeat.	Infrequent	3
Blood vessels:		
High blood pressure.	Rare	3
Muscles, bones, joints:		
Muscle twitching.	Infrequent	4
Genital, urinary:		
• Discolored or dark urine.	Infrequent	4
• Difficult urination.	Infrequent	4
Kidneys, liver, allergic:	None expected.	
Blood:		
Anemia	Rare	4
Others:		
• Tiredness	Infrequent	5
• Body odor.	Common	6

1- Life-threatening. Seek emergency treatment immediately.
2- Discontinue. Seek emergency treatment.
3- Discontinue. Call doctor right away.
4- Continue. Call doctor when convenient.
5- Continue. Tell doctor at next visit.
6- No action necessary.

WARNINGS & PRECAUTIONS

Don't take if:
- You are allergic to levodopa or carbidopa.
- You have taken MAO inhibitors in past 2 weeks.
- You have glaucoma (narrow-angle type).

Before you start, consult your doctor:
- If you have diabetes or epilepsy.
- If you have had high blood pressure, heart or lung disease.
- If you have had liver or kidney disease.
- If you have a peptic ulcer.
- If you have malignant melanoma.
- If you will have surgery within 2 months, including dental surgery, requiring general or spinal anesthesia.

Over age 60:
Adverse reactions and side effects may be more frequent and severe than in younger persons.

Pregnancy:
Risk to unborn child outweighs drug benefits. Don't use.

Breast-feeding:
Drug filters into milk. May harm child. Avoid.

Infants & children:
Not recommended.

Prolonged use:
May lead to uncontrolled movements of head, face, mouth, tongue, arms or legs.

Skin & sunlight:
No problems expected.

Driving, piloting or hazardous work:
Don't drive or pilot aircraft until you learn how medicine affects you. Don't work around dangerous machinery. Don't climb ladders or work in high places. Danger increases if you drink alcohol or take medicine affecting alertness and reflexes, such as antihistamines, tranquilizers, sedatives, pain medicine, narcotics and mind-altering drugs.

Airplane passengers:
No problems expected.

Discontinuing:
Don't discontinue without doctor's advice until you complete prescribed dose, even though symptoms diminish or disappear.

Others:
Expect to start with small dose and increase gradually to lessen frequency and severity of adverse reactions.

INTERACTION WITH OTHER DRUGS

GENERIC NAME OR DRUG CLASS	COMBINED EFFECT
Antiparkinsonism drugs (other)	Increased levodopa effect.
Haloperidol	Decreased levodopa effect.
MAO inhibitors	Dangerous rise in blood pressure.
Methyldopa	Decreased levodopa effect.
Papaverine	Decreased levodopa effect.
Phenothiazines	Decreased levodopa effect.
Pyridoxine (Vitamin B-6)	Decreased levodopa effect.
Rauwolfia alkaloids	Decreased levodopa effect.

INTERACTION WITH OTHER SUBSTANCES

INTERACTS WITH	COMBINED EFFECT
Alcohol:	None expected.
Beverages:	None expected.
Cocaine:	Decreased levodopa effect.
Foods:	None expected.
Marijuana:	Increased fatigue, lethargy, fainting.
Tobacco:	None expected.

LINCOMYCIN

BRAND NAMES

Lincocin

GENERAL INFORMATION

Habit forming? No
Prescription needed? Yes
Available as generic? No
Drug class: Antibiotic (lincomycin)

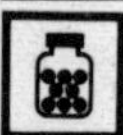

USES

Treatment of bacterial infections that are susceptible to lincomycin.

DOSAGE & USAGE INFORMATION

How to take:
Capsule or liquid—Swallow with liquid 1 hour before or 2 hours after eating.

When to take:
At the same times each day.

If you forget a dose:
Take as soon as you remember up to 2 hours late. If more than 2 hours, wait for next scheduled dose (don't double this dose).

What drug does:
Destroys susceptible bacteria. Does not kill viruses.

Time lapse before drug works:
3 to 5 days.

Don't take with:
See Interaction column and consult doctor.

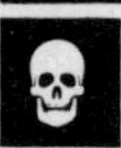

OVERDOSE

Symptoms:
Severe nausea, vomiting, diarrhea.

What to do:
Overdose unlikely to threaten life. If person takes much larger amount than prescribed, call doctor, poison-control center or hospital emergency room for instructions.

POSSIBLE ADVERSE REACTIONS OR SIDE EFFECTS

SYMPTOMS	FREQUENCY	WHAT TO DO
Brain & nervous system:	None expected.	
Skin:		
Rash, itch around groin, rectum or armpits.	Infrequent	4
Eyes:	None expected.	
Ears, nose, throat:		
• Unusual thirst.	Infrequent	3
• White patches in mouth.	Infrequent	4
Digestive:		
Vomiting, stomach cramps, severe and watery diarrhea with blood or mucus.	Infrequent	3
Heart & lungs:	None expected.	
Blood vessels:	None expected.	
Muscles, bones, joints:		
Painful, swollen joints.	Infrequent	3
Genital, urinary:		
Vaginal discharge, itching.	Infrequent	4
Kidneys:	None expected.	
Liver:		
Jaundice (yellow skin and eyes).	Infrequent	3
Allergic:	None expected.	
Blood:	None expected.	
Others:		
• Fever	Infrequent	3
• Tiredness, weakness, weight loss.	Infrequent	3

1- Life-threatening. Seek emergency treatment immediately.
2- Discontinue. Seek emergency treatment.
3- Discontinue. Call doctor right away.
4- Continue. Call doctor when convenient.

WARNINGS & PRECAUTIONS

Don't take if:
- You are allergic to lincomycins.
- You have had ulcerative colitis.
- Prescribed for infant under 1 month old.

Before you start, consult your doctor:
- If you have had yeast infections of mouth, skin or vagina.
- If you will have surgery within 2 months, including dental surgery, requiring general or spinal anesthesia.
- If you have kidney or liver disease.
- If you have allergies of any kind.

Over age 60:
Adverse reactions and side effects may be more frequent and severe than in younger persons.

Pregnancy:
Risk to unborn child outweighs drug benefits. Don't use.

Breast-feeding:
Drug passes into milk. Avoid drug or discontinue nursing until you finish medicine. Consult doctor for advice on maintaining milk supply.

Infants & children:
Don't give to infants younger than 1 month. Use for children only under medical supervision.

Prolonged use:
- Severe colitis with diarrhea and bleeding.
- You may become more susceptible to infections caused by germs not responsive to lincomycin.

Skin & sunlight:
No problems expected.

Driving, piloting or hazardous work:
No problems expected.

Airplane passengers:
No problems expected.

Discontinuing:
Don't discontinue without doctor's advice until you complete prescribed dose, even though symptoms diminish or disappear.

Others:
No problems expected.

INTERACTION WITH OTHER DRUGS

GENERIC NAME OR DRUG CLASS	COMBINED EFFECT
Antidiarrheal preparations	Decreased lincomycin effect.
Chloramphenicol	Decreased lincomycin effect.
Erythromycin	Decreased lincomycin effect.

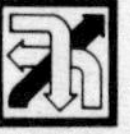

INTERACTION WITH OTHER SUBSTANCES

INTERACTS WITH	COMBINED EFFECT
Alcohol:	None expected.
Beverages:	None expected.
Cocaine:	None expected.
Foods:	None expected.
Marijuana:	None expected.
Tobacco:	None expected.

LIOTHYRONINE

BRAND NAMES

Cytomel
Ro-Thyronine
Tertroxin

GENERAL INFORMATION

Habit forming? No
Prescription needed? Yes
Available as generic? Yes
Drug class: Thyroid hormone

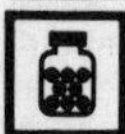

USES

Replacement for thyroid hormone deficiency.

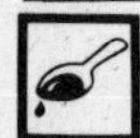

DOSAGE & USAGE INFORMATION

How to take:

- Tablet or capsule—Swallow with liquid.
- Extended-release tablets or capsules—Swallow each dose whole. If you take regular tablets, you may chew or crush them.

When to take:
At the same time each day before a meal or on awakening.

If you forget a dose:
Take as soon as you remember up to 12 hours late. If more than 12 hours, wait for next scheduled dose (don't double this dose).

What drug does:
Increases cell metabolism rate.

Time lapse before drug works:
48 hours.

Don't take with:
See Interaction column and consult doctor.

OVERDOSE

Symptoms:
"Hot" feeling, heart palpitations, nervousness, sweating, hand tremors, insomnia, rapid and irregular pulse, headache, irritability, diarrhea, weight loss, muscle cramps.

What to do:
Overdose unlikely to threaten life. If person takes much larger amount than prescribed, call doctor, poison-control center or hospital emergency room for instructions.

POSSIBLE ADVERSE REACTIONS OR SIDE EFFECTS

SYMPTOMS	FREQUENCY	WHAT TO DO
Brain & nervous system:		
Tremor, headache, irritability, insomnia.	Common	3
Skin:		
Hives, rash.	Infrequent	3
Eyes:	None expected.	
Ears, nose, throat:	None expected.	
Digestive:		
• Appetite change.	Common	4
• Diarrhea	Common	4
• Vomiting	Infrequent	3
Heart & lungs:		
Chest pain, rapid and irregular heartbeat, shortness of breath.	Infrequent	3
Blood vessels:	None expected.	
Muscles, bones, joints:		
Leg cramps.	Common	4
Genital, urinary:	None expected.	
Kidneys:	None expected.	
Liver:	None expected.	
Allergic:	None expected.	
Blood:	None expected.	
Others:		
• Change in menstrual periods.	Common	4
• Fever, heat sensitivity, unusual sweating.	Common	4
• Weight loss.	Common	4

1 - Life-threatening. Seek emergency treatment immediately.
2 - Discontinue. Seek emergency treatment.
3 - Discontinue. Call doctor right away.
4 - Continue. Call doctor when convenient.
5 - Continue. Tell doctor at next visit.
6 - No action necessary.

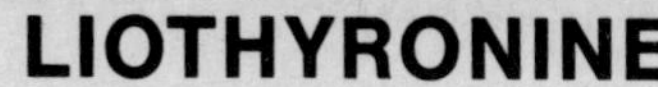

WARNINGS & PRECAUTIONS

Don't take if:
- You have had a heart attack within 6 weeks.
- You have no thyroid deficiency, but use this to lose weight.

Before you start, consult your doctor:
- If you have heart disease or high blood pressure.
- If you have diabetes.
- If you have Addison's disease, have had adrenal gland deficiency or use epinephrine, ephedrine or isoproterenol for asthma.

Over age 60:
More sensitive to thyroid hormone. May need smaller doses.

Pregnancy:
Considered safe if for thyroid deficiency only.

Breast-feeding:
Present in milk. Considered safe if dose is correct.

Infants & children:
Use only under medical supervision.

Prolonged use:
No problems expected, if dose is correct.

Skin & sunlight:
No problems expected.

Driving, piloting or hazardous work:
No problems expected.

Airplane passengers:
No problems expected.

Discontinuing:
Don't discontinue without consulting doctor. Dose may require gradual reduction if you have taken drug for a long time. Doses of other drugs may also require adjustment.

Others:
Digestive upsets, tremors, cramps, nervousness, insomnia or diarrhea may indicate need for dose adjustment.

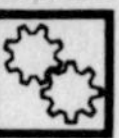

INTERACTION WITH OTHER DRUGS

GENERIC NAME OR DRUG CLASS	COMBINED EFFECT
Amphetamines	Increased amphetamine effect.
Anticoagulants (oral)	Increased anticoagulant effect.
Antidepressants (tricyclic)	Increased antidepressant effect.
Antidiabetics	Antidiabetic may require adjustment.
Aspirin (large doses, continuous use)	Increased liothyronine effect.
Barbiturates	Decreased barbiturate effect.
Cholestyramine	Decreased liothyronine effect.
Contraceptives (oral)	Decreased liothyronine effect.
Cortisone drugs	Requires dose adjustment to prevent cortisone deficiency.
Digitalis preparations	Increased digitalis effect.
Ephedrine	Increased ephedrine effect.
Epinephrine	Increased epinephrine effect.
Methylphenidate	Increased methylphenidate effect.
Phenytoin	Increased liothyronine effect.

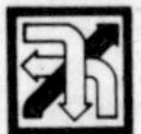

INTERACTION WITH OTHER SUBSTANCES

INTERACTS WITH	COMBINED EFFECT
Alcohol:	None expected.
Beverages:	None expected.
Cocaine:	Excess stimulation. Avoid.
Foods: Soybeans	Heavy consumption interferes with thyroid function.
Marijuana:	None expected.
Tobacco:	None expected.

LIOTRIX

BRAND NAMES

Euthroid
Thyrolar

GENERAL INFORMATION

Habit forming? No
Prescription needed? Yes
Available as generic? Yes
Drug class: Thyroid hormone

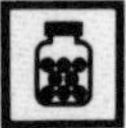

USES

Replacement for thyroid hormone deficiency.

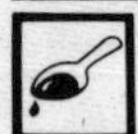

DOSAGE & USAGE INFORMATION

How to take:
- Tablet or capsule—Swallow with liquid.
- Extended-release tablets or capsules—Swallow each dose whole. If you take regular tablets, you may chew or crush them.

When to take:
At the same time each day before a meal or on awakening.

If you forget a dose:
Take as soon as you remember up to 12 hours late. If more than 12 hours, wait for next scheduled dose (don't double this dose).

What drug does:
Increases cell metabolism rate.

Time lapse before drug works:
48 hours.

Don't take with:
See Interaction column and consult doctor.

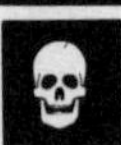

OVERDOSE

Symptoms:
"Hot" feeling, heart palpitations, nervousness, sweating, hand tremors, insomnia, rapid and irregular pulse, headache, irritability, diarrhea, weight loss, muscle cramps.

What to do:
Overdose unlikely to threaten life. If person takes much larger amount than prescribed, call doctor, poison-control center or hospital emergency room for instructions.

POSSIBLE ADVERSE REACTIONS OR SIDE EFFECTS

SYMPTOMS	FREQUENCY	WHAT TO DO
Brain & nervous system:		
Tremor, headache, irritability, insomnia.	Common	3
Skin:		
Hives, rash.	Infrequent	3
Eyes:	None expected.	
Ears, nose, throat:	None expected.	
Digestive:		
• Appetite change.	Common	4
• Diarrhea	Common	4
• Vomiting	Infrequent	3
Heart & lungs:		
Chest pain, rapid and irregular heartbeat, shortness of breath.	Infrequent	3
Blood vessels:	None expected.	
Muscles, bones, joints:		
Leg cramps.	Common	4
Genital, urinary:	None expected.	
Kidneys:	None expected.	
Liver:	None expected.	
Allergic:	None expected.	
Blood:	None expected.	
Others:		
• Change in menstrual periods.	Common	4
• Fever, heat sensitivity, unusual sweating.	Common	4
• Weight loss.	Common	4

1- Life-threatening. Seek emergency treatment immediately.
2- Discontinue. Seek emergency treatment.
3- Discontinue. Call doctor right away.
4- Continue. Call doctor when convenient.
5- Continue. Tell doctor at next visit.
6- No action necessary.

WARNINGS & PRECAUTIONS

Don't take if:
- You have had a heart attack within 6 weeks.
- You have no thyroid deficiency, but use this to lose weight.

Before you start, consult your doctor:
- If you have heart disease or high blood pressure.
- If you have diabetes.
- If you have Addison's disease, have had adrenal gland deficiency or use epinephrine, ephedrine or isoproterenol for asthma.

Over age 60:
More sensitive to thyroid hormone. May need smaller doses.

Pregnancy:
Considered safe if for thyroid deficiency only.

Breast-feeding:
Present in milk. Considered safe if dose is correct.

Infants & children:
Use only under medical supervision.

Prolonged use:
No problems expected, if dose is correct.

Skin & sunlight:
No problems expected.

Driving, piloting or hazardous work:
No problems expected.

Airplane passengers:
No problems expected.

Discontinuing:
Don't discontinue without consulting doctor. Dose may require gradual reduction if you have taken drug for a long time. Doses of other drugs may also require adjustment.

Others:
Digestive upsets, tremors, cramps, nervousness, insomnia or diarrhea may indicate need for dose adjustment.

INTERACTION WITH OTHER DRUGS

GENERIC NAME OR DRUG CLASS	COMBINED EFFECT
Amphetamines	Increased amphetamine effect.
Anticoagulants (oral)	Increased anticoagulant effect.
Antidepressants (tricyclic)	Increased antidepressant effect.
Antidiabetics	Antidiabetic may require adjustment.
Aspirin (large doses, continuous use)	Increased liotrix effect.
Barbiturates	Decreased barbiturate effect.
Cholestyramine	Decreased liotrix effect.
Contraceptives (oral)	Decreased liotrix effect.
Cortisone drugs	Requires dose adjustment to prevent cortisone deficiency.
Digitalis preparations	Increased digitalis effect.
Ephedrine	Increased ephedrine effect.
Epinephrine	Increased epinephrine effect.
Methylphenidate	Increased methylphenidate effect.
Phenytoin	Increased liotrix effect.

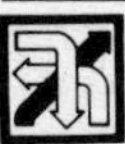

INTERACTION WITH OTHER SUBSTANCES

INTERACTS WITH	COMBINED EFFECT
Alcohol:	None expected.
Beverages:	None expected.
Cocaine:	Excess stimulation. Avoid.
Foods:	
Soybeans	Heavy consumption interferes with thyroid function.
Marijuana:	None expected.
Tobacco:	None expected.

LITHIUM

BRAND NAMES

Carbolith
Cibalith-S
Eskalith
Eskalith CR
Lithane
Lithizine
Lithobid
Lithonate
Lithotabs
Pfi-Lithium

GENERAL INFORMATION

Habit forming? No
Prescription needed? Yes
Available as generic? Yes
Drug class: Tranquilizer

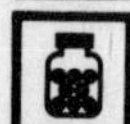

USES

Normalizes mood and behavior in manic-depressive illness.

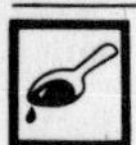

DOSAGE & USAGE INFORMATION

How to take:

- Tablet or capsule—Swallow with liquid or food to lessen stomach irritation. If you can't swallow whole, crumble tablet or open capsule and take with liquid or food. Drink 2 or 3 quarts liquid per day.
- Extended-release tablets or capsules—Swallow each dose whole.
- Syrup—Take at mealtime. Follow with 8 oz. water.

When to take:
At the same times each day, preferably mealtime.

If you forget a dose:
Take as soon as you remember up to 2 hours late. If more than 2 hours, wait for next scheduled dose (don't double this dose).

What drug does:
May correct chemical imbalance in brain's transmission of nerve impulses that influence mood and behavior.

Time lapse before drug works:
1 to 3 weeks. May require 3 months before depressive phase of illness improves.

Don't take with:
See Interaction column and consult doctor.

OVERDOSE

Symptoms:
Moderate overdose increases some side effects. Large overdose may cause convulsions, stupor and coma.

What to do:

- Dial 0 (operator) or 911 (emergency) for an ambulance or medical help. Then give first aid immediately.
- Additional emergency information on page 886.

POSSIBLE ADVERSE REACTIONS OR SIDE EFFECTS

SYMPTOMS	FREQUENCY	WHAT TO DO
Brain & nervous system:		
• Dizziness	Common	4
• Drowsiness, confusion.	Infrequent	5
Skin:		
Rash	Infrequent	3
Eyes:		
Blurred vision.	Rare	3
Ears, nose, throat:		
Dry mouth, thirst.	Common	5
Digestive:		
• Diarrhea, nausea, vomiting.	Common	4
• Stomach pain.	Infrequent	3
Heart & lungs, blood vessels, kidneys, liver, allergic, blood:	None expected.	
Muscles, bones, joints:		
• Shakiness, tremor.	Common	4
• Weakness	Infrequent	5
• Jerking of arms and legs.	Rare	4
• Swollen hands, feet.	Infrequent	4
Genital, urinary:		
Decreased sexual ability, increased urination.	Common	5
Others:		
• Slurred speech.	Infrequent	4
• Thyroid impairment—coldness; dry, puffy skin; muscle aches; headaches; weight gain; fatigue; menstrual changes.	Infrequent	4

1- Life-threatening. Seek emergency treatment immediately.
2- Discontinue. Seek emergency treatment.
3- Discontinue. Call doctor right away.
4- Continue. Call doctor when convenient.
5- Continue. Tell doctor at next visit.

WARNINGS & PRECAUTIONS

Don't take if:
- You are allergic to lithium.
- You have kidney or heart disease.
- Patient is younger than 12.

Before you start, consult your doctor:
- About all medications you take.
- If you plan to become pregnant within medication period.
- If you have diabetes, low thyroid function, epilepsy or any significant medical problem.
- If you are on a low-salt diet or drink more than 4 cups of coffee per day.
- If you plan surgery within 2 months.

Over age 60:
Adverse reactions and side effects may be more frequent and severe than in younger persons.

Pregnancy:
Risk to unborn child outweighs drug benefits. Don't use.

Breast-feeding:
Drug passes into milk. Avoid drug or discontinue nursing until you finish medicine. Consult doctor for advice on maintaining milk supply.

Infants & children:
Don't give to children younger than 12.

Prolonged use:
Enlarged thyroid with possible impaired function.

Skin & sunlight:
No problems expected.

Driving, piloting or hazardous work:
Don't drive or pilot aircraft until you learn how medicine affects you. Don't work around dangerous machinery. Don't climb ladders or work in high places. Danger increases if you drink alcohol or take medicine affecting alertness and reflexes.

Airplane passengers:
Consult doctor.

Discontinuing:
Don't discontinue without consulting doctor. Dose may require gradual reduction if you have taken drug for a long time. Doses of other drugs may also require adjustment.

Others:
- Regular checkups, periodic blood tests, and tests of lithium levels and thyroid function recommended.
- Avoid exercise in hot weather and other activities that cause heavy sweating. This contributes to lithium poisoning.

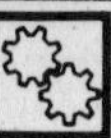

INTERACTION WITH OTHER DRUGS

GENERIC NAME OR DRUG CLASS	COMBINED EFFECT
Acetazolamide	Decreased lithium effect.
Aminophylline	Decreased lithium effect.
Diuretics	Increased lithium effect.
Haloperidol	Increased toxicity of both drugs.
Indomethacin	Increased lithium effect.
Methyldopa	Increased lithium effect.
Muscle relaxants (skeletal)	Increased skeletal-muscle relaxation.
Oxyphenbutazone	Increased lithium effect.
Phenothiazines	Decreased lithium effect.
Phentyoin	Increased lithium effect.
Phenylbutazone	Increased lithium effect.
Potassium iodide	Increased potassium iodide effect.
Sodium bicarbonate	Decreased lithium effect.
Tetracyclines	Increased lithium effect.

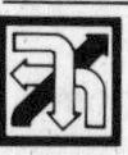

INTERACTION WITH OTHER SUBSTANCES

INTERACTS WITH	COMBINED EFFECT
Alcohol:	Possible lithium poisoning.
Beverages: Caffeine drinks	Increased lithium effect.
Cocaine:	Possible psychosis.
Foods: Salt	*Don't* restrict intake.
Marijuana:	Increased tremor and possible psychosis.
Tobacco:	None expected.

LORAZEPAM

BRAND NAMES

Ativan

GENERAL INFORMATION

Habit forming? Yes
Prescription needed? Yes
Available as generic? No
Drug class: Tranquilizer (benzodiazepine)

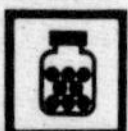

USES

Treatment for nervousness or tension.

DOSAGE & USAGE INFORMATION

How to take:
Tablet or capsule—Swallow with liquid. If you can't swallow whole, crumble tablet or open capsule and take with liquid or food.

When to take:
At the same time each day, according to instructions on prescription label.

If you forget a dose:
Take as soon as you remember up to 2 hours late. If more than 2 hours, wait for next scheduled dose (don't double this dose).

What drug does:
Affects limbic system of brain—part that controls emotions.

Time lapse before drug works:
2 hours. May take 6 weeks for full benefit.

Don't take with:
See Interaction column and consult doctor.

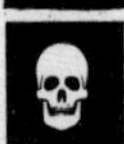

OVERDOSE

Symptoms:
Drowsiness, weakness, tremor, stupor, coma.

What to do:
- Dial 0 (operator) or 911 (emergency) for an ambulance or medical help. Then give first aid immediately.
- If patient is unconscious and not breathing, give mouth-to-mouth breathing. If there is no heartbeat, use cardiac massage and mouth-to-mouth breathing (CPR). Don't try to make patient vomit. If you can't get help quickly, take patient to nearest emergency facility.
- Additional emergency information on page 886.

POSSIBLE ADVERSE REACTIONS OR SIDE EFFECTS

SYMPTOMS	FREQUENCY	WHAT TO DO
Brain & nervous system:		
• Clumsiness, drowsiness, dizziness.	Common	4
• Hallucinations, confusion, depression, irritability.	Infrequent	3
Skin: Rash, itch.	Infrequent	3
Eyes: Vision changes.	Infrequent	3
Ears, nose, throat: Mouth, throat ulcers.	Rare	3
Digestive: Constipation or diarrhea, nausea, vomiting.	Infrequent	4
Heart & lungs: Slow heartbeat, breathing difficulty.	Rare	2
Blood vessels:	None expected.	
Muscles, bones, joints:	None expected.	
Genital, urinary: Urination difficulty.	Infrequent	4
Kidneys:	None expected.	
Liver: Jaundice (yellow eyes and skin).	Rare	3
Allergic:	None expected.	
Blood:	None expected.	
Others:	None expected.	

1- Life-threatening. Seek emergency treatment immediately.
2- Discontinue. Seek emergency treatment.
3- Discontinue. Call doctor right away.
4- Continue. Call doctor when convenient.
5- Continue. Tell doctor at next visit.
6- No action necessary.

WARNINGS & PRECAUTIONS

Don't take if:
- You are allergic to any benzodiazepine.
- You have myasthenia gravis.
- You are active or recovering alcoholic.
- Patient is younger than 6 months.

Before you start, consult your doctor:
- If you have liver, kidney or lung disease.
- If you have diabetes, epilepsy or porphyria.

Over age 60:
Adverse reactions and side effects may be more frequent and severe than in younger persons. You need smaller doses for shorter periods of time. May develop agitation, rage or "hangover effect."

Pregnancy:
Risk to unborn child outweighs drug benefits. Don't use.

Breast-feeding:
Drug passes into milk. Avoid drug or discontinue nursing until you finish medicine. Consult doctor for advice on maintaining milk supply.

Infants & children:
Use only under medical supervision for children older than 6 months.

Prolonged use:
May impair liver function.

Skin & sunlight:
No problems expected.

Driving, piloting or hazardous work:
Don't drive or pilot aircraft until you learn how medicine affects you. Don't work around dangerous machinery. Don't climb ladders or work in high places. Danger increases if you drink alcohol or take medicine affecting alertness and reflexes.

Airplane passengers:
No problems expected.

Discontinuing:
Don't discontinue without consulting doctor. Dose may require gradual reduction if you have taken drug for a long time. Doses of other drugs may also require adjustment.

Others:
- Hot weather, heavy exercise and profuse sweat may reduce excretion and cause overdose.
- Blood sugar may rise in diabetics, requiring insulin adjustment.

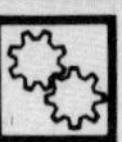

INTERACTION WITH OTHER DRUGS

GENERIC NAME OR DRUG CLASS	COMBINED EFFECT
Anticonvulsants	Change in seizure frequency or severity.
Antidepressants	Increased sedative effect of both drugs.
Antihistamines	Increased sedative effect of both drugs.
Antihypertensives	Excessively low blood pressure.
Cimetidine	Excess sedation.
Disulfiram	Increased lorazepam effect.
MAO inhibitors	Convulsions, deep sedation, rage.
Narcotics	Increased sedative effect of both drugs.
Sedatives	Increased sedative effect of both drugs.
Sleep inducers	Increased sedative effect of both drugs.
Tranquilizers	Increased sedative effect of both drugs.

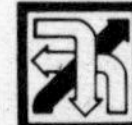

INTERACTION WITH OTHER SUBSTANCES

INTERACTS WITH	COMBINED EFFECT
Alcohol:	Heavy sedation. Avoid.
Beverages:	None expected.
Cocaine:	Decreased lorazepam effect.
Foods:	None expected.
Marijuana:	Heavy sedation. Avoid.
Tobacco:	Decreased lorazepam effect.

MAGNESIUM CARBONATE

BRAND NAMES

Alkets
Bisodol
De Witt's
Di-Gel
Estomul-M
Gaviscon
Magnagel
Marblen
Osti-Derm
Silain-Gel

GENERAL INFORMATION

Habit forming? No
Prescription needed? No
Available as generic? Yes
Drug class: Antacid, laxative

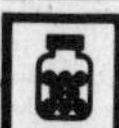

USES

- Treatment for hyperacidity in upper gastrointestinal tract, including stomach and esophagus. Symptoms may be heartburn or acid indigestion. Diseases include peptic ulcer, gastritis, esophagitis, hiatal hernia.
- Constipation relief.

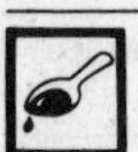

DOSAGE & USAGE INFORMATION

How to take:
- Tablet or capsule—Swallow with liquid.
- Chewable tablets or wafers—Chew well before swallowing.
- Liquid—Shake well and take undiluted.
- Powder—Mix with water and drink all liquid.

When to take:
1 to 3 hours after meals unless directed otherwise by your doctor.

If you forget a dose:
Take as soon as you remember.

What drug does:
- Neutralizes some of the hydrochloric acid in the stomach.
- Reduces action of pepsin, a digestive enzyme.
- Stimulates muscles in lower bowel wall.

Time lapse before drug works:
15 minutes.

Don't take with:
Other medicines at the same time. Decreases absorption of other drugs.

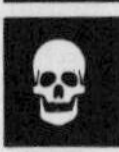

OVERDOSE

Symptoms:
Dry mouth, diarrhea, shallow breathing, stupor.

What to do:
- Dial 0 (operator) or 911 (emergency) for an ambulance or medical help. Then give first aid immediately.
- Additional emergency information on page 886.

POSSIBLE ADVERSE REACTIONS OR SIDE EFFECTS

SYMPTOMS	FREQUENCY	WHAT TO DO
Brain & nervous system:		
Mood changes.	Infrequent	4
Skin:	None expected.	
Eyes:	None expected.	
Ears, nose, throat:	None expected.	
Digestive:		
• Constipation, appetite loss.	Common	4
• Nausea, vomiting.	Infrequent	4
• Lower abdominal pain and swelling.	Infrequent	3
Heart & lungs:	None expected.	
Blood vessels:	None expected.	
Muscles, bones, joints:		
Bone pain, muscle weakness.	Infrequent	3
Genital, urinary:	None expected.	
Kidneys:	None expected.	
Liver:	None expected.	
Allergic:	None expected.	
Blood:	None expected.	
Others:		
• Swelling of wrists or ankles.	Infrequent	3
• Unusual weakness or tiredness.	Rare	3
• Weight loss.	Infrequent	4

1- Life-threatening. Seek emergency treatment immediately.
2- Discontinue. Seek emergency treatment.
3- Discontinue. Call doctor right away.
4- Continue. Call doctor when convenient.
5- Continue. Tell doctor at next visit.
6- No action necessary.

WARNINGS & PRECAUTIONS

Don't take if:
You are allergic to any antacid.

Before you start, consult your doctor:
- If you have kidney disease.
- If you have chronic constipation, colitis or diarrhea.
- If you have symptoms of appendicitis.
- If you have stomach or intestinal bleeding.

Over age 60:
Adverse reactions and side effects may be more frequent and severe than in younger persons. Diarrhea or constipation particularly likely.

Pregnancy:
Risk to unborn child outweighs drug benefits. Don't use.

Breast-feeding:
Drug passes into milk. Avoid drug or discontinue nursing until you finish medicine. Consult doctor for advice on maintaining milk supply.

Infants & children:
Use only under medical supervision.

Prolonged use:
No problems expected.

Skin & sunlight:
No problems expected.

Driving, piloting or hazardous work:
No problems expected.

Airplane passengers:
No problems expected.

Discontinuing:
May be unnecessary to finish medicine. Follow doctor's instructions.

Others:
Don't take longer than 2 weeks unless under medical supervision.

INTERACTION WITH OTHER DRUGS

GENERIC NAME OR DRUG CLASS	COMBINED EFFECT
Anticoagulants	Decreased anticoagulant effect.
Chlorpromazine	Decreased chlorpromazine effect.
Digitalis preparations	Decreased digitalis effect.
Iron supplements	Decreased iron effect.
Isoniazid	Decreased isoniazid effect.
Levodopa	Increased levodopa effect.
Meperidine	Increased meperidine effect.
Nalidixic acid	Decreased effect of nalidixic acid.
Oxyphenbutazone	Decreased oxyphenbutazone effect.
Para-aminosalicylic acid (PAS)	Decreased PAS effect.
Penicillins	Decreased penicillin effect.
Pentobarbital	Decreased pentobarbital effect.
Phenylbutazone	Decreased phenylbutazone effect.
Pseudoephedrine	Increased pseudoephedrine effect.

Additional interactions on page 838.

INTERACTION WITH OTHER SUBSTANCES

INTERACTS WITH	COMBINED EFFECT
Alcohol:	Decreased antacid effect.
Beverages:	No proven problems.
Cocaine:	No proven problems.
Foods:	Decreased antacid effect if taken with food. Wait 1 hour after eating.
Marijuana:	No proven problems.
Tobacco:	Decreased antacid effect.

MAGNESIUM CITRATE

BRAND NAMES

Citrate of Magnesia
Citroma
Citro-Mag
Citro-Nesia
Evac-Q-Kit
Evac-Q-Kwik
National

GENERAL INFORMATION

Habit forming? No
Prescription needed? No
Available as generic? Yes
Drug class: Laxative (hyperosmotic)

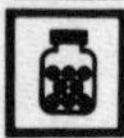

USES

Constipation relief.

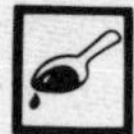

DOSAGE & USAGE INFORMATION

How to take:
Liquid—Dilute dose in beverage before swallowing.

When to take:
Usually once a day, preferably in the morning.

If you forget a dose:
Take as soon as you remember up to 8 hours before bedtime. If later, wait for next scheduled dose (don't double this dose). Don't take at bedtime.

What drug does:
Draws water into bowel from other body tissues. Causes distention through fluid accumulation, which promotes soft stool and accelerates bowel motion.

Time lapse before drug works:
30 minutes to 3 hours.

Don't take with:
See Interaction column and consult doctor.

OVERDOSE

Symptoms:
Fluid depletion, weakness, vomiting, fainting.

What to do:
Overdose unlikely to threaten life. If person takes much larger amount than prescribed, call doctor, poison-control center or hospital emergency room for instructions.

POSSIBLE ADVERSE REACTIONS OR SIDE EFFECTS

SYMPTOMS	FREQUENCY	WHAT TO DO
Brain & nervous system: Dizziness, confusion.	Rare	4
Skin:	None expected.	
Eyes:	None expected.	
Ears, nose, throat: Increased thirst.	Infrequent	5
Digestive: Cramps, nausea, diarrhea, gas.	Infrequent	5
Heart & lungs: Irregular heartbeat.	Infrequent	3
Blood vessels:	None expected.	
Muscles, bones, joints:	None expected.	
Genital, urinary:	None expected.	
Kidneys:	None expected.	
Liver:	None expected.	
Allergic:	None expected.	
Blood:	None expected.	
Others: Tiredness or weakness.	Rare	4

1-Life-threatening. Seek emergency treatment immediately.
2-Discontinue. Seek emergency treatment.
3-Discontinue. Call doctor right away.
4-Continue. Call doctor when convenient.
5-Continue. Tell doctor at next visit.
6-No action necessary.

WARNINGS & PRECAUTIONS

Don't take if:
- You are allergic to any hyperosmotic laxative.
- You have symptoms of appendicitis, inflamed bowel or intestinal blockage.
- You have missed a bowel movement for only 1 or 2 days.

Before you start, consult your doctor:
- If you have congestive heart disease.
- If you have diabetes.
- If you have high blood pressure.
- If you have a colostomy or ileostomy.
- If you have kidney disease.
- If you have a laxative habit.
- If you have rectal bleeding.
- If you take another laxative.

Over age 60:
Adverse reactions and side effects may be more frequent and severe than in younger persons.

Pregnancy:
Salt content may cause fluid retention and swelling. Avoid if possible.

Breast-feeding:
No problems expected.

Infants & children:
Use only under medical supervision.

Prolonged use:
Don't take for more than 1 week unless under a doctor's supervision. May cause laxative dependence.

Skin & sunlight:
No problems expected.

Driving, piloting or hazardous work:
No problems expected.

Airplane passengers:
No problems expected.

Discontinuing:
May be unnecessary to finish medicine. Follow doctor's instructions.

Others:
- Don't take to "flush out" your system or as a "tonic."
- Don't take within 2 hours of taking another medicine.

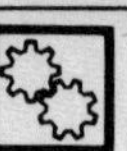

INTERACTION WITH OTHER DRUGS

GENERIC NAME OR DRUG CLASS	COMBINED EFFECT
Chlordiazepoxide	Decreased chlordiazepoxide effect.
Chlorpromazine	Decreased chlorpromazine effect.
Dicumarol	Decreased dicumarol effect.
Digoxin	Decreased digoxin effect.
Isoniazid	Decreased isoniazid effect.
Tetracyclines	Possible intestinal blockage.

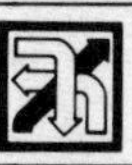

INTERACTION WITH OTHER SUBSTANCES

INTERACTS WITH	COMBINED EFFECT
Alcohol:	None expected.
Beverages:	None expected.
Cocaine:	None expected.
Foods:	None expected.
Marijuana:	None expected.
Tobacco:	None expected.

MAGNESIUM HYDROXIDE

BRAND NAMES

Aludrox
Arthritis Pain Formula
Camalox
Creamalin
Delcid
Di-Gel
Dolprn #3
Ducon
Gelusil
Kolantyl
Maalox
Magnatril
Maxamag
Milk of Magnesia
Mucotin
Mygel
Mylanta
Silain-Gel
Simeco
Univol
Vanquish
Win-Gel

GENERAL INFORMATION

Habit forming? No
Prescription needed? No
Available as generic? Yes
Drug class: Antacid, laxative

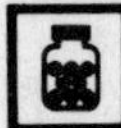

USES

- Treatment for hyperacidity in upper gastrointestinal tract, including stomach and esophagus. Symptoms may be heartburn or acid indigestion. Diseases include peptic ulcer, gastritis, esophagitis, hiatal hernia.
- Constipation relief.

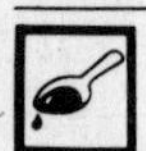

DOSAGE & USAGE INFORMATION

How to take:
- Tablet—Swallow with liquid.
- Liquid—Shake well and take undiluted.

When to take:
1 to 3 hours after meals unless directed otherwise by your doctor.

If you forget a dose:
Take as soon as you remember.

What drug does:
- Neutralizes some of the hydrochloric acid in the stomach.
- Reduces action of pepsin, a digestive enzyme.
- Stimulates muscles in lower bowel wall.

Time lapse before drug works:
15 minutes.

Don't take with:
Other medicines at the same time. Decreases absorption of other drugs.

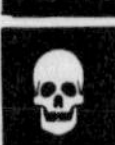

OVERDOSE

Symptoms:
Dry mouth, shallow breathing, diarrhea, stupor.

What to do:
- Dial 0 (operator) or 911 (emergency) for an ambulance or medical help. Then give first aid immediately.
- Additional emergency information on page 886.

POSSIBLE ADVERSE REACTIONS OR SIDE EFFECTS

SYMPTOMS	FREQUENCY	WHAT TO DO
Brain & nervous system:		
Mood changes.	Infrequent	4
Skin:	None expected.	
Eyes:	None expected.	
Ears, nose, throat:	None expected.	
Digestive:		
• Constipation, appetite loss.	Common	4
• Nausea, vomiting.	Infrequent	4
• Lower abdominal pain and swelling.	Infrequent	3
Heart & lungs:	None expected.	
Blood vessels:	None expected.	
Muscles, bones, joints:		
Bone pain, muscle weakness.	Infrequent	3
Genital, urinary:	None expected.	
Kidneys:	None expected.	
Liver:	None expected.	
Allergic:	None expected.	
Blood:	None expected.	
Others:		
• Swelling of wrists or ankles.	Infrequent	3
• Weight loss.	Infrequent	4

1-Life-threatening. Seek emergency treatment immediately.
2-Discontinue. Seek emergency treatment.
3-Discontinue. Call doctor right away.
4-Continue. Call doctor when convenient.
5-Continue. Tell doctor at next visit.
6-No action necessary.

WARNINGS & PRECAUTIONS

Don't take if:
You are allergic to any antacid.

Before you start, consult your doctor:
- If you have kidney disease.
- If you have chronic constipation, colitis or diarrhea.
- If you have symptoms of appendicitis.
- If you have stomach or intestinal bleeding.

Over age 60:
Adverse reactions and side effects may be more frequent and severe than in younger persons. Diarrhea or constipation particularly likely.

Pregnancy:
Risk to unborn child outweighs drug benefits. Don't use.

Breast-feeding:
Drug passes into milk. Avoid drug or discontinue nursing until you finish medicine. Consult doctor for advice on maintaining milk supply.

Infants & children:
Use only under medical supervision.

Prolonged use:
No problems expected.

Skin & sunlight:
No problems expected.

Driving, piloting or hazardous work:
No problems expected.

Airplane passengers:
No problems expected.

Discontinuing:
May be unnecessary to finish medicine. Follow doctor's instructions.

Others:
Don't take longer than 2 weeks unless under medical supervision.

INTERACTION WITH OTHER DRUGS

GENERIC NAME OR DRUG CLASS	COMBINED EFFECT
Anticoagulants	Decreased anticoagulant effect.
Chlorpromazine	Decreased chlorpromazine effect.
Digitalis preparations	Decreased digitalis effect.
Iron supplements	Decreased iron effect.
Isoniazid	Decreased isoniazid effect.
Levodopa	Increased levodopa effect.
Meperidine	Increased meperidine effect.
Nalidixic acid	Decreased effect of nalidixic acid.
Oxyphenbutazone	Decreased oxyphenbutazone effect.
Para-aminosalicylic acid (PAS)	Decreased PAS effect.
Penicillins	Decreased penicillin effect.
Pentobarbital	Decreased pentobarbital effect.
Phenylbutazone	Decreased phenylbutazone effect.
Pseudoephedrine	Increased pseudoephedrine effect.

Additional interactions on page 838.

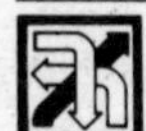

INTERACTION WITH OTHER SUBSTANCES

INTERACTS WITH	COMBINED EFFECT
Alcohol:	Decreased antacid effect.
Beverages:	No proven problems.
Cocaine:	No proven problems.
Foods:	Decreased antacid effect if taken with food. Wait 1 hour after eating.
Marijuana:	No proven problems.
Tobacco:	Decreased antacid effect.

MAGNESIUM SULFATE

BRAND NAMES

Eldercaps
Eldertonic
Epsom Salts
Glutofac
Vicon

GENERAL INFORMATION

Habit forming? No
Prescription needed? No
Available as generic? Yes
Drug class: Laxative (hyperosmotic)

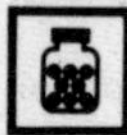

USES

Constipation relief.

DOSAGE & USAGE INFORMATION

How to take:
Powder or solid form—Dilute dose in beverage before swallowing. Solid form must be dissolved.

When to take:
Usually once a day, preferably in the morning.

If you forget a dose:
Take as soon as you remember up to 8 hours before bedtime. If later, wait for next scheduled dose (don't double this dose). Don't take at bedtime.

What drug does:
Draws water into bowel from other body tissues. Causes distention through fluid accumulation, which promotes soft stool and accelerates bowel motion.

Time lapse before drug works:
30 minutes to 3 hours.

Don't take with:
See Interaction column and consult doctor.

OVERDOSE

Symptoms:
Fluid depletion, weakness, vomiting, fainting.

What to do:
Overdose unlikely to threaten life. If person takes much larger amount than prescribed, call doctor, poison-control center or hospital emergency room for instructions.

POSSIBLE ADVERSE REACTIONS OR SIDE EFFECTS

SYMPTOMS	FREQUENCY	WHAT TO DO
Brain & nervous system: Dizziness, confusion.	Rare	4
Skin:	None expected.	
Eyes:	None expected.	
Ears, nose, throat: Increased thirst.	Infrequent	5
Digestive: Cramps, nausea, diarrhea, gas.	Infrequent	5
Heart & lungs: Irregular heartbeat.	Infrequent	3
Blood vessels:	None expected.	
Muscles, bones, joints:	None expected.	
Genital, urinary:	None expected.	
Kidneys:	None expected.	
Liver:	None expected.	
Allergic:	None expected.	
Blood:	None expected.	
Others: Tiredness or weakness.	Rare	4

1- Life-threatening. Seek emergency treatment immediately.
2- Discontinue. Seek emergency treatment.
3- Discontinue. Call doctor right away.
4- Continue. Call doctor when convenient.
5- Continue. Tell doctor at next visit.
6- No action necessary.

WARNINGS & PRECAUTIONS

Don't take if:
- You are allergic to any hyperosmotic laxative.
- You have symptoms of appendicitis, inflamed bowel or intestinal blockage.
- You have missed a bowel movement for only 1 or 2 days.

Before you start, consult your doctor:
- If you have congestive heart disease.
- If you have diabetes.
- If you have high blood pressure.
- If you have a colostomy or ileostomy.
- If you have kidney disease.
- If you have a laxative habit.
- If you have rectal bleeding.
- If you take another laxative.

Over age 60:
Adverse reactions and side effects may be more frequent and severe than in younger persons.

Pregnancy:
Salt content may cause fluid retention and swelling. Avoid if possible.

Breast-feeding:
No problems expected.

Infants & children:
Use only under medical supervision.

Prolonged use:
Don't take for more than 1 week unless under a doctor's supervision. May cause laxative dependence.

Skin & sunlight:
No problems expected.

Driving, piloting or hazardous work:
No problems expected.

Airplane passengers:
No problems expected.

Discontinuing:
May be unnecessary to finish medicine. Follow doctor's instructions.

Others:
- Don't take to "flush out" your system or as a "tonic."
- Don't take within 2 hours of taking another medicine.

INTERACTION WITH OTHER DRUGS

GENERIC NAME OR DRUG CLASS	COMBINED EFFECT
Chlordiazepoxide	Decreased chlordiazepoxide effect.
Chlorpromazine	Decreased chlorpromazine effect.
Dicumarol	Decreased dicumarol effect.
Digoxin	Decreased digoxin effect.
Isoniazid	Decreased isoniazid effect.
Tetracyclines	Possible intestinal blockage.

INTERACTION WITH OTHER SUBSTANCES

INTERACTS WITH	COMBINED EFFECT
Alcohol:	None expected.
Beverages:	None expected.
Cocaine:	None expected.
Foods:	None expected.
Marijuana:	None expected.
Tobacco:	None expected.

MAGNESIUM TRISILICATE

BRAND NAMES

A-M-T
Alma-Mag
Gaviscon
Gelusil
Gelusil-M
Magnatril
Mucotin
Neutrocomp
Sterazolidin
Trisogel

GENERAL INFORMATION

Habit forming? No
Prescription needed? No
Available as generic? Yes
Drug class: Antacid, laxative

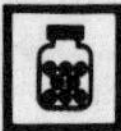

USES

- Treatment for hyperacidity in upper gastrointestinal tract, including stomach and esophagus. Symptoms may be heartburn or acid indigestion. Diseases include peptic ulcer, gastritis, esophagitis, hiatal hernia.
- Constipation relief.

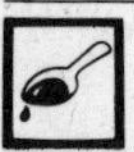

DOSAGE & USAGE INFORMATION

How to take:
- Tablet or capsule—Swallow with liquid.
- Chewable tablets or wafers—Chew well before swallowing.
- Liquid—Shake well and take undiluted.

When to take:
1 to 3 hours after meals unless directed otherwise by your doctor.

If you forget a dose:
Take as soon as you remember.

What drug does:
- Neutralizes some of the hydrochloric acid in the stomach.
- Reduces action of pepsin, a digestive enzyme.
- Stimulates muscles in lower bowel wall.

Time lapse before drug works:
15 minutes.

Don't take with:
Other medicines at the same time. Decreases absorption of other drugs.

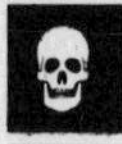

OVERDOSE

Symptoms:
Dry mouth, diarrhea, shallow breathing, stupor.

What to do:
- Dial 0 (operator) or 911 (emergency) for an ambulance or medical help. Then give first aid immediately.
- Additional emergency information on page 886.

POSSIBLE ADVERSE REACTIONS OR SIDE EFFECTS

SYMPTOMS	FREQUENCY	WHAT TO DO
Brain & nervous system:		
Mood changes.	Infrequent	4
Skin:	None expected.	
Eyes:	None expected.	
Ears, nose, throat:	None expected.	
Digestive:		
• Constipation, appetite loss.	Common	4
• Nausea, vomiting.	Infrequent	4
• Lower abdominal pain and swelling.	Infrequent	3
Heart & lungs:	None expected.	
Blood vessels:	None expected.	
Muscles, bones, joints:		
Bone pain, muscle weakness.	Infrequent	3
Genital, urinary:	None expected.	
Kidneys:	None expected.	
Liver:	None expected.	
Allergic:	None expected.	
Blood:	None expected.	
Others:		
• Swelling of wrists or ankles.	Infrequent	3
• Weight loss.	Infrequent	4

1-Life-threatening. Seek emergency treatment immediately.
2-Discontinue. Seek emergency treatment.
3-Discontinue. Call doctor right away.
4-Continue. Call doctor when convenient.
5-Continue. Tell doctor at next visit.
6-No action necessary.

WARNINGS & PRECAUTIONS

Don't take if:
You are allergic to any antacid.

Before you start, consult your doctor:
- If you have kidney disease.
- If you have chronic constipation, colitis or diarrhea.
- If you have symptoms of appendicitis.
- If you have stomach or intestinal bleeding.

Over age 60:
Adverse reactions and side effects may be more frequent and severe than in younger persons. Diarrhea or constipation particularly likely.

Pregnancy:
Risk to unborn child outweighs drug benefits. Don't use.

Breast-feeding:
Drug passes into milk. Avoid drug or discontinue nursing until you finish medicine. Consult doctor for advice on maintaining milk supply.

Infants & children:
Use only under medical supervision.

Prolonged use:
No problems expected.

Skin & sunlight:
No problems expected.

Driving, piloting or hazardous work:
No problems expected.

Airplane passengers:
No problems expected.

Discontinuing:
May be unnecessary to finish medicine. Follow doctor's instructions.

Others:
Don't take longer than 2 weeks unless under medical supervision.

INTERACTION WITH OTHER DRUGS

GENERIC NAME OR DRUG CLASS	COMBINED EFFECT
Anticoagulants	Decreased anticoagulant effect.
Chlorpromazine	Decreased chlorpromazine effect.
Digitalis preparations	Decreased digitalis effect.
Iron supplements	Decreased iron effect.
Isoniazid	Decreased isoniazid effect.
Levodopa	Increased levodopa effect.
Meperidine	Increased meperidine effect.
Nalidixic acid	Decreased effect of nalidixic acid.
Oxyphenbutazone	Decreased oxyphenbutazone effect.
Para-aminosalicylic acid (PAS)	Decreased PAS effect.
Penicillins	Decreased penicillin effect.
Pentobarbital	Decreased pentobarbital effect.
Phenylbutazone	Decreased phenylbutazone effect.
Pseudoephedrine	Increased pseudoephedrine effect.

Additional interactions on page 838.

INTERACTION WITH OTHER SUBSTANCES

INTERACTS WITH	COMBINED EFFECT
Alcohol:	Decreased antacid effect.
Beverages:	No proven problems.
Cocaine:	No proven problems.
Foods:	Decreased antacid effect if taken with food. Wait 1 hour after eating.
Marijuana:	No proven problems.
Tobacco:	Decreased antacid effect.

MALT SOUP EXTRACT

BRAND NAMES

Maltsupex

GENERAL INFORMATION

Habit forming? No
Prescription needed? No
Available as generic? Yes
Drug class: Laxative (bulk-forming)

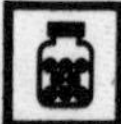

USES

Relieves constipation and prevents straining for bowel movement.

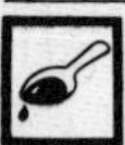

DOSAGE & USAGE INFORMATION

How to take:

- Liquid or powder—Dilute dose in 8 oz. cold water or fruit juice.
- Tablets—Swallow with 8 oz. cold liquid. Drink 6 to 8 glasses of water each day in addition to the one with each dose.

When to take:
At the same time each day, preferably morning.

If you forget a dose:
Take as soon as you remember. Resume regular schedule.

What drug does:
Absorbs water, stimulating the bowel to form a soft, bulky stool.

Time lapse before drug works:
May require 2 or 3 days to begin, then works in 12 to 24 hours.

Don't take with:

- See Interaction column and consult doctor.
- Don't take within 2 hours of taking another medicine.

OVERDOSE

Symptoms:
None expected.

What to do:
Overdose unlikely to threaten life. If person takes much larger amount than prescribed, call doctor, poison-control center or hospital emergency room for instructions.

POSSIBLE ADVERSE REACTIONS OR SIDE EFFECTS

SYMPTOMS	FREQUENCY	WHAT TO DO
Brain & nervous system:	None expected.	
Skin: Itch, rash.	Rare	3
Eyes:	None expected.	
Ears, nose, throat: Swallowing difficulty, "lump in throat" sensation.	Infrequent	4
Digestive:		
• Intestinal blockage.	Rare	3
• Nausea, vomiting, diarrhea.	Infrequent	4
Heart & lungs: Asthma	Rare	3
Blood vessels:	None expected.	
Muscles, bones, joints:	None expected.	
Genital, urinary:	None expected.	
Kidneys:	None expected.	
Liver:	None expected.	
Allergic:	None expected.	
Blood:	None expected.	
Others:	None expected.	

1-Life-threatening. Seek emergency treatment immediately.
2-Discontinue. Seek emergency treatment.
3-Discontinue. Call doctor right away.
4-Continue. Call doctor when convenient.
5-Continue. Tell doctor at next visit.
6-No action necessary.

WARNINGS & PRECAUTIONS

Don't take if:
- You are allergic to any bulk-forming laxative.
- You have symptoms of appendicitis, inflamed bowel or intestinal blockage.
- You have missed a bowel movement for only 1 or 2 days.

Before you start, consult your doctor:
- If you have diabetes.
- If you have a laxative habit.
- If you have rectal bleeding.
- If you have difficulty swallowing.
- If you take other laxatives.

Over age 60:
Adverse reactions and side effects may be more frequent and severe than in younger persons.

Pregnancy:
Most bulk-forming laxatives contain sodium or sugars which may cause fluid retention. Avoid if possible.

Breast-feeding:
No problems expected.

Infants & children:
Use only under medical supervision.

Prolonged use:
Don't take for more than 1 week unless under a doctor's supervision. May cause laxative dependence.

Skin & sunlight:
No problems expected.

Driving, piloting or hazardous work:
No problems expected.

Airplane passengers:
No problems expected.

Discontinuing:
May be unnecessary to finish medicine. Follow doctor's instructions.

Others:
Don't take to "flush out" your system or as a "tonic."

INTERACTION WITH OTHER DRUGS

GENERIC NAME OR DRUG CLASS	COMBINED EFFECT
Antibiotics	Decreased antibiotic effect.
Anticoagulants	Decreased anticoagulant effect.
Digitalis preparations	Decreased digitalis effect.
Salicylates (including aspirin)	Decreased salicylate effect.

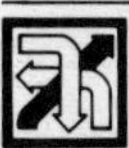

INTERACTION WITH OTHER SUBSTANCES

INTERACTS WITH	COMBINED EFFECT
Alcohol:	None expected.
Beverages:	None expected.
Cocaine:	None expected.
Foods:	None expected.
Marijuana:	None expected.
Tobacco:	None expected.

MAPROTILINE

BRAND NAMES

Ludiomil

GENERAL INFORMATION

Habit forming? No
Prescription needed? Yes
Available as generic? No
Drug class: Antidepressant

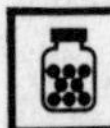

USES

Treatment for depression or anxiety associated with depression.

DOSAGE & USAGE INFORMATION

How to take:
Tablet or capsule—Swallow with liquid.

When to take:
At the same time each day, usually bedtime.

If you forget a dose:
Bedtime dose—If you forget your once-a-day bedtime dose, don't take it more than 3 hours late. If more than 3 hours, wait for next scheduled dose. Don't double this dose.

What drug does:
Probably affects part of brain that controls messages between nerve cells.

Time lapse before drug works:
Begins in 1 to 2 weeks. May require 4 to 6 weeks for maximum benefit.

Don't take with:
- Non-prescription drugs without consulting doctor.
- See Interaction column and consult doctor.

OVERDOSE

Symptoms:
Hallucinations, convulsions, coma.

What to do:
- Dial 0 (operator) or 911 (emergency) for an ambulance or medical help. Then give first aid immediately.
- If patient is unconscious and not breathing, give mouth-to-mouth breathing. If there is no heartbeat, use cardiac massage and mouth-to-mouth breathing (CPR). Don't try to make patient vomit. If you can't get help quickly, take patient to nearest emergency facility.
- Additional emergency information on page 886.

POSSIBLE ADVERSE REACTIONS OR SIDE EFFECTS

SYMPTOMS	FREQUENCY	WHAT TO DO
Brain & nervous system:		
• Hallucinations, shakiness, dizziness, fainting.	Infrequent	3
• Headache	Common	4
• Seizures	Rare	1
• Insomnia	Common	5
Skin:		
Rash, itch.	Rare	3
Eyes:		
Blurred vision, pain.	Infrequent	3
Ears, nose, throat:		
• Sore throat.	Rare	3
• Dry mouth or unpleasant taste.	Common	4
Digestive:		
• Constipation or diarrhea, nausea, indigestion.	Common	4
• Vomiting	Infrequent	3
• Craving sweets.	Common	5
Heart & lungs:		
Irregular heartbeat or slow pulse.	Infrequent	3
Blood vessels, muscles, bones, joints, kidneys, allergic, blood:	None expected.	
Genital, urinary:		
Difficulty urinating.	Infrequent	4
Liver:		
Jaundice (yellow skin and eyes).	Rare	3
Others:		
• Fever	Rare	3
• Fatigue, weakness.	Common	4

1- Life-threatening. Seek emergency treatment immediately.
2- Discontinue. Seek emergency treatment.
3- Discontinue. Call doctor right away.
4- Continue. Call doctor when convenient.
5- Continue. Tell doctor at next visit.

WARNINGS & PRECAUTIONS

Don't take if:

- You are allergic to any tricyclic antidepressant.
- You drink alcohol.
- You have had a heart attack within 6 weeks.
- You have glaucoma.
- You have taken MAO inhibitors within 2 weeks.
- Patient is younger than 12.

Before you start, consult your doctor:

- If you will have surgery within 2 months, including dental surgery, requiring general or spinal anesthesia.
- If you have an enlarged prostate.
- If you have heart disease or high blood pressure.
- If you have stomach or intestinal problems.
- If you have overactive thyroid.
- If you have asthma.
- If you have liver disease.

Over age 60:
More likely to develop urination difficulty and side effects listed under Brain & nervous system.

Pregnancy:
Studies inconclusive on harm to unborn child. Animal studies show fetal abnormalities. Decide with your doctor whether drug benefits justify risk to unborn child.

Breast-feeding:
Drug passes into milk. Avoid drug or discontinue nursing until you finish medicine. Consult doctor for advice on maintaining milk supply.

Infants & children:
Don't give to children younger than 12.

Prolonged use:
Request blood cell counts, liver-function studies, monitor blood pressure closely.

Skin & sunlight:
May cause rash or intensify sunburn in areas exposed to sun or sunlamp.

Driving, piloting or hazardous work:
Don't drive or pilot aircraft until you learn how medicine affects you. Don't work around dangerous machinery. Don't climb ladders or work in high places. Danger increases if you drink alcohol or take medicine affecting alertness and reflexes.

Airplane passengers:
No problems expected.

Discontinuing:
Don't discontinue without consulting doctor. Dose may require gradual reduction if you have taken drug for a long time. Doses of other drugs may also require adjustment.

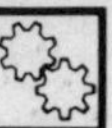

INTERACTION WITH OTHER DRUGS

GENERIC NAME OR DRUG CLASS	COMBINED EFFECT
Anticoagulants	Increased anticoagulant effect.
Anticholinergics	Increased sedation.
Antihistamines	Increased antihistamine effect.
Barbiturates	Decreased antidepressant effect.
Clonidine	Decreased clonidine effect.
Ethchlorvynol	Delirium
Guanethidine	Decreased guanethidine effect.
MAO inhibitors	Fever, delirium, convulsions.
Methyldopa	Decreased methyldopa effect.
Narcotics	Dangerous oversedation.
Phenytoin	Decreased phenytoin effect.
Quinidine	Irregular heartbeat.
Sedatives	Dangerous oversedation.
Sympathomimetics	Increased sympathomimetic effect.
Thiazide diuretics	Increased maprotiline effect.
Thyroid hormones	Irregular heartbeat.

INTERACTION WITH OTHER SUBSTANCES

INTERACTS WITH	COMBINED EFFECT
Alcohol: Beverages or medicines with alcohol.	Excessive intoxication. Avoid.
Beverages:	None expected.
Cocaine:	Excessive intoxication. Avoid.
Foods:	None expected.
Marijuana:	Excessive drowsiness. Avoid.
Tobacco:	May decrease absorption of maprotiline. Avoid.

MECLIZINE

BRAND NAMES

Antivert
Bonamine
Bonine
Motion Cure
Ru-Vert-M
Wehvert

GENERAL INFORMATION

Habit forming? No
Prescription needed? U.S.—Tablets: No
Liquid: Yes
Canada: Yes
Available as generic? No
Drug class: Antihistamine, antiemetic

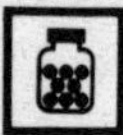

USES

Prevents motion sickness.

DOSAGE & USAGE INFORMATION

How to take:
Tablet—Swallow with liquid or food to lessen stomach irritation. If you can't swallow whole, crumble tablet and chew or take with liquid or food.

When to take:
30 minutes to 1 hour before traveling.

If you forget a dose:
Take as soon as you remember. Wait 4 hours for next dose.

What drug does:
Reduces sensitivity of nerve endings in inner ear, blocking messages to brain's vomiting center.

Time lapse before drug works:
30 to 60 minutes.

Don't take with:
See Interaction column and consult doctor.

OVERDOSE

Symptoms:
Drowsiness, confusion, incoordination, stupor, coma, weak pulse, shallow breathing.

What to do:
- Dial 0 (operator) or 911 (emergency) for an ambulance or medical help. Then give first aid immediately.
- Additional emergency information on page 886.

POSSIBLE ADVERSE REACTIONS OR SIDE EFFECTS

SYMPTOMS	FREQUENCY	WHAT TO DO
Brain & nervous system:		
• Drowsiness	Common	5
• Headache	Infrequent	4
• Restlessness, excitement, insomnia.	Rare	4
Skin:		
Rash or hives.	Rare	3
Eyes:		
Blurred vision.	Rare	4
Ears, nose, throat:		
Dry mouth, nose, throat.	Infrequent	5
Digestive:		
• Appetite loss, nausea.	Rare	5
• Diarrhea or constipation.	Infrequent	4
Heart & lungs:		
Fast heartbeat.	Infrequent	4
Blood vessels:	None expected.	
Muscles, bones, joints:	None expected.	
Genital, urinary:		
Urinary frequency, difficult urination.	Rare	4
Kidneys:	None expected.	
Liver:	None expected.	
Allergic:	None expected.	
Blood:	None expected.	
Others:	None expected.	

1- Life-threatening. Seek emergency treatment immediately.
2- Discontinue. Seek emergency treatment.
3- Discontinue. Call doctor right away.
4- Continue. Call doctor when convenient.
5- Continue. Tell doctor at next visit.

WARNINGS & PRECAUTIONS

Don't take if:
- You are allergic to meclizine, buclizine or cyclizine.
- You have taken MAO inhibitors in the past 2 weeks.

Before you start, consult your doctor:
- If you have glaucoma.
- If you have prostate enlargement.
- If you have reacted badly to any antihistamine.

Over age 60:
Adverse reactions and side effects may be more frequent and severe than in younger persons, especially impaired urination from enlarged prostate gland.

Pregnancy:
Studies inconclusive on harm to unborn child. Animal studies show fetal abnormalities. Decide with your doctor whether drug benefits justify risk to unborn child.

Breast-feeding:
Drug passes into milk. Avoid drug or discontinue nursing until you finish medicine. Consult doctor for advice on maintaining milk supply.

Infants & children:
No problems expected.

Prolonged use:
No problems expected.

Skin & sunlight:
No problems expected.

Driving, piloting or hazardous work:
Don't fly aircraft. Don't drive until you learn how medicine affects you. Don't work around dangerous machinery. Don't climb ladders or work in high places. Danger increases if you drink alcohol or take medicine affecting alertness and reflexes, such as antihistamines, tranquilizers, sedatives, pain medicine, narcotics and mind-altering drugs.

Airplane passengers:
Take 30 minutes before takeoff and every 4 hours while in the air.

Discontinuing:
No problems expected.

Others:
No problems expected.

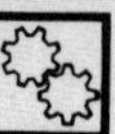

INTERACTION WITH OTHER DRUGS

GENERIC NAME OR DRUG CLASS	COMBINED EFFECT
Amphetamines	May decrease drowsiness caused by meclizine.
Anticholinergics	Increased effect of both drugs.
Antidepressants (tricyclic)	Increased effect of both drugs.
MAO inhibitors	Increased meclizine effect.
Narcotics	Increased effect of both drugs.
Pain relievers	Increased effect of both drugs.
Sedatives	Increased effect of both drugs.
Sleep inducers	Increased effect of both drugs.
Tranquilizers	Increased effect of both drugs.

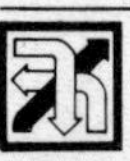

INTERACTION WITH OTHER SUBSTANCES

INTERACTS WITH	COMBINED EFFECT
Alcohol:	Increased sedation. Avoid.
Beverages: Caffeine drinks	May decrease drowsiness.
Cocaine:	None expected.
Foods:	None expected.
Marijuana:	Increased drowsiness, dry mouth.
Tobacco:	None expected.

MECLOFENAMATE

BRAND NAMES

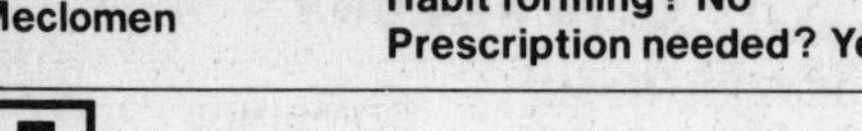

Meclomen

Habit forming? No
Prescription needed? Yes

GENERAL INFORMATION

Available as generic? No
Drug class: Antiinflammatory (non-steroid)

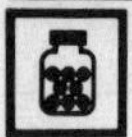

USES

Treatment for joint pain, stiffness, inflammation and swelling of arthritis and gout.

DOSAGE & USAGE INFORMATION

How to take:
Capsule—Swallow with liquid or food to lessen stomach irritation. If you can't swallow whole, open capsule and take with liquid or food.

When to take:
At the same times each day.

If you forget a dose:
Take as soon as you remember up to 2 hours late. If more than 2 hours, wait for next scheduled dose (don't double this dose).

What drug does:
Reduces tissue concentration of prostaglandins (hormones which produce inflammation and pain).

Time lapse before drug works:
Begins in 4 to 24 hours. May require 3 weeks regular use for maximum benefit.

Don't take with:
See Interaction column and consult doctor.

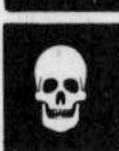

OVERDOSE

Symptoms:
Confusion, agitation, incoherence, convulsions, possible hemorrhage from stomach or intestine, coma.

What to do:
- Dial 0 (operator) or 911 (emergency) for an ambulance or medical help. Then give first aid immediately.
- Additional emergency information on page 886.

POSSIBLE ADVERSE REACTIONS OR SIDE EFFECTS

SYMPTOMS	FREQUENCY	WHAT TO DO
Brain & nervous system:		
• Depression, drowsiness.	Infrequent	4
• Convulsions, confusion.	Rare	3
• Dizziness	Common	4
• Headache	Common	5
Skin:		
Rash, hives or itch.	Rare	3
Eyes:		
Blurred vision.	Rare	3
Ears, nose, throat:		
Ringing in ears.	Infrequent	4
Digestive:		
• Bloody or black, tarry stools.	Rare	3
• Nausea, pain.	Common	4
• Constipation or diarrhea, vomiting.	Infrequent	4
Heart & lungs:		
Breathing difficulty, tightness in chest, rapid heartbeat.	Rare	3
Blood vessels:		
Unusual bleeding or bruising.	Rare	3
Muscles, bones, joints:		
Swollen feet, legs.	Infrequent	4
Genital, urinary:		
• Bloody urine.	Rare	3
• Difficult, painful or frequent urination.	Rare	4
Kidneys, allergic, blood:	None expected.	
Liver:		
Jaundice (yellow skin and eyes).	Rare	3
Others:		
Fatigue, weakness.	Rare	4

1- Life-threatening. Seek emergency treatment immediately.
2- Discontinue. Seek emergency treatment.
3- Discontinue. Call doctor right away.
4- Continue. Call doctor when convenient.
5- Continue. Tell doctor at next visit.

WARNINGS & PRECAUTIONS

Don't take if:
- You are allergic to aspirin or any non-steroid, antiinflammatory drug.
- You have gastritis, peptic ulcer, enteritis, ileitis, ulcerative colitis, asthma, heart failure, high blood pressure or bleeding problems.
- Patient is younger than 15.

Before you start, consult your doctor:
- If you have epilepsy.
- If you have Parkinson's disease.
- If you have been mentally ill.
- If you have had kidney disease or impaired kidney function.

Over age 60:
Adverse reactions and side effects may be more frequent and severe than in younger persons.

Pregnancy:
Studies inconclusive on harm to unborn child. Decide with your doctor whether drug benefits justify risk to unborn child.

Breast-feeding:
May harm child. Avoid.

Infants & children:
Not recommended for anyone younger than 15. Use only under medical supervision.

Prolonged use:
- Eye damage.
- Reduced hearing.
- Sore throat, fever.
- Weight gain.

Skin & sunlight:
No problems expected.

Driving, piloting or hazardous work:
Don't drive or pilot aircraft until you learn how medicine affects you. Don't work around dangerous machinery. Don't climb ladders or work in high places. Danger increases if you drink alcohol or take medicine affecting alertness and reflexes, such as antihistamines, tranquilizers, sedatives, pain medicine, narcotics and mind-altering drugs.

Airplane passengers:
No problems expected.

Discontinuing:
Don't discontinue without consulting doctor. Dose may require gradual reduction if you have taken drug for a long time. Doses of other drugs may also require adjustment.

Others:
No problems expected.

INTERACTION WITH OTHER DRUGS

GENERIC NAME OR DRUG CLASS	COMBINED EFFECT
Anticoagulants (oral)	Increased risk of bleeding.
Aspirin	Increased risk of stomach ulcer.
Cortisone drugs	Increased risk of stomach ulcer.
Furosemide	Decreased diuretic effect of furosemide.
Oxyphenbutazone	Possible stomach ulcer.
Phenylbutazone	Possible stomach ulcer.
Probenecid	Increased meclofenamate effect.
Thyroid hormones	Rapid heartbeat, blood-pressure rise.

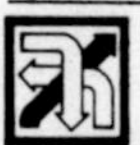

INTERACTION WITH OTHER SUBSTANCES

INTERACTS WITH	COMBINED EFFECT
Alcohol:	Possible stomach ulcer or bleeding.
Beverages:	None expected.
Cocaine:	None expected.
Foods:	None expected.
Marijuana:	Increased pain relief from meclofenamate.
Tobacco:	None expected.

MEDROXYPROGESTERONE

BRAND NAMES

Amen
Curretab
Depo-Provera
Provera

GENERAL INFORMATION

Habit forming? No
Prescription needed? Yes
Available as generic? No
Drug class: Female sex hormone (progestin)

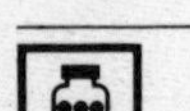

USES

- Treatment for menstrual or uterine disorders caused by progestin imbalance.
- Contraceptive
- Treatment for cancer of breast and uterus.

DOSAGE & USAGE INFORMATION

How to take:

- Tablet or capsule—Swallow with liquid or food to lessen stomach irritation. You may crumble tablet or open capsule.
- Injection—Take under doctor's supervision.

When to take:

Tablet, capsule—At the same time each day.

If you forget a dose:

- Menstrual disorders—Take up to 2 hours late. If more than 2 hours, wait for next dose (don't double this).
- Contraceptive—Consult your doctor. You may need to use another birth-control method until next period.

What drug does:

- Creates a uterine lining similar to pregnancy that prevents bleeding.
- Suppresses a pituitary gland hormone responsible for ovulation.
- Stimulates cervical mucus, which stops sperm penetration and prevents pregnancy.

Time lapse before drug works:

- Menstrual disorders—24 to 48 hours.
- Contraception—3 weeks.
- Cancer—May require 2 to 3 months regular use for maximum benefit.

Don't take with:

See Interaction column and consult doctor.

OVERDOSE

Symptoms:

Nausea, vomiting, fluid retention, breast discomfort or enlargement, vaginal bleeding.

What to do:

Overdose unlikely to threaten life. If person takes much larger amount than prescribed, call doctor, poison-control center or hospital emergency room for instructions.

POSSIBLE ADVERSE REACTIONS OR SIDE EFFECTS

SYMPTOMS	FREQUENCY	WHAT TO DO
Brain & nervous system:		
Depression	Infrequent	4
Skin:		
• Rash	Rare	3
• Acne, increased facial or body hair.	Infrequent	5
Eyes, ears, nose, throat, heart & lungs, muscles, bones, joints, kidneys, allergic, blood:	None expected.	
Digestive:		
• Stomach or side pain.	Rare	3
• Appetite or weight changes.	Common	5
• Nausea	Infrequent	5
Blood vessels:		
Blood clot in leg, brain or lung.	Rare	1
Muscles, bones, joints:		
Ankle, foot swelling.	Common	5
Genital, urinary:		
Prolonged vaginal bleeding.	Infrequent	3
Liver:		
Jaundice (yellow skin and eyes).	Rare	3
Others:		
• Breast tenderness.	Infrequent	5
• Unusual tiredness or weakness.	Common	5

1 - Life-threatening. Seek emergency treatment immediately.
2 - Discontinue. Seek emergency treatment.
3 - Discontinue. Call doctor right away.
4 - Continue. Call doctor when convenient.
5 - Continue. Tell doctor at next visit.

MEDROXYPROGESTERONE

WARNINGS & PRECAUTIONS

Don't take if:
- You are allergic to any progestin hormone.
- You may be pregnant.
- You have liver or gallbladder disease.
- You have had thrombophlebitis, embolism or stroke.
- You have unexplained vaginal bleeding.
- You have had breast or uterine cancer.

Before you start, consult your doctor:
- If you have heart or kidney disease.
- If you have diabetes.
- If you have a seizure disorder.
- If you suffer migraines.
- If you are easily depressed.

Over age 60:
Not recommended.

Pregnancy:
May harm child. Discontinue at first sign of pregnancy.

Breast-feeding:
Drug passes into milk. Avoid drug or discontinue nursing until you finish medicine. Consult doctor for advice on maintaining milk supply.

Infants & children:
Use only for female children under medical supervision.

Prolonged use:
No problems expected.

Skin & sunlight:
No problems expected.

Driving, piloting or hazardous work:
No problems expected.

Airplane passengers:
No problems expected.

Discontinuing:
Consult doctor. This medicine stays in the body and causes fetal abnormalities. Wait at least 3 months before becoming pregnant.

Others:
- Patients with diabetes must be monitored closely.
- Symptoms of blood clot in leg, brain or lung are: chest, groin, leg pain; sudden, severe headache; loss of coordination; vision change; shortness of breath; slurred speech.

INTERACTION WITH OTHER DRUGS

GENERIC NAME OR DRUG CLASS	COMBINED EFFECT
Antihistamines	Decreased medroxyprogesterone effect.
Oxyphenbutazone	Decreased medroxyprogesterone effect.
Phenobarbital	Decreased medroxyprogesterone effect.
Phenothiazines	Increased phenothiazine effect.
Phenylbutazone	Decreased medroxyprogesterone effect.
Rifampin	Decreased contraceptive effect.

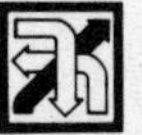

INTERACTION WITH OTHER SUBSTANCES

INTERACTS WITH	COMBINED EFFECT
Alcohol:	None expected.
Beverages:	None expected.
Cocaine:	Decreased medroxyprogesterone effect.
Foods: Salt	Fluid retention.
Marijuana:	Possible menstrual irregularities or bleeding between periods.
Tobacco: All forms.	Possible blood clots in lung, brain, legs. Avoid.

MEFENAMIC ACID

BRAND NAMES

Ponstan
Ponstel

GENERAL INFORMATION

Habit forming? No
Prescription needed? Yes
Available as generic? No
Drug class: Antiinflammatory (non-steroid)

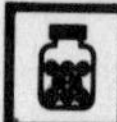

USES

- Pain reliever.
- Treatment for dysmenorrhea (painful or difficult menstruation).

DOSAGE & USAGE INFORMATION

How to take:
Capsule—Swallow with liquid or food to lessen stomach irritation. If you can't swallow whole, open capsule and take with liquid or food.

When to take:
At the same times each day.

If you forget a dose:
Take as soon as you remember up to 2 hours late. If more than 2 hours, wait for next scheduled dose (don't double this dose).

What drug does:
Reduces tissue concentration of prostaglandins (hormones which produce inflammation and pain).

Time lapse before drug works:
Begins in 4 to 24 hours. May require 3 weeks regular use for maximum benefit.

Don't take with:
See Interaction column and consult doctor.

OVERDOSE

Symptoms:
Confusion, agitation, incoherence, convulsions, possible hemorrhage from stomach or intestine, coma.

What to do:
- Dial 0 (operator) or 911 (emergency) for an ambulance or medical help. Then give first aid immediately.
- Additional emergency information on page 886.

POSSIBLE ADVERSE REACTIONS OR SIDE EFFECTS

SYMPTOMS	FREQUENCY	WHAT TO DO
Brain & nervous system:		
• Depression, drowsiness.	Infrequent	4
• Convulsions, confusion.	Rare	3
• Dizziness	Common	4
• Headache	Common	5
Skin:		
Rash, hives or itch.	Rare	3
Eyes:		
Blurred vision.	Rare	3
Ears, nose, throat:		
Ringing in ears.	Infrequent	4
Digestive:		
• Bloody or black, tarry stools.	Rare	3
• Nausea, pain.	Common	4
• Constipation or diarrhea, vomiting.	Infrequent	4
Heart & lungs:		
Breathing difficulty, tightness in chest, rapid heartbeat.	Rare	3
Blood vessels:		
Unusual bleeding or bruising.	Rare	3
Muscles, bones, joints:		
Swollen feet, legs.	Infrequent	4
Genital, urinary:		
• Bloody urine.	Rare	3
• Difficult, painful or frequent urination.	Rare	4
Kidneys, allergic, blood:	None expected.	
Liver:		
Jaundice (yellow skin and eyes).	Rare	3
Others:		
Fatigue, weakness.	Rare	4

1- Life-threatening. Seek emergency treatment immediately.
2- Discontinue. Seek emergency treatment.
3- Discontinue. Call doctor right away.
4- Continue. Call doctor when convenient.
5- Continue. Tell doctor at next visit.

WARNINGS & PRECAUTIONS

Don't take if:

- You are allergic to aspirin or any non-steroid, antiinflammatory drug.
- You have gastritis, peptic ulcer, enteritis, ileitis, ulcerative colitis, asthma, heart failure, high blood pressure or bleeding problems.
- Patient is younger than 15.

Before you start, consult your doctor:

- If you have epilepsy.
- If you have Parkinson's disease.
- If you have been mentally ill.
- If you have had kidney disease or impaired kidney function.

Over age 60:
Adverse reactions and side effects may be more frequent and severe than in younger persons.

Pregnancy:
Studies inconclusive on harm to unborn child. Decide with your doctor whether drug benefits justify risk to unborn child.

Breast-feeding:
May harm child. Avoid.

Infants & children:
Not recommended for anyone younger than 15. Use only under medical supervision.

Prolonged use:

- Eye damage.
- Reduced hearing.
- Sore throat, fever.
- Weight gain.

Skin & sunlight:
No problems expected.

Driving, piloting or hazardous work:
Don't drive or pilot aircraft until you learn how medicine affects you. Don't work around dangerous machinery. Don't climb ladders or work in high places. Danger increases if you drink alcohol or take medicine affecting alertness and reflexes, such as antihistamines, tranquilizers, sedatives, pain medicine, narcotics and mind-altering drugs.

Airplane passengers:
No problems expected.

Discontinuing:
Don't discontinue without consulting doctor. Dose may require gradual reduction if you have taken drug for a long time. Doses of other drugs may also require adjustment.

Others:
Don't take for more than 1 week.

INTERACTION WITH OTHER DRUGS

GENERIC NAME OR DRUG CLASS	COMBINED EFFECT
Anticoagulants (oral)	Increased risk of bleeding.
Aspirin	Increased risk of stomach ulcer.
Cortisone drugs	Increased risk of stomach ulcer.
Furosemide	Decreased diuretic effect of furosemide.
Oxyphenbutazone	Possible stomach ulcer.
Phenylbutazone	Possible stomach ulcer.
Probenecid	Increased effect of mefenamic acid.
Thyroid hormones	Rapid heartbeat, blood-pressure rise.

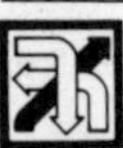

INTERACTION WITH OTHER SUBSTANCES

INTERACTS WITH	COMBINED EFFECT
Alcohol:	Possible stomach ulcer or bleeding.
Beverages:	None expected.
Cocaine:	None expected.
Foods:	None expected.
Marijuana:	Increased pain relief from mefenamic acid.
Tobacco:	None expected.

MELPHALAN (PAM, L-PAM, PHENYLALANINE MUSTARD)

BRAND NAMES

Alkeran

GENERAL INFORMATION

Habit forming? No
Prescription needed? Yes
Available as generic? No
Drug class: Antineoplastic, immunosuppressant

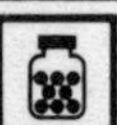

USES

- Treatment for some kinds of cancer.
- Suppresses immune response after transplant and in immune disorders.

DOSAGE & USAGE INFORMATION

How to take:
Tablet or capsule—Swallow with liquid after light meal. Don't drink fluids with meals. Drink extra fluids between meals. Avoid sweet or fatty foods.

When to take:
At the same time each day.

If you forget a dose:
Take as soon as you remember. Don't ever double dose.

What drug does:
Inhibits abnormal cell reproduction. May suppress immune system.

Time lapse before drug works:
Up to 6 weeks for full effect.

Don't take with:
See Interaction column and consult doctor.

OVERDOSE

Symptoms:
Bleeding, chills, fever, collapse, stupor, seizure.

What to do:
- Dial 0 (operator) or 911 (emergency) for an ambulance or medical help. Then give first aid immediately.
- If patient is unconscious and not breathing, give mouth-to-mouth breathing. If there is no heartbeat, use cardiac massage and mouth-to-mouth breathing (CPR). Don't try to make patient vomit. If you can't get help quickly, take patient to nearest emergency facility.
- Additional emergency information on page 886.

POSSIBLE ADVERSE REACTIONS OR SIDE EFFECTS

SYMPTOMS	FREQUENCY	WHAT TO DO
Brain & nervous system:		
Mental confusion.	Infrequent	4
Skin:		
• Unusual bleeding or bruising.	Common	3
• Hair loss.	Common	4
Eyes:	None expected.	
Ears, nose, throat:		
Mouth sores with sore throat, chills and fever.	Common	3
Digestive:		
• Black stools.	Common	3
• Sores in mouth and lips.	Common	3
• Nausea, vomiting, diarrhea (unavoidable).	Common	5
Heart & lungs:		
• Shortness of breath.	Infrequent	4
• Cough	Infrequent	5
Blood vessels:	None expected.	
Muscles, bones, joints:		
Joint pain.	Common	4
Genital, urinary:		
Menstrual changes.	Common	3
Kidneys, allergic, blood, liver:		
• Jaundice (yellow skin and eyes).	Rare	3
• May increase chance of developing leukemia.	Infrequent	4
Others:		
Tiredness, weakness.	Common	5

2- Discontinue. Seek emergency treatment.
3- Discontinue. Call doctor right away.
4- Continue. Call doctor when convenient.
5- Continue. Tell doctor at next visit.

MELPHALAN (PAM, L-PAM, PHENYLALANINE MUSTARD)

WARNINGS & PRECAUTIONS

Don't take if:

- You have had hypersensitivity to alkylating antineoplastic drugs.
- Your physician has not explained serious nature of your medical problem and risks of taking this medicine.

Before you start, consult your doctor:

- If you have gout.
- If you have had kidney stones.
- If you have active infection.
- If you have impaired kidney or liver function.
- If you have taken other antineoplastic drugs or had radiation treatment in last 3 weeks.

Over age 60:
Adverse reactions and side effects may be more frequent and severe than in younger persons.

Pregnancy:
Consult doctor. Risk to child is significant.

Breast-feeding:
Drug passes into milk. Don't nurse.

Infants & children:
Use only under special medical supervision at center experienced in anticancer drugs.

Prolonged use:
Adverse reactions more likely the longer drug is required.

Skin & sunlight:
No problems expected.

Driving, piloting or hazardous work:
No problems expected.

Airplane passengers:
No problems expected.

Discontinuing:
Don't discontinue without doctor's advice until you complete prescribed dose, even though symptoms diminish or disappear. Some side effects may follow discontinuing. Report to doctor blurred vision, convulsions, confusion, persistent headache.

Others:
May cause sterility.

INTERACTION WITH OTHER DRUGS

GENERIC NAME OR DRUG CLASS	COMBINED EFFECT
Antigout drugs	Decreased antigout effect.
Antineoplastic drugs (other)	Increased effect of all drugs, (may be beneficial).
Chloramphenicol	Increased likelihood of toxic effects of both drugs.

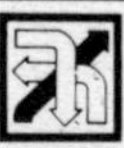

INTERACTION WITH OTHER SUBSTANCES

INTERACTS WITH	COMBINED EFFECT
Alcohol:	May increase chance of intestinal bleeding.
Beverages:	No problems expected.
Cocaine:	Increases chance of toxicity.
Foods:	Reduces irritation in stomach.
Marijuana:	No problems expected.
Tobacco:	Increases lung toxicity.

MEPHENYTOIN

BRAND NAMES

Mesantoin
Methoin

GENERAL INFORMATION

Habit forming? No
Prescription needed? Yes
Available as generic? Yes
Drug class: Anticonvulsant (hydantoin)

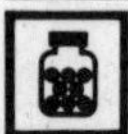

USES

- Prevents epileptic seizures.
- Stabilizes irregular heartbeat.

DOSAGE & USAGE INFORMATION

How to take:
- Tablet or capsule—Swallow with liquid.
- Extended-release tablets or capsules—Swallow each dose whole. If you take regular tablets, you may chew or crush them.

When to take:
At the same time each day.

If you forget a dose:
- If drug taken 1 time per day—Take as soon as you remember up to 12 hours late. If more than 12 hours, wait for next scheduled dose (don't double this dose).
- If taken several times per day—Take as soon as possible, then return to regular schedule.

What drug does:
Promotes sodium loss from nerve fibers. This lessens excitability and inhibits spread of nerve impulses.

Time lapse before drug works:
7 to 10 days continual use.

Don't take with:
See Interaction column and consult doctor.

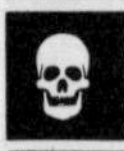

OVERDOSE

Symptoms:
Jerky eye movements; stagger; slurred speech; imbalance; drowsiness; blood-pressure drop; slow, shallow breathing; coma.

What to do:
- Dial 0 (operator) or 911 (emergency) for an ambulance or medical help. Then give first aid immediately.
- Additional emergency information on page 886.

POSSIBLE ADVERSE REACTIONS OR SIDE EFFECTS

SYMPTOMS	FREQUENCY	WHAT TO DO
Brain & nervous system:		
• Mild dizziness, drowsiness.	Common	4
• Headache, sleeplessness.	Infrequent	4
• Hallucinations, confusion, slurred speech, stagger.	Infrequent	3
Skin:		
Rash	Infrequent	3
Eyes:		
Vision changes.	Infrequent	3
Ears, nose, throat:		
Sore throat, fever.	Rare	3
Digestive:		
• Stomach pain.	Rare	3
• Constipation, nausea, vomiting.	Common	4
• Diarrhea	Infrequent	4
Heart & lungs, genital, urinary, kidneys, allergic blood:	None expected.	
Blood vessels:		
Unusual bleeding or bruising.	Rare	3
Muscles, bones, joints:		
Muscle twitching.	Infrequent	4
Liver:		
Jaundice (yellow skin and eyes).	Rare	3
Others:		
Increased body and facial hair.	Infrequent	5

1- Life-threatening. Seek emergency treatment immediately.
2- Discontinue. Seek emergency treatment.
3- Discontinue. Call doctor right away.
4- Continue. Call doctor when convenient.
5- Continue. Tell doctor at next visit.

WARNINGS & PRECAUTIONS

Don't take if:
You are allergic to any hydantoin anticonvulsant.

Before you start, consult your doctor:
- If you have had impaired liver function or disease.
- If you will have surgery within 2 months, including dental surgery, requiring general or spinal anesthesia.

Over age 60:
Adverse reactions and side effects may be more frequent and severe than in younger persons.

Pregnancy:
Risk to unborn child outweighs drug benefits. Don't use.

Breast-feeding:
Drug passes into milk. Avoid drug or discontinue nursing until you finish medicine. Consult doctor for advice on maintaining milk supply.

Infants & children:
Use only under medical supervision.

Prolonged use:
- Weakened bones.
- Lymph gland enlargement.
- Possible liver damage.
- Numbness and tingling of hands and feet.
- Continual back-and-forth eye movements.
- Bleeding, swollen or tender gums.

Skin & sunlight:
May cause rash or intensify sunburn in areas exposed to sun or sunlamp.

Driving, piloting or hazardous work:
Don't drive or pilot aircraft until you learn how medicine affects you. Don't work around dangerous machinery. Don't climb ladders or work in high places. Danger increases if you drink alcohol or take medicine affecting alertness and reflexes.

Airplane passengers:
No problems expected.

Discontinuing:
Don't discontinue without consulting doctor. Dose may require gradual reduction if you have taken drug for a long time. Doses of other drugs may also require adjustment.

INTERACTION WITH OTHER DRUGS

GENERIC NAME OR DRUG CLASS	COMBINED EFFECT
Anticoagulants	Increased effect of both drugs.
Antidepressants (tricyclic)	Need to adjust mephenytoin dose.
Antihypertensives	Increased effect of antihypertensive.
Aspirin	Increased mephenytoin effect.
Barbiturates	Changed seizure pattern.
Carbonic anhydrase inhibitors	Increased chance of bone disease.
Chloramphenicol	Increased mephenytoin effect.
Contraceptives (oral)	Increased seizures.
Cortisone drugs	Decreased cortisone effect.
Digitalis preparations	Decreased digitalis effect.
Disulfiram	Increased mephenytoin effect.
Estrogens	Increased mephenytoin effect.
Furosemide	Decreased furosemide effect.
Glutethimide	Decreased mephenytoin effect.
Griseofulvin	Increased griseofulvin effect.

Additional interactions on page 838.

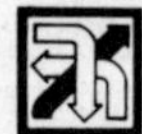

INTERACTION WITH OTHER SUBSTANCES

INTERACTS WITH	COMBINED EFFECT
Alcohol:	Possible decreased anticonvulsant effect. Use with caution.
Beverages:	None expected.
Cocaine:	Possible seizures.
Foods:	None expected.
Marijuana:	Drowsiness, unsteadiness, decreased anti-convulsant effect.
Tobacco:	None expected.

MEPHOBARBITAL

BRAND NAMES

Mebaral

GENERAL INFORMATION

Habit forming? Yes
Prescription needed? Yes
Available as generic? Yes
Drug class: Sedative, hypnotic (barbiturate)

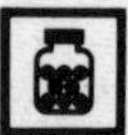

USES

- Reduces anxiety or nervous tension (low dose).
- Relieves insomnia (higher bedtime dose).
- Prevents seizures in epilepsy.

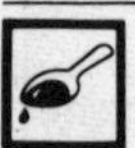

DOSAGE & USAGE INFORMATION

How to take:
Tablet—Swallow with liquid or food to lessen stomach irritation. If you can't swallow whole, crumble tablet and take with liquid or food.

When to take:
At the same times each day.

If you forget a dose:
Take as soon as you remember up to 2 hours late. If more than 2 hours, wait for next scheduled dose (don't double this dose).

What drug does:
May partially block nerve impulses at nerve-cell connections.

Time lapse before drug works:
60 minutes.

Don't take with:
- Non-prescription drugs without consulting doctor.
- See Interaction column and consult doctor.

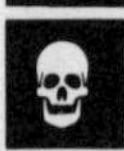

OVERDOSE

Symptoms:
Deep sleep, weak pulse, coma.

What to do:
- Dial 0 (operator) or 911 (emergency) for an ambulance or medical help. Then give first aid immediately.
- If patient is unconscious and not breathing, give mouth-to-mouth breathing. If there is no heartbeat use cardiac massage and mouth-to-mouth breathing (CPR). Don't try to make patient vomit. If you can't help quickly, take patient to nearest emergency facility.
- Additional emergency information on page 886.

POSSIBLE ADVERSE REACTIONS OR SIDE EFFECTS

SYMPTOMS	FREQUENCY	WHAT TO DO
Brain & nervous system:		
• Dizziness, drowsiness, "hangover effect."	Common	4
• Depression, confusion, slurred speech.	Infrequent	4
• Agitation	Rare	3
Skin:		
• Rash or hives.	Infrequent	3
• Face, lip swelling.	Infrequent	3
Eyes:		
Eyelid swelling.	Infrequent	3
Ears, nose, throat:		
Sore throat, fever.	Infrequent	3
Digestive:		
Diarrhea, nausea, vomiting.	Infrequent	4
Heart & lungs:		
• Slow heartbeat.	Rare	3
• Breathing difficulty.	Rare	3
Blood vessels:		
Unexplained bleeding or bruising.	Rare	4
Muscles, bones, joints:		
Joint or muscle pain.	Infrequent	4
Genital, urinary:	None expected.	
Kidneys:	None expected.	
Liver:		
Jaundice (yellow skin and eyes).	Rare	3
Allergic:	None expected.	
Blood:	None expected.	
Others:	None expected.	

1-Life-threatening. Seek emergency treatment immediately.
2-Discontinue. Seek emergency treatment.
3-Discontinue. Call doctor right away.
4-Continue. Call doctor when convenient.

WARNINGS & PRECAUTIONS

Don't take if:
- You are allergic to any barbiturate.
- You have porphyria.

Before you start, consult your doctor:
- If you have epilepsy.
- If you have kidney or liver damage.
- If you have asthma.
- If you have anemia.
- If you have chronic pain.
- If you will have surgery within 2 months, including dental surgery, requiring general or spinal anesthesia.

Over age 60:
Adverse reactions and side effects may be more frequent and severe than in younger persons. Use small doses.

Pregnancy:
Risk to unborn child outweighs drug benefits. Don't use.

Breast-feeding:
Drug passes into milk. Avoid drug or discontinue nursing until you finish medicine. Consult doctor for advice on maintaining milk supply.

Infants & children:
Use only under doctor's supervision.

Prolonged use:
- May cause addiction, anemia, chronic intoxication.
- May lower body temperature, making exposure to cold temperatures hazardous.

Skin & sunlight:
May cause rash or intensify sunburn in areas exposed to sun or sunlamp.

Driving, piloting or hazardous work:
Don't drive or pilot aircraft until you learn how medicine affects you. Don't work around dangerous machinery. Don't climb ladders or work in high places. Danger increases if you drink alcohol or take medicine affecting alertness and reflexes.

Airplane passengers:
No problems expected.

Discontinuing:
May be unnecessary to finish medicine. Follow doctor's instructions. If you develop withdrawal symptoms of hallucinations, agitation or sleeplessness after discontinuing, call doctor right away.

Others:
No problems expected.

INTERACTION WITH OTHER DRUGS

GENERIC NAME OR DRUG CLASS	COMBINED EFFECT
Anticoagulants (oral)	Decreased anticoagulant effect.
Anticonvulsants	Changed seizure patterns.
Antidepressants (tricyclic)	Decreased antidepressant effect.
Antidiabetics (oral)	Increased mephobarbital effect.
Antihistamines	Dangerous sedation. Avoid.
Antiinflammatory drugs (non-steroidal)	Decreased antiinflammatory effect.
Aspirin	Decreased aspirin effect.
Beta-adrenergic blockers	Decreased effect of beta-adrenergic blocker.
Contraceptives (oral)	Decreased contraceptive effect.
Cortisone drugs	Decreased cortisone effect.
Digitoxin	Decreased digitoxin effect.
Doxycycline	Decreased doxycycline effect.
Griseofulvin	Decreased griseofulvin effect.

Additional interactions on page 839.

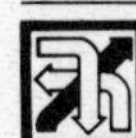

INTERACTION WITH OTHER SUBSTANCES

INTERACTS WITH	COMBINED EFFECT
Alcohol:	Possible fatal oversedation. Avoid.
Beverages:	None expected.
Cocaine:	Decreased mephobarbital effect.
Foods:	None expected.
Marijuana:	Excessive sedation. Avoid.
Tobacco:	None expected.

MEPROBAMATE

BRAND NAMES

Arcoban	Kalmn	Meprospan	Novo-Mepro
Bamate	Lan-Dol	Meprotabs	Pax 400
Bamo 400	Medi-Tran	Meribam	Quietal
Coprobate	Mep-E	Miltown	Robamate
Deprol	Meprocon	Neo-Tran	SK-Bamate

See complete brand names list, page 828.

GENERAL INFORMATION

Habit forming? Yes
Prescription needed? Yes
Available as generic? Yes
Drug class: Tranquilizer

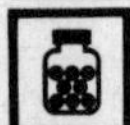

USES

Reduces mild anxiety, tension and insomnia.

DOSAGE & USAGE INFORMATION

How to take:

- Tablet or capsule—Swallow with liquid.
- Extended-release tablets or capsules—Swallow each dose whole. If you take regular tablets, you may chew or crush them.
- Liquid—Take as directed on label.

When to take:
At the same time each day.

If you forget a dose:
Take as soon as you remember up to 2 hours late. If more than 2 hours, wait for next scheduled dose (don't double this dose).

What drug does:
Sedates brain centers which control behavior and emotions.

Time lapse before drug works:
1 to 2 hours.

Don't take with:

- Non-prescription drugs containing alcohol or caffeine without consulting doctor.
- See Interaction column and consult doctor.

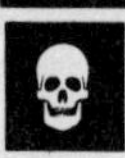

OVERDOSE

Symptoms:
Dizziness, slurred speech, stagger, depressed breathing and heart function, stupor, coma.

What to do:

- Dial 0 (operator) or 911 (emergency) for an ambulance or medical help. Then give first aid immediately.
- Additional emergency information on page 886.

POSSIBLE ADVERSE REACTIONS OR SIDE EFFECTS

SYMPTOMS	FREQUENCY	WHAT TO DO
Brain & nervous system:		
• Dizziness, confusion, agitation, drowiness, unsteadiness.	Common	5
• False sense of well-being, headache, slurred speech.	Infrequent	4
Skin:		
Rash, hives, itch.	Infrequent	3
Eyes:		
Vision changes.	Infrequent	3
Ears, nose, throat:		
Sore throat, fever.	Rare	3
Digestive:		
Diarrhea, nausea or vomiting.	Infrequent	3
Heart & lungs:		
Rapid, pounding, unusually slow or irregular heartbeat, breathing difficulty.	Rare	3
Blood vessels, muscles, bones, joints, genital, urinary, kidneys, liver, allergic:	None expected.	
Blood:		
Unusual bleeding or bruising.	Rare	3
Others:		
Fatigue, weakness.	Common	5

1- Life-threatening. Seek emergency treatment immediately.
2- Discontinue. Seek emergency treatment.
3- Discontinue. Call doctor right away.
4- Continue. Call doctor when convenient.
5- Continue. Tell doctor at next visit.

WARNINGS & PRECAUTIONS

Don't take if:

- You are allergic to meprobamate, tybanate, carbromal or carisoprodol.
- You have had porphyria.
- Patient is younger than 6.

Before you start, consult your doctor:

- If you have epilepsy.
- If you have impaired liver or kidney function.

Over age 60:
Adverse reactions and side effects may be more frequent and severe than in younger persons.

Pregnancy:
Risk to unborn child outweighs drug benefits. Don't use.

Breast-feeding:
Drug filters into milk. May harm child. Avoid.

Infants & children:
Not recommended.

Prolonged use:

- Habit forming.
- May impair blood-cell production.

Skin & sunlight:
No problems expected.

Driving, piloting or hazardous work:
Don't drive or pilot aircraft until you learn how medicine affects you. Don't work around dangerous machinery. Don't climb ladders or work in high places. Danger increases if you drink alcohol or take medicine affecting alertness and reflexes, such as antihistamines, tranquilizers, sedatives, pain medicine, narcotics and mind-altering drugs.

Airplane passengers:
No problems expected.

Discontinuing:
Don't discontinue without consulting doctor. Dose may require gradual reduction if you have taken drug for a long time. Doses of other drugs may also require adjustment.

Others:
No problems expected.

INTERACTION WITH OTHER DRUGS

GENERIC NAME OR DRUG CLASS	COMBINED EFFECT
Anticoagulants	Decreased anticoagulant effect.
Anticonvulsants	Change in seizure pattern.
Antidepressants	Increased antidepressant effect.
Contraceptives (oral)	Decreased contraceptive effect.
Estrogens	Decreased estrogen effect.
MAO inhibitors	Increased meprobamate effect.
Narcotics	Increased narcotic effect.
Sedatives	Increased sedative effect.
Sleep inducers	Increased effect of sleep inducer.
Tranquilizers	Increased tranquilizer effect.

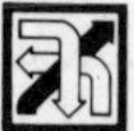

INTERACTION WITH OTHER SUBSTANCES

INTERACTS WITH	COMBINED EFFECT
Alcohol:	Dangerous increased effect of meprobamate.
Beverages: Caffeine drinks	Decreased calming effect of meprobamate.
Cocaine:	Decreased meprobamate effect.
Foods:	None expected.
Marijuana:	Increased sedative effect of meprobamate.
Tobacco:	None expected.

MERCAPTOPURINE

BRAND NAMES

Purinethol

GENERAL INFORMATION

Habit forming? No
Prescription needed? Yes
Available as generic? Yes
Drug class: Antineoplastic, immunosuppressant

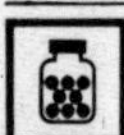

USES

- Treatment for some kinds of cancer.
- Treatment for regional enteritis and ulcerative colitis and other immune disorders.

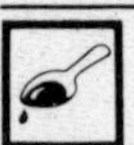

DOSAGE & USAGE INFORMATION

How to take:
Tablet—Swallow with liquid.

When to take:
At the same time each day.

If you forget a dose:
Skip the missed dose. Don't double the next dose.

What drug does:
Inhibits abnormal-cell reproduction.

Time lapse before drug works:
May require 6 weeks for maximum effect.

Don't take with:
See Interaction column and consult doctor.

OVERDOSE

Symptoms:
Headache, stupor, seizures.

What to do:
- Dial 0 (operator) or 911 (emergency) for an ambulance or medical help. Then give first aid immediately.
- If patient is unconscious and not breathing, give mouth-to-mouth breathing. If there is no heartbeat, use cardiac massage and mouth-to-mouth breathing (CPR). Don't try to make patient vomit. If you can't get help quickly, take patient to nearest emergency facility.
- Additional emergency information on page 886.

POSSIBLE ADVERSE REACTIONS OR SIDE EFFECTS

SYMPTOMS	FREQUENCY	WHAT TO DO
Brain & nervous system:		
• Seizures	Infrequent	2
• Dizziness, drowsiness, headache, confusion.	Infrequent	3
Skin:		
Acne, boils, hair loss, itch.	Infrequent	5
Eyes:		
Blurred vision.	Infrequent	3
Ears, nose, throat:		
Mouth sores, sore throat, fever, chills.	Common	3
Digestive:		
• Black stools or bloody vomit.	Common	2
• Stomach pain, nausea, vomiting.	Common	4
Heart & lungs:		
• Shortness or breath.	Infrequent	3
• Cough	Infrequent	4
Blood vessels:		
Unusual bleeding or bruising.	Common	3
Muscles, bones, joints:		
Joint pain.	Infrequent	3
Genital, urinary:		
Bloody urine.	Infrequent	3
Kidneys, allergic, blood, others:	None expected.	
Liver:		
Jaundice (yellow skin and eyes).	Infrequent	3

1- Life-threatening. Seek emergency treatment immediately.
2- Discontinue. Seek emergency treatment.
3- Discontinue. Call doctor right away.
4- Continue. Call doctor when convenient.
5- Continue. Tell doctor at next visit.

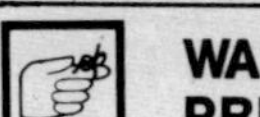

WARNINGS & PRECAUTIONS

Don't take if:
You are allergic to any antineoplastic.

Before you start, consult your doctor:
- If you are alcoholic.
- If you have blood, liver or kidney disease.
- If you have colitis or peptic ulcer.
- If you have gout.
- If you have an infection.
- If you plan to become pregnant within 3 months.

Over age 60:
Adverse reactions and side effects may be more frequent and severe than in younger persons.

Pregnancy:
Consult doctor.

Breast-feeding:
Drug passes into milk. Avoid drug or discontinue nursing.

Infants & children:
Use only under special medical supervision.

Prolonged use:
Adverse reactions more likely the longer drug is required.

Skin & sunlight:
No problems expected.

Driving, piloting or hazardous work:
Avoid if you feel dizzy, drowsy or confused. Otherwise, no problems expected.

Airplane passengers:
No problems expected.

Discontinuing:
Don't discontinue without doctor's advice until you complete prescribed dose, even though symptoms diminish or disappear. Some side effects may follow discontinuing. Report to doctor blurred vision, convulsions, confusion, persistent headache.

Others:
- Drink more water than usual to cause frequent urination.
- Don't give this medicine to anyone else for any purpose. It is a strong drug that requires close medical supervision.
- Report for frequent medical follow-up and laboratory studies.

INTERACTION WITH OTHER DRUGS

GENERIC NAME OR DRUG CLASS	COMBINED EFFECT
Allopurinol	Increased toxic effect of mercaptopurine.
Antineoplastic drugs (other)	Increased effect of both (may be desirable) or increase toxicity of each.
Acetaminophen	Increased likelihood of liver toxicity.
Isoniazid	Increased likelihood of liver toxicity.
Chloramphenicol	Increased toxicity of each.

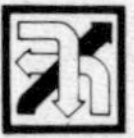

INTERACTION WITH OTHER SUBSTANCES

INTERACTS WITH	COMBINED EFFECT
Alcohol:	May increase chance of intestinal bleeding.
Beverages:	No problems expected.
Cocaine:	Increases chance of toxicity.
Foods:	Reduced irritation in stomach.
Marijuana:	No problems expected.
Tobacco:	Increases lung toxicity.

MESORIDAZINE

BRAND NAMES

Serentil

GENERAL INFORMATION

Habit forming? No
Prescription needed? Yes
Available as generic? Yes
Drug class: Tranquilizer, antiemetic (phenothiazine)

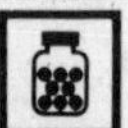

USES

- Stops nausea, vomiting.
- Reduces anxiety, agitation.

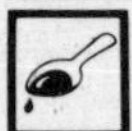

DOSAGE & USAGE INFORMATION

How to take:

- Tablet or capsule—Swallow with liquid or food to lessen stomach irritation.
- Suppositories—Remove wrapper and moisten suppository with water. Gently insert into rectum, large end first.
- Drops or liquid—Dilute dose in beverage.

When to take:

- Nervous and mental disorders—Take at the same times each day.
- Nausea and vomiting—Take as needed, no more often than every 4 hours.

If you forget a dose:

- Nervous and mental disorders—Take up to 2 hours late. If more than 2 hours, wait for next scheduled dose (don't double this).
- Nausea and vomiting—Take as soon as you remember. Wait 4 hours for next dose.

What drug does:

- Suppresses brain's vomiting center.
- Suppresses brain centers that control abnormal emotions and behavior.

Time lapse before drug works:

- Nausea and vomiting—1 hour or less.
- Nervous and mental disorders—4-6 weeks.

Don't take with:

- Antacid or medicine for diarrhea.
- Non-prescription drug for cough, cold or allergy.
- See Interaction column and consult doctor.

OVERDOSE

Symptoms:
Stupor, convulsions, coma.

What to do:

- Dial 0 (operator) or 911 (emergency) for an ambulance or medical help. Then give first aid immediately.
- Additional emergency information on page 886.

POSSIBLE ADVERSE REACTIONS OR SIDE EFFECTS

SYMPTOMS	FREQUENCY	WHAT TO DO
Brain & nervous system:		
• Restlessness, tremor.	Common	3
• Fainting	Infrequent	2
• Drowsiness	Common	3
Skin:		
• Rash	Infrequent	3
• Less perspiration.	Common	4
Eyes:		
Vision changes.	Rare	3
Ears, nose, throat:		
• Sore throat, fever.	Rare	3
• Dry mouth, nasal congestion.	Common	4
Digestive:		
Constipation	Common	4
Heart & lungs, blood vessels, kidneys, allergic, blood:	None expected.	
Muscles, bones, joints:		
Muscle spasms of face and neck, unsteady gait.	Common	2
Genital, urinary:		
Urination difficulty.	Infrequent	4
Liver:		
Jaundice (yellow eyes and skin).	Rare	3
Others:		
Less interest in sex, breast swelling, change in menstrual pattern.	Infrequent	4

1-Life-threatening. Seek emergency treatment immediately.
2-Discontinue. Seek emergency treatment.
3-Discontinue. Call doctor right away.
4-Continue. Call doctor when convenient.
5-Continue. Tell doctor at next visit.
6-No action necessary.

WARNINGS & PRECAUTIONS

Don't take if:
- You are allergic to any phenothiazine.
- You have a blood or bone-marrow disease.

Before you start, consult your doctor:
- If you will have surgery within 2 months, including dental surgery, requiring general or spinal anesthesia.
- If you have asthma, emphysema or other lung disorder.
- If you take non-prescription ulcer medicine, asthma medicine or amphetamines.

Over age 60:
Adverse reactions and side effects may be more frequent and severe than in younger persons. More likely to develop involuntary movement of jaws, lips, tongue, chewing. Report this to your doctor immediately. Early treatment can help.

Pregnancy:
Risk to unborn child outweighs drug benefits. Don't use.

Breast-feeding:
Drug passes into milk. Avoid drug or discontinue nursing until you finish medicine. Consult doctor for advice on maintaining milk supply.

Infants & children:
Don't give to children younger than 2.

Prolonged use:
May lead to tardive dyskinesia (involuntary movement of jaws, lips, tongue, chewing).

Skin & sunlight:
May cause rash or intensify sunburn in areas exposed to sun or sunlamp. Skin may remain sensitive for 3 months after discontinuing.

Driving, piloting or hazardous work:
Don't drive or pilot aircraft until you learn how medicine affects you. Don't work around dangerous machinery. Don't climb ladders or work in high places. Danger increases if you drink alcohol or take medicine affecting alertness and reflexes.

Airplane passengers:
No problems expected.

Discontinuing:
- Nervous and mental disorders—Don't discontinue without doctor's advice until you complete prescribed dose, even though symptoms diminish or disappear.
- Nausea and vomiting—May be unnecessary to finish medicine. Follow doctor's instructions.

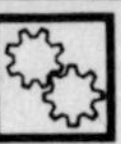

INTERACTION WITH OTHER DRUGS

GENERIC NAME OR DRUG CLASS	COMBINED EFFECT
Anticholinergics	Increased anticholinergic effect.
Antidepressants (tricyclic)	Increased mesoridazine effect.
Antihistamines	Increased antihistamine effect.
Appetite suppressants	Decreased suppressant effect.
Levodopa	Decreased levodopa effect.
Mind-altering drugs	Increased effect of mind-altering drugs.
Narcotics	Increased narcotic effect.
Phenytoin	Increased phenytoin effect.
Quinidine	Impaired heart function. Dangerous mixture.
Sedatives	Increased sedative effect.
Tranquilizers (other)	Increased tranquilizer effect.

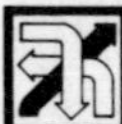

INTERACTION WITH OTHER SUBSTANCES

INTERACTS WITH	COMBINED EFFECT
Alcohol:	Dangerous oversedation.
Beverages:	None expected.
Cocaine:	Decreased effect of mesoridazine. Avoid.
Foods:	None expected.
Marijuana:	Drowsiness. May increase antinausea effect.
Tobacco:	None expected.

METAPROTERENOL

BRAND NAMES

Alupent
Metaprel

GENERAL INFORMATION

Habit forming? No
Prescription needed? Yes
Available as generic? No
Drug class: Bronchodilator, sympathomimetic

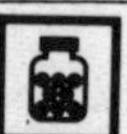

USES

Relieves wheezing and shortness of breath in bronchial asthma attacks, bronchitis and emphysema.

DOSAGE & USAGE INFORMATION

How to take:

- Tablet or liquid—Swallow with liquid or food to lessen stomach irritation.
- Inhaler—Follow instructions on package.

When to take:
When needed, according to doctor's instructions. Don't take more than 2 doses 1 hour apart.

If you forget a dose:
Take when you remember. Wait 2 hours for next dose.

What drug does:
Relaxes smooth muscles to relieve constriction of bronchial tubes.

Time lapse before drug works:
5 to 30 minutes.

Don't take with:
See Interaction column and consult doctor.

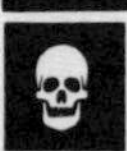

OVERDOSE

Symptoms:
Chest pain, irregular heartbeat, convulsions, coma.

What to do:

- Dial 0 (operator) or 911 (emergency) for an ambulance or medical help. Then give first aid immediately.
- If patient is unconscious and not breathing, give mouth-to-mouth breathing. If there is no heartbeat, use cardiac massage and mouth-to-mouth breathing (CPR). Don't try to make patient vomit. If you can't get help quickly, take patient to nearest emergency facility.
- Additional emergency information on page 886.

POSSIBLE ADVERSE REACTIONS OR SIDE EFFECTS

SYMPTOMS	FREQUENCY	WHAT TO DO
Brain & nervous system:		
Nervousness, restlessness, dizziness, weakness, headache, trembling.	Common	4
Skin:		
Paleness	Infrequent	4
Eyes:	None expected.	
Ears, nose, throat:		
Bad taste in mouth.	Infrequent	4
Digestive:		
Nausea or vomiting.	Infrequent	4
Heart & lungs:		
• Rapid or pounding heartbeat.	Common	3
• Chest pain.	Infrequent	3
Blood vessels:	None expected.	
Muscles, bones, joints:		
Muscle cramps in arms, hands, legs.	Infrequent	3
Genital, urinary:	None expected.	
Kidneys:	None expected.	
Liver:	None expected.	
Allergic:	None expected.	
Blood:	None expected.	
Others:		
Unusual sweating.	Infrequent	3

1- Life-threatening. Seek emergency treatment immediately.
2- Discontinue. Seek emergency treatment.
3- Discontinue. Call doctor right away.
4- Continue. Call doctor when convenient.
5- Continue. Tell doctor at next visit.
6- No action necessary.

WARNINGS & PRECAUTIONS

Don't take if:
You are allergic to any sympathomimetic.

Before you start, consult your doctor:
- If you have irregular or rapid heartbeat, congestive heart failure, coronary-artery disease or high blood pressure.
- If you have diabetes.
- If you have overactive thyroid.

Over age 60:
Adverse reactions and side effects may be more frequent and severe than in younger persons.

Pregnancy:
Risk to unborn child outweighs drug benefits. Don't use.

Breast-feeding:
Drug passes into milk. Avoid drug or discontinue nursing until you finish medicine. Consult doctor for advice on maintaining milk supply.

Infants & children:
Use only under medical supervision.

Prolonged use:
No problems expected.

Skin & sunlight:
No problems expected.

Driving, piloting or hazardous work:
Don't drive or pilot aircraft until you learn how medicine affects you. Don't work around dangerous machinery. Don't climb ladders or work in high places. Danger increases if you drink alcohol or take medicine affecting alertness and reflexes, such as antihistamines, tranquilizers, sedatives, pain medicine, narcotics and mind-altering drugs.

Airplane passengers:
No problems expected.

Discontinuing:
No problems expected.

Others:
Consult doctor immediately if breathing difficulty continues or worsens after using metaproterenol.

INTERACTION WITH OTHER DRUGS

GENERIC NAME OR DRUG CLASS	COMBINED EFFECT
Antidepressants (tricyclic)	Increased effect of both drugs.
Beta-adrenergic blockers	Decreased metaproterenol effect.
Hydralazine	Decreased hydralazine effect.
Sympathomimetics (other)	Increased effect of both drugs, especially harmful side effects.

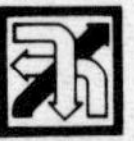

INTERACTION WITH OTHER SUBSTANCES

INTERACTS WITH	COMBINED EFFECT
Alcohol:	Decreased metaproterenol effect.
Beverages:	None expected.
Cocaine:	Possible metaproterenol toxicity.
Foods:	None expected.
Marijuana:	Overstimulation. Avoid.
Tobacco:	No proven problems.

METAXALONE

BRAND NAMES

Skelaxin

GENERAL INFORMATION

Habit forming? No
Prescription needed? Yes
Available as generic? Yes
Drug class: Muscle relaxant (skeletal)

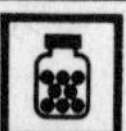

USES

Treatment for sprains, strains and muscle spasms.

DOSAGE & USAGE INFORMATION

How to take:
Tablet or capsule—Swallow with liquid.

When to take:
As needed, no more often than every 4 hours.

If you forget a dose:
Take as soon as you remember. Wait 4 hours for next dose.

What drug does:
Blocks body's pain messages to brain. May also sedate.

Time lapse before drug works:
60 minutes.

Don't take with:
See Interaction column and consult doctor.

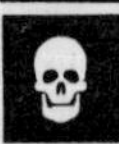

OVERDOSE

Symptoms:
Nausea, vomiting, diarrhea, headache. May progress to severe weakness, difficult breathing, sensation of paralysis, coma.

What to do:

- Dial 0 (operator) or 911 (emergency) for an ambulance or medical help. Then give first aid immediately.
- If patient is unconscious and not breathing, give mouth-to-mouth breathing. If there is no heartbeat, use cardiac massage and mouth-to-mouth breathing (CPR). Don't try to make patient vomit. If you can't get help quickly, take patient to nearest emergency facility.
- Additional emergency information on page 886.

POSSIBLE ADVERSE REACTIONS OR SIDE EFFECTS

SYMPTOMS	FREQUENCY	WHAT TO DO
Brain & nervous system:		
• Drowsiness, fainting, dizziness.	Common	4
• Agitation	Infrequent	3
Skin:		
Rash, hives or itch.	Rare	3
Eyes:	None expected.	
Ears, nose, throat:		
Sore throat, fever.	Rare	3
Digestive:		
• Constipation or diarrhea, nausea, cramps, vomiting.	Infrequent	3
• Bloody or tarry, black stool.	Rare	2
Heart & lungs:		
Wheezing, shortness of breath.	Infrequent	3
Blood vessels:	None expected.	
Muscles, bones, joints:	None expected.	
Genital, urinary:		
Orange or red-purple urine.	Common	6
Kidneys:	None expected.	
Liver:		
Jaundice (yellow eyes and skin).	Rare	3
Blood, allergic:	None expected.	
Others:		
Tiredness, weakness.	Rare	3

1- Life-threatening. Seek emergency treatment immediately.
2- Discontinue. Seek emergency treatment.
3- Discontinue. Call doctor right away.
4- Continue. Call doctor when convenient.
5- Continue. Tell doctor at next visit.
6- No action necessary.

WARNINGS & PRECAUTIONS

Don't take if:

- You are allergic to any skeletal-muscle relaxant.
- You have porphyria.

Before you start, consult your doctor:

- If you have had liver or kidney disease.
- If you plan pregnancy within medication period.

Over age 60:
Adverse reactions and side effects may be more frequent and severe than in younger persons.

Pregnancy:
No proven harm to unborn child. Avoid if possible.

Breast-feeding:
Drug passes into milk. Avoid drug or discontinue nursing until you finish medicine. Consult doctor for advice on maintaining milk supply.

Infants & children:
Not recommended.

Prolonged use:
Periodic liver-function tests recommended if you use this drug for a long time.

Skin & sunlight:
No problems expected.

Driving, piloting or hazardous work:
Don't drive or pilot aircraft until you learn how medicine affects you. Don't work around dangerous machinery. Don't climb ladders or work in high places. Danger increases if you drink alcohol or take medicine affecting alertness and reflexes, such as antihistamines, tranquilizers, sedatives, pain medicine, narcotics and mind-altering drugs.

Airplane passengers:
No problems expected.

Discontinuing:
Don't discontinue without doctor's advice until you complete prescribed dose, even though symptoms diminish or disappear.

Others:
No problems expected.

INTERACTION WITH OTHER DRUGS

GENERIC NAME OR DRUG CLASS	COMBINED EFFECT
Antidepressants	Increased sedation.
Antihistamines	Increased sedation.
Mind-altering drugs	Increased sedation.
Muscle relaxants (other)	Increased sedation.
Narcotics	Increased sedation.
Sedatives	Increased sedation.
Sleep inducers	Increased sedation.
Testosterone	Decreased metaxalone effect.
Tranquilizers	Increased sedation.

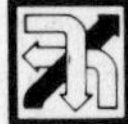

INTERACTION WITH OTHER SUBSTANCES

INTERACTS WITH	COMBINED EFFECT
Alcohol:	Increased sedation.
Beverages:	None expected.
Cocaine:	Lack of coordination, increased sedation.
Foods:	None expected.
Marijuana:	Lack of coordination, drowsiness, fainting.
Tobacco:	None expected.

METHAMPHETAMINE

BRAND NAMES

Desoxyn
Methampex

GENERAL INFORMATION

Habit forming? Yes
Prescription needed? Yes
Available as generic? Yes
Drug class: Central-nervous-system stimulant (amphetamine)

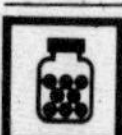

USES

- Prevents narcolepsy (attacks of uncontrollable sleepiness).
- Controls hyperactivity in children.

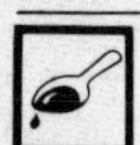

DOSAGE & USAGE INFORMATION

How to take:
- Tablet—Swallow with liquid.
- Extended-release tablets—Swallow each dose whole with liquid.

When to take:
- At the same times each day.
- Short-acting form—Don't take later than 6 hours before bedtime.
- Long-acting form—Take on awakening.

If you forget a dose:
- Short-acting form—Take up to 2 hours late. If more than 2 hours, wait for next dose (don't double this).
- Long-acting form—Take as soon as you remember. Wait 20 hours for next dose.

What drug does:
- Narcolepsy—Apparently affects brain centers to decrease fatigue or sleepiness and increase alertness and motor activity.
- Hyperactive children—Calms children, opposite to effect on narcoleptic adults.

Time lapse before drug works:
15 to 30 minutes.

Don't take with:
See Interaction column and consult doctor.

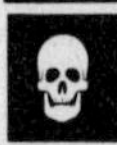

OVERDOSE

Symptoms:
Rapid heartbeat, hyperactivity, high fever, hallucinations, suicidal or homicidal feelings, convulsions, coma.

What to do:
- Dial 0 (operator) or 911 (emergency) for an ambulance or medical help. Then give first aid immediately.
- Additional emergency information on page 886.

POSSIBLE ADVERSE REACTIONS OR SIDE EFFECTS

SYMPTOMS	FREQUENCY	WHAT TO DO
Brain & nervous system:		
• Headache	Infrequent	4
• Dizziness, lack of alertness.	Infrequent	3
• Mood changes.	Rare	4
• Irritability, nervousness, insomnia.	Common	4
Skin:		
Rash, hives.	Rare	3
Eyes:		
Blurred vision.	Infrequent	3
Ears, nose, throat:		
Dry mouth.	Common	5
Digestive:		
Diarrhea or constipation, appetite loss, stomach pain, nausea, vomiting, weight loss.	Infrequent	5
Heart & lungs:		
• Fast, pounding heartbeat.	Infrequent	3
• Chest pain or irregular heartbeat.	Rare	3
Blood vessels, kidneys, liver, allergic, blood:	None expected.	
Muscles, bones, joints:		
Uncontrolled movements of head, neck, arms, legs.	Rare	3
Genital, urinary:		
Decreased sex drive, impotence.	Infrequent	5
Others:		
• Enlarged breasts.	Rare	4
• Unusual sweating.	Infrequent	3

1- Life-threatening. Seek emergency treatment immediately.
2- Discontinue. Seek emergency treatment.
3- Discontinue. Call doctor right away.
4- Continue. Call doctor when convenient.
5- Continue. Tell doctor at next visit.

METHAMPHETAMINE

WARNINGS & PRECAUTIONS

Don't take if:
- You are allergic to any methamphetamine.
- You will have surgery within 2 months, including dental surgery, requiring general or spinal anesthesia.

Before you start, consult your doctor:
- If you plan to become pregnant within medication period.
- If you have glaucoma.
- If you have heart or blood-vessel disease, or high blood pressure.
- If you have overactive thyroid, anxiety or tension.
- If you have a severe mental illness (especially children).

Over age 60:
Adverse reactions and side effects may be more frequent and severe than in younger persons.

Pregnancy:
Risk to unborn child outweighs drug benefits. Don't use.

Breast-feeding:
Drug passes into milk. Avoid drug or discontinue nursing.

Infants & children:
Not recommended for children under 12.

Prolonged use:
Habit forming.

Skin & sunlight:
No problems expected.

Driving, piloting or hazardous work:
Don't drive or pilot aircraft until you learn how medicine affects you. Don't work around dangerous machinery. Don't climb ladders or work in high places. Danger increases if you drink alcohol or take medicine affecting alertness and reflexes.

Airplane passengers:
No problems expected.

Discontinuing:
May be unnecessary to finish medicine. Follow doctor's instructions.

Others:
- This is a dangerous drug and must be closely supervised. Don't use for appetite control or depression. Potential for damage and abuse.
- During withdrawal phase, may cause prolonged sleep of several days.

INTERACTION WITH OTHER DRUGS

GENERIC NAME OR DRUG CLASS	COMBINED EFFECT
Anesthesias (general)	Irregular heartbeat.
Antidepressants (tricyclic)	Decreased methamphetamine effect.
Antihypertensives	Decreased antihypertensive effect.
Carbonic anhydrase inhibitors	Increased methamphetamine effect.
Guanethidine	Decreased guanethidine effect.
Haloperidol	Decreased methamphetamine effect.
MAO inhibitors	May severely increase blood pressure.
Phenothiazines	Decreased methamphetamine effect.
Sodium bicarbonate	Increased methamphetamine effect.

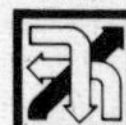

INTERACTION WITH OTHER SUBSTANCES

INTERACTS WITH	COMBINED EFFECT
Alcohol:	Decreased methamphetamine effect. Avoid.
Beverages:	
Caffeine drinks	Overstimulation. Avoid.
Cocaine:	Dangerous stimulation of nervous system. Avoid.
Foods:	None expected.
Marijuana:	Frequent use—Severely impaired mental function.
Tobacco:	None expected.

METHAQUALONE

BRAND NAMES

Mandrax
Mequelon
Mequin
Methadorm
Parest
Quaalude
Rouqualone-300
Sedalone
Sopor
Triador
Tualone
Tualone-300
Vitalone

GENERAL INFORMATION

Habit forming? Yes
Prescription needed? Yes
Available as generic? No
Drug class: Hypnotic

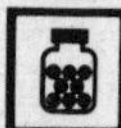

USES

Decreases anxiety, tension or insomnia.

DOSAGE & USAGE INFORMATION

How to take:
Tablet or capsule—Swallow with liquid. If you can't swallow whole, crumble tablet or open capsule and take with liquid or food.

When to take:
At the same time each day.

If you forget a dose:
Don't take missed dose. Wait for next scheduled dose. Don't double this dose.

What drug does:
Undetermined.

Time lapse before drug works:
20 to 30 minutes.

Don't take with:
- Alcohol or mind-altering drugs. Combinations can be fatal.
- Non-prescription drugs without consulting doctor.
- See Interaction column and consult doctor.

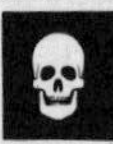

OVERDOSE

Symptoms:
Drowsiness, confusion, delirium, incoordination, vomiting, convulsions, abnormal bleeding, stupor, coma.

What to do:
- Dial 0 (operator) or 911 (emergency) for an ambulance or medical help. Then give first aid immediately.
- If patient is unconscious and not breathing, give mouth-to-mouth breathing. If there is no heartbeat, use cardiac massage and mouth-to-mouth breathing (CPR). Don't try to make patient vomit. If you can't get help quickly, take patient to nearest emergency facility.
- Additional emergency information on page 886.

POSSIBLE ADVERSE REACTIONS OR SIDE EFFECTS

SYMPTOMS	FREQUENCY	WHAT TO DO
Brain & nervous system:		
• Agitation	Infrequent	3
• Drowsiness	Common	4
• "Hangover-effect."	Common	6
Skin:		
Rash or hives.	Infrequent	3
Eyes:	None expected.	
Ears, nose, throat:	None expected.	
Digestive:		
Diarrhea, nausea, vomiting, stomach pain.	Common	3
Heart & lungs:		
Unusually slow heartbeat, breathing difficulty.	Infrequent	2
Blood vessels:	None expected.	
Muscles, bones, joints:		
Numbness, tingling, pain or weakness in hands or feet.	Infrequent	3
Genital, urinary:	None expected.	
Kidneys:	None expected.	
Liver:	None expected.	
Allergic:	None expected.	
Blood:	None expected.	
Others:		
• Sweating	Infrequent	3
• Tiredness or weakness.	Common	5

1 - Life-threatening. Seek emergency treatment immediately.
2 - Discontinue. Seek emergency treatment.
3 - Discontinue. Call doctor right away.
4 - Continue. Call doctor when convenient.
5 - Continue. Tell doctor at next visit.
6 - No action necessary.

WARNINGS & PRECAUTIONS

Don't take if:
- You are allergic to any hypnotic drug.
- You plan to become pregnant within medication period.
- Patient is younger than 12.

Before you start, consult your doctor:
- If you have had liver disease or impaired liver function.
- If you will have surgery within 2 months, including dental surgery, requiring general or spinal anesthesia.

Over age 60:
Adverse reactions and side effects may be more frequent and severe than in younger persons.

Pregnancy:
Risk to unborn child outweighs drug benefits. Don't use.

Breast-feeding:
Drug may filter into milk and harm child. Don't use.

Infants & children:
Not recommended.

Prolonged use:
Psychological and physical dependence.

Skin & sunlight:
No problems expected.

Driving, piloting or hazardous work:
Don't drive or pilot aircraft until you learn how medicine affects you. Don't work around dangerous machinery. Don't climb ladders or work in high places. Danger increases if you drink alcohol or take medicine affecting alertness and reflexes, such as antihistamines, tranquilizers, sedatives, pain medicine, narcotics and mind-altering drugs.

Airplane passengers:
Not recommended.

Discontinuing:
Don't discontinue without consulting doctor. Dose may require gradual reduction if you have taken drug for a long time. Doses of other drugs may also require adjustment.

Others:
No problems expected.

INTERACTION WITH OTHER DRUGS

GENERIC NAME OR DRUG CLASS	COMBINED EFFECT
Anticoagulants	Decreased anticoagulant effect.
Antihistamines	Increased sedation.
Narcotics	Increased narcotic effect.
Pain relievers	Increased effect of pain reliever.
Sedatives	Increased sedative effect.
Sleep inducers	Increased effect of sleep inducer.
Tranquilizers	Increased tranquilizer effect.

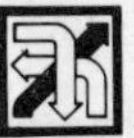

INTERACTION WITH OTHER SUBSTANCES

INTERACTS WITH	COMBINED EFFECT
Alcohol:	Dangerous depression of brain function. Avoid.
Beverages:	None expected.
Cocaine:	Decreased effect of both drugs. Avoid.
Foods:	None expected.
Marijuana:	Impairs physical performance. Avoid.
Tobacco:	None expected.

METHARBITAL

BRAND NAMES

Gemonil

GENERAL INFORMATION

Habit forming? Yes
Prescription needed? Yes
Available as generic? Yes
Drug class: Sedative, hypnotic (barbiturate)

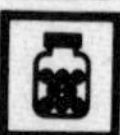

USES

Prevents convulsions.

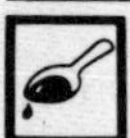

DOSAGE & USAGE INFORMATION

How to take:
Tablet—Swallow with liquid or food to lessen stomach irritation. If you can't swallow whole, crumble tablet and take with liquid or food.

When to take:
At the same times each day.

If you forget a dose:
Take as soon as you remember up to 2 hours late. If more than 2 hours, wait for next scheduled dose (don't double this dose).

What drug does:
May partially block nerve impulses at nerve-cell connections.

Time lapse before drug works:
60 minutes.

Don't take with:
- Non-prescription drugs without consulting doctor.
- See Interaction column and consult doctor.

OVERDOSE

Symptoms:
Deep sleep, weak pulse, coma.

What to do:
- Dial 0 (operator) or 911 (emergency) for an ambulance or medical help. Then give first aid immediately.
- If patient is unconscious and not breathing, give mouth-to-mouth breathing. If there is no heartbeat use cardiac massage and mouth-to-mouth breathing (CPR). Don't try to make patient vomit. If you can't help quickly, take patient to nearest emergency facility.
- Additional emergency information on page 886.

POSSIBLE ADVERSE REACTIONS OR SIDE EFFECTS

SYMPTOMS	FREQUENCY	WHAT TO DO
Brain & nervous system:		
• Dizziness, drowsiness, "hangover effect."	Common	4
• Depression, confusion, slurred speech.	Infrequent	4
• Agitation	Rare	3
Skin:		
• Rash or hives.	Infrequent	3
• Face, lip swelling.	Infrequent	3
Eyes:		
Eyelid swelling.	Infrequent	3
Ears, nose, throat:		
Sore throat, fever.	Infrequent	3
Digestive:		
Diarrhea, nausea, vomiting.	Infrequent	4
Heart & lungs:		
• Slow heartbeat.	Rare	3
• Breathing difficulty.	Rare	3
Blood vessels:		
Unexplained bleeding or bruising.	Rare	4
Muscles, bones, joints:		
Joint or muscle pain.	Infrequent	4
Genital, urinary:	None expected.	
Kidneys:	None expected.	
Liver:		
Jaundice (yellow skin and eyes).	Rare	3
Allergic:	None expected.	
Blood:	None expected.	
Others:	None expected.	

1 - Life-threatening. Seek emergency treatment immediately.
2 - Discontinue. Seek emergency treatment.
3 - Discontinue. Call doctor right away.
4 - Continue. Call doctor when convenient.

WARNINGS & PRECAUTIONS

Don't take if:
- You are allergic to any barbiturate.
- You have porphyria.

Before you start, consult your doctor:
- If you have epilepsy.
- If you have kidney or liver damage.
- If you have asthma.
- If you have anemia.
- If you have chronic pain.
- If you will have surgery within 2 months, including dental surgery, requiring general or spinal anesthesia.

Over age 60:
Adverse reactions and side effects may be more frequent and severe than in younger persons. Use small doses.

Pregnancy:
Risk to unborn child outweighs drug benefits. Don't use.

Breast-feeding:
Drug passes into milk. Avoid drug or discontinue nursing until you finish medicine. Consult doctor for advice on maintaining milk supply.

Infants & children:
Use only under doctor's supervision.

Prolonged use:
- May cause addiction, anemia, chronic intoxication.
- May lower body temperature, making exposure to cold temperatures hazardous.

Skin & sunlight:
May cause rash or intensify sunburn in areas exposed to sun or sunlamp.

Driving, piloting or hazardous work:
Don't drive or pilot aircraft until you learn how medicine affects you. Don't work around dangerous machinery. Don't climb ladders or work in high places. Danger increases if you drink alcohol or take medicine affecting alertness and reflexes.

Airplane passengers:
No problems expected.

Discontinuing:
May be unnecessary to finish medicine. Follow doctor's instructions. If you develop withdrawal symptoms of hallucinations, agitation or sleeplessness after discontinuing, call doctor right away.

Others:
Great potential for abuse.

INTERACTION WITH OTHER DRUGS

GENERIC NAME OR DRUG CLASS	COMBINED EFFECT
Anticoagulants (oral)	Decreased anticoagulant effect.
Anticonvulsants	Changed seizure patterns.
Antidepressants (tricyclic)	Decreased antidepressant effect.
Antidiabetics (oral)	Increased metharbital effect.
Antihistamines	Dangerous sedation. Avoid.
Antiinflammatory drugs (non-steroidal)	Decreased antiinflammatory effect.
Aspirin	Decreased aspirin effect.
Beta-adrenergic blockers	Decreased effect of beta-adrenergic blocker.
Contraceptives (oral)	Decreased contraceptive effect.
Cortisone drugs	Decreased cortisone effect.
Digitoxin	Decreased digitoxin effect.
Doxycycline	Decreased doxycycline effect.
Griseofulvin	Decreased griseofulvin effect.

Additional interactions on page 839.

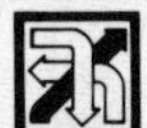

INTERACTION WITH OTHER SUBSTANCES

INTERACTS WITH	COMBINED EFFECT
Alcohol:	Possible fatal oversedation. Avoid.
Beverages:	None expected.
Cocaine:	Decreased metharbital effect.
Foods:	None expected.
Marijuana:	Excessive sedation. Avoid.
Tobacco:	None expected.

METHENAMINE

BRAND NAMES

Azo-Mandelamine
Hiprex
Mandelamine
Mandelets
Methandine
Prov-U-Sep
Renalgin
Sterine
Trac 2X
Urex
Urised
Uroblue
Uroquid-Acid
Uro-phosphate

GENERAL INFORMATION

Habit forming? No
Prescription needed? Yes
Available as generic? Yes
Drug class: Antiinfective (urinary)

USES

Suppresses chronic urinary-tract infections.

DOSAGE & USAGE INFORMATION

How to take:

- Tablet—Swallow with liquid or food to lessen stomach irritation. If you can't swallow whole, crumble tablet and take with liquid or food.
- Liquid form—Use a measuring spoon to ensure correct dose.
- Granules—Dissolve dose in 4 oz. of water. Drink all the liquid.

When to take:
At the same times each day.

If you forget a dose:
Take as soon as you remember up to 8 hours late. If more than 8 hours, wait for next scheduled dose (don't double this dose).

What drug does:
A chemical reaction in the urine changes methenamine into formaldehyde, which destroys certain bacteria.

Time lapse before drug works:
Continual use for 3 to 6 months.

Don't take with:
See Interaction column and consult doctor.

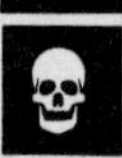

OVERDOSE

Symptoms:
Bloody urine, weakness, deep breathing, stupor, coma.

What to do:

- Dial 0 (operator) or 911 (emergency) for an ambulance or medical help. Then give first aid immediately.
- Additional emergency information on page 886.

POSSIBLE ADVERSE REACTIONS OR SIDE EFFECTS

SYMPTOMS	FREQUENCY	WHAT TO DO
Brain & nervous system:	None expected.	
Skin:		
Rash	Common	3
Eyes:	None expected.	
Ears, nose, throat:	None expected.	
Digestive:		
Nausea	Common	4
Heart & lungs:	None expected.	
Blood vessels:	None expected.	
Muscles, bones, joints:	None expected.	
Genital, urinary:		
• Urination difficulty.	Common	4
• Bloody urine.	Rare	3
• Burning on urination.	Rare	4
Kidneys:		
Lower back pain.	Rare	4
Liver:	None expected.	
Allergic:	None expected.	
Blood:	None expected.	
Others:	None expected.	

1- Life-threatening. Seek emergency treatment immediately.
2- Discontinue. Seek emergency treatment.
3- Discontinue. Call doctor right away.
4- Continue. Call doctor when convenient.
5- Continue. Tell doctor at next visit.
6- No action necessary.

WARNINGS & PRECAUTIONS

Don't take if:
- You are allergic to methenamine.
- You have a severe impairment of kidney or liver function.
- The urine cannot or should not be acidified (check with your doctor).

Before you start, consult your doctor:
- If you have had kidney or liver disease.
- If you plan to become pregnant within medication period.
- If you have had gout.

Over age 60:
Don't exceed recommended dose.

Pregnancy:
Studies inconclusive on harm to unborn child. Avoid if possible, especially first 3 months.

Breast-feeding:
Drug passes into milk in small amounts. Consult doctor.

Infants & children:
Use only under medical supervision.

Prolonged use:
No problems expected.

Skin & sunlight:
No problems expected.

Driving, piloting or hazardous work:
No problems expected.

Airplane passengers:
No problems expected.

Discontinuing:
Don't discontinue without doctor's advice until you complete prescribed dose, even though symptoms diminish or disappear.

Others:
Requires an acid urine to be effective. Eat more protein foods, cranberries, cranberry juice with vitamin C, plums, prunes.

INTERACTION WITH OTHER DRUGS

GENERIC NAME OR DRUG CLASS	COMBINED EFFECT
Antacids	Decreased methenamine effect.
Carbonic anhydrase inhibitors	Decreased methenamine effect.
Diuretics (thiazide)	Decreased urine acidity.
Sodium bicarbonate	Decreased methenamine effect.
Sulfa drugs	Possible kidney damage.
Vitamin C (1 to 4 grams per day)	Increased effect of methenamine, contributing to urine's acidity.

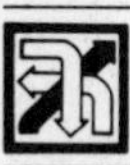

INTERACTION WITH OTHER SUBSTANCES

INTERACTS WITH	COMBINED EFFECT
Alcohol:	Possible brain depression. Avoid or use with caution.
Beverages:	
Milk	Decreased methenamine effect.
Cocaine:	None expected.
Foods:	None expected.
Marijuana:	Drowsiness, muscle weakness or blood-pressure drop.
Tobacco:	None expected.

METHICILLIN

BRAND NAMES

Azapen
Celbenin
Staphcillin

GENERAL INFORMATION

Habit forming? No
Prescription needed? Yes
Available as generic? Yes
Drug class: Antibiotic (penicillin)

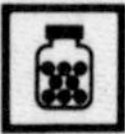

USES

Treatment of bacterial infections that are susceptible to methicillin.

DOSAGE & USAGE INFORMATION

How to take:
By injection only.

When to take:
Follow doctor's instructions.

If you forget a dose:
Consult doctor.

What drug does:
Destroys susceptible bacteria. Does not kill viruses.

Time lapse before drug works:
May be several days before medicine affects infection.

Don't take with:
See Interaction column and consult doctor.

OVERDOSE

Symptoms:
Severe diarrhea, nausea or vomiting.

What to do:
Overdose unlikely to threaten life. If person takes much larger amount than prescribed, call doctor, poison-control center or hospital emergency room for instructions.

POSSIBLE ADVERSE REACTIONS OR SIDE EFFECTS

SYMPTOMS	FREQUENCY	WHAT TO DO
Brain & nervous system:	None expected.	
Skin: Hives, rash, intense itch soon after a dose.	Rare	1
Eyes:	None expected.	
Ears, nose, throat: Dark or discolored tongue.	Common	5
Digestive: Mild nausea, vomiting, diarrhea.	Infrequent	4
Heart & lungs:	None expected.	
Blood vessels: Unexplained bleeding.	Rare	3
Muscles, bones, joints:	None expected.	
Genital, urinary:	None expected.	
Kidneys:	None expected.	
Liver:	None expected.	
Allergic: Life-threatening anaphylaxis may occur!	Rare	1 See page 888.
Blood:	None expected.	
Others:	None expected.	

1- Life-threatening. Seek emergency treatment immediately.
2- Discontinue. Seek emergency treatment.
3- Discontinue. Call doctor right away.
4- Continue. Call doctor when convenient.
5- Continue. Tell doctor at next visit.
6- No action necessary.

WARNINGS & PRECAUTIONS

Don't take if:
You are allergic to methicillin, cephalosporin antibiotics, other penicillins or penicillamine. Life-threatening reaction may occur.

Before you start, consult your doctor:
If you are allergic to any substance or drug.

Over age 60:
You may have skin reactions, particularly around genitals and anus.

Pregnancy:
Studies inconclusive on harm to unborn child. Animal studies show fetal abnormalities. Decide with your doctor whether drug benefits justify risk to unborn child.

Breast-feeding:
Drug passes into milk. Child may become sensitive to penicillins and have allergic reactions to penicillin drugs. Avoid methicillin or discontinue nursing until you finish medicine. Consult doctor for advice on maintaining milk supply.

Infants & children:
No problems expected.

Prolonged use:
- You may become more susceptible to infections caused by germs not responsive to methicillin.
- May cause kidney damage. Laboratory studies to detect damage recommended if you take for a long time.

Skin & sunlight:
No problems expected.

Driving, piloting or hazardous work:
Usually not dangerous. Most hazardous reactions likely to occur a few minutes after taking methicillin.

Airplane passengers:
No problems expected.

Discontinuing:
Don't discontinue without doctor's advice until you complete prescribed dose, even though symptoms diminish or disappear.

Others:
No problems expected.

INTERACTION WITH OTHER DRUGS

GENERIC NAME OR DRUG CLASS	COMBINED EFFECT
Chloramphenicol	Decreased effect of both drugs.
Erythromycins	Decreased effect of both drugs.
Paromomycin	Decreased effect of both drugs.
Tetracyclines	Decreased effect of both drugs.
Troleandomycin	Decreased effect of both drugs.

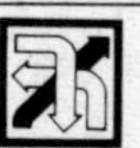

INTERACTION WITH OTHER SUBSTANCES

INTERACTS WITH	COMBINED EFFECT
Alcohol:	Occasional stomach irritation.
Beverages:	None expected.
Cocaine:	No proven problems.
Foods:	None expected.
Marijuana:	No proven problems.
Tobacco:	None expected.

METHOCARBAMOL

BRAND NAMES

Delaxin
Forbaxin
Marbaxin
Marbaxin-750
Metho-500
Robamol
Robaxin
Robaxisal
Spinaxin
Tumol

GENERAL INFORMATION

Habit forming? No
Prescription needed? Yes
Available as generic? Yes
Drug class: Muscle relaxant (skeletal)

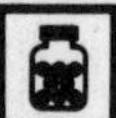

USES

Pain reliever for skeletal-muscle spasms.

DOSAGE & USAGE INFORMATION

How to take:
Tablet—Swallow with liquid. If you can't swallow whole, crumble tablet and take with liquid or food.

When to take:
As directed on label.

If you forget a dose:
Take as soon as you remember up to 2 hours late. If more than 2 hours, wait for next scheduled dose (don't double this dose).

What drug does:
Blocks reflex nerve impulses in brain and spinal cord.

Time lapse before drug works:
30 to 45 minutes.

Don't take with:
- Non-prescription drugs containing alcohol without consulting doctor.
- See Interaction column and consult doctor.

OVERDOSE

Symptoms:
Unsteadiness, lack of coordination, extreme weakness, paralysis, weak and rapid pulse, shallow breathing, cold and sweaty skin.

What to do:
- Dial 0 (operator) or 911 (emergency) for an ambulance or medical help. Then give first aid immediately.
- If patient is unconscious and not breathing, give mouth-to-mouth breathing. If there is no heartbeat, use cardiac massage and mouth-to-mouth breathing (CPR). Don't try to make patient vomit. If you can't get help quickly, take patient to nearest emergency facility.
- Additional emergency information on page 886.

POSSIBLE ADVERSE REACTIONS OR SIDE EFFECTS

SYMPTOMS	FREQUENCY	WHAT TO DO
Brain & nervous system:		
• Dizziness, drowsiness, lightheadedness.	Common	4
• Headache	Infrequent	4
Skin:		
Rash or itch.	Infrequent	3
Eyes:		
• Bloodshot eyes.	Infrequent	4
• Blurred or double vision.	Common	3
Ears, nose, throat:		
• Stuffy nose.	Infrequent	5
• Metallic taste.	Infrequent	4
Digestive:		
Nausea	Infrequent	5
Heart & lungs:	None expected.	
Blood vessels:	None expected.	
Muscles, bones, joints:	None expected.	
Genital, urinary:	None expected.	
Kidneys:	None expected.	
Liver:	None expected.	
Allergic:	None expected.	
Blood:	None expected.	
Others:		
Fever	Infrequent	4

1- Life-threatening. Seek emergency treatment immediately.
2- Discontinue. Seek emergency treatment.
3- Discontinue. Call doctor right away.
4- Continue. Call doctor when convenient.
5- Continue. Tell doctor at next visit.
6- No action necessary.

WARNINGS & PRECAUTIONS

Don't take if:
You are allergic to any muscle relaxant.

Before you start, consult your doctor:
- If you have epilepsy.
- If you have myasthenia gravis.
- If you have impaired kidney function.

Over age 60:
Adverse reactions and side effects may be more frequent and severe than in younger persons.

Pregnancy:
No proven harm to unborn child. Avoid if possible.

Breast-feeding:
Drug filters into milk. May harm child. Avoid.

Infants & children:
Not recommended.

Prolonged use:
No problems expected.

Skin & sunlight:
No problems expected.

Driving, piloting or hazardous work:
Don't drive or pilot aircraft until you learn how medicine affects you. Don't work around dangerous machinery. Don't climb ladders or work in high places. Danger increases if you drink alcohol or take medicine affecting alertness and reflexes, such as antihistamines, tranquilizers, sedatives, pain medicine, narcotics and mind-altering drugs.

Airplane passengers:
No problems expected.

Discontinuing:
May be unnecessary to finish medicine. Follow doctor's instructions.

Others:
No problems expected.

INTERACTION WITH OTHER DRUGS

GENERIC NAME OR DRUG CLASS	COMBINED EFFECT
Antidepressants (tricyclic)	Increased effect of both drugs.
Antimyasthenics	Decreased antimyasthenic effect.
Narcotics	Increased sedative effect.
Sedatives	Increased sedative effect.
Sleep inducers	Increased effect of sleep inducer.
Tranquilizers	Increased tranquilizer effect.

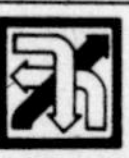

INTERACTION WITH OTHER SUBSTANCES

INTERACTS WITH	COMBINED EFFECT
Alcohol:	Depressed brain function. Avoid.
Beverages:	None expected.
Cocaine:	May increase muscle spasms.
Foods:	None expected.
Marijuana:	Drowsiness, muscle weakness, lack of coordination, fainting.
Tobacco:	None expected.

METHOTREXATE

BRAND NAMES

Mexate

GENERAL INFORMATION

Habit forming? No
Prescription needed? Yes
Available as generic? Yes
Drug class: Antimetabolite, antipsoriatic

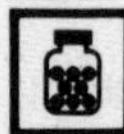

USES

- Treatment for some kinds of cancer.
- Treatment for psoriasis in patients with severe problems.

DOSAGE & USAGE INFORMATION

How to take:
Tablet—Swallow with liquid.

When to take:
At the same time each day.

If you forget a dose:
Skip the missed dose. Don't double the next dose.

What drug does:
Inhibits abnormal-cell reproduction.

Time lapse before drug works:
May require 6 weeks for maximum effect.

Don't take with:
See Interaction column and consult doctor.

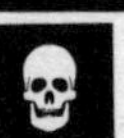

OVERDOSE

Symptoms:
Headache, stupor, seizures.

What to do:
- Dial 0 (operator) or 911 (emergency) for an ambulance or medical help. Then give first aid immediately.
- If patient is unconscious and not breathing, give mouth-to-mouth breathing. If there is no heartbeat, use cardiac massage and mouth-to-mouth breathing (CPR). Don't try to make patient vomit. If you can't get help quickly, take patient to nearest emergency facility.
- Additional emergency information on page 886.

POSSIBLE ADVERSE REACTIONS OR SIDE EFFECTS

SYMPTOMS	FREQUENCY	WHAT TO DO
Brain & nervous system:		
• Seizures	Infrequent	2
• Dizziness, drowsiness, headache, confusion.	Infrequent	3
Skin:		
Acne, boils, hair loss, itch.	Infrequent	5
Eyes:		
Blurred vision.	Infrequent	3
Ears, nose, throat:		
Mouth sores, sore throat, fever, chills.	Common	3
Digestive:		
• Black stools or bloody vomit.	Common	2
• Stomach pain, nausea, vomiting.	Common	4
Heart & lungs:		
• Shortness of breath.	Infrequent	3
• Cough	Infrequent	4
Blood vessels:		
Unusual bleeding or bruising.	Common	3
Muscles, bones, joints:		
Joint pain.	Infrequent	3
Genital, urinary:		
Bloody urine.	Infrequent	3
Kidneys, allergic, blood others:	None expected.	
Liver:		
Jaundice (yellow skin and eyes).	Infrequent	3

1- Life-threatening. Seek emergency treatment immediately.
2- Discontinue. Seek emergency treatment.
3- Discontinue. Call doctor right away.
4- Continue. Call doctor when convenient.
5- Continue. Tell doctor at next visit.

WARNINGS & PRECAUTIONS

Don't take if:
You are allergic to any antimetabolite.

Before you start, consult your doctor:
- If you are alcoholic.
- If you have blood, liver or kidney disease.
- If you have colitis or peptic ulcer.
- If you have gout.
- If you have an infection.
- If you plan to become pregnant within 3 months.

Over age 60:
Adverse reactions and side effects may be more frequent and severe than in younger persons.

Pregnancy:
- Psoriasis—Risk to unborn child outweighs drug benefits. Don't use.
- Cancer—Consult doctor.

Breast-feeding:
Drug passes into milk. Avoid drug or discontinue nursing.

Infants & children:
Use only under special medical supervision.

Prolonged use:
Adverse reactions more likely the longer drug is required.

Skin & sunlight:
No problems expected.

Driving, piloting or hazardous work:
Avoid if you feel dizzy, drowsy or confused. Otherwise, no problems expected.

Airplane passengers:
No problems expected.

Discontinuing:
Don't discontinue without doctor's advice until you complete prescribed dose, even though symptoms diminish or disappear. Some side effects may follow discontinuing. Report to doctor blurred vision, convulsions, confusion, persistent headache.

Others:
- Drink more water than usual to cause frequent urination.
- Don't give this medicine to anyone else for any purpose. It is a strong drug that requires close medical supervision.
- Report for frequent medical follow-up and laboratory studies.

INTERACTION WITH OTHER DRUGS

GENERIC NAME OR DRUG CLASS	COMBINED EFFECT
Anticoagulants (oral)	Increased anticoagulant effect.
Anticonvulsants (hydantoin)	Possible methotrexate toxicity.
Antigout drugs	Decreased antigout effect.
Asparaginase	Decreased methotrexate effect.
Flurouracil	Decreased methotrexate effect.
Oxyphenbutazone	Possible methotrexate toxicity.
Phenylbutazone	Possible methotrexate toxicity.
Probenecid	Possible methotrexate toxicity.
Pyrimethamine	Increased toxic effect of methotrexate.
Salicylates (including aspirin)	Possible methotrexate toxicity.
Sulfa drugs	Possible methotrexate toxicity.
Tetracyclines	Possible methotrexate toxicity.

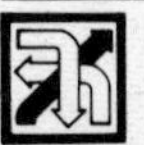

INTERACTION WITH OTHER SUBSTANCES

INTERACTS WITH	COMBINED EFFECT
Alcohol:	Likely liver damage. Avoid.
Beverages:	Extra fluid intake decreases chance of methotrexate toxicity.
Cocaine:	Increased chance of methotrexate adverse reactions. Avoid.
Foods:	None expected.
Marijuana:	None expected.
Tobacco:	None expected.

METHOXSALEN

BRAND NAMES

Oxsoralen

USES

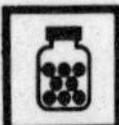

- Repigmenting skin affected with vitiligo (absence of skin pigment).
- Treatment for psoriasis, when other treatments haven't helped.
- Treatment for mycosis fungoides.

DOSAGE & USAGE INFORMATION

How to take:
Tablet or capsule—Swallow with liquid or food to lessen stomach irritation.

When to take:
2 to 4 hours before exposure to sunlight or sunlamp.

If you forget a dose:
Take as soon as you remember. Delay sun exposure for at least 2 hours after taking.

What drug does:
Helps pigment cells when used in conjunction with ultraviolet light.

Time lapse before drug works:
- For vitiligo, up to 6 months.
- For psoriasis, 10 weeks or longer.
- For tanning, 3 to 4 days.

Don't take with:
Any other medicine which causes skin sensitivity to sun. Ask pharmacist.

OVERDOSE

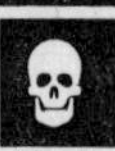

Symptoms:
Blistering skin, swelling feet and legs.

What to do:
Overdose unlikely to threaten life. If person takes much larger amount than prescribed, call doctor, poison-control center or hospital emergency room for instructions.

GENERAL INFORMATION

Habit forming? No
Prescription needed? Yes
Available as generic? No
Drug class: Repigmenting agent (psoralen)

POSSIBLE ADVERSE REACTIONS OR SIDE EFFECTS

SYMPTOMS	FREQUENCY	WHAT TO DO
Brain & nervous system:	None expected.	
Skin: Increased sensitivity to sun.	Always	Always protect from overexposure.
Eyes: Increased sensitivity to sunlight.	Always	Always protect with wrap-around sunglasses.
Ears, nose, throat:	None expected.	
Digestive:	None expected.	
Heart & lungs:	None expected.	
Blood vessels:	None expected.	
Muscles, bones, joints:	None expected.	
Genital, urinary:	None expected.	
Kidneys, allergic, blood:	None expected.	
Liver: Hepatitis with jaundice (yellow skin and eyes).	Rare	3

1-Life-threatening. Seek emergency treatment immediately.
2-Discontinue. Seek emergency treatment.
3-Discontinue. Call doctor right away.
4-Continue. Call doctor when convenient.
5-Continue. Tell doctor at next visit.
6-No action necessary.

WARNINGS & PRECAUTIONS

Don't take if:
- You are allergic to methoxsalen or any other psoralen.
- You are unwilling or unable to remain under close medical supervision.

Before you start, consult your doctor:
- If you have heart or liver disease.
- If you have allergy to sunlight.
- If you have cataracts.
- If you have albinism.
- If you have lupus erythematosis, porphyria, chronic infection, skin cancer or peptic ulcer.
- If you will have surgery within 2 months, including dental surgery, requiring general or spinal anesthesia.

Over age 60:
Adverse reactions and side effects may be more frequent and severe than in younger persons.

Pregnancy:
Risk to unborn child outweighs drug benefits. Don't use.

Breast-feeding:
Drug passes into milk. Avoid drug or discontinue nursing until you finish medicine. Consult doctor for advice on maintaining milk supply.

Infants & children:
Not recommended.

Prolonged use:
Increased chance of toxic effects.

Skin & sunlight:
Too much can burn skin. Cover skin for 24 hours before and 8 hours following treatments.

Driving, piloting or hazardous work:
No problems expected. Protect eyes and skin from bright light.

Airplane passengers:
Protect eyes from glaring bright light.

Discontinuing:
Skin may remain sensitive for some time after treatment stops. Use extra protection from sun.

Others:
Use sunblock on lips.

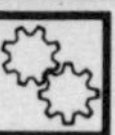

INTERACTION WITH OTHER DRUGS

GENERIC NAME OR DRUG CLASS	COMBINED EFFECT
Any medicine causing sensitization to sunlight, such as Acetohexamide, Amitriptyline, Anthralin, Barbiturates, Bendroflumethiazide, Carbamazepine, Chlordiazepoxide, Chloroquine, Chlorothiazide, Chloropromazine, Chloropropamide, Chlortetracycline, Chlorthalidone, Clindamycin, Coal tar derivatives, Cyproheptadine, Demeclocycline, Desipramine, Diethylstilbrestrol, Diphendydramine, Doxepin, Doxycycline, Estrogen, Fluphenazine, Gold preparations, Glyburide, Griseofulvin, Hydrochlorothiazide, Hydroflumethiazide, Imipramine, Lincomycin, Mesoridazine, Methacycline, Nalidixic acid, Nortriptyline, Oral contraceptive, Oxyphenbutazone, Oxytetracycline, Perphenazine, Phenobarbital, Phenylbutazone, Phenytoin, Prochlorperazine, Promazine, Promethazine, Protriptyline, Pyrazinamide, Sulfonamides, Tetracycline, Thioridazine, Thiazide diuretics, Tolazamide, Tolbutamide, Tranylcypromine, Triamterene, Trifluoperazine, Trimeprazine, Trimipramine, Triprolidine.	Greatly increased likelihood of extreme sensitivity to sunlight.

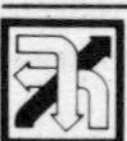

INTERACTION WITH OTHER SUBSTANCES

INTERACTS WITH	COMBINED EFFECT
Alcohol:	May increase chance of liver toxicity.
Beverages: Lime drinks.	Avoid—toxic.
Cocaine:	Increased change of toxicity. Avoid.
Foods: Those containing furocoumarin (limes, parsley, figs, parsnips, carrots, celery, mustard).	May cause toxic effects to psoralens.
Marijuana:	Increased chance of toxicity. Avoid.
Tobacco:	May cause uneven absorption of medicine. Avoid.

METHSUXIMIDE

BRAND NAMES

Celontin

GENERAL INFORMATION

Habit forming? No
Prescription needed? Yes
Available as generic? No
Drug class: Anticonvulsant (succinimide)

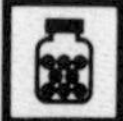

USES

Controls seizures in treatment of epilepsy.

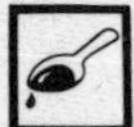

DOSAGE & USAGE INFORMATION

How to take:
Capsule—Swallow with liquid or food to lessen stomach irritation.

When to take:
Every day in regularly spaced doses, according to prescription.

If you forget a dose:
Take as soon as you remember up to 2 hours late. If more than 2 hours, wait for next scheduled dose (don't double this dose).

What drug does:
Depresses nerve transmissions in part of brain that controls muscles.

Time lapse before drug works:
3 hours.

Don't take with:
See Interaction column and consult doctor.

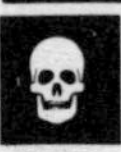

OVERDOSE

Symptoms:
Coma

What to do:
- Dial 0 (operator) or 911 (emergency) for an ambulance or medical help. Then give first aid immediately.
- If patient is unconscious and not breathing, give mouth-to-mouth breathing. If there is no heartbeat, use cardiac massage and mouth-to-mouth breathing (CPR). Don't try to make patient vomit. If you can't get help quickly, take patient to nearest emergency facility.
- Additional emergency information on page 886.

POSSIBLE ADVERSE REACTIONS OR SIDE EFFECTS

SYMPTOMS	FREQUENCY	WHAT TO DO
Brain & nervous system: Dizziness, drowsiness, headache, irritability, mood changes.	Infrequent	4
Skin: Rash	Rare	3
Eyes:	None expected.	
Ears, nose, throat: Sore throat, fever.	Rare	3
Digestive: Nausea, vomiting, stomach cramps, appetite loss.	Common	4
Heart & lungs:	None expected.	
Blood vessels:	None expected.	
Muscles, bones, joints:	None expected.	
Genital, urinary:	None expected.	
Kidneys:	None expected.	
Liver:	None expected.	
Allergic:	None expected.	
Blood: Unusual bleeding or bruising.	Rare	3
Others: Swollen lymph glands.	Rare	4

1- Life-threatening. Seek emergency treatment immediately.
2- Discontinue. Seek emergency treatment.
3- Discontinue. Call doctor right away.
4- Continue. Call doctor when convenient.
5- Continue. Tell doctor at next visit.
6- No action necessary.

WARNINGS & PRECAUTIONS

Don't take if:
You are allergic to any succinimide anticonvulsant.

Before you start, consult your doctor:
- If you plan to become pregnant within medication period.
- If you take other anticonvulsants.
- If you have blood disease.
- If you have kidney or liver disease.

Over age 60:
Adverse reactions and side effects may be more frequent and severe than in younger persons.

Pregnancy:
Risk to unborn child outweighs drug benefits. Don't use.

Breast-feeding:
Drug passes into milk. Avoid drug or discontinue nursing.

Infants & children:
Use only under medical supervision.

Prolonged use:
No problems expected.

Skin & sunlight:
No problems expected.

Driving, piloting or hazardous work:
Don't drive or pilot aircraft until you learn how medicine affects you. Don't work around dangerous machinery. Don't climb ladders or work in high places. Danger increases if you drink alcohol or take medicine affecting alertness and reflexes, such as antihistamines, tranquilizers, sedatives, pain medicine, narcotics and mind-altering drugs.

Airplane passengers:
No problems expected.

Discontinuing:
Don't discontinue without doctor's advice until you complete prescribed dose, even though symptoms diminish or disappear.

Others:
- Your response to medicine should be checked regularly by your doctor. Dose and schedule may have to be altered frequently to fit individual needs.
- Periodic blood-cell counts, kidney- and liver-function studies recommended.

INTERACTION WITH OTHER DRUGS

GENERIC NAME OR DRUG CLASS	COMBINED EFFECT
Anticonvulsants (other)	Increased effect of both drugs.
Antidepressants (tricyclic)	May provoke seizures.
Antipsychotics	May provoke seizures.

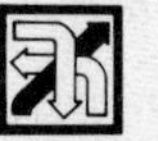

INTERACTION WITH OTHER SUBSTANCES

INTERACTS WITH	COMBINED EFFECT
Alcohol:	May provoke seizures.
Beverages:	None expected.
Cocaine:	May provoke seizures.
Foods:	None expected.
Marijuana:	May provoke seizures.
Tobacco:	None expected.

METHYCLOTHIAZIDE

BRAND NAMES

Aquatensen
Diutensen
Duretic
Enduron
Enduronyl

GENERAL INFORMATION

Habit forming? No
Prescription needed? Yes
Available as generic? Yes
Drug class: Antihypertensive, diuretic (thiazide)

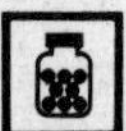

USES

- Controls, but doesn't cure, high blood pressure.
- Reduces fluid retention (edema) caused by conditions such as heart disorders and liver disease.

DOSAGE & USAGE INFORMATION

How to take:
Tablet or capsule—Swallow with liquid. If you can't swallow whole, crumble tablet or open capsule and take with liquid or food.
Don't exceed dose.

When to take:
At the same time each day.

If you forget a dose:
Take as soon as you remember up to 2 hours late. If more than 2 hours, wait for next scheduled dose (don't double this dose).

What drug does:
- Forces sodium and water excretion, reducing body fluid.
- Relaxes muscle cells of small arteries.
- Reduced body fluid and relaxed arteries lower blood pressure.

Time lapse before drug works:
4 to 6 hours. May require several weeks to lower blood pressure.

Don't take with:
- See Interaction column and consult doctor.
- Non-prescription drugs without consulting doctor.

OVERDOSE

Symptoms:
Cramps, weakness, drowsiness, weak pulse, coma.

What to do:
- Dial 0 (operator) or 911 (emergency) for an ambulance or medical help. Then give first aid immediately.
- Additional emergency information on page 886.

POSSIBLE ADVERSE REACTIONS OR SIDE EFFECTS

SYMPTOMS	FREQUENCY	WHAT TO DO
Brain & nervous system:		
• Dizziness	Infrequent	4
• Mood changes.	Infrequent	4
• Headaches	Infrequent	4
Skin:		
Rash or hives.	Rare	2
Eyes:		
Blurred vision.	Infrequent	3
Ears, nose, throat:		
• Sore throat, fever.	Rare	3
• Dry mouth, thirst.	Infrequent	5
Digestive:		
Severe abdominal pain, nausea, vomiting.	Infrequent	3
Heart & lungs:		
Irregular heartbeat, weak pulse.	Infrequent	3
Blood vessels:	None expected.	
Muscles, bones, joints:		
Weakness, tiredness.	Infrequent	4
Genital, urinary:	None expected.	
Kidneys:	None expected.	
Liver:		
Jaundice (yellow skin and eyes).	Rare	3
Allergic:	None expected.	
Blood:	None expected.	
Others:		
Weight changes.	Infrequent	4

1 - Life-threatening. Seek emergency treatment immediately.
2 - Discontinue. Seek emergency treatment.
3 - Discontinue. Call doctor right away.
4 - Continue. Call doctor when convenient.
5 - Continue. Tell doctor at next visit.
6 - No action necessary.

WARNINGS & PRECAUTIONS

Don't take if:
You are allergic to any thiazide diuretic drug.

Before you start, consult your doctor:
- If you are allergic to any sulfa drug.
- If you have gout.
- If you have liver, pancreas or kidney disorder.

Over age 60:
Adverse reactions and side effects may be more frequent and severe than in younger persons, especially dizziness and excessive potassium loss.

Pregnancy:
Risk to unborn child outweighs drug benefits. Don't use.

Breast-feeding:
Drug passes into milk. Avoid drug or discontinue nursing.

Infants & children:
No problems expected.

Prolonged use:
You may need medicine to treat high blood pressure for the rest of your life.

Skin & sunlight:
May cause rash or intensify sunburn in areas exposed to sun or sunlamp.

Driving, piloting or hazardous work:
Don't drive or pilot aircraft until you learn how medicine affects you. Don't work around dangerous machinery. Don't climb ladders or work in high places. Danger increases if you drink alcohol or take medicine affecting alertness and reflexes, such as antihistamines, tranquilizers, sedatives, pain medicine, narcotics and mind-altering drugs.

Airplane passengers:
No problems expected.

Discontinuing:
Don't discontinue without medical advice.

Others:
- Hot weather and fever may cause dehydration and drop in blood pressure. Dose may require temporary adjustment. Weigh daily and report any unexpected weight decreases to your doctor.
- May cause rise in uric acid, leading to gout.
- May cause blood-sugar rise in diabetics.

INTERACTION WITH OTHER DRUGS

GENERIC NAME OR DRUG CLASS	COMBINED EFFECT
Allopurinol	Decreased allopurinol effect.
Antidepressants (tricyclic)	Dangerous drop in blood pressure. Avoid combination unless under medical supervision.
Barbiturates	Increased methyclothiazide effect.
Cholestyramine	Decreased methyclothiazide effect.
Cortisone drugs	Excessive potassium loss that causes dangerous heart rhythms.
Digitalis preparations	Excessive potassium loss that causes dangerous heart rhythms.
Diuretics (thiazide)	Increased effect of other thiazide diuretics.
Lithium	Increased effect of lithium.
MAO inhibitors	Increased methyclothiazide effect.
Probenecid	Decreased probenecid effect.

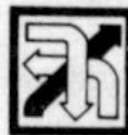

INTERACTION WITH OTHER SUBSTANCES

INTERACTS WITH	COMBINED EFFECT
Alcohol:	Dangerous blood-pressure drop.
Beverages:	None expected.
Cocaine:	None expected.
Foods:	
Licorice	Excessive potassium loss that causes dangerous heart rhythms.
Marijuana:	May increase blood pressure.
Tobacco:	None expected.

METHYLCELLULOSE

BRAND NAMES

Anorex-CCK
Cellothyl
Cologel
Gonio-Gel
Hydrolose
Lacril
Murocel

GENERAL INFORMATION

Habit forming? No
Prescription needed? No
Available as generic? Yes
Drug class: Laxative (bulk-forming)

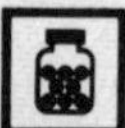

USES

Relieves constipation and prevents straining for bowel movement.

DOSAGE & USAGE INFORMATION

How to take:

- Liquid, powder, flakes, granules—Dilute dose in 8 oz. cold water or fruit juice.
- Capsules—Swallow with 8 oz. cold liquid. Drink 6 to 8 glasses of water each day in addition to the one with each dose.

When to take:
At the same time each day, preferably morning.

If you forget a dose:
Take as soon as you remember. Resume regular schedule.

What drug does:
Absorbs water, stimulating the bowel to form a soft, bulky stool.

Time lapse before drug works:
May require 2 or 3 days to begin, then works in 12 to 24 hours.

Don't take with:

- See Interaction column and consult doctor.
- Don't take within 2 hours of taking another medicine. Laxative interferes with medicine absorption.

OVERDOSE

Symptoms:
None expected.

What to do:
Overdose unlikely to threaten life. If person takes much larger amount than prescribed, call doctor, poison-control center or hospital emergency room for instructions.

POSSIBLE ADVERSE REACTIONS OR SIDE EFFECTS

SYMPTOMS	FREQUENCY	WHAT TO DO
Brain & nervous system:	None expected.	
Skin: Itch, rash.	Rare	3
Eyes:	None expected.	
Ears, nose, throat: Swallowing difficulty, "lump in throat" sensation.	Infrequent	4
Digestive:		
• Intestinal blockage.	Rare	3
• Nausea, vomiting, diarrhea.	Infrequent	4
Heart & lungs: Asthma	Rare	3
Blood vessels:	None expected.	
Muscles, bones, joints:	None expected.	
Genital, urinary:	None expected.	
Kidneys:	None expected.	
Liver:	None expected.	
Allergic:	None expected.	
Blood:	None expected.	
Others:	None expected.	

1- Life-threatening. Seek emergency treatment immediately.
2- Discontinue. Seek emergency treatment.
3- Discontinue. Call doctor right away.
4- Continue. Call doctor when convenient.
5- Continue. Tell doctor at next visit.
6- No action necessary.

WARNINGS & PRECAUTIONS

Don't take if:
- You are allergic to any bulk-forming laxative.
- You have symptoms of appendicitis, inflamed bowel or intestinal blockage.
- You have missed a bowel movement for only 1 or 2 days.

Before you start, consult your doctor:
- If you have diabetes.
- If you have a laxative habit.
- If you have rectal bleeding.
- If you have difficulty swallowing.
- If you take other laxatives.

Over age 60:
Adverse reactions and side effects may be more frequent and severe than in younger persons.

Pregnancy:
Most bulk-forming laxatives contain sodium or sugars which may cause fluid retention. Avoid if possible.

Breast-feeding:
No problems expected.

Infants & children:
Use only under medical supervision.

Prolonged use:
Don't take for more than 1 week unless under a doctor's supervision. May cause laxative dependence.

Skin & sunlight:
No problems expected.

Driving, piloting or hazardous work:
No problems expected.

Airplane passengers:
No problems expected.

Discontinuing:
May be unnecessary to finish medicine. Follow doctor's instructions.

Others:
Don't take to "flush out" your system or as a "tonic."

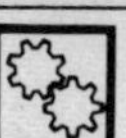

INTERACTION WITH OTHER DRUGS

GENERIC NAME OR DRUG CLASS	COMBINED EFFECT
Antibiotics	Decreased antibiotic effect.
Anticoagulants	Decreased anticoagulant effect.
Digitalis preparations	Decreased digitalis effect.
Salicylates (including aspirin)	Decreased salicylate effect.

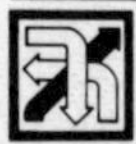

INTERACTION WITH OTHER SUBSTANCES

INTERACTS WITH	COMBINED EFFECT
Alcohol:	None expected.
Beverages:	None expected.
Cocaine:	None expected.
Foods:	None expected.
Marijuana:	None expected.
Tobacco:	None expected.

METHYLDOPA

BRAND NAMES

Aldomet
Aldoclor
Aldoril-15
Aldoril-25
Aldoril D30
Aldoril D50
Apo-Methyldopa
Dopamet
Medimet-250
Novomedopa
PMS Dopazide

GENERAL INFORMATION

Habit forming? No
Prescription needed? Yes
Available as generic? No
Drug class: Antihypertensive

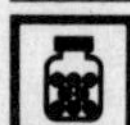

USES

Reduces high blood pressure.

DOSAGE & USAGE INFORMATION

How to take:
Liquid or tablet—Swallow with liquid. If you can't swallow whole, crumble tablet and take with liquid or food.

When to take:
At the same times each day.

If you forget a dose:
Take as soon as you remember up to 2 hours late. If more than 2 hours, wait for next scheduled dose (don't double this dose).

What drug does:
Relaxes walls of small arteries to decrease blood pressure.

Time lapse before drug works:
Continual use for 2 to 4 weeks may be necessary to determine effectiveness.

Don't take with:
See Interaction column and consult doctor.

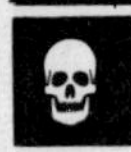

OVERDOSE

Symptoms:
Drowsiness; exhaustion; stupor; confusion; slow, weak pulse.

What to do:
- Dial 0 (operator) or 911 (emergency) for an ambulance or medical help. Then give first aid immediately.
- If patient is unconscious and not breathing, give mouth-to-mouth breathing. If there is no heartbeat, use cardiac massage and mouth-to-mouth breathing (CPR). Don't try to make patient vomit. If you can't get help quickly, take patient to nearest emergency facility.
- Additional emergency information on page 886.

POSSIBLE ADVERSE REACTIONS OR SIDE EFFECTS

SYMPTOMS	FREQUENCY	WHAT TO DO
Brain & nervous system:		
• Depression, nightmares, drowsiness, weakness.	Common	4
• Insomnia	Infrequent	4
Skin:		
Rash	Rare	3
Eyes:	None expected.	
Ears, nose, throat:		
Stuffy nose, dry mouth.	Common	4
Digestive:		
Nausea, vomiting, diarrhea.	Infrequent	4
Heart & lungs:		
Fast heartbeat.	Infrequent	3
Blood vessels:	None expected.	
Muscles, bones, joints:		
Swollen feet or legs.	Common	4
Genital, urinary:	None expected.	
Kidneys:	None expected.	
Liver:		
Jaundice (yellow skin and eyes).	Rare	3
Allergic:	None expected.	
Blood:	None expected.	
Others:		
• Unexplained fever.	Rare	3
• Fluid retention.	Common	4
• Breast swelling.	Infrequent	5
• Lower sex drive.	Infrequent	5

1-Life-threatening. Seek emergency treatment immediately.
2-Discontinue. Seek emergency treatment.
3-Discontinue. Call doctor right away.
4-Continue. Call doctor when convenient.
5-Continue. Tell doctor at next visit.
6-No action necessary.

WARNINGS & PRECAUTIONS

Don't take if:
You will have surgery within 2 months, including dental surgery, requiring general or spinal anesthesia.

Before you start, consult your doctor:
If you have liver disease.

Over age 60:
- Increased susceptibility to dizziness, unsteadiness, fainting, falling.
- Drug can produce or intensify Parkinson's disease.

Pregnancy:
No proven problems. Consult doctor.

Breast-feeding:
No proven problems. Consult doctor.

Infants & children:
Not used.

Prolonged use:
- May cause anemia.
- Severe edema (fluid retention).

Skin & sunlight:
No problems expected.

Driving, piloting or hazardous work:
Don't drive or pilot aircraft until you learn how medicine affects you. Don't work around dangerous machinery. Don't climb ladders or work in high places. Danger increases if you drink alcohol or take medicine affecting alertness and reflexes, such as antihistamines, tranquilizers, sedatives, pain medicine, narcotics and mind-altering drugs.

Airplane passengers:
No problems expected.

Discontinuing:
Don't discontinue without consulting doctor. Dose may require gradual reduction if you have taken drug for a long time. Doses of other drugs may also require adjustment.

Others:
Avoid heavy exercise, exertion, sweating.

INTERACTION WITH OTHER DRUGS

GENERIC NAME OR DRUG CLASS	COMBINED EFFECT
Amphetamines	Decreased methyldopa effect.
Anticoagulants (oral)	Increased anticoagulant effect.
Antidepressants (tricyclic)	Dangerous blood-pressure rise.
Antihypertensives	Increased antihypertensive effect.
Digitalis preparations	Excessively slow heartbeat.
Diuretics (thiazide)	Increased methyldopa effect.
Levodopa	Decreased levodopa effect.
MAO inhibitors	Dangerous blood-pressure rise.

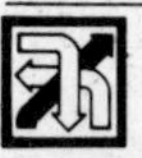

INTERACTION WITH OTHER SUBSTANCES

INTERACTS WITH	COMBINED EFFECT
Alcohol:	Increased sedation. Excessive blood-pressure drop. Avoid.
Beverages:	None expected.
Cocaine:	Decreased methyldopa effect.
Foods:	None expected.
Marijuana:	Possible fainting.
Tobacco:	Possible increased blood pressure.

METHYLERGONOVINE

BRAND NAMES

Methergine

GENERAL INFORMATION

Habit forming? No
Prescription needed? Yes
Available as generic? Yes
Drug class: Ergot preparation (uterine stimulant)

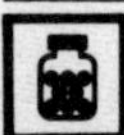

USES

Retards excessive post-delivery bleeding.

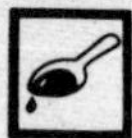

DOSAGE & USAGE INFORMATION

How to take:
Tablet—Swallow with liquid or food to lessen stomach irritation.

When to take:
At the same times each day.

If you forget a dose:
Don't take missed dose and don't double next one. Wait for next scheduled dose.

What drug does:
Causes smooth-muscle cells of uterine wall to contract and surround bleeding blood vessels of relaxed uterus.

Time lapse before drug works:
Tablets—20 to 30 minutes.

Don't take with:
See Interaction column and consult doctor.

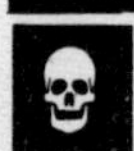

OVERDOSE

Symptoms:
Vomiting, diarrhea, weak pulse, low blood pressure, convulsions.

What to do:
- Dial 0 (operator) or 911 (emergency) for an ambulance or medical help. Then give first aid immediately.
- If patient is unconscious and not breathing, give mouth-to-mouth breathing. If there is no heartbeat, use cardiac massage and mouth-to-mouth breathing (CPR). Don't try to make patient vomit. If you can't get help quickly, take patient to nearest emergency facility.
- Additional emergency information on page 886.

POSSIBLE ADVERSE REACTIONS OR SIDE EFFECTS

SYMPTOMS	FREQUENCY	WHAT TO DO
Brain & nervous system:		
• Sudden, severe headache.	Rare	2
• Confusion	Infrequent	3
Skin:	None expected.	
Eyes:	None expected.	
Ears, nose, throat:		
Ringing in ears.	Infrequent	3
Digestive:		
• Nausea, vomiting.	Common	3
• Diarrhea	Infrequent	3
Heart & lungs:		
Shortness of breath, chest pain.	Rare	2
Blood vessels:	None expected.	
Muscles, bones, joints:		
• Muscle cramps.	Infrequent	3
• Numb, cold hands and feet.	Rare	2
Genital, urinary:	None expected.	
Kidneys:	None expected.	
Liver:	None expected.	
Allergic:	None expected.	
Blood:	None expected.	
Others:		
Unusual sweating.	Infrequent	4

1-Life-threatening. Seek emergency treatment immediately.
2-Discontinue. Seek emergency treatment.
3-Discontinue. Call doctor right away.
4-Continue. Call doctor when convenient.
5-Continue. Tell doctor at next visit.
6-No action necessary.

WARNINGS & PRECAUTIONS

Don't take if:
You are allergic to any ergot preparation.

Before you start, consult your doctor:
- If you have coronary-artery or blood-vessel disease.
- If you have liver or kidney disease.
- If you have high blood pressure.
- If you have postpartum infection.

Over age 60:
Not recommended.

Pregnancy:
Risk to unborn child outweighs drug benefits. Don't use.

Breast-feeding:
Drug passes into milk. Avoid drug or discontinue nursing until you finish medicine. Consult doctor for advice on maintaining milk supply.

Infants & children:
Not recommended.

Prolonged use:
Not recommended.

Skin & sunlight:
No problems expected.

Driving, piloting or hazardous work:
No problems expected.

Airplane passengers:
No problems expected.

Discontinuing:
May be unnecessary to finish medicine. Follow doctor's instructions.

Others:
Drug should be used for short time only following childbirth or miscarriage.

INTERACTION WITH OTHER DRUGS

GENERIC NAME OR DRUG CLASS	COMBINED EFFECT
Ergot preparations (other)	Increased methylergonovine effect.

INTERACTION WITH OTHER SUBSTANCES

INTERACTS WITH	COMBINED EFFECT
Alcohol:	None expected.
Beverages:	None expected.
Cocaine:	None expected.
Foods:	None expected.
Marijuana:	None expected.
Tobacco:	None expected.

METHYLPHENIDATE

BRAND NAMES

Methidate
Ritalin
Ritalin SR

GENERAL INFORMATION

Habit forming? Yes
Prescription needed? Yes
Available as generic? Yes
Drug class: Sympathomimetic

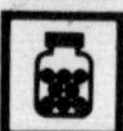

USES

- Treatment for hyperactive children.
- Treatment for drowsiness and fatigue in adults.
- Treatment for narcolepsy (uncontrollable attacks of sleepiness).

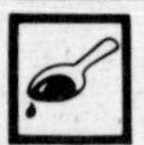

DOSAGE & USAGE INFORMATION

How to take:
Tablet or capsule—Swallow with liquid or food to lessen stomach irritation. If you can't swallow whole, crumble tablet or open capsule and take with liquid or food.

When to take:
At the same times each day.

If you forget a dose:
Take as soon as you remember up to 2 hours late. If more than 2 hours, wait for next scheduled dose (don't double this dose).

What drug does:
Stimulates brain to improve alertness, concentration and attention span. Calms the hyperactive child.

Time lapse before drug works:
- 1 month or more for maximum effect on child.
- 30 minutes to stimulate adults.

Don't take with:
See Interaction column and consult doctor.

OVERDOSE

Symptoms:
Rapid heartbeat; fever; confusion, hallucinations; convulsions; coma.

What to do:
- Dial 0 (operator) or 911 (emergency) for an ambulance or medical help. Then give first aid immediately.
- If patient is unconscious and not breathing, give mouth-to-mouth breathing. If there is no heartbeat, use cardiac massage and mouth-to-mouth breathing (CPR). Don't try to make patient vomit. If you can't get help quickly, take patient to nearest emergency facility.
- Additional emergency information on page 886.

POSSIBLE ADVERSE REACTIONS OR SIDE EFFECTS

SYMPTOMS	FREQUENCY	WHAT TO DO
Brain & nervous system:		
• Mood changes.	Common	4
• Nervousness, insomnia, dizziness, headache.	Common	5
Skin:		
Rash or hives.	Infrequent	3
Eyes:		
Blurred vision.	Rare	3
Ears, nose, throat:		
Sore throat, fever.	Rare	3
Digestive:		
• Appetite loss.	Common	5
• Nausea, abdominal pain.	Infrequent	4
Heart & lungs:		
Chest pain; fast, irregular heartbeat.	Infrequent	3
Blood vessels:		
Unusual bruising.	Infrequent	3
Muscles, bones, joints:		
Joint pain, uncontrolled movements.	Infrequent	3
Genital, urinary:	None expected.	
Kidneys:	None expected.	
Liver:	None expected.	
Allergic:	None expected.	
Blood:	None expected.	
Others:		
• Unexplained fever.	Infrequent	3
• Unusual tiredness.	Rare	4

1-Life-threatening. Seek emergency treatment immediately.
2-Discontinue. Seek emergency treatment.
3-Discontinue. Call doctor right away.
4-Continue. Call doctor when convenient.
5-Continue. Tell doctor at next visit.
6-No action necessary.

METHYLPHENIDATE

WARNINGS & PRECAUTIONS

Don't take if:
- You are allergic to methylphenidate.
- You have glaucoma.
- Patient is younger than 6.

Before you start, consult your doctor:
- If you have epilepsy.
- If you have high blood pressure.
- If you take MAO inhibitors.

Over age 60:
Adverse reactions and side effects may be more frequent and severe than in younger persons.

Pregnancy:
No proven harm to unborn child. Avoid if possible.

Breast-feeding:
No proven problems. Consult doctor.

Infants & children:
Use only under medical supervision for children 6 or older.

Prolonged use:
Rare possibility of physical growth retardation.

Skin & sunlight:
No problems expected.

Driving, piloting or hazardous work:
No problems expected.

Airplane passengers:
No problems expected.

Discontinuing:
Don't discontinue abruptly. Don't discontinue without doctor's advice until you complete prescribed dose, even though symptoms diminish or disappear.

Others:
Dose must be carefully adjusted by doctor.

INTERACTION WITH OTHER DRUGS

GENERIC NAME OR DRUG CLASS	COMBINED EFFECT
Anticholinergics	Increased anticholinergic effect.
Anticoagulants (oral)	Increased anticoagulant effect.
Anticonvulsants	Increased anticonvulsant effect.
Antidepressants (tricyclic)	Increased antidepressant effect.
Guanethidine	Decreased guanethidine effect.
MAO inhibitors	Dangerous rise in blood pressure.
Oxyphenbutazone	Increased oxyphenbutazone effect.
Phenylbutazone	Increased phenylbutazone effect.

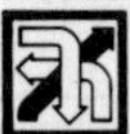

INTERACTION WITH OTHER SUBSTANCES

INTERACTS WITH	COMBINED EFFECT
Alcohol:	None expected.
Beverages:	
Caffeine drinks	May raise blood pressure.
Cocaine:	Overstimulation. Avoid.
Foods:	
Foods containing tyramine (see page 849).	May raise blood pressure.
Marijuana:	None expected.
Tobacco:	None expected.

METHYLPREDNISOLONE

BRAND NAMES

A-methaPred
Depo-Medrol
Depo-Pred-40
Depo-Pred-80
Duralone
Duralone-40
Duralone-80
Medralone
Medralone-40
Medralone-80
Medrol
Medrol Enpak
Medrone-80
Mepred-40
Methylone
Pro-Dep-40
Pro-Dep-80
Solu-Medrol

GENERAL INFORMATION

Habit forming? No
Prescription needed? Yes
Available as generic? Yes
Drug class: Cortisone drug (adrenal corticosteroid)

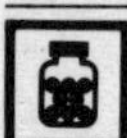

USES

- Reduces inflammation caused by many different medical problems.
- Treatment for some allergic diseases, blood disorders, kidney diseases, asthma and emphysema.
- Replaces corticosteroid deficiencies.

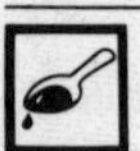

DOSAGE & USAGE INFORMATION

How to take:
Tablet—Swallow with liquid or food to lessen stomach irritation. If you can't swallow whole, crumble tablet and take with liquid or food.

When to take:
At the same times each day. Take once-a-day or once-every-other-day doses in mornings.

If you forget a dose:
- Several-doses-per-day prescription—Take as soon as you remember up to 2 hours late. If more than 2 hours, wait for next scheduled dose (don't double this dose).
- Once-a-day dose or less—Wait for next dose. Double this dose.

What drug does:
Decreases inflammatory responses.

Time lapse before drug works:
2 to 4 days.

Don't take with:
See Interaction column and consult doctor.

OVERDOSE

Symptoms:
Headache, convulsions, heart failure.

What to do:
- Dial 0 (operator) or 911 (emergency) for an ambulance or medical help. Then give first aid immediately.
- Additional emergency information on page 886.

POSSIBLE ADVERSE REACTIONS OR SIDE EFFECTS

SYMPTOMS	FREQUENCY	WHAT TO DO
Brain & nervous system:		
Mood changes, insomnia, restlessness.	Infrequent	4
Skin:		
• Acne	Common	4
• Rash	Rare	3
• Poor wound healing.	Common	4
Eyes:		
Blurred vision, halos around lights.	Infrequent	3
Ears, nose, throat:		
• Sore throat, fever.	Infrequent	3
• Thirst	Common	4
Digestive:		
• Indigestion, nausea, vomiting.	Common	4
• Bloody or black, tarry stool.	Infrequent	2
Heart & lungs:		
Irregular heartbeat.	Rare	2
Blood vessels, kidneys, liver, allergic, blood:	None expected.	
Muscles, bones, joints:		
Muscle cramps, swollen legs, feet.	Infrequent	3
Genital, urinary:		
Frequent urination.	Infrequent	4
Others:		
• Weight gain, round face.	Infrequent	4
• Fatigue, weakness.	Infrequent	4
• TB recurrence.	Infrequent	4
• Irregular menstrual periods.	Infrequent	4

1- Life-threatening. Seek emergency treatment immediately.
2- Discontinue. Seek emergency treatment.
3- Discontinue. Call doctor right away.
4- Continue. Call doctor when convenient.

WARNINGS & PRECAUTIONS

Don't take if:
- You are allergic to any cortisone drug.
- You have tuberculosis or fungus infection.
- You have herpes infection of eyes, lips or genitals.

Before you start, consult your doctor:
- If you have had tuberculosis.
- If you have congestive heart failure.
- If you have diabetes.
- If you have peptic ulcer.
- If you have glaucoma.
- If you have underactive thyroid.
- If you have high blood pressure.
- If you have myasthenia gravis.
- If you have blood clots in legs or lungs.

Over age 60:
Adverse reactions and side effects may be more frequent and severe than in younger persons. Likely to aggravate edema, diabetes or ulcers. Likely to cause cataracts and osteoporosis (softening of the bones).

Pregnancy:
Risk to unborn child outweighs drug benefits. Don't use.

Breast-feeding:
Drug passes into milk. Avoid drug or discontinue nursing until you finish medicine. Consult doctor for advice on maintaining milk supply.

Infants & children:
Use only under medical supervision.

Prolonged use:
- Retards growth in children.
- Possible glaucoma, cataracts, diabetes, fragile bones and thin skin.
- Functional dependence.

Skin & sunlight:
No problems expected.

Driving, piloting or hazardous work:
No problems expected.

Airplane passengers:
No problems expected.

Discontinuing:
- Don't discontinue without doctor's advice until you complete prescribed dose, even though symptoms diminish or disappear.
- Drug affects your response to surgery, illness, injury or stress for 2 years after discontinuing. Tell about drug to anyone who takes medical care of you within 2 years.

Others:
Avoid immunizations if possible.

INTERACTION WITH OTHER DRUGS

GENERIC NAME OR DRUG CLASS	COMBINED EFFECT
Amphoterecin B	Potassium depletion.
Anticholinergics	Possible glaucoma.
Anticoagulants (oral)	Decreased anticoagulant effect.
Anticonvulsants (hydantoin)	Decreased methylprednisolone effect.
Antidiabetics (oral)	Decreased antidiabetic effect.
Antihistamines	Decreased methylprednisolone effect.
Aspirin	Increased methylprednisolone effect.
Barbiturates	Decreased methylprednisolone effect. Oversedation.
Beta-adrenergic blockers	Decreased methylprednisolone effect.
Chloral hydrate	Decreased methylprednisolone effect.
Chlorthalidone	Potassium depletion.
Cholinergics	Decreased cholinergic effect.

Additional interactions on page 839.

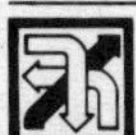

INTERACTION WITH OTHER SUBSTANCES

INTERACTS WITH	COMBINED EFFECT
Alcohol:	Risk of stomach ulcers.
Beverages:	No proven problems.
Cocaine:	Overstimulation. Avoid.
Foods:	No proven problems.
Marijuana:	Decreased immunity.
Tobacco:	Increased methylprednisolone effect. Possible toxicity.

METHYSERGIDE

BRAND NAMES

Sansert

GENERAL INFORMATION

Habit forming? Yes
Prescription needed? Yes
Available as generic? No
Drug class: Vasoconstrictor (antiserotonin)

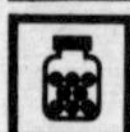

USES

Prevents migraine and other recurring vascular headaches.

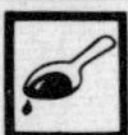

DOSAGE & USAGE INFORMATION

How to take:
Tablet—Swallow with liquid or with food to lessen stomach irritation. If you can't swallow whole, crumble tablet and take with liquid or food.

When to take:
At the same times each day.

If you forget a dose:
Don't take missed dose. Wait for next scheduled dose (don't double this dose).

What drug does:
Blocks the action of serotonin, a chemical that constricts blood vessels.

Time lapse before drug works:
About 3 weeks.

Don't take with:
See Interaction column and consult doctor.

OVERDOSE

Symptoms:
Nausea, vomiting, abdominal pain, severe diarrhea, lack of coordination, extreme thirst.

What to do:
Overdose unlikely to threaten life. If person takes much larger amount than prescribed, call doctor, poison-control center or hospital emergency room for instructions.

POSSIBLE ADVERSE REACTIONS OR SIDE EFFECTS

SYMPTOMS	FREQUENCY	WHAT TO DO
Brain & nervous system:		
• Drowsiness	Common	5
• Anxiety, agitation hallucinations.	Infrequent	3
Skin:		
Itching	Common	3
Eyes:		
Vision changes.	Infrequent	4
Ears, nose, throat:		
Extreme thirst.	Rare	3
Digestive:		
• Appetite loss.	Rare	3
• Nausea, vomiting, diarrhea.	Common	4
Heart & lungs:		
• Chest pain, shortness of breath.	Rare	3
• Unusually fast or slow heartbeat.	Infrequent	3
Blood vessels:		
• Fever, pale or swollen extremities.	Rare	3
• Numbness or tingling of extremities.	Common	4
Muscles, bones, joints:		
• Leg cramps, lower back pain.	Rare	3
• Leg weakness.	Common	4
Genital, urinary:		
Difficult or painful urination.	Rare	4
Kidneys:		
Side or groin pain.	Rare	3
Liver, allergic, blood:	None expected.	
Others:		
Weight change, hair loss.	Rare	5

1- Life-threatening. Seek emergency treatment immediately.
2- Discontinue. Seek emergency treatment.
3- Discontinue. Call doctor right away.
4- Continue. Call doctor when convenient.
5- Continue. Tell doctor at next visit.

WARNINGS & PRECAUTIONS

Don't take if:
- You are allergic to any antiserotonin.
- You plan to become pregnant within medication period.
- You have an infection.
- You have a heart or blood-vessel disease.
- You have a chronic lung disease.
- You have a collagen (connective tissue) disorder.
- You have impaired liver or kidney function.

Before you start, consult your doctor:
- If you have been allergic to any ergot preparation.
- If you have had a peptic ulcer.

Over age 60:
Adverse reactions and side effects may be more frequent and severe than in younger persons.

Pregnancy:
Manufacturer suggests risk to unborn child outweighs drug benefits, even though studies are inconclusive.

Breast-feeding:
Drug probably passes into milk. Avoid drug or discontinue nursing until you finish medicine. Consult doctor for advice on maintaining milk supply.

Infants & children:
Not recommended.

Prolonged use:
Possible fibrosis, a condition in which scar tissue is deposited on heart valves, in lung tissue, blood vessels and internal organs. After 6 months, decrease dose over 2 to 3 weeks. Then discontinue for at least 2 months for re-evaluation.

Skin & sunlight:
No problems expected.

Driving, piloting or hazardous work:
Avoid if you feel drowsy or dizzy. Otherwise, no problems expected.

Airplane passengers:
No problems expected.

Discontinuing:
- Don't discontinue without consulting doctor. Dose may require gradual reduction if you have taken drug for a long time. Doses of other drugs may also require adjustment.
- Probably should discontinue drug if you don't improve after 3 weeks' use.

Others:
- Periodic laboratory tests for liver function and blood counts recommended.
- Potential for abuse.

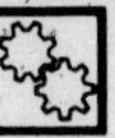

INTERACTION WITH OTHER DRUGS

GENERIC NAME OR DRUG CLASS	COMBINED EFFECT
Ergot preparations	Unpredictable increased or decreased effect of either drug.
Narcotics	Decreased narcotic effect.

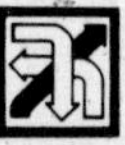

INTERACTION WITH OTHER SUBSTANCES

INTERACTS WITH	COMBINED EFFECT
Alcohol:	None expected. However, alcohol may trigger a migraine headache.
Beverages: Caffeine drinks	Decreased methysergide effect.
Cocaine:	May make headache worse.
Foods:	None expected. Avoid foods to which you are allergic.
Marijuana:	No proven problems.
Tobacco:	Blood-vessel constriction. Makes headache worse.

METOCLOPRAMIDE

BRAND NAMES

Maxeran
Reglan

GENERAL INFORMATION

Habit forming? No
Prescription needed? Yes
Available as generic? No
Drug class: Antiemetic; dopaminergic blocker

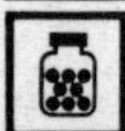

USES

- Relieves nausea and vomiting caused by chemotherapy and drug related postoperative factors.
- Relieves symptoms of esophagitis.

DOSAGE & USAGE INFORMATION

How to take:
Tablet or capsule—Swallow with liquid or food to lessen stomach irritation.

When to take:
30 minutes before symptoms expected, up to 4 times a day.

If you forget a dose:
Take as soon as you remember up to 2 hours late. If more than 2 hours, wait for next scheduled dose (don't double this dose).

What drug does:
- Prevents smooth muscle in stomach from relaxing.
- Affects vomiting center in brain.

Time lapse before drug works:
30 to 60 minutes.

Don't take with:
See Interaction column and consult doctor.

OVERDOSE

Symptoms:
Severe drowsiness, mental confusion, trembling, seizure, coma.

What to do:
- Dial O (operator) or 911 (emergency) for an ambulance or medical help. Then give first aid immediately.
- If patient is unconscious and not breathing, give mouth-to-mouth breathing. If there is no heartbeat, use cardiac massage and mouth-to-mouth breathing (CPR). Don't try to make patient vomit. If you can't get help quickly, take patient to nearest emergency facility.
- Additional emergency information on page 886.

POSSIBLE ADVERSE REACTIONS OR SIDE EFFECTS

SYMPTOMS	FREQUENCY	WHAT TO DO
Brain & nervous system:		
• Drowsiness	Common	4
• Restlessness	Common	4
• Dizziness	Infrequent	4
• Headache	Infrequent	4
• Insomnia	Infrequent	4
Skin:		
Rash	Frequent	4
Eyes:	Frequent	4
Ears, nose, throat:	Frequent	4
Digestive:		
• Constipation	Rare	4
• Diarrhea	Rare	4
• Nausea	Rare	4
Heart & lungs:	None expected.	
Blood vessels:	None expected.	
Muscles, bones, joints:	None expected.	
Genital, urinary:	None expected.	
Kidneys, allergic, blood, liver:	None expected.	
Others:		
• Breast tenderness and swelling.	Infrequent	4
• Increased milk flow.	Infrequent	4

1-Life-threatening. Seek emergency treatment immediately.
2-Discontinue. Seek emergency treatment.
3-Discontinue. Call doctor right away.
4-Continue. Call doctor when convenient.
5-Continue. Tell doctor at next visit.
6-No action necessary.

METOCLOPRAMIDE

WARNINGS & PRECAUTIONS

Don't take if:
You are allergic to procaine, procainamide or metoclopramide.

Before you start, consult your doctor:
- If you have Parkinson's disease.
- If you have liver or kidney disease.
- If you have epilepsy.
- If you have bleeding from gastrointestinal tract or intestinal obstruction.
- If you will have surgery within 2 months, including dental surgery, requiring general or spinal anesthesia.

Over age 60:
Adverse reactions and side effects may be more frequent and severe than in younger persons.

Pregnancy:
No proven harm to unborn child. Avoid if possible.

Breast-feeding:
Unknown effect.

Infants & children:
Adverse reactions more likely to occur than in adults.

Prolonged use:
Adverse reactions including muscle spasms and trembling hands more likely to occur.

Skin & sunlight:
No problems expected.

Driving, piloting or hazardous work:
Don't drive or pilot aircraft until you learn how medicine affects you. Don't work around dangerous machinery. Don't climb ladders or work in high places. Danger increases if you drink alcohol or take medicine affecting alertness and reflexes, such as antihistamines, tranquilizers, sedatives, pain medicine, narcotics and mind-altering drugs.

Airplane passengers:
No problems expected.

Discontinuing:
May be unnecessary to finish medicine. Follow doctor's instructions.

INTERACTION WITH OTHER DRUGS

GENERIC NAME OR DRUG CLASS	COMBINED EFFECT
Acetaminophen	Slow stomach emptying.
Levodopa	Slow stomach emptying.
Tetracycline	Slow stomach emptying.
Central nervous system depressants: **Sedatives** **Sleeping pills** **Tranquilizers** **Antidepressants** **Antihistamines** **Narcotics** **Muscle relaxants**	Excess sedation.
Bromocriptine	Decreased bromocriptine effect.
Digitalis preparations	Decreased absorption of digitalis.
Phenothiazines	Increased chance of muscle spasm and trembling.

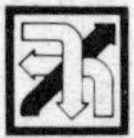

INTERACTION WITH OTHER SUBSTANCES

INTERACTS WITH	COMBINED EFFECT
Alcohol:	Excess sedation. Avoid.
Beverages: Coffee	Decreased metoclopramide effect.
Cocaine:	Decreased metoclopramide effect.
Foods:	No problems expected.
Marijuana:	Decreased metoclopramide effect.
Tobacco:	Decreased metoclopramide effect.

METOLAZONE

BRAND NAMES

Diulo
Zaroxolyn

GENERAL INFORMATION

Habit forming? No
Prescription needed? Yes
Available as generic? Yes
Drug class: Antihypertensive, diuretic (thiazide)

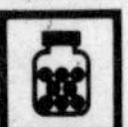

USES

- Controls, but doesn't cure, high blood pressure.
- Reduces fluid retention (edema) caused by conditions such as heart disorders and liver disease.

DOSAGE & USAGE INFORMATION

How to take:
Tablet or capsule—Swallow with 8 oz. of liquid. If you can't swallow whole, crumble tablet or open capsule and take with liquid or food. Don't exceed dose.

When to take:
At the same time each day.

If you forget a dose:
Take as soon as you remember up to 2 hours late. If more than 2 hours, wait for next scheduled dose (don't double this dose).

What drug does:
- Forces sodium and water excretion, reducing body fluid.
- Relaxes muscle cells of small arteries.
- Reduced body fluid and relaxed arteries lower blood pressure.

Time lapse before drug works:
4 to 6 hours. May require several weeks to lower blood pressure.

Don't take with:
- See Interaction column and consult doctor.
- Non-prescription drugs without consulting doctor.

OVERDOSE

Symptoms:
Cramps, weakness, drowsiness, weak pulse, coma.

What to do:
- Dial O (operator) or 911 (emergency) for an ambulance or medical help. Then give first aid immediately.
- Additional emergency information on page 886.

POSSIBLE ADVERSE REACTIONS OR SIDE EFFECTS

SYMPTOMS	FREQUENCY	WHAT TO DO
Brain & nervous system:		
• Dizziness	Infrequent	4
• Mood changes.	Infrequent	4
• Headaches	Infrequent	4
Skin:		
Rash or hives.	Rare	2
Eyes:		
Blurred vision.	Infrequent	3
Ears, nose, throat:		
• Sore throat, fever.	Rare	3
• Dry mouth, thirst.	Infrequent	5
Digestive:		
Severe abdominal pain, nausea, vomiting.	Infrequent	3
Heart & lungs:		
Irregular heartbeat, weak pulse.	Infrequent	3
Blood vessels:	None expected.	
Muscles, bones, joints:		
Weakness, tiredness.	Infrequent	4
Genital, urinary:	None expected.	
Kidneys:	None expected.	
Liver:		
Jaundice (yellow skin and eyes).	Rare	3
Allergic:	None expected.	
Blood:	None expected.	
Others:		
Weight changes.	Infrequent	4

1- Life-threatening. Seek emergency treatment immediately.
2- Discontinue. Seek emergency treatment.
3- Discontinue. Call doctor right away.
4- Continue. Call doctor when convenient.
5- Continue. Tell doctor at next visit.
6- No action necessary.

WARNINGS & PRECAUTIONS

Don't take if:
You are allergic to any thiazide diuretic drug.

Before you start, consult your doctor:
- If you are allergic to any sulfa drug.
- If you have gout.
- If you have liver, pancreas or kidney disorder.

Over age 60:
Adverse reactions and side effects may be more frequent and severe than in younger persons, especially dizziness and excessive potassium loss.

Pregnancy:
Risk to unborn child outweighs drug benefits. Don't use.

Breast-feeding:
Drug passes into milk. Avoid this medicine or discontinue nursing.

Infants & children:
No problems expected.

Prolonged use:
You may need medicine to treat high blood pressure for the rest of your life.

Skin & sunlight:
May cause rash or intensify sunburn in areas exposed to sun or sunlamp.

Driving, piloting or hazardous work:
Don't drive or pilot aircraft until you learn how medicine affects you. Don't work around dangerous machinery. Don't climb ladders or work in high places. Danger increases if you drink alcohol or take medicine affecting alertness and reflexes, such as antihistamines, tranquilizers, sedatives, pain medicine, narcotics and mind-altering drugs.

Airplane passengers:
No problems expected.

Discontinuing:
Don't discontinue without medical advice.

Others:
- Hot weather and fever may cause dehydration and drop in blood pressure. Dose may require temporary adjustment. Weigh daily and report any unexpected weight decreases to your doctor.
- May cause rise in uric acid, leading to gout.
- May cause blood-sugar rise in diabetics.

INTERACTION WITH OTHER DRUGS

GENERIC NAME OR DRUG CLASS	COMBINED EFFECT
Allopurinol	Decreased allopurinol effect.
Antidepressants (tricyclic)	Dangerous drop in blood pressure. Avoid combination unless under medical supervision.
Barbiturates	Increased metolazone effect.
Cholestyramine	Decreased metolazone effect.
Cortisone drugs	Excessive potassium loss that causes dangerous heart rhythms.
Digitalis preparations	Excessive potassium loss that causes dangerous heart rhythms.
Diuretics (thiazide)	Increased effect of other thiazide diuretics.
Lithium	Increased effect of lithium.
MAO inhibitors	Increased metolazone effect.
Probenecid	Decreased probenecid effect.

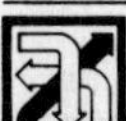

INTERACTIONS WITH OTHER SUBSTANCES

INTERACTS WITH	COMBINED EFFECT
Alcohol:	Dangerous blood-pressure drop.
Beverages:	None expected.
Cocaine:	None expected.
Foods:	
Licorice	Excessive potassium loss that causes dangerous heart rhythms.
Marijuana:	May increase blood pressure.
Tobacco:	None expected.

METOPROLOL

BRAND NAMES

Betaloc
Lopressor

GENERAL INFORMATION

Habit forming? No
Prescription needed? Yes
Available as generic? No
Drug class: Beta-adrenergic blocker

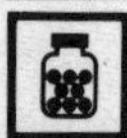

USES

- Reduces angina attacks.
- Stabilizes irregular heartbeat.
- Lowers blood pressure.
- Reduces frequency of migraine headaches. (Does not relieve headache pain.)
- Other uses prescribed by your doctor.

DOSAGE & USAGE INFORMATION

How to take:
Tablet or capsule—Swallow with liquid. If you can't swallow whole, crumble tablet or open capsule and take with liquid or food.

When to take:
With meals or immediately after.

If you forget a dose:
Take as soon as you remember. Return to regular schedule, but allow 3 hours between doses.

What drug does:
- Blocks certain actions of sympathetic nervous system.
- Lowers heart's oxygen requirements.
- Slows nerve impulses through heart.
- Reduces blood vessel contraction in heart, scalp and other body parts.

Time lapse before drug works:
1 to 4 hours.

Don't take with:
Non-prescription drugs or drugs in Interaction column without consulting doctor.

OVERDOSE

Symptoms:
Weakness, slow or weak pulse, blood pressure drop, fainting, convulsions, cold and sweaty skin.

What to do:
- Dial O (operator) or 911 (emergency) for an ambulance or medical help. Then give first aid immediately.
- Additional emergency information on page 886.

POSSIBLE ADVERSE REACTIONS OR SIDE EFFECTS

SYMPTOMS	FREQUENCY	WHAT TO DO
Brain & nervous system:		
• Hallucinations, nightmares, insomnia, headache.	Infrequent	3
• Confusion, depression, reduced alertness.	Infrequent	4
• Drowsiness, numbness or tingling of fingers or toes, dizziness.	Common	4
Skin:		
Rash	Rare	3
Eyes:	None expected.	
Ears, nose, throat:		
Sore throat, fever.	Rare	3
Digestive:		
• Diarrhea, nausea.	Common	4
• Constipation	Infrequent	5
Heart & lungs:		
• Pulse slower than 50 beats per minute.	Common	3
• Breathing difficulty.	Infrequent	3
Blood vessels:		
Cold hands, feet.	Common	5
Muscles, bones, joints, genital, urinary, kidneys, liver, allergic:	None expected.	
Blood:		
Unusual bleeding and bruising.	Rare	4
Others:		
• Fatigue, weakness.	Common	4
• Dry mouth, eyes, skin.	Common	5

1- Life-threatening. Seek emergency treatment immediately.
2- Discontinue. Seek emergency treatment.
3- Discontinue. Call doctor right away.
4- Continue. Call doctor when convenient.
5- Continue. Tell doctor at next visit.

WARNINGS & PRECAUTIONS

Don't take if:
- You are allergic to any beta-adrenergic blocker.
- You have asthma.
- You have hay fever symptoms.
- You have taken MAO inhibitors in past 2 weeks.

Before you start, consult your doctor:
- If you have heart disease or poor circulation to the extremities.
- If you have hay fever, asthma, chronic bronchitis, emphysema.
- If you have overactive thyroid function.
- If you have impaired liver or kidney function.
- If you will have surgery within 2 months, including dental surgery, requiring general or spinal anesthesia.
- If you have diabetes or hypoglycemia.

Over age 60:
Adverse reactions and side effects may be more frequent and severe than in younger persons.

Pregnancy:
Risk to unborn child outweighs drug benefits. Don't use.

Breast-feeding:
Drug passes into milk. Avoid drug or discontinue nursing until you finish medicine. Consult doctor for advice on maintaining milk supply.

Infants & children:
Not recommended.

Prolonged use:
Weakens heart muscle contractions.

Skin & sunlight:
No problems expected.

Driving, piloting or hazardous work:
Don't drive or pilot aircraft until you learn how medicine affects you. Don't work around dangerous machinery. Don't climb ladders or work in high places. Danger increases if you drink alcohol or take medicine affecting alertness and reflexes.

Airplane passengers:
No problems expected.

Discontinuing:
Don't discontinue without consulting doctor. Dose may require gradual reduction if you have taken drug for a long time. Doses of other drugs may also require adjustment.

Others:
May mask hypoglycemia.

INTERACTION WITH OTHER DRUGS

GENERIC NAME OR DRUG CLASS	COMBINED EFFECT
Antidiabetics	Increased antidiabetic effect.
Antihistamines	Decreased antihistamine effect.
Antihypertensives	Increased antihypertensive effect.
Antiinflammatory drugs	Decreased antiinflammatory effect.
Barbiturates	Increased barbiturate effect. Dangerous sedation.
Digitalis preparations	Can either increase or decrease heart rate. Improves irregular heartbeat.
Narcotics	Increased narcotic effect. Dangerous sedation.
Phenytoin	Increased metoprolol effect.
Quinidine	Slows heart excessively.
Reserpine	Increased reserpine effect. Excessive sedation and depression.

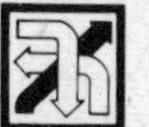

INTERACTION WITH OTHER SUBSTANCES

INTERACTS WITH	COMBINED EFFECT
Alcohol:	Excessive blood pressure drop. Avoid.
Beverages:	None expected.
Cocaine:	Irregular heartbeat. Avoid.
Foods:	None expected.
Marijuana:	Daily use—Impaired circulation to hands and feet.
Tobacco:	Possible irregular heartbeat.

METRONIDAZOLE

BRAND NAMES

Apo-Metronidazole
Flagyl
Metric 21
Metro I.V.
Metryl
Neo-Tric
Novonidazol
PMS Metronidazole
Protostat
Satric
SK-Metronidazole
Trikacide

GENERAL INFORMATION

Habit forming? No
Prescription needed? Yes
Available as generic? No
Drug class: Antiprotozoal

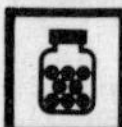

USES

Treatment for infections susceptible to metronidazole, such as trichomoniasis and amoebiasis.

DOSAGE & USAGE INFORMATION

How to take:

- Tablet or capsule—Swallow with liquid or food to lessen stomach irritation. If you can't swallow whole, crumble tablet or open capsule and take with liquid or food.
- Suppositories—Remove wrapper and moisten suppository with water. Gently insert larger end into vagina. Push well into vagina with finger or applicator.

When to take:
At the same times each day.

If you forget a dose:
Take as soon as you remember up to 2 hours late. If more than 2 hours, wait for next scheduled dose (don't double this dose).

What drug does:
Kills organisms causing the infection.

Time lapse before drug works:
Begins in 1 hour. May require regular use for 10 days to cure infection.

Don't take with:

- See Interaction column and consult doctor.
- Non-prescription medicines containing alcohol.

OVERDOSE

Symptoms:
Weakness, nausea, vomiting, diarrhea, confusion, seizures.

What to do:
Overdose unlikely to threaten life. If person takes much larger amount than prescribed, call doctor, poison-control center or hospital emergency room for instructions.

POSSIBLE ADVERSE REACTIONS OR SIDE EFFECTS

SYMPTOMS	FREQUENCY	WHAT TO DO
Brain & nervous system:		
• Mood changes, unsteadiness.	Rare	3
• Dizziness	Infrequent	3
• Headache	Infrequent	3
Skin:		
Rash, hives, redness, itch.	Infrequent	3
Eyes, heart & lungs, blood vessels, muscles, bones, joints, kidneys, liver, allergic, blood:	None expected.	
Ears, nose, throat:		
• Unpleasant taste.	Common	5
• Mouth irritation, soreness or infection.	Infrequent	3
• Sore throat, fever.	Infrequent	3
Digestive:		
• Appetite loss, nausea, stomach pain, diarrhea, vomiting.	Common	3
• Constipation	Infrequent	5
Genital, urinary:		
Vaginal irritation, discharge, dryness.	Infrequent	4
Others:		
• Numbness, tingling, weakness or pain in hands or feet.	Rare	3
• Fatigue, weakness.	Infrequent	4

1 - Life-threatening. Seek emergency treatment immediately.
2 - Discontinue. Seek emergency treatment.
3 - Discontinue. Call doctor right away.
4 - Continue. Call doctor when convenient.
5 - Continue. Tell doctor at next visit.

METRONIDAZOLE

WARNINGS & PRECAUTIONS

Don't take if:

- You are allergic to metronidazole.
- You have had a blood-cell or bone-marrow disorder.

Before you start, consult your doctor:

- If you plan to become pregnant within medication period.
- If you have a brain or nervous-system disorder.
- If you have liver or heart disease.
- If you drink alcohol.

Over age 60:
Adverse reactions and side effects may be more frequent and severe than in younger persons.

Pregnancy:
Risk to unborn child outweighs drug benefits. Manufacturer advises against use during first 3 months and only limited use after that. Don't use.

Breast-feeding:
Drug passes into milk. Avoid drug or discontinue nursing until you finish medicine. Consult doctor for advice on maintaining milk supply.

Infants & children:
Use in children for amoeba infection only under close medical supervision.

Prolonged use:
No problems expected.

Skin & sunlight:
No problems expected.

Driving, piloting or hazardous work:
Avoid if you feel dizzy or unsteady. Otherwise, no problems expected.

Airplane passengers:
No problems expected.

Discontinuing:
Don't discontinue without doctor's advice until you complete prescribed dose, even though symptoms diminish or disappear.

Others:
No problems expected.

INTERACTION WITH OTHER DRUGS

GENERIC NAME OR DRUG CLASS	COMBINED EFFECT
Anticoagulants (oral)	Decreased anticoagulant effect. Possible bleeding or bruising.
Disulfiram	Disulfiram reaction (see page 846). Avoid.
Oxytetracycline	Decreased metronidazole effect.

INTERACTION WITH OTHER SUBSTANCES

INTERACTS WITH	COMBINED EFFECT
Alcohol:	Possible disulfiram reaction (see page 846). Avoid alcohol in *any* form or amount.
Beverages:	None expected.
Cocaine:	Decreased metronidazole effect. Avoid.
Foods:	None expected.
Marijuana:	None expected.
Tobacco:	None expected.

MITOTANE

BRAND NAMES

Lysodren

GENERAL INFORMATION

Habit forming? No
Prescription needed? Yes
Available as generic? No
Drug class: Antineoplastic

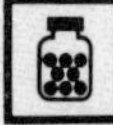

USES

- Treatment for some kinds of cancer.
- Treatment of Cushing's disease.

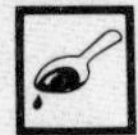

DOSAGE & USAGE INFORMATION

How to take:
Tablet or capsule—Take with liquid after light meal. Don't drink fluid with meals. Drink extra fluids between meals. Avoid sweet and fatty foods.

When to take:
At the same time each day.

If you forget a dose:
Take as soon as you remember. Don't ever double dose.

What drug does:
Suppresses adrenal cortex to prevent manufacture of excess cortisone.

Time lapse before drug works:
2 to 3 weeks for full effect.

Don't take with:
See Interaction column and consult doctor.

OVERDOSE

Symptoms:
Headache, vomiting blood, stupor, seizure.

What to do:
- Dial 0 (operator) or 911 (emergency) for an ambulance or medical help. Then give first aid immediately.
- If patient is unconscious and not breathing, give mouth-to-mouth breathing. If there is no heartbeat, use cardiac massage and mouth-to-mouth breathing (CPR). Don't try to make patient vomit. If you can't get help quickly, take patient to nearest emergency facility.
- Additional emergency information on page 886.

POSSIBLE ADVERSE REACTIONS OR SIDE EFFECTS

SYMPTOMS	FREQUENCY	WHAT TO DO
Brain & nervous system:		
• Dizziness when standing after sitting or lying.	Infrequent	4
• Mental depression.	Common	5
Skin:		
• Rash	Infrequent	4
• Hair loss.	Infrequent	4
• Purple bands on nails.	Infrequent	4
• Darkened skin.	Common	4
Eyes:		
Blurred vision, seeing double.	Infrequent	4
Ears, nose, throat:		
Fever, chills, sore throat.	Infrequent	2
Digestive:		
Appetite loss, nausea, vomiting.	Common	4
Heart & lungs:		
Cough, difficult breathing.	Infrequent	4
Blood vessels:		
Unusual bleeding or bruising.	Infrequent	3
Muscles, bones, joints:		
Numbness and tingling in feet and toes.	Infrequent	4
Genital, urinary:		
Blood in urine.	Rare	3
Kidneys, allergic, blood, liver:	None expected.	
Others:		
Tiredness, weakness.	Infrequent	4

2- Discontinue. Seek emergency treatment.
3- Discontinue. Call doctor right away.
4- Continue. Call doctor when convenient.
5- Continue. Tell doctor at next visit.

WARNINGS & PRECAUTIONS

Don't take if:
You are allergic to adrenocorticosteroids or any antineoplastic drug.

Before you start, consult your doctor:
- If you have liver disease.
- If you have infection.

Over age 60:
Adverse reactions and side effects may be more frequent and severe than in younger persons.

Pregnancy:
Consult doctor. Risk to child is significant.

Breast-feeding:
Drug passes into milk. Don't nurse.

Infants & children:
Use only under care of medical supervisors who are experienced in anticancer drugs.

Prolonged use:
Adverse reactions more likely the longer drug is required.

Skin & sunlight:
No problems expected.

Driving, piloting or hazardous work:
No problems expected.

Airplane passengers:
No problems expected.

Discontinuing:
- Don't discontinue without consulting doctor. Dose may require gradual reduction if you have taken drug for a long time. Doses of other drugs may also require adjustment.
- Some side effects may follow discontinuing. Report any new symptoms.

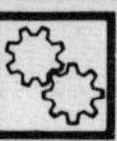

INTERACTION WITH OTHER DRUGS

GENERIC NAME OR DRUG CLASS	COMBINED EFFECT
Corticosteroids	Decreased effect of corticosteroid.
Sedatives	Increased central nervous system depression.
Sleeping pills	Increased central nervous system depression.
Tranquilizers	Increased central nervous system depression.
Antidepressants	Increased central nervous system depression.
Antihistamines	Increased central nervous system depression.
Narcotics	Increased central nervous system depression.
Mind-altering drugs (LSD, etc.)	Increased central nervous system depression.

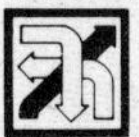

INTERACTION WITH OTHER SUBSTANCES

INTERACTS WITH	COMBINED EFFECT
Alcohol:	Increased depression. Avoid.
Beverages:	No problems expected.
Cocaine:	Increased toxicity. Avoid.
Foods:	Reduced irritation in stomach.
Marijuana:	No problems expected.
Tobacco:	Increased possibility of lung toxicity.

MONAMINE OXIDASE (MAO) INHIBITORS

BRAND AND GENERIC NAMES

Eutonyl
ISOCARBOXAZID
Marplan
Nardil
PARGYLINE
Parnate
PHENELZINE
TRANYLCYPROMINE

GENERAL INFORMATION

Habit forming? No
Prescription needed? Yes
Available as generic? No
Drug class: MAO inhibitor (monamine oxidase inhibitor), antidepressant

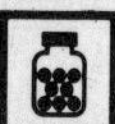

USES

- Treatment for depression.
- Pargyline sometimes used to lower blood pressure.

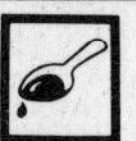

DOSAGE & USAGE INFORMATION

How to take:
Tablet—Swallow with liquid. If you can't swallow whole, crumble tablet and take with liquid or food.

When to take:
At the same times each day.

If you forget a dose:
Take as soon as you remember up to 2 hours late. If more than 2 hours, wait for next scheduled dose (don't double this dose).

What drug does:
Inhibits nerve transmissions in brain that may cause depression.

Time lapse before drug works:
4 to 6 weeks for maximum effect.

Don't take with:
- Non-prescription diet pills, nose drops, medicine for asthma, cough, cold or allergy, or medicine containing caffeine or alcohol.
- See Interaction column and consult doctor.

OVERDOSE

Symptoms:
Restlessness, agitation, fever, convulsions, coma.

What to do:
- Dial 0 (operator) or 911 (emergency) for an ambulance or medical help. Then give first aid immediately.
- Additional emergency information on page 886.

POSSIBLE ADVERSE REACTIONS OR SIDE EFFECTS

SYMPTOMS	FREQUENCY	WHAT TO DO
Brain & nervous system:		
• Fainting	Infrequent	2
• Severe headache.	Infrequent	3
• Dizziness when changing position.	Common	5
• Hallucinations, insomnia, nightmares.	Infrequent	4
Skin:		
Rash	Rare	3
Eyes, blood vessels, kidneys, allergic, blood:	None expected.	
Ears, nose, throat:		
Dry mouth.	Common	5
Digestive:		
• Diarrhea	Infrequent	4
• Constipation	Common	5
• Nausea, vomiting.	Rare	3
Heart & lungs:		
• Rapid or pounding heartbeat.	Infrequent	4
• Chest pain.	Infrequent	3
Muscles, bones, joints:		
Stiff neck.	Rare	3
Genital, urinary:		
Difficult urination.	Common	5
Liver:		
Jaundice (yellow skin and eyes).	Rare	3
Others:		
• Swollen feet, legs.	Infrequent	4
• Fever	Rare	3
• Lower sex drive.	Infrequent	5
• Fatigue, weakness.	Common	4

2- Discontinue. Seek emergency treatment.
3- Discontinue. Call doctor right away.
4- Continue. Call doctor when convenient.
5- Continue. Tell doctor at next visit.

MONAMINE OXIDASE (MAO) INHIBITORS

WARNINGS & PRECAUTIONS

Don't take if:
- You are allergic to any MAO inhibitor.
- You have heart disease, congestive heart failure, heart-rhythm irregularities or high blood pressure.
- You have liver or kidney disease.

Before you start, consult your doctor:
- If you are alcoholic.
- If you have asthma.
- If you have had a stroke.
- If you have diabetes or epilepsy.
- If you have overactive thyroid.
- If you have schizophrenia.
- If you have Parkinson's disease.
- If you have adrenal-gland tumor.
- If you will have surgery within 2 months, including dental surgery, requiring general or spinal anesthesia.

Over age 60:
Not recommended.

Pregnancy:
No proven harm to unborn child. Avoid if possible.

Breast-feeding:
Safety not established. Consult doctor.

Infants & children:
Not recommended.

Prolonged use:
May be toxic to liver.

Skin & sunlight:
May cause rash or intensify sunburn in areas exposed to sun or sunlamp.

Driving, piloting or hazardous work:
Don't drive or pilot aircraft until you learn how medicine affects you. Don't work around dangerous machinery. Don't climb ladders or work in high places. Danger increases if you drink alcohol or take medicine affecting alertness and reflexes.

Airplane passengers:
No problems expected.

Discontinuing:
- Don't discontinue without doctor's advice until you complete prescribed dose, even though symptoms diminish or disappear.
- Follow precautions regarding foods, drinks and other medicines for 2 weeks after discontinuing.

Others:
- May affect blood-sugar levels in patients with diabetes.
- Fever may indicate that MAO inhibitor dose requires adjustment.

INTERACTION WITH OTHER DRUGS

GENERIC NAME OR DRUG CLASS	COMBINED EFFECT
Amphetamines	Blood-pressure rise to life-threatening level.
Anticonvulsants	Changed seizure pattern.
Antidepressants (tricyclic)	Blood-pressure rise to life-threatening level.
Antidiabetics (oral and insulin)	Excessively low blood sugar.
Antihypertensives	Excessively low blood pressure.
Caffeine	Irregular heartbeat or high blood pressure.
Carbamazepine	Fever, seizures. Avoid.
Cyclobenzaprine	Fever, seizures. Avoid.
Diuretics	Excessively low blood pressure.
Guanethidine	Blood-pressure rise to life-threatening level.
Levodopa	Sudden, severe blood-pressure rise.
MAO inhibitors (other)	High fever, convulsions, death.

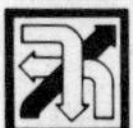

INTERACTION WITH OTHER SUBSTANCES

INTERACTS WITH	COMBINED EFFECT
Alcohol:	Increased sedation to dangerous level.
Beverages:	
Caffeine drinks	Irregular heartbeat or high blood pressure.
Drinks containing tyramine (see page 849).	Blood-pressure rise to life-threatening level.
Cocaine:	Overstimulation. Possibly fatal.
Foods:	
Foods containing tyramine (see page 849).	Blood-pressure rise to life-threatening level.
Marijuana:	Overstimulation. Avoid.
Tobacco:	No proven problems.

NADOLOL

BRAND NAMES

Corgard
Corzide

GENERAL INFORMATION

Habit forming? No
Prescription needed? Yes
Available as generic? No
Drug class: Beta-adrenergic blocker

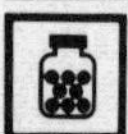

USES

- Reduces angina attacks.
- Stabilizes irregular heartbeat.
- Lowers blood pressure.
- Reduces frequency of migraine headaches. (Does not relieve headache pain.)
- Other uses prescribed by your doctor.

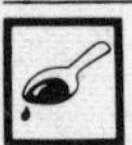

DOSAGE & USAGE INFORMATION

How to take:
Tablet or capsule—Swallow with liquid. If you can't swallow whole, crumble tablet or open capsule and take with liquid or food.

When to take:
With meals or immediately after.

If you forget a dose:
Take as soon as you remember. Return to regular schedule, but allow 3 hours between doses.

What drug does:
- Blocks certain actions of sympathetic nervous system.
- Lowers heart's oxygen requirements.
- Slows nerve impulses through heart.
- Reduces blood vessel contraction in heart, scalp and other body parts.

Time lapse before drug works:
1 to 4 hours.

Don't take with:
Non-prescription drugs or drugs in Interaction column without consulting doctor.

OVERDOSE

Symptoms:
Weakness, slow or weak pulse, blood pressure drop, fainting, convulsions, cold and sweaty skin.

What to do:
- Dial 0 (operator) or 911 (emergency) for an ambulance or medical help. Then give first aid immediately.
- Additional emergency information on page 886.

POSSIBLE ADVERSE REACTIONS OR SIDE EFFECTS

SYMPTOMS	FREQUENCY	WHAT TO DO
Brain & nervous system:		
• Hallucinations, nightmares, insomnia, headache.	Infrequent	3
• Confusion, depression, reduced alertness.	Infrequent	4
• Drowsiness, numbness or tingling of fingers or toes, dizziness.	Common	4
Skin:		
Rash	Rare	3
Eyes:	None expected.	
Ears, nose, throat:		
Sore throat, fever.	Rare	3
Digestive:		
• Diarrhea, nausea.	Common	4
• Constipation	Infrequent	5
Heart & lungs:		
• Pulse slower than 50 beats per minute.	Common	3
• Breathing difficulty.	Infrequent	3
Blood vessels:		
Cold hands, feet.	Common	5
Muscles, bones, joints, genital, urinary, kidneys, liver, allergic:	None expected.	
Blood:		
Unusual bleeding and bruising.	Rare	4
Others:		
• Fatigue, weakness.	Common	4
• Dry mouth, eyes, skin.	Common	5

1- Life-threatening. Seek emergency treatment immediately.
2- Discontinue. Seek emergency treatment.
3- Discontinue. Call doctor right away.
4- Continue. Call doctor when convenient.
5- Continue. Tell doctor at next visit.

WARNINGS & PRECAUTIONS

Don't take if:

- You are allergic to any beta-adrenergic blocker.
- You have asthma.
- You have hay fever symptoms.
- You have taken MAO inhibitors in past 2 weeks.

Before you start, consult your doctor:

- If you have heart disease or poor circulation to the extremities.
- If you have hay fever, asthma, chronic bronchitis, emphysema.
- If you have overactive thyroid function.
- If you have impaired liver or kidney function.
- If you will have surgery within 2 months, including dental surgery, requiring general or spinal anesthesia.
- If you have diabetes or hypoglycemia.

Over age 60:
Adverse reactions and side effects may be more frequent and severe than in younger persons.

Pregnancy:
Risk to unborn child outweighs drug benefits. Don't use.

Breast-feeding:
Drug passes into milk. Avoid drug or discontinue nursing until you finish medicine. Consult doctor for advice on maintaining milk supply.

Infants & children:
Not recommended.

Prolonged use:
Weakens heart muscle contractions.

Skin & sunlight:
No problems expected.

Driving, piloting or hazardous work:
Don't drive or pilot aircraft until you learn how medicine affects you. Don't work around dangerous machinery. Don't climb ladders or work in high places. Danger increases if you drink alcohol or take medicine affecting alertness and reflexes.

Airplane passengers:
No problems expected.

Discontinuing:
Don't discontinue without consulting doctor. Dose may require gradual reduction if you have taken drug for a long time. Doses of other drugs may also require adjustment.

Others:
May mask hypoglycemia.

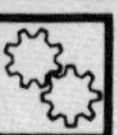

INTERACTION WITH OTHER DRUGS

GENERIC NAME OR DRUG CLASS	COMBINED EFFECT
Antidiabetics	Increased antidiabetic effect.
Antihistamines	Decreased antihistamine effect.
Antihypertensives	Increased antihypertensive effect.
Antiinflammatory drugs	Decreased antiinflammatory effect.
Barbiturates	Increased barbiturate effect. Dangerous sedation.
Digitalis preparations	Can either increase or decrease heart rate. Improves irregular heartbeat.
Narcotics	Increased narcotic effect. Dangerous sedation.
Phenytoin	Increased nadolol effect.
Quinidine	Slows heart excessively.
Reserpine	Increased reserpine effect. Excessive sedation and depression.

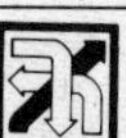

INTERACTION WITH OTHER SUBSTANCES

INTERACTS WITH	COMBINED EFFECT
Alcohol:	Excessive blood-pressure drop. Avoid.
Beverages:	None expected.
Cocaine:	Irregular heartbeat. Avoid.
Foods:	None expected.
Marijuana:	Daily use—Impaired circulation to hands and feet.
Tobacco:	Possible irregular heartbeat.

NAFCILLIN

BRAND NAMES

Nafcil
Nallpen
Unipen

GENERAL INFORMATION

Habit forming? No
Prescription needed? Yes
Available as generic? Yes
Drug class: Antibiotic (penicillin)

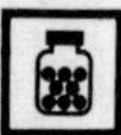

USES

Treatment of bacterial infections that are susceptible to nafcillin.

DOSAGE & USAGE INFORMATION

How to take:

- Tablets or capsules—Swallow with liquid on an empty stomach 1 hour before or 2 hours after eating.
- Liquid—Take with cold beverage. Liquid form is perishable and effective for only 7 days at room temperature. Effective for 14 days if stored in refrigerator. Don't freeze.

When to take:
Follow instructions on prescription label or side of package. Doses should be evenly spaced. For example, 4 times a day means every 6 hours.

If you forget a dose:
Take as soon as you remember. Continue regular schedule.

What drug does:
Destroys susceptible bacteria. Does not kill viruses.

Time lapse before drug works:
May be several days before medicine affects infection.

Don't take with:
See Interaction column and consult doctor.

OVERDOSE

Symptoms:
Severe diarrhea, nausea or vomiting.

What to do:
Overdose unlikely to threaten life. If person takes much larger amount than prescribed, call doctor, poison-control center or hospital emergency room for instructions.

POSSIBLE ADVERSE REACTIONS OR SIDE EFFECTS

SYMPTOMS	FREQUENCY	WHAT TO DO
Brain & nervous system:	None expected.	
Skin: Hives, rash, intense itch soon after a dose.	Rare	1
Eyes:	None expected.	
Ears, nose, throat: Dark or discolored tongue.	Common	5
Digestive: Mild nausea, vomiting, diarrhea.	Infrequent	4
Heart & lungs:	None expected.	
Blood vessels: Unexplained bleeding.	Rare	3
Muscles, bones, joints:	None expected.	
Genital, urinary:	None expected.	
Kidneys:	None expected.	
Liver:	None expected.	
Allergic: Life-threatening anaphylaxis may occur!	Rare	1 See page 888.
Blood:	None expected.	
Others:	None expected.	

1- Life-threatening. Seek emergency treatment immediately.
2- Discontinue. Seek emergency treatment.
3- Discontinue. Call doctor right away.
4- Continue. Call doctor when convenient.
5- Continue. Tell doctor at next visit.
6- No action necessary.

WARNINGS & PRECAUTIONS

Don't take if:
You are allergic to nafcillin, cephalosporin antibiotics, other penicillins or penicillamine. Life-threatening reaction may occur.

Before you start, consult your doctor:
If you are allergic to any substance or drug.

Over age 60:
You may have skin reactions, particularly around genitals and anus.

Pregnancy:
Studies inconclusive on harm to unborn child. Animal studies show fetal abnormalities. Decide with your doctor whether drug benefits justify risk to unborn child.

Breast-feeding:
Drug passes into milk. Child may become sensitive to penicillins and have allergic reactions to penicillin drugs. Avoid nafcillin or discontinue nursing until you finish medicine. Consult doctor for advice on maintaining milk supply.

Infants & children:
No problems expected.

Prolonged use:
You may become more susceptible to infections caused by germs not responsive to nafcillin.

Skin & sunlight:
No problems expected.

Driving, piloting or hazardous work:
Usually not dangerous. Most hazardous reactions likely to occur a few minutes after taking nafcillin.

Airplane passengers:
No problems expected.

Discontinuing:
Don't discontinue without doctor's advice until you complete prescribed dose, even though symptoms diminish or disappear.

Others:
Absorption of this drug in oral form is unpredictable. Injections are more reliable.

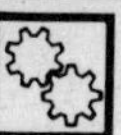

INTERACTION WITH OTHER DRUGS

GENERIC NAME OR DRUG CLASS	COMBINED EFFECT
Chloramphenicol	Decreased effect of both drugs.
Erythromycins	Decreased effect of both drugs.
Paromomycin	Decreased effect of both drugs.
Tetracyclines	Decreased effect of both drugs.
Troleandomycin	Decreased effect of both drugs.

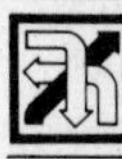

INTERACTION WITH OTHER SUBSTANCES

INTERACTS WITH	COMBINED EFFECT
Alcohol:	Occasional stomach irritation.
Beverages:	None expected.
Cocaine:	No proven problems.
Foods:	None expected.
Marijuana:	No proven problems.
Tobacco:	None expected.

NALIDIXIC ACID

BRAND NAMES

NegGram

GENERAL INFORMATION

Habit forming? No
Prescription needed? Yes
Available as generic? No
Drug class: Antimicrobial

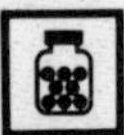

USES

Treatment for urinary-tract infections.

DOSAGE & USAGE INFORMATION

How to take:

- Tablet—Swallow with food or milk to lessen stomach irritation. If you can't swallow whole, crumble tablet and take with liquid or food.
- Liquid—Take with liquid or food.

When to take:
At the same times each day.

If you forget a dose:
Take as soon as you remember up to 2 hours late. If more than 2 hours, wait for next scheduled dose (don't double this dose).

What drug does:
Destroys bacteria susceptible to nalidixic acid.

Time lapse before drug works:
1 to 2 weeks.

Don't take with:
See Interaction column and consult doctor.

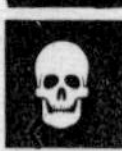

OVERDOSE

Symptoms:
Lethargy, stomach upset, behavioral changes, convulsions and stupor.

What to do:

- Dial 0 (operator) or 911 (emergency) for an ambulance or medical help. Then give first aid immediately.
- If patient is unconscious and not breathing, give mouth-to-mouth breathing. If there is no heartbeat, use cardiac massage and mouth-to-mouth breathing (CPR). Don't try to make patient vomit. If you can't get help quickly, take patient to nearest emergency facility.
- Additional emergency information on page 886.

POSSIBLE ADVERSE REACTIONS OR SIDE EFFECTS

SYMPTOMS	FREQUENCY	WHAT TO DO
Brain & nervous system:		
Dizziness, drowsiness.	Infrequent	4
Skin:		
• Rash, itch.	Common	3
• Paleness	Rare	3
Eyes:		
Decreased, blurred, or double vision; halos around lights or excess brightness; changes in color vision.	Common	3
Ears, nose, throat:		
Sore throat or fever.	Rare	3
Digestive:		
• Severe stomach pain, pale stool.	Rare	3
• Nausea, vomiting, diarrhea.	Common	3
Heart & lungs, muscles, bones, joints, genital, urinary, kidneys, allergic, blood:	None expected.	
Blood vessels:		
Unusual bruising or bleeding.	Rare	3
Liver:		
Jaundice (yellow skin and eyes).	Rare	3
Others:		
Fatigue, weakness.	Rare	3

1- Life-threatening. Seek emergency treatment immediately.
2- Discontinue. Seek emergency treatment.
3- Discontinue. Call doctor right away.
4- Continue. Call doctor when convenient.

WARNINGS & PRECAUTIONS

Don't take if:
- You are allergic to nalidixic acid.
- You have a seizure disorder (epilepsy, convulsions).

Before you start, consult your doctor:
- If you plan to become pregnant within medication period.
- If you have or have had kidney or liver disease.
- If you have impaired circulation of the brain (hardened arteries).
- If you have Parkinson's disease.
- If you have diabetes (it may affect urine-sugar tests).

Over age 60:
Adverse reactions and side effects may be more frequent and severe than in younger persons.

Pregnancy:
Risk to unborn child outweighs drug benefits. Don't use, especially during first 3 months.

Breast-feeding:
No problems expected, unless you have impaired kidney function. Consult doctor.

Infants & children:
Don't give to infants younger than 3 months.

Prolonged use:
No problems expected.

Skin & sunlight:
May cause rash or intensify sunburn in areas exposed to sun or sunlamp.

Driving, piloting or hazardous work:
Avoid if you feel drowsy, dizzy or have vision problems. Otherwise, no problems expected.

Airplane passengers:
No problems expected.

Discontinuing:
Don't discontinue without consulting doctor. Dose may require gradual reduction if you have taken drug for a long time. Doses of other drugs may also require adjustment.

Others:
Periodic blood counts and liver- and kidney-function tests recommended.

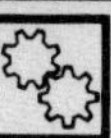

INTERACTION WITH OTHER DRUGS

GENERIC NAME OR DRUG CLASS	COMBINED EFFECT
Antacids	Decreased absorption of nalidixic acid.
Anticoagulants (oral)	Increased anticoagulant effect.
Nitrofurantoin	Decreased effect of nalidixic acid.
Probenecid	Decreased effect of nalidixic acid.
Vitamin C (in large doses)	Increased effect of nalidixic acid.

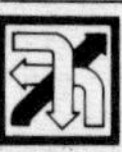

INTERACTION WITH OTHER SUBSTANCES

INTERACTS WITH	COMBINED EFFECT
Alcohol:	Impaired alertness, judgment and coordination.
Beverages:	None expected.
Cocaine:	Impaired judgment and coordination.
Foods:	None expected.
Marijuana:	Impaired alertness, judgment and coordination.
Tobacco:	None expected.

NAPROXEN

BRAND NAMES

Anaprox
Apo-Naproxen
Naprosyn
Novonaprox

GENERAL INFORMATION

Habit forming? No
Prescription needed? Yes
Available as generic? No
Drug class: Antiinflammatory (non-steroid)

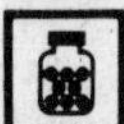

USES

- Treatment for joint pain, stiffness, inflammation and swelling of arthritis and gout.
- Pain reliever.
- Treatment for dysmenorrhea (painful or difficult menstruation).

DOSAGE & USAGE INFORMATION

How to take:
Tablet—Swallow with liquid or food to lessen stomach irritation. If you can't swallow whole, crumble tablet and take with liquid or food.

When to take:
At the same times each day.

If you forget a dose:
Take as soon as you remember up to 2 hours late. If more than 2 hours, wait for next scheduled dose (don't double this dose).

What drug does:
Reduces tissue concentration of prostaglandins (hormones which produce inflammation and pain).

Time lapse before drug works:
Begins in 4 to 24 hours. May require 3 weeks regular use for maximum benefit.

Don't take with:
See Interaction column and consult doctor.

OVERDOSE

Symptoms:
Confusion, agitation, incoherence, convulsions, possible hemorrhage from stomach or intestine, coma.

What to do:
- Dial 0 (operator) or 911 (emergency) for an ambulance or medical help. Then give first aid immediately.
- Additional emergency information on page 886.

POSSIBLE ADVERSE REACTIONS OR SIDE EFFECTS

SYMPTOMS	FREQUENCY	WHAT TO DO
Brain & nervous system:		
• Depression, drowsiness.	Infrequent	4
• Convulsions, confusion.	Rare	3
• Dizziness	Common	4
• Headache	Common	5
Skin:		
Rash, hives or itch.	Rare	3
Eyes:		
Blurred vision.	Rare	3
Ears, nose, throat:		
Ringing in ears.	Infrequent	4
Digestive:		
• Bloody or black, tarry stools.	Rare	3
• Nausea, pain.	Common	4
• Constipation or diarrhea, vomiting.	Infrequent	4
Heart & lungs:		
Breathing difficulty, tightness in chest, rapid heartbeat.	Rare	3
Blood vessels:		
Unusual bleeding or bruising.	Rare	3
Muscles, bones, joints:		
Swollen feet, legs.	Infrequent	4
Genital, urinary:		
• Bloody urine.	Rare	3
• Difficult, painful or frequent urination.	Rare	4
Kidneys, allergic, blood:	None expected.	
Liver:		
Jaundice (yellow skin and eyes).	Rare	3
Others:		
Fatigue, weakness.	Rare	4

3- Discontinue. Call doctor right away.
4- Continue. Call doctor when convenient.
5- Continue. Tell doctor at next visit.

WARNINGS & PRECAUTIONS

Don't take if:
- You are allergic to aspirin or any non-steroid, antiinflammatory drug.
- You have gastritis, peptic ulcer, enteritis, ileitis, ulcerative colitis, asthma, heart failure, high blood pressure or bleeding problems.
- You have had recent rectal bleeding and suppository form has been prescribed.
- Patient is younger than 15.

Before you start, consult your doctor:
- If you have epilepsy.
- If you have Parkinson's disease.
- If you have been mentally ill.
- If you have had kidney disease or impaired kidney function.

Over age 60:
Adverse reactions and side effects may be more frequent and severe than in younger persons.

Pregnancy:
Studies inconclusive on harm to unborn child. Decide with your doctor whether drug benefits justify risk to unborn child.

Breast-feeding:
May harm child. Avoid.

Infants & children:
Not recommended for anyone younger than 15. Use only under medical supervision.

Prolonged use:
- Eye damage.
- Reduced hearing.
- Sore throat, fever.
- Weight gain.

Skin & sunlight:
No problems expected.

Driving, piloting or hazardous work:
Don't drive or pilot aircraft until you learn how medicine affects you. Don't work around dangerous machinery. Don't climb ladders or work in high places. Danger increases if you drink alcohol or take medicine affecting alertness and reflexes, such as antihistamines, tranquilizers, sedatives, pain medicine, narcotics and mind-altering drugs.

Airplane passengers:
No problems expected.

Discontinuing:
Don't discontinue without consulting doctor. Dose may require gradual reduction if you have taken drug for a long time. Doses of other drugs may also require adjustment.

Others:
No problems expected.

INTERACTION WITH OTHER DRUGS

GENERIC NAME OR DRUG CLASS	COMBINED EFFECT
Anticoagulants, (oral)	Increased risk of bleeding.
Aspirin	Increased risk of stomach ulcer.
Cortisone drugs	Increased risk of stomach ulcer.
Furosemide	Decreased diuretic effect of furosemide.
Oxyphenbutazone	Possible stomach ulcer.
Phenylbutazone	Possible stomach ulcer.
Probenecid	Increased naproxen effect.
Thyroid hormones	Rapid heartbeat, blood-pressure rise.

INTERACTION WITH OTHER SUBSTANCES

INTERACTS WITH	COMBINED EFFECT
Alcohol:	Possible stomach ulcer or bleeding.
Beverages:	None expected.
Cocaine:	None expected.
Foods:	None expected.
Marijuana:	Increased pain relief from naproxen.
Tobacco:	None expected.

NARCOTIC ANALGESICS

BRAND AND GENERIC NAMES

Acetaminophen w/Codeine
Actifed-C Expectorant
A.P.C. w/Codeine Phosphate Tablets
Ascriptin w/Codeine
Calcidrine Syrup
Dimetane Expectorant-DC
Empirin w/Codeine
Fiorinal w/Codeine
Novahistine Expectorant

See complete brand and generic names list page 828.

GENERAL INFORMATION

Habit forming? Yes
Prescription needed? Yes
Available as generic? Yes
Drug class: Narcotic

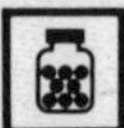

USES

- Relieves pain.
- Suppresses cough.

DOSAGE & USAGE INFORMATION

How to take:
- Tablet or capsule—Swallow with liquid. If you can't swallow whole, crumble tablet or open capsule and take with liquid or food.
- Drops or liquid—Dilute dose in beverage before swallowing.

When to take:
When needed. No more often than every 4 hours.

If you forget a dose:
Take as soon as you remember. Wait 4 hours for next dose.

What drug does:
- Blocks pain messages to brain and spinal cord.
- Reduces sensitivity of brain's cough-control center.

Time lapse before drug works:
30 minutes.

Don't take with:
See Interaction column and consult doctor.

OVERDOSE

Symptoms:
Deep sleep, slow breathing; slow pulse; flushed, warm skin; constricted pupils.

What to do:
- Dial 0 (operator) or 911 (emergency) for an ambulance or medical help. Then give first aid immediately.
- If patient is unconscious and not breathing, give mouth-to-mouth breathing. If there is no heartbeat, use cardiac massage and mouth-to-mouth breathing (CPR). Don't try to make patient vomit. If you can't get help quickly, take patient to nearest emergency facility.
- Additional emergency information on page 886.

POSSIBLE ADVERSE REACTIONS OR SIDE EFFECTS

SYMPTOMS	FREQUENCY	WHAT TO DO
Brain & nervous system:		
• Depression	Rare	4
• Dizziness	Common	4
Skin:		
• Hives, rash, itch, face swelling.	Rare	3
• Flushed face.	Common	4
Eyes:		
Blurred vision.	Rare	4
Ears, nose, throat:	None expected.	
Digestive:		
Severe constipation, abdominal pain, vomiting.	Infrequent	3
Heart & lungs:		
Slow heartbeat, irregular breathing.	Rare	3
Blood vessels:	None expected.	
Muscles, bones, joints:	None expected.	
Genital, urinary:		
Difficult urination.	Common	4
Kidneys:	None expected.	
Liver:	None expected.	
Allergic:	None expected.	
Blood:	None expected.	
Others:		
Unusual tiredness.	Common	4

1- Life-threatening. Seek emergency treatment immediately.
2- Discontinue. Seek emergency treatment.
3- Discontinue. Call doctor right away.
4- Continue. Call doctor when convenient.
5- Continue. Tell doctor at next visit.
6- No action necessary.

WARNINGS & PRECAUTIONS

Don't take if:
You are allergic to any narcotic.

Before you start, consult your doctor:
- If you have impaired liver or kidney function.
- If you will have surgery within 2 months, including dental surgery, requiring general or spinal anesthesia.

Over age 60:
More likely to be drowsy, dizzy, unsteady or constipated. Use only if absolutely necessary.

Pregnancy:
Decide with your doctor whether drug benefits justify risk to unborn child. Abuse by pregnant woman will result in addicted newborn. Withdrawal of newborn can be life-threatening.

Breast-feeding:
Drug filters into milk. May harm child. Avoid.

Infants & children:
Not recommended.

Prolonged use:
Causes psychological and physical dependence (addiction).

Skin & sunlight:
May cause rash or intensify sunburn in areas exposed to sun or sunlamp.

Driving, piloting or hazardous work:
Don't drive or pilot aircraft until you learn how medicine affects you. Don't work around dangerous machinery. Don't climb ladders or work in high places. Danger increases if you drink alcohol or take medicine affecting alertness and reflexes, such as antihistamines, tranquilizers, sedatives, pain medicine, narcotics and mind-altering drugs.

Airplane passengers:
No proven problems.

Discontinuing:
May be unnecessary to finish medicine. Follow doctor's instructions.

Others:
No problems expected.

INTERACTION WITH OTHER DRUGS

GENERIC NAME OR DRUG CLASS	COMBINED EFFECT
Analgesics (other)	Increased analgesic effect.
Antidepressants	Increased sedative effect.
Antihistamines	Increased sedative effect.
Mind-altering drugs	Increased sedative effect.
Narcotics (other)	Increased narcotic effect.
Phenothiazines	Increased phenothiazine effect.
Sedatives	Increased sedative effect.
Sleep inducers	Increased sedative effect.
Tranquilizers	Increased sedative effect.

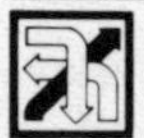

INTERACTION WITH OTHER SUBSTANCES

INTERACTS WITH	COMBINED EFFECT
Alcohol:	Increases alcohol's intoxicating effect. Avoid.
Beverages:	None expected.
Cocaine:	Increased cocaine toxic effects. Avoid.
Foods:	None expected.
Marijuana:	Impairs physical and mental performance. Avoid.
Tobacco:	None expected.

NEOMYCIN (ORAL)

BRAND NAMES

Mycifradin
Neobiotic

GENERAL INFORMATION

Habit forming? No
Prescription needed? Yes
Available as generic? Yes
Drug class: Antibiotic

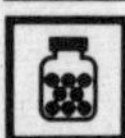

USES

- Clears intestinal tract of germs prior to surgery.
- Treats some causes of diarrhea.
- Lowers blood cholesterol.
- Lessens symptoms of hepatic coma.

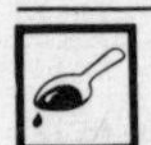

DOSAGE & USAGE INFORMATION

How to take:
Tablet or capsule—Swallow with liquid or food to lessen stomach irritation. If you can't swallow whole, crumble tablet or open capsule and take with liquid or food.

When to take:
According to directions on prescription.

If you forget a dose:
Take as soon as you remember up to 2 hours late. If more than 2 hours, wait for next scheduled dose (don't double this dose).

What drug does:
Kills germs susceptible to neomycin.

Time lapse before drug works:
2 to 3 days.

Don't take with:
See Interaction column and consult doctor.

OVERDOSE

Symptoms:
Loss of hearing, difficulty breathing, respiratory paralysis.

What to do:
- Dial 0 (operator) or 911 (emergency) for an ambulance or medical help. Then give first aid immediately.
- If patient is unconscious and not breathing, give mouth-to-mouth breathing. If there is no heartbeat, use cardiac massage and mouth-to-mouth breathing (CPR). Don't try to make patient vomit. If you can't get help quickly, take patient to nearest emergency facility.
- Additional emergency information on page 886.

POSSIBLE ADVERSE REACTIONS OR SIDE EFFECTS

SYMPTOMS	FREQUENCY	WHAT TO DO
Brain & nervous system:		
• Clumsiness	Rare	3
• Dizziness	Rare	3
Skin:		
Rash	Rare	3
Eyes:	None expected.	
Ears, nose, throat:		
• Hearing loss.	Rare	3
• Ringing or noises in ear.	Rare	3
Digestive:		
• Sore mouth.	Common	4
• Nausea, vomiting.	Common	4
• Frothy stools.	Rare	3
• Gaseousness	Rare	3
Heart & lungs:	None expected.	
Blood vessels:	None expected.	
Muscles, bones, joints:	None expected.	
Genital, urinary:		
Decreased frequency of urination.	Rare	3
Kidneys, allergic, blood, liver:	None expected.	

1- Life-threatening. Seek emergency treatment immediately.
2- Discontinue. Seek emergency treatment.
3- Discontinue. Call doctor right away.
4- Continue. Call doctor when convenient.
5- Continue. Tell doctor at next visit.
6- No action necessary.

WARNINGS & PRECAUTIONS

Don't take if:
You are allergic to neomycin or any aminoglycoside. (See Interactions column.)

Before you start, consult your doctor:
- If you will have surgery within 2 months, including dental surgery, requiring general or spinal anesthesia.
- If you have hearing loss or loss of balance secondary to 8th cranial nerve disease.
- If you have intestinal obstruction.
- If you have myasthenia gravis, Parkinson's disease, kidney disease, ulcers in intestines.

Over age 60:
Adverse reactions and side effects may be more frequent and severe than in younger persons.

Pregnancy:
No proven harm to unborn child. Avoid if possible.

Breast-feeding:
Avoid if possible.

Infants & children:
Only under close medical supervision.

Prolonged use:
Adverse effects more likely.

Skin & sunlight:
No problems expected.

Driving, piloting or hazardous work:
No problems expected.

Airplane passengers:
No problems expected.

Discontinuing:
May be unnecessary to finish medicine. Follow doctor's instructions.

INTERACTION WITH OTHER DRUGS

GENERIC NAME OR DRUG CLASS	COMBINED EFFECT
Aminoglycosides: Amikacin, Gentamicin, Kanamycin, Streptomycin, Tobramycin	Increases chance of toxic effect on hearing, kidney, muscles.
Vancomycin Mercaptomerin Furosemide Capreomycin Cisplatin Ethacrynic acid	Increases chance of toxic effects on hearing, kidneys.
Cephalothin	Increased chance of toxic effect on kidneys.

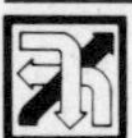

INTERACTION WITH OTHER SUBSTANCES

INTERACTS WITH	COMBINED EFFECT
Alcohol:	Increased chance of toxicity. Avoid.
Beverages:	No problems expected.
Cocaine:	Increased chance of toxicity. Avoid.
Foods:	No problems expected.
Marijuana:	Increased chance of toxicity. Avoid.
Tobacco:	No problems expected.

NEOSTIGMINE

BRAND NAMES

Prostigmin

GENERAL INFORMATION

Habit forming? No
Prescription needed? Yes
Available as generic? Yes
Drug class: Cholinergic (anticholinesterase)

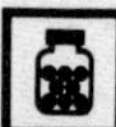

USES

- Treatment of myasthenia gravis.
- Treatment of urinary retention and abdominal distention.
- Antidote to adverse effects of muscle relaxants used in surgery.

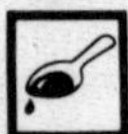

DOSAGE & USAGE INFORMATION

How to take:
Tablet—Swallow with liquid or food to lessen stomach irritation.

When to take:
As directed, usually 3 or 4 times a day.

If you forget a dose:
Take as soon as you remember up to 2 hours late. If more than 2 hours, wait for next scheduled dose (don't double this dose).

What drug does:
Inhibits the chemical activity of an enzyme (cholinesterase) so nerve impulses can cross the junction of nerves and muscles.

Time lapse before drug works:
3 hours.

Don't take with:
See Interaction column and consult doctor.

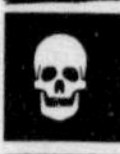

OVERDOSE

Symptoms:
Muscle weakness, cramps, twitching or clumsiness; severe diarrhea, nausea, vomiting, stomach cramps or pain; breathing difficulty; confusion, irritability, nervousness, restlessness, fear; unusually slow heartbeat; seizures.

What to do:
- Dial 0 (operator) or 911 (emergency) for an ambulance or medical help. Then give first aid immediately.
- Additional emergency information on page 886.

POSSIBLE ADVERSE REACTIONS OR SIDE EFFECTS

SYMPTOMS	FREQUENCY	WHAT TO DO
Brain & nervous system:		
Confusion, irritability.	Infrequent	2
Skin:	None expected.	
Eyes:		
Constricted pupils, watery eyes.	Infrequent	4
Ears, nose, throat:		
Excess saliva.	Common	4
Digestive:		
Mild diarrhea, nausea, vomiting, stomach cramps or pain.	Common	3
Heart & lungs:		
Lung congestion.	Infrequent	4
Blood vessels:	None expected.	
Muscles, bones, joints:	None expected.	
Genital, urinary:		
Frequent urge to urinate.	Infrequent	4
Kidneys:	None expected.	
Liver:	None expected.	
Allergic:	None expected.	
Blood:	None expected.	
Others:		
Unusual sweating.	Common	4

1-Life-threatening. Seek emergency treatment immediately.
2-Discontinue. Seek emergency treatment.
3-Discontinue. Call doctor right away.
4-Continue. Call doctor when convenient.
5-Continue. Tell doctor at next visit.
6-No action necessary.

WARNINGS & PRECAUTIONS

Don't take if:
- You are allergic to any cholinergic or bromide.
- You take mecamylamine.

Before you start, consult your doctor:
- If you plan to become pregnant within medication period.
- If you have bronchial asthma.
- If you have heartbeat irregularities.
- If you have urinary obstruction or urinary-tract infection.

Over age 60:
Adverse reactions and side effects may be more frequent and severe than in younger persons.

Pregnancy:
No proven harm to unborn child. Avoid if possible. May increase uterus contractions close to delivery.

Breast-feeding:
No problems expected, but consult doctor.

Infants & children:
Not recommended.

Prolonged use:
Medication may lose effectiveness. Discontinuing for a few days may restore effect.

Skin & sunlight:
No problems expected.

Driving, piloting or hazardous work:
Don't drive or pilot aircraft until you learn how medicine affects you. Don't work around dangerous machinery. Don't climb ladders or work in high places. Danger increases if you drink alcohol or take medicine affecting alertness and reflexes, such as antihistamines, tranquilizers, sedatives, pain medicine, narcotics and mind-altering drugs.

Airplane passengers:
No problems expected.

Discontinuing:
Don't discontinue without doctor's advice until you complete prescribed dose, even though symptoms diminish or disappear.

Others:
No problems expected.

INTERACTION WITH OTHER DRUGS

GENERIC NAME OR DRUG CLASS	COMBINED EFFECT
Anesthetics (local or general)	Decreased neostigmine effect.
Antiarrhythmics	Decreased neostigmine effect.
Antibiotics	Decreased neostigmine effect.
Anticholinergics	Decreased neostigmine effect. May mask severe side effects.
Cholinergics (other)	Reduced intestinal-tract function. Possible brain and nervous-system toxicity.
Mecamylamine	Decreased neostigmine effect.
Quinidine	Decreased neostigmine effect.

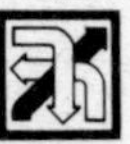

INTERACTION WITH OTHER SUBSTANCES

INTERACTS WITH	COMBINED EFFECT
Alcohol:	No proven problems with small doses.
Beverages:	None expected.
Cocaine:	Decreased neostigmine effect. Avoid.
Foods:	None expected.
Marijuana:	No proven problems.
Tobacco:	No proven problems.

NIACIN (NICOTINIC ACID)

BRAND NAMES

Diacin	Nico-Span	Nicotym
N-Caps	Nicobid	Novoniacin
Niac	Nicocap	Span-Niacin
Niacin	Nicolar	SK-Niacin
Nicalex	Nicotinex	Tega-Span
Nico-400	Nicotinyl alcohol	Vasotherm

Numerous other multiple vitamin-mineral supplements.

GENERAL INFORMATION

Habit forming? No
Prescription needed? Tablets: No
Liquid, capsules: Yes
Available as generic? Yes
Drug class: Vitamin supplement, vasodilator, antihyperlipidemic

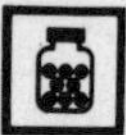

USES

- Replacement for niacin deficiency caused by inadequate diet.
- Treatment for vertigo (dizziness) and ringing in ears.
- Prevention of premenstrual headache.
- Reduction of blood levels of cholesterol and triglycerides.
- Treatment for pellagra.

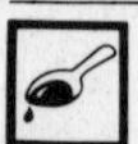

DOSAGE & USAGE INFORMATION

How to take:
- Tablet, capsule or liquid—Swallow with liquid or food to lessen stomach irritation.
- Extended-release tablets or capsules—Swallow each dose whole.

When to take:
At the same times each day.

If you forget a dose:
Take as soon as you remember. Wait 4 hours for next dose.

What drug does:
- Corrects niacin deficiency.
- Dilates blood vessels.
- In large doses, decreases cholesterol production.

Time lapse before drug works:
15 to 20 minutes.

Don't take with:
See Interaction column and consult doctor.

OVERDOSE

Symptoms:
Body flush, nausea, vomiting, abdominal cramps, diarrhea, weakness, lightheadedness, fainting, sweating.

What to do:
Overdose unlikely to threaten life. If person takes much larger amount than prescribed, call doctor, poison-control center or hospital emergency room for instructions.

POSSIBLE ADVERSE REACTIONS OR SIDE EFFECTS

SYMPTOMS	FREQUENCY	WHAT TO DO
Brain & nervous system: Headache, dizziness, faintness.	Infrequent	4
Skin: "Hot" feeling, flush.	Infrequent	6
Eyes:	None expected.	
Ears, nose, throat:	None expected.	
Digestive:	None expected.	
Heart & lungs:	None expected.	
Blood vessels:	None expected.	
Muscles, bones, joints: Temporary numbness and tingling in hands and feet.	Infrequent	4
Genital, urinary:	None expected.	
Kidneys:	None expected.	
Liver: Jaundice (yellow skin and eyes).	Rare	3
Allergic:	None expected.	
Blood:	None expected.	
Others:	None expected.	

1- Life-threatening. Seek emergency treatment immediately.
2- Discontinue. Seek emergency treatment.
3- Discontinue. Call doctor right away.
4- Continue. Call doctor when convenient.
5- Continue. Tell doctor at next visit.
6- No action necessary.

WARNINGS & PRECAUTIONS

Don't take if:
- You are allergic to niacin or any niacin-containing vitamin mixtures.
- You have impaired liver function.
- You have active peptic ulcer.

Before you start, consult your doctor:
- If you have diabetes.
- If you have gout.
- If you have gallbladder or liver disease.

Over age 60:
Response to drug cannot be predicted. Dose must be individualized.

Pregnancy:
Risk to unborn child outweighs drug benefits. Don't use.

Breast-feeding:
Studies inconclusive. Consult doctor.

Infants & children:
- Use only under supervision.
- Keep vitamin-mineral supplements out of children's reach.

Prolonged use:
Possible impaired liver function.

Skin & sunlight:
No problems expected.

Driving, piloting or hazardous work:
Avoid if you feel dizzy or faint. Otherwise, no problems expected.

Airplane passengers:
No problems expected.

Discontinuing:
May be unnecessary to finish medicine. Follow doctor's instructions.

Others:
- A balanced diet should provide all the niacin a healthy person needs and make supplements unnecessary. Best sources are meat, eggs and dairy products.
- Store in original container in cool, dry, dark place. Bathroom medicine chest too moist.
- Obesity reduces effectiveness.

INTERACTION WITH OTHER DRUGS

GENERIC NAME OR DRUG CLASS	COMBINED EFFECT
Antidiabetics	Decreased antidiabetic effect.
Beta-adrenergic blockers	Excessively low blood pressure.
Guanethidine	Increased guanethidine effect.
Isoniazid	Decreased niacin effect.
Mecamylamine	Excessively low blood pressure.
Methyldopa	Excessively low blood pressure.
Pargyline	Excessively low blood pressure.

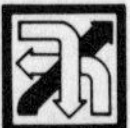

INTERACTION WITH OTHER SUBSTANCES

INTERACTS WITH	COMBINED EFFECT
Alcohol:	Excessively low blood pressure. Use caution.
Beverages:	None expected.
Cocaine:	Increased flushing.
Foods:	None expected.
Marijuana:	None expected.
Tobacco:	Decreased niacin effect.

NICOTINE RESIN COMPLEX

BRAND NAMES

Nicorette

GENERAL INFORMATION

Habit forming? Yes
Prescription needed? Yes
Available as generic? No
Drug class: Antismoking agent

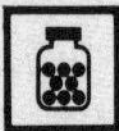

USES

Treats smoking addiction.

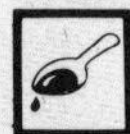

DOSAGE & USAGE INFORMATION

How to take:
Follow detailed instructions on patient instruction sheet provided with prescription.

When to take:
Follow detailed instructions on patient instruction sheet provided with prescription.

If you forget a dose:
Follow detailed instructions on patient instruction sheet provided with prescription.

What drug does:
Satisfies physical craving for nicotine in addicted persons and avoids peaks in blood nicotine level resulting from smoking.

Time lapse before drug works:
30 minutes.

Don't take with:
See Interaction column and consult doctor.

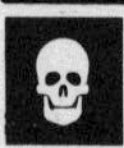

OVERDOSE

Symptoms:
Vomiting, irregular heartbeat.

What to do:
Overdose unlikely to threaten life. If person takes much larger amount than prescribed, call doctor, poison-control center or hospital emergency room for instructions.

POSSIBLE ADVERSE REACTIONS OR SIDE EFFECTS

SYMPTOMS	FREQUENCY	WHAT TO DO
Brain & nervous system:		
• Lightheadedness	Infrequent	4
• Headache	Infrequent	4
Skin:	None expected.	
Eyes:	None expected.	
Ears, nose, throat:		
• Injury to loose teeth.	Common	4
• Tingling in mouth.	Common	5
Digestive:		
• Belching	Common	5
• Mouth irritation.	Common	5
• Excessive salivation.	Common	5
• Nausea & vomiting.	Infrequent	3
• Hiccups	Infrequent	4
• Abdominal pain.	Infrequent	3
Heart & lungs:		
Increased irritability causing heartbeat irregularity.	Frequent	4
Blood vessels:	None expected.	
Muscles, bones, joints:		
Jaw muscle ache.	Common	4
Genital, urinary:	None expected.	
Kidneys, allergic, blood, liver:	None expected.	
Others:	None expected.	

1- Life-threatening. Seek emergency treatment immediately.
2- Discontinue. Seek emergency treatment.
3- Discontinue. Call doctor right away.
4- Continue. Call doctor when convenient.
5- Continue. Tell doctor at next visit.

WARNINGS & PRECAUTIONS

Don't take if:

- You are a non-smoker.
- You are pregnant or intend to become pregnant.
- You recently suffered a heart attack.

Before you start, consult your doctor:

- If you have coronary artery disease.
- If you have active temperomandibular joint disease.
- If you have severe angina.
- If you have peptic ulcer.

Over age 60:
Adverse reactions and side effects may be more frequent and severe than in younger persons.

Pregnancy:
Risk to unborn child outweighs drug benefits. Don't use.

Breast-feeding:
Drug passes into milk. Avoid drug or discontinue nursing until you finish medicine. Consult doctor for advice on maintaining milk supply.

Infants & children:
Don't use.

Prolonged use:
May cause addiction and greater likelihood of toxicity.

Skin & sunlight:
No problems expected.

Driving, piloting or hazardous work:
No problems expected.

Airplane passengers:
No problems expected.

Discontinuing:
May be unnecessary to finish medicine. Follow doctor's instructions.

INTERACTION WITH OTHER DRUGS

GENERIC NAME OR DRUG CLASS	COMBINED EFFECT
Beta-adrenergic blockers	Decreased blood pressure, (slight).
Caffeine	Increased effect of caffeine.
Cortisone drugs	Increased cortisone circulating in blood.
Furosemide	Increased effect of furosemide.
Glutethimide	Increased absorption of glutethimide.
Imipramine	Increased effect of imipramine.
Pentazocine	Increased effect of pentazocine.
Phenacetin	Increased effect of phenacetin.

Additional interactions on page 840.

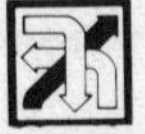

INTERACTION WITH OTHER SUBSTANCES

INTERACTS WITH	COMBINED EFFECT
Alcohol:	Increased cardiac irritability. Avoid.
Beverages:	
Caffeine	Increased cardiac irritability. Avoid any beverage with caffeine.
Cocaine:	Increased cardiac irritability. Avoid.
Foods:	No problems expected.
Marijuana:	Increased toxic effects. Avoid.
Tobacco:	Increased toxic effects. Avoid.

NIFEDIPINE

BRAND NAMES

Adalat
Procardia

GENERAL INFORMATION

Habit forming? No
Prescription needed? Yes
Available as generic? No
Drug class: Calcium-channel blocker, antiarrhythmic, antianginal

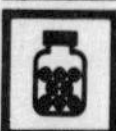

USES

Prevents angina attacks.

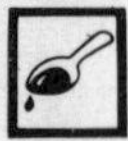

DOSAGE & USAGE INFORMATION

How to take:
Capsule—Swallow with liquid.

When to take:
At the same times each day 1 hour before or 2 hours after eating.

If you forget a dose:
Take as soon as you remember up to 2 hours late. If more than 2 hours, wait for next scheduled dose (don't double this dose).

What drug does:
- Reduces work that heart must perform.
- Reduces normal artery pressure.
- Increases oxygen to heart muscle.

Time lapse before drug works:
1 to 2 hours.

Don't take with:
See Interaction column and consult doctor.

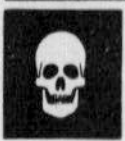

OVERDOSE

Symptoms:
Unusually fast or unusually slow heartbeat, loss of consciousness, cardiac arrest.

What to do:
- Dial 0 (operator) or 911 (emergency) for an ambulance or medical help. Then give first aid immediately.
- If patient is unconscious and not breathing, give mouth-to-mouth breathing. If there is no heartbeat, use cardiac massage and mouth-to-mouth breathing (CPR). Don't try to make patient vomit. If you can't get help quickly, take patient to nearest emergency facility.
- Additional emergency information on page 886.

POSSIBLE ADVERSE REACTIONS OR SIDE EFFECTS

SYMPTOMS	FREQUENCY	WHAT TO DO
Brain & nervous system:		
• Dizziness	Infrequent	4
• Headache	Rare	5
• Fainting	Rare	3
Skin:	None expected.	
Eyes:	None expected.	
Ears, nose, throat:	None expected.	
Digestive:		
Nausea, constipation.	Infrequent	5
Heart & lungs:		
• Unusually fast or unusually slow heartbeat.	Infrequent	3
• Wheezing, cough, shortness of breath.	Infrequent	3
• Chest pain.	Rare	3
Blood vessels:	None expected.	
Muscles, bones, joints:		
• Numbness, tingling in hands and feet.	Infrequent	4
• Swelling of ankles, feet, legs.	Infrequent	4
Genital, urinary:		
Difficult urination.	Infrequent	4
Kidneys:	None expected.	
Liver:	None expected.	
Allergic:	None expected.	
Blood:	None expected.	
Others:		
Tiredness	Common	5

1- Life-threatening. Seek emergency treatment immediately.
2- Discontinue. Seek emergency treatment.
3- Discontinue. Call doctor right away.
4- Continue. Call doctor when convenient.
5- Continue. Tell doctor at next visit.
6- No action necessary.

WARNINGS & PRECAUTIONS

Don't take if:
- You are allergic to nifedipine.
- You have very low blood pressure.

Before you start, consult your doctor:
- If you have kidney or liver disease.
- If you have high blood pressure.
- If you have heart disease other than coronary-artery disease.

Over age 60:
Adverse reactions and side effects may be more frequent and severe than in younger persons.

Pregnancy:
No proven harm to unborn child. Avoid if possible.

Breast-feeding:
Safety not established. Avoid if possible.

Infants & children:
Not recommended.

Prolonged use:
No problems expected.

Skin & sunlight:
No problems expected.

Driving, piloting or hazardous work:
Avoid if you feel dizzy. Otherwise, no problems expected.

Airplane passengers:
No problems expected.

Discontinuing:
Don't discontinue without doctor's advice until you complete prescribed dose, even though symptoms diminish or disappear.

Others:
- Learn to check your own pulse rate. If it drops to 50 beats per minute or lower, don't take nifedipine until you consult your doctor.
- Drug may lower blood-sugar level if daily dose is more than 60 mg.

INTERACTION WITH OTHER DRUGS

GENERIC NAME OR DRUG CLASS	COMBINED EFFECT
Anticoagulants (oral)	Increased anticoagulant effect.
Anticonvulsants (hydantoin)	Increased anticonvulsant effect.
Antihypertensives	Dangerous blood-pressure drop.
Beta-adrenergic blockers	Possible irregular heartbeat.
Calcium (large doses)	Decreased nifedipine effect.
Diuretics	Dangerous blood-pressure drop.
Digitalis preparations	Increased digitalis effect. May need to reduce dose.
Disopyramide	May cause dangerously slow, fast or irregular heartbeat.
Nitrates	Reduced angina attacks.
Quinidine	Increased quinidine effect.
Vitamin D (large doses)	Decreased nifedipine effect.

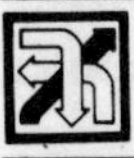

INTERACTION WITH OTHER SUBSTANCES

INTERACTS WITH	COMBINED EFFECT
Alcohol:	Dangerously low blood pressure. Avoid.
Beverages:	None expected.
Cocaine:	Possible irregular heartbeat. Avoid.
Foods:	None expected.
Marijuana:	Possible irregular heartbeat. Avoid.
Tobacco:	Possible rapid heartbeat. Avoid.

NITROFURANTOIN

BRAND NAMES

Apo-Nitrofurantoin
Cyantin
Furadantin
Furalan
Furaloid
Furantoin
Furatine
Macrodantin
Nephronex
Nifuran
Nitrex
Nitrodan
Novofuran
Sarodant
Trantoin
Urotoin

GENERAL INFORMATION

Habit forming? No
Prescription needed? Yes
Available as generic? Yes
Drug class: Antimicrobial

USES

Treatment for urinary-tract infections.

DOSAGE & USAGE INFORMATION

How to take:

- Tablet or capsule—Swallow with food or milk to lessen stomach irritation. If you can't swallow whole, crumble tablet or open capsule and take with liquid or food.
- Liquid—Shake well and take with food. Use a measuring spoon to ensure accuracy.

When to take:
At the same times each day.

If you forget a dose:
Take as soon as you remember up to 2 hours late. If more than 2 hours, wait for next scheduled dose (don't double this dose).

What drug does:
Prevents susceptible bacteria in the urinary tract from growing and multiplying.

Time lapse before drug works:
1 to 2 weeks.

Don't take with:
See Interaction column and consult doctor.

OVERDOSE

Symptoms:
Nausea, vomiting, abdominal pain, diarrhea.

What to do:
Overdose unlikely to threaten life. If person takes much larger amount than prescribed, call doctor, poison-control center or hospital emergency room for instructions.

POSSIBLE ADVERSE REACTIONS OR SIDE EFFECTS

SYMPTOMS	FREQUENCY	WHAT TO DO
Brain & nervous system:		
Dizziness, drowsiness, headache.	Infrequent	4
Skin:		
• Rash, itch.	Infrequent	3
• Numbness, tingling or burning of face or mouth.	Infrequent	3
• Paleness	Infrequent	4
Ears, nose, throat:		
In children, discolored teeth (liquid).	Infrequent	4
Digestive:		
Diarrhea, appetite loss, nausea, vomiting.	Common	3
Heart & lungs:		
Chest pain, cough, breathing difficulty.	Common	3
Eyes, blood vessels, muscles, bones, joints, kidneys, blood:	None expected.	
Genital, urinary:		
Rusty-color or brown urine.	Common	6
Liver:		
Jaundice (yellow skin and eyes).	Rare	3
Allergic:		
Life-threatening anaphylaxis may occur!	Rare	1 See page 888.
Others:		
• Chills or unexplained fever.	Common	3
• Fatigue, weakness	Infrequent	3

1-Life-threatening. Seek emergency treatment immediately.
2-Discontinue. Seek emergency treatment.
3-Discontinue. Call doctor right away.
4-Continue. Call doctor when convenient.
5-Continue. Tell doctor at next visit.
6-No action necessary.

WARNINGS & PRECAUTIONS

Don't take if:
- You are allergic to nitrofurantoin.
- You have impaired kidney function.
- You drink alcohol.

Before you start, consult your doctor:
- If you are prone to allergic reactions.
- If you are pregnant and within 2 weeks of delivery.
- If you have had kidney disease, lung disease, anemia, nerve damage, or G6PD deficiency (a metabolic deficiency).
- If you have diabetes. Drug may affect urine sugar tests.

Over age 60:
Adverse reactions and side effects may be more frequent and severe than in younger persons.

Pregnancy:
Risk to unborn child outweighs drug benefits, especially in last month of pregnancy. Don't use.

Breast-feeding:
Drug passes into milk. Avoid drug or discontinue nursing until you finish medicine. Consult doctor for advice on maintaining milk supply.

Infants & children:
Don't give to infants younger than 1 month. Use only under medical supervision for older children.

Prolonged use:
Chest pain, cough, shortness of breath.

Skin & sunlight:
No problems expected.

Driving, piloting or hazardous work:
Avoid if you feel dizzy or drowsy. Otherwise, no problems expected.

Airplane passengers:
No problems expected.

Discontinuing:
Don't discontinue without consulting doctor. Dose may require gradual reduction if you have taken drug for a long time. Doses of other drugs may also require adjustment.

Others:
Periodic blood counts, liver-function tests, and chest X-rays recommended.

INTERACTION WITH OTHER DRUGS

GENERIC NAME OR DRUG CLASS	COMBINED EFFECT
Nalidixic acid	Decreased nitrofurantoin effect.
Phenobarbital	Decreased nitrofurantoin effect.
Probenecid	Increased nitrofurantoin effect.
Sulfinpyrazone	Possible nitrofurantoin toxicity.

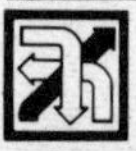

INTERACTION WITH OTHER SUBSTANCES

INTERACTS WITH	COMBINED EFFECT
Alcohol:	Possible disulfiram reaction (see page 846). Avoid.
Beverages:	None expected.
Cocaine:	No proven problems.
Foods:	None expected.
Marijuana:	None expected.
Tobacco:	None expected.

NITROGLYCERIN (GLYCERYL TRINITRATE)

BRAND NAMES

Glyceryl Trinitrate
Nitro-Bid
Nitro-Dur
Nitrodisc
Nitrogard-SR
Nitroglyn
Nitrol
Nitrolin
Nitrong
Nitrospan
Nitrostabilin
Nitrostat
Susadrin
Transderm-Nitro
Tridil
Vasoglyn

GENERAL INFORMATION

Habit forming? No
Prescription needed? Yes
Available as generic? Yes
Drug class: Vasodilator, antianginal (nitrate)

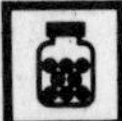

USES

Treatment for angina pain caused by temporary lack of oxygen to heart muscle.

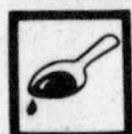

DOSAGE & USAGE INFORMATION

How to take:
- Tablet or capsule—Swallow whole with liquid. Don't crush, chew or open.
- Ointment—Apply as directed.
- Sublingual tablets—Place under tongue every 3 to 5 minutes at earliest sign of angina. If discomfort is not angina, nitroglycerin will not bring relief. If you don't have complete relief with 3 or 4 tablets, call doctor.

When to take:
Swallowed tablets or capsules—Take at the same time every day.

If you forget a dose:
Swallowed tablets or capsules—Take up to 2 hours late. If more than 2 hours, wait for next dose (don't double this).

What drug does:
Relaxes and expands muscles of arteries to heart, increasing blood and oxygen supply.

Time lapse before drug works:
- Sublingual tablets—1 to 3 minutes.
- Other forms—15 to 30 minutes. Will not stop an attack, but may prevent attacks.

Don't take with:
See Interaction column and consult doctor.

OVERDOSE

Symptoms:
Flushed face, vomiting, weakness, sweating, fainting, shortness of breath, coma.

What to do:
- Dial 0 (operator) or 911 (emergency) for an ambulance or medical help. Then give first aid immediately.
- Additional emergency information on page 886.

POSSIBLE ADVERSE REACTIONS OR SIDE EFFECTS

SYMPTOMS	FREQUENCY	WHAT TO DO
Brain & nervous system:		
Faintness, dizziness, headache.	Common	5
Skin:		
• Flushed or pale face.	Common	5
• Rash	Infrequent	3
• Severe irritation, peeling.	Rare	4
Eyes:	None expected.	
Ears, nose, throat:	None expected.	
Digestive:		
Nausea, vomiting.	Common	3
Heart & lungs:		
Rapid heartbeat.	Common	5
Blood vessels:	None expected.	
Muscles, bones, joints:	None expected.	
Genital, urinary:	None expected.	
Kidneys:	None expected.	
Liver:	None expected.	
Allergic:	None expected.	
Blood:	None expected.	
Others:	None expected.	

1- Life-threatening. Seek emergency treatment immediately.
2- Discontinue. Seek emergency treatment.
3- Discontinue. Call doctor right away.
4- Continue. Call doctor when convenient.
5- Continue. Tell doctor at next visit.
6- No action necessary.

NITROGLYCERIN (GLYCERYL TRINITRATE)

WARNINGS & PRECAUTIONS

Don't take if:
You are allergic to any nitrate.

Before you start, consult your doctor:
- If you are taking non-prescription drugs.
- If you plan to become pregnant within medication period.
- If you have glaucoma.
- If you have reacted badly to any vasodilator drug.
- If you drink alcoholic beverages or smoke marijuana.

Over age 60:
Adverse reactions and side effects may be more frequent and severe than in younger persons. Likely to lower blood pressure excessively.

Pregnancy:
No proven harm to unborn child. Avoid if possible.

Breast-feeding:
No problems expected, but consult doctor.

Infants & children:
Not recommended.

Prolonged use:
No problems expected.

Skin & sunlight:
No problems expected.

Driving, piloting or hazardous work:
Avoid if you feel dizzy or faint. Otherwise, no problems expected.

Airplane passengers:
No problems expected.

Discontinuing:
Don't discontinue without doctor's advice (except sublingual tablets) until you complete prescribed dose, even though symptoms diminish or disappear.

Others:
Keep sublingual tablets in original container. Always carry them with you, but keep from body heat if possible.

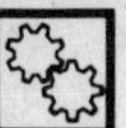

INTERACTION WITH OTHER DRUGS

GENERIC NAME OR DRUG CLASS	COMBINED EFFECT
Anticholinergics	Increased pressure within the eye.
Antidepressants (tricyclic)	Severe blood-pressure drop.
Antihypertensives	Severe blood-pressure drop.
Beta-adrenergic blockers	Dangerous blood-pressure drop.
Cholinergics	Decreased cholinergic effect.
Ephedrine	Decreased nitroglycerin effect.

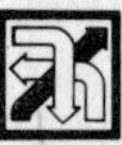

INTERACTION WITH OTHER SUBSTANCES

INTERACTS WITH	COMBINED EFFECT
Alcohol:	Increased headache severity and likely fainting. Avoid.
Beverages:	None expected.
Cocaine:	Flushed face and headache. Avoid.
Foods:	None expected.
Marijuana:	Decreased nitroglycerin effect, increased angina pain. Avoid.
Tobacco:	Decreased nitroglycerin effect.

NORETHINDRONE

BRAND NAMES

Micronor
Modicon 21
Norinyl 1+35
21-Day Tablets
Norlestrin
Norlutate Acetate
Norlutin
Nor-Q.D.
Ortho-Novum 1/35
Ovcon
Tri-Norinyl

GENERAL INFORMATION

Habit forming? No
Prescription needed? Yes
Available as generic? No
Drug class: Female sex hormone (progestin)

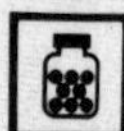

USES

- Treatment for menstrual or uterine disorders caused by progestin imbalance.
- Contraceptive

DOSAGE & USAGE INFORMATION

How to take:
Tablet or capsule—Swallow with liquid or food to lessen stomach irritation. You may crumble tablet or open capsule.

When to take:
At the same time each day.

If you forget a dose:
- Menstrual disorders—Take up to 2 hours late. If more than 2 hours, wait for next dose (don't double this).
- Contraceptive—Consult your doctor. You may need to use another birth-control method until next period.

What drug does:
- Creates a uterine lining similar to pregnancy that prevents bleeding.
- Suppresses a pituitary gland hormone responsible for ovulation.
- Stimulates cervical mucus, which stops sperm penetration and prevents pregnancy.

Time lapse before drug works:
- Menstrual disorders—24 to 48 hours.
- Contraception—3 weeks.

Don't take with:
See Interaction column and consult doctor.

OVERDOSE

Symptoms:
Nausea, vomiting, fluid retention, breast discomfort or enlargement, vaginal bleeding.

What to do:
Overdose unlikely to threaten life. If person takes much larger amount than prescribed, call doctor, poison-control center or hospital emergency room for instructions.

POSSIBLE ADVERSE REACTIONS OR SIDE EFFECTS

SYMPTOMS	FREQUENCY	WHAT TO DO
Brain & nervous system:		
Depression	Infrequent	4
Skin:		
• Rash	Rare	3
• Acne, increased facial or body hair.	Infrequent	5
Eyes, ears, nose, throat, heart & lungs, muscles, bones, joints, kidneys, allergic, blood:	None expected.	
Digestive:		
• Stomach or side pain.	Rare	3
• Appetite or weight changes.	Common	5
• Nausea	Infrequent	5
Blood vessels:		
Blood clot in leg, brain or lung.	Rare	1
Muscles, bones, joints:		
Ankle, foot swelling.	Common	5
Genital, urinary:		
Prolonged vaginal bleeding.	Infrequent	3
Liver:		
Jaundice (yellow skin and eyes).	Rare	3
Others:		
• Breast tenderness.	Infrequent	5
• Unusual tiredness or weakness.	Common	5

1 - Life-threatening. Seek emergency treatment immediately.
2 - Discontinue. Seek emergency treatment.
3 - Discontinue. Call doctor right away.
4 - Continue. Call doctor when convenient.
5 - Continue. Tell doctor at next visit.

WARNINGS & PRECAUTIONS

Don't take if:
- You are allergic to any progestin hormone.
- You may be pregnant.
- You have liver or gallbladder disease.
- You have had thrombophlebitis, embolism or stroke.
- You have unexplained vaginal bleeding.
- You have had breast or uterine cancer.

Before you start, consult your doctor:
- If you have heart or kidney disease.
- If you have diabetes.
- If you have a seizure disorder.
- If you suffer migraines.
- If you are easily depressed.

Over age 60:
Not recommended.

Pregnancy:
May harm child. Discontinue at first sign of pregnancy.

Breast-feeding:
Drug passes into milk. Avoid drug or discontinue nursing until you finish medicine. Consult doctor for advice on maintaining milk supply.

Infants & children:
Use only for female children under medical supervision.

Prolonged use:
No problems expected.

Skin & sunlight:
No problems expected.

Driving, piloting or hazardous work:
No problems expected.

Airplane passengers:
No problems expected.

Discontinuing:
Consult doctor. This medicine stays in the body and causes fetal abnormalities. Wait at least 3 months before becoming pregnant.

Others:
- Patients with diabetes must be monitored closely.
- Symptoms of blood clot in leg, brain or lung are: chest, groin, leg pain; sudden, severe headache; loss of coordination; vision change; shortness of breath; slurred speech.

INTERACTION WITH OTHER DRUGS

GENERIC NAME OR DRUG CLASS	COMBINED EFFECT
Antihistamines	Decreased norethindrone effect.
Oxyphenbutazone	Decreased norethindrone effect.
Phenobarbital	Decreased norethindrone effect.
Phenothiazines	Increased phenothiazine effect.
Phenylbutazone	Decreased norethindrone effect.

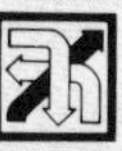

INTERACTION WITH OTHER SUBSTANCES

INTERACTS WITH	COMBINED EFFECT
Alcohol:	None expected.
Beverages:	None expected.
Cocaine:	Decreased norethindrone effect.
Foods: Salt	Fluid retention.
Marijuana:	Possible menstrual irregularities or bleeding between periods.
Tobacco:	Possible blood clots in lung, brain, legs. Avoid.

NORETHINDRONE ACETATE

BRAND NAMES

Norlutate

GENERAL INFORMATION

Habit forming? No
Prescription needed? Yes
Available as generic? No
Drug class: Female sex hormone (progestin)

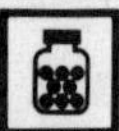

USES

- Treatment for menstrual or uterine disorders caused by progestin imbalance.
- Contraceptive
- Treatment for cancer of breast and uterus.

DOSAGE & USAGE INFORMATION

How to take:
Tablet or capsule—Swallow with liquid or food to lessen stomach irritation. You may crumble tablet or open capsule.

When to take:
At the same time each day.

If you forget a dose:
- Menstrual disorders—Take up to 2 hours late. If more than 2 hours, wait for next dose (don't double this).
- Contraceptive—Consult your doctor. You may need to use another birth-control method until next period.

What drug does:
- Creates a uterine lining similar to pregnancy that prevents bleeding.
- Suppresses a pituitary gland hormone responsible for ovulation.
- Stimulates cervical mucus, which stops sperm penetration and prevents pregnancy.

Time lapse before drug works:
- Menstrual disorders—24 to 48 hours.
- Contraception—3 weeks.
- Cancer—May require 2 to 3 months.

Don't take with:
See Interaction column and consult doctor.

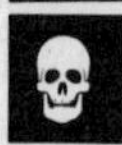

OVERDOSE

Symptoms:
Nausea, vomiting, fluid retention, breast discomfort or enlargement, vaginal bleeding.

What to do:
Overdose unlikely to threaten life. If person takes much larger amount than prescribed, call doctor, poison-control center or hospital emergency room for instructions.

POSSIBLE ADVERSE REACTIONS OR SIDE EFFECTS

SYMPTOMS	FREQUENCY	WHAT TO DO
Brain & nervous system:		
Depression	Infrequent	4
Skin:		
• Rash	Rare	3
• Acne, increased facial or body hair.	Infrequent	5
Eyes, ears, nose, throat, heart & lungs, muscles, bones, joints, kidneys, allergic, blood:	None expected.	
Digestive:		
• Stomach or side pain.	Rare	3
• Appetite or weight changes.	Common	5
• Nausea	Infrequent	5
Blood vessels:		
Blood clot in leg, brain or lung.	Rare	1
Muscles, bones, joints:		
Ankle, foot swelling.	Common	5
Genital, urinary:		
Prolonged vaginal bleeding.	Infrequent	3
Liver:		
Jaundice (yellow skin and eyes).	Rare	3
Others:		
• Breast tenderness.	Infrequent	5
• Unusual tiredness or weakness.	Common	5

1- Life-threatening. Seek emergency treatment immediately.
2- Discontinue. Seek emergency treatment.
3- Discontinue. Call doctor right away.
4- Continue. Call doctor when convenient.
5- Continue. Tell doctor at next visit.

WARNINGS & PRECAUTIONS

Don't take if:
- You are allergic to any progestin hormone.
- You may be pregnant.
- You have liver or gallbladder disease.
- You have had thrombophlebitis, embolism or stroke.
- You have unexplained vaginal bleeding.
- You have had breast or uterine cancer.

Before you start, consult your doctor:
- If you have heart or kidney disease.
- If you have diabetes.
- If you have a seizure disorder.
- If you suffer migraines.
- If you are easily depressed.

Over age 60:
Not recommended.

Pregnancy:
May harm child. Discontinue at first sign of pregnancy.

Breast-feeding:
Drug passes into milk. Avoid drug or discontinue nursing until you finish medicine. Consult doctor for advice on maintaining milk supply.

Infants & children:
Use only for female children under medical supervision.

Prolonged use:
No problems expected.

Skin & sunlight:
No problems expected.

Driving, piloting or hazardous work:
No problems expected.

Airplane passengers:
No problems expected.

Discontinuing:
Consult doctor. This medicine stays in the body and causes fetal abnormalities. Wait at least 3 months before becoming pregnant.

Others:
- Patients with diabetes must be monitored closely.
- Symptoms of blood clot in leg, brain or lung are: chest, groin, leg pain; sudden, severe headache; loss of coordination; vision change; shortness of breath; slurred speech.

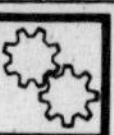

INTERACTION WITH OTHER DRUGS

GENERIC NAME OR DRUG CLASS	COMBINED EFFECT
Antihistamines	Decreased norethindrone acetate effect.
Oxyphenbutazone	Decreased norethindrone acetate effect.
Phenobarbital	Decreased norethindrone acetate effect.
Phenothiazines	Increased phenothiazine effect.
Phenylbutazone	Decreased norethindrone acetate effect.

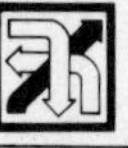

INTERACTION WITH OTHER SUBSTANCES

INTERACTS WITH	COMBINED EFFECT
Alcohol:	None expected.
Beverages:	None expected.
Cocaine:	Decreased norethindrone acetate effect.
Foods: Salt	Fluid retention.
Marijuana:	Possible menstrual irregularities or bleeding between periods.
Tobacco:	Possible blood clots in lung, brain, legs. Avoid.

NORGESTREL

BRAND NAMES

Lo-Ovral
Ovral
Ovrette

GENERAL INFORMATION

Habit forming? No
Prescription needed? Yes
Available as generic? No
Drug class: Female sex hormone (progestin)

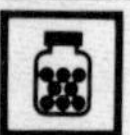

USES

Contraceptive

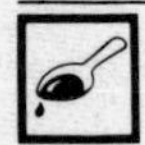

DOSAGE & USAGE INFORMATION

How to take:
Tablet or capsule—Swallow with liquid or food to lessen stomach irritation. You may crumble tablet or open capsule.

When to take:
At the same time each day.

If you forget a dose:
Consult your doctor. You may need to use another birth-control method until next period, then resume norgestrel.

What drug does:
- Creates a uterine lining similar to pregnancy that prevents bleeding.
- Suppresses a pituitary gland hormone responsible for ovulation.
- Stimulates cervical mucus, which stops sperm penetration and prevents pregnancy.

Time lapse before drug works:
3 weeks. Use another method of birth control until then.

Don't take with:
See Interaction column and consult doctor.

OVERDOSE

Symptoms:
Nausea, vomiting, fluid retention, breast discomfort or enlargement, vaginal bleeding.

What to do:
Overdose unlikely to threaten life. If person takes much larger amount than prescribed, call doctor, poison-control center or hospital emergency room for instructions.

POSSIBLE ADVERSE REACTIONS OR SIDE EFFECTS

SYMPTOMS	FREQUENCY	WHAT TO DO
Brain & nervous system:		
Depression	Infrequent	4
Skin:		
• Rash	Rare	3
• Acne, increased facial or body hair.	Infrequent	5
Eyes, ears, nose, throat, heart & lungs, muscles, bones, joints, kidneys, allergic, blood:	None expected.	
Digestive:		
• Stomach or side pain.	Rare	3
• Appetite or weight changes.	Common	5
• Nausea	Infrequent	5
Blood vessels:		
Blood clot in leg, brain or lung.	Rare	1
Muscles, bones, joints:		
Ankle, foot swelling.	Common	5
Genital, urinary:		
Prolonged vaginal bleeding.	Infrequent	3
Liver:		
Jaundice (yellow skin and eyes).	Rare	3
Others:		
• Breast tenderness.	Infrequent	5
• Unusual tiredness or weakness.	Common	5

1-Life-threatening. Seek emergency treatment immediately.
2-Discontinue. Seek emergency treatment.
3-Discontinue. Call doctor right away.
4-Continue. Call doctor when convenient.
5-Continue. Tell doctor at next visit.

WARNINGS & PRECAUTIONS

Don't take if:
- You are allergic to any progestin hormone.
- You may be pregnant.
- You have liver or gallbladder disease.
- You have had thrombophlebitis, embolism or stroke.
- You have unexplained vaginal bleeding.
- You have had breast or uterine cancer.

Before you start, consult your doctor:
- If you have heart or kidney disease.
- If you have diabetes.
- If you have a seizure disorder.
- If you suffer migraines.
- If you are easily depressed.

Over age 60:
Not recommended.

Pregnancy:
May harm child. Discontinue at first sign of pregnancy.

Breast-feeding:
Drug passes into milk. Avoid drug or discontinue nursing until you finish medicine. Consult doctor for advice on maintaining milk supply.

Infants & children:
Use only for female children under medical supervision.

Prolonged use:
No problems expected.

Skin & sunlight:
No problems expected.

Driving, piloting or hazardous work:
No problems expected.

Airplane passengers:
No problems expected.

Discontinuing:
Consult doctor. This medicine stays in the body and causes fetal abnormalities. Wait at least 3 months before becoming pregnant.

Others:
- Patients with diabetes must be monitored closely.
- Symptoms of blood clot in leg, brain or lung are: chest, groin, leg pain; sudden, severe headache; loss of coordination; vision change; shortness of breath; slurred speech.

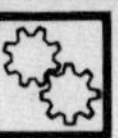

INTERACTION WITH OTHER DRUGS

GENERIC NAME OR DRUG CLASS	COMBINED EFFECT
Antihistamines	Decreased norgestrel effect.
Oxyphenbutazone	Decreased norgestrel effect.
Phenobarbital	Decreased norgestrel effect.
Phenothiazines	Increased phenothiazine effect.
Phenylbutazone	Decreased norgestrel effect.

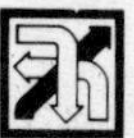

INTERACTION WITH OTHER SUBSTANCES

INTERACTS WITH	COMBINED EFFECT
Alcohol:	None expected.
Beverages:	None expected.
Cocaine:	Decreased norgestrel effect.
Foods: Salt	Fluid retention.
Marijuana:	Possible menstrual irregularities or bleeding between periods.
Tobacco:	Possible blood clots in lung, brain, legs. Avoid.

NORTRIPTYLINE

BRAND NAMES

Aventyl
Pamelor

GENERAL INFORMATION

Habit forming? No
Prescription needed? Yes
Available as generic? Yes
Drug class: Antidepressant (tricyclic)

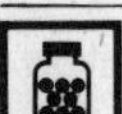

USES

Gradually relieves, but doesn't cure, symptoms of depression.

DOSAGE & USAGE INFORMATION

How to take:

- Capsule—Swallow with liquid.
- Liquid—Use measuring spoon.

When to take:
At the same time each day, usually bedtime.

If you forget a dose:
Bedtime dose—If you forget your once-a-day bedtime dose, don't take it more than 3 hours late. If more than 3 hours, wait for next scheduled dose. Don't double this dose.

What drug does:
Probably affects part of brain that controls messages between nerve cells.

Time lapse before drug works:
Begins in 1 to 2 weeks. May require 4 to 6 weeks for maximum benefit.

Don't take with:

- Non-prescription drugs without consulting doctor.
- See Interaction column and consult doctor.

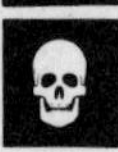

OVERDOSE

Symptoms:
Hallucinations, convulsions, coma.

What to do:

- Dial 0 (operator) or 911 (emergency) for an ambulance or medical help. Then give first aid immediately.
- If patient is unconscious and not breathing, give mouth-to-mouth breathing. If there is no heartbeat, use cardiac massage and mouth-to-mouth breathing (CPR). Don't try to make patient vomit. If you can't get help quickly, take patient to nearest emergency facility.
- Additional emergency information on page 886.

POSSIBLE ADVERSE REACTIONS OR SIDE EFFECTS

SYMPTOMS	FREQUENCY	WHAT TO DO
Brain & nervous system:		
• Hallucinations, shakiness, dizziness, fainting.	Infrequent	3
• Headache	Common	4
• Seizures	Rare	1
• Insomnia	Common	5
Skin:		
Rash, itch.	Rare	3
Eyes:		
Blurred vision, pain.	Infrequent	3
Ears, nose, throat:		
• Sore throat.	Rare	3
• Dry mouth or unpleasant taste.	Common	4
Digestive:		
• Constipation or diarrhea, nausea, indigestion.	Common	4
• Vomiting	Infrequent	3
• "Sweet tooth"	Common	5
Heart & lungs:		
Irregular heartbeat or slow pulse.	Infrequent	3
Blood vessels, muscles, bones, joints, kidneys, allergic, blood:	None expected.	
Genital, urinary:		
Difficulty urinating.	Infrequent	4
Liver:		
Jaundice (yellow skin and eyes).	Rare	3
Others:		
• Fever	Rare	3
• Fatigue, weakness.	Common	4

1- Life-threatening. Seek emergency treatment immediately.
2- Discontinue. Seek emergency treatment.
3- Discontinue. Call doctor right away.
4- Continue. Call doctor when convenient.
5- Continue. Tell doctor at next visit.

WARNINGS & PRECAUTIONS

Don't take if:
- You are allergic to any tricyclic antidepressant.
- You drink alcohol.
- You have had a heart attack within 6 weeks.
- You have glaucoma.
- You have taken MAO inhibitors within 2 weeks.
- Patient is younger than 12.

Before you start, consult your doctor:
- If you will have surgery within 2 months, including dental surgery, requiring general or spinal anesthesia.
- If you have an enlarged prostate.
- If you have heart disease or high blood pressure.
- If you have stomach or intestinal problems.
- If you have an overactive thyroid.
- If you have asthma.
- If you have liver disease.

Over age 60:
More likely to develop urination difficulty and side effects under *Brain & nervous system*, opposite.

Pregnancy:
Studies inconclusive on harm to unborn child. Animal studies show fetal abnormalities. Decide with your doctor whether drug benefits justify risk to unborn child.

Breast-feeding:
Drug passes into milk. Avoid drug or discontinue nursing until you finish medicine. Consult doctor for advice on maintaining milk supply.

Infants & children:
Don't give to children younger than 12.

Prolonged use:
No problems expected.

Skin & sunlight:
May cause rash or intensify sunburn in areas exposed to sun or sunlamp.

Driving, piloting or hazardous work:
Don't drive or pilot aircraft until you learn how medicine affects you. Don't work around dangerous machinery. Don't climb ladders or work in high places. Danger increases if you drink alcohol or take medicine affecting alertness and reflexes.

Airplane passengers:
No problems expected.

Discontinuing:
Don't discontinue without consulting doctor. Dose may require gradual reduction if you have taken drug for a long time. Doses of other drugs may also require adjustment.

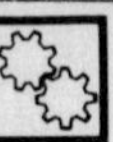

INTERACTION WITH OTHER DRUGS

GENERIC NAME OR DRUG CLASS	COMBINED EFFECT
Anticoagulants (oral)	Increased anticoagulant effect.
Anticholinergics	Increased sedation.
Antihistamines	Increased antihistamine effect.
Barbiturates	Decreased antidepressant effect.
Clonidine	Decreased clonidine effect.
Diuretics (thiazide)	Increased nortriptyline effect.
Ethchlorvynol	Delirium
Guanethidine	Decreased guanethidine effect.
MAO inhibitors	Fever, delirium, convulsions.
Methyldopa	Decreased methyldopa effect.
Narcotics	Dangerous oversedation.
Phenytoin	Decreased phenytoin effect.
Quinidine	Irregular heartbeat.
Sedatives	Dangerous oversedation.
Sympathomimetics	Increased sympathomimetic effect.
Thyroid hormones	Irregular heartbeat.

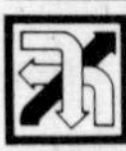

INTERACTION WITH OTHER SUBSTANCES

INTERACTS WITH	COMBINED EFFECT
Alcohol: Beverages or medicines with alcohol.	Excessive intoxication. Avoid.
Beverages:	None expected.
Cocaine:	Excessive intoxication. Avoid.
Foods:	None expected.
Marijuana:	Excessive drowsiness. Avoid.
Tobacco:	None expected.

NYLIDRIN

BRAND NAMES

Arlidin
Arlidin Forte
Circlidrin
Pervadil
PMS Nylidrin
Rolidrin

GENERAL INFORMATION

Habit forming? No
Prescription needed? Yes
Available as generic? Yes
Drug class: Vasodilator

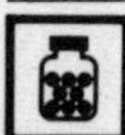

USES

- Improves poor circulation in extremities.
- Reduces dizziness caused by poor circulation in inner ear.

DOSAGE & USAGE INFORMATION

How to take:
Tablet—Swallow with liquid or food to lessen stomach irritation. If you can't swallow whole, crumble tablet and take with liquid or food.

When to take:
At the same times each day.

If you forget a dose:
Take as soon as you remember up to 2 hours late. If more than 2 hours, wait for next scheduled dose (don't double this dose).

What drug does:
Stimulates nerves that dilate blood vessels, increasing oxygen and nutrients.

Time lapse before drug works:
10 to 30 minutes.

Don't take with:
See Interaction column and consult doctor.

OVERDOSE

Symptoms:
Blood-pressure drop; nausea, vomiting; rapid, irregular heartbeat, chest pain; blurred vision; metallic taste.

What to do:
- Dial 0 (operator) or 911 (emergency) for an ambulance or medical help. Then give first aid immediately.
- If patient is unconscious and not breathing, give mouth-to-mouth breathing. If there is no heartbeat, use cardiac massage and mouth-to-mouth breathing (CPR). Don't try to make patient vomit. If you can't get help quickly, take patient to nearest emergency facility.
- Additional emergency information on page 886.

POSSIBLE ADVERSE REACTIONS OR SIDE EFFECTS

SYMPTOMS	FREQUENCY	WHAT TO DO
Brain & nervous system:		
• Dizziness	Infrequent	4
• Headache, nervousness.	Rare	4
• Trembling	Rare	3
Skin:		
Flushed face.	Rare	4
Eyes:		
Blurred vision.	Common	4
Ears, nose, throat:		
Metallic taste.	Common	5
Digestive:		
Nausea, vomiting.	Rare	4
Heart & lungs:		
• Chest pain.	Common	3
• Rapid or irregular heartbeat.	Infrequent	3
Blood vessels:		
• Fever	Common	4
• Chills	Rare	3
• Low blood pressure on standing.	Common	4
Muscles, bones, joints:	None expected.	
Genital, urinary:		
Decreased or difficult urination.	Common	4
Kidneys:	None expected.	
Liver:	None expected.	
Allergic:	None expected.	
Blood:	None expected.	
Others:		
Weakness, tiredness.	Infrequent	4

1-Life-threatening. Seek emergency treatment immediately.
2-Discontinue. Seek emergency treatment.
3-Discontinue. Call doctor right away.
4-Continue. Call doctor when convenient.
5-Continue. Tell doctor at next visit.
6-No action necessary.

WARNINGS & PRECAUTIONS

Don't take if:
- You are allergic to any vasodilator drugs.
- You have had a heart attack or stroke within 4 weeks.
- You have an active peptic ulcer.

Before you start, consult your doctor:
- If you have had heart disease, heart-rhythm disorders (especially rapid heartbeat), a stroke or poor circulation to the brain.
- If you have glaucoma.
- If you have an overactive thyroid gland.
- If you plan to become pregnant within medication period.
- If you use tobacco.

Over age 60:
Adverse reactions and side effects may be more frequent and severe than in younger persons.

Pregnancy:
No proven harm to unborn child. Avoid if possible.

Breast-feeding:
No proven problems. Consult doctor.

Infants & children:
Not recommended.

Prolonged use:
No problems expected.

Skin & sunlight:
No problems expected.

Driving, piloting or hazardous work:
Don't drive or pilot aircraft until you learn how medicine affects you. Don't work around dangerous machinery. Don't climb ladders or work in high places. Danger increases if you drink alcohol or take medicine affecting alertness and reflexes, such as antihistamines, tranquilizers, sedatives, pain medicine, narcotics and mind-altering drugs.

Airplane passengers:
No problems expected.

Discontinuing:
Don't discontinue without consulting doctor. If your condition worsens, contact your doctor immediately. Dose may require gradual reduction if you have taken drug for a long time. Doses of other drugs may also require adjustment.

Others:
No problems expected.

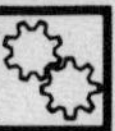

INTERACTION WITH OTHER DRUGS

GENERIC NAME OR DRUG CLASS	COMBINED EFFECT
Beta-adrenergic blockers	Decreased effect of nylidrin.
Phenothiazines	Increased blood level of phenothiazines.

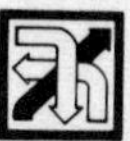

INTERACTION WITH OTHER SUBSTANCES

INTERACTS WITH	COMBINED EFFECT
Alcohol:	Possible increased stomach-acid secretion. Use with caution.
Beverages:	None expected.
Cocaine:	Increased adverse effects of nylidrin.
Foods:	None expected.
Marijuana:	None expected.
Tobacco:	Decreased nylidrin effect. Worsens circulation. Avoid.

NYSTATIN

BRAND NAMES

Achrostatin V
Candex
Declostatin
Korostatin
Mycolog
Mycostatin
Myco-Triacet
Mykinac
Mytrex
Nadostine
Nilstat
Nyaderm
Nystaform
Nystex
O-V statin
Terrastatin

GENERAL INFORMATION

Habit forming? No
Prescription needed? Yes
Available as generic? Yes
Drug class: Antifungal

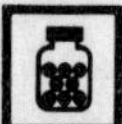

USES

Treatment of fungus infections susceptible to nystatin.

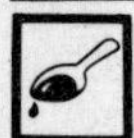

DOSAGE & USAGE INFORMATION

How to take:

- Tablet or capsule—Swallow with liquid. If you can't swallow whole, crumble tablet or open capsule and take with liquid or food.
- Suppositories—Remove wrapper and moisten suppository with water. Gently insert larger end into vagina. Push well into vagina with finger.
- Ointment, cream or lotion—Use as directed by doctor and label.
- Liquid—Take as directed. Instruction varies by preparation.

When to take:
At the same time each day.

If you forget a dose:
Take as soon as you remember up to 2 hours late. If more than 2 hours, wait for next scheduled dose (don't double this dose).

What drug does:
Prevents growth and reproduction of fungus.

Time lapse before drug works:
Begins immediately. May require 3 weeks for maximum benefit, depending on location and severity of infection.

Don't take with:
See Interaction column and consult doctor.

OVERDOSE

Symptoms:
Mild overdose may cause nausea, vomiting, diarrhea.

What to do:
Overdose unlikely to threaten life. If person takes much larger amount than prescribed, call doctor, poison-control center or hospital emergency room for instructions.

POSSIBLE ADVERSE REACTIONS OR SIDE EFFECTS

SYMPTOMS	FREQUENCY	WHAT TO DO
Brain & nervous system:	None expected.	
Skin: Mild irritation, itch at application site.	Infrequent	3
Eyes:	None expected.	
Ears, nose, throat:	None expected.	
Digestive: Nausea, stomach pain, vomiting, diarrhea.	Common (at high doses)	3
Heart & lungs:	None expected.	
Blood vessels:	None expected.	
Muscles, bones, joints:	None expected.	
Genital, urinary:	None expected.	
Kidneys:	None expected.	
Liver:	None expected.	
Allergic:	None expected.	
Blood:	None expected.	
Others:	None expected.	

1-Life-threatening. Seek emergency treatment immediately.
2-Discontinue. Seek emergency treatment.
3-Discontinue. Call doctor right away.
4-Continue. Call doctor when convenient.
5-Continue. Tell doctor at next visit.
6-No action necessary.

WARNINGS & PRECAUTIONS

Don't take if:
You are allergic to nystatin.

Before you start, consult your doctor:
If you plan to become pregnant within medication period.

Over age 60:
No problems expected.

Pregnancy:
No proven harm to unborn child. Avoid if possible.

Breast-feeding:
No proven problems. Consult doctor.

Infants & children:
No problems expected.

Prolonged use:
No problems expected.

Skin & sunlight:
No problems expected.

Driving, piloting or hazardous work:
No problems expected.

Airplane passengers:
No problems expected.

Discontinuing:
Don't discontinue without doctor's advice until you complete prescribed dose, even though symptoms diminish or disappear.

Others:
No problems expected.

INTERACTION WITH OTHER DRUGS

GENERIC NAME OR DRUG CLASS	COMBINED EFFECT
None	

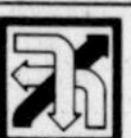

INTERACTION WITH OTHER SUBSTANCES

INTERACTS WITH	COMBINED EFFECT
Alcohol:	None expected.
Beverages:	None expected.
Cocaine:	None expected.
Foods:	None expected.
Marijuana:	None expected.
Tobacco:	None expected.

ORPHENADRINE

BRAND NAMES

Banflex
Disipal
Flexoject
Flexon
K-Flex
Marflex
Myolin
Neocyten
Norflex
Norgesic
Norgesic Forte
O-Flex
Ro-Orphena
Tega-Flex
X-Otag

GENERAL INFORMATION

Habit forming? No
Prescription needed? U.S.: Yes
Canada: No
Available as generic? Yes
Drug class: Muscle relaxant, anticholinergic, antihistamine, antiparkinsonism

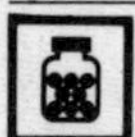

USES

- Reduces muscle-strain discomfort.
- Relieves symptoms of Parkinson's disease.

DOSAGE & USAGE INFORMATION

How to take:
Tablet—Swallow with liquid. If you can't swallow whole, crumble tablet and take with liquid or food.

When to take:
At the same times each day.

If you forget a dose:
Take as soon as you remember up to 6 hours late. If more than 6 hours, wait for next scheduled dose (don't double this dose).

What drug does:
Sedative and analgesic effects reduce spasm and pain in skeletal muscles.

Time lapse before drug works:
1 to 2 hours.

Don't take with:
See Interaction column and consult doctor.

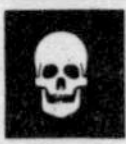

OVERDOSE

Symptoms:
Fainting, confusion, widely dilated pupils, rapid pulse, convulsions, coma.

What to do:
- Dial 0 (operator) or 911 (emergency) for an ambulance or medical help. Then give first aid immediately.
- Additional emergency information on page 886.

POSSIBLE ADVERSE REACTIONS OR SIDE EFFECTS

SYMPTOMS	FREQUENCY	WHAT TO DO
Brain & nervous system: Weakness, headache, dizziness, drowsiness, agitation, tremor, confusion.	Infrequent	3
Skin: Rash or itch.	Rare	3
Eyes: Blurred vision, dilated pupils.	Rare	3
Ears, nose, throat: Dry mouth.	Infrequent	4
Digestive: Nausea, vomiting, constipation.	Infrequent	4
Heart & lungs: Rapid or pounding heartbeat.	Infrequent	3
Blood vessels:	None expected.	
Muscles, bones, joints:	None expected.	
Genital, urinary: Urinary hesitancy or retention.	Infrequent	4
Kidneys:	None expected.	
Liver:	None expected.	
Allergic:	None expected.	
Blood:	None expected.	
Others:	None expected.	

1- Life-threatening. Seek emergency treatment immediately.
2- Discontinue. Seek emergency treatment.
3- Discontinue. Call doctor right away.
4- Continue. Call doctor when convenient.
5- Continue. Tell doctor at next visit.
6- No action necessary.

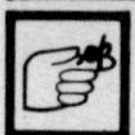

WARNINGS & PRECAUTIONS

Don't take if:
You are allergic to orphenadrine.

Before you start, consult your doctor:
- If you have glaucoma.
- If you have myasthenia gravis.
- If you have difficulty emptying bladder.
- If you have had heart disease or heart-rhythm disturbance.
- If you have had a peptic ulcer.

Over age 60:
Adverse reactions and side effects may be more frequent and severe than in younger persons.

Pregnancy:
No proven harm to unborn child. Avoid if possible.

Breast-feeding:
No proven problems. Consult doctor.

Infants & children:
Not recommended for children younger than 12.

Prolonged use:
Increased internal-eye pressure.

Skin & sunlight:
No problems expected.

Driving, piloting or hazardous work:
Don't drive or pilot aircraft until you learn how medicine affects you. Don't work around dangerous machinery. Don't climb ladders or work in high places. Danger increases if you drink alcohol or take medicine affecting alertness and reflexes, such as antihistamines, tranquilizers, sedatives, pain medicine, narcotics and mind-altering drugs.

Airplane passengers:
No problems expected.

Discontinuing:
May be unnecessary to finish medicine. Follow doctor's instructions.

Others:
No problems expected.

INTERACTION WITH OTHER DRUGS

GENERIC NAME OR DRUG CLASS	COMBINED EFFECT
Anticholinergics	Increased anticholinergic effect.
Chlorpromazine	Hypoglycemia (low blood sugar).
Griseofulvin	Decreased griseofulvin effect.
Levodopa	Increased effect of levodopa. (Improves effectiveness in treating Parkinson's disease.)
Phenylbutazone	Decreased phenylbutazone effect.
Propoxyphene	Possible confusion, nervousness, tremors.

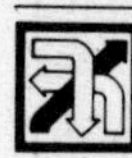

INTERACTION WITH OTHER SUBSTANCES

INTERACTS WITH	COMBINED EFFECT
Alcohol:	Increased drowsiness. Avoid.
Beverages:	None expected.
Cocaine:	Decreased orphenadrine effect. Avoid.
Foods:	None expected.
Marijuana:	Increased drowsiness, mouth dryness, muscle weakness, fainting.
Tobacco:	None expected.

OXACILLIN

BRAND NAMES

Bactocill
Prostaphlin

GENERAL INFORMATION

Habit forming? No
Prescription needed? Yes
Available as generic? Yes
Drug class: Antibiotic (penicillin)

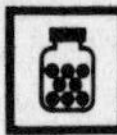

USES

Treatment of bacterial infections that are susceptible to oxacillin.

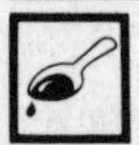

DOSAGE & USAGE INFORMATION

How to take:

- Tablets or capsules—Swallow with liquid on an empty stomach 1 hour before or 2 hours after eating.
- Liquid—Take with cold beverage. Liquid form is perishable and effective for only 7 days at room temperature. Effective for 14 days if stored in refrigerator. Don't freeze.

When to take:
Follow instructions on prescription label or side of package. Doses should be evenly spaced. For example, 4 times a day means every 6 hours.

If you forget a dose:
Take as soon as you remember. Continue regular schedule.

What drug does:
Destroys susceptible bacteria. Does not kill viruses.

Time lapse before drug works:
May be several days before medicine affects infection.

Don't take with:
See Interaction column and consult doctor.

OVERDOSE

Symptoms:
Severe diarrhea, nausea or vomiting.

What to do:
Overdose unlikely to threaten life. If person takes much larger amount than prescribed, call doctor, poison-control center or hospital emergency room for instructions.

POSSIBLE ADVERSE REACTIONS OR SIDE EFFECTS

SYMPTOMS	FREQUENCY	WHAT TO DO
Brain & nervous system:	None expected.	
Skin: Hives, rash, intense itch soon after a dose.	Rare	1
Eyes:	None expected.	
Ears, nose, throat: Dark or discolored tongue.	Common	5
Digestive: Mild nausea, vomiting, diarrhea.	Infrequent	4
Heart & lungs:	None expected.	
Blood vessels: Unexplained bleeding.	Rare	3
Muscles, bones, joints:	None expected.	
Genital, urinary:	None expected.	
Kidneys:	None expected.	
Liver:	None expected.	
Allergic: Life-threatening anaphylaxis may occur!	Rare	1 See page 888.
Blood:	None expected.	
Others:	None expected.	

1- Life-threatening. Seek emergency treatment immediately.
2- Discontinue. Seek emergency treatment.
3- Discontinue. Call doctor right away.
4- Continue. Call doctor when convenient.
5- Continue. Tell doctor at next visit.
6- No action necessary.

WARNINGS & PRECAUTIONS

Don't take if:
You are allergic to oxacillin, cephalosporin antibiotics, other penicillins or penicillamine. Life-threatening reaction may occur.

Before you start, consult your doctor:
If you are allergic to any substance or drug.

Over age 60:
You may have skin reactions, particularly around genitals and anus.

Pregnancy:
Studies inconclusive on harm to unborn child. Animal studies show fetal abnormalities. Decide with your doctor whether drug benefits justify risk to unborn child.

Breast-feeding:
Drug passes into milk. Child may become sensitive to penicillins and have allergic reactions to penicillin drugs. Avoid oxacillin or discontinue nursing until you finish medicine. Consult doctor for advice on maintaining milk supply.

Infants & children:
No problems expected.

Prolonged use:
You may become more susceptible to infections caused by germs not responsive to oxacillin.

Skin & sunlight:
No problems expected.

Driving, piloting or hazardous work:
Usually not dangerous. Most hazardous reactions likely to occur a few minutes after taking oxacillin.

Airplane passengers:
No problems expected.

Discontinuing:
Don't discontinue without doctor's advice until you complete prescribed dose, even though symptoms diminish or disappear.

Others:
No problems expected.

INTERACTION WITH OTHER DRUGS

GENERIC NAME OR DRUG CLASS	COMBINED EFFECT
Chloramphenicol	Decreased effect of both drugs.
Erythromycins	Decreased effect of both drugs.
Paromomycin	Decreased effect of both drugs.
Tetracyclines	Decreased effect of both drugs.
Troleandomycin	Decreased effect of both drugs.

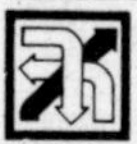

INTERACTION WITH OTHER SUBSTANCES

INTERACTS WITH	COMBINED EFFECT
Alcohol:	Occasional stomach irritation.
Beverages:	None expected.
Cocaine:	No proven problems.
Foods:	None expected.
Marijuana:	No proven problems.
Tobacco:	None expected.

OXAZEPAM

BRAND NAMES

Apo-Oxazepam
Ox-Pam
Serax
Zapex

GENERAL INFORMATION

Habit forming? Yes
Prescription needed? Yes
Available as generic? No
Drug class: Tranquilizer (benzodiazepine)

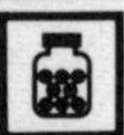

USES

Treatment for nervousness or tension.

DOSAGE & USAGE INFORMATION

How to take:
Tablet or capsule—Swallow with liquid. If you can't swallow whole, crumble tablet or open capsule and take with liquid or food.

When to take:
At the same time each day, according to instructions on prescription label.

If you forget a dose:
Take as soon as you remember up to 2 hours late. If more than 2 hours, wait for next scheduled dose (don't double this dose).

What drug does:
Affects limbic system of brain—part that controls emotions.

Time lapse before drug works:
2 hours. May take 6 weeks for full benefit.

Don't take with:
See Interaction column and consult doctor.

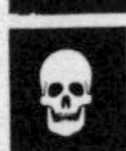

OVERDOSE

Symptoms:
Drowsiness, weakness, tremor, stupor, coma.

What to do:
- Dial 0 (operator) or 911 (emergency) for an ambulance or medical help. Then give first aid immediately.
- If patient is unconscious and not breathing, give mouth-to-mouth breathing. If there is no heartbeat, use cardiac massage and mouth-to-mouth breathing (CPR). Don't try to make patient vomit. If you can't get help quickly, take patient to nearest emergency facility.
- Additional emergency information on page 886.

POSSIBLE ADVERSE REACTIONS OR SIDE EFFECTS

SYMPTOMS	FREQUENCY	WHAT TO DO
Brain & nervous system:		
• Clumsiness, drowsiness, dizziness.	Common	4
• Hallucinations, confusion, depression, irritability.	Infrequent	3
Skin:		
Rash, itch.	Infrequent	3
Eyes:		
Vision changes.	Infrequent	3
Ears, nose, throat:		
Mouth, throat ulcers.	Rare	3
Digestive:		
Constipation or diarrhea, nausea, vomiting.	Infrequent	4
Heart & lungs:		
Slow heartbeat, breathing difficulty.	Rare	2
Blood vessels:	None expected.	
Muscles, bones, joints:	None expected.	
Genital, urinary:		
Urination difficulty.	Infrequent	4
Kidneys:	None expected.	
Liver:		
Jaundice (yellow eyes and skin).	Rare	3
Allergic:	None expected.	
Blood:	None expected.	
Others:	None expected.	

1- Life-threatening. Seek emergency treatment immediately.
2- Discontinue. Seek emergency treatment.
3- Discontinue. Call doctor right away.
4- Continue. Call doctor when convenient.
5- Continue. Tell doctor at next visit.
6- No action necessary.

WARNINGS & PRECAUTIONS

Don't take if:
- You are allergic to any benzodiazepine.
- You have myasthenia gravis.
- You are active or recovering alcoholic.
- Patient is younger than 6 months.

Before you start, consult your doctor:
- If you have liver, kidney or lung disease.
- If you have diabetes, epilepsy or porphyria.

Over age 60:
Adverse reactions and side effects may be more frequent and severe than in younger persons. You need smaller doses for shorter periods of time. May develop agitation, rage or "hangover effect."

Pregnancy:
Risk to unborn child outweighs drug benefits. Don't use.

Breast-feeding:
Drug passes into milk. Avoid drug or discontinue nursing until you finish medicine. Consult doctor for advice on maintaining milk supply.

Infants & children:
Use only under medical supervision for children older than 6 months.

Prolonged use:
May impair liver function.

Skin & sunlight:
No problems expected.

Driving, piloting or hazardous work:
Don't drive or pilot aircraft until you learn how medicine affects you. Don't work around dangerous machinery. Don't climb ladders or work in high places. Danger increases if you drink alcohol or take medicine affecting alertness and reflexes.

Airplane passengers:
No problems expected.

Discontinuing:
Don't discontinue without consulting doctor. Dose may require gradual reduction if you have taken drug for a long time. Doses of other drugs may also require adjustment.

Others:
- Hot weather, heavy exercise and profuse sweat may reduce excretion and cause overdose.
- Blood sugar may rise in diabetics, requiring insulin adjustment.

INTERACTION WITH OTHER DRUGS

GENERIC NAME OR DRUG CLASS	COMBINED EFFECT
Anticonvulsants	Change in seizure frequency or severity.
Antidepressants	Increased sedative effect of both drugs.
Antihistamines	Increased sedative effect of both drugs.
Antihypertensives	Excessively low blood pressure.
Cimetidine	Excess sedation.
Disulfiram	Increased oxazepam effect.
MAO inhibitors	Convulsions, deep sedation, rage.
Narcotics	Increased sedative effect of both drugs.
Sedatives	Increased sedative effect of both drugs.
Sleep inducers	Increased sedative effect of both drugs.
Tranquilizers	Increased sedative effect of both drugs.

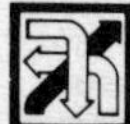

INTERACTION WITH OTHER SUBSTANCES

INTERACTS WITH	COMBINED EFFECT
Alcohol:	Heavy sedation. Avoid.
Beverages:	None expected.
Cocaine:	Decreased oxazepam effect.
Foods:	None expected.
Marijuana:	Heavy sedation. Avoid.
Tobacco:	Decreased oxazepam effect.

OXTRIPHYLLINE

BRAND NAMES

Apo-Oxtriphylline
Brondecon
Choledyl
Choledyl SA
Chophylline
Novotriphyl
Theophylline Choline

GENERAL INFORMATION

Habit forming? No
Prescription needed? Canada—No
U.S: High strength—Yes
Low strength—No
Available as generic? Yes
Drug class: Bronchodilator (xanthine)

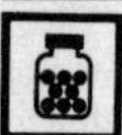

USES

Treatment for bronchial asthma symptoms.

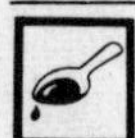

DOSAGE & USAGE INFORMATION

How to take:

- Tablet or capsule—Swallow with liquid.
- Extended-release tablets or capsules—Swallow each dose whole. If you take regular tablets, you may chew or crush them.
- Suppositories—Remove wrapper and moisten suppository with water. Gently insert larger end into rectum. Push well into rectum with finger.
- Syrup—Take as directed on bottle.
- Enema—Use as directed on label.

When to take:
Most effective taken on empty stomach 1 hour before or 2 hours after eating. However, may take with food to lessen stomach upset.

If you forget a dose:
Take as soon as you remember up to 2 hours late. If more than 2 hours, wait for next scheduled dose (don't double this dose).

What drug does:
Relaxes and expands bronchial tubes.

Time lapse before drug works:
15 to 30 minutes.

Don't take with:
See Interaction column and consult doctor.

OVERDOSE

Symptoms:
Restlessness, irritability, confusion, delirium, convulsions, rapid pulse, coma.

What to do:

- Dial 0 (operator) or 911 (emergency) for an ambulance or medical help. Then give first aid immediately.
- Additional emergency information on page 886.

POSSIBLE ADVERSE REACTIONS OR SIDE EFFECTS

SYMPTOMS	FREQUENCY	WHAT TO DO
Brain & nervous system:		
• Headache, irritability, nervousness, restlessness, insomnia.	Common	4
• Dizziness or lightheadedness.	Infrequent	4
Skin:		
• Rash or hives.	Infrequent	3
• Flushed face.	Infrequent	4
Eyes:	None expected.	
Ears, nose, throat:	None expected.	
Digestive:		
• Nausea, vomiting, stomach pain.	Common	4
• Diarrhea, appetite loss.	Infrequent	3
Heart & lungs:		
• Rapid breathing.	Infrequent	3
• Irregular heartbeat.	Infrequent	3
Blood vessels:	None expected.	
Muscles, bones, joints:	None expected.	
Genital, urinary:	None expected.	
Kidneys:	None expected.	
Liver:	None expected.	
Allergic:	None expected.	
Blood:	None expected.	
Others:	None expected.	

1- Life-threatening. Seek emergency treatment immediately.
2- Discontinue. Seek emergency treatment.
3- Discontinue. Call doctor right away.
4- Continue. Call doctor when convenient.
5- Continue. Tell doctor at next visit.
6- No action necessary.

WARNINGS & PRECAUTIONS

Don't take if:
- You are allergic to any bronchodilator.
- You have an active peptic ulcer.

Before you start, consult your doctor:
- If you have had impaired kidney or liver function.
- If you have gastritis.
- If you have a peptic ulcer.
- If you have high blood pressure or heart disease.
- If you take medication for gout.

Over age 60:
Adverse reactions and side effects may be more frequent and severe than in younger persons.

Pregnancy:
Risk to unborn child outweighs drug benefits. Don't use.

Breast-feeding:
Drug passes into milk. Avoid drug or discontinue nursing until you finish medicine. Consult doctor for advice on maintaining milk supply.

Infants & children:
Use only under medical supervision.

Prolonged use:
Stomach irritation.

Skin & sunlight:
No problems expected.

Driving, piloting or hazardous work:
Avoid if lightheaded or dizzy. Otherwise, no problems expected.

Airplane passengers:
No problems expected.

Discontinuing:
May be unnecessary to finish medicine. Follow doctor's instructions.

Others:
No problems expected.

INTERACTION WITH OTHER DRUGS

GENERIC NAME OR DRUG CLASS	COMBINED EFFECT
Allopurinol	Decreased allopurinol effect.
Ephedrine	Increased effect of both drugs.
Epinephrine	Increased effect of both drugs.
Erythromycin	Increased oxtriphylline effect.
Furosemide	Increased furosemide effect.
Lincomycins	Increased oxtriphylline effect.
Lithium	Decreased lithium effect.
Probenecid	Decreased effect of both drugs.
Propranolol	Decreased oxtriphylline effect.
Rauwolfia alkaloids	Rapid heartbeat.
Sulfinpyrazone	Decreased sulfinpyrazone effect.
Troleandomycin	Increased oxtriphylline effect.

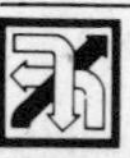

INTERACTION WITH OTHER SUBSTANCES

INTERACTS WITH	COMBINED EFFECT
Alcohol:	None expected.
Beverages:	
Caffeine drinks	Nervousness and insomnia.
Cocaine:	Excess stimulation. Avoid.
Foods:	None expected.
Marijuana:	Slightly increased antiasthmatic effect of oxtriphylline.
Tobacco:	Decreased oxtriphylline effect.

OXYMETAZOLINE

BRAND NAMES

Afrin
Bayfrin
Dristan Long Lasting
Duramist Plus
Duration
Nafrine
Neo-Synephrine 12 Hour
Nostrilla
Ocuclear
Otrivin
Oxymeta-12 Nasal Spray
Sinex Long-Lasting
St. Joseph Decongestant for Children

GENERAL INFORMATION

Habit forming? No
Prescription needed? No
Available as generic? No
Drug class: Sympathomimetic

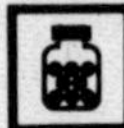

USES

Relieves congestion of nose, sinuses and throat from allergies and infections.

DOSAGE & USAGE INFORMATION

How to take:
Nasal solution, nasal spray—Use as directed on label. Avoid contamination. Don't use same container for more than 1 person.

When to take:
When needed, no more often than every 4 hours.

If you forget a dose:
Take as soon as you remember. Wait 4 hours for next dose.

What drug does:
Constricts walls of small arteries in nose, sinuses and eustachian tubes.

Time lapse before drug works:
5 to 30 minutes.

Don't take with:
- Non-prescription drugs for allergy, cough or cold without consulting doctor.
- See Interaction column and consult doctor.

OVERDOSE

Symptoms:
Headache, sweating, anxiety, agitation, rapid and irregular heartbeat.

What to do:
- Dial 0 (operator) or 911 (emergency) for an ambulance or medical help. Then give first aid immediately.
- If patient is unconscious and not breathing, give mouth-to-mouth breathing. If there is no heartbeat, use cardiac massage and mouth-to-mouth breathing (CPR). If you can't get help quickly, take patient to nearest emergency facility.
- Additional emergency information on page 886.

POSSIBLE ADVERSE REACTIONS OR SIDE EFFECTS

SYMPTOMS	FREQUENCY	WHAT TO DO
Brain & nervous system:		
Headache or lightheadedness, insomnia, nervousness.	Infrequent	4
Skin:	None expected.	
Eyes:	None expected.	
Ears, nose, throat:		
Runny, stuffy, burning, dry or stinging nose, sneezing.	Common	4
Digestive:	None expected.	
Heart & lungs:		
Fast, irregular or pounding heartbeat.	Common	4
Blood vessels:	None expected.	
Muscles, bones, joints:	None expected.	
Genital, urinary:	None expected.	
Kidneys:	None expected.	
Liver:	None expected.	
Allergic:	None expected.	
Blood:	None expected.	
Others:	None expected.	

1- Life-threatening. Seek emergency treatment immediately.
2- Discontinue. Seek emergency treatment.
3- Discontinue. Call doctor right away.
4- Continue. Call doctor when convenient.
5- Continue. Tell doctor at next visit.
6- No action necessary.

WARNINGS & PRECAUTIONS

Don't take if:
You are allergic to any sympathomimetic nasal spray.

Before you start, consult your doctor:
- If you have heart disease or high blood pressure.
- If you have diabetes.
- If you have overactive thyroid.
- If you have taken MAO inhibitors in past 2 weeks.

Over age 60:
Adverse reactions and side effects may be more frequent and severe than in younger persons.

Pregnancy:
No proven harm to unborn child. Avoid if possible.

Breast-feeding:
No proven problems. Consult doctor.

Infants & children:
Don't give to children younger than 2.

Prolonged use:
Drug may lose effectiveness, cause increased congestion ("rebound effect," see page 849) and irritate nasal membranes.

Skin & sunlight:
No problems expected.

Driving, piloting or hazardous work:
No problems expected.

Airplane passengers:
No problems expected.

Discontinuing:
May be unnecessary to finish medicine. Follow doctor's instructions.

Others:
No problems expected.

INTERACTION WITH OTHER DRUGS

GENERIC NAME OR DRUG CLASS	COMBINED EFFECT
MAO inhibitors	Dangerous blood-pressure rise.
Sympathomimetics	Increased effect of both drugs, especially harmful side effects.

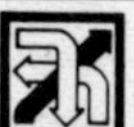

INTERACTION WITH OTHER SUBSTANCES

INTERACTS WITH	COMBINED EFFECT
Alcohol:	None expected.
Beverages:	
Caffeine drinks	Nervousness or insomnia.
Cocaine:	Overstimulation. Avoid.
Foods:	None expected.
Marijuana:	Overstimulation. Avoid.
Tobacco:	None expected.

OXYPHENBUTAZONE

BRAND NAMES

Oxalid
Oxybutazone
Tandearil

GENERAL INFORMATION

Habit forming? No
Prescription needed? Yes
Available as generic? Yes
Drug class: Antiinflammatory (non-steroid)

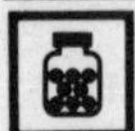

USES

- Treatment for joint pain, stiffness, inflammation and swelling of arthritis and gout.
- Pain reliever.
- Treatment for dysmenorrhea (painful or difficult menstruation).

DOSAGE & USAGE INFORMATION

How to take:
Tablet or capsule—Swallow with liquid or food to lessen stomach irritation. If you can't swallow whole, crumble tablet or open capsule and take with liquid or food.

When to take:
At the same times each day.

If you forget a dose:
Take as soon as you remember up to 2 hours late. If more than 2 hours, wait for next scheduled dose (don't double this dose).

What drug does:
Reduces tissue concentration of prostaglandins (hormones which produce inflammation and pain).

Time lapse before drug works:
Begins in 4 to 24 hours. May require 3 weeks regular use for maximum benefit.

Don't take with:
See Interaction column and consult doctor.

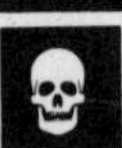

OVERDOSE

Symptoms:
Confusion, agitation, incoherence, convulsions, possible hemorrhage from stomach or intestine, coma.

What to do:
- Dial 0 (operator) or 911 (emergency) for an ambulance or medical help. Then give first aid immediately.
- Additional emergency information on page 886.

POSSIBLE ADVERSE REACTIONS OR SIDE EFFECTS

SYMPTOMS	FREQUENCY	WHAT TO DO
Brain & nervous system:		
• Depression, drowsiness.	Infrequent	4
• Convulsions, confusion.	Rare	3
• Dizziness	Common	4
• Headache	Common	5
Skin:		
Rash, hives or itch.	Rare	3
Eyes:		
Blurred vision.	Rare	3
Ears, nose, throat:		
• Ringing in ears.	Infrequent	4
• Sore throat, fever, mouth ulcers.	Rare	3
Digestive:		
• Black stools, vomiting blood.	Rare	3
• Stomach upset.	Common	4
• Constipation or diarrhea, vomiting.	Infrequent	4
Heart & lungs:		
Breathing difficulty, tightness in chest.	Rare	3
Blood vessels:		
Unusual bleeding or bruising.	Rare	3
Muscles, bones, joints:		
Swollen feet, legs.	Infrequent	4
Genital, urinary:		
• Bloody urine.	Rare	3
• Difficult, painful or frequent urination.	Rare	4
Kidneys, allergic, blood, liver:	None expected.	
Others:		
• Fatigue, weakness.	Rare	4
• Weight gain.	Rare	4

1- Life-threatening. Seek emergency treatment immediately.
2- Discontinue. Seek emergency treatment.
3- Discontinue. Call doctor right away.
4- Continue. Call doctor when convenient.
5- Continue. Tell doctor at next visit.

WARNINGS & PRECAUTIONS

Don't take if:
- You are allergic to aspirin or any non-steroid, antiinflammatory drug.
- You have gastritis, peptic ulcer, enteritis, ileitis, ulcerative colitis.
- Patient is younger than 15.

Before you start, consult your doctor:
- If you have epilepsy.
- If you have Parkinson's disease.
- If you have been mentally ill.
- If you have had kidney disease or impaired kidney function, asthma, high blood pressure, heart failure, temporal arthritis, or polymyalgia rheumatica.

Over age 60:
Adverse reactions and side effects may be more frequent and severe than in younger persons.

Pregnancy:
Studies inconclusive on harm to unborn child. Animal studies show fetal abnormalities. Decide with your doctor whether drug benefits justify risk to unborn child.

Breast-feeding:
Drug filters into milk. May harm child. Avoid.

Infants & children:
Not recommended for those younger than 15. Use only under medical supervision.

Prolonged use:
- Eye damage.
- May cause rare bone-marrow damage, jaundice (yellow skin and eyes), reduced hearing.
- Periodic blood counts recommended if you use a long time.

Skin & sunlight:
No problems expected.

Driving, piloting or hazardous work:
Don't drive or pilot aircraft until you learn how medicine affects you. Don't work around dangerous machinery. Don't climb ladders or work in high places. Danger increases if you drink alcohol or take medicine affecting alertness and reflexes, such as antihistamines, tranquilizers, sedatives, pain medicine, narcotics and mind-altering drugs.

Airplane passengers:
No problems expected.

Discontinuing:
Don't discontinue without consulting doctor. Dose may require gradual reduction if you have taken drug for a long time. Doses of other drugs may also require adjustment.

INTERACTION WITH OTHER DRUGS

GENERIC NAME OR DRUG CLASS	COMBINED EFFECT
Anticoagulants (oral)	Increased anticoagulant effect.
Aspirin	Possible stomach ulcer.
Antidiabetics (oral)	Increased antidiabetic effect.
Chloroquine	Possible skin toxicity.
Digitoxin	Decreased digitoxin effect.
Gold compounds	Increased toxicity to skin and bone marrow.
Hydroxychloroquine	Possible skin toxicity.
Methotrexate	Increased toxicity of both drugs to bone marrow.
Penicillamine	Possible toxicity.
Phenytoin	Possible toxic phenytoin effect.
Trimethoprim	Possible bone-marrow toxicity.

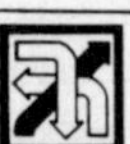

INTERACTION WITH OTHER SUBSTANCES

INTERACTS WITH	COMBINED EFFECT
Alcohol:	Possible stomach ulcer or bleeding.
Beverages:	None expected.
Cocaine:	None expected.
Foods:	None expected.
Marijuana:	Increased pain relief from oxyphenbutazone.
Tobacco:	None expected.

PANCRELIPASE

BRAND NAMES

Cotazym
Ilozyme
Ku-Zyme HP
Pancrease

GENERAL INFORMATION

Habit forming? No
Prescription needed? Yes
Available as generic? No
Drug class: Enzyme (pancreatic)

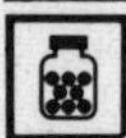

USES

- Replaces pancreatic enzyme deficiency caused by surgery or disease.
- Treats fatty stools (steatorrhea).

DOSAGE & USAGE INFORMATION

How to take:

- Capsules—swallow whole. Do not take with milk or milk products.
- Powder—sprinkle on liquid or soft food.

When to take:
Before meals.

If you forget a dose:
Take as soon as you remember up to 2 hours late. If more than 2 hours, wait for next scheduled dose (don't double this dose).

What drug does:
Enhances digestion of proteins, carbohydrates and fats.

Time lapse before drug works:
30 minutes.

Don't take with:
See Interaction column and consult doctor.

OVERDOSE

Symptoms:
Shortness of breath, wheezing, diarrhea.

What to do:
Overdose unlikely to threaten life. If person takes much larger amount than prescribed, call doctor, poison-control center or hospital emergency room for instructions.

POSSIBLE ADVERSE REACTIONS OR SIDE EFFECTS

SYMPTOMS	FREQUENCY	WHAT TO DO
Brain & nervous system:	None expected.	
Skin:		
Rash, hives.	Rare	3
Eyes:	None expected.	
Ears, nose, throat:	None expected.	
Digestive:		
Nausea.	Rare	4
Heart & lungs:	None expected.	
Blood vessels:	None expected.	
Muscles, bones, joints:		
Joint pain.	Rare	4
Genital, urinary:		
Bloody urine.	Rare	3
Kidneys, allergic, blood, liver:	None expected.	
Others:		
Swollen feet or legs.	Rare	3

1- Life-threatening. Seek emergency treatment immediately.
2- Discontinue. Seek emergency treatment.
3- Discontinue. Call doctor right away.
4- Continue. Call doctor when convenient.
5- Continue. Tell doctor at next visit.
6- No action necessary.

WARNINGS & PRECAUTIONS

Don't take if:
You are allergic to pancreatin, pancrelipase, or pork.

Before you start, consult your doctor:
If you take any other medicines.

Over age 60:
Adverse reactions and side effects may be more frequent and severe than in younger persons.

Pregnancy:
Risk to unborn child outweighs drug benefits. Don't use.

Breast-feeding:
Drug passes into milk. Avoid drug or discontinue nursing until you finish medicine. Consult doctor for advice on maintaining milk supply.

Infants & children:
Under close medical supervision only.

Prolonged use:
No additional problems expected.

Skin & sunlight:
No problems expected.

Driving, piloting or hazardous work:
No problems expected.

Airplane passengers:
No problems expected.

Discontinuing:
Don't discontinue without consulting doctor. Dose may require gradual reduction if you have taken drug for a long time. Doses of other drugs may also require adjustment.

Others:
If you take powder form, avoid inhaling.

INTERACTION WITH OTHER DRUGS

GENERIC NAME OR DRUG CLASS	COMBINED EFFECT
Calcium carbonate antacids.	Decreased effect of pancrelipase.
Magnesium hydroxide antacids	Decreased effect of pancrelipase.
Iron preparations	Decreased iron absorption.

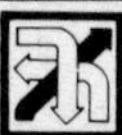

INTERACTION WITH OTHER SUBSTANCES

INTERACTS WITH	COMBINED EFFECT
Alcohol:	Unknown.
Beverages: Milk	Decreased effect of pancrelipase.
Cocaine:	Unknown.
Foods: Ice cream, milk products.	Decreased effect of pancrelipase.
Marijuana:	Decreased absorption of pancrelipase.
Tobacco:	Decreased absorption of pancrelipase.

PANTOTHENIC ACID (VITAMIN B-5)

BRAND AND GENERIC NAMES

CALCIUM PATOTHENATE
Durasil
Pantholin
PANTOTHENIC ACID
Ingredients in numerous multiple vitamin-mineral supplements.

GENERAL INFORMATION

Habit forming? No
Prescription needed? No
Available as generic? Yes
Drug class: Vitamin supplement

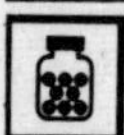

USES

Prevents and treats vitamin B-5 deficiency.

DOSAGE & USAGE INFORMATION

How to take:
- Tablet or capsule—Swallow with liquid.
- Extended-release tablets—Swallow each dose whole with liquid.

When to take:
At the same times each day.

If you forget a dose:
Take as soon as you remember, then resume regular schedule.

What drug does:
Acts as co-enzyme in carbohydrate, protein and fat metabolism.

Time lapse before drug works:
15 to 20 minutes.

Don't take with:
- Levodopa—Small amounts of pantothenic acid will nullify levodopa effect. Carbidopa-levodopa combination not affected by this interaction.
- See Interaction column and consult doctor.

OVERDOSE

Symptoms:
None expected.

What to do:
Overdose unlikely to threaten life.

POSSIBLE ADVERSE REACTIONS OR SIDE EFFECTS

SYMPTOMS	FREQUENCY	WHAT TO DO
Brain & nervous system:	None expected.	
Skin:	None expected.	
Eyes:	None expected.	
Ears, nose, throat:	None expected.	
Digestive:	None expected.	
Heart & lungs:	None expected.	
Blood vessels:	None expected.	
Muscles, bones, joints:	None expected.	
Genital, urinary:	None expected.	
Kidneys, allergic, blood, liver:	None expected.	

1 - Life-threatening. Seek emergency treatment immediately.
2 - Discontinue. Seek emergency treatment.
3 - Discontinue. Call doctor right away.
4 - Continue. Call doctor when convenient.
5 - Continue. Tell doctor at next visit.
6 - No action necessary.

PANTOTHENIC ACID (VITAMIN B-5)

WARNINGS & PRECAUTIONS

Don't take if:
You are allergic to pantothenic acid.

Before you start, consult your doctor:
If you have hemophilia.

Over age 60:
No problems expected.

Pregnancy:
Don't exceed recommended dose.

Breast-feeding:
Don't exceed recommended dose.

Infants & children:
Don't exceed recommended dose.

Prolonged use:
Large doses for more than 1 month may cause toxicity.

Skin & sunlight:
No problems expected.

Driving, piloting or hazardous work:
No problems expected.

Airplane passengers:
No problems expected.

Discontinuing:
No problems expected.

Others:
Regular pantothenic acid supplements are recommended if you take chloramphenicol, cycloserine, ethionamide, hydralazine, immunosuppressants, isoniazid or penicillamine. These decrease pantothenic acid absorption and can cause anemia or tingling and numbness in hands and feet.

INTERACTION WITH OTHER DRUGS

GENERIC NAME OR DRUG CLASS	COMBINED EFFECT
None expected.	

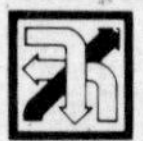

INTERACTION WITH OTHER SUBSTANCES

INTERACTS WITH	COMBINED EFFECT
Alcohol:	None expected.
Beverages:	None expected.
Cocaine:	None expected.
Foods:	None expected.
Marijuana:	None expected.
Tobacco:	May decrease pantothenic acid absorption. Decreased pantothenic acid effect.

PAPAVERINE

BRAND NAMES

Cerebid	Kavrin	Pavacap	Pavatran
Cerespan	Myobid	Pavadon	Paverolan
Copavin	Octapav	Pavagen	Ro-Papan
Durapav	P-200	Pavased	Sustaverine
Dylate	P-A-V	Pavasule	Vasospan

See complete brand names list, page 829.

GENERAL INFORMATION

Habit forming? No
Prescription needed? Yes
Available as generic? Yes
Drug class: Vasodilator

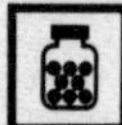

USES

Improves poor circulation in the extremities or brain.

DOSAGE & USAGE INFORMATION

How to take:
- Tablet or capsule—Swallow with liquid or food to lessen stomach irritation. If you can't swallow whole, crumble tablet or open capsule and take with liquid or food.
- Extended-release tablets or capsules—Swallow whole with liquid.
- Liquid—Follow label instructions.

When to take:
At the same times each day.

If you forget a dose:
Take as soon as you remember up to 2 hours late. If more than 2 hours, wait for next scheduled dose (don't double this dose).

What drug does:
Relaxes and expands blood-vessel walls, allowing better distribution of oxygen and nutrients.

Time lapse before drug works:
30 to 60 minutes.

Don't take with:
- Non-prescription drugs without consulting doctor.
- See Interaction column and consult doctor.

OVERDOSE

Symptoms:
Weakness, fainting, flush, sweating, stupor, irregular heartbeat.

What to do:
- Dial 0 (operator) or 911 (emergency) for an ambulance or medical help. Then give first aid immediately.
- Additional emergency information on page 886.

POSSIBLE ADVERSE REACTIONS OR SIDE EFFECTS

SYMPTOMS	FREQUENCY	WHAT TO DO
Brain & nervous system:		
Drowsiness, dizziness, headache.	Common	4
Skin:		
• Flushed face.	Common	4
• Rash, itch.	Infrequent	3
Eyes:		
Blurred or double vision.	Infrequent	3
Ears, nose, throat:		
Dry mouth, throat.	Common	5
Digestive:		
Stomach irritation, indigestion, nausea, mild constipation.	Common	4
Heart & lungs:		
Deep breathing, rapid heartbeat.	Infrequent	4
Blood vessels:		
Low blood pressure, causing lethargy or dizziness (especially on change of position).	Common	4
Muscles, bones, joints, genital, urinary, kidneys, allergic, blood:	None expected.	
Liver:		
Jaundice (yellow skin and eyes).	Rare	3
Others:		
Weakness	Infrequent	3

1-Life-threatening. Seek emergency treatment immediately.
2-Discontinue. Seek emergency treatment.
3-Discontinue. Call doctor right away.
4-Continue. Call doctor when convenient.
5-Continue. Tell doctor at next visit.

WARNINGS & PRECAUTIONS

Don't take if:
You are allergic to any narcotic.

Before you start, consult your doctor:
- If you plan to become pregnant within medication period.
- If you have had a heart attack, heart disease, angina or stroke.
- If you have Parkinson's disease.

Over age 60:
Adverse reactions and side effects may be more frequent and severe than in younger persons.

Pregnancy:
No proven harm to unborn child. Avoid if possible.

Breast-feeding:
Drug filters into milk. May harm child. Avoid.

Infants & children:
Not recommended.

Prolonged use:
No problems expected.

Skin & sunlight:
No problems expected.

Driving, piloting or hazardous work:
Don't drive or pilot aircraft until you learn how medicine affects you. Don't work around dangerous machinery. Don't climb ladders or work in high places. Danger increases if you drink alcohol or take medicine affecting alertness and reflexes, such as antihistamines, tranquilizers, sedatives, pain medicine, narcotics and mind-altering drugs.

Airplane passengers:
No problems expected.

Discontinuing:
May be unnecessary to finish medicine. If drug does not help in 1 to 2 weeks, consult doctor about discontinuing.

Others:
- Periodic liver-function tests recommended.
- Internal eye-pressure measurements recommended if you have glaucoma.

INTERACTION WITH OTHER DRUGS

GENERIC NAME OR DRUG CLASS	COMBINED EFFECT
Levodopa	Decreased levodopa effect.
Narcotics	Increased papaverine effect.
Pain relievers	Increased papaverine effect.
Sedatives	Increased papaverine effect.
Tranquilizers	Increased papaverine effect.

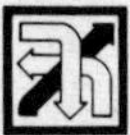

INTERACTION WITH OTHER SUBSTANCES

INTERACTS WITH	COMBINED EFFECT
Alcohol:	None expected.
Beverages:	None expected.
Cocaine:	Decreased papaverine effect.
Foods:	None expected.
Marijuana:	None expected.
Tobacco:	Decrease in papaverine's dilation of blood vessels.

PARA-AMINOSALICYLIC ACID (PAS)

BRAND NAMES

Nemasol
Parasal
P.A.S.
P.A.S. Acid
Pasna
Teebacin

GENERAL INFORMATION

Habit forming? No
Prescription needed? Yes
Available as generic? Yes
Drug class: Antitubercular

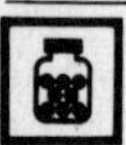

USES

Treatment for tuberculosis.

DOSAGE & USAGE INFORMATION

How to take:
- Tablet—Swallow with liquid or food to lessen stomach irritation.
- Powder—Dissolve dose in water. Stir well and drink all liquid.

When to take:
At the same times each day.

If you forget a dose:
Take as soon as you remember up to 2 hours late. If more than 2 hours, wait for next scheduled dose (don't double this dose).

What drug does:
- Prevents growth of TB germs.
- Makes TB germs more susceptible to other antituberculosis drugs.

Time lapse before drug works:
6 months.

Don't take with:
See Interaction column and consult doctor.

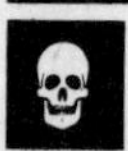

OVERDOSE

Symptoms:
Nausea, vomiting, diarrhea; rapid breathing; convulsions.

What to do:
- Dial 0 (operator) or 911 (emergency) for an ambulance or medical help. Then give first aid immediately.
- Additional emergency information on page 886.

POSSIBLE ADVERSE REACTIONS OR SIDE EFFECTS

SYMPTOMS	FREQUENCY	WHAT TO DO
Brain & nervous system:		
• Headache	Infrequent	4
• Confusion	Infrequent	3
Skin:		
Itching, dry, puffy skin.	Infrequent	4
Eyes:		
Light sensitivity.	Infrequent	4
Ears, nose, throat:		
Sore throat, fever.	Infrequent	4
Digestive:		
• Constipation or vomiting.	Infrequent	4
• Diarrhea or stomach pain.	Common	4
Heart & lungs, blood vessels, muscles, bones, joints, allergic, blood:	None expected.	
Genital, urinary:		
• Painful urination.	Common	3
• Bloody urine.	Infrequent	3
Kidneys:		
Low back pain.	Common	3
Liver:		
Jaundice (yellow skin and eyes).	Rare	3
Others:		
• Chills	Common	3
• Swelling in front of neck.	Infrequent	4
• Changed menstrual pattern.	Infrequent	5
• Decreased sex drive in men.	Infrequent	4
• Fatigue, weakness.	Infrequent	4

1- Life-threatening. Seek emergency treatment immediately.
2- Discontinue. Seek emergency treatment.
3- Discontinue. Call doctor right away.
4- Continue. Call doctor when convenient.
5- Continue. Tell doctor at next visit.

PARA-AMINOSALICYLIC ACID (PAS)

WARNINGS & PRECAUTIONS

Don't take if:

- You are allergic to PAS, aspirin or other salicylates.
- Tablets have turned brownish or purplish.

Before you start, consult your doctor:

- If you have ulcers in stomach or duodenum.
- If you have liver or kidney disease.
- If you have epilepsy.
- If you have adrenal insufficiency.
- If you have heart disease or congestive heart failure.
- If you have cancer.
- If you have overactive thyroid.

Over age 60:
Adverse reactions and side effects may be more frequent and severe than in younger persons.

Pregnancy:
Risk to unborn child outweighs drug benefits. Don't use.

Breast-feeding:
No proven problems. Consult doctor.

Infants & children:
Use only under medical supervision.

Prolonged use:
Enlarged thyroid gland and decreased function.

Skin & sunlight:
No problems expected.

Driving, piloting or hazardous work:
No problems expected.

Airplane passengers:
No problems expected.

Discontinuing:
No problems expected.

Others:

- Treatment may need to continue for several years or indefinitely.
- Periodic blood tests and liver- and kidney-function studies recommended.

INTERACTION WITH OTHER DRUGS

GENERIC NAME OR DRUG CLASS	COMBINED EFFECT
Aminobenzoic acid (PABA)	Decreased effect of PAS.
Anticoagulants (oral)	Increased anticoagulant effect.
Anticonvulsants (hydantoin)	Increased anticonvulsant effect.
Aspirin	Stomach irritation.
Barbiturates	Oversedation.
Folic acid	Decreased effect of folic acid.
Probenecid	Increased PAS effect. Possible toxicity.
Rifampin	Decreased rifampin effect.
Sulfa drugs	Decreased effect of sulfa drugs.
Sulfinpyrazone	Increased PAS effect. Possible toxicity.
Tetracyclines	Reduced absorption of PAS. Space doses 3 hours apart.

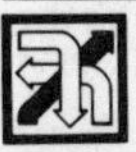

INTERACTION WITH OTHER SUBSTANCES

INTERACTS WITH	COMBINED EFFECT
Alcohol:	Possible liver disease.
Beverages:	None expected
Cocaine:	None expected.
Foods:	None expected.
Marijuana:	None expected.
Tobacco:	None expected, but tobacco smoking may slow recovery. Avoid.

PARAMETHASONE

BRAND NAMES

Haldrone

GENERAL INFORMATION

Habit forming? No
Prescription needed? Yes
Available as generic? No
Drug class: Cortisone drug (adrenal corticosteroid)

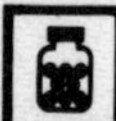

USES

- Reduces inflammation caused by many different medical problems.
- Treatment for some allergic diseases, blood disorders, kidney diseases, asthma and emphysema.
- Replaces corticosteroid deficiencies.

DOSAGE & USAGE INFORMATION

How to take:
Tablet—Swallow with liquid or food to lessen stomach irritation. If you can't swallow whole, crumble tablet and take with liquid or food.

When to take:
At the same times each day. Take once-a-day or once-every-other-day doses in mornings.

If you forget a dose:
- Several-doses-per-day prescription—Take as soon as you remember up to 2 hours late. If more than 2 hours, wait for next scheduled dose (don't double this dose).
- Once-a-day dose or less—Wait for next dose. Double this dose.

What drug does:
Decreases inflammatory responses.

Time lapse before drug works:
2 to 4 days.

Don't take with:
See Interaction column and consult doctor.

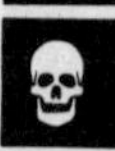

OVERDOSE

Symptoms:
Headache, convulsions, heart failure.

What to do:
- Dial 0 (operator) or 911 (emergency) for an ambulance or medical help. Then give first aid immediately.
- Additional emergency information on page 886.

POSSIBLE ADVERSE REACTIONS OR SIDE EFFECTS

SYMPTOMS	FREQUENCY	WHAT TO DO
Brain & nervous system:		
Mood changes, insomnia, restlessness.	Infrequent	4
Skin:		
• Acne	Common	4
• Rash	Rare	3
• Poor wound healing.	Common	4
Eyes:		
Blurred vision, halos around lights.	Infrequent	3
Ears, nose, throat:		
• Sore throat, fever.	Infrequent	3
• Thirst	Common	4
Digestive:		
• Indigestion, nausea, vomiting.	Common	4
• Bloody or black, tarry stool.	Infrequent	2
Heart & lungs:		
Irregular heartbeat.	Rare	2
Blood vessels, kidneys, liver, allergic, blood:	None expected.	
Muscles, bones, joints:		
Muscle cramps, swollen legs, feet.	Infrequent	3
Genital, urinary:		
Frequent urination.	Infrequent	4
Others:		
• Weight gain, round face.	Infrequent	4
• Fatigue, weakness.	Infrequent	4
• TB recurrence.	Infrequent	4
• Irregular menstrual periods.	Infrequent	4

1-Life-threatening. Seek emergency treatment immediately.
2-Discontinue. Seek emergency treatment.
3-Discontinue. Call doctor right away.
4-Continue. Call doctor when convenient.

WARNINGS & PRECAUTIONS

Don't take if:
- You are allergic to any cortisone drug.
- You have tuberculosis or fungus infection.
- You have herpes infection of eyes, lips or genitals.

Before you start, consult your doctor:
- If you have had tuberculosis.
- If you have congestive heart failure.
- If you have diabetes.
- If you have peptic ulcer.
- If you have glaucoma.
- If you have underactive thyroid.
- If you have high blood pressure.
- If you have myasthenia gravis.
- If you have blood clots in legs or lungs.

Over age 60:
Adverse reactions and side effects may be more frequent and severe than in younger persons. Likely to aggravate edema, diabetes or ulcers. Likely to cause cataracts and osteoporosis (softening of the bones).

Pregnancy:
Risk to unborn child outweighs drug benefits. Don't use.

Breast-feeding:
Drug passes into milk. Avoid drug or discontinue nursing until you finish medicine. Consult doctor for advice on maintaining milk supply.

Infants & children:
Use only under medical supervision.

Prolonged use:
- Retards growth in children.
- Possible glaucoma, cataracts, diabetes, fragile bones and thin skin.
- Functional dependence.

Skin & sunlight:
No problems expected.

Driving, piloting or hazardous work:
No problems expected.

Airplane passengers:
No problems expected.

Discontinuing:
- Don't discontinue without doctor's advice until you complete prescribed dose, even though symptoms diminish or disappear.
- Drug affects your response to surgery, illness, injury or stress for 2 years after discontinuing. Tell about drug to anyone who takes medical care of you within 2 years.

Others:
Avoid immunizations if possible.

INTERACTION WITH OTHER DRUGS

GENERIC NAME OR DRUG CLASS	COMBINED EFFECT
Amphoterecin B	Potassium depletion.
Anticholinergics	Possible glaucoma.
Anticoagulants (oral)	Decreased anticoagulant effect.
Anticonvulsants (hydantoin)	Decreased paramethasone effect.
Antidiabetics (oral)	Decreased antidiabetic effect.
Antihistamines	Decreased paramethasone effect.
Aspirin	Increased paramethasone effect.
Barbiturates	Decreased paramethasone effect. Oversedation.
Beta-adrenergic blockers	Decreased paramethasone effect.
Chloral hydrate	Decreased paramethasone effect.
Chlorthalidone	Potassium depletion.
Cholinergics	Decreased cholinergic effect.
Contraceptives (oral)	Increased paramethasone effect.
Digitalis preparations	Dangerous potassium depletion. Possible digitalis toxicity.

Additional interactions on page 840.

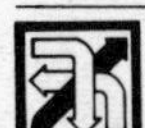

INTERACTION WITH OTHER SUBSTANCES

INTERACTS WITH	COMBINED EFFECT
Alcohol:	Risk of stomach ulcers.
Beverages:	No proven problems.
Cocaine:	Overstimulation. Avoid.
Foods:	No proven problems.
Marijuana:	Decreased immunity.
Tobacco:	Increased paramethasone effect. Possible toxicity.

PAREGORIC

BRAND NAMES

Brown Mixture
CM with Paregoric
Diban
Donnagel-PG
Kaoparin
Opium Tincture
Parepectolin
Pomalin

GENERAL INFORMATION

Habit forming? Yes
Prescription needed? Yes
Available as generic? Yes
Drug class: Narcotic, antidiarrheal

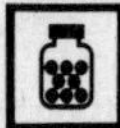

USES

Reduces intestinal cramps and diarrhea.

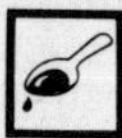

DOSAGE & USAGE INFORMATION

How to take:
Drops or liquid—Dilute dose in beverage before swallowing.

When to take:
As needed for diarrhea, no more often than every 4 hours.

If you forget a dose:
Take as soon as you remember. Wait 4 hours for next dose.

What drug does:
Anesthetizes surface membranes of intestines and blocks nerve impulses.

Time lapse before drug works:
2 to 6 hours.

Don't take with:
See Interaction column and consult doctor.

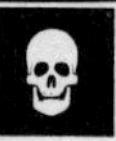

OVERDOSE

Symptoms:
Deep sleep; slow breathing; slow pulse; flushed, warm skin; constricted pupils.

What to do:
- Dial 0 (operator) or 911 (emergency) for an ambulance or medical help. Then give first aid immediately.
- If patient is unconscious and not breathing, give mouth-to-mouth breathing. If there is no heartbeat, use cardiac massage and mouth-to-mouth breathing (CPR). Don't try to make patient vomit. If you can't get help quickly, take patient to nearest emergency facility.
- Additional emergency information on page 886.

POSSIBLE ADVERSE REACTIONS OR SIDE EFFECTS

SYMPTOMS	FREQUENCY	WHAT TO DO
Brain & nervous system:		
• Depression	Rare	4
• Dizziness	Common	4
Skin:		
• Hives, itch, rash.	Rare	3
• Flushed face.	Common	4
Eyes:	None expected.	
Ears, nose, throat:	None expected.	
Digestive:		
Severe constipation, abdominal pain, vomiting.	Infrequent	3
Heart & lungs:		
Slow heartbeat, irregular breathing.	Rare	3
Blood vessels:	None expected.	
Muscles, bones, joints:	None expected.	
Genital, urinary:		
Difficult urination.	Common	4
Kidneys:	None expected.	
Liver:	None expected.	
Allergic:	None expected.	
Blood:	None expected.	
Others:		
Unusual tiredness.	Common	4

1 - Life-threatening. Seek emergency treatment immediately.
2 - Discontinue. Seek emergency treatment.
3 - Discontinue. Call doctor right away.
4 - Continue. Call doctor when convenient.
5 - Continue. Tell doctor at next visit.
6 - No action necessary.

WARNINGS & PRECAUTIONS

Don't take if:
You are allergic to any narcotic.

Before you start, consult your doctor:
If you have impaired liver or kidney function.

Over age 60:
More likely to be drowsy, dizzy, unsteady or constipated.

Pregnancy:
No proven harm to unborn child. Avoid if possible.

Breast-feeding:
Drug filters into milk. May depress infant. Avoid.

Infants & children:
Use only under medical supervision.

Prolonged use:
Causes psychological and physical dependence.

Skin & sunlight:
No problems expected.

Driving, piloting or hazardous work:
Don't drive or pilot aircraft until you learn how medicine affects you. Don't work around dangerous machinery. Don't climb ladders or work in high places. Danger increases if you drink alcohol or take medicine affecting alertness and reflexes, such as antihistamines, tranquilizers, sedatives, pain medicine, narcotics and mind-altering drugs.

Airplane passengers:
No problems expected.

Discontinuing:
May be unnecessary to finish medicine. Follow doctor's instructions.

Others:
Great potential for abuse.

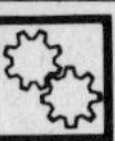

INTERACTION WITH OTHER DRUGS

GENERIC NAME OR DRUG CLASS	COMBINED EFFECT
Analgesics	Increased analgesic effect.
Antidepressants	Increased sedative effect.
Antihistamines	Increased sedative effect.
Mind-altering drugs	Increased sedative effect.
Narcotics (other)	Increased narcotic effect.
Phenothiazines	Increased sedative effect of paregoric.
Sedatives	Excessive sedation.
Sleep inducers	Increased effect of sleep inducers.
Tranquilizers	Increased tranquilizer effect.

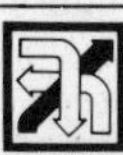

INTERACTION WITH OTHER SUBSTANCES

INTERACTS WITH	COMBINED EFFECT
Alcohol:	Increases alcohol's intoxicating effect. Avoid.
Beverages:	None expected.
Cocaine:	None expected.
Foods:	None expected.
Marijuana:	Impairs physical and mental performance.
Tobacco:	None expected.

PEMOLINE

BRAND NAMES

Cyclert

GENERAL INFORMATION

Habit forming? Yes
Prescription needed? Yes
Available as generic? No
Drug class: Central-nervous-system stimulant

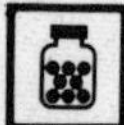

USES

- Decreases overactivity and lengthens attention span in hyperactive children.
- Treatment of minimal brain dysfunction.

DOSAGE & USAGE INFORMATION

How to take:
Tablet or capsule—Swallow with liquid or food to lessen stomach irritation. If you can't swallow whole, crumble tablet or open capsule and take with liquid or food.

When to take:
At the same times each day.

If you forget a dose:
Take as soon as you remember up to 2 hours late. If more than 2 hours, wait for next scheduled dose (don't double this dose).

What drug does:
Stimulates brain to improve alertness, concentration and attention span. Calms the hyperactive child.

Time lapse before drug works:
- 1 month or more for maximum effect on child.
- 30 minutes to stimulate adults.

Don't take with:
See Interaction column and consult doctor.

OVERDOSE

Symptoms:
Rapid heartbeat, hallucinations, fever, confusion, convulsions, coma.

What to do:
- Dial 0 (operator) or 911 (emergency) for an ambulance or medical help. Then give first aid immediately.
- If patient is unconscious and not breathing, give mouth-to-mouth breathing. If there is no heartbeat, use cardiac massage and mouth-to-mouth breathing (CPR). Don't try to make patient vomit. If you can't get help quickly, take patient to nearest emergency facility.
- Additional emergency information on page 886.

POSSIBLE ADVERSE REACTIONS OR SIDE EFFECTS

SYMPTOMS	FREQUENCY	WHAT TO DO
Brain & nervous system:		
• Insomnia	Common	4
• Irritability, depression, dizziness, headache, drowsiness.	Infrequent	3
Skin:		
Rash	Infrequent	4
Eyes:		
Unusual movement of eyes.	Infrequent	3
Ears, nose, throat:		
Unusual movements of tongue.	Infrequent	4
Digestive:		
• Appetite loss.	Infrequent	4
• Abdominal pain.	Infrequent	4
• Nausea	Infrequent	4
Heart & lungs:		
Rapid heartbeat.	Infrequent	3
Blood vessels:	None expected.	
Muscles, bones, joints:	None expected.	
Genital, urinary:	None expected.	
Kidneys, allergic, blood, liver:		
Jaundice (yellow skin and eyes).	Rare	3
Others:		
Weight loss.	Infrequent	4

1-Life-threatening. Seek emergency treatment immediately.
2-Discontinue. Seek emergency treatment.
3-Discontinue. Call doctor right away.
4-Continue. Call doctor when convenient.
5-Continue. Tell doctor at next visit.

WARNINGS & PRECAUTIONS

Don't take if:
You are allergic to pemoline.

Before you start, consult your doctor:
- If you have liver disease.
- If you have kidney disease.
- If patient younger than 6 years.
- If there is marked emotional instability.

Over age 60:
Adverse reactions and side effects may be more frequent and severe than in younger persons.

Pregnancy:
No proven harm to unborn child. Avoid if possible.

Breast-feeding:
No problems expected. Consult doctor.

Infants & children:
Use only under close medical supervision for children 6 or older.

Prolonged use:
Rare possibility of physical growth retardation.

Skin & sunlight:
No problems expected.

Driving, piloting or hazardous work:
Don't drive or pilot aircraft until you learn how medicine affects you. Don't work around dangerous machinery. Don't climb ladders or work in high places. Danger increases if you drink alcohol or take medicine affecting alertness and reflexes, such as antihistamines, tranquilizers, sedatives, pain medicine, narcotics and mind-altering drugs.

Airplane passengers:
No problems expected.

Discontinuing:
Don't discontinue without consulting doctor. Dose may require gradual reduction if you have taken drug for a long time. Doses of other drugs may also require adjustment.

Others:
Dose must be carefully adjusted by doctor.

INTERACTION WITH OTHER DRUGS

GENERIC NAME OR DRUG CLASS	COMBINED EFFECT
None identified.	

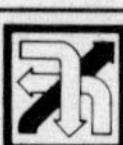

INTERACTION WITH OTHER SUBSTANCES

INTERACTS WITH	COMBINED EFFECT
Alcohol:	More chance of depression. Avoid.
Beverages: Caffeine drinks.	May raise blood pressure. Avoid.
Cocaine:	Overstimulation. Avoid.
Foods:	No problems expected.
Marijuana:	Unknown
Tobacco:	Unknown

PENICILLAMINE

BRAND NAMES

Cuprimine
Depen

GENERAL INFORMATION

Habit forming? No
Prescription needed? Yes
Available as generic? Yes
Drug class: Chelating agent, antirheumatic, antidote (heavy-metal)

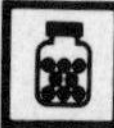

USES

- Treatment for rheumatoid arthritis.
- Prevention of kidney stones.
- Treatment for heavy-metal poisoning.

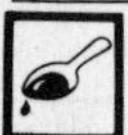

DOSAGE & USAGE INFORMATION

How to take:
Tablets or capsules—With liquid on an empty stomach 1 hour before or 2 hours after eating.

When to take:
At the same times each day.

If you forget a dose:
- 1 dose a day—Take as soon as you remember up to 12 hours late. If more than 12 hours, wait for next scheduled dose (don't double this dose).
- More than 1 dose a day—Take as soon as you remember up to 2 hours late. If more than 2 hours, wait for next scheduled dose (don't double this dose).

What drug does:
- Combines with heavy metals so kidney can excrete them.
- Combines with cysteine (amino acid found in many foods) to prevent cysteine kidney stones.
- May improve protective function of some white-blood cells against rheumatoid arthritis.

Time lapse before drug works:
2 to 3 months.

Don't take with:
See Interaction column and consult doctor.

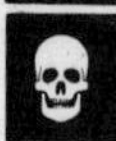

OVERDOSE

Symptoms:
Ulcers, sores, convulsions, coughing up blood, coma.

What to do:
- Dial 0 (operator) or 911 (emergency) for an ambulance or medical help. Then give first aid immediately.
- Additional emergency information on page 886.

POSSIBLE ADVERSE REACTIONS OR SIDE EFFECTS

SYMPTOMS	FREQUENCY	WHAT TO DO
Brain & nervous system:	None expected.	
Skin:		
Rash, itch.	Common	3
Eyes:		
Double or blurred vision, pain.	Rare	3
Ears, nose, throat:		
• Sore throat, fever.	Infrequent	3
• Ringing in ears.	Rare	3
• Ulcer, sores, white spots in mouth.	Rare	3
Digestive:		
Appetite loss, nausea, diarrhea, vomiting.	Infrequent	4
Heart & lungs:		
Breathing difficulty, coughing up blood.	Rare	3
Blood vessels:		
Unusual bruising.	Infrequent	3
Muscles, bones, joints:		
• Joint pain.	Common	3
• Swollen feet, legs.	Infrequent	3
Genital, urinary:		
Bloody or cloudy urine.	Infrequent	3
Kidneys, allergic, blood:	None expected.	
Liver:		
Jaundice (yellow skin and eyes).	Rare	3
Others:		
• Fever, swollen lymph glands.	Common	3
• Weight gain.	Infrequent	3
• Fatigue, weakness.	Infrequent	3

1- Life-threatening. Seek emergency treatment immediately.
2- Discontinue. Seek emergency treatment.
3- Discontinue. Call doctor right away.
4- Continue. Call doctor when convenient.

WARNINGS & PRECAUTIONS

Don't take if:
- You are allergic to penicillamine.
- You have severe anemia.

Before you start, consult your doctor:
- If you have kidney disease.
- If you are allergic to any pencillin antibiotic.

Over age 60:
More likely to damage blood cells and kidneys.

Pregnancy:
Risk to unborn child outweighs drug benefits. Don't use.

Breast-feeding:
Drug filters into milk. May harm child. Avoid.

Infants & children:
Use only under medical supervision.

Prolonged use:
May damage blood cells, kidney, liver.

Skin & sunlight:
No problems expected.

Driving, piloting or hazardous work:
No problems expected.

Airplane passengers:
No problems expected.

Discontinuing:
No problems expected.

Others:
Request laboratory studies on blood and urine every 2 weeks. Kidney- and liver-function studies recommended every 6 months.

INTERACTION WITH OTHER DRUGS

GENERIC NAME OR DRUG CLASS	COMBINED EFFECT
Gold compounds	Damage to blood cells and kidney.
Immunosuppressants	Damage to blood cells and kidney.
Iron supplements	Decreased effect of penicillamine. Wait 2 hours between doses.
Oxyphenbutazone	Damage to blood cells and kidney.
Phenylbutazone	Damage to blood cells and kidney.
Quinine	Damage to blood cells and kidney.

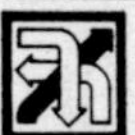

INTERACTION WITH OTHER SUBSTANCES

INTERACTS WITH	COMBINED EFFECT
Alcohol:	Increased side effects of penicillamine.
Beverages:	None expected.
Cocaine:	Increased side effects of penicillamine.
Foods:	None expected.
Marijuana:	Increased side effects of penicillamine.
Tobacco:	None expected.

PENICILLIN G

BRAND NAMES

Bicillin
Crystapen
Crysticillin
Duracillin
Megacillin
Penioral
Pentids
Permapen
Pfizerpen-AS
Pfizerpen G
SK-Penicillin G
Wycillin

GENERAL INFORMATION

Habit forming? No
Prescription needed? Yes
Available as generic? Yes
Drug class: Antibiotic (penicillin)

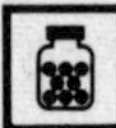

USES

Treatment of bacterial infections that are susceptible to penicillin G.

DOSAGE & USAGE INFORMATION

How to take:

- Tablets or capsules—Swallow with liquid on an empty stomach 1 hour before or 2 hours after eating.
- Liquid—Take with cold beverage. Liquid form is perishable and effective for only 7 days at room temperature. Effective for 14 days if stored in refrigerator. Don't freeze.

When to take:
Follow instructions on prescription label or side of package. Doses should be evenly spaced. For example, 4 times a day means every 6 hours.

If you forget a dose:
Take as soon as you remember. Continue regular schedule.

What drug does:
Destroys susceptible bacteria. Does not kill viruses.

Time lapse before drug works:
May be several days before medicine affects infection.

Don't take with:
See Interaction column and consult doctor.

OVERDOSE

Symptoms:
Severe diarrhea, nausea or vomiting.

What to do:
Overdose unlikely to threaten life. If person takes much larger amount than prescribed, call doctor, poison-control center or hospital emergency room for instructions.

POSSIBLE ADVERSE REACTIONS OR SIDE EFFECTS

SYMPTOMS	FREQUENCY	WHAT TO DO
Brain & nervous system:	None expected.	
Skin: Hives, rash, intense itch soon after a dose.	Rare	1
Eyes:	None expected.	
Ears, nose, throat: Dark or discolored tongue.	Common	5
Digestive: Mild nausea, vomiting, diarrhea.	Infrequent	4
Heart & lungs:	None expected.	
Blood vessels: Unexplained bleeding.	Rare	3
Muscles, bones, joints:	None expected.	
Genital, urinary:	None expected.	
Kidneys:	None expected.	
Liver:	None expected.	
Allergic: Life-threatening anaphylaxis may occur!	Rare	1 See page 888.
Blood:	None expected.	
Others:	None expected.	

1 - Life-threatening. Seek emergency treatment immediately.
2 - Discontinue. Seek emergency treatment.
3 - Discontinue. Call doctor right away.
4 - Continue. Call doctor when convenient.
5 - Continue. Tell doctor at next visit.
6 - No action necessary.

WARNINGS & PRECAUTIONS

Don't take if:
You are allergic to penicillin G, cephalosporin antibiotics, other penicillins or penicillamine. Life-threatening reaction may occur.

Before you start, consult your doctor:
If you are allergic to any substance or drug.

Over age 60:
You may have skin reactions, particularly around genitals and anus.

Pregnancy:
Studies inconclusive on harm to unborn child. Animal studies show fetal abnormalities. Decide with your doctor whether drug benefits justify risk to unborn child.

Breast-feeding:
Drug passes into milk. Child may become sensitive to penicillins and have allergic reactions to penicillin drugs. Avoid penicillin G or discontinue nursing until you finish medicine. Consult doctor for advice on maintaining milk supply.

Infants & children:
No problems expected.

Prolonged use:
You may become more susceptible to infections caused by germs not responsive to penicillin G.

Skin & sunlight:
No problems expected.

Driving, piloting or hazardous work:
Usually not dangerous. Most hazardous reactions likely to occur a few minutes after taking penicillin G.

Airplane passengers:
No problems expected.

Discontinuing:
Don't discontinue without doctor's advice until you complete prescribed dose, even though symptoms diminish or disappear.

Others:
Urine sugar test for diabetes may show false positive result.

INTERACTION WITH OTHER DRUGS

GENERIC NAME OR DRUG CLASS	COMBINED EFFECT
Chloramphenicol	Decreased effect of both drugs.
Erythromycins	Decreased effect of both drugs.
Paromomycin	Decreased effect of both drugs.
Tetracyclines	Decreased effect of both drugs.
Troleandomycin	Decreased effect of both drugs.

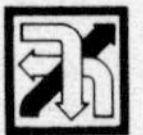

INTERACTION WITH OTHER SUBSTANCES

INTERACTS WITH	COMBINED EFFECT
Alcohol:	Occasional stomach irritation.
Beverages:	None expected.
Cocaine:	No proven problems.
Foods:	Decreased effect of penicillin G.
Marijuana:	No proven problems.
Tobacco:	None expected.

PENICILLIN V

BRAND NAMES

Betapen-VK
Compocillin VK
Ledercillin VK
Novapen V
Pen-Vee K
Penapar VK
Pfizerpen VK
Robicillin VK
SK-Penicillin VK
Uticillin VK
V-Cillin
Veetids

GENERAL INFORMATION

Habit forming? No
Prescription needed? Yes
Available as generic? Yes
Drug class: Antibiotic (penicillin)

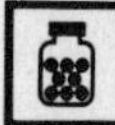

USES

- Treatment of bacterial infections that are susceptible to penicillin V.
- Prevention of streptococcal infections in susceptible persons such as those with heart valves damaged by rheumatic fever.

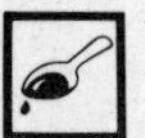

DOSAGE & USAGE INFORMATION

How to take:

- Tablets or capsules—Swallow with liquid on an empty stomach 1 hour before meals or 2 hours after eating.
- Liquid—Take with cold beverage. Liquid form is perishable and effective for only 7 days at room temperature. Effective for 14 days if stored in refrigerator. Don't freeze.

When to take:
Follow instructions on prescription label or side of package. Doses should be evenly spaced. For example, 4 times a day means every 6 hours.

If you forget a dose:
Take as soon as you remember. Continue regular schedule.

What drug does:
Destroys susceptible bacteria. Does not kill viruses.

Time lapse before drug works:
May be several days before penicillin V affects infection.

Don't take with:
See Interaction column and consult doctor.

OVERDOSE

Symptoms:
Severe diarrhea, nausea or vomiting.

What to do:
Overdose unlikely to threaten life. If person takes much larger amount than prescribed, call doctor, poison-control center or hospital emergency room for instructions.

POSSIBLE ADVERSE REACTIONS OR SIDE EFFECTS

SYMPTOMS	FREQUENCY	WHAT TO DO
Brain & nervous system:	None expected.	
Skin: Hives, rash, intense itch soon after a dose.	Rare	1
Eyes:	None expected.	
Ears, nose, throat: Dark or discolored tongue.	Common	5
Digestive: Mild nausea, vomiting, diarrhea.	Infrequent	4
Heart & lungs:	None expected.	
Blood vessels: Unexplained bleeding.	Rare	3
Muscles, bones, joints:	None expected.	
Genital, urinary:	None expected.	
Kidneys:	None expected.	
Liver:	None expected.	
Allergic: Life-threatening anaphylaxis may occur!	Rare	1 See page 888.
Blood:	None expected.	
Others:	None expected.	

1- Life-threatening. Seek emergency treatment immediately.
2- Discontinue. Seek emergency treatment.
3- Discontinue. Call doctor right away.
4- Continue. Call doctor when convenient.
5- Continue. Tell doctor at next visit.
6- No action necessary.

WARNINGS & PRECAUTIONS

Don't take if:
You are allergic to penicillin V, cephalosporin antibiotics, other penicillins or penicillamine. Life-threatening reaction may occur.

Before you start, consult your doctor:
If you are allergic to any substance or drug.

Over age 60:
You may have skin reactions, particularly around genitals and anus.

Pregnancy:
Studies inconclusive on danger to unborn child. Decide with your doctor whether drug benefits justify risk to unborn child.

Breast-feeding:
Drug passes into milk. Child may become sensitive to penicillin. Child more likely to have future allergic reactions to penicillin. Avoid penicillin V or discontinue nursing until you finish medicine. Consult doctor for advice on maintaining milk supply.

Infants & children:
No problems expected.

Prolonged use:
You may become more susceptible to infections caused by germs not responsive to penicillin V.

Skin & sunlight:
No problems expected.

Driving, piloting or hazardous work:
Usually not dangerous. Most hazardous reactions likely to occur a few minutes after taking penicillin V.

Airplane passengers:
No problems expected.

Discontinuing:
Don't discontinue without doctor's advice until you have finished prescribed dose, even if symptoms diminish or disappear.

Others:
No problems expected.

INTERACTION WITH OTHER DRUGS

GENERIC NAME OR DRUG CLASS	COMBINED EFFECT
Chloramphenicol	Decreased effect of both drugs.
Erythromycins	Decreased effect of both drugs.
Paromomycin	Decreased effect of both drugs.
Tetracyclines	Decreased effect of both drugs.
Troleandomycin	Decreased effect of both drugs.

INTERACTION WITH OTHER SUBSTANCES

INTERACTS WITH	COMBINED EFFECT
Alcohol:	Occasional stomach irritation.
Beverages:	None expected.
Cocaine:	No proven problems.
Foods:	Decreased effect of penicillin V.
Marijuana:	No proven problems.
Tobacco:	None expected.

PENTAERYTHRITOL TETRANITRATE

BRAND NAMES

Duotrate
Kaytrate
Naptrate
Pentestan
Pentraspan
Pentritol
Peritrate
P.E.T.N.

GENERAL INFORMATION

Habit forming? No
Prescription needed? Yes
Available as generic? Yes
Drug class: Antianginal (nitrate)

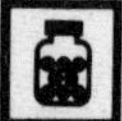

USES

Reduces frequency and severity of angina attacks.

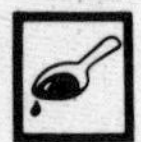

DOSAGE & USAGE INFORMATION

How to take:

- Regular tablet—Swallow with liquid. You may chew or crush it.
- Extended-release tablets or capsules—Swallow each dose whole with liquid.

When to take:
Take at the same times each day, 1 or 2 hours after meals.

If you forget a dose:
Take as soon as you remember up to 2 hours late. If more than 2 hours, wait for next scheduled dose (don't double this dose).

What drug does:
Relaxes blood vessels, increasing blood flow to heart muscle.

Time lapse before drug works:
30 minutes.

Don't take with:
See Interaction column and consult doctor.

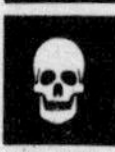

OVERDOSE

Symptoms:
Vomiting, sweating, shortness of breath, loss of consciousness.

What to do:

- Dial 0 (operator) or 911 (emergency) for an ambulance or medical help. Then give first aid immediately.
- Additional emergency information on page 886.

POSSIBLE ADVERSE REACTIONS OR SIDE EFFECTS

SYMPTOMS	FREQUENCY	WHAT TO DO
Brain & nervous system:		
• Headache	Common	5
• Fainting	Infrequent	3
Skin:		
• Rash	Rare	3
• Flushed face and neck.	Common	5
Eyes:	None expected.	
Ears, nose, throat:	None expected.	
Digestive:		
Nausea, vomiting.	Common	5
Heart & lungs:		
Rapid heartbeat.	Common	5
Blood vessels:	None expected.	
Muscles, bones, joints:	None expected.	
Genital, urinary:	None expected.	
Kidneys:	None expected.	
Liver:	None expected.	
Allergic:	None expected.	
Blood:	None expected.	
Others:	None expected.	

1 - Life-threatening. Seek emergency treatment immediately.
2 - Discontinue. Seek emergency treatment.
3 - Discontinue. Call doctor right away.
4 - Continue. Call doctor when convenient.
5 - Continue. Tell doctor at next visit.
6 - No action necessary.

PENTAERYTHRITOL TETRANITRATE

WARNINGS & PRECAUTIONS

Don't take if:
You are allergic to nitrates, including nitroglycerin.

Before you start, consult your doctor:
If you have glaucoma.

Over age 60:
Adverse reactions and side effects may be more frequent and severe than in younger persons.

Pregnancy:
No proven harm to unborn child. Avoid if possible.

Breast-feeding:
No proven problems. Consult your doctor.

Infants & children:
Not recommended.

Prolonged use:
Drug may become less effective and require higher doses.

Skin & sunlight:
No problems expected.

Driving, piloting or hazardous work:
Don't drive or pilot aircraft until you learn how medicine affects you. Don't work around dangerous machinery. Don't climb ladders or work in high places. Danger increases if you drink alcohol or take medicine affecting alertness and reflexes, such as antihistamines, tranquilizers, sedatives, pain medicine, narcotics and mind-altering drugs.

Airplane passengers:
No problems expected.

Discontinuing:
Don't discontinue without doctor's advice until you complete prescribed dose, even though symptoms diminish or disappear.

Others:
Periodic laboratory blood studies recommended if you take pentaerythritol tetranitrate.

INTERACTION WITH OTHER DRUGS

GENERIC NAME OR DRUG CLASS	COMBINED EFFECT
Anticholinergics	Increased internal eye pressure.
Antidepressants (tricyclic)	Excessive blood-pressure drop.
Antihypertensives	Excessive blood-pressure drop.
Beta-adrenergic blockers	Excessive blood-pressure drop.
Cholinergics	Decreased cholinergic effect.
Ephedrine	Decreased effect of pentaerythritol tetranitrate.

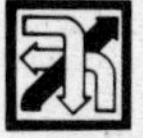

INTERACTION WITH OTHER SUBSTANCES

INTERACTS WITH	COMBINED EFFECT
Alcohol:	Excessive blood-pressure drop.
Beverages:	None expected.
Cocaine:	Flushed face and headache. Avoid.
Foods:	None expected.
Marijuana:	Decreased effect of pentaerythritol tetranitrate.
Tobacco:	Decreased effect of pentaerythritol tetranitrate.

PENTOBARBITAL

BRAND NAMES

Carbrital
Nembutal
Nova-Rectal
Novopentobarb
Pentogen
Quless
Wigraine-PB

GENERAL INFORMATION

Habit forming? Yes
Prescription needed? Yes
Available as generic? Yes
Drug class: Sedative, hypnotic (barbiturate)

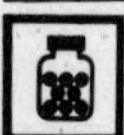

USES

- Reduces anxiety or nervous tension (low dose).
- Relieves insomnia (higher bedtime dose).

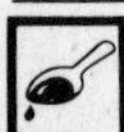

DOSAGE & USAGE INFORMATION

How to take:
- Tablet, capsule or liquid—Swallow with food or liquid to lessen stomach irritation. If you can't swallow whole, crumble tablet or open capsule and take with liquid or food.
- Suppositories—Remove wrapper and moisten suppository with water. Gently insert larger end into rectum. Push well into rectum with finger.

When to take:
At the same times each day.

If you forget a dose:
Take as soon as you remember up to 2 hours late. If more than 2 hours, wait for next scheduled dose (don't double this dose).

What drug does:
May partially block nerve impulses at nerve-cell connections.

Time lapse before drug works:
60 minutes.

Don't take with:
- Non-prescription drugs without consulting doctor.
- See Interaction column and consult doctor.

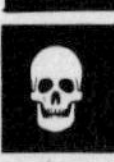

OVERDOSE

Symptoms:
Deep sleep, weak pulse, coma.

What to do:
- Dial 0 (operator) or 911 (emergency) for an ambulance or medical help. Then give first aid immediately.
- Additional emergency information on page 886.

POSSIBLE ADVERSE REACTIONS OR SIDE EFFECTS

SYMPTOMS	FREQUENCY	WHAT TO DO
Brain & nervous system:		
• Dizziness, drowsiness, "hangover effect."	Common	4
• Depression, confusion, slurred speech.	Infrequent	4
• Agitation	Rare	3
Skin:		
• Rash or hives.	Infrequent	3
• Face, lip swelling.	Infrequent	3
Eyes:		
Eyelid swelling.	Infrequent	3
Ears, nose, throat:		
Sore throat, fever.	Infrequent	3
Digestive:		
Diarrhea, nausea, vomiting.	Infrequent	4
Heart & lungs:		
• Slow heartbeat.	Rare	3
• Breathing difficulty.	Rare	3
Blood vessels:		
Unexplained bleeding or bruising.	Rare	4
Muscles, bones, joints:		
Joint or muscle pain.	Infrequent	4
Genital, urinary:	None expected.	
Kidneys:	None expected.	
Liver:		
Jaundice (yellow skin and eyes).	Rare	3
Allergic:	None expected.	
Blood:	None expected.	
Others:	None expected.	

1- Life-threatening. Seek emergency treatment immediately.
2- Discontinue. Seek emergency treatment.
3- Discontinue. Call doctor right away.
4- Continue. Call doctor when convenient.

WARNINGS & PRECAUTIONS

Don't take if:
- You are allergic to any barbiturate.
- You have porphyria.

Before you start, consult your doctor:
- If you have epilepsy.
- If you have kidney or liver damage.
- If you have asthma.
- If you have anemia.
- If you have chronic pain.
- If you will have surgery within 2 months, including dental surgery, requiring general or spinal anesthesia.

Over age 60:
Adverse reactions and side effects may be more frequent and severe than in younger persons. Use small doses.

Pregnancy:
Risk to unborn child outweighs drug benefits. Don't use.

Breast-feeding:
Drug passes into milk. Avoid drug or discontinue nursing until you finish medicine. Consult doctor for advice on maintaining milk supply.

Infants & children:
Use only under doctor's supervision.

Prolonged use:
- May cause addiction, anemia, chronic intoxication.
- May lower body temperature, making exposure to cold temperatures hazardous.

Skin & sunlight:
May cause rash or intensify sunburn in areas exposed to sun or sunlamp.

Driving, piloting or hazardous work:
Don't drive or pilot aircraft until you learn how medicine affects you. Don't work around dangerous machinery. Don't climb ladders or work in high places. Danger increases if you drink alcohol or take medicine affecting alertness and reflexes.

Airplane passengers:
No problems expected.

Discontinuing:
May be unnecessary to finish medicine. Follow doctor's instructions. If you develop withdrawal symptoms of hallucinations, agitation or sleeplessness after discontinuing, call doctor right away.

Others:
Great potential for abuse.

INTERACTION WITH OTHER DRUGS

GENERIC NAME OR DRUG CLASS	COMBINED EFFECT
Anticoagulants (oral)	Decreased anticoagulant effect.
Anticonvulsants	Changed seizure patterns.
Antidepressants (tricyclic)	Decreased antidepressant effect.
Antidiabetics (oral)	Increased pentobarbital effect.
Antihistamines	Dangerous sedation. Avoid.
Antiinflammatory drugs (non-steroidal)	Decreased antiinflammatory effect.
Aspirin	Decreased aspirin effect.
Beta-adrenergic blockers	Decreased effect of beta-adrenergic blocker.
Contraceptives (oral)	Decreased contraceptive effect.
Cortisone drugs	Decreased cortisone effect.
Digitoxin	Decreased digitoxin effect.
Doxycycline	Decreased doxycycline effect.
Griseofulvin	Decreased griseofulvin effect.

Additional interactions on page 840.

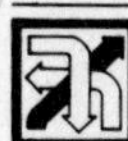

INTERACTION WITH OTHER SUBSTANCES

INTERACTS WITH	COMBINED EFFECT
Alcohol:	Possible fatal oversedation. Avoid.
Beverages:	None expected.
Cocaine:	Decreased pentobarbital effect.
Foods:	None expected.
Marijuana:	Excessive sedation. Avoid.
Tobacco:	None expected.

PERPHENAZINE

BRAND NAMES

Apo-Perphenazine
Etrafon
Phenazine
Triavil
Trilafon

GENERAL INFORMATION

Habit forming? No
Prescription needed? Yes
Available as generic? Yes
Drug class: Tranquilizer, antiemetic (phenothiazine)

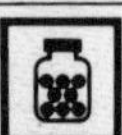

USES

- Stops nausea, vomiting.
- Reduces anxiety, agitation.

DOSAGE & USAGE INFORMATION

How to take:
- Tablet or capsule—Swallow with liquid or food to lessen stomach irritation.
- Suppositories—Remove wrapper and moisten suppository with water. Gently insert into rectum, large end first.
- Drops or liquid—Dilute dose in beverage.

When to take:
- Nervous and mental disorders—Take at the same times each day.
- Nausea and vomiting—Take as needed, no more often than every 4 hours.

If you forget a dose:
- Nervous and mental disorders—Take up to 2 hours late. If more than 2 hours, wait for next scheduled dose (don't double this).
- Nausea and vomiting—Take as soon as you remember. Wait 4 hours for next dose.

What drug does:
- Suppresses brain's vomiting center.
- Suppresses brain centers that control abnormal emotions and behavior.

Time lapse before drug works:
- Nausea and vomiting—1 hour or less.
- Nervous and mental disorders—4-6 weeks.

Don't take with:
- Antacid or medicine for diarrhea.
- Non-prescription drug for cough, cold or allergy.
- See Interaction column and consult doctor.

OVERDOSE

Symptoms:
Stupor, convulsions, coma.

What to do:
- Dial 0 (operator) or 911 (emergency) for an ambulance or medical help. Then give first aid immediately.
- Additional emergency information on page 886.

POSSIBLE ADVERSE REACTIONS OR SIDE EFFECTS

SYMPTOMS	FREQUENCY	WHAT TO DO
Brain & nervous system:		
• Restlessness, tremor.	Common	3
• Fainting	Infrequent	2
• Drowsiness	Common	3
Skin:		
• Rash	Infrequent	3
• Less perspiration.	Common	4
Eyes:		
Vision changes.	Rare	3
Ears, nose, throat:		
• Sore throat, fever.	Rare	3
• Dry mouth, nasal congestion.	Common	4
Digestive:		
Constipation	Common	4
Heart & lungs, blood vessels, kidneys, allergic, blood:	None expected.	
Muscles, bones, joints:		
Muscle spasms of face and neck, unsteady gait.	Common	2
Genital, urinary:		
Urination difficulty.	Infrequent	4
Liver:		
Jaundice (yellow eyes and skin).	Rare	3
Others:		
Less interest in sex, breast swelling, change in menstrual pattern.	Infrequent	4

1-Life-threatening. Seek emergency treatment immediately.
2-Discontinue. Seek emergency treatment.
3-Discontinue. Call doctor right away.
4-Continue. Call doctor when convenient.
5-Continue. Tell doctor at next visit.
6-No action necessary.

WARNINGS & PRECAUTIONS

Don't take if:

- You are allergic to any phenothiazine.
- You have a blood or bone-marrow disease.

Before you start, consult your doctor:

- If you will have surgery within 2 months, including dental surgery, requiring general or spinal anesthesia.
- If you have asthma, emphysema or other lung disorder.
- If you take non-prescription ulcer medicine, asthma medicine or amphetamines.

Over age 60:
Adverse reactions and side effects may be more frequent and severe than in younger persons. More likely to develop involuntary movement of jaws, lips, tongue, chewing. Report this to your doctor immediately. Early treatment can help.

Pregnancy:
Risk to unborn child outweighs drug benefits. Don't use.

Breast-feeding:
Drug passes into milk. Avoid drug or discontinue nursing until you finish medicine. Consult doctor for advice on maintaining milk supply.

Infants & children:
Don't give to children younger than 2.

Prolonged use:
May lead to tardive dyskinesia (involuntary movement of jaws, lips, tongue, chewing).

Skin & sunlight:
May cause rash or intensify sunburn in areas exposed to sun or sunlamp. Skin may remain sensitive for 3 months after discontinuing.

Driving, piloting or hazardous work:
Don't drive or pilot aircraft until you learn how medicine affects you. Don't work around dangerous machinery. Don't climb ladders or work in high places. Danger increases if you drink alcohol or take medicine affecting alertness and reflexes.

Airplane passengers:
No problems expected.

Discontinuing:

- Nervous and mental disorders—Don't discontinue without doctor's advice until you complete prescribed dose, even though symptoms diminish or disappear.
- Nausea and vomiting—May be unnecessary to finish medicine. Follow doctor's instructions.

INTERACTION WITH OTHER DRUGS

GENERIC NAME OR DRUG CLASS	COMBINED EFFECT
Anticholinergics	Increased anticholinergic effect.
Antidepressants (tricyclic)	Increased perphenazine effect.
Antihistamines	Increased antihistamine effect.
Appetite suppressants	Decreased suppressant effect.
Levodopa	Decreased levodopa effect.
Mind-altering drugs	Increased effect of mind-altering drugs.
Narcotics	Increased narcotic effect.
Phenytoin	Increased phenytoin effect.
Quinidine	Impaired heart function. Dangerous mixture.
Sedatives	Increased sedative effect.
Tranquilizers (other)	Increased tranquilizer effect.

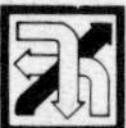

INTERACTION WITH OTHER SUBSTANCES

INTERACTS WITH	COMBINED EFFECT
Alcohol:	Dangerous oversedation.
Beverages:	None expected.
Cocaine:	Decreased perphenazine effect. Avoid.
Foods:	None expected.
Marijuana:	Drowsiness. May increase antinausea effect.
Tobacco:	None expected.

PHENACETIN

BRAND NAMES

A.P.C. Tablets
Aspirin Compound with Codeine
Emprazil
Fiorinal
P.A.C. Compound
Percodan
Propoxyphene Compound 65
Sinubid
SK-65 Compound
Soma Compound
Synalgos

GENERAL INFORMATION

Habit forming? No
Prescription needed? No
Available as generic? Yes
Drug class: Analgesic, fever reducer

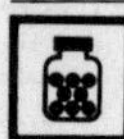

USES

- Relieves pain.
- Reduces fever.

DOSAGE & USAGE INFORMATION

How to take:
- Tablet or capsule—Swallow with liquid or food to lessen stomach irritation. You may chew or crush tablets.
- Extended-release tablets or capsules—Swallow each dose whole with liquid.

When to take:
At the same times each day.

If you forget a dose:
Take as soon as you remember up to 2 hours late. If more than 2 hours, wait for next scheduled dose (don't double this dose).

What drug does:
Reduces level of prostaglandins, a chemical involved in producing inflammation, fever, pain.

Time lapse before drug works:
15 minutes.

Don't take with:
See Interaction column and consult doctor.

OVERDOSE

Symptoms:
Sweating, bloody urine, convulsions, coma.

What to do:
- Dial 0 (operator) or 911 (emergency) for an ambulance or medical help. Then give first aid immediately.
- Additional emergency information on page 886.

POSSIBLE ADVERSE REACTIONS OR SIDE EFFECTS

SYMPTOMS	FREQUENCY	WHAT TO DO
Brain & nervous system:		
Confusion, drowsiness.	Infrequent	4
Skin:		
Rash, itch, hives.	Infrequent	3
Eyes:	None expected.	
Ears, nose, throat:		
Sore throat, fever, sores in mouth.	Infrequent	3
Digestive:		
• Nausea	Infrequent	4
• Black, tarry or bloody stools.	Rare	2
Heart & lungs:	None expected.	
Blood vessels:		
Easy bruising.	Rare	3
Muscles, bones, joints:		
Swollen feet, legs.	Rare	3
Genital, urinary:		
Bloody urine.	Rare	3
Kidneys:	None expected.	
Liver:	None expected.	
Allergic:	None expected.	
Blood:		
Anemia	Rare	3
Others:		
• Blue fingernails.	Rare	3
• Fatigue, weakness.	Rare	3

1- Life-threatening. Seek emergency treatment immediately.
2- Discontinue. Seek emergency treatment.
3- Discontinue. Call doctor right away.
4- Continue. Call doctor when convenient.
5- Continue. Tell doctor at next visit.
6- No action necessary.

WARNINGS & PRECAUTIONS

Don't take if:
You are allergic to phenacetin, aspirin or any of the many mixtures which contain either.

Before you start, consult your doctor:
- If you have kidney or liver disease.
- If you have G6PD deficiency.

Over age 60:
Adverse reactions and side effects may be more frequent and severe than in younger persons.

Pregnancy:
May cause anemia in newborn. Avoid if possible.

Breast-feeding:
Drug passes into milk. Avoid drug or discontinue nursing until you finish medicine. Consult doctor for advice on maintaining milk supply.

Infants & children:
Not recommended.

Prolonged use:
Kidney damage. Don't take regularly without medical advice.

Skin & sunlight:
No problems expected.

Driving, piloting or hazardous work:
No problems expected.

Airplane passengers:
No problems expected.

Discontinuing:
May be unnecessary to finish medicine. Follow doctor's instructions.

Others:
No problems expected.

INTERACTION WITH OTHER DRUGS

GENERIC NAME OR DRUG CLASS	COMBINED EFFECT
Phenobarbital	Decreased phenacetin effect.

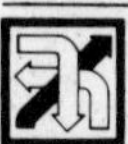

INTERACTION WITH OTHER SUBSTANCES

INTERACTS WITH	COMBINED EFFECT
Alcohol:	None expected.
Beverages:	None expected.
Cocaine:	None expected.
Foods:	None expected.
Marijuana:	Increased pain relief.
Tobacco:	None expected.

PHENAZOPYRIDINE

BRAND NAMES

Azo-100
Azodine
Azo-Gantanol
Azo-Gantrisin
Azo-Mandelamine
Azo-Standard
Azotrex
Di-Azo
Phen-Azo
Phenazodine
Pyridiate
Pyridium
Pyridium Plus
Pyrodine
Pyronium
Thiosulfil-A
Urobiotic

GENERAL INFORMATION

Habit forming? No
Prescription needed? Yes
Available as generic? Yes
Drug class: Analgesic (urinary)

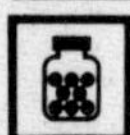

USES

Relieves pain of lower urinary-tract irritation, as in cystitis, urethritis or prostatitis.
Relieves symptoms only. Phenazopyridine alone does not cure infections.

DOSAGE & USAGE INFORMATION

How to take:
Tablet or capsule—Swallow with liquid or food to lessen stomach irritation.

When to take:
At the same times each day.

If you forget a dose:
Take as soon as you remember up to 2 hours late. If more than 2 hours, wait for next scheduled dose (don't double this dose).

What drug does:
Anesthetizes lower urinary tract. Relieves pain, burning, pressure and urgency to urinate.

Time lapse before drug works:
1 to 2 hours.

Don't take with:
No restrictions.

OVERDOSE

Symptoms:
Shortness of breath, weakness.

What to do:
Overdose unlikely to threaten life. If person takes much larger amount than prescribed, call doctor, poison-control center or hospital emergency room for instructions.

POSSIBLE ADVERSE REACTIONS OR SIDE EFFECTS

SYMPTOMS	FREQUENCY	WHAT TO DO
Brain & nervous system:		
Headache	Rare	4
Skin:		
Rash	Rare	3
Eyes:	None expected.	
Ears, nose, throat:	None expected.	
Digestive:		
Indigestion	Infrequent	4
Heart & lungs:	None expected.	
Blood vessels:	None expected.	
Muscles, bones, joints:	None expected.	
Genital, urinary:		
Red-orange urine.	Common	6
Kidneys:	None expected.	
Liver:		
Jaundice (yellow skin and eyes).	Rare	3
Allergic:	None expected.	
Blood:		
Anemia	Rare	4
Others:		
Fatigue, weakness.	Infrequent	4

1-Life-threatening. Seek emergency treatment immediately.
2-Discontinue. Seek emergency treatment.
3-Discontinue. Call doctor right away.
4-Continue. Call doctor when convenient.
5-Continue. Tell doctor at next visit.
6-No action necessary.

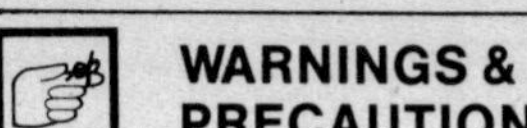

WARNINGS & PRECAUTIONS

Don't take if:
- You have hepatitis.
- You are allergic to any urinary analgesic.

Before you start, consult your doctor:
If you have kidney or liver disease.

Over age 60:
Adverse reactions and side effects may be more frequent and severe than in younger persons.

Pregnancy:
No proven harm to unborn child. Avoid if possible.

Breast-feeding:
No problems expected.

Infants & children:
Not recommended.

Prolonged use:
- Orange or yellow skin.
- Anemia. Occasional blood studies recommended.

Skin & sunlight:
No problems expected.

Driving, piloting or hazardous work:
No problems expected.

Airplane passengers:
No problems expected.

Discontinuing:
May be unnecessary to finish medicine. Follow doctor's instructions.

Others:
No problems expected.

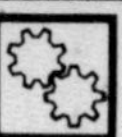

INTERACTION WITH OTHER DRUGS

GENERIC NAME OR DRUG CLASS	COMBINED EFFECT
None	

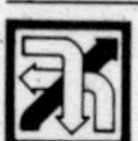

INTERACTION WITH OTHER SUBSTANCES

INTERACTS WITH	COMBINED EFFECT
Alcohol:	None expected.
Beverages:	None expected.
Cocaine:	None expected.
Foods:	None expected.
Marijuana:	None expected.
Tobacco:	None expected.

PHENIRAMINE

BRAND NAMES

Citra Capsules
Fiogesic
Inhistor
Robitussin-AC
Triaminic
Triaminicin
Triaminicol
Tussagesic
Tussaminic
Ursinus

See complete brand names list, page 829.

GENERAL INFORMATION

Habit forming? No
Prescription needed? High strength: Yes
Low strength: No
Available as generic? Yes
Drug class: Antihistamine

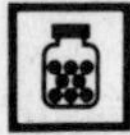

USES

Reduces allergic symptoms such as hay fever, hives, rash or itching.

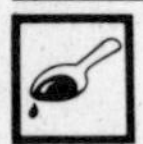

DOSAGE & USAGE INFORMATION

How to take:

- Tablet, syrup or capsule—Swallow with liquid or food to lessen stomach irritation.
- Extended-release tablets or capsules—Swallow each dose whole.

When to take:
Varies with form. Follow label directions.

If you forget a dose:
Take as soon as you remember up to 2 hours late. If more than 2 hours, wait for next scheduled dose (don't double this dose).

What drug does:
Blocks action of histamine after an allergic response triggers histamine release in sensitive cells.

Time lapse before drug works:
30 minutes.

Don't take with:
See Interaction column and consult doctor.

OVERDOSE

Symptoms:
Convulsions, red face, hallucinations, coma.

What to do:

- Dial 0 (operator) or 911 (emergency) for an ambulance or medical help. Then give first aid immediately.
- Additional emergency information on page 886.

POSSIBLE ADVERSE REACTIONS OR SIDE EFFECTS

SYMPTOMS	FREQUENCY	WHAT TO DO
Brain & nervous system:		
• Nightmares, agitation, irritability.	Rare	3
• Drowsiness, dizziness.	Common	5
Skin:	None expected.	
Eyes:		
• Vision changes.	Infrequent	3
• Less tolerance for contact lenses.	Infrequent	4
Ears, nose, throat:		
• Sore throat, fever.	Rare	3
• Dry mouth, nose, throat.	Common	5
Digestive:		
• Nausea	Common	5
• Appetite loss.	Infrequent	5
Heart & lungs:		
Rapid heartbeat.	Rare	3
Blood vessels:		
Unusual bleeding or bruising.	Rare	3
Muscles, bones, joints, kidneys, liver, allergic, blood:	None expected.	
Genital, urinary:		
Urination difficulty.	Infrequent	4
Others:		
Fatigue, weakness.	Rare	3

1- Life-threatening. Seek emergency treatment immediately.
2- Discontinue. Seek emergency treatment.
3- Discontinue. Call doctor right away.
4- Continue. Call doctor when convenient.
5- Continue. Tell doctor at next visit.
6- No action necessary.

WARNINGS & PRECAUTIONS

Don't take if:
You are allergic to any antihistamine.

Before you start, consult your doctor:
- If you have glaucoma.
- If you have enlarged prostate.
- If you have asthma.
- If you have kidney disease.
- If you have peptic ulcer.
- If you will have surgery within 2 months, including dental surgery, requiring general or spinal anesthesia.

Over age 60:
Don't exceed recommended dose. Adverse reactions and side effects may be more frequent and severe than in younger persons, especially urination difficulty, diminished alertness and other brain and nervous-system symptoms.

Pregnancy:
No proven harm to unborn child. Avoid if possible.

Breast-feeding:
Drug passes into milk. Avoid drug or discontinue nursing until you finish medicine. Consult doctor for advice on maintaining milk supply.

Infants & children:
Not recommended for premature or newborn infants. Otherwise, no problems expected.

Prolonged use:
Avoid. May damage bone-marrow and nerve cells.

Skin & sunlight:
May cause rash or intensify sunburn in areas exposed to sun or sunlamp.

Driving, piloting or hazardous work:
Don't drive or pilot aircraft until you learn how medicine affects you. Don't work around dangerous machinery. Don't climb ladders or work in high places. Danger increases if you drink alcohol or take medicine affecting alertness and reflexes, such as antihistamines, tranquilizers, sedatives, pain medicine, narcotics and mind-altering drugs.

Airplane passengers:
No problems expected.

Discontinuing:
No problems expected.

Others:
May mask symptoms of hearing damage from aspirin, other salicylates, cisplatin, paromomycin, vancomycin or anticonvulsants. Consult doctor if you use these.

INTERACTION WITH OTHER DRUGS

GENERIC NAME OR DRUG CLASS	COMBINED EFFECT
Anticholinergics	Increased anticholinergic effect.
Antidepressants	Excess sedation. Avoid.
Antihistamines (other)	Excess sedation. Avoid.
Hypnotics	Excess sedation. Avoid.
MAO inhibitors	Increased pheniramine effect.
Mind-altering drugs	Excess sedation. Avoid.
Narcotics	Excess sedation. Avoid.
Sedatives	Excess sedation. Avoid.
Sleep inducers	Excess sedation. Avoid.
Tranquilizers	Excess sedation. Avoid.

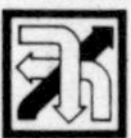

INTERACTION WITH OTHER SUBSTANCES

INTERACTS WITH	COMBINED EFFECT
Alcohol:	Excess sedation. Avoid.
Beverages: Caffeine drinks	Less pheniramine sedation.
Cocaine:	Decreased pheniramine effect. Avoid.
Foods:	None expected.
Marijuana:	Excess sedation. Avoid.
Tobacco:	None expected.

PHENOBARBITAL

BRAND NAMES

Anaspaz-PB
Eskabarb
Gardenal
Nova-Pheno
Probital
Sedadrops
SK-Phenobarbital
Solfoton
See complete brand names list, page 829.

GENERAL INFORMATION

Habit forming? Yes
Prescription needed? Yes
Available as generic? Yes
Drug class: Sedative, hypnotic (barbiturate), anticonvulsant

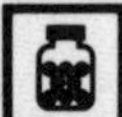

USES

- Reduces anxiety or nervous tension (low dose).
- Relieves insomnia (higher bedtime dose).
- Prevents convulsions or seizures, such as epilepsy.

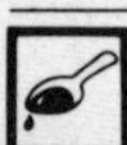

DOSAGE & USAGE INFORMATION

How to take:

- Tablet, liquid or capsule—Swallow with liquid or food to lessen stomach irritation. If you can't swallow whole, crumble tablet or open capsule and take with liquid or food.
- Extended-release tablets or capsules—Swallow each dose whole.
- Drops—Dilute dose in beverage before swallowing.

When to take:
At the same times each day.

If you forget a dose:
Take as soon as you remember up to 2 hours late. If more than 2 hours, wait for next scheduled dose (don't double this dose).

What drug does:
May partially block nerve impulses at nerve-cell connections.

Time lapse before drug works:
60 minutes.

Don't take with:

- Non-prescription drugs without consulting doctor.
- See Interaction column and consult doctor.

OVERDOSE

Symptoms:
Deep sleep, weak pulse, coma.

What to do:

- Dial 0 (operator) or 911 (emergency) for an ambulance or medical help. Then give first aid immediately.
- Additional emergency information on page 886.

POSSIBLE ADVERSE REACTIONS OR SIDE EFFECTS

SYMPTOMS	FREQUENCY	WHAT TO DO
Brain & nervous system:		
• Dizziness, drowsiness, "hangover effect."	Common	4
• Depression, confusion, slurred speech.	Infrequent	4
• Agitation	Rare	3
Skin:		
• Rash or hives.	Infrequent	3
• Face, lip swelling.	Infrequent	3
Eyes:		
Eyelid swelling.	Infrequent	3
Ears, nose, throat:		
Sore throat, fever.	Infrequent	3
Digestive:		
Diarrhea, nausea, vomiting.	Infrequent	4
Heart & lungs:		
• Slow heartbeat.	Rare	3
• Breathing difficulty.	Rare	3
Blood vessels:		
Unexplained bleeding or bruising.	Rare	4
Muscles, bones, joints:		
Joint or muscle pain.	Infrequent	4
Genital, urinary:	None expected.	
Kidneys:	None expected.	
Liver:		
Jaundice (yellow skin and eyes).	Rare	3
Allergic:	None expected.	
Blood:	None expected.	
Others:	None expected.	

1- Life-threatening. Seek emergency treatment immediately.
2- Discontinue. Seek emergency treatment.
3- Discontinue. Call doctor right away.
4- Continue. Call doctor when convenient.

WARNINGS & PRECAUTIONS

Don't take if:
- You are allergic to any barbiturate.
- You have porphyria.

Before you start, consult your doctor:
- If you have epilepsy.
- If you have kidney or liver damage.
- If you have asthma.
- If you have anemia.
- If you have chronic pain.
- If you will have surgery within 2 months, including dental surgery, requiring general or spinal anesthesia.

Over age 60:
Adverse reactions and side effects may be more frequent and severe than in younger persons. Use small doses.

Pregnancy:
Risk to unborn child outweighs drug benefits. Don't use.

Breast-feeding:
Drug passes into milk. Avoid drug or discontinue nursing until you finish medicine. Consult doctor for advice on maintaining milk supply.

Infants & children:
Use only under doctor's supervision.

Prolonged use:
- May cause addiction, anemia, chronic intoxication.
- May lower body temperature, making exposure to cold temperatures hazardous.

Skin & sunlight:
May cause rash or intensify sunburn in areas exposed to sun or sunlamp.

Driving, piloting or hazardous work:
Don't drive or pilot aircraft until you learn how medicine affects you. Don't work around dangerous machinery. Don't climb ladders or work in high places. Danger increases if you drink alcohol or take medicine affecting alertness and reflexes.

Airplane passengers:
No problems expected.

Discontinuing:
May be unnecessary to finish medicine. Follow doctor's instructions. If you develop withdrawal symptoms of hallucinations, agitation or sleeplessness after discontinuing, call doctor right away.

Others:
Great potential for abuse.

INTERACTION WITH OTHER DRUGS

GENERIC NAME OR DRUG CLASS	COMBINED EFFECT
Anticoagulants (oral)	Decreased anticoagulant effect.
Anticonvulsants	Changed seizure patterns.
Antidepressants (tricyclic)	Decreased antidepressant effect.
Antidiabetics (oral)	Increased phenobarbital effect.
Antihistamines	Dangerous sedation. Avoid.
Antiinflammatory drugs (non-steroidal)	Decreased antiinflammatory effect.
Aspirin	Decreased aspirin effect.
Beta-adrenergic blockers	Decreased effect of beta-adrenergic blocker.
Contraceptives (oral)	Decreased contraceptive effect.
Cortisone drugs	Decreased cortisone effect.
Digitoxin	Decreased digitoxin effect.
Doxycycline	Decreased doxycycline effect.
Griseofulvin	Decreased griseofulvin effect.

Additional interactions on page 840.

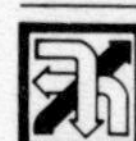

INTERACTION WITH OTHER SUBSTANCES

INTERACTS WITH	COMBINED EFFECT
Alcohol:	Possible fatal oversedation. Avoid.
Beverages:	None expected.
Cocaine:	Decreased phenobarbital effect.
Foods:	None expected.
Marijuana:	Excessive sedation. Avoid.
Tobacco:	None expected.

PHENOLPHTHALEIN

BRAND NAMES

Agoral
Alophen
Correctol
Espotabs
Evac-Q-Kit
Evac-Q-Kwik
Evac-U-Gen
Evac-U-Lax
Ex-Lax
Feen-A-Mint
Fructines-Vichy
Phenolax
Prulet
Trilax

GENERAL INFORMATION

Habit forming? No
Prescription needed? No
Available as generic? Yes
Drug class: Laxative (stimulant)

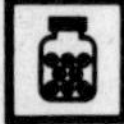

USES

Constipation relief.

DOSAGE & USAGE INFORMATION

How to take:

- Tablet or wafer—Swallow with liquid. If you can't swallow whole, chew or crumble and take with liquid or food.
- Liquid—Drink 6 to 8 glasses of water each day, in addition to one taken with each dose.
- Chewable tablets—Chew thoroughly before swallowing.

When to take:
Usually at bedtime with a snack, unless directed otherwise.

If you forget a dose:
Take as soon as you remember.

What drug does:
Acts on smooth muscles of intestine wall to cause vigorous bowel movement.

Time lapse before drug works:
6 to 10 hours.

Don't take with:

- See Interaction column and consult doctor.
- Don't take within 2 hours of taking another medicine. Laxative interferes with medicine absorption.

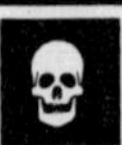

OVERDOSE

Symptoms:
Vomiting, electrolyte depletion.

What to do:
Overdose unlikely to threaten life. If person takes much larger amount than prescribed, call doctor, poison-control center or hospital emergency room for instructions.

POSSIBLE ADVERSE REACTIONS OR SIDE EFFECTS

SYMPTOMS	FREQUENCY	WHAT TO DO
Brain & nervous system:		
Irritability, confusion, headache.	Rare	3
Skin:		
Rash	Rare	3
Eyes:	None expected.	
Ears, nose, throat:	None expected.	
Digestive:		
Belching, cramps, nausea.	Infrequent	4
Heart & lungs:		
Breathing difficulty, irregular heartbeat.	Rare	3
Blood vessels:	None expected.	
Muscles, bones, joints:		
Muscle cramps.	Rare	3
Genital, urinary:		
Pink to orange urine.	Common	6
Kidneys:		
Burning on urination.	Rare	4
Liver:	None expected.	
Allergic:	None expected.	
Blood:	None expected.	
Others:		
• Rectal irritation.	Common	4
• Dangerous potassium loss.	Infrequent	3
• Unusual tiredness or weakness.	Rare	3

1 - Life-threatening. Seek emergency treatment immediately.
2 - Discontinue. Seek emergency treatment.
3 - Discontinue. Call doctor right away.
4 - Continue. Call doctor when convenient.
5 - Continue. Tell doctor at next visit.
6 - No action necessary.

WARNINGS & PRECAUTIONS

Don't take if:
- You have symptoms of appendicitis, inflamed bowel or intestinal blockage.
- You are allergic to a stimulant laxative.
- You have missed a bowel movement for only 1 or 2 days.

Before you start, consult your doctor:
- If you have a colostomy or ileostomy.
- If you have congestive heart disease.
- If you have diabetes.
- If you have high blood pressure.
- If you have a laxative habit.
- If you have rectal bleeding.
- If you take other laxatives.

Over age 60:
Adverse reactions and side effects may be more frequent and severe than in younger persons.

Pregnancy:
Risk to mother and unborn child outweighs drug benefits. Don't use.

Breast-feeding:
Drug passes into milk. Avoid drug or discontinue nursing until you finish medicine. Consult doctor for advice on maintaining milk supply.

Infants & children:
Use only under medical supervision.

Prolonged use:
Don't take for more than 1 week unless under a doctor's supervision. May cause laxative dependence.

Skin & sunlight:
No problems expected.

Driving, piloting or hazardous work:
No problems expected.

Airplane passengers:
No problems expected.

Discontinuing:
May be unnecessary to finish medicine. Follow doctor's instructions.

Others:
Don't take to "flush out" your system or as a "tonic."

INTERACTION WITH OTHER DRUGS

GENERIC NAME OR DRUG CLASS	COMBINED EFFECT
Antacids	Tablet coating may dissolve too rapidly, irritating stomach or bowel.
Antihypertensives	May cause dangerous low potassium level.
Diuretics	May cause dangerous low potassium level.

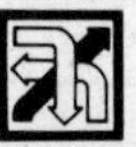

INTERACTION WITH OTHER SUBSTANCES

INTERACTS WITH	COMBINED EFFECT
Alcohol:	None expected.
Beverages:	
Milk	Tablet coating may dissolve too rapidly, irritating stomach or bowel.
Cocaine:	None expected.
Foods:	None expected.
Marijuana:	None expected.
Tobacco:	None expected.

PHENPROCOUMON

BRAND NAMES

Liquamar
Marcumar

GENERAL INFORMATION

Habit forming? No
Prescription needed? Yes
Available as generic? Yes
Drug class: Anticoagulant

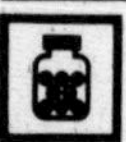

USES

Reduces blood clots. Used for abnormal clotting inside blood vessels.

DOSAGE & USAGE INFORMATION

How to take:
Tablet—Swallow with liquid. If you can't swallow whole, crumble tablet and take with liquid or food.

When to take:
At the same time each day.

If you forget a dose:
Take as soon as you remember up to 12 hours late. If more than 12 hours, wait for next scheduled dose (don't double this dose). Inform your doctor of any missed doses.

What drug does:
Blocks action of vitamin K necessary for blood clotting.

Time lapse before drug works:
36 to 48 hours.

Don't take with:
See Interaction column and consult doctor.

OVERDOSE

Symptoms:
Bloody vomit and bloody or black stools, red urine.

What to do:
- Dial 0 (operator) or 911 (emergency) for an ambulance or medical help. Then give first aid immediately.
- Additional emergency information on page 886.

POSSIBLE ADVERSE REACTIONS OR SIDE EFFECTS

SYMPTOMS	FREQUENCY	WHAT TO DO
Brain & nervous system:		
Dizziness, headache.	Rare	3
Skin:		
Rash, hives, itch.	Infrequent	3
Eyes:		
Blurred vision.	Infrequent	3
Ears, nose, throat:		
• Sore throat.	Infrequent	3
• Mouth sores.	Rare	3
Digestive:		
• Black stools or bloody vomit.	Infrequent	2
• Diarrhea, cramps, nausea, vomiting.	Infrequent	4
• Bloating, gas.	Common	5
Heart & lungs:		
Coughing up blood.	Infrequent	2
Blood vessels:		
Easy bruising, bleeding.	Infrequent	3
Muscles, bones, joints:		
Swollen feet, legs.	Infrequent	4
Genital, urinary:		
Cloudy or red urine.	Infrequent	3
Kidneys:		
Back pain.	Infrequent	3
Liver:		
Jaundice (yellow skin and eyes).	Infrequent	3
Allergic, blood:	None expected.	
Others:		
• Fever, chills.	Infrequent	3
• Hair loss.	Infrequent	4
• Fatigue, weakness.	Infrequent	3

1-Life-threatening. Seek emergency treatment immediately.
2-Discontinue. Seek emergency treatment.
3-Discontinue. Call doctor right away.
4-Continue. Call doctor when convenient.
5-Continue. Tell doctor at next visit.

WARNINGS & PRECAUTIONS

Don't take if:
- You have been allergic to any oral anticoagulant.
- You have a bleeding disorder.
- You have an active peptic ulcer.
- You have ulcerative colitis.

Before you start, consult your doctor:
- If you take any other drugs, including non-prescription drugs.
- If you have high blood pressure.
- If you have heavy or prolonged menstrual periods.
- If you have diabetes.
- If you have a bladder catheter.
- If you have serious liver or kidney disease.
- If you will have surgery within 2 months, including dental surgery, requiring general or spinal anesthesia.

Over age 60:
Adverse reactions and side effects may be more frequent and severe than in younger persons.

Pregnancy:
Risk to unborn child outweighs drug benefits. Don't use.

Breast-feeding:
Drug filters into milk. May harm child. Avoid.

Infants & children:
Use only under doctor's supervision.

Prolonged use:
No problems expected.

Skin & sunlight:
No problems expected.

Driving, piloting or hazardous work:
- Avoid hazardous activities that could cause injury.
- Don't drive if you feel dizzy or have blurred vision.

Airplane passengers:
No problems expected.

Discontinuing:
Don't discontinue without consulting doctor. Dose may require gradual reduction if you have taken drug for a long time. Doses of other drugs may also require adjustment.

Others:
Carry identification to state you take anticoagulants.

INTERACTION WITH OTHER DRUGS

GENERIC NAME OR DRUG CLASS	COMBINED EFFECT
Acetaminophen	Increased phenprocoumon effect.
Allopurinol	Increased phenprocoumon effect.
Androgens	Increased phenprocoumon effect.
Antacids (large doses)	Decreased phenprocoumon effect.
Antibiotics	Increased phenprocoumon effect.
Anticonvulsants (hydantoin)	Increased effect of both drugs.
Antidepressants (tricyclic)	Increased phenprocoumon effect.
Antidiabetics (oral)	Increased phenprocoumon effect.
Antihistamines	Unpredictable increased or decreased anticoagulant effect.
Barbiturates	Decreased phenprocoumon effect.

Additional interactions on page 840.

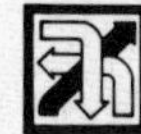

INTERACTION WITH OTHER SUBSTANCES

INTERACTS WITH	COMBINED EFFECT
Alcohol:	Can increase or decrease effect of anticoagulant. Use with caution.
Beverages:	None expected.
Cocaine:	None expected.
Foods: High in vitamin K such as fish, liver, spinach, cabbage.	May decrease anticoagulant effect.
Marijuana:	None expected.
Tobacco:	None expected.

PHENSUXIMIDE

BRAND NAMES

Milontin

GENERAL INFORMATION

Habit forming? No
Prescription needed? Yes
Available as generic? No
Drug class: Anticonvulsant (succinimide)

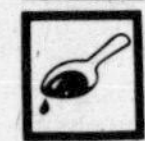

USES

Controls seizures in treatment of epilepsy.

DOSAGE & USAGE INFORMATION

How to take:
Capsule or syrup—Swallow with liquid or food to lessen stomach irritation.

When to take:
Every day in regularly-spaced doses, according to prescription.

If you forget a dose:
Take as soon as you remember up to 2 hours late. If more than 2 hours, wait for next scheduled dose (don't double this dose).

What drug does:
Depresses nerve transmissions in part of brain that controls muscles.

Time lapse before drug works:
3 hours.

Don't take with:
See Interaction column and consult doctor.

OVERDOSE

Symptoms:
Coma

What to do:
- Dial 0 (operator) or 911 (emergency) for an ambulance or medical help. Then give first aid immediately.
- If patient is unconscious and not breathing, give mouth-to-mouth breathing. If there is no heartbeat, use cardiac massage and mouth-to-mouth breathing (CPR). Don't try to make patient vomit. If you can't get help quickly, take patient to nearest emergency facility.
- Additional emergency information on page 886.

POSSIBLE ADVERSE REACTIONS OR SIDE EFFECTS

SYMPTOMS	FREQUENCY	WHAT TO DO
Brain & nervous system:		
Dizziness, drowsiness, headache, irritability, mood changes.	Infrequent	4
Skin:		
Rash	Rare	3
Eyes:	None expected.	
Ears, nose, throat:		
Sore throat, fever.	Rare	3
Digestive:		
Nausea, vomiting, stomach cramps, appetite loss.	Common	4
Heart & lungs:	None expected.	
Blood vessels:	None expected.	
Muscles, bones, joints:	None expected.	
Genital, urinary:	None expected.	
Kidneys:	None expected.	
Liver:	None expected.	
Allergic:	None expected.	
Blood:		
Unusual bleeding or bruising.	Rare	3
Others:		
Swollen lymph glands.	Rare	4

1-Life-threatening. Seek emergency treatment immediately.
2-Discontinue. Seek emergency treatment.
3-Discontinue. Call doctor right away.
4-Continue. Call doctor when convenient.
5-Continue. Tell doctor at next visit.
6-No action necessary.

WARNINGS & PRECAUTIONS

Don't take if:
You are allergic to any succinimide anticonvulsant.

Before you start, consult your doctor:
- If you plan to become pregnant within medication period.
- If you take other anticonvulsants.
- If you have blood disease.
- If you have kidney or liver disease.

Over age 60:
Adverse reactions and side effects may be more frequent and severe than in younger persons.

Pregnancy:
Risk to unborn child outweighs drug benefits. Don't use.

Breast-feeding:
Drug passes into milk. Avoid drug or discontinue nursing.

Infants & children:
Use only under medical supervision.

Prolonged use:
No problems expected.

Skin & sunlight:
No problems expected.

Driving, piloting or hazardous work:
Don't drive or pilot aircraft until you learn how medicine affects you. Don't work around dangerous machinery. Don't climb ladders or work in high places. Danger increases if you drink alcohol or take medicine affecting alertness and reflexes, such as antihistamines, tranquilizers, sedatives, pain medicine, narcotics and mind-altering drugs.

Airplane passengers:
No problems expected.

Discontinuing:
Don't discontinue without doctor's advice until you complete prescribed dose, even though symptoms diminish or disappear.

Others:
- Your response to medicine should be checked regularly by your doctor. Dose and schedule may have to be altered frequently to fit individual needs.
- Periodic blood-cell counts, kidney- and liver-function studies recommended.

INTERACTION WITH OTHER DRUGS

GENERIC NAME OR DRUG CLASS	COMBINED EFFECT
Anticonvulsants (other)	Increased effect of both drugs.
Antidepressants (tricyclic)	May provoke seizures.
Antipsychotics	May provoke seizures.

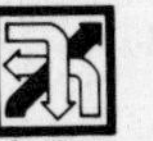

INTERACTION WITH OTHER SUBSTANCES

INTERACTS WITH	COMBINED EFFECT
Alcohol:	May provoke seizures.
Beverages:	None expected.
Cocaine:	May provoke seizures.
Foods:	None expected.
Marijuana:	May provoke seizures.
Tobacco:	None expected.

PHENYLBUTAZONE

BRAND NAMES

Butagesic
Sterazolidin
Phenbutazone

See complete brand names list, page 829.

GENERAL INFORMATION

Habit forming? No
Prescription needed? Yes
Available as generic? Yes
Drug class: Antiinflammatory (non-steroid)

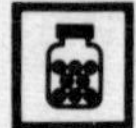

USES

- Treatment for joint pain, stiffness, inflammation and swelling of arthritis and gout.
- Pain reliever.
- Treatment for dysmenorrhea (painful or difficult menstruation).

DOSAGE & USAGE INFORMATION

How to take:
Tablet or capsule—Swallow with liquid or food to lessen stomach irritation. If you can't swallow whole, crumble tablet or open capsule and take with liquid or food.

When to take:
At the same times each day.

If you forget a dose:
Take as soon as you remember up to 2 hours late. If more than 2 hours, wait for next scheduled dose (don't double this dose).

What drug does:
Reduces tissue concentration of prostaglandins (hormones which produce inflammation and pain).

Time lapse before drug works:
Begins in 4 to 24 hours. May require 3 weeks regular use for maximum benefit.

Don't take with:
See Interaction column and consult doctor.

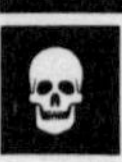

OVERDOSE

Symptoms:
Confusion, agitation, incoherence, convulsions, possible hemorrhage from stomach or intestine, coma.

What to do:
- Dial 0 (operator) or 911 (emergency) for an ambulance or medical help. Then give first aid immediately.
- Additional emergency information on page 886.

POSSIBLE ADVERSE REACTIONS OR SIDE EFFECTS

SYMPTOMS	FREQUENCY	WHAT TO DO
Brain & nervous system:		
• Depression, drowsiness.	Infrequent	4
• Convulsions, confusion.	Rare	3
• Dizziness	Common	4
• Headache	Common	5
Skin:		
Rash, hives or itch.	Rare	3
Eyes:		
Blurred vision.	Rare	3
Ears, nose, throat:		
• Ringing in ears.	Infrequent	4
• Sore throat, fever, mouth ulcers.	Rare	3
Digestive:		
• Black stools, vomiting blood.	Rare	3
• Stomach upset.	Common	4
• Constipation or diarrhea, vomiting.	Infrequent	4
Heart & lungs:		
Breathing difficulty, tightness in chest.	Rare	3
Blood vessels:		
Unusual bleeding or bruising.	Rare	3
Muscles, bones, joints:		
Swollen feet, legs.	Infrequent	4
Genital, urinary:		
• Bloody urine.	Rare	3
• Difficult, painful or frequent urination.	Rare	4
Kidneys, allergic, blood, liver:	None expected.	
Others:		
• Fatigue, weakness.	Rare	4
• Weight gain.	Rare	4

1- Life-threatening. Seek emergency treatment immediately.
2- Discontinue. Seek emergency treatment.
3- Discontinue. Call doctor right away.
4- Continue. Call doctor when convenient.
5- Continue. Tell doctor at next visit.

WARNINGS & PRECAUTIONS

Don't take if:

- You are allergic to aspirin or any non-steroid, antiinflammatory drug.
- You have gastritis, peptic ulcer, enteritis, ileitis, ulcerative colitis.
- Patient is younger than 15.

Before you start, consult your doctor:

- If you have epilepsy.
- If you have Parkinson's disease.
- If you have been mentally ill.
- If you have had kidney disease or impaired kidney function, asthma, high blood pressure, heart failure, temporal arthritis, or polymyalgia rheumatica.

Over age 60:
Adverse reactions and side effects may be more frequent and severe than in younger persons.

Pregnancy:
Studies inconclusive on harm to unborn child. Animal studies show fetal abnormalities. Decide with your doctor whether drug benefits justify risk to unborn child.

Breast-feeding:
Drug filters into milk. May harm child. Avoid.

Infants & children:
Not recommended for those younger than 15. Use only under medical supervision.

Prolonged use:

- Eye damage.
- May cause rare bone-marrow damage, jaundice (yellow skin and eyes), reduced hearing.
- Periodic blood counts recommended if you use a long time.

Skin & sunlight:
No problems expected.

Driving, piloting or hazardous work:
Don't drive or pilot aircraft until you learn how medicine affects you. Don't work around dangerous machinery. Don't climb ladders or work in high places. Danger increases if you drink alcohol or take medicine affecting alertness and reflexes, such as antihistamines, tranquilizers, sedatives, pain medicine, narcotics and mind-altering drugs.

Airplane passengers:
No problems expected.

Discontinuing:
Don't discontinue without consulting doctor. Dose may require gradual reduction if you have taken drug for a long time. Doses of other drugs may also require adjustment.

INTERACTION WITH OTHER DRUGS

GENERIC NAME OR DRUG CLASS	COMBINED EFFECT
Anticoagulants (oral)	Increased anticoagulant effect.
Aspirin	Possible stomach ulcer.
Antidiabetics (oral)	Increased antidiabetic effect.
Chloroquine	Possible skin toxicity.
Digitoxin	Decreased digitoxin effect.
Gold compounds	Increased toxicity to skin and bone marrow.
Hydroxychloroquine	Possible skin toxicity.
Methotrexate	Increased toxicity of both drugs to bone marrow.
Penicillamine	Possible toxicity.
Phenytoin	Possible toxic phenytoin effect.
Trimethoprim	Possible bone-marrow toxicity.

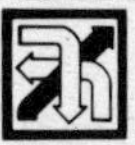

INTERACTION WITH OTHER SUBSTANCES

INTERACTS WITH	COMBINED EFFECT
Alcohol:	Possible stomach ulcer or bleeding.
Beverages:	None expected.
Cocaine:	None expected.
Foods:	None expected.
Marijuana:	Increased pain relief from phenylbutazone.
Tobacco:	None expected.

PHENYLEPHRINE

BRAND NAMES

4-Way Tablets
4-Way Nasal Spray
Chlor-Trimeton
Contac
Coricidin Mist
Coryban-D Cough Syrup
Co-Tylenol
Dristan Nasal Spray
Duo-Medihaler
Isophrin
Neo-Synephrine
Super Anahist

See complete brand names list, page 829.

GENERAL INFORMATION

Habit forming? No
Prescription needed? No
Available as generic? Yes
Drug class: Sympathomimetic

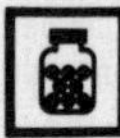

USES

Temporary relief of congestion of nose, sinuses and throat caused by allergies, colds or sinusitis.

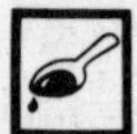

DOSAGE & USAGE INFORMATION

How to take:

- Syrup, tablet or capsule—Swallow with liquid or food to lessen stomach irritation.
- Extended-release tablets or capsules—Swallow each dose whole.
- Nasal solution, nasal spray, nasal jelly—Take as directed on package.

When to take:
As needed, no more often than every 4 hours.

If you forget a dose:
Take when you remember. Wait 4 hours for next dose. Never double a dose.

What drug does:
Contracts blood-vessel walls of nose, sinus and throat tissues, enlarging airways.

Time lapse before drug works:
5 to 30 minutes.

Don't take with:

- Non-prescription drugs for asthma, cough, cold, allergy, appetite suppressants, sleeping pills or drugs containing caffeine without consulting doctor.
- See Interaction column and consult doctor.

OVERDOSE

Symptoms:
Headache, heart palpitations, vomiting, blood-pressure rise, slow and forceful pulse.

What to do:

- Dial 0 (operator) or 911 (emergency) for an ambulance or medical help. Then give first aid immediately.
- Additional emergency information on page 886.

POSSIBLE ADVERSE REACTIONS OR SIDE EFFECTS

SYMPTOMS	FREQUENCY	WHAT TO DO
Brain & nervous system: Headache or dizziness, trembling, insomnia, nervousness.	Common	4
Skin: Paleness	Infrequent	4
Eyes:	None expected.	
Ears, nose, throat: Burning, dryness, stinging inside nose.	Common	4
Digestive:	None expected.	
Heart & lungs: Fast or pounding heartbeat.	Common	3
Blood vessels:	None expected.	
Muscles, bones, joints:	None expected.	
Genital, urinary:	None expected.	
Kidneys:	None expected.	
Liver:	None expected.	
Allergic:	None expected.	
Blood:	None expected.	
Others: Unusual sweating.	Rare	3

1- Life-threatening. Seek emergency treatment immediately.
2- Discontinue. Seek emergency treatment.
3- Discontinue. Call doctor right away.
4- Continue. Call doctor when convenient.
5- Continue. Tell doctor at next visit.
6- No action necessary.

WARNINGS & PRECAUTIONS

Don't take if:
You are allergic to any sympathomimetic.

Before you start, consult your doctor:
- If you have high blood pressure.
- If you have heart disease.
- If you have diabetes.
- If you have overactive thyroid.
- If you have taken MAO inhibitors in past 2 weeks.

Over age 60:
Adverse reactions and side effects may be more frequent and severe than in younger persons.

Pregnancy:
Risk to unborn child outweighs drug benefits. Don't use.

Breast-feeding:
Drug passes into milk. Avoid drug or discontinue nursing until you finish medicine. Consult doctor for advice on maintaining milk supply.

Infants & children:
Use only under close supervision.

Prolonged use:
- "Rebound" congestion (see page 849) and chemical irritation of nasal membranes.
- May cause functional dependence.

Skin & sunlight:
No problems expected.

Driving, piloting or hazardous work:
No problems expected.

Airplane passengers:
No problems expected.

Discontinuing:
May be unnecessary to finish medicine. Follow doctor's instructions.

Others:
No problems expected.

INTERACTION WITH OTHER DRUGS

GENERIC NAME OR DRUG CLASS	COMBINED EFFECT
Amphetamines	Increased nervousness.
Antiasthmatics	Nervous stimulation.
Antihypertensives	Decreased antihypertensive effect.
MAO inhibitors	Dangerous blood-pressure rise.
Sedatives	Decreased sedative effect.
Tranquilizers	Decreased tranquilizer effect.

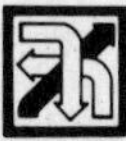

INTERACTION WITH OTHER SUBSTANCES

INTERACTS WITH	COMBINED EFFECT
Alcohol:	None expected.
Beverages: Caffeine drinks	Excess brain stimulation.
Cocaine:	Excess brain stimulation.
Foods:	None expected.
Marijuana:	None expected.
Tobacco:	None expected.

PHENYLPROPANOLAMINE

BRAND NAMES

Alka-Seltzer Plus	Dietac	Sine-Off
Allerest	Dimetapp	Sinubid
Caldecon	4-Way Nasal Spray	Sinutab
Coffee-Break		Triaminicin
Contac	Naldecon	Triaminicol
Control	Sinarest	Tussagesic

See complete brand names list, page 830.

GENERAL INFORMATION

Habit forming? No
Prescription needed? Low strength: No
High strength: Yes
Available as generic? Yes
Drug class: Sympathomimetic

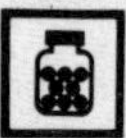

USES

- Relieves bronchial asthma.
- Decreases congestion of breathing passages.
- Suppresses allergic reactions.
- Decreases appetite.

DOSAGE & USAGE INFORMATION

How to take:
- Tablet or capsule—Swallow with liquid. You may chew or crush tablet.
- Extended-release tablets or capsules—Swallow each dose whole.
- Syrup—Take as directed on bottle.

When to take:
As needed, no more often than every 4 hours.

If you forget a dose:
Take up to 2 hours late. If more than 2 hours, wait for next dose (don't double this dose).

What drug does:
- Prevents cells from releasing allergy-causing chemicals (histamines).
- Relaxes muscles of bronchial tubes.
- Decreases blood-vessel size and blood flow, thus causing decongestion.

Time lapse before drug works:
30 to 60 minutes.

Don't take with:
- Non-prescription drugs for cough, cold, allergy or asthma without consulting doctor.
- See Interaction column and consult doctor.

OVERDOSE

Symptoms:
Severe anxiety, confusion, delirium, muscle tremors, rapid and irregular pulse.

What to do:
- Dial 0 (operator) or 911 (emergency) for an ambulance or medical help. Then give first aid immediately.
- Additional emergency information on page 886.

POSSIBLE ADVERSE REACTIONS OR SIDE EFFECTS

SYMPTOMS	FREQUENCY	WHAT TO DO
Brain & nervous system:		
• Nervousness, headache.	Common	4
• Dizziness	Infrequent	4
Skin:		
Paleness	Common	4
Eyes:	None expected.	
Ears, nose, throat:	None expected.	
Digestive:		
Appetite loss, nausea, vomiting.	Infrequent	4
Heart & lungs:		
• Irregular heartbeat.	Infrequent	3
• Rapid heartbeat.	Common	3
• Tightness in chest.	Rare	3
Blood vessels:	None expected.	
Muscles, bones, joints:	None expected.	
Genital, urinary:		
Difficult urination.	Infrequent	4
Kidneys:	None expected.	
Liver:	None expected.	
Allergic:	None expected.	
Blood:	None expected.	
Others:		
Insomnia	Common	5

1- Life-threatening. Seek emergency treatment immediately.
2- Discontinue. Seek emergency treatment.
3- Discontinue. Call doctor right away.
4- Continue. Call doctor when convenient.
5- Continue. Tell doctor at next visit.
6- No action necessary.

PHENYLPROPANOLAMINE

WARNINGS & PRECAUTIONS

Don't take if:
You are allergic to any sympathomimetic drug.

Before you start, consult your doctor:
- If you have high blood pressure.
- If you have diabetes.
- If you have overactive thyroid gland.
- If you have difficulty urinating.
- If you have taken any MAO inhibitors in past 2 weeks.
- If you have taken digitalis preparations in the last 7 days.
- If you will have surgery within 2 months, including dental surgery, requiring general or spinal anesthesia.

Over age 60:
More likely to develop high blood pressure, heart-rhythm disturbances, angina and to feel drug's stimulant effects.

Pregnancy:
No proven harm to unborn child. Avoid if possible.

Breast-feeding:
Drug passes into milk. Avoid drug or discontinue nursing until you finish medicine. Consult doctor for advice on maintaining milk supply.

Infants & children:
No special problems expected.

Prolonged use:
- Excessive doses—Rare toxic psychosis.
- Men with enlarged prostate gland may have more urination difficulty.

Skin & sunlight:
No known problems.

Driving, piloting or hazardous work:
No restrictions unless you feel dizzy.

Airplane passengers:
No problems expected.

Discontinuing:
May be unnecessary to finish medicine. Follow doctor's instructions.

Others:
No problems expected.

INTERACTION WITH OTHER DRUGS

GENERIC NAME OR DRUG CLASS	COMBINED EFFECT
Anesthetics (general)	Increased phenylpropanolamine effect.
Antidepressants (tricyclic)	Increased effect of phenylpropanolamine. Excessive stimulation of heart and blood pressure.
Antihypertensives	Decreased antihypertensive effect.
Digitalis preparations	Serious heart-rhythm disturbances.
Epinephrine	Increased epinephrine effect.
Ergot preparations	Serious blood-pressure rise.
Guanethidine	Decreased effect of both drugs.
MAO inhibitors	Increased phenylpropanolamine effect. Dangerous blood-pressure rise.

INTERACTION WITH OTHER SUBSTANCES

INTERACTS WITH	COMBINED EFFECT
Alcohol:	None expected.
Beverages: Caffeine drinks	Nervousness or insomnia.
Cocaine:	Rapid heartbeat. Avoid.
Foods:	None expected.
Marijuana:	Rapid heartbeat, possible heart-rhythm disturbance. Avoid.
Tobacco:	None expected.

PHENYLTOLOXAMINE

BRAND NAMES

Amaril D
Amaril D Spantab
Comhist
Condecal
Decongestabs
Kutrase
Magsal
Naldecol
Naldecon
Naldelate
Percogesic
Poly-Histine-D
Quadra Hist
Sinocon
Sinubid
Sinutab
Trihista-Phen-25
Tri-Phen-Chlor
Tudecon
Tussionex

GENERAL INFORMATION

Habit forming? No
Prescription needed? No
Available as generic? No
Drug class: Antihistamine

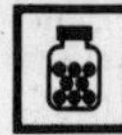

USES

Relieves symptoms of hay fever, allergic reactions and infections of nose and throat.

DOSAGE & USAGE INFORMATION

How to take:

- Extended-release tablets or capsules—Swallow each dose whole with liquid.
- Syrup—Take as directed on label.
- Pediatric drops—Dilute dose in beverage before swallowing.

When to take:
As needed, no more often than every 3 hours.

If you forget a dose:
Take as soon as you remember. Wait 3 hours for next dose (don't double this dose).

What drug does:
Blocks histamine action in sensitized tissues.

Time lapse before drug works:
30 minutes.

Don't take with:

- Non-prescription drugs containing alcohol without consulting doctor.
- See Interaction column and consult doctor.

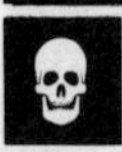

OVERDOSE

Symptoms:

- Adults—Drowsiness, confusion, incoordination, unsteadiness, muscle tremors, stupor, coma.
- Children—Excitement, hallucinations, overactivity, convulsions.

What to do:

- Dial 0 (operator) or 911 (emergency) for an ambulance or medical help. Then give first aid immediately.
- Additional emergency information on page 886.

POSSIBLE ADVERSE REACTIONS OR SIDE EFFECTS

SYMPTOMS	FREQUENCY	WHAT TO DO
Brain & nervous system:		
• Nightmares agitation, irritability, (especially children).	Rare	3
• Drowsiness	Common	5
• Confusion	Infrequent	4
Skin:	None expected.	
Eyes:		
Vision changes.	Rare	3
Ears, nose, throat:		
• Sore throat, fever.	Rare	3
• Dry mouth, nose, throat, ringing or buzzing in ears.	Infrequent	4
Digestive:		
• Appetite loss.	Infrequent	4
• Stomach upset or pain.	Infrequent	3
Heart & lungs:		
• Thick bronchial secretions.	Common	5
• Rapid heartbeat.	Infrequent	3
Blood vessels:		
Unusual bleeding or bruising.	Rare	3
Muscles, bones, joints, kidneys, liver, allergic, blood:	None expected.	
Genital, urinary:		
Difficult or painful urination.	Infrequent	4
Others:		
• Unusual sweating.	Rare	4
• Fatigue, weakness.	Rare	3

1-Life-threatening. Seek emergency treatment immediately.
2-Discontinue. Seek emergency treatment.
3-Discontinue. Call doctor right away.
4-Continue. Call doctor when convenient.
5-Continue. Tell doctor at next visit.

WARNINGS & PRECAUTIONS

Don't take if:
- You are allergic to any antihistamine.
- You have asthma attacks.
- You have glaucoma.
- You have urination difficulty.

Before you start, consult your doctor:
- If you have reacted badly to any antihistamine.
- If you have had peptic ulcer disease.
- If you will have surgery within 2 months, including dental surgery, requiring general or spinal anesthesia.

Over age 60:
Likely to be drowsy, dizzy or lethargic and have impaired thinking, judgment and memory. Increases urination problems from enlarged prostate gland.

Pregnancy:
No proven problems. Consult doctor.

Breast-feeding:
Drug passes into milk. Avoid drug or discontinue nursing until you finish medicine. Consult doctor for advice on maintaining milk supply.

Infants & children:
Use only under medical supervision.

Prolonged use:
No problems expected.

Skin & sunlight:
May cause rash or intensify sunburn in areas exposed to sun or sunlamp.

Driving, piloting or hazardous work:
Don't drive or pilot aircraft until you learn how medicine affects you. Don't work around dangerous machinery. Don't climb ladders or work in high places. Danger increases if you drink alcohol or take medicine affecting alertness and reflexes.

Airplane passengers:
Take 30 to 60 minutes before departure.

Discontinuing:
May be unnecessary to finish medicine. Follow doctor's instructions.

Others:
No problems expected.

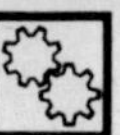

INTERACTION WITH OTHER DRUGS

GENERIC NAME OR DRUG CLASS	COMBINED EFFECT
Amphetamines	Decreased effect of phenyltoloxamine, especially drowsiness.
Anticholinergics	Increased anticholinergic effect.
Anticonvulsants (hydantoin)	Changed pattern of epileptic seizures.
Antidepressants	Increased antidepressant effect.
Narcotics	Increased sedation.
Pain relievers	Increased sedation.
Sedatives	Increased sedation.
Sleep inducers	Increased sedation.
Tranquilizers	Increased sedation.

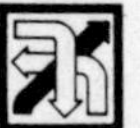

INTERACTION WITH OTHER SUBSTANCES

INTERACTS WITH	COMBINED EFFECT
Alcohol:	Rapid, excessive sedation. Use caution.
Beverages:	None expected.
Cocaine:	Decreased phenyltoloxamine effect.
Foods:	None expected.
Marijuana:	Excessive sedation.
Tobacco:	None expected.

PHENYTOIN

BRAND NAMES

Dantoin
Dilantin
Dilantin Infatabs
Dilantin Kapseals
Di-Phen
Diphenylan
Diphenylhydantoin
Novophenytoin

GENERAL INFORMATION

Habit forming? No
Prescription needed? Yes
Available as generic? Yes
Drug class: Anticonvulsant (hydantoin)

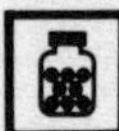

USES

- Prevents epileptic seizures.
- Stabilizes irregular heartbeat.

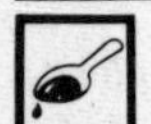

DOSAGE & USAGE INFORMATION

How to take:

- Tablet or capsule—Swallow with liquid.
- Extended-release tablets or capsules—Swallow each dose whole. If you take regular tablets, you may chew or crush them.

When to take:
At the same time each day.

If you forget a dose:

- If drug taken 1 time per day—Take as soon as you remember up to 12 hours late. If more than 12 hours, wait for next scheduled dose (don't double this dose).
- If taken several times per day—Take as soon as possible, then return to regular schedule.

What drug does:
Promotes sodium loss from nerve fibers. This lessens excitability and inhibits spread of nerve impulses.

Time lapse before drug works:
7 to 10 days continual use.

Don't take with:
See Interaction column and consult doctor.

OVERDOSE

Symptoms:
Jerky eye movements; stagger; slurred speech; imbalance; drowsiness; blood-pressure drop; slow, shallow breathing; coma.

What to do:

- Dial 0 (operator) or 911 (emergency) for an ambulance or medical help. Then give first aid immediately.
- Additional emergency information on page 886.

POSSIBLE ADVERSE REACTIONS OR SIDE EFFECTS

SYMPTOMS	FREQUENCY	WHAT TO DO
Brain & nervous system:		
• Mild dizziness, drowsiness.	Common	4
• Headache, sleeplessness.	Infrequent	4
• Hallucinations, confusion, slurred speech, stagger.	Infrequent	3
Skin:		
Rash	Infrequent	3
Eyes:		
Vision changes.	Infrequent	3
Ears, nose, throat:		
Sore throat, fever.	Rare	3
Digestive:		
• Stomach pain.	Rare	3
• Constipation, nausea, vomiting.	Common	4
• Diarrhea	Infrequent	4
Heart & lungs, genital, urinary, kidneys, allergic blood:	None expected.	
Blood vessels:		
Unusual bleeding or bruising.	Rare	3
Muscles, bones, joints:		
Muscle twitching.	Infrequent	4
Liver:		
Jaundice (yellow skin and eyes).	Rare	3
Others:		
Increased body and facial hair.	Infrequent	5

1 - Life-threatening. Seek emergency treatment immediately.
2 - Discontinue. Seek emergency treatment.
3 - Discontinue. Call doctor right away.
4 - Continue. Call doctor when convenient.
5 - Continue. Tell doctor at next visit.

WARNINGS & PRECAUTIONS

Don't take if:
You are allergic to any hydantoin anticonvulsant.

Before you start, consult your doctor:
- If you have had impaired liver function or disease.
- If you will have surgery within 2 months, including dental surgery, requiring general or spinal anesthesia.

Over age 60:
Adverse reactions and side effects may be more frequent and severe than in younger persons.

Pregnancy:
Risk to unborn child outweighs drug benefits. Don't use.

Breast-feeding:
Drug passes into milk. Avoid drug or discontinue nursing until you finish medicine. Consult doctor for advice on maintaining milk supply.

Infants & children:
Use only under medical supervision.

Prolonged use:
- Weakened bones.
- Lymph gland enlargement.
- Possible liver damage.
- Numbness and tingling of hands and feet.
- Continual back-and-forth eye movements.
- Bleeding, swollen or tender gums.

Skin & sunlight:
May cause rash or intensify sunburn in areas exposed to sun or sunlamp.

Driving, piloting or hazardous work:
Don't drive or pilot aircraft until you learn how medicine affects you. Don't work around dangerous machinery. Don't climb ladders or work in high places. Danger increases if you drink alcohol or take medicine affecting alertness and reflexes.

Airplane passengers:
No problems expected.

Discontinuing:
Don't discontinue without consulting doctor. Dose may require gradual reduction if you have taken drug for a long time. Doses of other drugs may also require adjustment.

INTERACTION WITH OTHER DRUGS

GENERIC NAME OR DRUG CLASS	COMBINED EFFECT
Anticoagulants	Increased effect of both drugs.
Antidepressants (tricyclic)	Need to adjust phenytoin dose.
Antihypertensives	Increased effect of antihypertensive.
Aspirin	Increased phenytoin effect.
Barbiturates	Changed seizure pattern.
Carbonic anhydrase inhibitors	Increased chance of bone disease.
Chloramphenicol	Increased phenytoin effect.
Contraceptives (oral)	Increased seizures.
Cortisone drugs	Decreased cortisone effect.
Digitalis preparations	Decreased digitalis effect.
Disulfiram	Increased phenytoin effect.
Estrogens	Increased phenytoin effect.
Furosemide	Decreased furosemide effect.
Glutethimide	Decreased phenytoin effect.

See additional Interactions, page 842.

INTERACTION WITH OTHER SUBSTANCES

INTERACTS WITH	COMBINED EFFECT
Alcohol:	Possible decreased anticonvulsant effect. Use with caution.
Beverages:	None expected.
Cocaine:	Possible seizures.
Foods:	None expected.
Marijuana:	Drowsiness, unsteadiness, decreased anti-convulsant effect.
Tobacco:	None expected.

PILOCARPINE

BRAND NAMES

Adsorbocarpine
Akarpine
Almocarpine
Isopto Carpine
Minims
Miocarpine
Nova-Carpine
Pilocar
Pilocel
Pilomiotin
Piloptic
P.V. Carpine
P.V. Carpine Liquifilm

GENERAL INFORMATION

Habit forming? No
Prescription needed? U.S.: Yes; Canada: No
Available as generic? Yes
Drug class: Antiglaucoma

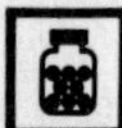

USES

Treatment for glaucoma.

DOSAGE & USAGE INFORMATION

How to take:
- Drops—Apply to eyes. Close eyes for 1 or 2 minutes to absorb medicine.
- Eye system—Follow label directions.

When to take:
As directed on label.

If you forget a dose:
Apply as soon as possible and return to prescribed schedule. Don't double dose.

What drug does:
Reduces internal eye pressure.

Time lapse before drug works:
15 to 30 minutes.

Don't take with:
See Interaction column and consult doctor.

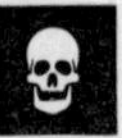

OVERDOSE

Symptoms:
If swallowed—Nausea, vomiting, diarrhea, forceful urination, profuse sweating, rapid pulse, breathing difficulty, loss of consciousness.

What to do:
- Dial 0 (operator) or 911 (emergency) for an ambulance or medical help. Then give first aid immediately.
- If patient is unconscious and not breathing, give mouth-to-mouth breathing. If there is no heartbeat, use cardiac massage and mouth-to-mouth breathing (CPR). Don't try to make patient vomit. If you can't get help quickly, take patient to nearest emergency facility.
- Additional emergency information on page 886.

POSSIBLE ADVERSE REACTIONS OR SIDE EFFECTS

SYMPTOMS	FREQUENCY	WHAT TO DO
Brain & nervous system:		
Headache	Infrequent	3
Skin:		
Profuse sweating.	Infrequent	4
Eyes:		
• Pain, blurred or altered vision.	Common	4
• Eye irritation or twitching.	Infrequent	3
Ears, nose, throat:		
Unusual saliva flow.	Infrequent	4
Digestive:		
Nausea, vomiting, diarrhea.	Infrequent	3
Heart & lungs:		
Breathing difficulty.	Infrequent	3
Blood vessels:	None expected.	
Muscles, bones, joints:		
Muscle tremors.	Infrequent	3
Genital, urinary:	None expected.	
Kidneys:	None expected.	
Liver:	None expected.	
Allergic:	None expected.	
Blood:	None expected.	
Others:	None expected.	

1- Life-threatening. Seek emergency treatment immediately.
2- Discontinue. Seek emergency treatment.
3- Discontinue. Call doctor right away.
4- Continue. Call doctor when convenient.
5- Continue. Tell doctor at next visit.
6- No action necessary.

WARNINGS & PRECAUTIONS

Don't take if:
You are allergic to pilocarpine.

Before you start, consult your doctor:
- If you take sedatives, sleeping pills, tranquilizers, antidepressants, antihistamines, narcotics or mind-altering drugs.
- If you have asthma.
- If you have conjunctivitis (pink eye).

Over age 60:
Adverse reactions and side effects may be more frequent and severe than in younger persons.

Pregnancy:
No proven harm to unborn child. Avoid if possible.

Breast-feeding:
No proven problems. Consult doctor.

Infants & children:
Not recommended.

Prolonged use:
You may develop tolerance for drug, making it ineffective.

Skin & sunlight:
No problems expected.

Driving, piloting or hazardous work:
Don't drive or pilot aircraft until you learn how medicine affects you. Don't work around dangerous machinery. Don't climb ladders or work in high places. Danger increases if you drink alcohol or take medicine affecting alertness and reflexes, such as antihistamines, tranquilizers, sedatives, pain medicine, narcotics and mind-altering drugs.

Airplane passengers:
No problems expected.

Discontinuing:
Doctor may discontinue and substitute another drug to keep treatment effective.

Others:
- Can provoke asthma attack in susceptible individuals.
- Drops may impair vision for 2 to 3 hours.

INTERACTION WITH OTHER DRUGS

GENERIC NAME OR DRUG CLASS	COMBINED EFFECT
Amphetamines	Decreased pilocarpine effect.
Anticholinergics	Decreased pilocarpine effect.
Appetite suppressants	Decreased pilocarpine effect.
Cortisone drugs	Decreased pilocarpine effect.
Phenothiazines	Decreased pilocarpine effect.

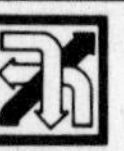

INTERACTION WITH OTHER SUBSTANCES

INTERACTS WITH	COMBINED EFFECT
Alcohol:	May prolong alcohol's effect on brain.
Beverages:	None expected.
Cocaine:	Decreased pilocarpine effect. Avoid.
Foods:	None expected.
Marijuana:	Used once or twice weekly—May help lower internal eye pressure.
Tobacco:	None expected.

PINDOLOL

BRAND NAMES

Pindolol
Visken

GENERAL INFORMATION

Habit forming? No
Prescription needed? Yes
Available as generic? No
Drug class: Beta-adrenergic blocker

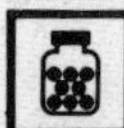

USES

- Reduces angina attacks.
- Stabilizes irregular heartbeat.
- Lowers blood pressure.
- Reduces frequency of migraine headaches. (Does not relieve headache pain.)
- Other uses prescribed by your doctor.

DOSAGE & USAGE INFORMATION

How to take:
Tablet or capsule—Swallow with liquid. If you can't swallow whole, crumble tablet or open capsule and take with liquid or food.

When to take:
With meals or immediately after.

If you forget a dose:
Take as soon as you remember. Return to regular schedule, but allow 3 hours between doses.

What drug does:
- Blocks certain actions of sympathetic nervous system.
- Lowers heart's oxygen requirements.
- Slows nerve impulses through heart.
- Reduces blood vessel contraction in heart, scalp and other body parts.

Time lapse before drug works:
1 to 4 hours.

Don't take with:
Non-prescription drugs or drugs in Interaction column without consulting doctor.

OVERDOSE

Symptoms:
Weakness, slow or weak pulse, blood pressure drop, fainting, convulsions, cold and sweaty skin.

What to do:
- Dial 0 (operator) or 911 (emergency) for an ambulance or medical help. Then give first aid immediately.
- Additional emergency information on page 886.

POSSIBLE ADVERSE REACTIONS OR SIDE EFFECTS

SYMPTOMS	FREQUENCY	WHAT TO DO
Brain & nervous system:		
• Hallucinations, nightmares, insomnia, headache.	Infrequent	3
• Confusion, depression, reduced alertness.	Infrequent	4
• Drowsiness, numbness or tingling of fingers or toes, dizziness.	Common	4
Skin:		
Rash	Rare	3
Eyes:	None expected.	
Ears, nose, throat:		
Sore throat, fever.	Rare	3
Digestive:		
• Diarrhea, nausea.	Common	4
• Constipation	Infrequent	5
Heart & lungs:		
• Pulse slower than 50 beats per minute.	Common	3
• Breathing difficulty.	Infrequent	3
Blood vessels:		
Cold hands, feet.	Common	5
Muscles, bones, joints, genital, urinary, kidneys, liver, allergic:	None expected.	
Blood:		
Unusual bleeding and bruising.	Rare	4
Others:		
• Fatigue, weakness.	Common	4
• Dry mouth, eyes, skin.	Common	5

1- Life-threatening. Seek emergency treatment immediately.
2- Discontinue. Seek emergency treatment.
3- Discontinue. Call doctor right away.
4- Continue. Call doctor when convenient.
5- Continue. Tell doctor at next visit.

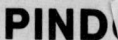

WARNINGS & PRECAUTIONS

Don't take if:

- You are allergic to any beta-adrenergic blocker.
- You have asthma.
- You have hay fever symptoms.
- You have taken MAO inhibitors in past 2 weeks.

Before you start, consult your doctor:

- If you have heart disease or poor circulation to the extremities.
- If you have hay fever, asthma, chronic bronchitis, emphysema.
- If you have overactive thyroid function.
- If you have impaired liver or kidney function.
- If you will have surgery within 2 months, including dental surgery, requiring general or spinal anesthesia.
- If you have diabetes or hypoglycemia.

Over age 60:
Adverse reactions and side effects may be more frequent and severe than in younger persons.

Pregnancy:
Risk to unborn child outweighs drug benefits. Don't use.

Breast-feeding:
Drug passes into milk. Avoid drug or discontinue nursing until you finish medicine. Consult doctor for advice on maintaining milk supply.

Infants & children:
Not recommended.

Prolonged use:
Weakens heart muscle contractions.

Skin & sunlight:
No problems expected.

Driving, piloting or hazardous work:
Don't drive or pilot aircraft until you learn how medicine affects you. Don't work around dangerous machinery. Don't climb ladders or work in high places. Danger increases if you drink alcohol or take medicine affecting alertness and reflexes.

Airplane passengers:
No problems expected.

Discontinuing:
Don't discontinue without consulting doctor. Dose may require gradual reduction if you have taken drug for a long time. Doses of other drugs may also require adjustment.

Others:
May mask hypoglycemia.

INTERACTION WITH OTHER DRUGS

GENERIC NAME OR DRUG CLASS	COMBINED E
Antidiabetics	Increased antic effect.
Antihistamines	Decreased antihistamine effect.
Antihypertensives	Increased antihypertensive effect.
Antiinflammatory drugs	Decreased antiinflammatory effect.
Barbiturates	Increased barbiturate effect. Dangerous sedation.
Digitalis preparations	Can either increase or decrease heart rate. Improves irregular heartbeat.
Narcotics	Increased narcotic effect. Dangerous sedation.
Phenytoin	Increased pindolol effect.
Quinidine	Slows heart excessively.
Reserpine	Increased reserpine effect. Excessive sedation and depression.

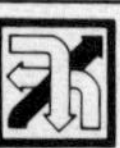

INTERACTION WITH OTHER SUBSTANCES

INTERACTS WITH	COMBINED EFFECT
Alcohol:	Excessive blood-pressure drop. Avoid.
Beverages:	None expected.
Cocaine:	Irregular heartbeat. Avoid.
Foods:	None expected.
Marijuana:	Daily use—Impaired circulation to hands and feet.
Tobacco:	Possible irregular heartbeat.

PIPERACETAZINE

BRAND NAMES

Quide

GENERAL INFORMATION

Habit forming? No
Prescription needed? Yes
Available as generic? Yes
Drug class: Tranquilizer, antiemetic (phenothiazine)

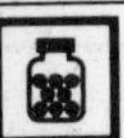

USES

- Stops nausea, vomiting.
- Reduces anxiety, agitation.

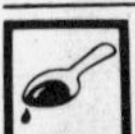

DOSAGE & USAGE INFORMATION

How to take:
- Tablet or capsule—Swallow with liquid or food to lessen stomach irritation.
- Suppositories—Remove wrapper and moisten suppository with water. Gently insert into rectum, large end first.
- Drops or liquid—Dilute dose in beverage.

When to take:
- Nervous and mental disorders—Take at the same times each day.
- Nausea and vomiting—Take as needed, no more often than every 4 hours.

If you forget a dose:
- Nervous and mental disorders—Take up to 2 hours late. If more than 2 hours, wait for next scheduled dose (don't double this).
- Nausea and vomiting—Take as soon as you remember. Wait 4 hours for next dose.

What drug does:
- Suppresses brain's vomiting center.
- Suppresses brain centers that control abnormal emotions and behavior.

Time lapse before drug works:
- Nausea and vomiting—1 hour or less.
- Nervous and mental disorders—4-6 weeks.

Don't take with:
- Antacid or medicine for diarrhea.
- Non-prescription drug for cough, cold or allergy.
- See Interaction column and consult doctor.

OVERDOSE

Symptoms:
Stupor, convulsions, coma.

What to do:
- Dial 0 (operator) or 911 (emergency) for an ambulance or medical help. Then give first aid immediately.
- Additional emergency information on page 886.

POSSIBLE ADVERSE REACTIONS OR SIDE EFFECTS

SYMPTOMS	FREQUENCY	WHAT TO DO
Brain & nervous system:		
• Restlessness, tremor.	Common	3
• Fainting	Infrequent	2
• Drowsiness	Common	3
Skin:		
• Rash	Infrequent	3
• Less perspiration.	Common	4
Eyes:		
Vision changes.	Rare	3
Ears, nose, throat:		
• Sore throat, fever.	Rare	3
• Dry mouth, nasal congestion.	Common	4
Digestive:		
Constipation	Common	4
Heart & lungs, blood vessels, kidneys, allergic, blood:	None expected.	
Muscles, bones, joints:		
Muscle spasms of face and neck, unsteady gait.	Common	2
Genital, urinary:		
Urination difficulty.	Infrequent	4
Liver:		
Jaundice (yellow eyes and skin).	Rare	3
Others:		
Less interest in sex, breast swelling, change in menstrual pattern.	Infrequent	4

1-Life-threatening. Seek emergency treatment immediately.
2-Discontinue. Seek emergency treatment.
3-Discontinue. Call doctor right away.
4-Continue. Call doctor when convenient.
5-Continue. Tell doctor at next visit.
6-No action necessary.

WARNINGS & PRECAUTIONS

Don't take if:
- You are allergic to any phenothiazine.
- You have a blood or bone-marrow disease.

Before you start, consult your doctor:
- If you will have surgery within 2 months, including dental surgery, requiring general or spinal anesthesia.
- If you have asthma, emphysema or other lung disorder.
- If you take non-prescription ulcer medicine, asthma medicine or amphetamines.

Over age 60:
Adverse reactions and side effects may be more frequent and severe than in younger persons. More likely to develop involuntary movement of jaws, lips, tongue, chewing. Report this to your doctor immediately. Early treatment can help.

Pregnancy:
Risk to unborn child outweighs drug benefits. Don't use.

Breast-feeding:
Drug passes into milk. Avoid drug or discontinue nursing until you finish medicine. Consult doctor for advice on maintaining milk supply.

Infants & children:
Don't give to children younger than 2.

Prolonged use:
May lead to tardive dyskinesia (involuntary movement of jaws, lips, tongue, chewing).

Skin & sunlight:
May cause rash or intensify sunburn in areas exposed to sun or sunlamp. Skin may remain sensitive for 3 months after discontinuing.

Driving, piloting or hazardous work:
Don't drive or pilot aircraft until you learn how medicine affects you. Don't work around dangerous machinery. Don't climb ladders or work in high places. Danger increases if you drink alcohol or take medicine affecting alertness and reflexes.

Airplane passengers:
No problems expected.

Discontinuing:
- Nervous and mental disorders—Don't discontinue without doctor's advice until you complete prescribed dose, even though symptoms diminish or disappear.
- Nausea and vomiting—May be unnecessary to finish medicine. Follow doctor's instructions.

INTERACTION WITH OTHER DRUGS

GENERIC NAME OR DRUG CLASS	COMBINED EFFECT
Anticholinergics	Increased anticholinergic effect.
Antidepressants (tricyclic)	Increased piperacetazine effect.
Antihistamines	Increased antihistamine effect.
Appetite suppressants	Decreased suppressant effect.
Levodopa	Decreased levodopa effect.
Mind-altering drugs	Increased effect of mind-altering drugs.
Narcotics	Increased narcotic effect.
Phenytoin	Increased phenytoin effect.
Quinidine	Impaired heart function. Dangerous mixture.
Sedatives	Increased sedative effect.
Tranquilizers (other)	Increased tranquilizer effect.

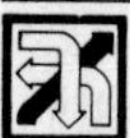

INTERACTION WITH OTHER SUBSTANCES

INTERACTS WITH	COMBINED EFFECT
Alcohol:	Dangerous oversedation.
Beverages:	None expected.
Cocaine:	Decreased piperacetazine effect. Avoid.
Foods:	None expected.
Marijuana:	Drowsiness. May increase antinausea effect.
Tobacco:	None expected.

PIROXICAM

BRAND NAMES

Feldene

GENERAL INFORMATION

Habit forming? No
Prescription needed? Yes
Available as generic? No
Drug class: Antiinflammatory (non-steroid)

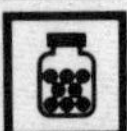

USES

- Relieves symptoms of rheumatoid arthritis, osteoarthritis and gout.
- Relieves symptoms of ankylosing spondylitis.

DOSAGE & USAGE INFORMATION

How to take:
Tablet—Swallow with liquid of food to lessen stomach irritation. If you can't swallow whole, crumble tablet and take with liquid or food.

When to take:
At the same times each day.

If you forget a dose:
Take as soon as you remember up to 2 hours late. If more than 2 hours, wait for next scheduled dose (don't double this dose).

What drug does:
Reduces tissue concentration of prostaglandins (hormones that produce inflammation and pain).

Time lapse before drug works:
Begins in 4 to 24 hours. May require 3 weeks regular use for maximum benefit.

Don't take with:
See Interaction column and consult doctor.

OVERDOSE

Symptoms:
Confusion, agitation, incoherence, convulsions, possible hemorrhage from stomach or intestine, coma.

What to do:
- Dial 0 (operator) or 911 (emergency) for an ambulance or medical help. Then give first aid immediately.
- Additional emergency information on page 886.

POSSIBLE ADVERSE REACTIONS OR SIDE EFFECTS

SYMPTOMS	FREQUENCY	WHAT TO DO
Brain & nervous system:		
• Depression, drowsiness.	Infrequent	4
• Convulsions, confusion.	Rare	3
• Dizziness	Common	4
• Headache	Common	5
Skin:		
Rash, hives or itch.	Rare	3
Eyes:		
Blurred vision.	Rare	3
Ears, nose, throat:		
Ringing in ears.	Infrequent	4
Digestive:		
• Bloody or black, tarry stools.	Rare	3
• Nausea, pain.	Common	4
• Constipation or diarrhea, vomiting.	Infrequent	4
Heart & lungs:		
Breathing difficulty, tightness in chest, rapid heartbeat.	Rare	3
Blood vessels:		
Unusual bleeding or bruising.	Rare	3
Muscles, bones, joints:		
Swollen feet, legs.	Infrequent	4
Genital, urinary:		
• Bloody urine.	Rare	3
• Difficult, painful or frequent urination.	Rare	4
Kidneys, allergic, blood:	None expected.	
Liver:		
Jaundice (yellow skin and eyes).	Rare	3
Others:		
Fatigue, weakness.	Rare	4

3- Discontinue. Call doctor right away.
4- Continue. Call doctor when convenient.
5- Continue. Tell doctor at next visit.

WARNINGS & PRECAUTIONS

Don't take if:
- You are allergic to aspirin or any non-steroid, antiinflammatory drug.
- You have gastritis, peptic ulcer, enteritis, ileitis, ulcerative colitis, asthma, heart failure, high blood pressure or bleeding problems.
- Patient is younger than 15.

Before you start, consult your doctor:
- If you have epilepsy.
- If you have Parkinson's disease.
- If you have been mentally ill.
- If you have had kidney disease or impaired kidney function.
- If you will have surgery within 2 months, including dental surgery, requiring general or spinal anesthesia.

Over age 60:
Adverse reactions and side effects may be more frequent and severe than in younger persons. Smaller than average doses may reduce unpleasant side effects.

Pregnancy:
Studies inconclusive on harm to unborn child. Animal studies show fetal abnormalities. Decide with your doctor whether drug benefits justify risk to unborn child.

Breast-feeding:
May harm child. Avoid.

Infants & children:
Not recommended for anyone younger than 15. Use only under medical supervision.

Prolonged use:
- Eye damage, reduced hearing, sore throat, fever.
- Weight gain.
- Request liver-function and bleeding time studies.

Skin & sunlight:
No problems expected.

Driving, piloting or hazardous work:
Don't drive or pilot aircraft until you learn how medicine affects you. Don't work around dangerous machinery. Don't climb ladders or work in high places. Danger increases if you drink alcohol or take medicine affecting alertness and reflexes, such as antihistamines, tranquilizers, sedatives, pain medicine, narcotics and mind-altering drugs.

Airplane passengers:
No problems expected.

Discontinuing:
Don't discontinue without consulting doctor. Dose may require gradual reduction if you have taken drug for a long time. Doses of other drugs may also require adjustment.

INTERACTION WITH OTHER DRUGS

GENERIC NAME OR DRUG CLASS	COMBINED EFFECT
Anticoagulants (oral)	Increased risk of bleeding.
Aspirin	Increased risk of stomach ulcer.
Cortisone drugs	Increased risk of stomach ulcer.
Furosemide	Decreased diuretic effect of furosemide.
Oxyphenbutazone	Possible stomach ulcer.
Phenylbutazone	Possible stomach ulcer.
Probenecid	Increased piroxicam effect.
Thyroid hormones	Rapid heartbeat, blood-pressure rise.

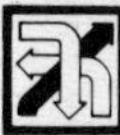

INTERACTION WITH OTHER SUBSTANCES

INTERACTS WITH	COMBINED EFFECT
Alcohol:	Possible stomach ulcer or bleeding.
Beverages:	None expected.
Cocaine:	Depression following cocaine use. Avoid.
Foods:	None expected.
Marijuana:	Increased pain relief from piroxicam, but may be depressing.
Tobacco:	Decreased absorption of piroxicam. Avoid tobacco.

POLOXAMER 188

BRAND NAMES

Alaxin

GENERAL INFORMATION

Habit forming? No
Prescription needed? No
Available as generic? Yes
Drug class: Laxative (emollient)

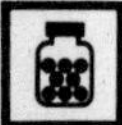

USES

Constipation relief.

DOSAGE & USAGE INFORMATION

How to take:

- Tablet or capsule—Swallow with liquid. Don't open capsules.
- Drops—Dilute dose in beverage before swallowing.
- Syrup—Take as directed on bottle.

When to take:
At the same time each day, preferably bedtime.

If you forget a dose:
Take as soon as you remember. Wait 12 hours for next dose. Return to regular schedule.

What drug does:
Makes stool hold fluid so it is easier to pass.

Time lapse before drug works:
2 to 3 days of continual use.

Don't take with:

- Other medicines at same time. Wait 2 hours.
- See Interaction column and consult doctor.

OVERDOSE

Symptoms:
Appetite loss, nausea, vomiting, diarrhea.

What to do:
Overdose unlikely to threaten life. If person takes much larger amount than prescribed, call doctor, poison-control center or hospital emergency room for instructions.

POSSIBLE ADVERSE REACTIONS OR SIDE EFFECTS

SYMPTOMS	FREQUENCY	WHAT TO DO
Brain & nervous system:	None expected.	
Skin:		
Rash	Rare	3
Eyes:	None expected.	
Ears, nose, throat:		
Throat irritation (liquid only).	Infrequent	4
Digestive:		
Intestinal and stomach cramps.	Infrequent	4
Heart & lungs:	None expected.	
Blood vessels:	None expected.	
Muscles, bones, joints:	None expected.	
Genital, urinary:	None expected.	
Kidneys:	None expected.	
Liver:	None expected.	
Allergic:	None expected.	
Blood:	None expected.	
Others:	None expected.	

1 - Life-threatening. Seek emergency treatment immediately.
2 - Discontinue. Seek emergency treatment.
3 - Discontinue. Call doctor right away.
4 - Continue. Call doctor when convenient.
5 - Continue. Tell doctor at next visit.
6 - No action necessary.

WARNINGS & PRECAUTIONS

Don't take if:
- You are allergic to any emollient laxative.
- You have abdominal pain and fever that might be appendicitis.

Before you start, consult your doctor:
- If you are taking other laxatives.
- To be sure constipation isn't a sign of a serious disorder.

Over age 60:
You must drink 6 to 8 glasses of fluid every 24 hours for drug to work.

Pregnancy:
No problems expected. Consult doctor.

Breast-feeding:
No problems expected.

Infants & children:
No problems expected.

Prolonged use:
Avoid. Overuse of laxatives may damage intestine lining.

Skin & sunlight:
No problems expected.

Driving, piloting or hazardous work:
No problems expected.

Airplane passengers:
No problems expected.

Discontinuing:
May be unnecessary to finish medicine. Follow doctor's instructions.

Others:
No problems expected.

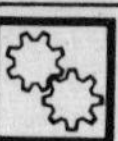

INTERACTION WITH OTHER DRUGS

GENERIC NAME OR DRUG CLASS	COMBINED EFFECT
Danthron	Possible liver damage.
Digitalis preparations	Toxic absorption of digitalis.
Mineral oil	Increased mineral oil absorption into bloodstream. Avoid.
Phenolphthalein	Increased phenolphthalein absorption. Possible toxicity.

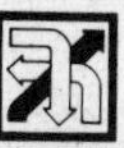

INTERACTION WITH OTHER SUBSTANCES

INTERACTS WITH	COMBINED EFFECT
Alcohol:	None expected.
Beverages:	None expected.
Cocaine:	None expected.
Foods:	None expected.
Marijuana:	None expected.
Tobacco:	None expected.

POLYCARBOPHIL CALCIUM

BRAND NAMES

Mitrolan

GENERAL INFORMATION

Habit forming? No
Prescription needed? No
Available as generic? No
Drug class: Laxative (bulk-forming), antidiarrheal

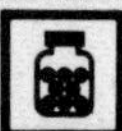

USES

- Relieves constipation and prevents straining for bowel movement.
- Stops diarrhea.

DOSAGE & USAGE INFORMATION

How to take:
- Tablets (laxative)—Swallow with 8 oz. cold liquid. Drink 6 to 8 glasses of water each day in addition to the one with each dose.
- Tablets (diarrhea)—Take without water at half-hour intervals.

When to take:
At the same times each day.

If you forget a dose:
Take as soon as you remember. Resume regular schedule.

What drug does:
Absorbs water, stimulating the bowel to form a soft, bulky stool and decreasing watery diarrhea.

Time lapse before drug works:
May require 2 or 3 days to begin, then works in 12 to 24 hours.

Don't take with:
- See Interaction column and consult doctor.
- Don't take within 2 hours of taking another medicine.

OVERDOSE

Symptoms:
None expected.

What to do:
Overdose unlikely to threaten life. If person takes much larger amount than prescribed, call doctor, poison-control center or hospital emergency room for instructions.

POSSIBLE ADVERSE REACTIONS OR SIDE EFFECTS

SYMPTOMS	FREQUENCY	WHAT TO DO
Brain & nervous system:	None expected.	
Skin:		
Itch, rash.	Rare	3
Eyes:	None expected.	
Ears, nose, throat:		
Swallowing difficulty, "lump in throat" sensation.	Infrequent	4
Digestive:		
• Intestinal blockage.	Rare	3
• Nausea, vomiting, diarrhea.	Infrequent	4
Heart & lungs:		
Asthma	Rare	3
Blood vessels:	None expected.	
Muscles, bones, joints:	None expected.	
Genital, urinary:	None expected.	
Kidneys:	None expected.	
Liver:	None expected.	
Allergic:	None expected.	
Blood:	None expected.	
Others:	None expected.	

1 - Life-threatening. Seek emergency treatment immediately.
2 - Discontinue. Seek emergency treatment.
3 - Discontinue. Call doctor right away.
4 - Continue. Call doctor when convenient.
5 - Continue. Tell doctor at next visit.
6 - No action necessary.

WARNINGS & PRECAUTIONS

Don't take if:
- You are allergic to any bulk-forming laxative.
- You have symptoms of appendicitis, inflamed bowel or intestinal blockage.
- You have missed a bowel movement for only 1 or 2 days.

Before you start, consult your doctor:
- If you have diabetes.
- If you have a laxative habit.
- If you have rectal bleeding.
- If you have difficulty swallowing.
- If you take other laxatives.

Over age 60:
Adverse reactions and side effects may be more frequent and severe than in younger persons.

Pregnancy:
Most bulk-forming laxatives contain sodium or sugars which may cause fluid retention. Avoid if possible.

Breast-feeding:
No problems expected.

Infants & children:
Use only under medical supervision.

Prolonged use:
Don't take for more than 1 week unless under a doctor's supervision. May cause laxative dependence.

Skin & sunlight:
No problems expected.

Driving, piloting or hazardous work:
No problems expected.

Airplane passengers:
No problems expected.

Discontinuing:
May be unnecessary to finish medicine. Follow doctor's instructions.

Others:
Don't take to "flush out" your system or as a "tonic."

INTERACTION WITH OTHER DRUGS

GENERIC NAME OR DRUG CLASS	COMBINED EFFECT
Antibiotics	Decreased antibiotic effect.
Anticoagulants	Decreased anticoagulant effect.
Digitalis preparations	Decreased digitalis effect.
Salicylates (including aspirin)	Decreased salicylate effect.

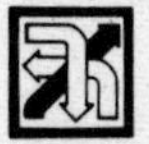

INTERACTION WITH OTHER SUBSTANCES

INTERACTS WITH	COMBINED EFFECT
Alcohol:	None expected.
Beverages:	None expected.
Cocaine:	None expected.
Foods:	None expected.
Marijuana:	None expected.
Tobacco:	None expected.

POLYTHIAZIDE

BRAND NAMES

Renese

GENERAL INFORMATION

Habit forming? No
Prescription needed? Yes
Available as generic? Yes
Drug class: Antihypertensive, diuretic (thiazide)

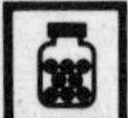

USES

- Controls, but doesn't cure, high blood pressure.
- Reduces fluid retention (edema) caused by conditions such as heart disorders and liver disease.

DOSAGE & USAGE INFORMATION

How to take:
Tablet or capsule—Swallow with 8 oz. of liquid. If you can't swallow whole, crumble tablet or open capsule and take with liquid or food. Don't exceed dose.

When to take:
At the same time each day.

If you forget a dose:
Take as soon as you remember up to 2 hours late. If more than 2 hours, wait for next scheduled dose (don't double this dose).

What drug does:
- Forces sodium and water excretion, reducing body fluid.
- Relaxes muscle cells of small arteries.
- Reduced body fluid and relaxed arteries lower blood pressure.

Time lapse before drug works:
4 to 6 hours. May require several weeks to lower blood pressure.

Don't take with:
- See Interaction column and consult doctor.
- Non-prescription drugs without consulting doctor.

OVERDOSE

Symptoms:
Cramps, weakness, drowsiness, weak pulse, coma.

What to do:
- Dial 0 (operator) or 911 (emergency) for an ambulance or medical help. Then give first aid immediately.
- Additional emergency information on page 886.

POSSIBLE ADVERSE REACTIONS OR SIDE EFFECTS

SYMPTOMS	FREQUENCY	WHAT TO DO
Brain & nervous system:		
• Dizziness	Infrequent	4
• Mood changes.	Infrequent	4
• Headaches	Infrequent	4
Skin:		
Rash or hives.	Rare	2
Eyes:		
Blurred vision.	Infrequent	3
Ears, nose, throat:		
• Sore throat, fever.	Rare	3
• Dry mouth, thirst.	Infrequent	5
Digestive:		
Severe abdominal pain, nausea, vomiting.	Infrequent	3
Heart & lungs:		
Irregular heartbeat, weak pulse.	Infrequent	3
Blood vessels:	None expected.	
Muscles, bones, joints:		
Weakness, tiredness.	Infrequent	4
Genital, urinary:	None expected.	
Kidneys:	None expected.	
Liver:		
Jaundice (yellow skin and eyes).	Rare	3
Allergic:	None expected.	
Blood:	None expected.	
Others:		
Weight changes.	Infrequent	4

1-Life-threatening. Seek emergency treatment immediately.
2-Discontinue. Seek emergency treatment.
3-Discontinue. Call doctor right away.
4-Continue. Call doctor when convenient.
5-Continue. Tell doctor at next visit.
6-No action necessary.

WARNINGS & PRECAUTIONS

Don't take if:
You are allergic to any thiazide diuretic drug.

Before you start, consult your doctor:
- If you are allergic to any sulfa drug.
- If you have gout.
- If you have liver, pancreas or kidney disorder.

Over age 60:
Adverse reactions and side effects may be more frequent and severe than in younger persons, especially dizziness and excessive potassium loss.

Pregnancy:
Risk to unborn child outweighs drug benefits. Don't use.

Breast-feeding:
Drug passes into milk. Avoid drug or discontinue nursing.

Infants & children:
No problems expected.

Prolonged use:
You may need medicine to treat high blood pressure for the rest of your life.

Skin & sunlight:
May cause rash or intensify sunburn in areas exposed to sun or sunlamp.

Driving, piloting or hazardous work:
Don't drive or pilot aircraft until you learn how medicine affects you. Don't work around dangerous machinery. Don't climb ladders or work in high places. Danger increases if you drink alcohol or take medicine affecting alertness and reflexes, such as antihistamines, tranquilizers, sedatives, pain medicine, narcotics and mind-altering drugs.

Airplane passengers:
No problems expected.

Discontinuing:
Don't discontinue without medical advice.

Others:
- Hot weather and fever may cause dehydration and drop in blood pressure. Dose may require temporary adjustment. Weigh daily and report any unexpected weight decreases to your doctor.
- May cause rise in uric acid, leading to gout.
- May cause blood-sugar rise in diabetics.

INTERACTION WITH OTHER DRUGS

GENERIC NAME OR DRUG CLASS	COMBINED EFFECT
Allopurinol	Decreased allopurinol effect.
Antidepressants (tricyclic)	Dangerous drop in blood pressure. Avoid combination unless under medical supervision.
Barbiturates	Increased polythiazide effect.
Cholestyramine	Decreased polythiazide effect.
Cortisone drugs	Excessive potassium loss that causes dangerous heart rhythms.
Digitalis preparations	Excessive potassium loss that causes dangerous heart rhythms.
Diuretics (thiazide)	Increased effect of other thiazide diuretics.
Lithium	Increased effect of lithium.
MAO inhibitors	Increased polythiazide effect.
Probenecid	Decreased probenecid effect.

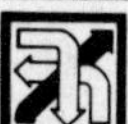

INTERACTION WITH OTHER SUBSTANCES

INTERACTS WITH	COMBINED EFFECT
Alcohol:	Dangerous blood-pressure drop.
Beverages:	None expected.
Cocaine:	None expected.
Foods:	
Licorice	Excessive potassium loss that causes dangerous heart rhythms.
Marijuana:	May increase blood pressure.
Tobacco:	None expected.

POTASSIUM ACETATE, POTASSIUM BICARBONATE & POTASSIUM CITRATE

BRAND NAMES

Potassium Triplex
Tri-K
Trikates

GENERAL INFORMATION

Habit forming? No
Prescription needed? Yes
Available as generic? Yes
Drug class: Mineral supplement (potassium)

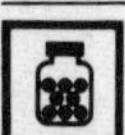

USES

Treatment for potassium deficiency from illness, diuretics, cortisone drugs or digitalis preparations.

DOSAGE & USAGE INFORMATION

How to take:

- Tablet or capsule—Swallow with liquid or food to lessen stomach irritation. You may chew or crush tablet.
- Extended-release tablets or capsules—Swallow each dose whole with liquid.
- Effervescent tablets, granules, powder or liquid—Dilute dose in water.

When to take:
At the same times each day, preferably with food or immediately after meals.

If you forget a dose:
Take as soon as you remember. Don't double next dose.

What drug does:
Preserves or restores normal function of nerve cells, heart and skeletal-muscle cells, kidneys and stomach-juice secretion.

Time lapse before drug works:
12 to 24 hours.

Don't take with:
See Interaction column and consult doctor.

OVERDOSE

Symptoms:
Paralysis of arms and legs, irregular heartbeat, blood-pressure drop, convulsions, coma, cardiac arrest.

What to do:

- Dial 0 (operator) or 911 (emergency) for an ambulance or medical help. Then give first aid immediately.
- Additional emergency information on page 886.

POSSIBLE ADVERSE REACTIONS OR SIDE EFFECTS

SYMPTOMS	FREQUENCY	WHAT TO DO
Brain & nervous system:		
• Numbness and tingling in hands and feet.	Rare	4
• Confusion	Rare	3
Skin:	None expected.	
Eyes:	None expected.	
Ears, nose, throat:	None expected.	
Digestive: Diarrhea, nausea, vomiting, stomach discomfort.	Infrequent	4
Heart & lungs: Irregular heartbeat, breathing difficulty.	Rare	3
Blood vessels:	None expected.	
Muscles, bones, joints: Unusual fatigue, weakness, heaviness of legs.	Rare	3
Genital, urinary:	None expected.	
Kidneys:	None expected.	
Liver:	None expected.	
Allergic:	None expected.	
Blood:	None expected.	
Others:	None expected.	

1- Life-threatening. Seek emergency treatment immediately.
2- Discontinue. Seek emergency treatment.
3- Discontinue. Call doctor right away.
4- Continue. Call doctor when convenient.
5- Continue. Tell doctor at next visit.
6- No action necessary.

POTASSIUM ACETATE, POTASSIUM BICARBONATE & POTASSIUM CITRATE

WARNINGS & PRECAUTIONS

Don't take if:

- You are allergic to any potassium supplement.
- You have kidney disease.

Before you start, consult your doctor:

- If you have Addison's disease.
- If you have heart disease.
- If you have intestinal blockage.
- If you have a stomach ulcer.
- If you use diuretics.
- If you use heart medicine.
- If you use laxatives or have chronic diarrhea.
- If you use salt substitutes or low-salt milk.

Over age 60:
Observe dose schedule strictly. Potassium balance is critical. Deviation above or below normal can have serious results.

Pregnancy:
No problems expected if you adhere strictly to prescribed dose.

Breast-feeding:
Studies inconclusive on harm to infant. Consult doctor.

Infants & children:
Use only under doctor's supervision.

Prolonged use:
Slows absorption of vitamin B-12. May cause anemia.

Skin & sunlight:
No problems expected.

Driving, piloting or hazardous work:
No problems expected.

Airplane passengers:
No problems expected.

Discontinuing:
Don't discontinue without consulting doctor. Dose may require gradual reduction if you have taken drug for a long time. Doses of other drugs may also require adjustment.

Others:
Overdose or underdose serious. Frequent laboratory blood studies recommended.

INTERACTION WITH OTHER DRUGS

GENERIC NAME OR DRUG CLASS	COMBINED EFFECT
Digitalis preparations	Possible irregular heartbeat.
Diuretics (thiazide)	Decreased potassium effect.
Spironolactone	Dangerous rise in blood potassium.
Triamterene	Dangerous rise in blood potassium.

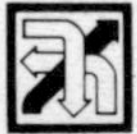

INTERACTION WITH OTHER SUBSTANCES

INTERACTS WITH	COMBINED EFFECT
Alcohol:	None expected.
Beverages: Salty drinks such as tomato juice, commercial thirst quenchers.	Increased fluid retention.
Cocaine:	May cause irregular heartbeat.
Foods: Salty foods.	Increased fluid retention.
Marijuana:	May cause irregular heartbeat.
Tobacco:	None expected.

POTASSIUM BICARBONATE & CITRIC ACID

BRAND NAMES

K-Lyte
K-Lyte DS

GENERAL INFORMATION

Habit forming? No
Prescription needed? Yes
Available as generic? Yes
Drug class: Mineral supplement (potassium)

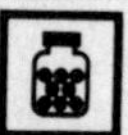

USES

Treatment for potassium deficiency from illness, diuretics, cortisone drugs or digitalis preparations.

DOSAGE & USAGE INFORMATION

How to take:

- Tablet or capsule—Swallow with liquid or food to lessen stomach irritation. You may chew or crush tablet.
- Extended-release tablets or capsules—Swallow each dose whole with liquid.
- Effervescent tablets, granules, powder or liquid—Dilute dose in water.

When to take:
At the same times each day, preferably with food or immediately after meals.

If you forget a dose:
Take as soon as you remember. Don't double next dose.

What drug does:
Preserves or restores normal function of nerve cells, heart and skeletal-muscle cells, kidneys and stomach-juice secretion.

Time lapse before drug works:
12 to 24 hours.

Don't take with:
See Interaction column and consult doctor.

OVERDOSE

Symptoms:
Paralysis of arms and legs, irregular heartbeat, blood-pressure drop, convulsions, coma, cardiac arrest.

What to do:

- Dial 0 (operator) or 911 (emergency) for an ambulance or medical help. Then give first aid immediately.
- Additional emergency information on page 886.

POSSIBLE ADVERSE REACTIONS OR SIDE EFFECTS

SYMPTOMS	FREQUENCY	WHAT TO DO
Brain & nervous system:		
• Numbness and tingling in hands and feet.	Rare	4
• Confusion.	Rare	3
Skin:	None expected.	
Eyes:	None expected.	
Ears, nose, throat:	None expected.	
Digestive:		
Diarrhea, nausea, vomiting, stomach discomfort.	Infrequent	4
Heart & lungs:		
Irregular heartbeat, breathing difficulty.	Rare	3
Blood vessels:	None expected.	
Muscles, bones, joints:		
Unusual fatigue, weakness, heaviness of legs.	Rare	3
Genital, urinary:	None expected.	
Kidneys:	None expected.	
Liver:	None expected.	
Allergic:	None expected.	
Blood:	None expected.	
Others:	None expected.	

1- Life-threatening. Seek emergency treatment immediately.
2- Discontinue. Seek emergency treatment.
3- Discontinue. Call doctor right away.
4- Continue. Call doctor when convenient.
5- Continue. Tell doctor at next visit.
6- No action necessary.

POTASSIUM BICARBONATE & CITRIC ACID

WARNINGS & PRECAUTIONS

Don't take if:

- You are allergic to any potassium supplement.
- You have kidney disease.

Before you start, consult your doctor:

- If you have Addison's disease.
- If you have heart disease.
- If you have intestinal blockage.
- If you have a stomach ulcer.
- If you use diuretics.
- If you use heart medicine.
- If you use laxatives or have chronic diarrhea.
- If you use salt substitutes or low-salt milk.

Over age 60:
Observe dose schedule strictly. Potassium balance is critical. Deviation above or below normal can have serious results.

Pregnancy:
No problems expected if you adhere strictly to prescribed dose.

Breast-feeding:
Studies inconclusive on harm to infant. Consult doctor.

Infants & children:
Use only under doctor's supervision.

Prolonged use:
Slows absorption of vitamin B-12. May cause anemia.

Skin & sunlight:
No problems expected.

Driving, piloting or hazardous work:
No problems expected.

Airplane passengers:
No problems expected.

Discontinuing:
Don't discontinue without consulting doctor. Dose may require gradual reduction if you have taken drug for a long time. Doses of other drugs may also require adjustment.

Others:
Overdose or underdose serious. Frequent laboratory blood studies recommended.

INTERACTION WITH OTHER DRUGS

GENERIC NAME OR DRUG CLASS	COMBINED EFFECT
Digitalis preparations	Possible irregular heartbeat.
Diuretics (thiazide)	Decreased potassium effect.
Spironolactone	Dangerous rise in blood potassium.
Triamterene	Dangerous rise in blood potassium.

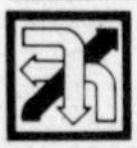

INTERACTION WITH OTHER SUBSTANCES

INTERACTS WITH	COMBINED EFFECT
Alcohol:	None expected.
Beverages: Salty drinks such as tomato juice, commercial thirst quenchers.	Increased fluid retention.
Cocaine:	May cause irregular heartbeat.
Foods: Salty foods.	Increased fluid retention.
Marijuana:	May cause irregular heartbeat.
Tobacco:	None expected.

POTASSIUM BICARBONATE, POTASSIUM CARBONATE & POTASSIUM CHLORIDE

BRAND NAMES

KEFF

GENERAL INFORMATION

Habit forming? No
Prescription needed? Yes
Available as generic? Yes
Drug class: Mineral supplement (potassium)

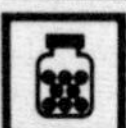

USES

Treatment for potassium deficiency from illness, diuretics, cortisone drugs or digitalis preparations.

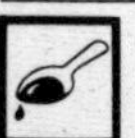

DOSAGE & USAGE INFORMATION

How to take:

- Tablet or capsule—Swallow with liquid or food to lessen stomach irritation. You may chew or crush tablet.
- Extended-release tablets or capsules—Swallow each dose whole with liquid.
- Effervescent tablets, granules, powder or liquid—Dilute dose in water.

When to take:
At the same times each day, preferably with food or immediately after meals.

If you forget a dose:
Take as soon as you remember. Don't double next dose.

What drug does:
Preserves or restores normal function of nerve cells, heart and skeletal-muscle cells, kidneys and stomach-juice secretion.

Time lapse before drug works:
12 to 24 hours.

Don't take with:
See Interaction column and consult doctor.

OVERDOSE

Symptoms:
Paralysis of arms and legs, irregular heartbeat, blood-pressure drop, convulsions, coma, cardiac arrest.

What to do:

- Dial 0 (operator) or 911 (emergency) for an ambulance or medical help. Then give first aid immediately.
- Additional emergency information on page 886.

POSSIBLE ADVERSE REACTIONS OR SIDE EFFECTS

SYMPTOMS	FREQUENCY	WHAT TO DO
Brain & nervous system:		
• Numbness and tingling in hands and feet.	Rare	4
• Confusion	Rare	3
Skin:	None expected.	
Eyes:	None expected.	
Ears, nose, throat:	None expected.	
Digestive: Diarrhea, nausea, vomiting, stomach discomfort.	Infrequent	4
Heart & lungs: Irregular heartbeat, breathing difficulty.	Rare	3
Blood vessels:	None expected.	
Muscles, bones, joints: Unusual fatigue, weakness, heaviness of legs.	Rare	3
Genital, urinary:	None expected.	
Kidneys:	None expected.	
Liver:	None expected.	
Allergic:	None expected.	
Blood:	None expected.	
Others:	None expected.	

1- Life-threatening. Seek emergency treatment immediately.
2- Discontinue. Seek emergency treatment.
3- Discontinue. Call doctor right away.
4- Continue. Call doctor when convenient.
5- Continue. Tell doctor at next visit.
6- No action necessary.

POTASSIUM BICARBONATE, POTASSIUM CARBONATE & POTASSIUM CHLORIDE

WARNINGS & PRECAUTIONS

Don't take if:
- You are allergic to any potassium supplement.
- You have kidney disease.

Before you start, consult your doctor:
- If you have Addison's disease.
- If you have heart disease.
- If you have intestinal blockage.
- If you have a stomach ulcer.
- If you use diuretics.
- If you use heart medicine.
- If you use laxatives or have chronic diarrhea.
- If you use salt substitutes or low-salt milk.

Over age 60:
Observe dose schedule strictly. Potassium balance is critical. Deviation above or below normal can have serious results.

Pregnancy:
No problems expected if you adhere strictly to prescribed dose.

Breast-feeding:
Studies inconclusive on harm to infant. Consult doctor.

Infants & children:
Use only under doctor's supervision.

Prolonged use:
Slows absorption of vitamin B-12. May cause anemia.

Skin & sunlight:
No problems expected.

Driving, piloting or hazardous work:
No problems expected.

Airplane passengers:
No problems expected.

Discontinuing:
Don't discontinue without consulting doctor. Dose may require gradual reduction if you have taken drug for a long time. Doses of other drugs may also require adjustment.

Others:
Overdose or underdose serious. Frequent laboratory blood studies recommended.

INTERACTION WITH OTHER DRUGS

GENERIC NAME OR DRUG CLASS	COMBINED EFFECT
Digitalis preparations	Possible irregular heartbeat.
Diuretics (thiazide)	Decreased potassium effect.
Spironolactone	Dangerous rise in blood potassium.
Triamterene	Dangerous rise in blood potassium.

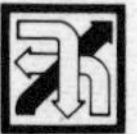

INTERACTION WITH OTHER SUBSTANCES

INTERACTS WITH	COMBINED EFFECT
Alcohol:	None expected.
Beverages: Salty drinks such as tomato juice, commercial thirst quenchers.	Increased fluid retention.
Cocaine:	May cause irregular heartbeat.
Foods: Salty foods.	Increased fluid retention.
Marijuana:	May cause irregular heartbeat.
Tobacco:	None expected.

POTASSIUM BICARBONATE & POTASSIUM CHLORIDE

BRAND NAMES

Klorvess

GENERAL INFORMATION

Habit forming? No
Prescription needed? Yes
Available as generic? Yes
Drug class: Mineral supplement (potassium)

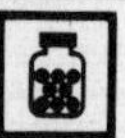

USES

Treatment for potassium deficiency from illness, diuretics, cortisone drugs or digitalis preparations.

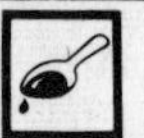

DOSAGE & USAGE INFORMATION

How to take:

- Tablet or capsule—Swallow with liquid or food to lessen stomach irritation. You may chew or crush tablet.
- Extended-release tablets or capsules—Swallow each dose whole with liquid.
- Effervescent tablets, granules, powder or liquid—Dilute dose in water.

When to take:
At the same times each day, preferably with food or immediately after meals.

If you forget a dose:
Take as soon as you remember. Don't double next dose.

What drug does:
Preserves or restores normal function of nerve cells, heart and skeletal-muscle cells, kidneys and stomach-juice secretion.

Time lapse before drug works:
12 to 24 hours.

Don't take with:
See Interaction column and consult doctor.

OVERDOSE

Symptoms:
Paralysis of arms and legs, irregular heartbeat, blood-pressure drop, convulsions, coma, cardiac arrest.

What to do:

- Dial 0 (operator) or 911 (emergency) for an ambulance or medical help. Then give first aid immediately.
- Additional emergency information on page 886.

POSSIBLE ADVERSE REACTIONS OR SIDE EFFECTS

SYMPTOMS	FREQUENCY	WHAT TO DO
Brain & nervous system:		
• Numbness and tingling in hands and feet.	Rare	4
• Confusion	Rare	3
Skin:	None expected.	
Eyes:	None expected.	
Ears, nose, throat:	None expected.	
Digestive:		
Diarrhea, nausea, vomiting, stomach discomfort.	Infrequent	4
Heart & lungs:		
Irregular heartbeat, breathing difficulty.	Rare	3
Blood vessels:	None expected.	
Muscles, bones, joints:		
Unusual fatigue, weakness, heaviness of legs.	Rare	3
Genital, urinary:	None expected.	
Kidneys:	None expected.	
Liver:	None expected.	
Allergic:	None expected.	
Blood:	None expected.	
Others:	None expected.	

1- Life-threatening. Seek emergency treatment immediately.
2- Discontinue. Seek emergency treatment.
3- Discontinue. Call doctor right away.
4- Continue. Call doctor when convenient.
5- Continue. Tell doctor at next visit.
6- No action necessary.

POTASSIUM BICARBONATE & POTASSIUM CHLORIDE

WARNINGS & PRECAUTIONS

Don't take if:

- You are allergic to any potassium supplement.
- You have kidney disease.

Before you start, consult your doctor:

- If you have Addison's disease.
- If you have heart disease.
- If you have intestinal blockage.
- If you have a stomach ulcer.
- If you use diuretics.
- If you use heart medicine.
- If you use laxatives or have chronic diarrhea.
- If you use salt substitutes or low-salt milk.

Over age 60:
Observe dose schedule strictly. Potassium balance is critical. Deviation above or below normal can have serious results.

Pregnancy:
No problems expected if you adhere strictly to prescribed dose.

Breast-feeding:
Studies inconclusive on harm to infant. Consult doctor.

Infants & children:
Use only under doctor's supervision.

Prolonged use:
Slows absorption of vitamin B-12. May cause anemia.

Skin & sunlight:
No problems expected.

Driving, piloting or hazardous work:
No problems expected.

Airplane passengers:
No problems expected.

Discontinuing:
Don't discontinue without consulting doctor. Dose may require gradual reduction if you have taken drug for a long time. Doses of other drugs may also require adjustment.

Others:
Overdose or underdose serious. Frequent laboratory blood studies recommended.

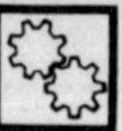

INTERACTION WITH OTHER DRUGS

GENERIC NAME OR DRUG CLASS	COMBINED EFFECT
Digitalis preparations	Possible irregular heartbeat.
Diuretics (thiazide)	Decreased potassium effect.
Spironolactone	Dangerous rise in blood potassium.
Triamterene	Dangerous rise in blood potassium.

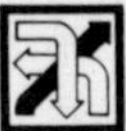

INTERACTION WITH OTHER SUBSTANCES

INTERACTS WITH	COMBINED EFFECT
Alcohol:	None expected.
Beverages: Salty drinks such as tomato juice, commercial thirst quenchers.	Increased fluid retention.
Cocaine:	May cause irregular heartbeat.
Foods: Salty foods.	Increased fluid retention.
Marijuana:	May cause irregular heartbeat.
Tobacco:	None expected.

POTASSIUM BICARBONATE, POTASSIUM CHLORIDE & CITRIC ACID

BRAND NAMES

K-Lyte/Cl

GENERAL INFORMATION

Habit forming? No
Prescription needed? Yes
Available as generic? Yes
Drug class: Mineral supplement (potassium)

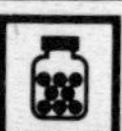

USES

Treatment for potassium deficiency from illness, diuretics, cortisone drugs or digitalis preparations.

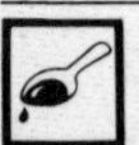

DOSAGE & USAGE INFORMATION

How to take:

- Tablet or capsule—Swallow with liquid or food to lessen stomach irritation. You may chew or crush tablet.
- Extended-release tablets or capsules—Swallow each dose whole with liquid.
- Effervescent tablets, granules, powder or liquid—Dilute dose in water.

When to take:
At the same times each day, preferably with food or immediately after meals.

If you forget a dose:
Take as soon as you remember. Don't double next dose.

What drug does:
Preserves or restores normal function of nerve cells, heart and skeletal-muscle cells, kidneys and stomach-juice secretion.

Time lapse before drug works:
12 to 24 hours.

Don't take with:
See Interaction column and consult doctor.

OVERDOSE

Symptoms:
Paralysis of arms and legs, irregular heartbeat, blood-pressure drop, convulsions, coma, cardiac arrest.

What to do:

- Dial 0 (operator) or 911 (emergency) for an ambulance or medical help. Then give first aid immediately.
- Additional emergency information on page 886.

POSSIBLE ADVERSE REACTIONS OR SIDE EFFECTS

SYMPTOMS	FREQUENCY	WHAT TO DO
Brain & nervous system:		
• Numbness and tingling in hands and feet.	Rare	4
• Confusion	Rare	3
Skin:	None expected.	
Eyes:	None expected.	
Ears, nose, throat:	None expected.	
Digestive: Diarrhea, nausea, vomiting, stomach discomfort.	Infrequent	4
Heart & lungs: Irregular heartbeat, breathing difficulty.	Rare	3
Blood vessels:	None expected.	
Muscles, bones, joints: Unusual fatigue, weakness, heaviness of legs.	Rare	3
Genital, urinary:	None expected.	
Kidneys:	None expected.	
Liver:	None expected.	
Allergic:	None expected.	
Blood:	None expected.	
Others:	None expected.	

1- Life-threatening. Seek emergency treatment immediately.
2- Discontinue. Seek emergency treatment.
3- Discontinue. Call doctor right away.
4- Continue. Call doctor when convenient.
5- Continue. Tell doctor at next visit.
6- No action necessary.

POTASSIUM BICARBONATE, POTASSIUM CHLORIDE & CITRIC ACID

WARNINGS & PRECAUTIONS

Don't take if:
- You are allergic to any potassium supplement.
- You have kidney disease.

Before you start, consult your doctor:
- If you have Addison's disease.
- If you have heart disease.
- If you have intestinal blockage.
- If you have a stomach ulcer.
- If you use diuretics.
- If you use heart medicine.
- If you use laxatives or have chronic diarrhea.
- If you use salt substitutes or low-salt milk.

Over age 60:
Observe dose schedule strictly. Potassium balance is critical. Deviation above or below normal can have serious results.

Pregnancy:
No problems expected if you adhere strictly to prescribed dose.

Breast-feeding:
Studies inconclusive on harm to infant. Consult doctor.

Infants & children:
Use only under doctor's supervision.

Prolonged use:
Slows absorption of vitamin B-12. May cause anemia.

Skin & sunlight:
No problems expected.

Driving, piloting or hazardous work:
No problems expected.

Airplane passengers:
No problems expected.

Discontinuing:
Don't discontinue without consulting doctor. Dose may require gradual reduction if you have taken drug for a long time. Doses of other drugs may also require adjustment.

Others:
Overdose or underdose serious. Frequent laboratory blood studies recommended.

INTERACTION WITH OTHER DRUGS

GENERIC NAME OR DRUG CLASS	COMBINED EFFECT
Digitalis preparations	Possible irregular heartbeat.
Diuretics (thiazide)	Decreased potassium effect.
Spironolactone	Dangerous rise in blood potassium.
Triamterene	Dangerous rise in blood potassium.

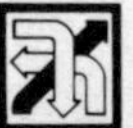

INTERACTION WITH OTHER SUBSTANCES

INTERACTS WITH	COMBINED EFFECT
Alcohol:	None expected.
Beverages: Salty drinks such as tomato juice, commercial thirst quenchers.	Increased fluid retention.
Cocaine:	May cause irregular heartbeat.
Foods: Salty foods.	Increased fluid retention.
Marijuana:	May cause irregular heartbeat.
Tobacco:	None expected.

POTASSIUM BICARBONATE, POTASSIUM CHLORIDE & POTASSIUM CITRATE

BRAND NAMES

Kaochlor-Eff

GENERAL INFORMATION

Habit forming? No
Prescription needed? Yes
Available as generic? Yes
Drug class: Mineral supplement (potassium)

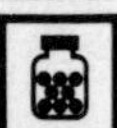

USES

Treatment for potassium deficiency from illness, diuretics, cortisone drugs or digitalis preparations.

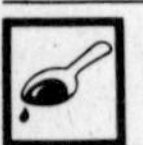

DOSAGE & USAGE INFORMATION

How to take:

- Tablet or capsule—Swallow with liquid or food to lessen stomach irritation. You may chew or crush tablet.
- Extended-release tablets or capsules—Swallow each dose whole with liquid.
- Effervescent tablets, granules, powder or liquid—Dilute dose in water.

When to take:
At the same times each day, preferably with food or immediately after meals.

If you forget a dose:
Take as soon as you remember. Don't double next dose.

What drug does:
Preserves or restores normal function of nerve cells, heart and skeletal-muscle cells, kidneys and stomach-juice secretion.

Time lapse before drug works:
12 to 24 hours.

Don't take with:
See Interaction column and consult doctor.

OVERDOSE

Symptoms:
Paralysis of arms and legs, irregular heartbeat, blood-pressure drop, convulsions, coma, cardiac arrest.

What to do:

- Dial 0 (operator) or 911 (emergency) for an ambulance or medical help. Then give first aid immediately.
- Additional emergency information on page 886.

POSSIBLE ADVERSE REACTIONS OR SIDE EFFECTS

SYMPTOMS	FREQUENCY	WHAT TO DO
Brain & nervous system:		
• Numbness and tingling in hands and feet.	Rare	4
• Confusion	Rare	3
Skin:	None expected.	
Eyes:	None expected.	
Ears, nose, throat:	None expected.	
Digestive:		
Diarrhea, nausea, vomiting, stomach discomfort.	Infrequent	4
Heart & lungs:		
Irregular heartbeat, breathing difficulty.	Rare	3
Blood vessels:	None expected.	
Muscles, bones, joints:		
Unusual fatigue, weakness, heaviness of legs.	Rare	3
Genital, urinary:	None expected.	
Kidneys:	None expected.	
Liver:	None expected.	
Allergic:	None expected.	
Blood:	None expected.	
Others:	None expected.	

1- Life-threatening. Seek emergency treatment immediately.
2- Discontinue. Seek emergency treatment.
3- Discontinue. Call doctor right away.
4- Continue. Call doctor when convenient.
5- Continue. Tell doctor at next visit.
6- No action necessary.

POTASSIUM BICARBONATE, POTASSIUM CHLORIDE & POTASSIUM CITRATE

WARNINGS & PRECAUTIONS

Don't take if:
- You are allergic to any potassium supplement.
- You have kidney disease.

Before you start, consult your doctor:
- If you have Addison's disease.
- If you have heart disease.
- If you have intestinal blockage.
- If you have a stomach ulcer.
- If you use diuretics.
- If you use heart medicine.
- If you use laxatives or have chronic diarrhea.
- If you use salt substitutes or low-salt milk.

Over age 60:
Observe dose schedule strictly. Potassium balance is critical. Deviation above or below normal can have serious results.

Pregnancy:
No problems expected if you adhere strictly to prescribed dose.

Breast-feeding:
Studies inconclusive on harm to infant. Consult doctor.

Infants & children:
Use only under doctor's supervision.

Prolonged use:
Slows absorption of vitamin B-12. May cause anemia.

Skin & sunlight:
No problems expected.

Driving, piloting or hazardous work:
No problems expected.

Airplane passengers:
No problems expected.

Discontinuing:
Don't discontinue without consulting doctor. Dose may require gradual reduction if you have taken drug for a long time. Doses of other drugs may also require adjustment.

Others:
Overdose or underdose serious. Frequent laboratory blood studies recommended.

INTERACTION WITH OTHER DRUGS

GENERIC NAME OR DRUG CLASS	COMBINED EFFECT
Digitalis preparations	Possible irregular heartbeat.
Diuretics (thiazide)	Decreased potassium effect.
Spironolactone	Dangerous rise in blood potassium.
Triamterene	Dangerous rise in blood potassium.

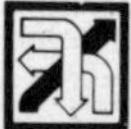

INTERACTION WITH OTHER SUBSTANCES

INTERACTS WITH	COMBINED EFFECT
Alcohol:	None expected.
Beverages: Salty drinks such as tomato juice, commercial thirst quenchers.	Increased fluid retention.
Cocaine:	May cause irregular heartbeat.
Foods: Salty foods.	Increased fluid retention.
Marijuana:	May cause irregular heartbeat.
Tobacco:	None expected.

POTASSIUM CHLORIDE

BRAND NAMES

Infalyte
Kaochlor
Kaon-Cl
KATO
Kay-Ciel
K-Lor
KLOR-10%
KLOR-CON
Klorvess
Klotrix
K-Tabs
Micro-K
Pfiklor
Potage
Run-K
Slow-K

GENERAL INFORMATION

Habit forming? No
Prescription needed? Yes
Available as generic? Yes
Drug class: Mineral supplement (potassium)

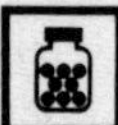

USES

Treatment for potassium deficiency from illness, diuretics, cortisone drugs or digitalis preparations.

DOSAGE & USAGE INFORMATION

How to take:
- Tablet or capsule—Swallow with liquid or food to lessen stomach irritation. You may chew or crush tablet.
- Extended-release tablets or capsules—Swallow each dose whole with liquid.
- Effervescent tablets, granules, powder or liquid—Dilute dose in water.

When to take:
At the same times each day, preferably with food or immediately after meals.

If you forget a dose:
Take as soon as you remember. Don't double next dose.

What drug does:
Preserves or restores normal function of nerve cells, heart and skeletal-muscle cells, kidneys and stomach-juice secretion.

Time lapse before drug works:
12 to 24 hours.

Don't take with:
See Interaction column and consult doctor.

OVERDOSE

Symptoms:
Paralysis of arms and legs, irregular heartbeat, blood-pressure drop, convulsions, coma, cardiac arrest.

What to do:
- Dial 0 (operator) or 911 (emergency) for an ambulance or medical help. Then give first aid immediately.
- Additional emergency information on page 886.

POSSIBLE ADVERSE REACTIONS OR SIDE EFFECTS

SYMPTOMS	FREQUENCY	WHAT TO DO
Brain & nervous system:		
• Numbness and tingling in hands and feet.	Rare	4
• Confusion	Rare	3
Skin:	None expected.	
Eyes:	None expected.	
Ears, nose, throat:	None expected.	
Digestive:		
Diarrhea, nausea, vomiting, stomach discomfort.	Infrequent	4
Heart & lungs:		
Irregular heartbeat, breathing difficulty.	Rare	3
Blood vessels:	None expected.	
Muscles, bones, joints:		
Unusual fatigue, weakness, heaviness of legs.	Rare	3
Genital, urinary:	None expected.	
Kidneys:	None expected.	
Liver:	None expected.	
Allergic:	None expected.	
Blood:	None expected.	
Others:	None expected.	

1- Life-threatening. Seek emergency treatment immediately.
2- Discontinue. Seek emergency treatment.
3- Discontinue. Call doctor right away.
4- Continue. Call doctor when convenient.
5- Continue. Tell doctor at next visit.
6- No action necessary.

WARNINGS & PRECAUTIONS

Don't take if:
- You are allergic to any potassium supplement.
- You have kidney disease.

Before you start, consult your doctor:
- If you have Addison's disease.
- If you have heart disease.
- If you have intestinal blockage.
- If you have a stomach ulcer.
- If you use diuretics.
- If you use heart medicine.
- If you use laxatives or have chronic diarrhea.
- If you use salt substitutes or low-salt milk.

Over age 60:
Observe dose schedule strictly. Potassium balance is critical. Deviation above or below normal can have serious results.

Pregnancy:
No problems expected if you adhere strictly to prescribed dose.

Breast-feeding:
Studies inconclusive on harm to infant. Consult doctor.

Infants & children:
Use only under doctor's supervision.

Prolonged use:
Slows absorption of vitamin B-12. May cause anemia.

Skin & sunlight:
No problems expected.

Driving, piloting or hazardous work:
No problems expected.

Airplane passengers:
No problems expected.

Discontinuing:
Don't discontinue without consulting doctor. Dose may require gradual reduction if you have taken drug for a long time. Doses of other drugs may also require adjustment.

Others:
Overdose or underdose serious. Frequent laboratory blood studies recommended.

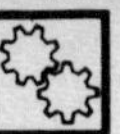

INTERACTION WITH OTHER DRUGS

GENERIC NAME OR DRUG CLASS	COMBINED EFFECT
Digitalis preparations	Possible irregular heartbeat.
Diuretics (thiazide)	Decreased potassium effect.
Spironolactone	Dangerous rise in blood potassium.
Triamterene	Dangerous rise in blood potassium.

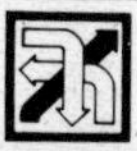

INTERACTION WITH OTHER SUBSTANCES

INTERACTS WITH	COMBINED EFFECT
Alcohol:	None expected.
Beverages: Salty drinks such as tomato juice, commercial thirst quenchers.	Increased fluid retention.
Cocaine:	May cause irregular heartbeat.
Foods: Salty foods.	Increased fluid retention.
Marijuana:	May cause irregular heartbeat.
Tobacco:	None expected.

POTASSIUM CHLORIDE & POTASSIUM GLUCONATE

BRAND NAMES

Kolyum

GENERAL INFORMATION

Habit forming? No
Prescription needed? Yes
Available as generic? Yes
Drug class: Mineral supplement (potassium)

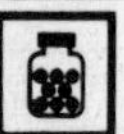

USES

Treatment for potassium deficiency from illness, diuretics, cortisone drugs or digitalis preparations.

DOSAGE & USAGE INFORMATION

How to take:

- Tablet or capsule—Swallow with liquid or food to lessen stomach irritation. You may chew or crush tablet.
- Extended-release tablets or capsules—Swallow each dose whole with liquid.
- Effervescent tablets, granules, powder or liquid—Dilute dose in water.

When to take:
At the same times each day, preferably with food or immediately after meals.

If you forget a dose:
Take as soon as you remember. Don't double next dose.

What drug does:
Preserves or restores normal function of nerve cells, heart and skeletal-muscle cells, kidneys and stomach-juice secretion.

Time lapse before drug works:
12 to 24 hours.

Don't take with:
See Interaction column and consult doctor.

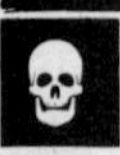

OVERDOSE

Symptoms:
Paralysis of arms and legs, irregular heartbeat, blood-pressure drop, convulsions, coma, cardiac arrest.

What to do:

- Dial 0 (operator) or 911 (emergency) for an ambulance or medical help. Then give first aid immediately.
- Additional emergency information on page 886.

POSSIBLE ADVERSE REACTIONS OR SIDE EFFECTS

SYMPTOMS	FREQUENCY	WHAT TO DO
Brain & nervous system:		
• Numbness and tingling in hands and feet.	Rare	4
• Confusion	Rare	3
Skin:	None expected.	
Eyes:	None expected.	
Ears, nose, throat:	None expected.	
Digestive:		
Diarrhea, nausea, vomiting, stomach discomfort.	Infrequent	4
Heart & lungs:		
Irregular heartbeat, breathing difficulty.	Rare	3
Blood vessels:	None expected.	
Muscles, bones, joints:		
Unusual fatigue, weakness, heaviness of legs.	Rare	3
Genital, urinary:	None expected.	
Kidneys:	None expected.	
Liver:	None expected.	
Allergic:	None expected.	
Blood:	None expected.	
Others:	None expected.	

1- Life-threatening. Seek emergency treatment immediately.
2- Discontinue. Seek emergency treatment.
3- Discontinue. Call doctor right away.
4- Continue. Call doctor when convenient.
5- Continue. Tell doctor at next visit.
6- No action necessary.

POTASSIUM CHLORIDE & POTASSIUM GLUCONATE

WARNINGS & PRECAUTIONS

Don't take if:
- You are allergic to any potassium supplement.
- You have kidney disease.

Before you start, consult your doctor:
- If you have Addison's disease.
- If you have heart disease.
- If you have intestinal blockage.
- If you have a stomach ulcer.
- If you use diuretics.
- If you use heart medicine.
- If you use laxatives or have chronic diarrhea.
- If you use salt substitutes or low-salt milk.

Over age 60:
Observe dose schedule strictly. Potassium balance is critical. Deviation above or below normal can have serious results.

Pregnancy:
No problems expected if you adhere strictly to prescribed dose.

Breast-feeding:
Studies inconclusive on harm to infant. Consult doctor.

Infants & children:
Use only under doctor's supervision.

Prolonged use:
Slows absorption of vitamin B-12. May cause anemia.

Skin & sunlight:
No problems expected.

Driving, piloting or hazardous work:
No problems expected.

Airplane passengers:
No problems expected.

Discontinuing:
Don't discontinue without consulting doctor. Dose may require gradual reduction if you have taken drug for a long time. Doses of other drugs may also require adjustment.

Others:
Overdose or underdose serious. Frequent laboratory blood studies recommended.

INTERACTION WITH OTHER DRUGS

GENERIC NAME OR DRUG CLASS	COMBINED EFFECT
Digitalis preparations	Possible irregular heartbeat.
Diuretics (thiazide)	Decreased potassium effect.
Spironolactone	Dangerous rise in blood potassium.
Triamterene	Dangerous rise in blood potassium.

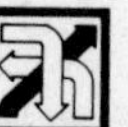

INTERACTION WITH OTHER SUBSTANCES

INTERACTS WITH	COMBINED EFFECT
Alcohol:	None expected.
Beverages: Salty drinks such as tomato juice, commercial thirst quenchers.	Increased fluid retention.
Cocaine:	May cause irregular heartbeat.
Foods: Salty foods.	Increased fluid retention.
Marijuana:	May cause irregular heartbeat.
Tobacco:	None expected.

POTASSIUM CITRATE & POTASSIUM GLUCONATE

BRAND NAMES

Alka-Seltzer
Bi-K
K-Lyte
Polycitra
Twin-K

GENERAL INFORMATION

Habit forming? No
Prescription needed? Yes
Available as generic? Yes
Drug class: Mineral supplement (potassium)

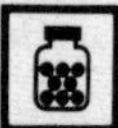

USES

Treatment for potassium deficiency from illness, diuretics, cortisone drugs or digitalis preparations.

DOSAGE & USAGE INFORMATION

How to take:

- Tablet or capsule—Swallow with liquid or food to lessen stomach irritation. You may chew or crush tablet.
- Extended-release tablets or capsules—Swallow each dose whole with liquid.
- Effervescent tablets, granules, powder or liquid—Dilute dose in water.

When to take:
At the same times each day, preferably with food or immediately after meals.

If you forget a dose:
Take as soon as you remember. Don't double next dose.

What drug does:
Preserves or restores normal function of nerve cells, heart and skeletal-muscle cells, kidneys and stomach-juice secretion.

Time lapse before drug works:
12 to 24 hours.

Don't take with:
See Interaction column and consult doctor.

OVERDOSE

Symptoms:
Paralysis of arms and legs, irregular heartbeat, blood-pressure drop, convulsions, coma, cardiac arrest.

What to do:

- Dial 0 (operator) or 911 (emergency) for an ambulance or medical help. Then give first aid immediately.
- Additional emergency information on page 886.

POSSIBLE ADVERSE REACTIONS OR SIDE EFFECTS

SYMPTOMS	FREQUENCY	WHAT TO DO
Brain & nervous system:		
• Numbness and tingling in hands and feet.	Rare	4
• Confusion	Rare	3
Skin:	None expected.	
Eyes:	None expected.	
Ears, nose, throat:	None expected.	
Digestive: Diarrhea, nausea, vomiting, stomach discomfort.	Infrequent	4
Heart & lungs: Irregular heartbeat, breathing difficulty.	Rare	3
Blood vessels:	None expected.	
Muscles, bones, joints: Unusual fatigue, weakness, heaviness of legs.	Rare	3
Genital, urinary:	None expected.	
Kidneys:	None expected.	
Liver:	None expected.	
Allergic:	None expected.	
Blood:	None expected.	
Others:	None expected.	

1- Life-threatening. Seek emergency treatment immediately.
2- Discontinue. Seek emergency treatment.
3- Discontinue. Call doctor right away.
4- Continue. Call doctor when convenient.
5- Continue. Tell doctor at next visit.
6- No action necessary.

POTASSIUM CITRATE & POTASSIUM GLUCONATE

WARNINGS & PRECAUTIONS

Don't take if:
- You are allergic to any potassium supplement.
- You have kidney disease.

Before you start, consult your doctor:
- If you have Addison's disease.
- If you have heart disease.
- If you have intestinal blockage.
- If you have a stomach ulcer.
- If you use diuretics.
- If you use heart medicine.
- If you use laxatives or have chronic diarrhea.
- If you use salt substitutes or low-salt milk.

Over age 60:
Observe dose schedule strictly. Potassium balance is critical. Deviation above or below normal can have serious results.

Pregnancy:
No problems expected if you adhere strictly to prescribed dose.

Breast-feeding:
Studies inconclusive on harm to infant. Consult doctor.

Infants & children:
Use only under doctor's supervision.

Prolonged use:
Slows absorption of vitamin B-12. May cause anemia.

Skin & sunlight:
No problems expected.

Driving, piloting or hazardous work:
No problems expected.

Airplane passengers:
No problems expected.

Discontinuing:
Don't discontinue without consulting doctor. Dose may require gradual reduction if you have taken drug for a long time. Doses of other drugs may also require adjustment.

Others:
Overdose or underdose serious. Frequent laboratory blood studies recommended.

INTERACTION WITH OTHER DRUGS

GENERIC NAME OR DRUG CLASS	COMBINED EFFECT
Digitalis preparations	Possible irregular heartbeat.
Diuretics (thiazide)	Decreased potassium effect.
Spironolactone	Dangerous rise in blood potassium.
Triamterene	Dangerous rise in blood potassium.

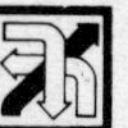

INTERACTION WITH OTHER SUBSTANCES

INTERACTS WITH	COMBINED EFFECT
Alcohol:	None expected.
Beverages: Salty drinks such as tomato juice, commercial thirst quenchers.	Increased fluid retention.
Cocaine:	May cause irregular heartbeat.
Foods: Salty foods.	Increased fluid retention.
Marijuana:	May cause irregular heartbeat.
Tobacco:	None expected.

POTASSIUM GLUCONATE

BRAND NAMES

Bi-K
Kaon
K-10
Twin-K

GENERAL INFORMATION

Habit forming? No
Prescription needed? Yes
Available as generic? Yes
Drug class: Mineral supplement (potassium)

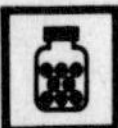

USES

Treatment for potassium deficiency from illness, diuretics, cortisone drugs or digitalis preparations.

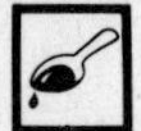

DOSAGE & USAGE INFORMATION

How to take:
- Tablet or capsule—Swallow with liquid or food to lessen stomach irritation. You may chew or crush tablet.
- Extended-release tablets or capsules—Swallow each dose whole with liquid.
- Effervescent tablets, granules, powder or liquid—Dilute dose in water.

When to take:
At the same times each day, preferably with food or immediately after meals.

If you forget a dose:
Take as soon as you remember. Don't double next dose.

What drug does:
Preserves or restores normal function of nerve cells, heart and skeletal-muscle cells, kidneys and stomach-juice secretion.

Time lapse before drug works:
12 to 24 hours.

Don't take with:
See Interaction column and consult doctor.

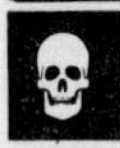

OVERDOSE

Symptoms:
Paralysis of arms and legs, irregular heartbeat, blood-pressure drop, convulsions, coma, cardiac arrest.

What to do:
- Dial 0 (operator) or 911 (emergency) for an ambulance or medical help. Then give first aid immediately.
- Additional emergency information on page 886.

POSSIBLE ADVERSE REACTIONS OR SIDE EFFECTS

SYMPTOMS	FREQUENCY	WHAT TO DO
Brain & nervous system:		
• Numbness and tingling in hands and feet.	Rare	4
• Confusion	Rare	3
Skin:	None expected.	
Eyes:	None expected.	
Ears, nose, throat:	None expected.	
Digestive:		
Diarrhea, nausea, vomiting, stomach discomfort.	Infrequent	4
Heart & lungs:		
Irregular heartbeat, breathing difficulty.	Rare	3
Blood vessels:	None expected.	
Muscles, bones, joints:		
Unusual fatigue, weakness, heaviness of legs.	Rare	3
Genital, urinary:	None expected.	
Kidneys:	None expected.	
Liver:	None expected.	
Allergic:	None expected.	
Blood:	None expected.	
Others:	None expected.	

1- Life-threatening. Seek emergency treatment immediately.
2- Discontinue. Seek emergency treatment.
3- Discontinue. Call doctor right away.
4- Continue. Call doctor when convenient.
5- Continue. Tell doctor at next visit.
6- No action necessary.

POTASSIUM GLUCONATE

WARNINGS & PRECAUTIONS

Don't take if:
- You are allergic to any potassium supplement.
- You have kidney disease.

Before you start, consult your doctor:
- If you have Addison's disease.
- If you have heart disease.
- If you have intestinal blockage.
- If you have a stomach ulcer.
- If you use diuretics.
- If you use heart medicine.
- If you use laxatives or have chronic diarrhea.
- If you use salt substitutes or low-salt milk.

Over age 60:
Observe dose schedule strictly. Potassium balance is critical. Deviation above or below normal can have serious results.

Pregnancy:
No problems expected if you adhere strictly to prescribed dose.

Breast-feeding:
Studies inconclusive on harm to infant. Consult doctor.

Infants & children:
Use only under doctor's supervision.

Prolonged use:
Slows absorption of vitamin B-12. May cause anemia.

Skin & sunlight:
No problems expected.

Driving, piloting or hazardous work:
No problems expected.

Airplane passengers:
No problems expected.

Discontinuing:
Don't discontinue without consulting doctor. Dose may require gradual reduction if you have taken drug for a long time. Doses of other drugs may also require adjustment.

Others:
Overdose or underdose serious. Frequent laboratory blood studies recommended.

INTERACTION WITH OTHER DRUGS

GENERIC NAME OR DRUG CLASS	COMBINED EFFECT
Digitalis preparations	Possible irregular heartbeat.
Diuretics (thiazide)	Decreased potassium effect.
Spironolactone	Dangerous rise in blood potassium.
Triamterene	Dangerous rise in blood potassium.

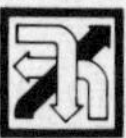

INTERACTION WITH OTHER SUBSTANCES

INTERACTS WITH	COMBINED EFFECT
Alcohol:	None expected.
Beverages: Salty drinks such as tomato juice, commercial thirst quenchers.	Increased fluid retention.
Cocaine:	May cause irregular heartbeat.
Foods: Salty foods.	Increased fluid retention.
Marijuana:	May cause irregular heartbeat.
Tobacco:	None expected.

PRAZEPAM

BRAND NAMES

Centrax

GENERAL INFORMATION

Habit forming? Yes
Prescription needed? Yes
Available as generic? No
Drug class: Tranquilizer (benzodiazepine)

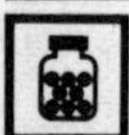

USES

Treatment for nervousness or tension.

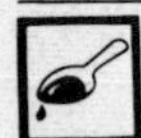

DOSAGE & USAGE INFORMATION

How to take:
Tablet or capsule—Swallow with liquid. If you can't swallow whole, crumble tablet or open capsule and take with liquid or food.

When to take:
At the same time each day, according to instructions on prescription label.

If you forget a dose:
Take as soon as you remember up to 2 hours late. If more than 2 hours, wait for next scheduled dose (don't double this dose).

What drug does:
Affects limbic system of brain—part that controls emotions.

Time lapse before drug works:
2 hours. May take 6 weeks for full benefit.

Don't take with:
See Interaction column and consult doctor.

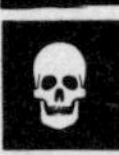

OVERDOSE

Symptoms:
Drowsiness, weakness, tremor, stupor, coma.

What to do:
- Dial 0 (operator) or 911 (emergency) for an ambulance or medical help. Then give first aid immediately.
- If patient is unconscious and not breathing, give mouth-to-mouth breathing. If there is no heartbeat, use cardiac massage and mouth-to-mouth breathing (CPR). Don't try to make patient vomit. If you can't get help quickly, take patient to nearest emergency facility.
- Additional emergency information on page 886.

POSSIBLE ADVERSE REACTIONS OR SIDE EFFECTS

SYMPTOMS	FREQUENCY	WHAT TO DO
Brain & nervous system:		
• Clumsiness, drowsiness, dizziness.	Common	4
• Hallucinations, confusion, depression, irritability.	Infrequent	3
Skin:		
Rash, itch.	Infrequent	3
Eyes:		
Vision changes.	Infrequent	3
Ears, nose, throat:		
Mouth, throat ulcers.	Rare	3
Digestive:		
Constipation or diarrhea, nausea, vomiting.	Infrequent	4
Heart & lungs:		
Slow heartbeat, breathing difficulty.	Rare	2
Blood vessels:	None expected.	
Muscles, bones, joints:	None expected.	
Genital, urinary:		
Urination difficulty.	Infrequent	4
Kidneys:	None expected.	
Liver:		
Jaundice (yellow eyes and skin).	Rare	3
Allergic:	None expected.	
Blood:	None expected.	
Others:	None expected.	

1- Life-threatening. Seek emergency treatment immediately.
2- Discontinue. Seek emergency treatment.
3- Discontinue. Call doctor right away.
4- Continue. Call doctor when convenient.
5- Continue. Tell doctor at next visit.
6- No action necessary.

WARNINGS & PRECAUTIONS

Don't take if:

- You are allergic to any benzodiazepine.
- You have myasthenia gravis.
- You have glaucoma.
- You are active or recovering alcoholic.
- Patient is younger than 6 months.

Before you start, consult your doctor:

- If you have liver, kidney or lung disease.
- If you have diabetes, epilepsy or porphyria.

Over age 60:
Adverse reactions and side effects may be more frequent and severe than in younger persons. You need smaller doses for shorter periods of time. May develop agitation, rage or "hangover effect."

Pregnancy:
Risk to unborn child outweighs drug benefits. Don't use.

Breast-feeding:
Drug passes into milk. Avoid drug or discontinue nursing until you finish medicine. Consult doctor for advice on maintaining milk supply.

Infants & children:
Use only under medical supervision for children older than 6 months.

Prolonged use:
May impair liver function.

Skin & sunlight:
No problems expected.

Driving, piloting or hazardous work:
Don't drive or pilot aircraft until you learn how medicine affects you. Don't work around dangerous machinery. Don't climb ladders or work in high places. Danger increases if you drink alcohol or take medicine affecting alertness and reflexes.

Airplane passengers:
No problems expected.

Discontinuing:
Don't discontinue without consulting doctor. Dose may require gradual reduction if you have taken drug for a long time. Doses of other drugs may also require adjustment.

Others:

- Hot weather, heavy exercise and profuse sweat may reduce excretion and cause overdose.
- Blood sugar may rise in diabetics, requiring insulin adjustment.

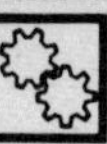

INTERACTION WITH OTHER DRUGS

GENERIC NAME OR DRUG CLASS	COMBINED EFFECT
Anticonvulsants	Change in seizure frequency or severity.
Antidepressants	Increased sedative effect of both drugs.
Antihistamines	Increased sedative effect of both drugs.
Antihypertensives	Excessively low blood pressure.
Cimetidine	Excess sedation.
Disulfiram	Increased prazepam effect.
MAO inhibitors	Convulsions, deep sedation, rage.
Narcotics	Increased sedative effect of both drugs.
Sedatives	Increased sedative effect of both drugs.
Sleep inducers	Increased sedative effect of both drugs.
Tranquilizers	Increased sedative effect of both drugs.

INTERACTION WITH OTHER SUBSTANCES

INTERACTS WITH	COMBINED EFFECT
Alcohol:	Heavy sedation. Avoid.
Beverages:	None expected.
Cocaine:	Decreased prazepam effect.
Foods:	None expected.
Marijuana:	Heavy sedation. Avoid.
Tobacco:	Decreased prazepam effect.

PRAZOSIN

BRAND NAMES

Minipress
Minizide

GENERAL INFORMATION

Habit forming? No
Prescription needed? Yes
Available as generic? No
Drug class: Antihypertensive

USES

- Treatment for high blood pressure.
- Improves congestive heart failure.

DOSAGE & USAGE INFORMATION

How to take:
Tablet or capsule—Swallow with liquid. If you can't swallow whole, crumble tablet or open capsule and take with liquid or food.

When to take:
At the same times each day.

If you forget a dose:
Take as soon as you remember up to 2 hours late. If more than 2 hours, wait for next scheduled dose (don't double this dose).

What drug does:
Expands and relaxes blood-vessel walls to lower blood pressure.

Time lapse before drug works:
30 minutes.

Don't take with:
See Interaction column and consult doctor.

OVERDOSE

Symptoms:
Extreme weakness; loss of consciousness; cold, sweaty skin; weak, rapid pulse; coma.

What to do:
- Dial 0 (operator) or 911 (emergency) for an ambulance or medical help. Then give first aid immediately.
- If patient is unconscious and not breathing, give mouth-to-mouth breathing. If there is no heartbeat, use cardiac massage and mouth-to-mouth breathing (CPR). Don't try to make patient vomit. If you can't get help quickly, take patient to nearest emergency facility.
- Additional emergency information on page 886.

POSSIBLE ADVERSE REACTIONS OR SIDE EFFECTS

SYMPTOMS	FREQUENCY	WHAT TO DO
Brain & nervous system:		
• Vivid dreams, drowsiness, dizziness.	Common	4
• Headache, irritability, depression.	Infrequent	5
Skin:		
Rash or itch.	Infrequent	3
Eyes:		
Blurred vision.	Infrequent	3
Ears, nose, throat:		
Dry mouth, stuffy nose.	Infrequent	5
Digestive:		
Appetite loss, constipation or diarrhea, stomach pain, nausea, vomiting.	Infrequent	4
Heart & lungs:		
• Rapid heartbeat.	Common	3
• Shortness of breath, chest pain.	Infrequent	3
Blood vessels, kidneys, liver, allergic, blood:	None expected.	
Muscles, bones, joints:		
• Fluid retention.	Infrequent	4
• Joint, muscle aches.	Infrequent	4
Genital, urinary:		
• More urination.	Infrequent	5
• Decreased sexual function.	Rare	4

1-Life-threatening. Seek emergency treatment immediately.
2-Discontinue. Seek emergency treatment.
3-Discontinue. Call doctor right away.
4-Continue. Call doctor when convenient.
5-Continue. Tell doctor at next visit.

WARNINGS & PRECAUTIONS

Don't take if:
- You are allergic to prazosin.
- You are depressed.
- You will have surgery within 2 months, including dental surgery, requiring general or spinal anesthesia.

Before you start, consult your doctor:
- If you experience lightheadedness or fainting with other antihypertensive drugs.
- If you are easily depressed.
- If you have impaired brain circulation or have had a stroke.
- If you have coronary heart disease (with or without angina).
- If you have kidney disease or impaired liver function.

Over age 60:
Begin with no more than 1 mg. per day for first 3 days. Increases should be gradual and supervised by your doctor. Don't stand while taking. Sudden changes in position may cause falls. Sit or lie down promptly if you feel dizzy. If you have impaired brain circulation or coronary heart disease, excessive lowering of blood pressure should be avoided. Report problems to your doctor immediately.

Pregnancy:
Studies inconclusive on harm to unborn child. Animal studies show fetal abnormalities. Decide with your doctor whether drug benefits justify risk to child.

Breast-feeding:
No proven problems. Consult doctor.

Infants & children:
Not recommended.

Prolonged use:
No problems expected.

Skin & sunlight:
No problems expected.

Driving, piloting or hazardous work:
Don't drive or pilot aircraft until you learn how medicine affects you. Don't work around dangerous machinery. Don't climb ladders or work in high places.

Airplane passengers:
No problems expected.

Discontinuing:
Don't discontinue without doctor's advice until you complete prescribed dose, even though symptoms diminish or disappear.

Others:
First dose likely to cause fainting. Take it at night and get out of bed slowly next morning.

INTERACTION WITH OTHER DRUGS

GENERIC NAME OR DRUG CLASS	COMBINED EFFECT
Amitriptyline	Acute agitation.
Amphetamines	Decreased prazosin effect.
Antihypertensives (other)	Increased effect of other drugs.
Chlorpromazine	Acute agitation.
MAO inhibitors	Blood-pressure drop.
Nitroglycerin	Prolonged effect of prazosin.

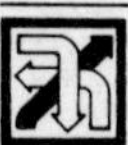

INTERACTION WITH OTHER SUBSTANCES

INTERACTS WITH	COMBINED EFFECT
Alcohol:	Excessive blood-pressure drop.
Beverages:	None expected.
Cocaine:	Decreased prazosin effect. Avoid.
Foods:	None expected.
Marijuana:	Possible fainting. Avoid.
Tobacco:	Possible spasm of coronary arteries. Avoid.

PREDNISOLONE

BRAND NAMES

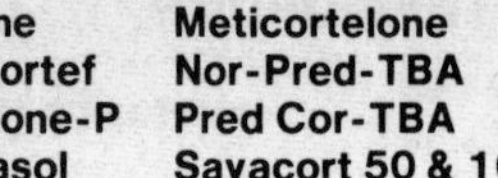

Cortalone
Delta-Cortef
Fernisolone-P
Hydeltrasol
Hydeltra-TBA
Meticortelone
Nor-Pred-TBA
Pred Cor-TBA
Savacort 50 & 100
Sterane

See complete brand names list, page 830.

GENERAL INFORMATION

Habit forming? No
Prescription needed? Yes
Available as generic? Yes
Drug class: Cortisone drug (adrenal corticosteroid)

USES

- Reduces inflammation caused by many different medical problems.
- Treatment for some allergic diseases, blood disorders, kidney diseases, asthma and emphysema.
- Replaces corticosteroid deficiencies.

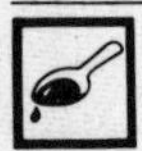

DOSAGE & USAGE INFORMATION

How to take:
Tablet—Swallow with liquid or food to lessen stomach irritation. If you can't swallow whole, crumble tablet and take with liquid or food.

When to take:
At the same times each day. Take once-a-day or once-every-other-day doses in mornings.

If you forget a dose:
- Several-doses-per-day prescription—Take as soon as you remember up to 2 hours late. If more than 2 hours, wait for next scheduled dose (don't double this dose).
- Once-a-day dose or less—Wait for next dose. Double this dose.

What drug does:
Decreases inflammatory responses.

Time lapse before drug works:
2 to 4 days.

Don't take with:
See Interaction column and consult doctor.

OVERDOSE

Symptoms:
Headache, convulsions, heart failure.

What to do:
- Dial 0 (operator) or 911 (emergency) for an ambulance or medical help. Then give first aid immediately.
- Additional emergency information on page 886.

POSSIBLE ADVERSE REACTIONS OR SIDE EFFECTS

SYMPTOMS	FREQUENCY	WHAT TO DO
Brain & nervous system:		
Mood changes, insomnia, restlessness.	Infrequent	4
Skin:		
• Acne	Common	4
• Rash	Rare	3
• Poor wound healing.	Common	4
Eyes:		
Blurred vision, halos around lights.	Infrequent	3
Ears, nose, throat:		
• Sore throat, fever.	Infrequent	3
• Thirst	Common	4
Digestive:		
• Indigestion, nausea, vomiting.	Common	4
• Bloody or black, tarry stool.	Infrequent	2
Heart & lungs:		
Irregular heartbeat.	Rare	2
Blood vessels, kidneys, liver, allergic, blood:	None expected.	
Muscles, bones, joints:		
Muscle cramps, swollen legs, feet.	Infrequent	3
Genital, urinary:		
Frequent urination.	Infrequent	4
Others:		
• Weight gain, round face.	Infrequent	4
• Fatigue, weakness.	Infrequent	4
• TB recurrence.	Infrequent	4
• Irregular menstrual periods.	Infrequent	4

1-Life-threatening. Seek emergency treatment immediately.
2-Discontinue. Seek emergency treatment.
3-Discontinue. Call doctor right away.
4-Continue. Call doctor when convenient.

WARNINGS & PRECAUTIONS

Don't take if:
- You are allergic to any cortisone drug.
- You have tuberculosis or fungus infection.
- You have herpes infection of eyes, lips or genitals.

Before you start, consult your doctor:
- If you have had tuberculosis.
- If you have congestive heart failure.
- If you have diabetes.
- If you have peptic ulcer.
- If you have glaucoma.
- If you have underactive thyroid.
- If you have high blood pressure.
- If you have myasthenia gravis.
- If you have blood clots in legs or lungs.

Over age 60:
Adverse reactions and side effects may be more frequent and severe than in younger persons. Likely to aggravate edema, diabetes or ulcers. Likely to cause cataracts and osteoporosis (softening of the bones).

Pregnancy:
Risk to unborn child outweighs drug benefits. Don't use.

Breast-feeding:
Drug passes into milk. Avoid drug or discontinue nursing until you finish medicine. Consult doctor for advice on maintaining milk supply.

Infants & children:
Use only under medical supervision.

Prolonged use:
- Retards growth in children.
- Possible glaucoma, cataracts, diabetes, fragile bones and thin skin.
- Functional dependence.

Skin & sunlight:
No problems expected.

Driving, piloting or hazardous work:
No problems expected.

Airplane passengers:
No problems expected.

Discontinuing:
- Don't discontinue without doctor's advice until you complete prescribed dose, even though symptoms diminish or disappear.
- Drug affects your response to surgery, illness, injury or stress for 2 years after discontinuing. Tell about drug to anyone who takes medical care of you within 2 years.

Others:
Avoid immunizations if possible.

INTERACTION WITH OTHER DRUGS

GENERIC NAME OR DRUG CLASS	COMBINED EFFECT
Amphoterecin B	Potassium depletion.
Anticholinergics	Possible glaucoma.
Anticoagulants (oral)	Decreased anticoagulant effect.
Anticonvulsants (hydantoin)	Decreased prednisolone effect.
Antidiabetics (oral)	Decreased antidiabetic effect.
Antihistamines	Decreased prednisolone effect.
Aspirin	Increased prednisolone effect.
Barbiturates	Decreased prednisolone effect. Oversedation.
Beta-adrenergic blockers	Decreased prednisolone effect.
Chloral hydrate	Decreased prednisolone effect.
Chlorthalidone	Potassium depletion.
Cholinergics	Decreased cholinergic effect.
Contraceptives (oral)	Increased prednisolone effect.
Digitalis preparations	Dangerous potassium depletion. Possible digitalis toxicity.
Diuretics (thiazide)	Potassium depletion.

Additional interactions on page 842.

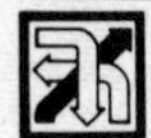

INTERACTION WITH OTHER SUBSTANCES

INTERACTS WITH	COMBINED EFFECT
Alcohol:	Risk of stomach ulcers.
Beverages:	No proven problems.
Cocaine:	Overstimulation. Avoid.
Foods:	No proven problems.
Marijuana:	Decreased immunity.
Tobacco:	Increased prednisolone effect. Possible toxicity.

PREDNISONE

BRAND NAMES

Apo-Prednisone
Colisone
Cortan
Deltasone
Liquid-Pred
Meticorten
Novoprednisone
Orasone
Paracort
SK-Prednisone
Sterapred
Sterazolidin
Winpred

GENERAL INFORMATION

Habit forming? No
Prescription needed? Yes
Available as generic? Yes
Drug class: Cortisone drug (adrenal corticosteroid)

USES

- Reduces inflammation caused by many different medical problems.
- Treatment for some allergic diseases, blood disorders, kidney diseases, asthma and emphysema.
- Replaces corticosteroid deficiencies.

DOSAGE & USAGE INFORMATION

How to take:
Tablet or syrup—Swallow with liquid or food to lessen stomach irritation. If you can't swallow whole, crumble tablet.

When to take:
At the same times each day. Take once-a-day or once-every-other-day doses in mornings.

If you forget a dose:
- Several-doses-per-day prescription—Take as soon as you remember up to 2 hours late. If more than 2 hours, wait for next scheduled dose (don't double this dose).
- Once-a-day dose or less—Wait for next dose. Double this dose.

What drug does:
Decreases inflammatory responses.

Time lapse before drug works:
2 to 4 days.

Don't take with:
See Interaction column and consult doctor.

OVERDOSE

Symptoms:
Headache, convulsions, heart failure.

What to do:
- Dial 0 (operator) or 911 (emergency) for an ambulance or medical help. Then give first aid immediately.
- Additional emergency information on page 886.

POSSIBLE ADVERSE REACTIONS OR SIDE EFFECTS

SYMPTOMS	FREQUENCY	WHAT TO DO
Brain & nervous system:		
Mood changes, insomnia, restlessness.	Infrequent	4
Skin:		
• Acne	Common	4
• Rash	Rare	3
• Poor wound healing.	Common	4
Eyes:		
Blurred vision, halos around lights.	Infrequent	3
Ears, nose, throat:		
• Sore throat, fever.	Infrequent	3
• Thirst	Common	4
Digestive:		
• Indigestion, nausea, vomiting.	Common	4
• Bloody or black, tarry stool.	Infrequent	2
Heart & lungs:		
Irregular heartbeat.	Rare	2
Blood vessels, kidneys, liver, allergic, blood:	None expected.	
Muscles, bones, joints:		
Muscle cramps, swollen legs, feet.	Infrequent	3
Genital, urinary:		
Frequent urination.	Infrequent	4
Others:		
• Weight gain, round face.	Infrequent	4
• Fatigue, weakness.	Infrequent	4
• TB recurrence.	Infrequent	4
• Irregular menstrual periods.	Infrequent	4

1 - Life-threatening. Seek emergency treatment immediately.
2 - Discontinue. Seek emergency treatment.
3 - Discontinue. Call doctor right away.
4 - Continue. Call doctor when convenient.

WARNINGS & PRECAUTIONS

Don't take if:
- You are allergic to any cortisone drug.
- You have tuberculosis or fungus infection.
- You have herpes infection of eyes, lips or genitals.

Before you start, consult your doctor:
- If you have had tuberculosis.
- If you have congestive heart failure.
- If you have diabetes.
- If you have peptic ulcer.
- If you have glaucoma.
- If you have underactive thyroid.
- If you have high blood pressure.
- If you have myasthenia gravis.
- If you have blood clots in legs or lungs.

Over age 60:
Adverse reactions and side effects may be more frequent and severe than in younger persons. Likely to aggravate edema, diabetes or ulcers. Likely to cause cataracts and osteoporosis (softening of the bones).

Pregnancy:
Risk to unborn child outweighs drug benefits. Don't use.

Breast-feeding:
Drug passes into milk. Avoid drug or discontinue nursing until you finish medicine. Consult doctor for advice on maintaining milk supply.

Infants & children:
Use only under medical supervision.

Prolonged use:
- Retards growth in children.
- Possible glaucoma, cataracts, diabetes, fragile bones and thin skin.
- Functional dependence.

Skin & sunlight:
No problems expected.

Driving, piloting or hazardous work:
No problems expected.

Airplane passengers:
No problems expected.

Discontinuing:
- Don't discontinue without doctor's advice until you complete prescribed dose, even though symptoms diminish or disappear.
- Drug affects your response to surgery, illness, injury or stress for 2 years after discontinuing. Tell about drug to anyone who takes medical care of you within 2 years.

Others:
Avoid immunizations if possible.

INTERACTION WITH OTHER DRUGS

GENERIC NAME OR DRUG CLASS	COMBINED EFFECT
Amphoterecin B	Potassium depletion.
Anticholinergics	Possible glaucoma.
Anticoagulants (oral)	Decreased anticoagulant effect.
Anticonvulsants (hydantoin)	Decreased prednisone effect.
Antidiabetics (oral)	Decreased antidiabetic effect.
Antihistamines	Decreased prednisone effect.
Aspirin	Increased prednisone effect.
Barbiturates	Decreased prednisone effect. Oversedation.
Beta-adrenergic blockers	Decreased prednisone effect.
Chloral hydrate	Decreased prednisone effect.
Chlorthalidone	Potassium depletion.
Cholinergics	Decreased cholinergic effect.
Contraceptives (oral)	Increased prednisone effect.
Digitalis preparations	Dangerous potassium depletion. Possible digitalis toxicity.
Diuretics (thiazide)	Potassium depletion.

Additional interactions on page 842.

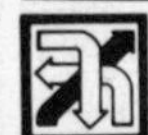

INTERACTION WITH OTHER SUBSTANCES

INTERACTS WITH	COMBINED EFFECT
Alcohol:	Risk of stomach ulcers.
Beverages:	No proven problems.
Cocaine:	Overstimulation. Avoid.
Foods:	No proven problems.
Marijuana:	Decreased immunity.
Tobacco:	Increased prednisone effect. Possible toxicity.

PRIMIDONE

BRAND NAMES

Apo-Primidone
Mysoline
Sertan

GENERAL INFORMATION

Habit forming? No
Prescription needed? Yes
Available as generic? Yes
Drug class: Anticonvulsant

USES

Prevents epileptic seizures.

DOSAGE & USAGE INFORMATION

How to take:

- Tablet or capsule—Swallow with liquid. If you can't swallow whole, crumble tablet or open capsule and take with liquid or food.
- Liquid—If desired, dilute dose in beverage before swallowing.

When to take:
Daily in regularly spaced doses, according to doctor's prescription.

If you forget a dose:
Take as soon as you remember up to 2 hours late. If more than 2 hours, wait for next scheduled dose (don't double this dose).

What drug does:
Probably inhibits repetitious spread of impulses along nerve pathways.

Time lapse before drug works:
2 to 3 weeks.

Don't take with:
See Interaction column and consult doctor.

OVERDOSE

Symptoms:
Slow, shallow breathing; weak, rapid pulse; confusion, deep sleep, coma.

What to do:

- Dial 0 (operator) or 911 (emergency) for an ambulance or medical help. Then give first aid immediately.
- If patient is unconscious and not breathing, give mouth-to-mouth breathing. If there is no heartbeat, use cardiac massage and mouth-to-mouth breathing (CPR). Don't try to make patient vomit. If you can't get help quickly, take patient to nearest emergency facility.
- Additional emergency information on page 886.

POSSIBLE ADVERSE REACTIONS OR SIDE EFFECTS

SYMPTOMS	FREQUENCY	WHAT TO DO
Brain & nervous system:		
• Confusion	Common	4
• Clumsiness, dizziness, drowsiness.	Common	5
• Headache	Infrequent	4
Skin:		
Rash or hives.	Rare	3
Eyes:		
• Vision change.	Common	4
• Eyelid swelling.	Rare	4
Ears, nose, throat:	None expected.	
Digestive:		
Nausea, vomiting, appetite loss.	Infrequent	4
Heart & lungs:		
Breathing difficulty.	Common	3
Blood vessels:	None expected.	
Muscles, bones, joints:	None expected.	
Genital, urinary:		
Decreased sexual ability.	Rare	5
Kidneys:	None expected.	
Liver:	None expected.	
Allergic:	None expected.	
Blood:	None expected.	
Others:		
• Unusual excitement, particularly in children.	Infrequent	3
• Fatigue, weakness.	Rare	3

1- Life-threatening. Seek emergency treatment immediately.
2- Discontinue. Seek emergency treatment.
3- Discontinue. Call doctor right away.
4- Continue. Call doctor when convenient.
5- Continue. Tell doctor at next visit.
6- No action necessary.

WARNINGS & PRECAUTIONS

Don't take if:
- You are allergic to any barbiturate.
- You have had porphyria.

Before you start, consult your doctor:
- If you have had liver, kidney or lung disease or asthma.
- If you have lupus.

Over age 60:
Adverse reactions and side effects may be more frequent and severe than in younger persons.

Pregnancy:
Studies inconclusive on harm to unborn child. Animal studies show fetal abnormalities. Decide with your doctor whether drug benefits justify risk to unborn child.

Breast-feeding:
Drug filters into milk. May harm child. Avoid.

Infants & children:
Use only under medical supervision.

Prolonged use:
- Enlarged lymph and thyroid glands.
- Anemia
- Rickets in children and osteomalacia (insufficient calcium to bones) in adults.

Skin & sunlight:
None expected.

Driving, piloting or hazardous work:
Don't drive or pilot aircraft until you learn how medicine affects you. Don't work around dangerous machinery. Don't climb ladders or work in high places. Danger increases if you drink alcohol or take medicine affecting alertness and reflexes.

Airplane passengers:
No problems expected.

Discontinuing:
Don't discontinue abruptly or without doctor's advice until you complete prescribed dose, even though symptoms diminish or disappear.

Others:
- Tell doctor if you become ill or injured and must interrupt dose schedule.
- Periodic laboratory blood tests of drug level recommended.

INTERACTION WITH OTHER DRUGS

GENERIC NAME OR DRUG CLASS	COMBINED EFFECT
Anticoagulants (oral)	Decreased primidone effect.
Anticonvulsants (other)	Changed seizure pattern.
Antidepressants	Increased antidepressant effect.
Antidiabetics	Increased effect of primidone sedation.
Antihistamines	Increased effect of primidone sedation.
Aspirin	Decreased aspirin effect.
Contraceptives (oral)	Decreased contraceptive effect.
Cortisone drugs	Decreased cortisone effect.
Digitalis preparations	Decreased digitalis effect.
Griseofulvin	Decreased griseofulvin effect.
Isoniazid	Increased isoniazid effect.
MAO inhibitors	Increased effect of primidone sedation.
Mind-altering drugs	Increased effect of mind-altering drugs.

Additional interactions on page 842.

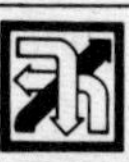

INTERACTION WITH OTHER SUBSTANCES

INTERACTS WITH	COMBINED EFFECT
Alcohol:	Dangerous sedative effect. Avoid.
Beverages:	None expected.
Cocaine:	Decreased primidone effect.
Foods:	Possible need for more vitamin D.
Marijuana:	Decreased anticonvulsant effect of primidone. Drowsiness, unsteadiness.
Tobacco:	None expected.

PROBENECID

BRAND NAMES

Benacen
Benemid
Benuryl
ColBENEMID
Col-Probenecid
Polycillin-PRB
Probalan
SK-Probenecid

GENERAL INFORMATION

Habit forming? No
Prescription needed? Yes
Available as generic? Yes
Drug class: Antigout (uricosuric)

USES

- Treatment for chronic gout.
- Increases blood levels of penicillins and cephalosporins.

DOSAGE & USAGE INFORMATION

How to take:
Tablet or capsule—Swallow with liquid or food to lessen stomach irritation. If you can't swallow whole, crumble tablet or open capsule and take with liquid or food.

When to take:
At the same time each day.

If you forget a dose:
Take as soon as you remember up to 12 hours late. If more than 12 hours, wait for next scheduled dose (don't double this dose).

What drug does:
- Forces kidneys to excrete uric acid.
- Reduces amount of penicillin excreted in urine.

Time lapse before drug works:
May require several months of regular use to prevent acute gout.

Don't take with:
- Non-prescription drugs containing aspirin or caffeine.
- See Interaction column and consult doctor.

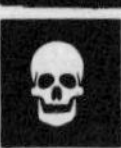

OVERDOSE

Symptoms:
Breathing difficulty, severe nervous agitation, convulsions, delirium, coma.

What to do:
- Dial 0 (operator) or 911 (emergency) for an ambulance or medical help. Then give first aid immediately.
- Additional emergency information on page 886.

POSSIBLE ADVERSE REACTIONS OR SIDE EFFECTS

SYMPTOMS	FREQUENCY	WHAT TO DO
Brain & nervous system:		
• Headache	Common	4
• Dizziness	Infrequent	4
Skin:		
Flushed face, itching.	Infrequent	4
Eyes:	None expected.	
Ears, nose, throat:		
Sore throat.	Rare	3
Digestive:		
Appetite loss, nausea, vomiting.	Common	4
Heart & lungs:		
Breathing difficulty.	Rare	3
Blood vessels:		
Unusual bleeding or bruising.	Rare	3
Muscles, bones, joints:		
Red, painful joint.	Rare	3
Genital, urinary:		
• Bloody urine.	Infrequent	3
• Painful or frequent urination.	Infrequent	5
Kidneys:		
Low back pain.	Infrequent	3
Liver:		
Jaundice (yellow skin and eyes).	Rare	3
Allergic:	None expected.	
Blood:	None expected.	
Others:		
Fever	Rare	3

1- Life-threatening. Seek emergency treatment immediately.
2- Discontinue. Seek emergency treatment.
3- Discontinue. Call doctor right away.
4- Continue. Call doctor when convenient.
5- Continue. Tell doctor at next visit.

WARNINGS & PRECAUTIONS

Don't take if:

- You are allergic to any uricosuric.
- You have acute gout.
- Patient is younger than 2.

Before you start, consult your doctor:

- If you have had kidney stones or kidney disease.
- If you have a peptic ulcer.
- If you have bone-marrow or blood-cell disease.

Over age 60:
Adverse reactions and side effects may be more frequent and severe than in younger persons.

Pregnancy:
Studies inconclusive on harm to unborn child. Animal studies show fetal abnormalities. Decide with your doctor whether drug benefits justify risk to unborn child.

Breast-feeding:
No proven problems.

Infants & children:
Not recommended.

Prolonged use:
Possible kidney damage.

Skin & sunlight:
No problems expected.

Driving, piloting or hazardous work:
Avoid if you feel dizzy. Otherwise, no problems expected.

Airplane passengers:
No problems expected.

Discontinuing:
Don't discontinue without consulting doctor. Dose may require gradual reduction if you have taken drug for a long time. Doses of other drugs may also require adjustment.

Others:
If signs of gout attack develop while taking medicine, consult doctor.

INTERACTION WITH OTHER DRUGS

GENERIC NAME OR DRUG CLASS	COMBINED EFFECT
Acetohexamide	Increased acetohexamide effect.
Anticoagulants (oral)	Increased anticoagulant effect.
Aspirin	Decreased probenecid effect.
Cephalosporins	Increased cephalosporin effect.
Dapsone	Increased dapsone effect. Increased toxicity.
Diuretics (thiazide)	Decreased probenecid effect.
Indomethacin	Increased adverse effects of indomethacin.
Methotrexate	Increased methotrexate toxicity.
Nitrofurantoin	Increased effect of nitrofurantoin.
Para-aminosalicylic acid (PAS)	Increased effect of para-aminosalicylic acid.
Penicillins	Enhanced penicillin effect.
Pyrazinamide	Decreased probenecid effect.

Additional interactions on page 843.

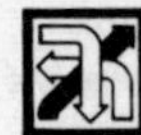

INTERACTION WITH OTHER SUBSTANCES

INTERACTS WITH	COMBINED EFFECT
Alcohol:	Decreased probenecid effect.
Beverages:	
Caffeine drinks	Loss of probenecid effectiveness.
Cocaine:	None expected.
Foods:	None expected.
Marijuana:	Daily use—Decreased probenecid effect.
Tobacco:	None expected.

PROCAINAMIDE

BRAND NAMES

Procan
Procan SR
Procamide
Procapan
Pronestyl
Pronestyl SR
Sub-Quin

GENERAL INFORMATION

Habit forming? No
Prescription needed? Yes
Available as generic? Yes
Drug class: Antiarrhythmic

USES

Stabilizes irregular heartbeat.

DOSAGE & USAGE INFORMATION

How to take:

- Tablet or capsule—Swallow with liquid.
- Extended-release tablets or capsules—Swallow each dose whole. If you take regular tablets, you may chew or crush them.

When to take:
Best taken on empty stomach, 1 hour before or 2 hours after meals. If necessary, may be taken with food or milk to lessen stomach upset.

If you forget a dose:
Take as soon as you remember up to 2 hours late. If more than 2 hours, wait for next scheduled dose (don't double this dose).

What drug does:
Slows activity of pacemaker (rhythm-control center of heart) and delays transmission of electrical impulses.

Time lapse before drug works:
30 to 60 minutes.

Don't take with:
See Interaction column and consult doctor.

OVERDOSE

Symptoms:
Fast and irregular heartbeat, stupor, fainting, cardiac arrest.

What to do:

- Dial 0 (operator) or 911 (emergency) for an ambulance or medical help. Then give first aid immediately.
- Additional emergency information on page 886.

POSSIBLE ADVERSE REACTIONS OR SIDE EFFECTS

SYMPTOMS	FREQUENCY	WHAT TO DO
Brain & nervous system:		
• Hallucinations, confusion, depression.	Rare	3
• Dizziness	Infrequent	4
Skin:		
Itch, rash.	Rare	3
Eyes:	None expected.	
Ears, nose, throat:		
Sore throat, fever.	Rare	3
Digestive:		
Diarrhea, appetite loss, nausea, vomiting.	Common	4
Heart & lungs:		
Painful breathing.	Infrequent	3
Blood vessels:	None expected.	
Muscles, bones, joints:		
Joint pain.	Infrequent	3
Genital, urinary:	None expected.	
Kidneys:	None expected.	
Liver:	None expected.	
Allergic:	None expected.	
Blood:	None expected.	
Others:		
• Fever	Rare	3
• Fatigue	Rare	4

1-Life-threatening. Seek emergency treatment immediately.
2-Discontinue. Seek emergency treatment.
3-Discontinue. Call doctor right away.
4-Continue. Call doctor when convenient.
5-Continue. Tell doctor at next visit.
6-No action necessary.

WARNINGS & PRECAUTIONS

Don't take if:
- You are allergic to procainamide.
- You have myasthenia gravis.

Before you start, consult your doctor:
- If you are allergic to local anesthetics that end in "caine."
- If you have had liver or kidney disease or impaired kidney function.
- If you have had lupus.
- If you take digitalis preparations.
- If you will have surgery within 2 months, including dental surgery, requiring general or spinal anesthesia.

Over age 60:
Adverse reactions and side effects may be more frequent and severe than in younger persons.

Pregnancy:
No proven harm to unborn child. Avoid if possible.

Breast-feeding:
No proven problems. Consult doctor.

Infants & children:
Not recommended.

Prolonged use:
May cause lupus-like illness.

Skin & sunlight:
No problems expected.

Driving, piloting or hazardous work:
Use caution if you feel dizzy or weak. Otherwise, no problems expected.

Airplane passengers:
No problems expected.

Discontinuing:
Don't discontinue without doctor's advice until you complete prescribed dose, even though symptoms diminish or disappear.

Others:
No problems expected.

INTERACTION WITH OTHER DRUGS

GENERIC NAME OR DRUG CLASS	COMBINED EFFECT
Acetazolamide	Increased procainamide effect.
Ambenonium	Decreased ambenonium effect.
Antihypertensives	Increased antihypertensive effect.
Antimyasthenics	Decreased antimyasthenic effect.
Anticholinergics	Increased anticholinergic effect.
Kanamycin	Severe muscle weakness, impaired breathing.
Neomycin	Severe muscle weakness, impaired breathing.

INTERACTION WITH OTHER SUBSTANCES

INTERACTS WITH	COMBINED EFFECT
Alcohol:	None expected.
Beverages: Caffeine drinks, iced drinks.	Irregular heartbeat.
Cocaine:	Decreased procainamide effect.
Foods:	None expected.
Marijuana:	None expected.
Tobacco:	Decreased procainamide effect.

PROCARBAZINE

BRAND NAMES

Matulane
Natulan

GENERAL INFORMATION

Habit forming? No
Prescription needed? Yes
Available as generic? No
Drug class: Antineoplastic

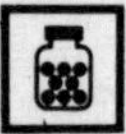

USES

Treatment for some kinds of cancer.

DOSAGE & USAGE INFORMATION

How to take:
Tablet or capsule—Swallow with liquid after light meal. Don't drink fluids with meals. Drink extra fluids between meals. Avoid sweet or fatty foods.

When to take:
At the same time each day.

If you forget a dose:
Take as soon as you remember. Don't double dose ever.

What drug does:
Inhibits abnormal cell reproduction. Procarbazine is an alkylating agent and a MAO inhibitor.

Time lapse before drug works:
Up to 6 weeks for full effect.

Don't take with:
See Interaction column and consult doctor.

OVERDOSE

Symptoms:
Restlessness, agitation, fever, convulsions, bleeding.

What to do:
- Dial 0 (operator) or 911 (emergency) for an ambulance or medical help. Then give first aid immediately.
- If patient is unconscious and not breathing, give mouth-to-mouth breathing. If there is no heartbeat, use cardiac massage and mouth-to-mouth breathing (CPR). Don't try to make patient vomit. If you can't get help quickly, take patient to nearest emergency facility.
- Additional emergency information on page 886.

POSSIBLE ADVERSE REACTIONS OR SIDE EFFECTS

SYMPTOMS	FREQUENCY	WHAT TO DO
Brain & nervous system:		
• Fainting	Infrequent	2
• Severe headache.	Infrequent	3
• Dizziness when changing position.	Common	5
• Hallucinations, insomnia, nightmares.	Infrequent	4
Skin:		
Rash	Rare	3
Eyes, blood vessels, kidneys, allergic, blood:		
Abnormal bleeding. or bruising.	Infrequent	3
Ears, nose, throat:		
Dry mouth.	Common	5
Digestive:		
• Diarrhea	Infrequent	4
• Constipation	Common	5
• Nausea, vomiting.	Rare	3
Heart & lungs:		
• Rapid or pounding heartbeat.	Infrequent	4
• Chest pain.	Infrequent	3
Muscles, bones, joints:		
Stiff neck.	Rare	3
Genital, urinary:		
Difficult urination.	Common	5
Liver:		
Jaundice (yellow skin and eyes).	Rare	3
Others:		
• Swollen feet, legs.	Infrequent	4
• Fever	Rare	3
• Lower sex drive.	Infrequent	5
• Fatigue, weakness.	Common	4

1- Life-threatening. Seek emergency treatment immediately.
2- Discontinue. Seek emergency treatment.
3- Discontinue. Call doctor right away.
4- Continue. Call doctor when convenient.
5- Continue. Tell doctor at next visit.

WARNINGS & PRECAUTIONS

Don't take if:
- You are allergic to any MAO inhibitor.
- You have heart disease, congestive heart failure, heart-rhythm irregularities or high blood pressure.
- You have liver or kidney disease.

Before you start, consult your doctor:
- If you are alcoholic.
- If you have asthma.
- If you have had a stroke.
- If you have diabetes or epilepsy.
- If you have overactive thyroid.
- If you have schizophrenia.
- If you have Parkinson's disease.
- If you have adrenal-gland tumor.
- If you will have surgery within 2 months, including dental surgery, requiring general or spinal anesthesia.

Over age 60:
Not recommended.

Pregnancy:
Avoid if possible.

Breast-feeding:
Safety not established. Consult doctor.

Infants & children:
Not recommended.

Prolonged use:
May be toxic to liver.

Skin & sunlight:
May cause rash or intensify sunburn in areas exposed to sun or sunlamp.

Driving, piloting or hazardous work:
Don't drive or pilot aircraft until you learn how medicine affects you. Don't work around dangerous machinery. Don't climb ladders or work in high places. Danger increases if you drink alcohol or take medicine affecting alertness and reflexes.

Airplane passengers:
No problems expected.

Discontinuing:
- Don't discontinue without doctor's advice until you complete prescribed dose, even though symptoms diminish or disappear.
- Follow precautions regarding foods, drinks and other medicines for 2 weeks after discontinuing.

Others:
- May affect blood-sugar levels in patients with diabetes.
- Fever may indicate that MAO inhibitor dose requires adjustment.

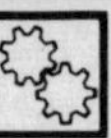

INTERACTION WITH OTHER DRUGS

GENERIC NAME OR DRUG CLASS	COMBINED EFFECT
Amphetamines	Blood-pressure rise to life-threatening level.
Anticonvulsants	Changed seizure pattern.
Antidepressants (tricyclic)	Blood-pressure rise to life-threatening level.
Antidiabetics (oral and insulin)	Excessively low blood sugar.
Caffeine	Irregular heartbeat or high blood pressure.
Carbamazepine	Fever, seizures. Avoid.
Cyclobenzaprine	Fever, seizures. Avoid.
Diuretics	Excessively low blood pressure.
Guanethidine	Blood-pressure rise to life-threatening level.
Levodopa	Sudden, severe blood-pressure rise.
MAO inhibitors (other)	High fever, convulsions, death.

INTERACTION WITH OTHER SUBSTANCES

INTERACTS WITH	COMBINED EFFECT
Alcohol:	Increased sedation to dangerous level.
Beverages:	
Caffeine drinks	Irregular heartbeat or high blood pressure.
Drinks containing tyramine (see page 849).	Blood-pressure rise to life-threatening level.
Cocaine:	Overstimulation. Possibly fatal.
Foods:	
Foods containing tyramine (see page 849).	Blood-pressure rise to life-threatening level.
Marijuana:	Overstimulation. Avoid.
Tobacco:	No proven problems.

PROCHLORPERAZINE

BRAND NAMES

Combid
Compazine
Eskatrol
Prochlor-Iso
Pro-Iso
Stemetil

GENERAL INFORMATION

Habit forming? No
Prescription needed? Yes
Available as generic? Yes
Drug class: Tranquilizer, antiemetic (phenothiazine)

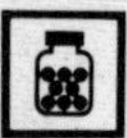

USES

- Stops nausea, vomiting.
- Reduces anxiety, agitation.

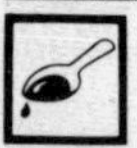

DOSAGE & USAGE INFORMATION

How to take:
- Tablet or capsule—Swallow with liquid or food to lessen stomach irritation.
- Suppositories—Remove wrapper and moisten suppository with water. Gently insert into rectum, large end first.
- Drops or liquid—Dilute dose in beverage.

When to take:
- Nervous and mental disorders—Take at the same times each day.
- Nausea and vomiting—Take as needed, no more often than every 4 hours.

If you forget a dose:
- Nervous and mental disorders—Take up to 2 hours late. If more than 2 hours, wait for next scheduled dose (don't double this).
- Nausea and vomiting—Take as soon as you remember. Wait 4 hours for next dose.

What drug does:
- Suppresses brain's vomiting center.
- Suppresses brain centers that control abnormal emotions and behavior.

Time lapse before drug works:
- Nausea and vomiting—1 hour or less.
- Nervous and mental disorders—4-6 weeks.

Don't take with:
- Antacid or medicine for diarrhea.
- Non-prescription drug for cough, cold or allergy.
- See Interaction column and consult doctor.

OVERDOSE

Symptoms:
Stupor, convulsions, coma.

What to do:
- Dial 0 (operator) or 911 (emergency) for an ambulance or medical help. Then give first aid immediately.
- Additional emergency information on page 886.

POSSIBLE ADVERSE REACTIONS OR SIDE EFFECTS

SYMPTOMS	FREQUENCY	WHAT TO DO
Brain & nervous system:		
• Restlessness, tremor.	Common	3
• Fainting	Infrequent	2
• Drowsiness	Common	3
Skin:		
• Rash	Infrequent	3
• Less perspiration.	Common	4
Eyes:		
Vision changes.	Rare	3
Ears, nose, throat:		
• Sore throat, fever.	Rare	3
• Dry mouth, nasal congestion.	Common	4
Digestive:		
Constipation	Common	4
Heart & lungs, blood vessels, kidneys, allergic, blood:	None expected.	
Muscles, bones, joints:		
Muscle spasms of face and neck, unsteady gait.	Common	2
Genital, urinary:		
Urination difficulty.	Infrequent	4
Liver:		
Jaundice (yellow eyes and skin).	Rare	3
Others:		
Less interest in sex, breast swelling, change in menstrual pattern.	Infrequent	4

1-Life-threatening. Seek emergency treatment immediately.
2-Discontinue. Seek emergency treatment.
3-Discontinue. Call doctor right away.
4-Continue. Call doctor when convenient.
5-Continue. Tell doctor at next visit.
6-No action necessary.

WARNINGS & PRECAUTIONS

Don't take if:
- You are allergic to any phenothiazine.
- You have a blood or bone-marrow disease.

Before you start, consult your doctor:
- If you will have surgery within 2 months, including dental surgery, requiring general or spinal anesthesia.
- If you have asthma, emphysema or other lung disorder.
- If you take non-prescription ulcer medicine, asthma medicine or amphetamines.

Over age 60:
Adverse reactions and side effects may be more frequent and severe than in younger persons. More likely to develop involuntary movement of jaws, lips, tongue, chewing. Report this to your doctor immediately. Early treatment can help.

Pregnancy:
Risk to unborn child outweighs drug benefits. Don't use.

Breast-feeding:
Drug passes into milk. Avoid drug or discontinue nursing until you finish medicine. Consult doctor for advice on maintaining milk supply.

Infants & children:
Don't give to children younger than 2.

Prolonged use:
May lead to tardive dyskinesia (involuntary movement of jaws, lips, tongue, chewing).

Skin & sunlight:
May cause rash or intensify sunburn in areas exposed to sun or sunlamp. Skin may remain sensitive for 3 months after discontinuing.

Driving, piloting or hazardous work:
Don't drive or pilot aircraft until you learn how medicine affects you. Don't work around dangerous machinery. Don't climb ladders or work in high places. Danger increases if you drink alcohol or take medicine affecting alertness and reflexes.

Airplane passengers:
No problems expected.

Discontinuing:
- Nervous and mental disorders—Don't discontinue without doctor's advice until you complete prescribed dose, even though symptoms diminish or disappear.
- Nausea and vomiting—May be unnecessary to finish medicine. Follow doctor's instructions.

INTERACTION WITH OTHER DRUGS

GENERIC NAME OR DRUG CLASS	COMBINED EFFECT
Anticholinergics	Increased anticholinergic effect.
Antidepressants (tricyclic)	Increased prochlorperazine effect.
Antihistamines	Increased antihistamine effect.
Appetite suppressants	Decreased suppressant effect.
Levodopa	Decreased levodopa effect.
Mind-altering drugs	Increased effect of mind-altering drugs.
Narcotics	Increased narcotic effect.
Phenytoin	Increased phenytoin effect.
Quinidine	Impaired heart function. Dangerous mixture.
Sedatives	Increased sedative effect.
Tranquilizers (other)	Increased tranquilizer effect.

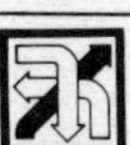

INTERACTION WITH OTHER SUBSTANCES

INTERACTS WITH	COMBINED EFFECT
Alcohol:	Dangerous oversedation.
Beverages:	None expected.
Cocaine:	Decreased prochlorperazine effect. Avoid.
Foods:	None expected.
Marijuana:	Drowsiness. May increase antinausea effect.
Tobacco:	None expected.

PROCYCLIDINE

BRAND NAMES

Kemadrin

GENERAL INFORMATION

Habit forming? No
Prescription needed? Yes
Available as generic? No
Drug class: Antidyskinetic, antiparkinsonism

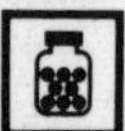

USES

- Treatment of Parkinson's disease.
- Treatment of adverse effects of phenothiazines.

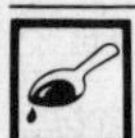

DOSAGE & USAGE INFORMATION

How to take:
Tablets or capsules—Take with food to lessen stomach irritation.

When to take:
At the same times each day.

If you forget a dose:
Take as soon as you remember up to 2 hours late. If more than 2 hours, wait for next scheduled dose (don't double this dose).

What drug does:
- Balances chemical reactions necessary to send nerve impulses within base of brain.
- Improves muscle control and reduces stiffness.

Time lapse before drug works:
1 to 2 hours.

Don't take with:
- Non-prescription drugs for colds, cough or allergy.
- See Interaction column and consult doctor.

OVERDOSE

Symptoms:
Agitation, dilated pupils, hallucinations, dry mouth, rapid heartbeat, sleepiness.

What to do:
- Dial 0 (operator) or 911 (emergency) for an ambulance or medical help. Then give first aid immediately.
- If patient is unconscious and not breathing, give mouth-to-mouth breathing. If there is no heartbeat, use cardiac massage and mouth-to-mouth breathing (CPR). Don't try to make patient vomit. If you can't get help quickly, take patient to nearest emergency facility.
- Additional emergency information on page 886.

POSSIBLE ADVERSE REACTIONS OR SIDE EFFECTS

SYMPTOMS	FREQUENCY	WHAT TO DO
Brain & nervous system:		
Confusion, dizziness.	Rare	4
Skin:		
Rash	Rare	3
Eyes:		
• Pain	Rare	3
• Blurred vision, light sensitivity.	Common	4
Ears, nose, throat:		
Sore mouth or tongue.	Rare	4
Digestive:		
• Constipation	Common	4
• Nausea, vomiting.	Common	4
Heart & lungs:	None expected.	
Blood vessels:	None expected.	
Muscles, bones, joints:		
• Muscle cramps.	Rare	4
• Numbness, weakness in hands or feet.	Rare	4
Genital, urinary:		
Difficult or painful urination.	Common	5
Kidneys:	None expected.	
Liver:	None expected.	
Allergic:	None expected.	
Blood:	None expected.	
Others:	None expected.	

1 - Life-threatening. Seek emergency treatment immediately.
2 - Discontinue. Seek emergency treatment.
3 - Discontinue. Call doctor right away.
4 - Continue. Call doctor when convenient.
5 - Continue. Tell doctor at next visit.
6 - No action necessary.

WARNINGS & PRECAUTIONS

Don't take if:
You are allergic to any antidyskinetic.

Before you start, consult your doctor:
- If you have had glaucoma.
- If you have had high blood pressure or heart disease.
- If you have had impaired liver function.
- If you have had kidney disease or urination difficulty.

Over age 60:
More sensitive to drug. Aggravates symptoms of enlarged prostate. Causes impaired thinking, hallucinations, nightmares. Consult doctor about any of these.

Pregnancy:
Studies inconclusive on harm to unborn child. Animal studies show fetal abnormalities. Decide with your doctor whether drug benefits justify risk to unborn child.

Breast-feeding:
No problems expected.

Infants & children:
Not recommended for children 3 and younger. Use for older children only under doctor's supervision.

Prolonged use:
Possible glaucoma.

Skin & sunlight:
No problems expected.

Driving, piloting or hazardous work:
Don't drive or pilot aircraft until you learn how medicine affects you. Don't work around dangerous machinery. Don't climb ladders or work in high places. Danger increases if you drink alcohol or take medicine affecting alertness and reflexes, such as antihistamines, tranquilizers, sedatives, pain medicine, narcotics and mind-altering drugs.

Airplane passengers:
No problems expected.

Discontinuing:
Don't discontinue without consulting doctor. Dose may require gradual reduction if you have taken drug for a long time. Doses of other drugs may also require adjustment.

Others:
- Internal eye pressure should be measured regularly.
- Avoid becoming overheated.

INTERACTION WITH OTHER DRUGS

GENERIC NAME OR DRUG CLASS	COMBINED EFFECT
Amantadine	Increased amantadine effect.
Antidepressants (tricyclic)	Increased procyclidine effect. May cause glaucoma.
Antihistamines	Increased procyclidine effect.
Levodopa	Increased levodopa effect. Improved results in treating Parkinson's disease.
Meperidine	Increased procyclidine effect.
MAO inhibitors	Increased procyclidine effect.
Orphenadrine	Increased procyclidine effect.
Phenothiazines	Behavior changes.
Primidone	Excessive sedation.
Procainamide	Increased procainamide effect.
Quinidine	Increased procyclidine effect.
Tranquilizers	Excessive sedation.

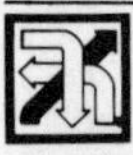

INTERACTION WITH OTHER SUBSTANCES

INTERACTS WITH	COMBINED EFFECT
Alcohol:	None expected.
Beverages:	None expected.
Cocaine:	Decreased procyclidine effect. Avoid.
Foods:	None expected.
Marijuana:	None expected.
Tobacco:	None expected.

PROMAZINE

BRAND NAMES

Norzine
Promanyl
Sparine

GENERAL INFORMATION

Habit forming? No
Prescription needed? Yes
Available as generic? Yes
Drug class: Tranquilizer, antiemetic (phenothiazine)

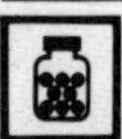

USES

- Stops nausea, vomiting.
- Reduces anxiety, agitation.

DOSAGE & USAGE INFORMATION

How to take:
- Tablet or capsule—Swallow with liquid or food to lessen stomach irritation.
- Suppositories—Remove wrapper and moisten suppository with water. Gently insert into rectum, large end first.
- Drops or liquid—Dilute dose in beverage.

When to take:
- Nervous and mental disorders—Take at the same times each day.
- Nausea and vomiting—Take as needed, no more often than every 4 hours.

If you forget a dose:
- Nervous and mental disorders—Take up to 2 hours late. If more than 2 hours, wait for next scheduled dose (don't double this).
- Nausea and vomiting—Take as soon as you remember. Wait 4 hours for next dose.

What drug does:
- Suppresses brain's vomiting center.
- Suppresses brain centers that control abnormal emotions and behavior.

Time lapse before drug works:
- Nausea and vomiting—1 hour or less.
- Nervous and mental disorders—4-6 weeks.

Don't take with:
- Antacid or medicine for diarrhea.
- Non-prescription drug for cough, cold or allergy.
- See Interaction column and consult doctor.

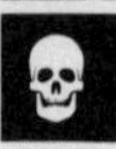

OVERDOSE

Symptoms:
Stupor, convulsions, coma.

What to do:
- Dial 0 (operator) or 911 (emergency) for an ambulance or medical help. Then give first aid immediately.
- Additional emergency information on page 886.

POSSIBLE ADVERSE REACTIONS OR SIDE EFFECTS

SYMPTOMS	FREQUENCY	WHAT TO DO
Brain & nervous system:		
• Restlessness, tremor.	Common	3
• Fainting	Infrequent	2
• Drowsiness	Common	3
Skin:		
• Rash	Infrequent	3
• Less perspiration.	Common	4
Eyes:		
Vision changes.	Rare	3
Ears, nose, throat:		
• Sore throat, fever.	Rare	3
• Dry mouth, nasal congestion.	Common	4
Digestive:		
Constipation	Common	4
Heart & lungs, blood vessels, kidneys, allergic, blood:	None expected.	
Muscles, bones, joints:		
Muscle spasms of face and neck, unsteady gait.	Common	2
Genital, urinary:		
Urination difficulty.	Infrequent	4
Liver:		
Jaundice (yellow eyes and skin).	Rare	3
Others:		
Less interest in sex, breast swelling, change in menstrual pattern.	Infrequent	4

1- Life-threatening. Seek emergency treatment immediately.
2- Discontinue. Seek emergency treatment.
3- Discontinue. Call doctor right away.
4- Continue. Call doctor when convenient.
5- Continue. Tell doctor at next visit.
6- No action necessary.

WARNINGS & PRECAUTIONS

Don't take if:
- You are allergic to any phenothiazine.
- You have a blood or bone-marrow disease.

Before you start, consult your doctor:
- If you will have surgery within 2 months, including dental surgery, requiring general or spinal anesthesia.
- If you have asthma, emphysema or other lung disorder.
- If you take non-prescription ulcer medicine, asthma medicine or amphetamines.

Over age 60:
Adverse reactions and side effects may be more frequent and severe than in younger persons. More likely to develop involuntary movement of jaws, lips, tongue, chewing. Report this to your doctor immediately. Early treatment can help.

Pregnancy:
Risk to unborn child outweighs drug benefits. Don't use.

Breast-feeding:
Drug passes into milk. Avoid drug or discontinue nursing until you finish medicine. Consult doctor for advice on maintaining milk supply.

Infants & children:
Don't give to children younger than 2.

Prolonged use:
May lead to tardive dyskinesia (involuntary movement of jaws, lips, tongue, chewing).

Skin & sunlight:
May cause rash or intensify sunburn in areas exposed to sun or sunlamp. Skin may remain sensitive for 3 months after discontinuing.

Driving, piloting or hazardous work:
Don't drive or pilot aircraft until you learn how medicine affects you. Don't work around dangerous machinery. Don't climb ladders or work in high places. Danger increases if you drink alcohol or take medicine affecting alertness and reflexes.

Airplane passengers:
No problems expected.

Discontinuing:
- Nervous and mental disorders—Don't discontinue without doctor's advice until you complete prescribed dose, even though symptoms diminish or disappear.
- Nausea and vomiting—May be unnecessary to finish medicine. Follow doctor's instructions.

INTERACTION WITH OTHER DRUGS

GENERIC NAME OR DRUG CLASS	COMBINED EFFECT
Anticholinergics	Increased anticholinergic effect.
Antidepressants (tricyclic)	Increased promazine effect.
Antihistamines	Increased antihistamine effect.
Appetite suppressants	Decreased suppressant effect.
Levodopa	Decreased levodopa effect.
Mind-altering drugs	Increased effect of mind-altering drugs.
Narcotics	Increased narcotic effect.
Phenytoin	Increased phenytoin effect.
Quinidine	Impaired heart function. Dangerous mixture.
Sedatives	Increased sedative effect.
Tranquilizers (other)	Increased tranquilizer effect.

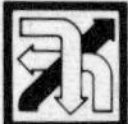

INTERACTION WITH OTHER SUBSTANCES

INTERACTS WITH	COMBINED EFFECT
Alcohol:	Dangerous oversedation.
Beverages:	None expected.
Cocaine:	Decreased promazine effect. Avoid.
Foods:	None expected.
Marijuana:	Drowsiness. May increase antinausea effect.
Tobacco:	None expected.

PROMETHAZINE

BRAND NAMES

Baymethazine
Dihydrocodeine Compound
Fellozine
Ganphen
Histanil
Historest
K-Phen
Mepergan Fortis
Pentazine
Phenergan
Phenerhist
Promet 50
Prorex
Prosedin
Provigan
Remsed
Synalgos
Synalgos-DC
ZiPan

GENERAL INFORMATION

Habit forming? No
Prescription needed? Yes
Available as generic? Yes
Drug class: Antihistamine, tranquilizer (phenothiazine)

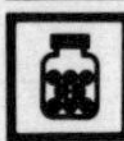

USES

- Stops nausea, vomiting and dizziness of motion sickness.
- Produces mild sedation and light sleep.
- Reduces allergic symptoms of hay fever and hives.

DOSAGE & USAGE INFORMATION

How to take:
- Tablets or liquid—Swallow with water.
- Suppositories—Remove wrapper and moisten suppository with water. Gently insert larger end into rectum. Push well into rectum with finger.

When to take:
Take as needed, no more often than every 12 hours.

If you forget a dose:
Take as soon as you remember. Wait 12 hours for next dose.

What drug does:
- Blocks stimulation of brain's vomiting center.
- Suppresses brain centers that control abnormal emotions and behavior.
- Blocks histamine action in sensitized cells.

Time lapse before drug works:
1 to 2 hours.

Don't take with:
- Antacid or medicine for diarrhea.
- Non-prescription drug for cough, cold or allergy.
- See Interaction column and consult doctor.

OVERDOSE

Symptoms:
Stupor, convulsions, coma.

What to do:
- Dial 0 (operator) or 911 (emergency) for an ambulance or medical help. Then give first aid immediately.
- Additional emergency information on page 886.

POSSIBLE ADVERSE REACTIONS OR SIDE EFFECTS

SYMPTOMS	FREQUENCY	WHAT TO DO
Brain & nervous system:		
• Restlessness, tremor, drowsiness.	Common	3
• Fainting	Infrequent	2
Skin:		
• Rash	Infrequent	3
• Less perspiration.	Common	4
Eyes:		
Vision changes.	Rare	3
Ears, nose, throat:		
• Sore throat, fever.	Rare	3
• Dry mouth, nasal congestion.	Common	4
Digestive:		
Constipation	Common	4
Heart & lungs:	None expected.	
Blood vessels:	None expected.	
Muscles, bones, joints:		
Muscle spasms of face and neck, unsteady gait.	Infrequent	3
Genital, urinary:		
Urination difficulty.	Infrequent	4
Kidneys:	None expected.	
Liver:		
Jaundice (yellow eyes and skin).	Rare	3
Allergic:	None expected.	
Blood:	None expected.	
Others:		
Less interest in sex, breast swelling, menstrual changes.	Infrequent	4

1 - Life-threatening. Seek emergency treatment immediately.
2 - Discontinue. Seek emergency treatment.
3 - Discontinue. Call doctor right away.
4 - Continue. Call doctor when convenient.

WARNINGS & PRECAUTIONS

Don't take if:
- You are allergic to any phenothiazine.
- You have a blood or bone-marrow disease.

Before you start, consult your doctor:
- If you will have surgery within 2 months, including dental surgery, requiring general or spinal anesthesia.
- If you have asthma, emphysema or other lung disorder.
- If you take non-prescription ulcer medicine, asthma medicine or amphetamines.

Over age 60:
Adverse reactions and side effects may be more frequent and severe than in younger persons. More likely to develop tardive dyskinesia (involuntary movement of jaws, lips, tongue, chewing). Report this to your doctor immediately. Early treatment can help.

Pregnancy:
Risk to unborn child outweighs drug benefits. Don't use.

Breast-feeding:
Drug passes into milk. Avoid drug or discontinue nursing until you finish medicine. Consult doctor for advice on maintaining milk supply.

Infants & children:
Don't give to children younger than 2.

Prolonged use:
May lead to tardive dyskinesia (involuntary movement of jaws, lips, tongue, chewing).

Skin & sunlight:
May cause rash or intensify sunburn in areas exposed to sun or sunlamp. Skin may remain sensitive for 3 months after discontinuing.

Driving, piloting or hazardous work:
Don't drive or pilot aircraft until you learn how medicine affects you. Don't work around dangerous machinery. Don't climb ladders or work in high places. Danger increases if you drink alcohol or take medicine affecting alertness and reflexes.

Airplane passengers:
No problems expected.

Discontinuing:
- Nervous and mental disorders—Don't discontinue without doctor's advice until you complete prescribed dose, even though symptoms diminish or disappear.
- Nausea, vomiting or allergy—May be unnecessary to finish medicine. Follow doctor's instructions.

INTERACTION WITH OTHER DRUGS

GENERIC NAME OR DRUG CLASS	COMBINED EFFECT
Antacids	Decreased promethazine effect.
Anticholinergics	Increased anticholinergic effect.
Anticonvulsants (hydantoin)	Increased anticonvulsant effect.
Antidepressants (tricyclic)	Increased promethazine effect.
Antihistamines (other)	Increased antihistamine effect.
Appetite suppressants	Decreased suppressant effect.
Barbiturates	Oversedation.
Guanethidine	Decreased guanethidine effect.
Levodopa	Decreased levodopa effect.
MAO inhibitors	Increased promethazine effect.
Mind-altering drugs	Increased effect of mind-altering drugs.
Narcotics	Increased narcotic effect.
Sedatives	Increased sedative effect.
Tranquilizers (other)	Increased tranquilizer effect.

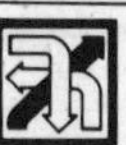

INTERACTION WITH OTHER SUBSTANCES

INTERACTS WITH	COMBINED EFFECT
Alcohol:	Dangerous oversedation.
Beverages:	None expected.
Cocaine:	Decreased promethazine effect. Avoid.
Foods:	None expected.
Marijuana:	Drowsiness. May increase antinausea effect.
Tobacco:	None expected.

PROPANTHELINE

BRAND NAMES

Banlin
Norpanth
Novopropanthil
Pro-Banthine
Pro-Banthine with Phenobarbital
Propanthel
Ropanth
SK-Propantheline

GENERAL INFORMATION

Habit forming? No
Prescription needed? Low strength: No
High strength: Yes
Available as generic? Yes
Drug class: Antispasmodic, anticholinergic

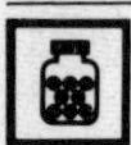

USES

Reduces spasms of digestive system, bladder and urethra.

DOSAGE & USAGE INFORMATION

How to take:
Tablet—Swallow with liquid or food to lessen stomach irritation.

When to take:
30 minutes before meals (unless directed otherwise by doctor).

If you forget a dose:
Take as soon as you remember up to 2 hours late. If more than 2 hours, wait for next scheduled dose (don't double this dose).

What drug does:
Blocks nerve impulses at parasympathetic nerve endings, preventing muscle contractions and gland secretions of organs involved.

Time lapse before drug works:
15 to 30 minutes.

Don't take with:
See Interaction column and consult doctor.

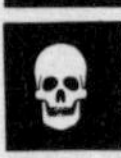

OVERDOSE

Symptoms:
Dilated pupils; rapid pulse and breathing; dizziness; fever; hallucinations; confusion; slurred speech; agitation; flushed face; convulsions; coma.

What to do:
- Dial 0 (operator) or 911 (emergency) for an ambulance or medical help. Then give first aid immediately.
- Additional emergency information on page 886.

POSSIBLE ADVERSE REACTIONS OR SIDE EFFECTS

SYMPTOMS	FREQUENCY	WHAT TO DO
Brain & nervous system:		
• Headache	Infrequent	4
• Confusion, delirium.	Common	3
Skin:		
Rash or hives.	Rare	3
Eyes:		
Pain, blurred vision.	Rare	3
Ears, nose, throat:		
Dryness	Common	6
Digestive:		
• Constipation	Common	5
• Nausea, vomiting.	Common	4
Heart & lungs:		
Rapid heartbeat.	Common	3
Blood vessels:	None expected.	
Muscles, bones, joints:	None expected.	
Genital, urinary:		
Difficult urination.	Infrequent	4
Kidneys:	None expected.	
Liver:	None expected.	
Allergic:	None expected.	
Blood:	None expected.	
Others:		
Less perspiration.	Common	4

1- Life-threatening. Seek emergency treatment immediately.
2- Discontinue. Seek emergency treatment.
3- Discontinue. Call doctor right away.
4- Continue. Call doctor when convenient.
5- Continue. Tell doctor at next visit.
6- No action necessary.

WARNINGS & PRECAUTIONS

Don't take if:

- You are allergic to any anticholinergic.
- You have trouble with stomach bloating.
- You have difficulty emptying your bladder completely.
- You have narrow-angle glaucoma.
- You have severe ulcerative colitis.

Before you start, consult your doctor:

- If you have open-angle glaucoma.
- If you have angina.
- If you have chronic bronchitis or asthma.
- If you have hiatal hernia.
- If you have liver disease.
- If you have enlarged prostate.
- If you have myasthenia gravis.
- If you have peptic ulcer.
- If you will have surgery within 2 months, including dental surgery, requiring general or spinal anesthesia.

Over age 60:
Adverse reactions and side effects may be more frequent and severe than in younger persons.

Pregnancy:
Studies inconclusive on harm to unborn child. Animal studies show fetal abnormalities. Decide with your doctor whether drug benefits justify risk to unborn child.

Breast-feeding:
Drug passes into milk and decreases milk flow. Avoid drug or discontinue nursing until you finish medicine. Consult doctor for advice on maintaining milk supply.

Infants & children:
Use only under medical supervision.

Prolonged use:
Chronic constipation, possible fecal impaction. Consult doctor immediately.

Skin & sunlight:
No problems expected.

Driving, piloting or hazardous work:
Use disqualifies you for piloting aircraft. Otherwise, no problems expected.

Airplane passengers:
No problems expected.

Discontinuing:
May be unnecessary to finish medicine. Follow doctor's instructions.

Others:
No problems expected.

INTERACTION WITH OTHER DRUGS

GENERIC NAME OR DRUG CLASS	COMBINED EFFECT
Amantadine	Increased propantheline effect.
Anticholinergics (other)	Increased propantheline effect.
Antidepressants (tricyclic)	Increased propantheline effect.
Antihistamines	Increased propantheline effect.
Cortisone drugs	Increased internal eye pressure.
Haloperidol	Increased internal eye pressure.
MAO inhibitors	Increased propantheline effect.
Meperidine	Increased propantheline effect.
Methylphenidate	Increased propantheline effect.
Orphenadrine	Increased propantheline effect.
Phenothiazines	Increased propantheline effect.
Pilocarpine	Loss of pilocarpine effect in glaucoma treatment.
Vitamin C	Decreased propantheline effect. Avoid large doses of vitamin C.

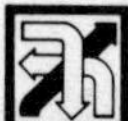

INTERACTION WITH OTHER SUBSTANCES

INTERACTS WITH	COMBINED EFFECT
Alcohol:	None expected.
Beverages:	None expected.
Cocaine:	Excessively rapid heartbeat. Avoid.
Foods:	None expected.
Marijuana:	Drowsiness and dry mouth.
Tobacco:	None expected.

PROPRANOLOL

BRAND NAMES

Apo-Propranolol
Detensol
Inderal
Inderide
Novopranol
Panolol

GENERAL INFORMATION

Habit forming? No
Prescription needed? Yes
Available as generic? No
Drug class: Beta-adrenergic blocker

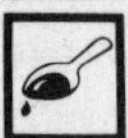

USES

- Reduces angina attacks.
- Stabilizes irregular heartbeat.
- Lowers blood pressure.
- Reduces frequency of migraine headaches. (Does not relieve headache pain.)
- Other uses prescribed by your doctor.

DOSAGE & USAGE INFORMATION

How to take:
Tablet or capsule—Swallow with liquid. If you can't swallow whole, crumble tablet or open capsule and take with liquid or food.

When to take:
With meals or immediately after.

If you forget a dose:
Take as soon as you remember. Return to regular schedule, but allow 3 hours between doses.

What drug does:
- Blocks certain actions of sympathetic nervous system.
- Lowers heart's oxygen requirements.
- Slows nerve impulses through heart.
- Reduces blood vessel contraction in heart, scalp and other body parts.

Time lapse before drug works:
1 to 4 hours.

Don't take with:
Non-prescription drugs or drugs in Interaction column without consulting doctor.

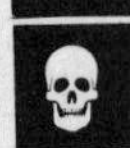

OVERDOSE

Symptoms:
Weakness, slow or weak pulse, blood pressure drop, fainting, convulsions, cold and sweaty skin.

What to do:
- Dial O (operator) or 911 (emergency) for an ambulance or medical help. Then give first aid immediately.
- Additional emergency information on page 886.

POSSIBLE ADVERSE REACTIONS OR SIDE EFFECTS

SYMPTOMS	FREQUENCY	WHAT TO DO
Brain & nervous system:		
• Hallucinations, nightmares, insomnia, headache.	Infrequent	3
• Confusion, depression, reduced alertness.	Infrequent	4
• Drowsiness, numbness or tingling of fingers or toes, dizziness.	Common	4
Skin:		
Rash	Rare	3
Eyes:	None expected.	
Ears, nose, throat:		
Sore throat, fever.	Rare	3
Digestive:		
• Diarrhea, nausea.	Common	4
• Constipation	Infrequent	5
Heart & lungs:		
• Pulse slower than 50 beats per minute.	Common	3
• Breathing difficulty.	Infrequent	3
Blood vessels:		
Cold hands, feet.	Common	5
Muscles, bones, joints, genital, urinary, kidneys, liver, allergic:	None expected.	
Blood:		
Unusual bleeding and bruising.	Rare	4
Others:		
• Fatigue, weakness.	Common	4
• Dry mouth, eyes, skin.	Common	5

1-Life-threatening. Seek emergency treatment immediately.
2-Discontinue. Seek emergency treatment.
3-Discontinue. Call doctor right away.
4-Continue. Call doctor when convenient.
5-Continue. Tell doctor at next visit.

WARNINGS & PRECAUTIONS

Don't take if:
- You are allergic to any beta-adrenergic blocker.
- You have asthma.
- You have hay fever symptoms.
- You have taken MAO inhibitors in past 2 weeks.

Before you start, consult your doctor:
- If you have heart disease or poor circulation to the extremities.
- If you have hay fever, asthma, chronic bronchitis, emphysema.
- If you have overactive thyroid function.
- If you have impaired liver or kidney function.
- If you will have surgery within 2 months, including dental surgery, requiring general or spinal anesthesia.
- If you have diabetes or hypoglycemia.

Over age 60:
Adverse reactions and side effects may be more frequent and severe than in younger persons.

Pregnancy:
Risk to unborn child outweighs drug benefits. Don't use.

Breast-feeding:
Drug passes into milk. Avoid drug or discontinue nursing until you finish medicine. Consult doctor for advice on maintaining milk supply.

Infants & children:
Not recommended.

Prolonged use:
Weakens heart muscle contractions.

Skin & sunlight:
No problems expected.

Driving, piloting or hazardous work:
Don't drive or pilot aircraft until you learn how medicine affects you. Don't work around dangerous machinery. Don't climb ladders or work in high places. Danger increases if you drink alcohol or take medicine affecting alertness and reflexes.

Airplane passengers:
No problems expected.

Discontinuing:
Don't discontinue without consulting doctor. Dose may require gradual reduction if you have taken drug for a long time. Doses of other drugs may also require adjustment.

Others:
May mask hypoglycemia.

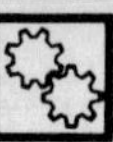

INTERACTION WITH OTHER DRUGS

GENERIC NAME OR DRUG CLASS	COMBINED EFFECT
Antidiabetics	Increased antidiabetic effect.
Antihistamines	Decreased antihistamine effect.
Antihypertensives	Increased antihypertensive effect.
Antiinflammatory drugs	Decreased antiinflammatory effect.
Barbiturates	Increased barbiturate effect. Dangerous sedation.
Digitalis preparations	Can either increase or decrease heart rate. Improves irregular heartbeat.
Narcotics	Increased narcotic effect. Dangerous sedation.
Phenytoin	Increased propranolol effect.
Quinidine	Slows heart excessively.
Reserpine	Increased reserpine effect. Excessive sedation and depression.

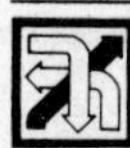

INTERACTION WITH OTHER SUBSTANCES

INTERACTS WITH	COMBINED EFFECT
Alcohol:	Excessive blood-pressure drop. Avoid.
Beverages:	None expected.
Cocaine:	Irregular heartbeat. Avoid.
Foods:	None expected.
Marijuana:	Daily use—Impaired circulation to hands and feet.
Tobacco:	Possible irregular heartbeat.

PROTRIPTYLINE

BRAND NAMES

Triptil
Vivactil

GENERAL INFORMATION

Habit forming? No
Prescription needed? Yes
Available as generic? No
Drug class: Antidepressant (tricyclic)

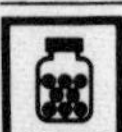

USES

Gradually relieves, but doesn't cure, symptoms of depression.

DOSAGE & USAGE INFORMATION

How to take:
Tablet—Swallow with liquid.

When to take:
At the same time each day, usually bedtime.

If you forget a dose:
Bedtime dose—If you forget your once-a-day bedtime dose, don't take it more than 3 hours late. If more than 3 hours, wait for next scheduled dose. Don't double this dose.

What drug does:
Probably affects part of brain that controls messages between nerve cells.

Time lapse before drug works:
Begins in 1 to 2 weeks. May require 4 to 6 weeks for maximum benefit.

Don't take with:
- Non-prescription drugs without consulting doctor.
- See Interaction column and consult doctor.

OVERDOSE

Symptoms:
Hallucinations, convulsions, coma.

What to do:
- Dial 0 (operator) or 911 (emergency) for an ambulance or medical help. Then give first aid immediately.
- If patient is unconscious and not breathing, give mouth-to-mouth breathing. If there is no heartbeat, use cardiac massage and mouth-to-mouth breathing (CPR). Don't try to make patient vomit. If you can't get help quickly, take patient to nearest emergency facility.
- Additional emergency information on page 886.

POSSIBLE ADVERSE REACTIONS OR SIDE EFFECTS

SYMPTOMS	FREQUENCY	WHAT TO DO
Brain & nervous system:		
• Hallucinations, shakiness, dizziness, fainting.	Infrequent	3
• Headache	Common	4
• Seizures	Rare	1
• Insomnia	Common	5
Skin:		
Rash, itch.	Rare	3
Eyes:		
Blurred vision, pain.	Infrequent	3
Ears, nose, throat:		
• Sore throat.	Rare	3
• Dry mouth or unpleasant taste.	Common	4
Digestive:		
• Constipation or diarrhea, nausea, indigestion.	Common	4
• Vomiting	Infrequent	3
• "Sweet tooth"	Common	5
Heart & lungs:		
Irregular heartbeat or slow pulse.	Infrequent	3
Blood vessels, muscles, bones, joints, kidneys, allergic, blood:	None expected.	
Genital, urinary:		
Difficulty urinating.	Infrequent	4
Liver:		
Jaundice (yellow skin and eyes).	Rare	3
Others:		
• Fever	Rare	3
• Fatigue, weakness.	Common	4

1- Life-threatening. Seek emergency treatment immediately.
2- Discontinue. Seek emergency treatment.
3- Discontinue. Call doctor right away.
4- Continue. Call doctor when convenient.
5- Continue. Tell doctor at next visit.

WARNINGS & PRECAUTIONS

Don't take if:
- You are allergic to any tricyclic antidepressant.
- You drink alcohol.
- You have had a heart attack within 6 weeks.
- You have glaucoma.
- You have taken MAO inhibitors within 2 weeks.
- Patient is younger than 12.

Before you start, consult your doctor:
- If you will have surgery within 2 months, including dental surgery, requiring general or spinal anesthesia.
- If you have an enlarged prostate.
- If you have heart disease or high blood pressure.
- If you have stomach or intestinal problems.
- If you have an overactive thyroid.
- If you have asthma.
- If you have liver disease.

Over age 60:
More likely to develop urination difficulty and side effects under Brain & nervous system.

Pregnancy:
Studies inconclusive on harm to unborn child. Animal studies show fetal abnormalities. Decide with your doctor whether drug benefits justify risk to unborn child.

Breast-feeding:
Drug passes into milk. Avoid drug or discontinue nursing until you finish medicine. Consult doctor for advice on maintaining milk supply.

Infants & children:
Don't give to children younger than 12.

Prolonged use:
No problems expected.

Skin & sunlight:
May cause rash or intensify sunburn in areas exposed to sun or sunlamp.

Driving, piloting or hazardous work:
Don't drive or pilot aircraft until you learn how medicine affects you. Don't work around dangerous machinery. Don't climb ladders or work in high places. Danger increases if you drink alcohol or take medicine affecting alertness and reflexes.

Airplane passengers:
No problems expected.

Discontinuing:
Don't discontinue without consulting doctor. Dose may require gradual reduction if you have taken drug for a long time. Doses of other drugs may also require adjustment.

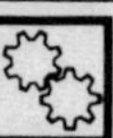

INTERACTION WITH OTHER DRUGS

GENERIC NAME OR DRUG CLASS	COMBINED EFFECT
Anticoagulants (oral)	Increased anticoagulant effect.
Anticholinergics	Increased sedation.
Antihistamines	Increased antihistamine effect.
Barbiturates	Decreased antidepressant effect.
Clonidine	Decreased clonidine effect.
Diuretics (thiazide)	Increased protriptyline effect.
Ethchlorvynol	Delirium
Guanethidine	Decreased guanethidine effect.
MAO inhibitors	Fever, delirium, convulsions.
Methyldopa	Decreased methyldopa effect.
Narcotics	Dangerous oversedation.
Phenytoin	Decreased phenytoin effect.
Quinidine	Irregular heartbeat.
Sedatives	Dangerous oversedation.
Sympathomimetics	Increased sympathomimetic effect.
Thyroid hormones	Irregular heartbeat.

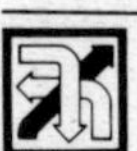

INTERACTION WITH OTHER SUBSTANCES

INTERACTS WITH	COMBINED EFFECT
Alcohol: Beverages or medicines with alcohol.	Excessive intoxication. Avoid.
Beverages:	None expected.
Cocaine:	Excessive intoxication. Avoid.
Foods:	None expected.
Marijuana:	Excessive drowsiness. Avoid.
Tobacco:	None expected.

PSEUDOEPHEDRINE

BRAND NAMES

Actifed
Afrinol
Cenafed
D-Feda
Deconamine
Dimacol
Disophrol
Drixoral
Eltor
Emprazil
Fedahist
Fedrazil
Neobid
Novafed
Sudafed

See complete brand names list, page 831.

GENERAL INFORMATION

Habit forming? No
Prescription needed?
U.S.: Low strength—No
High strength—Yes
Canada: No
Available as generic? Yes
Drug class: Sympathomimetic

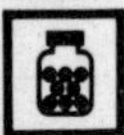

USES

Reduces congestion of nose, sinuses and throat from allergies and infections.

DOSAGE & USAGE INFORMATION

How to take:
- Tablet or capsule—Swallow with liquid. You may chew or crush tablet.
- Extended-release tablets or capsules—Swallow each dose whole.
- Syrup—Take as directed on label.

When to take:
- At the same times each day.
- To prevent insomnia, take last dose of day a few hours before bedtime.

If you forget a dose:
Take up to 2 hours late. If more than 2 hours, wait for next dose (don't double this).

What drug does:
Decreases blood volume in nasal tissues, shrinking tissues and enlarging airways.

Time lapse before drug works:
15 to 20 minutes.

Don't take with:
- See Interaction column and consult doctor.
- Non-prescription drugs with caffeine without consulting doctor.

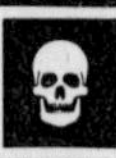

OVERDOSE

Symptoms:
Nervousness, restlessness, headache, rapid or irregular heartbeat, sweating, nausea, vomiting, anxiety, confusion, delirium, muscle tremors.

What to do:
- Dial 0 (operator) or 911 (emergency) for an ambulance or medical help. Then give first aid immediately.
- Additional emergency information on page 886.

POSSIBLE ADVERSE REACTIONS OR SIDE EFFECTS

SYMPTOMS	FREQUENCY	WHAT TO DO
Brain & nervous system:		
• Hallucinations, seizures.	Rare	2
• Agitation, insomnia.	Common	5
• Dizziness, headache, trembling, weakness.	Infrequent	4
Skin, eyes, ears, nose, throat, blood vessels, muscles, bones, joints, kidneys, liver, allergic, blood:	None expected.	
Digestive:		
Nausea or vomiting.	Infrequent	3
Heart & lungs:		
Irregular or slow heartbeat, breathing difficulty, unusually fast or pounding heartbeat.	Infrequent	3
Genital, urinary:		
Difficult or painful urination.	Infrequent	3
Others:		
• Increased sweating.	Infrequent	3
• Paleness	Infrequent	5

1 - Life-threatening. Seek emergency treatment immediately.
2 - Discontinue. Seek emergency treatment.
3 - Discontinue. Call doctor right away.
4 - Continue. Call doctor when convenient.
5 - Continue. Tell doctor at next visit.

WARNINGS & PRECAUTIONS

Don't take if:
You are allergic to any sympathomimetic drug.

Before you start, consult your doctor:
- If you have overactive thyroid or diabetes.
- If you have taken any MAO inhibitors in past 2 weeks.
- If you take digitalis preparations or have high blood pressure or heart disease.
- If you will have surgery within 2 months, including dental surgery, requiring general or spinal anesthesia.
- If you have urination difficulty.

Over age 60:
Adverse reactions and side effects may be more frequent and severe than in younger persons.

Pregnancy:
No proven harm to unborn child. Avoid if possible.

Breast-feeding:
Drug passes into milk. Avoid drug or discontinue nursing until you finish medicine. Consult doctor for advice on maintaining milk supply.

Infants & children:
Keep dose low or avoid.

Prolonged use:
No proven problems.

Skin & sunlight:
No problems expected.

Driving, piloting or hazardous work:
Avoid if you feel dizzy. Otherwise, no problems expected..

Airplane passengers:
Use 30 minutes before departure. Repeat every 4 hours.

Discontinuing:
May be unnecessary to finish medicine. Follow doctor's instructions.

Others:
No problems expected.

INTERACTION WITH OTHER DRUGS

GENERIC NAME OR DRUG CLASS	COMBINED EFFECT
Antidepressants (tricyclic)	Increased pseudoephedrine effect.
Antihypertensives	Decreased antihypertensive effect.
Beta-adrenergic blockers	Decreased effect of beta-adrenergic blockers.
Digitalis preparations	Irregular heartbeat.
Epinephrine	Increased epinephrine effect. Excessive heart stimulation and blood-pressure increase.
Ergot preparations	Serious blood-pressure rise.
Guanethidine	Decreased effect of both drugs.
MAO inhibitors	Increased pseudoephedrine effect.

INTERACTION WITH OTHER SUBSTANCES

INTERACTS WITH	COMBINED EFFECT
Alcohol:	None expected.
Beverages: Caffeine drinks	Nervousness or insomnia.
Cocaine:	Dangerous stimulation. Avoid.
Foods:	None expected.
Marijuana:	Rapid heartbeat.
Tobacco:	None expected.

PSYLLIUM

BRAND NAMES

Effersyllium
Fiberall
Hydrocil
Konsyl
L.A. Formula
Metamucil
Modane Bulk
Mucillium
Mucilose
Naturacil
Plova
Prompt
Regacilium
Reguloid
Saraka
Senokot with Psyllium
Serutan
Siblin
Sof-Cil
Syllact
V-Lax

GENERAL INFORMATION

Habit forming? No
Prescription needed? No
Available as generic? Yes
Drug class: Laxative (bulk-forming)

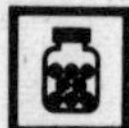

USES

Relieves constipation and prevents straining for bowel movement.

DOSAGE & USAGE INFORMATION

How to take:
Powder, flakes or granules—Dilute dose in 8 oz. cold water or fruit juice.

When to take:
At the same time each day, preferably morning.

If you forget a dose:
Take as soon as you remember. Resume regular schedule.

What drug does:
Absorbs water, stimulating the bowel to form a soft, bulky stool.

Time lapse before drug works:
May require 2 or 3 days to begin, then works in 12 to 24 hours.

Don't take with:
- See Interaction column and consult doctor.
- Don't take within 2 hours of taking another medicine.

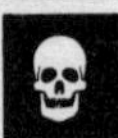

OVERDOSE

Symptoms:
None expected.

What to do:
Overdose unlikely to threaten life. If person takes much larger amount than prescribed, call doctor, poison-control center or hospital emergency room for instructions.

POSSIBLE ADVERSE REACTIONS OR SIDE EFFECTS

SYMPTOMS	FREQUENCY	WHAT TO DO
Brain & nervous system:	None expected.	
Skin: Itch, rash.	Rare	3
Eyes:	None expected.	
Ears, nose, throat: Swallowing difficulty, "lump in throat" sensation.	Infrequent	4
Digestive: Intestinal blockage.	Rare	3
Heart & lungs: Asthma	Rare	3
Blood vessels:	None expected.	
Muscles, bones, joints:	None expected.	
Genital, urinary:	None expected.	
Kidneys:	None expected.	
Liver:	None expected.	
Allergic:	None expected.	
Blood:	None expected.	
Others:	None expected.	

1- Life-threatening. Seek emergency treatment immediately.
2- Discontinue. Seek emergency treatment.
3- Discontinue. Call doctor right away.
4- Continue. Call doctor when convenient.
5- Continue. Tell doctor at next visit.
6- No action necessary.

WARNINGS & PRECAUTIONS

Don't take if:
- You are allergic to any bulk-forming laxative.
- You have symptoms of appendicitis, inflamed bowel or intestinal blockage.
- You have missed a bowel movement for only 1 or 2 days.

Before you start, consult your doctor:
- If you have diabetes.
- If you have kidney disease.
- If you have a laxative habit.
- If you have rectal bleeding.
- If you have difficulty swallowing.
- If you take other laxatives.

Over age 60:
Adverse reactions and side effects may be more frequent and severe than in younger persons.

Pregnancy:
Most bulk-forming laxatives contain sodium or sugars which may cause fluid retention. Avoid if possible.

Breast-feeding:
No problems expected.

Infants & children:
Use only under medical supervision.

Prolonged use:
Don't take for more than 1 week unless under a doctor's supervision. May cause laxative dependence.

Skin & sunlight:
No problems expected.

Driving, piloting or hazardous work:
No problems expected.

Airplane passengers:
No problems expected.

Discontinuing:
May be unnecessary to finish medicine. Follow doctor's instructions.

Others:
Don't take to "flush out" your system, or as a "tonic."

INTERACTION WITH OTHER DRUGS

GENERIC NAME OR DRUG CLASS	COMBINED EFFECT
Antibiotics	Decreased antibiotic effect.
Anticoagulants	Decreased anticoagulant effect.
Digitalis preparations	Decreased digitalis effect.
Salicylates (including aspirin)	Decreased salicylate effect.

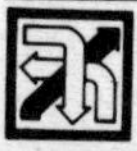

INTERACTION WITH OTHER SUBSTANCES

INTERACTS WITH	COMBINED EFFECT
Alcohol:	None expected.
Beverages:	None expected.
Cocaine:	None expected.
Foods:	None expected.
Marijuana:	None expected.
Tobacco:	None expected.

PYRIDOSTIGMINE

BRAND NAMES

Mestinon
Regonol

GENERAL INFORMATION

Habit forming? No
Prescription needed? Yes
Available as generic? Yes
Drug class: Cholinergic (anticholinesterase)

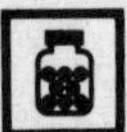

USES

- Treatment of myasthenia gravis.
- Treatment of urinary retention and abdominal distention.
- Antidote to adverse effects of muscle relaxants used in surgery.

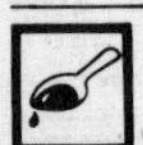

DOSAGE & USAGE INFORMATION

How to take:
- Tablet or syrup—Swallow with liquid or food to lessen stomach irritation.
- Extended-release tablets or capsules—Swallow each dose whole. If you take regular tablets, you may chew or crush them.

When to take:
As directed, usually 3 or 4 times a day.

If you forget a dose:
Take as soon as you remember up to 2 hours late. If more than 2 hours, wait for next scheduled dose (don't double this dose).

What drug does:
Inhibits the chemical activity of an enzyme (cholinesterase) so nerve impulses can cross the junction of nerves and muscles.

Time lapse before drug works:
3 hours.

Don't take with:
See Interaction column and consult doctor.

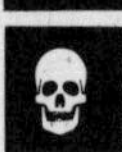

OVERDOSE

Symptoms:
Muscle weakness, cramps, twitching or clumsiness; severe diarrhea, nausea, vomiting, stomach cramps or pain; breathing difficulty; confusion, irritability, nervousness, restlessness, fear; unusually slow heartbeat; seizures.

What to do:
- Dial 0 (operator) or 911 (emergency) for an ambulance or medical help. Then give first aid immediately.
- Additional emergency information on page 886.

POSSIBLE ADVERSE REACTIONS OR SIDE EFFECTS

SYMPTOMS	FREQUENCY	WHAT TO DO
Brain & nervous system:		
Confusion, irritability.	Infrequent	2
Skin:	None expected.	
Eyes:		
Constricted pupils, watery eyes.	Infrequent	4
Ears, nose, throat:		
Excess saliva.	Common	4
Digestive:		
Mild diarrhea, nausea, vomiting, stomach cramps or pain.	Common	3
Heart & lungs:		
Lung congestion.	Infrequent	4
Blood vessels:	None expected.	
Muscles, bones, joints:	None expected.	
Genital, urinary:		
Frequent urge to urinate.	Infrequent	4
Kidneys:	None expected.	
Liver:	None expected.	
Allergic:	None expected.	
Blood:	None expected.	
Others:		
Unusual sweating.	Common	4

1- Life-threatening. Seek emergency treatment immediately.
2- Discontinue. Seek emergency treatment.
3- Discontinue. Call doctor right away.
4- Continue. Call doctor when convenient.
5- Continue. Tell doctor at next visit.
6- No action necessary.

WARNINGS & PRECAUTIONS

Don't take if:
- You are allergic to any cholinergic or bromide.
- You take mecamylamine.

Before you start, consult your doctor:
- If you plan to become pregnant within medication period.
- If you have bronchial asthma.
- If you have heartbeat irregularities.
- If you have urinary obstruction or urinary-tract infection.

Over age 60:
Adverse reactions and side effects may be more frequent and severe than in younger persons.

Pregnancy:
No proven harm to unborn child. Avoid if possible. May increase uterus contractions close to delivery.

Breast-feeding:
No problems expected, but consult doctor.

Infants & children:
Not recommended.

Prolonged use:
Medication may lose effectiveness. Discontinuing for a few days may restore effect.

Skin & sunlight:
No problems expected.

Driving, piloting or hazardous work:
Don't drive or pilot aircraft until you learn how medicine affects you. Don't work around dangerous machinery. Don't climb ladders or work in high places. Danger increases if you drink alcohol or take medicine affecting alertness and reflexes, such as antihistamines, tranquilizers, sedatives, pain medicine, narcotics and mind-altering drugs.

Airplane passengers:
No problems expected.

Discontinuing:
Don't discontinue without doctor's advice until you complete prescribed dose, even though symptoms diminish or disappear.

Others:
No problems expected.

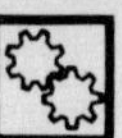

INTERACTION WITH OTHER DRUGS

GENERIC NAME OR DRUG CLASS	COMBINED EFFECT
Anesthetics (local or general)	Decreased pyridostigmine effect.
Antiarrhythmics	Decreased pyridostigmine effect.
Antibiotics	Decreased pyridostigmine effect.
Anticholinergics	Decreased pyridostigmine effect. May mask severe side effects.
Cholinergics (other)	Reduced intestinal-tract function. Possible brain and nervous-system toxicity.
Mecamylamine	Decreased pyridostigmine effect.
Quinidine	Decreased pyridostigmine effect.

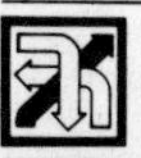

INTERACTION WITH OTHER SUBSTANCES

INTERACTS WITH	COMBINED EFFECT
Alcohol:	No proven problems with small doses.
Beverages:	None expected.
Cocaine:	Decreased pyridostigmine effect. Avoid.
Foods:	None expected.
Marijuana:	No proven problems.
Tobacco:	No proven problems.

PYRIDOXINE (VITAMIN B-6)

BRAND NAMES

Alba-Lybe
Al-Vite
Beelith
Beesix
Bendectin
Eldertonic
Glutofac
Hemo-vite
Herpecin-L
Hexa-Betalin
Hexacrest
Hexavibex
Mega-B
Nu-Iron-V
Pyroxine
Rodex
Tex Six T.R.
Vicon

GENERAL INFORMATION

Habit forming? No
Prescription needed? High strength: Yes
Low strength: No
Available as generic? Yes
Drug class: Vitamin supplement

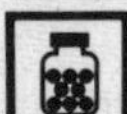

USES

- Prevention and treatment of pyridoxine deficiency.
- Treatment of some forms of anemia.

DOSAGE & USAGE INFORMATION

How to take:
- Tablets—Swallow with liquid.
- Extended-release tablets—Swallow each dose whole with liquid.

When to take:
At the same times each day.

If you forget a dose:
Take as soon as you remember, then resume regular schedule.

What drug does:
Acts as co-enzyme in carbohydrate, protein and fat metabolism.

Time lapse before drug works:
15 to 20 minutes.

Don't take with:
- Levodopa—Small amounts of pyridoxine will nullify levodopa effect. Carbidopa-levodopa combination not affected by this interaction.
- See Interaction column and consult doctor.

OVERDOSE

Symptoms:
None expected.

What to do:
Overdose unlikely to threaten life.

POSSIBLE ADVERSE REACTIONS OR SIDE EFFECTS

SYMPTOMS	FREQUENCY	WHAT TO DO
Brain & nervous system:	None expected.	
Skin:	None expected.	
Eyes:	None expected.	
Ears, nose, throat:	None expected.	
Digestive:	None expected.	
Heart & lungs:	None expected.	
Blood vessels:	None expected.	
Muscles, bones, joints:	None expected.	
Genital, urinary:	None expected.	
Kidneys:	None expected.	
Liver:	None expected.	
Allergic:	None expected.	
Blood:	None expected.	
Others:	None expected.	

1-Life-threatening. Seek emergency treatment immediately.
2-Discontinue. Seek emergency treatment.
3-Discontinue. Call doctor right away.
4-Continue. Call doctor when convenient.
5-Continue. Tell doctor at next visit.
6-No action necessary.

WARNINGS & PRECAUTIONS

Don't take if:
You are allergic to pyridoxine.

Before you start, consult your doctor:
If you are pregnant or breast-feeding.

Over age 60:
No problems expected.

Pregnancy:
Don't exceed recommended dose.

Breast-feeding:
Don't exceed recommended dose.

Infants & children:
Don't exceed recommended dose.

Prolonged use:
Large doses for more than 1 month may cause toxicity.

Skin & sunlight:
No problems expected.

Driving, piloting or hazardous work:
No problems expected.

Airplane passengers:
No problems expected.

Discontinuing:
No problems expected.

Others:
Regular pyridoxine supplements recommended if you take chloramphenicol, cycloserine, ethionamide, hydralazine, immunosuppressants, isoniazid or penicillamine. These decrease pyridoxine absorption and can cause anemia or tingling and numbness in hands and feet.

INTERACTION WITH OTHER DRUGS

GENERIC NAME OR DRUG CLASS	COMBINED EFFECT
Chloramphenicol	Decreased pyridoxine effect.
Contraceptives (oral)	Decreased pyridoxine effect.
Cycloserine	Decreased pyridoxine effect.
Ethionamide	Decreased pyridoxine effect.
Hydralazine	Decreased pyridoxine effect.
Immunosuppressants	Decreased pyridoxine effect.
Isoniazid	Decreased pyridoxine effect.
Penicillamine	Decreased pyridoxine effect.
Levodopa	Decreased levodopa effect.

INTERACTION WITH OTHER SUBSTANCES

INTERACTS WITH	COMBINED EFFECT
Alcohol:	None expected.
Beverages:	None expected.
Cocaine:	None expected.
Foods:	None expected.
Marijuana:	None expected.
Tobacco:	May decrease pyridoxine absorption. Decreased pyridoxine effect.

PYRILAMINE

BRAND NAMES

Allertoc
Allerstat
Covanamine
Dormarex
Duphrene
Histalet Forte
Napril Plateau
Panadyl
Relemine
Rynatan
Somnicaps
Triaminic
Trihista-Phen-25
Tussanil

See complete brand names list, page 831.

GENERAL INFORMATION

Habit forming? No
Prescription needed? No
Available as generic? Yes
Drug class: Antihistamine

USES

- Reduces allergic symptoms such as hay fever, hives, rash or itching.
- Prevents motion sickness, nausea, vomiting.
- Induces sleep.

DOSAGE & USAGE INFORMATION

How to take:
Tablet or capsule—Swallow with liquid or food to lessen stomach irritation.

When to take:
Varies with form. Follow label directions.

If you forget a dose:
Take as soon as you remember up to 2 hours late. If more than 2 hours, wait for next scheduled dose (don't double this dose).

What drug does:
Blocks action of histamine after an allergic response triggers histamine release in sensitive cells.

Time lapse before drug works:
30 minutes.

Don't take with:
See Interaction column and consult doctor.

OVERDOSE

Symptoms:
Convulsions, red face, hallucinations, coma.

What to do:
- Dial 0 (operator) or 911 (emergency) for an ambulance or medical help. Then give first aid immediately.
- If patient is unconscious and not breathing, give mouth-to-mouth breathing. If there is no heartbeat, use cardiac massage and mouth-to-mouth breathing (CPR). Don't try to make patient vomit. If you can't get help quickly, take patient to nearest emergency facility.
- Additional emergency information on page 886.

POSSIBLE ADVERSE REACTIONS OR SIDE EFFECTS

SYMPTOMS	FREQUENCY	WHAT TO DO
Brain & nervous system:		
• Nightmares, agitation, irritability.	Rare	3
• Drowsiness, dizziness.	Common	5
Skin:	None expected.	
Eyes:		
• Vision changes.	Infrequent	3
• Less tolerance for contact lenses.	Infrequent	4
Ears, nose, throat:		
• Sore throat, fever.	Rare	3
• Dry mouth, nose, throat.	Common	5
Digestive:		
• Nausea	Common	5
• Appetite loss.	Infrequent	5
Heart & lungs:		
Rapid heartbeat.	Rare	3
Blood vessels:		
Unusual bleeding or bruising.	Rare	3
Muscles, bones, joints, kidneys, liver, allergic, blood:	None expected.	
Genital, urinary:		
Urination difficulty.	Infrequent	4
Others:		
Fatigue, weakness.	Rare	3

1-Life-threatening. Seek emergency treatment immediately.
2-Discontinue. Seek emergency treatment.
3-Discontinue. Call doctor right away.
4-Continue. Call doctor when convenient.
5-Continue. Tell doctor at next visit.
6-No action necessary.

WARNINGS & PRECAUTIONS

Don't take if:
You are allergic to any antihistamine.

Before you start, consult your doctor:
- If you have glaucoma.
- If you have enlarged prostate.
- If you have asthma.
- If you have kidney disease.
- If you have peptic ulcer.
- If you will have surgery within 2 months, including dental surgery, requiring general or spinal anesthesia.

Over age 60:
Don't exceed recommended dose. Adverse reactions and side effects may be more frequent and severe than in younger persons, especially urination difficulty, diminished alertness and other brain and nervous-system symptoms.

Pregnancy:
No proven harm to unborn child. Avoid if possible.

Breast-feeding:
Drug passes into milk. Avoid drug or discontinue nursing until you finish medicine. Consult doctor for advice on maintaining milk supply.

Infants & children:
Not recommended for premature or newborn infants. Otherwise, no problems expected.

Prolonged use:
Avoid. May damage bone marrow and nerve cells.

Skin & sunlight:
May cause rash or intensify sunburn in areas exposed to sun or sunlamp.

Driving, piloting or hazardous work:
Don't drive or pilot aircraft until you learn how medicine affects you. Don't work around dangerous machinery. Don't climb ladders or work in high places. Danger increases if you drink alcohol or take medicine affecting alertness and reflexes, such as antihistamines, tranquilizers, sedatives, pain medicine, narcotics and mind-altering drugs.

Airplane passengers:
No problems expected.

Discontinuing:
No problems expected.

Others:
May mask symptoms of hearing damage from aspirin, other salicylates, cisplatin, paromomycin, vancomycin or anticonvulsants. Consult doctor if you use these.

INTERACTION WITH OTHER DRUGS

GENERIC NAME OR DRUG CLASS	COMBINED EFFECT
Anticholinergics	Increased anticholinergic effect.
Antidepressants	Excess sedation. Avoid.
Antihistamines (other)	Excess sedation. Avoid.
Hypnotics	Excess sedation. Avoid.
MAO inhibitors	Increased pyrilamine effect.
Mind-altering drugs	Excess sedation. Avoid.
Narcotics	Excess sedation. Avoid.
Sedatives	Excess sedation. Avoid.
Sleep inducers	Excess sedation. Avoid.
Tranquilizers	Excess sedation. Avoid.

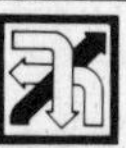

INTERACTION WITH OTHER SUBSTANCES

INTERACTS WITH	COMBINED EFFECT
Alcohol:	Excess sedation. Avoid.
Beverages:	
Caffeine drinks	Less pyrilamine sedation.
Cocaine:	Decreased pyrilamine effect. Avoid.
Foods:	None expected.
Marijuana:	Excess sedation. Avoid.
Tobacco:	None expected.

PYRVINIUM

BRAND NAMES

Pamovin
Povan
Pyr-pam
Vanquin

GENERAL INFORMATION

Habit forming? No
Prescription needed? Yes
Available as generic? No
Drug class: Antihelminthic (antiworm medication)

USES

Treatment for pinworm infestation.

DOSAGE & USAGE INFORMATION

How to take:
- Tablet—Swallow whole with food or liquid. Don't crush or chew tablet.
- Liquid—Take with food or liquid.

When to take:
According to label instructions. Usually a single dose, which may be repeated in 2 or 3 weeks.

If you forget a dose:
Take when remembered.

What drug does:
Interferes with a metabolic process in the infecting parasite and kills it.

Time lapse before drug works:
12 hours.

Don't take with:
Non-prescription drugs for pinworms.

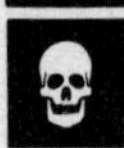

OVERDOSE

Symptoms:
Increased severity of adverse reactions and side effects.

What to do:
Overdose unlikely to threaten life. If person takes much larger amount than prescribed, call doctor, poison-control center or hospital emergency room for instructions.

POSSIBLE ADVERSE REACTIONS OR SIDE EFFECTS

SYMPTOMS	FREQUENCY	WHAT TO DO
Brain & nervous system:		
Dizziness	Rare	4
Skin:		
Rash	Rare	3
Eyes:	None expected.	
Ears, nose, throat:	None expected.	
Digestive:		
Stomach cramps, nausea, vomiting.	Rare	4
Heart & lungs:	None expected.	
Blood vessels:	None expected.	
Muscles, bones, joints:	None expected.	
Genital, urinary:	None expected.	
Kidneys:	None expected.	
Liver:	None expected.	
Allergic:	None expected.	
Blood:	None expected.	
Others:	None expected.	

1- Life-threatening. Seek emergency treatment immediately.
2- Discontinue. Seek emergency treatment.
3- Discontinue. Call doctor right away.
4- Continue. Call doctor when convenient.
5- Continue. Tell doctor at next visit.
6- No action necessary.

WARNINGS & PRECAUTIONS

Don't take if:
You are allergic to any antihelminthic drug.

Before you start, consult your doctor:
- If you have kidney or liver disease.
- If you have a bowel disease or inflammation.

Over age 60:
Adverse reactions and side effects may be more frequent and severe than in younger persons.

Pregnancy:
No proven harm to unborn child. Avoid if possible.

Breast-feeding:
No problems expected, but consult doctor.

Infants & children:
No problems expected.

Prolonged use:
Not recommended.

Skin & sunlight:
May cause rash or intensify sunburn in areas exposed to sun or sunlamp.

Driving, piloting or hazardous work:
Avoid if you feel dizzy. Otherwise, no problems expected.

Airplane passengers:
No problems expected.

Discontinuing:
Don't discontinue without doctor's advice until you complete prescribed dose, even though symptoms diminish or disappear.

Others:
- This medicine is a dye that permanently stains most materials. Teeth will be stained a few days. Stool and vomit may be red.
- Pinworm infestations are highly contagious. All family members should be treated at the same time.

INTERACTION WITH OTHER DRUGS

GENERIC NAME OR DRUG CLASS	COMBINED EFFECT
None	

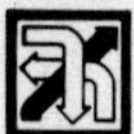

INTERACTION WITH OTHER SUBSTANCES

INTERACTS WITH	COMBINED EFFECT
Alcohol:	None expected.
Beverages:	None expected.
Cocaine:	None expected.
Foods:	None expected.
Marijuana:	None expected.
Tobacco:	None expected.

QUINESTROL

BRAND NAMES

Estrovis

GENERAL INFORMATION

Habit forming? No
Prescription needed? Yes
Available as generic? Yes
Drug class: Female sex hormone (estrogen)

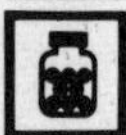

USES

- Treatment for symptoms of menopause and menstrual-cycle irregularity.
- Replacement for female hormone deficiency.

DOSAGE & USAGE INFORMATION

How to take:
Tablet—Swallow with liquid. If you can't swallow whole, crumble tablet and take with liquid or food.

When to take:
At the same time each day.

If you forget a dose:
Take as soon as you remember up to 12 hours late. If more than 12 hours, wait for next scheduled dose (don't double this dose).

What drug does:
Restores normal estrogen level in tissues.

Time lapse before drug works:
10 to 20 days.

Don't take with:
See Interaction column and consult doctor.

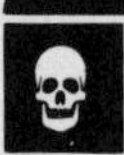

OVERDOSE

Symptoms:
Nausea, vomiting, fluid retention, breast enlargement and discomfort, abnormal vaginal bleeding.

What to do:
Overdose unlikely to threaten life. If person takes much larger amount than prescribed, call doctor, poison-control center or hospital emergency room for instructions.

POSSIBLE ADVERSE REACTIONS OR SIDE EFFECTS

SYMPTOMS	FREQUENCY	WHAT TO DO
Brain & nervous system:		
Depression, dizziness, irritability.	Infrequent	4
Skin:		
• Rash	Infrequent	3
• Brown blotches.	Infrequent	5
• Hair loss.	Infrequent	5
Eyes, ears, nose, throat, heart & lungs, muscles, bones, joints, kidneys, allergic, blood:	None expected.	
Digestive:		
• Stomach or side pain.	Infrequent	3
• Stomach cramps.	Common	3
• Appetite loss.	Common	4
• Nausea, diarrhea.	Common	5
• Vomiting	Infrequent	4
Blood vessels:		
Swollen ankles, feet.	Common	5
Genital, urinary:		
Vaginal discharge or bleeding.	Infrequent	5
Liver:		
Jaundice (yellow skin and eyes).	Rare	3
Others:		
• Breast lumps.	Infrequent	4
• Swollen, tender breasts.	Common	5
• Changes in sex drive.	Infrequent	5

1- Life-threatening. Seek emergency treatment immediately.
2- Discontinue. Seek emergency treatment.
3- Discontinue. Call doctor right away.
4- Continue. Call doctor when convenient.
5- Continue. Tell doctor at next visit.

WARNINGS & PRECAUTIONS

Don't take if:
- You are allergic to any estrogen-containing drugs.
- You have impaired liver function.
- You have had blood clots, stroke or heart attack.
- You have unexplained vaginal bleeding.

Before you start, consult your doctor:
- If you have had cancer of breast or reproductive organs, fibrocystic breast disease, fibroid tumors of the uterus or endometriosis.
- If you have had migraine headaches, epilepsy or porphyria.
- If you have diabetes, high blood pressure, asthma, congestive heart failure, kidney disease or gallstones.
- If you plan to become pregnant within 3 months.

Over age 60:
Controversial. You and your doctor must decide if drug risks outweigh benefits.

Pregnancy:
Risk to unborn child outweighs drug benefits. Don't use.

Breast-feeding:
Drug filters into milk. May harm child. Avoid.

Infants & children:
Not recommended.

Prolonged use:
Increased growth of fibroid tumors of uterus. Possible association with cancer of uterus.

Skin & sunlight:
May cause rash or intensify sunburn in areas exposed to sun or sunlamp.

Driving, piloting or hazardous work:
No problems expected.

Airplane passengers:
No problems expected.

Discontinuing:
You may need to discontinue quinestrol periodically. Consult your doctor.

Others:
In rare instances, may cause blood clot in lung, brain or leg. Symptoms are *sudden* severe headache, coordination loss, vision change, chest pain, breathing difficulty, slurred speech, pain in legs or groin. Seek emergency treatment immediately.

INTERACTION WITH OTHER DRUGS

GENERIC NAME OR DRUG CLASS	COMBINED EFFECT
Anticoagulants (oral)	Decreased anticoagulant effect.
Anticonvulsants (hydantoin)	Increased seizures.
Antidiabetics (oral)	Unpredictable increase or decrease in blood sugar.
Clofibrate	Decreased clofibrate effect.
Carbamazepine	Increased seizures.
Meprobamate	Increased quinestrol effect.
Phenobarbital	Decreased quinestrol effect.
Primidone	Decreased quinestrol effect.
Rifampin	Decreased quinestrol effect.
Thyroid hormones	Decreased thyroid effect.

INTERACTION WITH OTHER SUBSTANCES

INTERACTS WITH	COMBINED EFFECT
Alcohol:	None expected.
Beverages:	None expected.
Cocaine:	No proven problems.
Foods:	None expected.
Marijuana:	Possible menstrual irregularities and bleeding between periods.
Tobacco:	Increased risk of blood clots leading to stroke or heart attack.

QUINETHAZONE

BRAND NAMES

Aquamox
Hydromox

GENERAL INFORMATION

Habit forming? No
Prescription needed? Yes
Available as generic? Yes
Drug class: Antihypertensive, diuretic (thiazide)

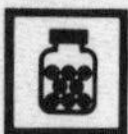

USES

- Controls, but doesn't cure, high blood pressure.
- Reduces fluid retention (edema) caused by conditions such as heart disorders and liver disease.

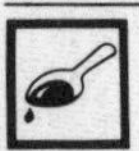

DOSAGE & USAGE INFORMATION

How to take:
Tablet or capsule—Swallow with liquid. If you can't swallow whole, crumble tablet or open capsule and take with liquid or food. Don't exceed dose.

When to take:
At the same time each day.

If you forget a dose:
Take as soon as you remember up to 2 hours late. If more than 2 hours, wait for next scheduled dose (don't double this dose).

What drug does:
- Forces sodium and water excretion, reducing body fluid.
- Relaxes muscle cells of small arteries.
- Reduced body fluid and relaxed arteries lower blood pressure.

Time lapse before drug works:
4 to 6 hours. May require several weeks to lower blood pressure.

Don't take with:
- See Interaction column and consult doctor.
- Non-prescription drugs without consulting doctor.

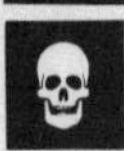

OVERDOSE

Symptoms:
Cramps, weakness, drowsiness, weak pulse, coma.

What to do:
- Dial 0 (operator) or 911 (emergency) for an ambulance or medical help. Then give first aid immediately.
- Additional emergency information on page 886.

POSSIBLE ADVERSE REACTIONS OR SIDE EFFECTS

SYMPTOMS	FREQUENCY	WHAT TO DO
Brain & nervous system:		
• Dizziness	Infrequent	4
• Mood changes.	Infrequent	4
• Headaches	Infrequent	4
Skin:		
Rash or hives.	Rare	2
Eyes:		
Blurred vision.	Infrequent	3
Ears, nose, throat:		
• Sore throat, fever.	Rare	3
• Dry mouth, thirst.	Infrequent	5
Digestive:		
Severe abdominal pain, nausea, vomiting.	Infrequent	3
Heart & lungs:		
Irregular heartbeat, weak pulse.	Infrequent	3
Blood vessels:	None expected.	
Muscles, bones, joints:		
Weakness, tiredness.	Infrequent	4
Genital, urinary:	None expected.	
Kidneys:	None expected.	
Liver:		
Jaundice (yellow skin and eyes).	Rare	3
Allergic:	None expected.	
Blood:	None expected.	
Others:		
Weight changes.	Infrequent	4

1 - Life-threatening. Seek emergency treatment immediately.
2 - Discontinue. Seek emergency treatment.
3 - Discontinue. Call doctor right away.
4 - Continue. Call doctor when convenient.
5 - Continue. Tell doctor at next visit.
6 - No action necessary.

WARNINGS & PRECAUTIONS

Don't take if:
You are allergic to any thiazide diuretic drug.

Before you start, consult your doctor:
- If you are allergic to any sulfa drug.
- If you have gout.
- If you have liver, pancreas or liver disorder.

Over age 60:
Adverse reactions and side effects may be more frequent and severe than in younger persons, especially dizziness and excessive potassium loss.

Pregnancy:
Risk to unborn child outweighs drug benefits. Don't use.

Breast-feeding:
Drug passes into milk. Avoid drug or discontinue nursing.

Infants & children:
No problems expected.

Prolonged use:
You may need medicine to treat high blood pressure for the rest of your life.

Skin & sunlight:
May cause rash or intensify sunburn in areas exposed to sun or sunlamp.

Driving, piloting or hazardous work:
Don't drive or pilot aircraft until you learn how medicine affects you. Don't work around dangerous machinery. Don't climb ladders or work in high places. Danger increases if you drink alcohol or take medicine affecting alertness and reflexes, such as antihistamines, tranquilizers, sedatives, pain medicine, narcotics and mind-altering drugs.

Airplane passengers:
No problems expected.

Discontinuing:
Don't discontinue without medical advice.

Others:
- Hot weather and fever may cause dehydration and drop in blood pressure. Dose may require temporary adjustment. Weigh daily and report any unexpected weight decreases to your doctor.
- May cause rise in uric acid, leading to gout.
- May cause blood-sugar rise in diabetics.

INTERACTION WITH OTHER DRUGS

GENERIC NAME OR DRUG CLASS	COMBINED EFFECT
Allopurinol	Decreased allopurinol effect.
Antidepressants (tricyclic)	Dangerous drop in blood pressure. Avoid combination unless under medical supervision.
Barbiturates	Increased quinethazone effect.
Cholestyramine	Decreased quinethazone effect.
Cortisone drugs	Excessive potassium loss that causes dangerous heart rhythms.
Digitalis preparations	Excessive potassium loss that causes dangerous heart rhythms.
Diuretics (thiazide)	Increased effect of other thiazide diuretics.
Lithium	Increased effect of lithium.
MAO inhibitors	Increased quinethazone effect.
Probenecid	Decreased probenecid effect.

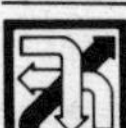

INTERACTION WITH OTHER SUBSTANCES

INTERACTS WITH	COMBINED EFFECT
Alcohol:	Dangerous blood-pressure drop.
Beverages:	None expected.
Cocaine:	None expected.
Foods:	
Licorice	Excessive potassium loss that causes dangerous heart rhythms.
Marijuana:	May increase blood pressure.
Tobacco:	None expected.

QUINIDINE

BRAND NAMES

Apo-Quinidine
Biquin Durules
Cardioquin
Cin-Quin
Duraquin
Novoquinidin
Quinaglute Dura-Tabs
Quinate
Quinidex Extentabs
Quinobarb
Quinora
SK-Quinidine Sulfate

GENERAL INFORMATION

Habit forming? No
Prescription needed? U.S.: Yes, Canada: No
Available as generic? Yes
Drug class: Antiarrhythmic

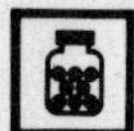

USES

Corrects heart-rhythm disorders.

DOSAGE & USAGE INFORMATION

How to take:

- Tablet or capsule—Swallow liquid or with food to lessen stomach irritation.
- Extended-release tablets or capsules—Swallow each dose whole. If you take regular tablets, you may chew or crush them.

When to take:
At the same times each day.

If you forget a dose:
Take as soon as you remember up to 2 hours late. If more than 2 hours, wait for next scheduled dose (don't double this dose).

What drug does:
Delays nerve impulses to the heart to regulate heartbeat.

Time lapse before drug works:
2 to 4 hours.

Don't take with:
See Interaction column and consult doctor.

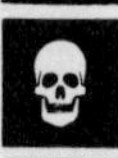

OVERDOSE

Symptoms:
Confusion, severe blood-pressure drop, breathing difficulty, fainting.

What to do:

- Dial 0 (operator) or 911 (emergency) for an ambulance or medical help. Then give first aid immediately.
- If patient is unconscious and not breathing, give mouth-to-mouth breathing. If there is no heartbeat, use cardiac massage and mouth-to-mouth breathing (CPR). Don't try to make patient vomit. If you can't get help quickly, take patient to nearest emergency facility.
- Additional emergency information on page 886.

POSSIBLE ADVERSE REACTIONS OR SIDE EFFECTS

SYMPTOMS	FREQUENCY	WHAT TO DO
Brain & nervous system:		
Dizziness, lightheadedness, fainting, headache, confusion.	Infrequent	3
Skin:		
Rash	Infrequent	3
Eyes:		
Vision changes.	Infrequent	3
Ears, nose, throat:		
Ringing in ears.	Infrequent	4
Digestive:		
Bitter taste, diarrhea, nausea, vomiting.	Common	3
Heart & lungs:		
Breathing difficulty, rapid heartbeat.	Infrequent	3
Blood vessels:		
Unusual bleeding or bruising.	Rare	3
Muscles, bones, joints:	None expected.	
Genital, urinary:	None expected.	
Kidneys:	None expected.	
Liver:	None expected.	
Allergic:	None expected.	
Blood:	None expected.	
Others:		
Weakness	Rare	4

1- Life-threatening. Seek emergency treatment immediately.
2- Discontinue. Seek emergency treatment.
3- Discontinue. Call doctor right away.
4- Continue. Call doctor when convenient.
5- Continue. Tell doctor at next visit.
6- No action necessary.

WARNINGS & PRECAUTIONS

Don't take if:
- You are allergic to quinidine.
- You have an active infection.

Before you start, consult your doctor:
About any drug you take, including non-prescription drugs.

Over age 60:
Adverse reactions and side effects may be more frequent and severe than in younger persons.

Pregnancy:
Risk to unborn child outweighs drug benefits. Don't use.

Breast-feeding:
Drug filters into milk. May harm child. Avoid.

Infants & children:
No problems expected.

Prolonged use:
No problems expected.

Skin & sunlight:
No problems expected.

Driving, piloting or hazardous work:
Don't drive or pilot aircraft until you learn how medicine affects you. Don't work around dangerous machinery. Don't climb ladders or work in high places. Danger increases if you drink alcohol or take medicine affecting alertness and reflexes, such as antihistamines, tranquilizers, sedatives, pain medicine, narcotics and mind-altering drugs.

Airplane passengers:
No problems expected.

Discontinuing:
Don't discontinue without doctor's advice until you complete prescribed dose, even though symptoms diminish or disappear.

Others:
No problems expected.

INTERACTION WITH OTHER DRUGS

GENERIC NAME OR DRUG CLASS	COMBINED EFFECT
Anticholinergics	Increased anticholinergic effect.
Anticoagulants	Increased anticoagulant effect.
Antihypertensives	Increased antihypertensive effect.
Cholinergics	Decreased cholinergic effect.
Digitalis preparations	Slows heartbeat excessively.
Phenytoin	Increased quinidine effect.
Propranolol	Slows heartbeat excessively.
Pyrimethamine	Increased quinidine effect.
Rauwolfia alkaloids	Seriously disturbs heart rhythms.

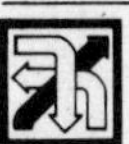

INTERACTION WITH OTHER SUBSTANCES

INTERACTS WITH	COMBINED EFFECT
Alcohol:	None expected.
Beverages:	
Caffeine drinks	Causes rapid heartbeat. Use sparingly.
Cocaine:	Irregular heartbeat. Avoid.
Foods:	None expected.
Marijuana:	Can cause fainting.
Tobacco:	Irregular heartbeat. Avoid.

QUININE

BRAND NAMES

Coco-Quinine
Kinine
NovoQuinie
Quinamm
Quindan
Quine
Quinite
Streme

GENERAL INFORMATION

Habit forming? No
Prescription needed? High strength: Yes
Low strength: No
Available as generic? Yes
Drug class: Antiprotozoal

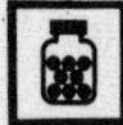

USES

- Treatment or prevention of malaria.
- Relief of muscle cramps

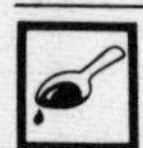

DOSAGE & USAGE INFORMATION

How to take:
Liquid, tablet or capsule—Swallow with liquid or food to lessen stomach irritation.

When to take:
- Prevention—At the same time each day, usually at bedtime.
- Treatment—At the same times each day in evenly spaced doses.

If you forget a dose:
- Prevention—Take as soon as you remember up to 12 hours late. If more than 12 hours, wait for next scheduled dose (don't double this dose).
- Treatment—Take as soon as you remember up to 2 hours late. If more than 2 hours, wait for next scheduled dose (don't double this dose).

What drug does:
- Reduces contractions of skeletal muscles.
- Increases blood flow.
- Interferes with genes in malaria microorganisms.

Time lapse before drug works:
May require several days or weeks for maximum effect.

Don't take with:
See Interaction column and consult doctor.

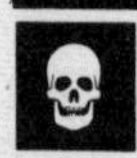

OVERDOSE

Symptoms:
Severe impairment of vision and hearing; severe nausea, vomiting, diarrhea; shallow breathing, fast heartbeat; apprehension, confusion, delirium.

What to do:
Dial 0 (operator) or 911 (emergency) for an ambulance or medical help. Then give first aid immediately.

POSSIBLE ADVERSE REACTIONS OR SIDE EFFECTS

SYMPTOMS	FREQUENCY	WHAT TO DO
Brain & nervous system: Dizziness, headache.	Common	4
Skin: Rash, hives, itch.	Infrequent	3
Eyes: Blurred or changed vision.	Common	3
Ears, nose, throat: • Ringing or buzzing in ears, impaired hearing.	Common	5
• Sore throat, fever.	Rare	3
Digestive: Stomach discomfort, mild nausea, vomiting, diarrhea.	Common	4
Heart & lungs: Breathing difficulty.	Infrequent	3
Blood vessels: Unusual bleeding or bruising.	Rare	3
Muscles, bones, joints: Unusual tiredness or weakness.	Rare	3
Genital, urinary:	None expected.	
Kidneys:	None expected.	
Liver:	None expected.	
Allergic:	None expected.	
Blood:	None expected.	
Others:	None expected.	

1- Life-threatening. Seek emergency treatment immediately.
2- Discontinue. Seek emergency treatment.
3- Discontinue. Call doctor right away.
4- Continue. Call doctor when convenient.
5- Continue. Tell doctor at next visit.
6- No action necessary.

WARNINGS & PRECAUTIONS

Don't take if:
You are allergic to quinine or quinidine.

Before you start, consult your doctor:
- If you plan to become pregnant within medication period.
- If you have asthma.
- If you have eye disease, hearing problems or ringing in the ears.
- If you have heart disease.
- If you have myasthenia gravis.

Over age 60:
Adverse reactions and side effects may be more frequent and severe than in younger persons.

Pregnancy:
Risk to unborn child outweighs drug benefits. Don't use.

Breast-feeding:
Drug filters into milk. May harm child. Avoid.

Infants & children:
Use only under medical supervision.

Prolonged use:
May develop headache, blurred vision, nausea, temporary hearing loss, but seldom need to discontinue because of these symptoms.

Skin & sunlight:
No problems expected.

Driving, piloting or hazardous work:
Avoid if you feel dizzy or have blurred vision. Otherwise, no problems expected.

Airplane passengers:
No problems expected.

Discontinuing:
Don't discontinue without doctor's advice until you complete prescribed dose, even though symptoms diminish or disappear.

Others:
Don't confuse with quinidine, a medicine for heart-rhythm problems.

INTERACTION WITH OTHER DRUGS

GENERIC NAME OR DRUG CLASS	COMBINED EFFECT
Antacids (with aluminum hydroxide)	Decreased quinine effect.
Anticoagulants	Increased anticoagulant effect.
Quinidine	Possible toxic effects of quinine.
Sodium bicarbonate	Possible toxic effects of quinine.

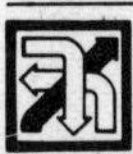

INTERACTION WITH OTHER SUBSTANCES

INTERACTS WITH	COMBINED EFFECT
Alcohol:	No proven problems.
Beverages:	None expected.
Cocaine:	No proven problems.
Foods:	None expected.
Marijuana:	No proven problems.
Tobacco:	None expected.

RANITIDINE

BRAND NAMES

Zantac

GENERAL INFORMATION

Habit forming? No
Prescription needed? Yes
Available as generic? No
Drug class: Histamine H2 antagonist

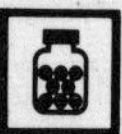

USES

- Treatment for duodenal ulcer.
- Decreases acid in stomach.

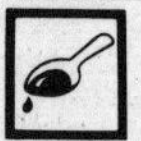

DOSAGE & USAGE INFORMATION

How to take:
Tablets—Swallow with liquid.

When to take:
At same times each day.

If you forget a dose:
Take as soon as you remember up to 2 hours late. If more than 2 hours, wait for next scheduled dose (don't double this dose).

What drug does:
Decreases stomach-acid production.

Time lapse before drug works:
2 to 3 hours.

Don't take with:
- Alcohol
- See Interaction column and consult doctor.

OVERDOSE

Symptoms:
Muscular tremors, vomiting, rapid breathing, coma.

What to do:
- Dial 0 (operator) or 911 (emergency) for an ambulance or medical help. Then give first aid immediately.
- If patient is unconscious and not breathing, give mouth-to-mouth breathing. If there is no heartbeat, use cardiac massage and mouth-to-mouth breathing (CPR). Don't try to make patient vomit. If you can't get help quickly, take patient to nearest emergency facility.
- Additional emergency information on page 886.

POSSIBLE ADVERSE REACTIONS OR SIDE EFFECTS

SYMPTOMS	FREQUENCY	WHAT TO DO
Brain & nervous system: Headache, dizziness.	Infrequent	4
Skin: Rash	Infrequent	3
Eyes:	None expected.	
Ears, nose, throat:	None expected.	
Digestive: Constipation, abdominal pain, nausea.	Infrequent	4
Heart & lungs:	None expected.	
Blood vessels:	None expected.	
Muscles, bones, joints:	None expected.	
Genital, urinary:	None expected.	
Kidneys:	None expected.	
Liver: Jaundice (yellow skin and eyes).	Rare	3
Allergic:	None expected.	
Blood:	None expected.	
Others:	None expected.	

1- Life-threatening. Seek emergency treatment immediately.
2- Discontinue. Seek emergency treatment.
3- Discontinue. Call doctor right away.
4- Continue. Call doctor when convenient.
5- Continue. Tell doctor at next visit.
6- No action necessary.

WARNINGS & PRECAUTIONS

Don't take if:
You are allergic to any histamine H2 antagonist.

Before you start, consult your doctor:
If you have kidney disease.

Over age 60:
Adverse reactions and side effects may be more frequent and severe than in younger persons.

Pregnancy:
No proven harm to unborn child. Avoid if possible.

Breast-feeding:
Drug passes into milk. Avoid drug or discontinue nursing until you finish medicine. Consult doctor for advice on maintaining milk supply.

Infants & children:
Not recommended.

Prolonged use:
Not recommended. Use for short term only.

Skin & sunlight:
No problems expected.

Driving, piloting or hazardous work:
Avoid if you feel dizzy. Otherwise, no problems expected.

Airplane passengers:
No problems expected.

Discontinuing:
Don't discontinue without consulting doctor until you finish prescribed dose, even though symptoms diminish or disappear.

Others:
No problems expected.

INTERACTION WITH OTHER DRUGS

GENERIC NAME OR DRUG CLASS	COMBINED EFFECT
Antacids	Decreased absorption of ranitidine if taken simultaneously.
Ketoconazole	Decreased absorption of ranitidine.

INTERACTION WITH OTHER SUBSTANCES

INTERACTS WITH	COMBINED EFFECT
Alcohol:	Decreased ranitidine effect.
Beverages:	None expected.
Cocaine:	No proven problems.
Foods:	None expected.
Marijuana:	No proven problems.
Tobacco:	Decreased ranitidine effect.

RAUWOLFIA ALKALOIDS

BRAND AND GENERIC NAMES

Alkarau	**Metatensin**	**Reserpoid**
Broserpine	**Naquival**	**Sandril**
Dralserp	**Oreticyl**	**Serpasil**
Harmonyl-D	**Rau-Sed**	

See complete brand and generic names list, page 831.

GENERAL INFORMATION

Habit forming? No
Prescription needed? Yes
Available as generic? Yes
Drug class: Antihypertensive, tranquilizer (rauwolfia alkaloid)

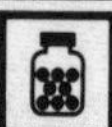

USES

- Treatment for high blood pressure.
- Tranquilizer for mental and emotional disturbances.

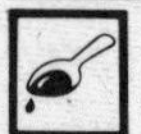

DOSAGE & USAGE INFORMATION

How to take:
Tablet—Swallow with liquid or food to lessen stomach irritation. If you can't swallow whole, crumble tablet and take with liquid or food.

When to take:
At the same times each day.

If you forget a dose:
Take as soon as you remember up to 2 hours late. If more than 2 hours, wait for next scheduled dose (don't double this dose).

What drug does:
- Interferes with nerve impulses and relaxes blood-vessel muscles, reducing blood pressure.
- Suppresses brain centers that control emotions.

Time lapse before drug works:
3 weeks continual use required to determine effectiveness.

Don't take with:
See Interaction column and consult doctor.

OVERDOSE

Symptoms:
Drowsiness; slow, weak pulse; slow, shallow breathing; diarrhea; coma; flush; low body temperature.

What to do:
- Dial 0 (operator) or 911 (emergency) for an ambulance or medical help. Then give first aid immediately.
- Additional emergency information on page 886.

POSSIBLE ADVERSE REACTIONS OR SIDE EFFECTS

SYMPTOMS	FREQUENCY	WHAT TO DO
Brain & nervous system:		
• Trembling hands.	Infrequent	4
• Headache, drowsiness or faintness, lethargy.	Common	5
• Depression	Common	4
Skin:		
Rash or itch.	Rare	3
Eyes:		
Redness	Common	5
Ears, nose, throat:		
• Sore throat, fever.	Rare	3
• Stuffy nose.	Common	5
Digestive:		
• Stomach pain, nausea, vomiting.	Rare	3
• Black stool, bloody vomit.	Infrequent	3
Heart & lungs:		
Chest pain, shortness of breath, irregular or slow heartbeat.	Infrequent	3
Blood vessels:		
Unusual bleeding or bruising.	Rare	3
Muscles, bones, joints:		
Stiffness	Infrequent	3
Genital, urinary:		
• Painful urination.	Rare	4
• Impotence, lower sex drive.	Common	5
Kidneys, allergic, blood, others:	None expected.	
Liver:		
Jaundice (yellow skin and eyes).	Rare	3

1- Life-threatening. Seek emergency treatment immediately.
2- Discontinue. Seek emergency treatment.
3- Discontinue. Call doctor right away.
4- Continue. Call doctor when convenient.
5- Continue. Tell doctor at next visit.

WARNINGS & PRECAUTIONS

Don't take if:

- You are allergic to any rauwolfia alkaloid.
- You are depressed.
- You have active peptic ulcer.
- You have ulcerative colitis.

Before you start, consult your doctor:

- If you have been depressed.
- If you have had peptic ulcer, ulcerative colitis or gallstones.
- If you have epilepsy.
- If you will have surgery within 2 months, including dental surgery, requiring general or spinal anesthesia.

Over age 60:
Adverse reactions and side effects may be more frequent and severe than in younger persons.

Pregnancy:
Studies inconclusive on harm to unborn child. Animal studies show fetal abnormalities. Decide with your doctor whether drug benefits justify risk to unborn child.

Breast-feeding:
Drug passes into milk. Avoid drug or discontinue nursing until you finish medicine. Consult doctor for advice on maintaining milk supply.

Infants & children:
Not recommended.

Prolonged use:
Causes cancer in laboratory animals. Consult your doctor if you have family or personal history of cancer.

Skin & sunlight:
No problems expected.

Driving, piloting or hazardous work:
Avoid if you feel drowsy, dizzy or faint. Otherwise, no problems expected.

Airplane passengers:
No problems expected.

Discontinuing:
Don't discontinue without consulting doctor. Dose may require gradual reduction if you have taken drug for a long time. Doses of other drugs may also require adjustment.

Others:
Consult your doctor if you do isometric exercises. These raise blood pressure. Drug may intensify blood-pressure rise.

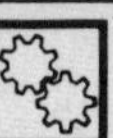

INTERACTION WITH OTHER DRUGS

GENERIC NAME OR DRUG CLASS	COMBINED EFFECT
Anticoagulants (oral)	Unpredictable increased or decreased effect of anticoagulant.
Anticonvulsants	Serious change in seizure pattern.
Antidepressants	Increased antidepressant effect.
Antihistamines	Increased antihistamine effect.
Aspirin	Decreased aspirin effect.
Beta-adrenergic blockers	Increased effect of rauwolfia alkaloids. Excessive sedation.
Digitalis preparations	Irregular heartbeat.
Levodopa	Decreased levodopa effect.
MAO inhibitors	Severe depression.
Mind-altering drugs	Excessive sedation.

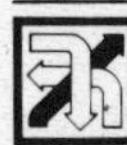

INTERACTION WITH OTHER SUBSTANCES

INTERACTS WITH	COMBINED EFFECT
Alcohol:	Increased intoxication. Use with extreme caution.
Beverages:	
Carbonated drinks	Decreased rauwolfia alkaloids effect.
Cocaine:	Decreased rauwolfia alkaloids effect.
Foods:	
Spicy foods	Possible digestive upset.
Marijuana:	Occasional use—Mild drowsiness. Daily use—Moderate drowsiness, low blood pressure, depression.
Tobacco:	No problems expected.

RIBOFLAVIN (VITAMIN B-2)

BRAND NAMES

Riobin-50
Many multivitamin preparations.

GENERAL INFORMATION

Habit forming? No
Prescription needed? No
Available as generic? Yes
Drug class: Vitamin supplement

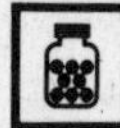

USES

- Dietary supplement to ensure normal growth and health.
- Dietary supplement to treat symptoms caused by deficiency of B-2: sores in mouth, eyes sensitive to light, itching and peeling skin.
- Infections, stomach problems, burns, alcoholism, liver disease.
- Overactive thyroid may cause need for extra Vitamin B-2.

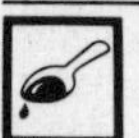

DOSAGE & USAGE INFORMATION

How to take:
Tablet or capsule—Swallow with liquid or food to lessen stomach irritation. If you can't swallow whole, crumble tablet or open capsule and take with liquid or food.

When to take:
At the same times each day.

If you forget a dose:
Take as soon as you remember. Resume regular schedule. Don't double dose.

What drug does:
Promotes normal growth and health.

Time lapse before drug works:
Requires continual intake.

Don't take with:
See Interaction column and consult doctor.

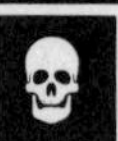

OVERDOSE

Symptoms:
Dark urine, nausea, vomiting.

What to do:
Overdose unlikely to threaten life. If person takes much larger amount than prescribed, call doctor, poison-control center or hospital emergency room for instructions.

POSSIBLE ADVERSE REACTIONS OR SIDE EFFECTS

SYMPTOMS	FREQUENCY	WHAT TO DO
Brain & nervous system:	None expected.	
Skin:	None expected.	
Eyes:	None expected.	
Ears, nose, throat:	None expected.	
Digestive:	None expected.	
Heart & lungs:	None expected.	
Blood vessels:	None expected.	
Muscles, bones, joints:	None expected.	
Genital, urinary:		
Urine yellow in color.	Common	6
Kidneys, allergic, blood, liver:	None expected.	

1 - Life-threatening. Seek emergency treatment immediately.
2 - Discontinue. Seek emergency treatment.
3 - Discontinue. Call doctor right away.
4 - Continue. Call doctor when convenient.
5 - Continue. Tell doctor at next visit.
6 - No action necessary.

RIBOFLAVIN (VITAMIN B-2)

WARNINGS & PRECAUTIONS

Don't take if:
- You are allergic to any B vitamin.
- You have chronic kidney failure.

Before you start, consult your doctor:
If you are pregnant or plan pregnancy.

Over age 60:
No problems expected.

Pregnancy:
Recommended. Consult doctor.

Breast-feeding:
Recommended. Consult doctor.

Infants & children:
Consult doctor.

Prolonged use:
No problems expected.

Skin & sunlight:
No problems expected.

Driving, piloting or hazardous work:
No problems expected.

Airplane passengers:
No problems expected.

Discontinuing:
No problems expected.

Others:
A balanced diet should provide all the vitamin B-2 a healthy person needs and make supplements unnecessary during periods of good health. Best sources are milk, meats and green leafy vegetables.

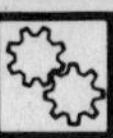

INTERACTION WITH OTHER DRUGS

GENERIC NAME OR DRUG CLASS	COMBINED EFFECT
Antidepressants (tricyclic)	Decreased riboflavin effect.
Phenothiazines	Decreased riboflavin effect.
Probenecid	Decreased riboflavin effect.

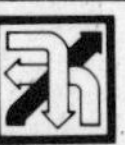

INTERACTION WITH OTHER SUBSTANCES

INTERACTS WITH	COMBINED EFFECT
Alcohol:	Prevents uptake and absorption of Vitamin B-2.
Beverages:	No problems expected.
Cocaine:	No problems expected.
Foods:	No problems expected.
Marijuana:	No problems expected.
Tobacco:	Prevents absorption of vitamin B-2 and other vitamins and nutrients.

RIFAMPIN

BRAND NAMES

Rifadin
Rifomycin
Rifamate
Rimactane
Rofact

GENERAL INFORMATION

Habit forming? No
Prescription needed? Yes
Available as generic? No
Drug class: Antibiotic (rifamycin)

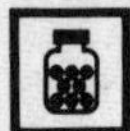

USES

Treatment for tuberculosis and other infections. Requires daily use for 1 to 2 years.

DOSAGE & USAGE INFORMATION

How to take:
Capsule—Swallow with liquid. If you can't swallow whole, open capsule and take with liquid or small amount of food. For child, mix with small amount of applesauce or jelly.

When to take:
1 hour before or 2 hours after a meal.

If you forget a dose:
Take as soon as you remember up to 2 hours late. If more than 2 hours, wait for next scheduled dose (don't double this dose).

What drug does:
Prevents multiplication of tuberculosis germs.

Time lapse before drug works:
Usually 2 weeks. May require 1 to 2 years without missed doses for maximum benefit.

Don't take with:
See Interaction column and consult doctor.

OVERDOSE

Symptoms:
Slow, shallow breathing; weak, rapid pulse; cold, sweaty skin; coma.

What to do:
- Dial 0 (operator) or 911 (emergency) for an ambulance or medical help. Then give first aid immediately.
- If patient is unconscious and not breathing, give mouth-to-mouth breathing. If there is no heartbeat, use cardiac massage and mouth-to-mouth breathing (CPR). Don't try to make patient vomit. If you can't get help quickly, take patient to nearest emergency facility.
- Additional emergency information on page 886.

POSSIBLE ADVERSE REACTIONS OR SIDE EFFECTS

SYMPTOMS	FREQUENCY	WHAT TO DO
Brain & nervous system:		
• Headache	Infrequent	5
• Dizziness, unsteady gait, confusion.	Infrequent	4
Skin:		
Rash, itch.	Infrequent	3
Eyes:		
Blurred vision.	Infrequent	3
Ears, nose, throat:		
Sore throat, mouth or tongue.	Rare	3
Digestive:		
• Diarrhea	Common	4
• Appetite loss, vomiting.	Rare	4
Heart & lungs:		
Breathing difficulty.	Infrequent	3
Blood vessels:	None expected.	
Muscles, bones, joints:		
Muscle, bone pain.	Infrequent	4
Genital, urinary:		
Less urination.	Rare	4
Kidneys:	None expected.	
Liver:		
Jaundice (yellow skin and eyes).	Rare	3
Allergic:	None expected.	
Blood:	None expected.	
Others:		
Reddish urine, stool, saliva, sweat and tears.	Common	4

1-Life-threatening. Seek emergency treatment immediately.
2-Discontinue. Seek emergency treatment.
3-Discontinue. Call doctor right away.
4-Continue. Call doctor when convenient.
5-Continue. Tell doctor at next visit.
6-No action necessary.

WARNINGS & PRECAUTIONS

Don't take if:
- You are allergic to rifampin.
- You wear soft contact lenses.

Before you start, consult your doctor:
If you are alcoholic or have liver disease.

Over age 60:
Adverse reactions and side effects may be more frequent and severe than in younger persons.

Pregnancy:
Studies inconclusive on harm to unborn child. Animal studies show fetal abnormalities. Decide with your doctor whether drug benefits justify risk to unborn child.

Breast-feeding:
No proven problems. Consult doctor.

Infants & children:
Use only under medical supervision.

Prolonged use:
You may become more susceptible to infections caused by germs not responsive to rifampin.

Skin & sunlight:
No problems expected.

Driving, piloting or hazardous work:
Don't drive or pilot aircraft until you learn how medicine affects you. Don't work around dangerous machinery. Don't climb ladders or work in high places. Danger increases if you drink alcohol or take medicine affecting alertness and reflexes, such as antihistamines, tranquilizers, sedatives, pain medicine, narcotics and mind-altering drugs.

Airplane passengers:
No problems expected.

Discontinuing:
Don't discontinue without doctor's advice until you complete prescribed dose, even though symptoms diminish or disappear.

Others:
No problems expected.

INTERACTION WITH OTHER DRUGS

GENERIC NAME OR DRUG CLASS	COMBINED EFFECT
Anticoagulants (oral)	Decreased anticoagulant effect.
Barbiturates	Decreased barbiturate effect.
Contraceptives (oral)	Decreased contraceptive effect.
Cortisone drugs	Decreased effect of cortisone drugs.
Dapsone	Decreased dapsone effect.
Digitoxin	Decreased digitoxin effect.
Isoniazid	Possible toxicity to liver.
Methadone	Decreased methadone effect.
Para-aminosalicylic acid (PAS)	Decreased rifampin effect.
Probenecid	Possible toxicity to liver.
Tolbutamide	Decreased tolbutamide effect.
Trimethoprim	Decreased trimethoprim effect.

INTERACTION WITH OTHER SUBSTANCES

INTERACTS WITH	COMBINED EFFECT
Alcohol:	Possible toxicity to liver.
Beverages:	None expected.
Cocaine:	No proven problems.
Foods:	None expected.
Marijuana:	No proven problems.
Tobacco:	None expected.

RITODRINE

BRAND NAMES

Yutopar

GENERAL INFORMATION

Habit forming? No
Prescription needed? Yes
Available as generic? No
Drug class: Labor inhibitor; Beta-adrenergic stimulator

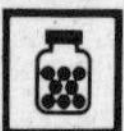

USES

Halts premature labor in pregnancies of 20 or more weeks.

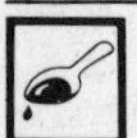

DOSAGE & USAGE INFORMATION

How to take:
Tablet or capsule—Swallow with liquid or food to lessen stomach irritation. If you can't swallow whole, crumble tablet or open capsule and take with liquid or food.

When to take:
Every 4 to 6 hours until term.

If you forget a dose:
Take as soon as you remember up to 2 hours late. If more than 2 hours, wait for next scheduled dose (don't double this dose).

What drug does:
Inhibits contractions of uterus (womb).

Time lapse before drug works:
30 to 60 minutes (oral form). Faster intravenously.

Don't take with:
See Interaction column and consult doctor.

OVERDOSE

Symptoms:
Rapid, irregular heartbeat to 120 or more; shortness of breath.

What to do:
- Dial 0 (operator) or 911 (emergency) for an ambulance or medical help. Then give first aid immediately.
- If patient is unconscious and not breathing, give mouth-to-mouth breathing. If there is no heartbeat, use cardiac massage and mouth-to-mouth breathing (CPR). Don't try to make patient vomit. If you can't get help quickly, take patient to nearest emergency facility.
- Additional emergency information on page 886.

POSSIBLE ADVERSE REACTIONS OR SIDE EFFECTS

SYMPTOMS	FREQUENCY	WHAT TO DO
Brain & nervous system:		
• Nervousness, trembling.	Infrequent	4
• Headache	Infrequent	4
Skin:		
Skin rash.	Rare	3
Eyes:	None expected.	
Ears, nose, throat:	None expected.	
Digestive:		
Nausea, vomiting.	Infrequent	4
Heart & lungs:		
• Increased heart rate.	Always	4
• Irregular heartbeat.	Common	3
• Shortness of breath.	Infrequent	3
Blood vessels:	None expected.	
Muscles, bones, joints:	None expected.	
Genital, urinary:	None expected.	
Kidneys, allergic, blood, liver:	None expected.	
Others:		
Increased systolic blood pressure.	Common	5

1- Life-threatening. Seek emergency treatment immediately.
2- Discontinue. Seek emergency treatment.
3- Discontinue. Call doctor right away.
4- Continue. Call doctor when convenient.
5- Continue. Tell doctor at next visit.
6- No action necessary.

WARNINGS & PRECAUTIONS

Don't take if:
- You have heart disease.
- You have eclampsia.
- You have lung congestion.
- You have infection in the uterus.
- You have an overactive thyroid.
- You have a bleeding disorder.

Before you start, consult your doctor:
- If you have asthma.
- If you have diabetes.
- If you have high blood pressure.
- If you have pre-eclampsia.

Over age 60:
Not used.

Pregnancy:
Ritodrine crosses placenta, but animal studies show that it causes no effects on fetuses. Benefits versus risks must be assessed by you and your doctor.

Breast-feeding:
Not applicable.

Infants & children:
Not used.

Prolonged use:
Request blood sugar and electrolytes measurements.

Skin & sunlight:
No problems expected.

Driving, piloting or hazardous work:
Don't drive or pilot aircraft until you learn how medicine affects you. Don't work around dangerous machinery. Don't climb ladders or work in high places. Danger increases if you drink alcohol or take medicine affecting alertness and reflexes, such as antihistamines, tranquilizers, sedatives, pain medicine, narcotics and mind-altering drugs.

Airplane passengers:
No problems expected.

Discontinuing:
Don't discontinue without consulting doctor. Dose may require gradual reduction if you have taken drug for a long time. Doses of other drugs may also require adjustment.

INTERACTION WITH OTHER DRUGS

GENERIC NAME OR DRUG CLASS	COMBINED EFFECT
Beta blockers	Decreased effect of ritodrine.
Adrenal corticosteroids	Increased chance of fluid in lungs of mother. Avoid.
Sympathomimetics	Increased side effects of both.

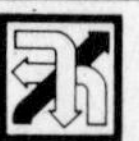

INTERACTION WITH OTHER SUBSTANCES

INTERACTS WITH	COMBINED EFFECT
Alcohol:	Increased adverse effects. Avoid.
Beverages:	No problems expected.
Cocaine:	Injury to fetus. Avoid.
Foods:	No problems expected.
Marijuana:	Injury to fetus. Avoid.
Tobacco:	Injury to fetus. Avoid.

SALICYLATES

BRAND AND GENERIC NAMES

Arcylate DIFLUNISAL Mobidin
Arthropan Disalcid S-60

See complete brand and generic names list, page 831.

GENERAL INFORMATION

Habit forming? No
Prescription needed? No
Available as generic? Yes
Drug class: Analgesic, antiinflammatory (salicylate)

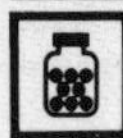

USES

- Reduces pain, fever, inflammation.
- Relieves swelling, stiffness, joint pain of arthritis or rheumatism.

DOSAGE & USAGE INFORMATION

How to take:

- Tablet or capsule—Swallow with liquid.
- Extended-release tablets or capsules—Swallow each dose whole.
- Suppositories—Remove wrapper and moisten suppository with water. Gently insert into rectum, large end first.

When to take:
Pain, fever, inflammation—As needed, no more often than every 4 hours.

If you forget a dose:

- Pain, fever—Take as soon as you remember. Wait 4 hours for next dose.
- Arthritis—Take as soon as you remember up to 2 hours late. Return to regular schedule.

What drug does:

- Affects hypothalamus, part of brain that regulates temperature by dilating small blood vessels in skin.
- Prevents clumping of platelets (small blood cells) so blood vessels remain open.
- Decreases prostaglandin effect.
- Suppresses body's pain messages.

Time lapse before drug works:
30 minutes for pain, fever, arthritis.

Don't take with:

- Tetracyclines. Space doses 1 hour apart.
- See Interaction column and consult doctor.

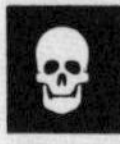

OVERDOSE

Symptoms:
Ringing in ears; nausea; vomiting; dizziness; fever; deep, rapid breathing; hallucinations; convulsions; coma.

What to do:

- Dial 0 (operator) or 911 (emergency) for an ambulance or medical help. Then give first aid immediately. See page 886.

POSSIBLE ADVERSE REACTIONS OR SIDE EFFECTS

SYMPTOMS	FREQUENCY	WHAT TO DO
Brain & nervous system:		
Drowsiness	Rare	4
Skin:		
Rash, hives, itch.	Rare	3
Eyes:		
Diminished vision.	Rare	3
Ears, nose, throat:		
Ringing in ears.	Common	5
Digestive:		
• Nausea, vomiting, abdominal pain.	Common	2
• Black stools.	Rare	2
• Black or bloody vomit.	Rare	1
• Heartburn, indigestion.	Common	4
Heart & lungs:		
Shortness of breath, wheezing.	Rare	3
Blood vessels, muscles, bones, joints, kidneys, blood:	None expected.	
Genital, urinary:		
Blood in urine.	Rare	1
Liver:		
Jaundice (yellow eyes and skin).	Rare	3
Allergic:		
Life-threatening anaphylaxis may occur!	Rare	1 See page 888.
Others:		
Unexplained fever.	Rare	2

1- Life-threatening. Seek emergency treatment immediately.
2- Discontinue. Seek emergency treatment.
3- Discontinue. Call doctor right away.
4- Continue. Call doctor when convenient.
5- Continue. Tell doctor at next visit.
6- No action necessary.

WARNINGS & PRECAUTIONS

Don't take if:
- You need to restrict sodium in your diet. Buffered effervescent tablets and sodium salicylate are high in sodium.
- Salicylates have a strong vinegar-like odor, which means it has decomposed.
- You have a peptic ulcer of stomach or duodenum.
- You have a bleeding disorder.

Before you start, consult your doctor:
- If you have had stomach or duodenal ulcers.
- If you have had gout.
- If you have asthma or nasal polyps.

Over age 60:
More likely to cause hidden bleeding in stomach or intestines. Watch for dark stools.

Pregnancy:
Risk to unborn child outweighs drug benefits. Don't use.

Breast-feeding:
Drug passes into milk. Avoid drug or discontinue nursing until you finish medicine. Consult doctor for advice on maintaining milk supply.

Infants & children:
Overdose frequent and severe. Keep bottles out of children's reach.

Prolonged use:
Kidney damage. Periodic kidney-function test recommended.

Skin & sunlight:
Aspirin combined with sunscreen may decrease sunburn.

Driving, piloting or hazardous work:
No restrictions unless you feel drowsy.

Airplane passengers:
No problems expected.

Discontinuing:
For chronic illness—Don't discontinue without doctor's advice until you complete prescribed dose, even though symptoms diminish or disappear.

Others:
- Salicylates can complicate surgery, pregnancy, labor and delivery, and illness.
- For arthritis—Don't change dose without consulting doctor.
- Urine tests for blood sugar may be inaccurate.

INTERACTION WITH OTHER DRUGS

GENERIC NAME OR DRUG CLASS	COMBINED EFFECT
Allopurinol	Decreased allopurinol effect.
Antacids	Decreased salicylate effect.
Anticoagulants	Increased anticoagulant effect. Abnormal bleeding.
Antidiabetics (oral)	Low blood sugar.
Antiinflammatory drugs (non-steroid)	Risk of stomach bleeding and ulcers.
Aspirin (other)	Likely salicylate toxicity.
Cortisone drugs	Increased cortisone effect. Risk of ulcers and stomach bleeding.
Furosemide	Possible salicylate toxicity.
Indomethacin	Risk of stomach bleeding and ulcers.
Methotrexate	Increased methotrexate effect.
Para-aminosalicylic acid (PAS)	Possible salicylate toxicity.
Penicillins	Increased effect of both drugs.
Phenobarbital	Decreased salicylate effect.

Additional interactions on page 843.

INTERACTION WITH OTHER SUBSTANCES

INTERACTS WITH	COMBINED EFFECT
Alcohol:	Possible stomach irritation and bleeding. Avoid.
Beverages:	None expected.
Cocaine:	None expected.
Foods:	None expected.
Marijuana:	Possible increased pain relief, but marijuana may slow body's recovery. Avoid.
Tobacco:	None expected.

SCOPOLAMINE (HYOSCINE)

BRAND NAMES

Barbidonna
Donnatal
Kinesed
Levamine
Omnibel
Vonodonnal

See complete brand names list, page 831.

GENERAL INFORMATION

Habit forming? No
Prescription needed? Low strength: No
High strength: Yes
Available as generic? Yes
Drug class: Antispasmodic, anticholinergic

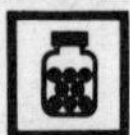

USES

- Reduces spasms of digestive system, bladder and urethra.
- Relieves painful menstruation.
- Prevents motion sickness.

DOSAGE & USAGE INFORMATION

How to take:
- Tablet or capsule—Swallow with liquid or food to lessen stomach irritation.
- Extended-release tablets or capsules—Swallow each dose whole.
- Drops—Dilute dose in beverage.
- Skin discs—Clean application site. Change application sites with each dose.

When to take:
- Motion sickness—Apply disc 30 minutes before departure.
- Other uses—Take 30 minutes before meals (unless directed otherwise by doctor).

If you forget a dose:
Take up to 2 hours late. If more than 2 hours, wait for next dose (don't double this).

What drug does:
Blocks nerve impulses at parasympathetic nerve endings, preventing muscle contractions and gland secretions of organs involved.

Time lapse before drug works:
15 to 30 minutes.

Don't take with:
See Interaction column and consult doctor.

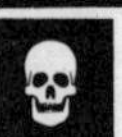

OVERDOSE

Symptoms:
Dilated pupils; rapid pulse and breathing; dizziness; fever; hallucinations; confusion; slurred speech; agitation; flushed face; convulsions; coma.

What to do:
- Dial 0 (operator) or 911 (emergency) for an ambulance or medical help. Then give first aid immediately.
- Additional emergency information on page 886.

POSSIBLE ADVERSE REACTIONS OR SIDE EFFECTS

SYMPTOMS	FREQUENCY	WHAT TO DO
Brain & nervous system:		
• Headache	Infrequent	4
• Confusion, delirium.	Common	3
Skin:		
Rash or hives.	Rare	3
Eyes:		
Pain, blurred vision.	Rare	3
Ears, nose, throat:		
Dryness	Common	6
Digestive:		
• Constipation	Common	5
• Nausea, vomiting.	Common	4
Heart & lungs:		
Rapid heartbeat.	Common	3
Blood vessels:	None expected.	
Muscles, bones, joints:	None expected.	
Genital, urinary:		
Difficult urination.	Infrequent	4
Kidneys:	None expected.	
Liver:	None expected.	
Allergic:	None expected.	
Blood:	None expected.	
Others:		
Less perspiration.	Common	4

1- Life-threatening. Seek emergency treatment immediately.
2- Discontinue. Seek emergency treatment.
3- Discontinue. Call doctor right away.
4- Continue. Call doctor when convenient.
5- Continue. Tell doctor at next visit.
6- No action necessary.

SCOPOLAMINE (HYOSCINE)

WARNINGS & PRECAUTIONS

Don't take if:
- You are allergic to any anticholinergic.
- You have trouble with stomach bloating.
- You have difficulty emptying your bladder completely.
- You have narrow-angle glaucoma.
- You have severe ulcerative colitis.

Before you start, consult your doctor:
- If you have open-angle glaucoma.
- If you have angina.
- If you have chronic bronchitis or asthma.
- If you have hiatal hernia.
- If you have liver disease.
- If you have enlarged prostate.
- If you have myasthenia gravis.
- If you have peptic ulcer.
- If you will have surgery within 2 months, including dental surgery, requiring general or spinal anesthesia.

Over age 60:
Adverse reactions and side effects may be more frequent and severe than in younger persons.

Pregnancy:
Studies inconclusive on harm to unborn child. Animal studies show fetal abnormalities. Decide with your doctor whether drug benefits justify risk to unborn child.

Breast-feeding:
Drug passes into milk and decreases milk flow. Avoid drug or discontinue nursing until you finish medicine. Consult doctor for advice on maintaining milk supply.

Infants & children:
Use only under medical supervision.

Prolonged use:
Chronic constipation, possible fecal impaction. Consult doctor immediately.

Skin & sunlight:
No problems expected.

Driving, piloting or hazardous work:
Use disqualifies you for piloting aircraft. Otherwise, no problems expected.

Airplane passengers:
No problems expected.

Discontinuing:
May be unnecessary to finish medicine. Follow doctor's instructions.

Others:
No problems expected.

INTERACTION WITH OTHER DRUGS

GENERIC NAME OR DRUG CLASS	COMBINED EFFECT
Amantadine	Increased scopolamine effect.
Anticholinergics (other)	Increased scopolamine effect.
Antidepressants (tricyclic)	Increased scopolamine effect.
Antihistamines	Increased scopolamine effect.
Cortisone drugs	Increased internal-eye pressure.
Haloperidol	Increased internal-eye pressure.
MAO inhibitors	Increased scopolamine effect.
Meperidine	Increased scopolamine effect.
Methylphenidate	Increased scopolamine effect.
Orphenadrine	Increased scopolamine effect.
Phenothiazines	Increased scopolamine effect.
Pilocarpine	Loss of pilocarpine effect in glaucoma treatment.
Vitamin C	Decreased scopolamine effect. Avoid large doses of vitamin C.

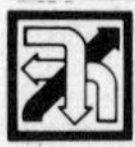

INTERACTION WITH OTHER SUBSTANCES

INTERACTS WITH	COMBINED EFFECT
Alcohol:	None expected.
Beverages:	None expected.
Cocaine:	Excessively rapid heartbeat. Avoid.
Foods:	None expected.
Marijuana:	Drowsiness and dry mouth.
Tobacco:	None expected.

SECOBARBITAL

BRAND NAMES

Novo Secobarb
Secogen
Seconal
Seral
Tuinal

GENERAL INFORMATION

Habit forming? Yes
Prescription needed? Yes
Available as generic? Yes
Drug class: Sedative, hypnotic (barbiturate)

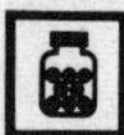

USES

- Reduces anxiety or nervous tension (low dose).
- Relieves insomnia (higher bedtime dose).

DOSAGE & USAGE INFORMATION

How to take:
- Tablet, capsule or liquid—Swallow with food or liquid to lessen stomach irritation. If you can't swallow whole, crumble tablet or open capsule and take with liquid or food.
- Suppositories—Remove wrapper and moisten suppository with water. Gently insert larger end into rectum. Push well into rectum with finger.

When to take:
At the same times each day.

If you forget a dose:
Take as soon as you remember up to 2 hours late. If more than 2 hours, wait for next scheduled dose (don't double this dose).

What drug does:
May partially block nerve impulses at nerve-cell connections.

Time lapse before drug works:
60 minutes.

Don't take with:
- Non-prescription drugs without consulting doctor.
- See Interaction column and consult doctor.

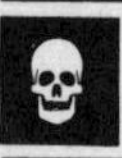

OVERDOSE

Symptoms:
Deep sleep, weak pulse, coma.

What to do:
- Dial 0 (operator) or 911 (emergency) for an ambulance or medical help. Then give first aid immediately.
- Additional emergency information on page 886.

POSSIBLE ADVERSE REACTIONS OR SIDE EFFECTS

SYMPTOMS	FREQUENCY	WHAT TO DO
Brain & nervous system:		
• Dizziness, drowsiness, "hangover effect."	Common	4
• Depression, confusion, slurred speech.	Infrequent	4
• Agitation	Rare	3
Skin:		
• Rash or hives.	Infrequent	3
• Face, lip swelling.	Infrequent	3
Eyes:		
Eyelid swelling.	Infrequent	3
Ears, nose, throat:		
Sore throat, fever.	Infrequent	3
Digestive:		
Diarrhea, nausea, vomiting.	Infrequent	4
Heart & lungs:		
• Slow heartbeat.	Rare	3
• Breathing difficulty.	Rare	3
Blood vessels:		
Unexplained bleeding or bruising.	Rare	4
Muscles, bones, joints:		
Joint or muscle pain.	Infrequent	4
Genital, urinary:	None expected.	
Kidneys:	None expected.	
Liver:		
Jaundice (yellow skin and eyes).	Rare	3
Allergic:	None expected.	
Blood:	None expected.	
Others:	None expected.	

1- Life-threatening. Seek emergency treatment immediately.
2- Discontinue. Seek emergency treatment.
3- Discontinue. Call doctor right away.
4- Continue. Call doctor when convenient.

WARNINGS & PRECAUTIONS

Don't take if:
- You are allergic to any barbiturate.
- You have porphyria.

Before you start, consult your doctor:
- If you have epilepsy.
- If you have kidney or liver damage.
- If you have asthma.
- If you have anemia.
- If you have chronic pain.
- If you will have surgery within 2 months, including dental surgery, requiring general or spinal anesthesia.

Over age 60:
Adverse reactions and side effects may be more frequent and severe than in younger persons. Use small doses.

Pregnancy:
Risk to unborn child outweighs drug benefits. Don't use.

Breast-feeding:
Drug passes into milk. Avoid drug or discontinue nursing until you finish medicine. Consult doctor for advice on maintaining milk supply.

Infants & children:
Use only under doctor's supervision.

Prolonged use:
- May cause addiction, anemia, chronic intoxication.
- May lower body temperature, making exposure to cold temperatures hazardous.

Skin & sunlight:
May cause rash or intensify sunburn in areas exposed to sun or sunlamp.

Driving, piloting or hazardous work:
Don't drive or pilot aircraft until you learn how medicine affects you. Don't work around dangerous machinery. Don't climb ladders or work in high places. Danger increases if you drink alcohol or take medicine affecting alertness and reflexes.

Airplane passengers:
No problems expected.

Discontinuing:
May be unnecessary to finish medicine. Follow doctor's instructions. If you develop withdrawal symptoms of hallucinations, agitation or sleeplessness after discontinuing, call doctor right away.

Others:
Great potential for abuse.

INTERACTION WITH OTHER DRUGS

GENERIC NAME OR DRUG CLASS	COMBINED EFFECT
Anticoagulants (oral)	Decreased anticoagulant effect.
Anticonvulsants	Changed seizure patterns.
Antidepressants (tricyclic)	Decreased antidepressant effect.
Antidiabetics (oral)	Increased secobarbital effect.
Antihistamines	Dangerous sedation. Avoid.
Antiinflammatory drugs (non-steroidal)	Decreased antiinflammatory effect.
Aspirin	Decreased aspirin effect.
Beta-adrenergic blockers	Decreased effect of beta-adrenergic blocker.
Contraceptives (oral)	Decreased contraceptive effect.
Cortisone drugs	Decreased cortisone effect.
Digitoxin	Decreased digitoxin effect.
Doxycycline	Decreased doxycycline effect.
Griseofulvin	Decreased griseofulvin effect.

Additional interactions on page 843.

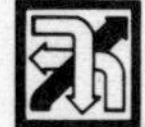

INTERACTION WITH OTHER SUBSTANCES

INTERACTS WITH	COMBINED EFFECT
Alcohol:	Possible fatal oversedation. Avoid.
Beverages:	None expected.
Cocaine:	Decreased secobarbital effect.
Foods:	None expected.
Marijuana:	Excessive sedation. Avoid.
Tobacco:	None expected.

SENNA

BRAND NAMES

Black Draught
Casa-Fru
Dr. Caldwell's Senna Laxative
Fletcher's Castoria
Senexon
Senokot
Senolax
Swiss Kriss
X-Prep

GENERAL INFORMATION

Habit forming? No
Prescription needed? No
Available as generic? Yes
Drug class: Laxative (stimulant)

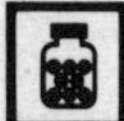

USES

Constipation relief.

DOSAGE & USAGE INFORMATION

How to take:

- Tablet—Swallow with liquid. If you can't swallow whole, chew or crumble tablet and take with liquid or food.
- Liquid, granules—Drink 6 to 8 glasses of water each day, in addition to one taken with each dose.

When to take:
Usually at bedtime with a snack, unless directed otherwise.

If you forget a dose:
Take as soon as you remember.

What drug does:
Acts on smooth muscles of intestine wall to cause vigorous bowel movement.

Time lapse before drug works:
6 to 10 hours.

Don't take with:

- See Interaction column and consult doctor.
- Don't take within 2 hours of taking another medicine. Laxative interferes with medicine absorption.

OVERDOSE

Symptoms:
Vomiting, electrolyte depletion.

What to do:
Overdose unlikely to threaten life. If person takes much larger amount than prescribed, call doctor, poison-control center or hospital emergency room for instructions.

POSSIBLE ADVERSE REACTIONS OR SIDE EFFECTS

SYMPTOMS	FREQUENCY	WHAT TO DO
Brain & nervous system:		
Irritability, confusion, headache.	Rare	3
Skin:		
Rash	Rare	3
Eyes:	None expected.	
Ears, nose, throat:	None expected.	
Digestive:		
Belching, cramps, nausea.	Infrequent	4
Heart & lungs:		
Breathing difficulty, irregular heartbeat.	Rare	3
Blood vessels:	None expected.	
Muscles, bones, joints:		
Muscle cramps.	Rare	3
Genital, urinary:		
Yellow-brown or red-violet urine.	Common	6
Kidneys:		
Burning on urination.	Rare	4
Liver:	None expected.	
Allergic:	None expected.	
Blood:	None expected.	
Others:		
• Rectal irritation.	Common	4
• Dangerous potassium loss.	Infrequent	3
• Unusual tiredness or weakness.	Rare	3

1- Life-threatening. Seek emergency treatment immediately.
2- Discontinue. Seek emergency treatment.
3- Discontinue. Call doctor right away.
4- Continue. Call doctor when convenient.
5- Continue. Tell doctor at next visit.
6- No action necessary.

WARNINGS & PRECAUTIONS

Don't take if:
- You have symptoms of appendicitis, inflamed bowel or intestinal blockage.
- You are allergic to a stimulant laxative.
- You have missed a bowel movement for only 1 or 2 days.

Before you start, consult your doctor:
- If you have a colostomy or ileostomy.
- If you have congestive heart disease.
- If you have diabetes.
- If you have high blood pressure.
- If you have a laxative habit.
- If you have rectal bleeding.
- If you take other laxatives.

Over age 60:
Adverse reactions and side effects may be more frequent and severe than in younger persons.

Pregnancy:
Risk to mother and unborn child outweighs drug benefits. Don't use.

Breast-feeding:
Drug passes into milk. Avoid drug or discontinue nursing until you finish medicine. Consult doctor for advice on maintaining milk supply.

Infants & children:
Use only under medical supervision.

Prolonged use:
Don't take for more than 1 week unless under a doctor's supervision. May cause laxative dependence.

Skin & sunlight:
No problems expected.

Driving, piloting or hazardous work:
No problems expected.

Airplane passengers:
No problems expected.

Discontinuing:
May be unnecessary to finish medicine. Follow doctor's instructions.

Others:
Don't take to "flush out" your system or as a "tonic."

INTERACTION WITH OTHER DRUGS

GENERIC NAME OR DRUG CLASS	COMBINED EFFECT
Antihypertensives	May cause dangerous low potassium level.
Diuretics	May cause dangerous low potassium level.

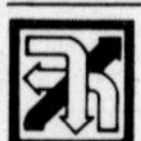

INTERACTION WITH OTHER SUBSTANCES

INTERACTS WITH	COMBINED EFFECT
Alcohol:	None expected.
Beverages:	None expected.
Cocaine:	None expected.
Foods:	None expected.
Marijuana:	None expected.
Tobacco:	None expected.

SENNOSIDES A & B

BRAND NAMES

Glysennid
Nytilax
Senokot
X-Prep

GENERAL INFORMATION

Habit forming? No
Prescription needed? No
Available as generic? Yes
Drug class: Laxative (stimulant)

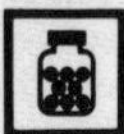

USES

Constipation relief.

DOSAGE & USAGE INFORMATION

How to take:

- Tablet—Swallow with liquid. If you can't swallow whole, chew or crumble tablet and take with liquid or food.
- Liquid, granules—Drink 6 to 8 glasses of water each day, in addition to one taken with each dose.

When to take:
Usually at bedtime with a snack, unless directed otherwise.

If you forget a dose:
Take as soon as you remember.

What drug does:
Acts on smooth muscles of intestine wall to cause vigorous bowel movement.

Time lapse before drug works:
6 to 10 hours.

Don't take with:

- See Interaction column and consult doctor.
- Don't take within 2 hours of taking another medicine. Laxative interferes with medicine absorption.

OVERDOSE

Symptoms:
Vomiting, electrolyte depletion.

What to do:
Overdose unlikely to threaten life. If person takes much larger amount than prescribed, call doctor, poison-control center or hospital emergency room for instructions.

POSSIBLE ADVERSE REACTIONS OR SIDE EFFECTS

SYMPTOMS	FREQUENCY	WHAT TO DO
Brain & nervous system:		
Irritability, confusion, headache.	Rare	3
Skin:		
Rash	Rare	3
Eyes:	None expected.	
Ears, nose, throat:	None expected.	
Digestive:		
Belching, cramps, nausea.	Infrequent	4
Heart & lungs:		
Breathing difficulty, irregular heartbeat.	Rare	3
Blood vessels:	None expected.	
Muscles, bones, joints:		
Muscle cramps.	Rare	3
Genital, urinary:		
Yellow-brown or red-violet urine.	Common	6
Kidneys:		
Burning on urination.	Rare	4
Liver:	None expected.	
Allergic:	None expected.	
Blood:	None expected.	
Others:		
• Rectal irritation.	Common	4
• Dangerous potassium loss.	Infrequent	3
• Unusual tiredness or weakness.	Rare	3

1- Life-threatening. Seek emergency treatment immediately.
2- Discontinue. Seek emergency treatment.
3- Discontinue. Call doctor right away.
4- Continue. Call doctor when convenient.
5- Continue. Tell doctor at next visit.
6- No action necessary.

WARNINGS & PRECAUTIONS

Don't take if:
- You have symptoms of appendicitis, inflamed bowel or intestinal blockage.
- You are allergic to a stimulant laxative.
- You have missed a bowel movement for only 1 or 2 days.

Before you start, consult your doctor:
- If you have a colostomy or ileostomy.
- If you have congestive heart disease.
- If you have diabetes.
- If you have high blood pressure.
- If you have a laxative habit.
- If you have rectal bleeding.
- If you take other laxatives.

Over age 60:
Adverse reactions and side effects may be more frequent and severe than in younger persons.

Pregnancy:
Risk to mother and unborn child outweighs drug benefits. Don't use.

Breast-feeding:
Drug passes into milk. Avoid drug or discontinue nursing until you finish medicine. Consult doctor for advice on maintaining milk supply.

Infants & children:
Use only under medical supervision.

Prolonged use:
Don't take for more than 1 week unless under a doctor's supervision. May cause laxative dependence.

Skin & sunlight:
No problems expected.

Driving, piloting or hazardous work:
No problems expected.

Airplane passengers:
No problems expected.

Discontinuing:
May be unnecessary to finish medicine. Follow doctor's instructions.

Others:
Don't take to "flush out" your system or as a "tonic."

INTERACTION WITH OTHER DRUGS

GENERIC NAME OR DRUG CLASS	COMBINED EFFECT
Antihypertensives	May cause dangerous low potassium level.
Diuretics	May cause dangerous low potassium level.

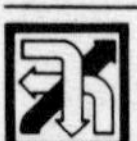

INTERACTION WITH OTHER SUBSTANCES

INTERACTS WITH	COMBINED EFFECT
Alcohol:	None expected.
Beverages:	None expected.
Cocaine:	None expected.
Foods:	None expected.
Marijuana:	None expected.
Tobacco:	None expected.

SIMETHICONE

BRAND NAMES

Barriere
Celluzyme
Di-Gel
Gas-X
Gelusil
Mygel
Mylanta
Mylicon
Ovol
Phazyme
Riopan Plus
Simeco
Silain
Tri-Cone

GENERAL INFORMATION

Habit forming? No
Prescription needed? No
Available as generic? Yes
Drug class: Antiflatulent

USES

- Treatment for retention of abdominal gas.
- Used prior to x-ray of abdomen to reduce gas shadows.

DOSAGE & USAGE INFORMATION

How to take:

- Tablet—Swallow with liquid.
- Liquid—Dissolve in water. Drink complete dose.
- Chewable tablets—Chew completely. Don't swallow whole.

When to take:
After meals and at bedtime.

If you forget a dose:
Take when remembered if needed.

What drug does:
Reduces surface tension of gas bubbles in stomach.

Time lapse before drug works:
10 minutes.

Don't take with:
No restrictions.

OVERDOSE

Symptoms:
None expected.

What to do:
Overdose unlikely to threaten life.

POSSIBLE ADVERSE REACTIONS OR SIDE EFFECTS

SYMPTOMS	FREQUENCY	WHAT TO DO
Brain & nervous system:	None expected.	
Skin:	None expected.	
Eyes:	None expected.	
Ears, nose, throat:	None expected.	
Digestive:	None expected.	
Heart & lungs:	None expected.	
Blood vessels:	None expected.	
Muscles, bones, joints:	None expected.	
Genital, urinary:	None expected.	
Kidneys:	None expected.	
Liver:	None expected.	
Allergic:	None expected.	
Blood:	None expected.	
Others:	None expected.	

1- Life-threatening. Seek emergency treatment immediately.
2- Discontinue. Seek emergency treatment.
3- Discontinue. Call doctor right away.
4- Continue. Call doctor when convenient.
5- Continue. Tell doctor at next visit.
6- No action necessary.

WARNINGS & PRECAUTIONS

Don't take if:
You are allergic to simethicone.

Before you start, consult your doctor:
No problems expected.

Over age 60:
No problems expected.

Pregnancy:
No proven harm to unborn child. Avoid if possible.

Breast-feeding:
No problems expected.

Infants & children:
Not recommended.

Prolonged use:
No problems expected.

Skin & sunlight:
No problems expected.

Driving, piloting or hazardous work:
No problems expected.

Airplane passengers:
No problems expected.

Discontinuing:
May be unnecessary to finish medicine. Discontinue when symptoms disappear.

Others:
No problems expected.

INTERACTION WITH OTHER DRUGS

GENERIC NAME OR DRUG CLASS	COMBINED EFFECT
None	

INTERACTION WITH OTHER SUBSTANCES

INTERACTS WITH	COMBINED EFFECT
Alcohol:	None expected.
Beverages:	None expected.
Cocaine:	None expected.
Foods:	None expected.
Marijuana:	None expected.
Tobacco:	None expected.

SODIUM BICARBONATE

BRAND NAMES

Alka-Citrate Compound
Alka-Seltzer Antacid
Arm and Hammer
Baking Soda
Bell/ans
Bisodol
Bisodol Powder
Brioschi
Bromo Seltzer
Ceo-Two
Chembicarb
Citrocarbonate
Eno
Fizrin
Infalyte
Seidlitz Powder
Soda Mint

GENERAL INFORMATION

Habit forming? No
Prescription needed? No
Available as generic? Yes
Drug class: Antacid

USES

Treatment for hyperacidity in upper gastrointestinal tract, including stomach and esophagus. Symptoms may be heartburn or acid indigestion. Diseases include peptic ulcer, gastritis, esophagitis, hiatal hernia.

DOSAGE & USAGE INFORMATION

How to take:

- Tablet—Swallow with liquid.
- Chewable tablets or wafers—Chew well before swallowing.
- Powder—Dilute dose in beverage before swallowing.

When to take:
1 to 3 hours after meals unless directed otherwise by your doctor.

If you forget a dose:
Take as soon as you remember.

What drug does:

- Neutralizes some of the hydrochloric acid in the stomach.
- Reduces action of pepsin, a digestive enzyme.

Time lapse before drug works:
15 minutes.

Don't take with:
Other medicines at the same time. Decreases absorption of other drugs.

OVERDOSE

Symptoms:
Weakness, fatigue, dizziness.

What to do:
Overdose unlikely to threaten life. If person takes much larger amount than prescribed, call doctor, poison-control center or hospital emergency room for instructions.

POSSIBLE ADVERSE REACTIONS OR SIDE EFFECTS

SYMPTOMS	FREQUENCY	WHAT TO DO
Brain & nervous system:		
Mood changes.	Infrequent	4
Skin:	None expected.	
Eyes:	None expected.	
Ears, nose, throat:	None expected.	
Digestive:		
• Constipation, appetite loss.	Common	4
• Nausea, vomiting.	Infrequent	4
• Lower abdominal pain and swelling.	Infrequent	3
• Belching	Common	5
Heart & lungs:	None expected.	
Blood vessels:	None expected.	
Muscles, bones, joints:		
Bone pain, muscle weakness.	Infrequent	3
Genital, urinary:	None expected.	
Kidneys:	None expected.	
Liver:	None expected.	
Allergic:	None expected.	
Blood:	None expected.	
Others:		
• Swelling of wrists or ankles.	Infrequent	3
• Weight loss.	Infrequent	4
• Weight gain.	Common	4

1- Life-threatening. Seek emergency treatment immediately.
2- Discontinue. Seek emergency treatment.
3- Discontinue. Call doctor right away.
4- Continue. Call doctor when convenient.
5- Continue. Tell doctor at next visit.
6- No action necessary.

WARNINGS & PRECAUTIONS

Don't take if:
You are allergic to any antacid.

Before you start, consult your doctor:
- If you have kidney disease, liver disease, high blood pressure or congestive heart failure.
- If you have chronic constipation or diarrhea.
- If you have symptoms of appendicitis.
- If you have stomach or intestinal bleeding.

Over age 60:
Adverse reactions and side effects may be more frequent and severe than in younger persons. Diarrhea or constipation particularly likely.

Pregnancy:
Risk to unborn child outweighs drug benefits. Don't use.

Breast-feeding:
Drug passes into milk. Avoid drug or discontinue nursing until you finish medicine. Consult doctor for advice on maintaining milk supply.

Infants & children:
Use only under medical supervision.

Prolonged use:
Prolonged use with calcium supplements or milk leads to too much calcium in blood.

Skin & sunlight:
No problems expected.

Driving, piloting or hazardous work:
No problems expected.

Airplane passengers:
No problems expected.

Discontinuing:
May be unnecessary to finish medicine. Follow doctor's instructions.

Others:
Don't take longer than 2 weeks unless under medical supervision.

INTERACTION WITH OTHER DRUGS

GENERIC NAME OR DRUG CLASS	COMBINED EFFECT
Amphetamine	Increased amphetamine effect.
Anticoagulants	Decreased anticoagulant effect.
Iron supplements	Decreased iron effect.
Meperidine	Increased meperidine effect.
Nalidixic acid	Decreased effect of nalidixic acid.
Oxyphenbutazone	Decreased oxyphenbutazone effect.
Para-aminosalicylic acid (PAS)	Decreased PAS effect.
Penicillins	Decreased penicillin effect.
Pentobarbital	Decreased pentobarbital effect.
Phenylbutazone	Decreased phenylbutazone effect.
Pseudoephedrine	Increased pseudoephedrine effect.
Quinidine	Increased quinidine effect.
Salicylates	Decreased salicylate effect.
Sulfa drugs	Decreased sulfa effect.
Tetracyclines	Decreased tetracycline effect.

INTERACTION WITH OTHER SUBSTANCES

INTERACTS WITH	COMBINED EFFECT
Alcohol:	Decreased antacid effect.
Beverages:	No proven problems.
Cocaine:	No proven problems.
Foods:	Decreased antacid effect. Wait 1 hour after eating.
Marijuana:	No proven problems.
Tobacco:	Decreased antacid effect.

SODIUM CARBONATE

BRAND NAMES

Rolaids

GENERAL INFORMATION

Habit forming? No
Prescription needed? No
Available as generic? Yes
Drug class: Antacid

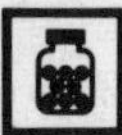

USES

Treatment for hyperacidity in upper gastrointestinal tract, including stomach and esophagus. Symptoms may be heartburn or acid indigestion. Diseases include peptic ulcer, gastritis, esophagitis, hiatal hernia.

DOSAGE & USAGE INFORMATION

How to take:
Chewable tablets or wafers—Chew well before swallowing.

When to take:
1 to 3 hours after meals unless directed otherwise by your doctor.

If you forget a dose:
Take as soon as you remember.

What drug does:

- Neutralizes some of the hydrochloric acid in the stomach.
- Reduces action of pepsin, a digestive enzyme.

Time lapse before drug works:
15 minutes.

Don't take with:
Other medicines at the same time. Decreases absorption of other drugs.

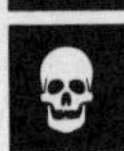

OVERDOSE

Symptoms:
Weakness, fatigue, dizziness.

What to do:
Overdose unlikely to threaten life. If person takes much larger amount than prescribed, call doctor, poison-control center or hospital emergency room for instructions.

POSSIBLE ADVERSE REACTIONS OR SIDE EFFECTS

SYMPTOMS	FREQUENCY	WHAT TO DO
Brain & nervous system:		
Mood changes.	Infrequent	4
Skin:	None expected.	
Eyes:	None expected.	
Ears, nose, throat:	None expected.	
Digestive:		
• Constipation, appetite loss.	Common	4
• Nausea, vomiting.	Infrequent	4
• Lower abdominal pain and swelling.	Infrequent	3
Heart & lungs:	None expected.	
Blood vessels:	None expected.	
Muscles, bones, joints:		
Bone pain, muscle weakness.	Infrequent	3
Genital, urinary:	None expected.	
Kidneys:	None expected.	
Liver:	None expected.	
Allergic:	None expected.	
Blood:	None expected.	
Others:		
• Swelling of wrists or ankles.	Infrequent	3
• Weight loss.	Infrequent	4

1- Life-threatening. Seek emergency treatment immediately.
2- Discontinue. Seek emergency treatment.
3- Discontinue. Call doctor right away.
4- Continue. Call doctor when convenient.
5- Continue. Tell doctor at next visit.
6- No action necessary.

WARNINGS & PRECAUTIONS

Don't take if:
You are allergic to any antacid.

Before you start, consult your doctor:
- If you have kidney disease, liver disease, high blood pressure or congestive heart failure.
- If you have chronic constipation or diarrhea.
- If you have symptoms of appendicitis.
- If you have stomach or intestinal bleeding.

Over age 60:
Adverse reactions and side effects may be more frequent and severe than in younger persons. Diarrhea or constipation particularly likely.

Pregnancy:
Risk to unborn child outweighs drug benefits. Don't use.

Breast-feeding:
Drug passes into milk. Avoid drug or discontinue nursing until you finish medicine. Consult doctor for advice on maintaining milk supply.

Infants & children:
Use only under medical supervision.

Prolonged use:
Fluid retention.

Skin & sunlight:
No problems expected.

Driving, piloting or hazardous work:
No problems expected.

Airplane passengers:
No problems expected.

Discontinuing:
May be unnecessary to finish medicine. Follow doctor's instructions.

Others:
Don't take longer than 2 weeks unless under medical supervision.

INTERACTION WITH OTHER DRUGS

GENERIC NAME OR DRUG CLASS	COMBINED EFFECT
Anticoagulants	Decreased anticoagulant effect.
Chlorpromazine	Decreased chlorpromazine effect.
Digitalis preparations	Decreased digitalis effect.
Iron supplements	Decreased iron effect.
Meperidine	Increased meperidine effect.
Nalidixic acid	Decreased effect of nalidixic acid.
Oxyphenbutazone	Decreased oxyphenbutazone effect.
Para-aminosalicylic acid (PAS)	Decreased PAS effect.
Penicillins	Decreased penicillin effect.
Pentobarbital	Decreased pentobarbital effect.
Phenylbutazone	Decreased phenylbutazone effect.
Pseudoephedrine	Increased pseudoephedrine effect.
Sulfa drugs	Decreased sulfa effect.
Tetracyclines	Decreased tetracycline effect.
Vitamins A and C	Decreased vitamin effect.

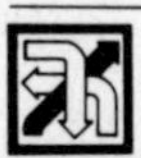

INTERACTION WITH OTHER SUBSTANCES

INTERACTS WITH	COMBINED EFFECT
Alcohol:	Decreased antacid effect.
Beverages:	No proven problems.
Cocaine:	No proven problems.
Foods:	Decreased antacid effect. Wait 1 hour after eating.
Marijuana:	No proven problems.
Tobacco:	Decreased antacid effect.

SODIUM FLUORIDE

BRAND NAMES

Denta-Fl
Flo-Tab
Fluorident
Fluoritab
Fluorodex
Flura
Karidium
Luride
Luride-SF
Nafeen
Pediaflor
Pedi-Dent
Stay-Flo
Studaflor
Thera-Flur

Numerous other multiple vitamin-mineral supplements.

GENERAL INFORMATION

Habit forming? No
Prescription needed? Yes
Available as generic? Yes
Drug class: Mineral supplement (fluoride)

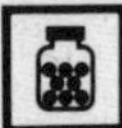

USES

Reduces tooth cavities.

DOSAGE & USAGE INFORMATION

How to take:

- Tablet—Swallow with liquid or crumble tablet and take with liquid (*not* milk) or food.
- Liquid—Measure with dropper and take directly or with liquid.
- Chewable tablets—Chew slowly and thoroughly before swallowing.

When to take:
Usually at bedtime after teeth are thoroughly brushed.

If you forget a dose:
Take as soon as you remember. Don't double a forgotten dose. Return to schedule.

What drug does:
Provides supplemental fluoride to combat tooth decay.

Time lapse before drug works:
8 weeks to provide maximum effect.

Don't take with:

- Other medicine simultaneously.
- See Interaction column.

OVERDOSE

Symptoms:
Stomach cramps or pain, nausea, faintness, vomiting (possibly bloody), diarrhea, black stools, shallow breathing.

What to do:

- Dial 0 (operator) or 911 (emergency) for an ambulance or medical help. Then give first aid immediately.
- Additional emergency information on page 886.

POSSIBLE ADVERSE REACTIONS OR SIDE EFFECTS

SYMPTOMS	FREQUENCY	WHAT TO DO
Brain & nervous system:	None expected.	
Skin: Rash	Infrequent	3
Eyes:	None expected.	
Ears, nose, throat: Sores in mouth and lips.	Rare	3
Digestive: Severe upsets only with overdose.	Rare	2
Heart & lungs:	None expected.	
Blood vessels:	None expected.	
Muscles, bones, joints:	None expected.	
Genital, urinary:	None expected.	
Kidneys:	None expected.	
Liver:	None expected.	
Allergic:	None expected.	
Blood:	None expected.	
Others:	None expected.	

1-Life-threatening. Seek emergency treatment immediately.
2-Discontinue. Seek emergency treatment.
3-Discontinue. Call doctor right away.
4-Continue. Call doctor when convenient.
5-Continue. Tell doctor at next visit.
6-No action necessary.

SODIUM FLUORIDE

WARNINGS & PRECAUTIONS

Don't take if:
- Your water supply contains 0.7 parts fluoride per million. Too much fluoride stains teeth permanently.
- You are allergic to any fluoride-containing product.
- You have underactive thyroid.

Before you start, consult your doctor:
Not necessary.

Over age 60:
No problems expected.

Pregnancy:
No problems expected.

Breast-feeding:
No problems expected.

Infants & children:
No problems expected except accidental overdose. Keep vitamin-mineral supplements out of children's reach.

Prolonged use:
Excess may cause discolored teeth and decreased calcium in blood.

Skin & sunlight:
No problems expected.

Driving, piloting or hazardous work:
No problems expected.

Airplane passengers:
No problems expected.

Discontinuing:
No problems expected.

Others:
Store in original plastic container. Fluoride decomposes glass.

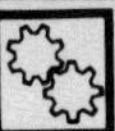

INTERACTION WITH OTHER DRUGS

GENERIC NAME OR DRUG CLASS	COMBINED EFFECT
None	

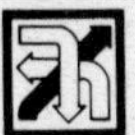

INTERACTION WITH OTHER SUBSTANCES

INTERACTS WITH	COMBINED EFFECT
Alcohol:	None expected.
Beverages:	
Milk	Prevents absorption of fluoride. Space dose 2 hours before or after milk.
Cocaine:	None expected.
Foods:	None expected.
Marijuana:	None expected.
Tobacco:	None expected.

SODIUM PHOSPHATE

BRAND NAMES

Phospho-Soda
Sal Hepatica

GENERAL INFORMATION

Habit forming? No
Prescription needed? No
Available as generic? Yes
Drug class: Laxative (hyperosmotic)

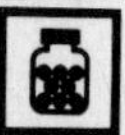

USES

Constipation relief.

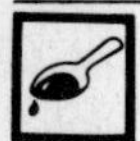

DOSAGE & USAGE INFORMATION

How to take:
Liquid, effervescent tablet or powder—Dilute dose in beverage before swallowing.

When to take:
Usually once a day, preferably in the morning.

If you forget a dose:
Take as soon as you remember up to 8 hours before bedtime. If later, wait for next scheduled dose (don't double this dose). Don't take at bedtime.

What drug does:
Draws water into bowel from other body tissues. Causes distention through fluid accumulation, which promotes soft stool and accelerates bowel motion.

Time lapse before drug works:
30 minutes to 3 hours.

Don't take with:
See Interaction column and consult doctor.

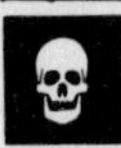

OVERDOSE

Symptoms:
Fluid depletion, weakness, vomiting, fainting.

What to do:
Overdose unlikely to threaten life. If person takes much larger amount than prescribed, call doctor, poison-control center or hospital emergency room for instructions.

POSSIBLE ADVERSE REACTIONS OR SIDE EFFECTS

SYMPTOMS	FREQUENCY	WHAT TO DO
Brain & nervous system: Dizziness, confusion.	Rare	4
Skin:	None expected.	
Eyes:	None expected.	
Ears, nose, throat: Increased thirst.	Infrequent	5
Digestive: Cramps, nausea, diarrhea, gas.	Infrequent	5
Heart & lungs: Irregular heartbeat.	Infrequent	3
Blood vessels:	None expected.	
Muscles, bones, joints:	None expected.	
Genital, urinary:	None expected.	
Kidneys:	None expected.	
Liver:	None expected.	
Allergic:	None expected.	
Blood:	None expected.	
Others: Tiredness or weakness.	Rare	4

1-Life-threatening. Seek emergency treatment immediately.
2-Discontinue. Seek emergency treatment.
3-Discontinue. Call doctor right away.
4-Continue. Call doctor when convenient.
5-Continue. Tell doctor at next visit.
6-No action necessary.

SODIUM PHOSPHATE

WARNINGS & PRECAUTIONS

Don't take if:
- You are allergic to any hyperosmotic laxative.
- You have symptoms of appendicitis, inflamed bowel or intestinal blockage.
- You have missed a bowel movement for only 1 or 2 days.

Before you start, consult your doctor:
- If you have congestive heart disease.
- If you have diabetes.
- If you have high blood pressure.
- If you have a colostomy or ileostomy.
- If you have kidney disease.
- If you have a laxative habit.
- If you have rectal bleeding.
- If you take another laxative.

Over age 60:
Adverse reactions and side effects may be more frequent and severe than in younger persons.

Pregnancy:
Salt content may cause fluid retention and swelling. Avoid if possible.

Breast-feeding:
No problems expected.

Infants & children:
Use only under medical supervision.

Prolonged use:
Don't take for more than 1 week unless under a doctor's supervision. May cause laxative dependence.

Skin & sunlight:
No problems expected.

Driving, piloting or hazardous work:
No problems expected.

Airplane passengers:
No problems expected.

Discontinuing:
May be unnecessary to finish medicine. Follow doctor's instructions.

Others:
- Don't take to "flush out" your system or as a "tonic."
- Don't take within 2 hours of taking another medicine.

INTERACTION WITH OTHER DRUGS

GENERIC NAME OR DRUG CLASS	COMBINED EFFECT
Chlordiazepoxide	Decreased chlordiazepoxide effect.
Chlorpromazine	Decreased chlorpromazine effect.
Dicumarol	Decreased dicumarol effect.
Digoxin	Decreased digoxin effect.
Isoniazid	Decreased isoniazid effect.
Tetracyclines	Possible intestinal blockage.

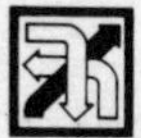

INTERACTION WITH OTHER SUBSTANCES

INTERACTS WITH	COMBINED EFFECT
Alcohol:	None expected.
Beverages:	None expected.
Cocaine:	None expected.
Foods:	None expected.
Marijuana:	None expected.
Tobacco:	None expected.

SPIRONOLACTONE

BRAND NAMES

Aldactazide
Aldactone
Spironazide

GENERAL INFORMATION

Habit forming? No
Prescription needed? Yes
Available as generic? No
Drug class: Antihypertensive, diuretic

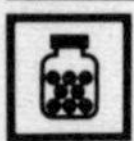

USES

- Reduces high blood pressure.
- Prevents fluid retention.

DOSAGE & USAGE INFORMATION

How to take:
Tablet—Swallow with liquid or food to lessen stomach irritation. If you can't swallow whole, crumble tablet and take with liquid or food.

When to take:
- 1 dose a day—Take after breakfast.
- More than 1 dose a day—Take last dose no later than 6 p.m.

If you forget a dose:
- 1 dose a day—Take as soon as you remember up to 12 hours late. If more than 12 hours, wait for next scheduled dose (don't double this dose).
- More than 1 dose a day—Take as soon as you remember. Wait 6 hours for next dose.

What drug does:
- Increases sodium and water excretion through increased urine production, decreasing body fluid and blood pressure.
- Retains potassium.

Time lapse before drug works:
3 to 5 days.

Don't take with:
See Interaction column and consult doctor.

OVERDOSE

Symptoms:
Thirst, drowsiness, confusion, fatigue, weakness, nausea, vomiting, irregular heartbeat, excessive blood-pressure drop.

What to do:
- Dial 0 (operator) or 911 (emergency) for an ambulance or medical help. Then give first aid immediately.
- Additional emergency information on page 886.

POSSIBLE ADVERSE REACTIONS OR SIDE EFFECTS

SYMPTOMS	FREQUENCY	WHAT TO DO
Brain & nervous system:		
Drowsiness or headache.	Common	4
Skin:		
• Rash or itch.	Rare	3
• Confusion	Infrequent	3
Eyes:	None expected.	
Ears, nose, throat:		
• Deep voice in women.	Rare	5
• Thirst	Common	4
Digestive:		
Nausea, vomiting, diarrhea.	Common	4
Heart & lungs:		
Irregular heartbeat, shortness of breath.	Infrequent	3
Blood vessels:	None expected.	
Muscles, bones, joints:		
Numbness, tingling in hands or feet.	Infrequent	4
Genital, urinary:	None expected.	
Kidneys:	None expected.	
Liver:	None expected.	
Allergic:	None expected.	
Blood:	None expected.	
Others:		
• Irregular menstruation, breast tenderness, change in sex drive.	Infrequent	4
• Unusual sweating.	Infrequent	3

1- Life-threatening. Seek emergency treatment immediately.
2- Discontinue. Seek emergency treatment.
3- Discontinue. Call doctor right away.
4- Continue. Call doctor when convenient.
5- Continue. Tell doctor at next visit.
6- No action necessary.

WARNINGS & PRECAUTIONS

Don't take if:
- You are allergic to spironolactone.
- You have impaired kidney function.
- Your serum potassium level is high.

Before you start, consult your doctor:
- If you have had kidney or liver disease.
- If you will have surgery within 2 months, including dental surgery, requiring general or spinal anesthesia.

Over age 60:
- Limit use to 2 to 3 weeks if possible.
- Adverse reactions and side effects may be more frequent and severe than in younger persons.
- Heat or fever can reduce blood pressure. May require dose adjustment.
- Overdose and extended use may cause blood clots.

Pregnancy:
No proven harm to unborn child. Avoid if possible.

Breast-feeding:
No proven problems. Consult doctor.

Infants & children:
Use only under medical supervision.

Prolonged use:
Potassium retention with irregular heartbeat, unusual weakness and confusion.

Skin & sunlight:
No problems expected.

Driving, piloting or hazardous work:
Avoid if you feel drowsy. Otherwise, no problems expected.

Airplane passengers:
No problems expected.

Discontinuing:
Consult doctor about adjusting doses of other drugs.

Others:
No problems expected.

INTERACTION WITH OTHER DRUGS

GENERIC NAME OR DRUG CLASS	COMBINED EFFECT
Anticoagulants (oral)	Decreased anticoagulant effect.
Antihypertensives (other)	Increased antihypertensive effect.
Aspirin	Decreased spironolactone effect.
Digitalis preparations	Decreased digitalis effect.
Diuretics (other)	Increased effect of both drugs. Beneficial if needed and dose correct.
Laxatives	Reduced potassium levels.
Lithium	Likely lithium toxicity.
Potassium supplements	Dangerous potassium retention.
Sodium bicarbonate	Reduces high potassium levels.
Triamterene	Dangerous potassium retention.

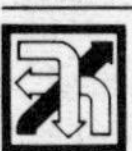

INTERACTION WITH OTHER SUBSTANCES

INTERACTS WITH	COMBINED EFFECT
Alcohol:	None expected.
Beverages:	
Low-salt milk	Possible potassium toxicity.
Cocaine:	Decreased spironolactone effect.
Foods:	
Salt	Don't restrict unless directed by doctor.
Salt substitutes	Possible potassium toxicity.
Marijuana:	Increased thirst, fainting.
Tobacco:	None expected.

SUCRALFATE

BRAND NAMES

Carafate

GENERAL INFORMATION

Habit forming? No
Prescription needed? Yes
Available as generic? No
Drug class: Anti-ulcer

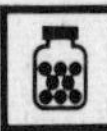

USES

Treatment of duodenal ulcer.

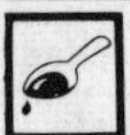

DOSAGE & USAGE INFORMATION

How to take:
Tablet or capsule—Swallow with liquid or food to lessen stomach irritation. If you can't swallow whole, crumble tablet or open capsule and take with liquid or food.

When to take:
1 hour before meals and at bedtime. Allow 2 hours to elapse before taking other prescription medicines.

If you forget a dose:
Take as soon as you remember up to 2 hours late. If more than 2 hours, wait for next scheduled dose (don't double this dose).

What drug does:
Covers ulcer site and protects from acid, enzymes and bile salts.

Time lapse before drug works:
Begins in 30 minutes. May require several days to relieve pain.

Don't take with:
See Interaction column and consult doctor.

OVERDOSE

Symptoms:
No data available yet for this new drug.

What to do:
Overdose unlikely to threaten life. If person takes much larger amount than prescribed, call doctor, poison-control center or hospital emergency room for instructions.

POSSIBLE ADVERSE REACTIONS OR SIDE EFFECTS

SYMPTOMS	FREQUENCY	WHAT TO DO
Brain & nervous system:		
Dizziness, sleepiness.	Infrequent	4
Skin:		
Rash, itching.	Infrequent	4
Eyes:	None expected.	
Ears, nose, throat:	None expected.	
Digestive:		
• Abdominal pain.	Infrequent	4
• Nausea, vomiting.	Infrequent	4
• Indigestion	Infrequent	4
• Constipation	Common	4
Heart & lungs:	None expected.	
Blood vessels:	None expected.	
Muscles, bones, joints:		
Back pain.	Infrequent	4
Genital, urinary:	None expected.	
Kidneys, allergic, blood, liver:	None expected.	
Others:	None expected.	

1- Life-threatening. Seek emergency treatment immediately.
2- Discontinue. Seek emergency treatment.
3- Discontinue. Call doctor right away.
4- Continue. Call doctor when convenient.
5- Continue. Tell doctor at next visit.
6- No action necessary.

WARNINGS & PRECAUTIONS

Don't take if:
You are allergic to sucralfate.

Before you start, consult your doctor:
If you will have surgery within 2 months, including dental surgery, requiring general or spinal anesthesia.

Over age 60:
Adverse reactions and side effects may be more frequent and severe than in younger persons.

Pregnancy:
No proven harm to unborn child. Avoid if possible.

Breast-feeding:
Unknown effects.

Infants & children:
Safety not established.

Prolonged use:
Request blood counts if medicine needed longer than 8 weeks.

Skin & sunlight:
No problems expected.

Driving, piloting or hazardous work:
Don't drive or pilot aircraft until you learn how medicine affects you. Don't work around dangerous machinery. Don't climb ladders or work in high places. Danger increases if you drink alcohol or take medicine affecting alertness and reflexes, such as antihistamines, tranquilizers, sedatives, pain medicine, narcotics and mind-altering drugs.

Airplane passengers:
No problems expected.

Discontinuing:
Don't discontinue without consulting doctor. Dose may require gradual reduction if you have taken drug for a long time. Doses of other drugs may also require adjustment.

INTERACTION WITH OTHER DRUGS

GENERIC NAME OR DRUG CLASS	COMBINED EFFECT
Tetracyclines	Decreased absorption of tetracycline if taken simultaneously.
Phenytoin	Decreased absorption of phenytoin if taken simultaneously.
Cimetidine	Decreased absorption of cimetidine if taken simultaneously.

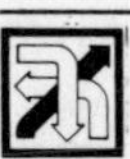

INTERACTION WITH OTHER SUBSTANCES

INTERACTS WITH	COMBINED EFFECT
Alcohol:	Irritates ulcer. Avoid.
Beverages: Caffeine	Irritates ulcer. Avoid.
Cocaine:	May make ulcer worse. Avoid.
Foods:	No problems expected.
Marijuana:	May make ulcer worse. Avoid.
Tobacco:	May make ulcer worse. Avoid.

SULFACYTINE

BRAND NAMES

Renoquid

GENERAL INFORMATION

Habit forming? No
Prescription needed? Yes
Available as generic? Yes
Drug class: Sulfa (sulfonamide)

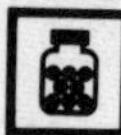

USES

Treatment for infections responsive to this drug.

DOSAGE & USAGE INFORMATION

How to take:
Tablet—Swallow with liquid. Instructions to take on empty stomach mean 1 hour before or 2 hours after eating.

When to take:
At the same times each day, evenly spaced.

If you forget a dose:
Take as soon as you remember up to 2 hours late. If more than 2 hours, wait for next scheduled dose (don't double this dose).

What drug does:
Interferes with a nutrient (folic acid) necessary for growth and reproduction of bacteria. Will not attack viruses.

Time lapse before drug works:
2 to 5 days to affect infection.

Don't take with:
See Interaction column and consult doctor.

OVERDOSE

Symptoms:
Less urine; bloody urine; coma.

What to do:
- Dial O (operator) or 911 (emergency) for an ambulance or medical help. Then give first aid immediately.
- Additional emergency information on page 886.

POSSIBLE ADVERSE REACTIONS OR SIDE EFFECTS

SYMPTOMS	FREQUENCY	WHAT TO DO
Brain & nervous system:		
Headache, dizziness.	Common	4
Skin:		
• Itch, rash.	Common	3
• Redness, peeling, blistering.	Infrequent	3
Eyes:	None expected.	
Ears, nose, throat:		
Sore throat, fever.	Infrequent	3
Digestive:		
• Swallowing difficulty.	Infrequent	3
• Appetite loss, nausea, vomiting, diarrhea.	Common	4
Heart & lungs:	None expected.	
Blood vessels:		
Unusual bruising.	Infrequent	3
Muscles, bones, joints:		
Aching joints, muscles.	Infrequent	3
Genital, urinary:		
Painful urination.	Rare	3
Kidneys:		
Low back pain.	Rare	3
Liver:		
Jaundice (yellow skin and eyes).	Infrequent	3
Allergic:	None expected.	
Blood:	None expected.	
Others:	None expected.	

1-Life-threatening. Seek emergency treatment immediately.
2-Discontinue. Seek emergency treatment.
3-Discontinue. Call doctor right away.
4-Continue. Call doctor when convenient.

WARNINGS & PRECAUTIONS

Don't take if:
You are allergic to any sulfa drug.

Before you start, consult your doctor:
- If you are allergic to carbonic anhydrase inhibitors, oral antidiabetics or thiazide diuretics.
- If you are allergic by nature.
- If you have liver or kidney disease.
- If you have porphyria.
- If you have developed anemia from use of any drug.

Over age 60:
Adverse reactions and side effects may be more frequent and severe than in younger persons.

Pregnancy:
Risk to unborn child outweighs drug benefits. Don't use.

Breast-feeding:
Drug passes into milk. Avoid drug or discontinue nursing until you finish medicine. Consult doctor for advice on maintaining milk supply.

Infants & children:
Don't give to infants younger than 1 month.

Prolonged use:
- May enlarge thyroid gland.
- You may become more susceptible to infections caused by germs not responsive to this drug.
- Request frequent blood counts, liver- and kidney-function studies.

Skin & sunlight:
May cause rash or intensify sunburn in areas exposed to sun or sunlamp.

Driving, piloting or hazardous work:
Avoid if you feel dizzy. Otherwise, no problems expected.

Airplane passengers:
No problems expected.

Discontinuing:
Don't discontinue without doctor's advice until you complete prescribed dose, even though symptoms diminish or disappear.

Others:
- Drink 2 quarts of liquid each day to prevent adverse reactions.
- If you require surgery, tell anesthetist you take sulfa. Pentothal anesthesia should not be used.

INTERACTION WITH OTHER DRUGS

GENERIC NAME OR DRUG CLASS	COMBINED EFFECT
Anticoagulants (oral)	Increased anticoagulant effect.
Anticonvulsants (hydantoin)	Toxic effect on brain.
Aspirin	Increased sulfa effect.
Isoniazid	Possible anemia.
Methenamine	Possible kidney blockage.
Methotrexate	Increased methotrexate effect.
Oxyphenbutazone	Increased sulfa effect.
Para-aminosalicylic acid (PAS)	Decreased sulfa effect.
Penicillins	Decreased penicillin effect.
Phenylbutazone	Increased sulfa effect.
Probenecid	Increased sulfa effect.
Sulfinpyrazone	Increased sulfa effect.
Trimethoprim	Increased sulfa effect.
Vitamin C	Possible kidney damage. Avoid large doses of vitamin C.

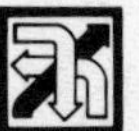

INTERACTION WITH OTHER SUBSTANCES

INTERACTS WITH	COMBINED EFFECT
Alcohol:	Increased alcohol effect.
Beverages: Less than 2 quarts of fluid daily.	Kidney damage.
Cocaine:	None expected.
Foods:	None expected.
Marijuana:	None expected.
Tobacco:	None expected.

SULFAMETHOXAZOLE

BRAND NAMES

Apo-Sulfamethoxazole
Azo Gantanol
Bactrim
Cetamide
Cotrim D.S.
Gantanol
Gantrisin
Methoxanol
Septra
SMZ-TMP

GENERAL INFORMATION

Habit forming? No
Prescription needed? Yes
Available as generic? Yes
Drug class: Sulfa (sulfonamide)

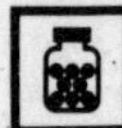

USES

Treatment for infections responsive to this drug.

DOSAGE & USAGE INFORMATION

How to take:

- Tablet—Swallow with liquid. Instructions to take on empty stomach mean 1 hour before or 2 hours after eating.
- Liquid—Shake carefully before measuring.

When to take:
At the same times each day, evenly spaced.

If you forget a dose:
Take as soon as you remember up to 2 hours late. If more than 2 hours, wait for next scheduled dose (don't double this dose).

What drug does:
Interferes with a nutrient (folic acid) necessary for growth and reproduction of bacteria. Will not attack viruses.

Time lapse before drug works:
2 to 5 days to affect infection.

Don't take with:
See Interaction column and consult doctor.

OVERDOSE

Symptoms:
Less urine; bloody urine; coma.

What to do:

- Dial O (operator) or 911 (emergency) for an ambulance or medical help. Then give first aid immediately.
- Additional emergency information on page 886.

POSSIBLE ADVERSE REACTIONS OR SIDE EFFECTS

SYMPTOMS	FREQUENCY	WHAT TO DO
Brain & nervous system:		
Headache, dizziness.	Common	4
Skin:		
• Itch, rash.	Common	3
• Redness, peeling, blistering.	Infrequent	3
Eyes:	None expected.	
Ears, nose, throat:		
Sore throat, fever.	Infrequent	3
Digestive:		
• Swallowing difficulty.	Infrequent	3
• Appetite loss, nausea, vomiting, diarrhea.	Common	4
Heart & lungs:	None expected.	
Blood vessels:		
Unusual bruising.	Infrequent	3
Muscles, bones, joints:		
Aching joints, muscles.	Infrequent	3
Genital, urinary:		
Painful urination.	Rare	3
Kidneys:		
Low back pain.	Rare	3
Liver:		
Jaundice (yellow skin and eyes).	Infrequent	3
Allergic:	None expected.	
Blood:	None expected.	
Others:	None expected.	

1 - Life-threatening. Seek emergency treatment immediately.
2 - Discontinue. Seek emergency treatment.
3 - Discontinue. Call doctor right away.
4 - Continue. Call doctor when convenient.

WARNINGS & PRECAUTIONS

Don't take if:
You are allergic to any sulfa drug.

Before you start, consult your doctor:
- If you are allergic to carbonic anhydrase inhibitors, oral antidiabetics or thiazide diuretics.
- If you are allergic by nature.
- If you have liver or kidney disease.
- If you have porphyria.
- If you have developed anemia from use of any drug.

Over age 60:
Adverse reactions and side effects may be more frequent and severe than in younger persons.

Pregnancy:
Risk to unborn child outweighs drug benefits. Don't use.

Breast-feeding:
Drug passes into milk. Avoid drug or discontinue nursing until you finish medicine. Consult doctor for advice on maintaining milk supply.

Infants & children:
Don't give to infants younger than 1 month.

Prolonged use:
- May enlarge thyroid gland.
- You may become more susceptible to infections caused by germs not responsive to this drug.
- Request frequent blood counts, liver- and kidney-function studies.

Skin & sunlight:
May cause rash or intensify sunburn in areas exposed to sun or sunlamp.

Driving, piloting or hazardous work:
Avoid if you feel dizzy. Otherwise, no problems expected.

Airplane passengers:
No problems expected.

Discontinuing:
Don't discontinue without doctor's advice until you complete prescribed dose, even though symptoms diminish or disappear.

Others:
- Drink 2 quarts of liquid each day to prevent adverse reactions.
- If you require surgery, tell anesthetist you take sulfa. Pentothal anesthesia should not be used.

INTERACTION WITH OTHER DRUGS

GENERIC NAME OR DRUG CLASS	COMBINED EFFECT
Anticoagulants (oral)	Increased anticoagulant effect.
Anticonvulsants (hydantoin)	Toxic effect on brain.
Aspirin	Increased sulfa effect.
Isoniazid	Possible anemia.
Methenamine	Possible kidney blockage.
Methotrexate	Increased methotrexate effect.
Oxyphenbutazone	Increased sulfa effect.
Para-aminosalicylic acid (PAS)	Decreased sulfa effect.
Penicillins	Decreased penicillin effect.
Phenylbutazone	Increased sulfa effect.
Probenecid	Increased sulfa effect.
Sulfinpyrazone	Increased sulfa effect.
Trimethoprim	Increased sulfa effect.
Vitamin C	Possible kidney damage. Avoid large doses of vitamin C.

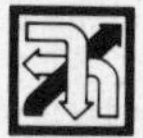

INTERACTION WITH OTHER SUBSTANCES

INTERACTS WITH	COMBINED EFFECT
Alcohol:	Increased alcohol effect.
Beverages: Less than 2 quarts of fluid daily.	Kidney damage.
Cocaine:	None expected.
Foods:	None expected.
Marijuana:	None expected.
Tobacco:	None expected.

SULFASALAZINE

BRAND NAMES

Azulfidine
Salazopyrin
SAS-500

GENERAL INFORMATION

Habit forming? No
Prescription needed? Yes
Available as generic? Yes
Drug class: Sulfa (sulfonamide)

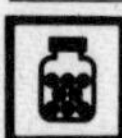

USES

Treatment for ulceration and bleeding during active phase of ulcerative colitis.

DOSAGE & USAGE INFORMATION

How to take:

- Tablet—Swallow with liquid. Instructions to take on empty stomach mean 1 hour before or 2 hours after eating.
- Liquid—Shake carefully before measuring.

When to take:
At the same times each day, evenly spaced.

If you forget a dose:
Take as soon as you remember up to 2 hours late. If more than 2 hours, wait for next scheduled dose (don't double this dose).

What drug does:
Antiinflammatory action reduces tissue destruction in colon.

Time lapse before drug works:
2 to 5 days.

Don't take with:
See Interaction column and consult doctor.

OVERDOSE

Symptoms:
Less urine; bloody urine; coma.

What to do:

- Dial O (operator) or 911 (emergency) for an ambulance or medical help. Then give first aid immediately.
- Additional emergency information on page 886.

POSSIBLE ADVERSE REACTIONS OR SIDE EFFECTS

SYMPTOMS	FREQUENCY	WHAT TO DO
Brain & nervous system:		
Headache, dizziness.	Common	4
Skin:		
• Itch, rash.	Common	3
• Redness, peeling, blistering.	Infrequent	3
Eyes:	None expected.	
Ears, nose, throat:		
Sore throat, fever.	Infrequent	3
Digestive:		
• Swallowing difficulty.	Infrequent	3
• Appetite loss, nausea, vomiting, diarrhea.	Common	4
Heart & lungs:	None expected.	
Blood vessels:		
Unusual bruising.	Infrequent	3
Muscles, bones, joints:		
Aching joints, muscles.	Infrequent	3
Genital, urinary:		
• Painful urination.	Rare	3
• Orange urine.	Common	5
Kidneys:		
Low back pain.	Rare	3
Liver:		
Jaundice (yellow skin and eyes).	Infrequent	3
Allergic:	None expected.	
Blood:	None expected.	
Others:	None expected.	

1- Life-threatening. Seek emergency treatment immediately.
2- Discontinue. Seek emergency treatment.
3- Discontinue. Call doctor right away.
4- Continue. Call doctor when convenient.
5- Continue. Tell doctor at next visit.

WARNINGS & PRECAUTIONS

Don't take if:
You are allergic to any sulfa drug.

Before you start, consult your doctor:
- If you are allergic to carbonic anhydrase inhibitors, oral antidiabetics or thiazide diuretics.
- If you are allergic by nature.
- If you have liver or kidney disease.
- If you have porphyria.
- If you have developed anemia from use of any drug.

Over age 60:
Adverse reactions and side effects may be more frequent and severe than in younger persons.

Pregnancy:
Risk to unborn child outweighs drug benefits. Don't use.

Breast-feeding:
Drug passes into milk. Avoid drug or discontinue nursing until you finish medicine. Consult doctor for advice on maintaining milk supply.

Infants & children:
Don't give to infants younger than 1 month.

Prolonged use:
- May enlarge thyroid gland.
- You may become more susceptible to infections caused by germs not responsive to this drug.
- Request frequent blood counts, liver- and kidney-function studies.

Skin & sunlight:
May cause rash or intensify sunburn in areas exposed to sun or sunlamp.

Driving, piloting or hazardous work:
Avoid if you feel dizzy. Otherwise, no problems expected.

Airplane passengers:
No problems expected.

Discontinuing:
Don't discontinue without doctor's advice until you complete prescribed dose, even though symptoms diminish or disappear.

Others:
- Drink 2 quarts of liquid each day to prevent adverse reactions.
- If you require surgery, tell anesthetist you take sulfa. Pentothal anesthesia should not be used.

INTERACTION WITH OTHER DRUGS

GENERIC NAME OR DRUG CLASS	COMBINED EFFECT
Antibiotics	Decreased sulfasalazine effect.
Anticoagulants (oral)	Increased anticoagulant effect.
Anticonvulsants (hydantoin)	Toxic effect on brain.
Aspirin	Increased sulfa effect.
Digoxin	Decreased digoxin effect.
Iron supplements	Decreased sulfa effect.
Isoniazid	Possible anemia.
Methenamine	Possible kidney blockage.
Methotrexate	Increased methotrexate effect.
Oxyphenbutazone	Increased sulfa effect.
Para-aminosalicylic acid (PAS)	Decreased sulfa effect.
Penicillins	Decreased penicillin effect.
Phenylbutazone	Increased sulfa effect.
Probenecid	Increased sulfa effect.
Sulfinpyrazone	Increased sulfa effect.
Trimethoprim	Increased sulfa effect.
Vitamin C	Possible kidney damage. Avoid large doses of vitamin C.

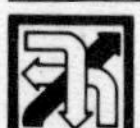

INTERACTION WITH OTHER SUBSTANCES

INTERACTS WITH	COMBINED EFFECT
Alcohol:	Increased alcohol effect.
Beverages: Less than 2 quarts of fluid daily.	Kidney damage.
Cocaine:	None expected.
Foods:	None expected.
Marijuana:	None expected.
Tobacco:	None expected.

SULFINPYRAZONE

BRAND NAMES

Antazone
Anturan
Anturane
Apo-Sulfinpyrazone
Novopyrazone
Zynol

GENERAL INFORMATION

Habit forming? No
Prescription needed? Yes
Available as generic? No
Drug class: Antigout (uricosuric)

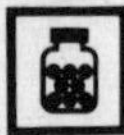

USES

- Treatment for chronic gout.
- Reduces severity of recurrent heart attack. (This use is experimental and not yet approved by F.D.A.)

DOSAGE & USAGE INFORMATION

How to take:
Tablet or capsule—Swallow with liquid or food to lessen stomach irritation. If you can't swallow whole, crumble tablet or open capsule and take with liquid or food.

When to take:
At the same times each day.

If you forget a dose:
Take as soon as you remember up to 2 hours late. If more than 2 hours, wait for next scheduled dose (don't double this dose).

What drug does:
Reduces uric-acid level in blood and tissues by increasing amount of uric acid secreted in urine by kidneys.

Time lapse before drug works:
May require 6 months to prevent gout attacks.

Don't take with:
See Interaction column and consult doctor.

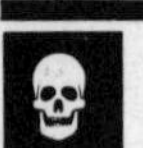

OVERDOSE

Symptoms:
Breathing difficulty, imbalance, convulsions, coma.

What to do:
- Dial 0 (operator) or 911 (emergency) for an ambulance or medical help. Then give first aid immediately.
- If patient is unconscious and not breathing, give mouth-to-mouth breathing. If there is no heartbeat, use cardiac massage and mouth-to-mouth breathing (CPR). Don't try to make patient vomit. If you can't get help quickly, take patient to nearest emergency facility.
- Additional emergency information on page 886.

POSSIBLE ADVERSE REACTIONS OR SIDE EFFECTS

SYMPTOMS	FREQUENCY	WHAT TO DO
Brain & nervous system:	None expected.	
Skin:		
Rash	Infrequent	4
Eyes:	None expected.	
Ears, nose, throat:		
Sore throat, fever.	Rare	3
Digestive:		
• Bloody or black, tarry stools.	Rare	2
• Nausea, vomiting, stomach pain.	Infrequent	4
Heart & lungs:	None expected.	
Blood vessels:		
Unusual bleeding or bruising.	Rare	3
Muscles, bones, joints:		
Red, painful joint.	Rare	3
Genital, urinary:		
• Bloody urine.	Rare	3
• Difficult or painful urination.	Infrequent	3
Kidneys:		
Low back pain.	Infrequent	4
Liver:	None expected.	
Allergic:	None expected.	
Blood:	None expected.	
Others:		
Fatigue or weakness.	Rare	3

1- Life-threatening. Seek emergency treatment immediately.
2- Discontinue. Seek emergency treatment.
3- Discontinue. Call doctor right away.
4- Continue. Call doctor when convenient.
5- Continue. Tell doctor at next visit.
6- No action necessary.

WARNINGS & PRECAUTIONS

Don't take if:
- You are allergic to any uricosuric.
- You have acute gout.
- You have active ulcers (stomach or duodenal), enteritis or ulcerative colitis.
- You have blood-cell disorders.
- You are allergic to oxyphenbutazone or phenylbutazone.

Before you start, consult your doctor:
If you have kidney or blood disease.

Over age 60:
Adverse reactions and side effects may be more frequent and severe than in younger persons. You require lower dose because of decreased kidney function.

Pregnancy:
Studies inconclusive on harm to unborn child. Animal studies show fetal abnormalities. Decide with your doctor whether drug benefits justify risk to unborn child.

Breast-feeding:
No proven problems. Consult doctor.

Infants & children:
Not recommended.

Prolonged use:
Possible kidney damage.

Skin & sunlight:
No problems expected.

Driving, piloting or hazardous work:
No problems expected.

Airplane passengers:
No problems expected.

Discontinuing:
Don't discontinue without consulting doctor. Dose may require gradual reduction if you have taken drug for a long time. Doses of other drugs may also require adjustment.

Others:
- Drink 10 to 12 glasses of water each day you take this medicine.
- Periodic blood and urine laboratory tests recommended.

INTERACTION WITH OTHER DRUGS

GENERIC NAME OR DRUG CLASS	COMBINED EFFECT
Anticoagulants (oral)	Increased anticoagulant effect.
Antidiabetics (oral)	Increased antidiabetic effect.
Aspirin	Bleeding tendency. Decreased sulfinpyrazone effect.
Cephalexin	Increased effect of cephalexin.
Cephradine	Increased effect of cephradine.
Contraceptives (oral)	Increased bleeding between menstrual periods.
Diuretics	Decreased sulfinpyrazone effect.
Insulin	Increased insulin effect.
Penicillins	Increased penicillin effect.
Probenecid	Possible increased sulfinpyrazone effect.
Salicylates	Bleeding tendency. Decreased sulfinpyrazone effect.
Sulfa drugs	Increased effect of sulfa drugs.

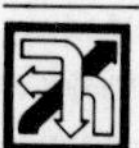

INTERACTION WITH OTHER SUBSTANCES

INTERACTS WITH	COMBINED EFFECT
Alcohol:	Decreased sulfinpyrazone effect.
Beverages: Caffeine drinks	Decreased sulfinpyrazone effect.
Cocaine:	None expected.
Foods:	None expected.
Marijuana:	Occasional use—None expected. Daily use—May increase blood level of uric acid.
Tobacco:	None expected.

SULFISOXAZOLE

BRAND NAMES

Apo-Sulfisoxazole
Azo-Gantrisin
Azo-Soxazole
Barazole
Chemovag
Gantrisin
G-Sox
Lipo Gantrisin
Koro-Sulf
Novosoxazole
Pediazole
Rosoxol
SK-Soxazole
Sosol
Soxa
Sulfagen
Sulfizin
Sulfizole
Urisoxin

GENERAL INFORMATION

Habit forming? No
Prescription needed? Yes
Available as generic? Yes
Drug class: Sulfa (sulfonamide)

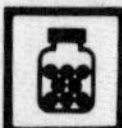

USES

Treatment for infections responsive to this drug.

DOSAGE & USAGE INFORMATION

How to take:

- Tablet—Swallow with liquid. Instructions to take on empty stomach mean 1 hour before or 2 hours after eating.
- Liquid—Shake carefully before measuring.

When to take:
At the same times each day, evenly spaced.

If you forget a dose:
Take as soon as you remember up to 2 hours late. If more than 2 hours, wait for next scheduled dose (don't double this dose).

What drug does:
Interferes with a nutrient (folic acid) necessary for growth and reproduction of bacteria. Will not attack viruses.

Time lapse before drug works:
2 to 5 days to affect infection.

Don't take with:
See Interaction column and consult doctor.

OVERDOSE

Symptoms:
Less urine; bloody urine; coma.

What to do:

- Dial O (operator) or 911 (emergency) for an ambulance or medical help. Then give first aid immediately.
- Additional emergency information on page 886.

POSSIBLE ADVERSE REACTIONS OR SIDE EFFECTS

SYMPTOMS	FREQUENCY	WHAT TO DO
Brain & nervous system:		
Headache, dizziness.	Common	4
Skin:		
• Itch, rash.	Common	3
• Redness, peeling, blistering.	Infrequent	3
Eyes:	None expected.	
Ears, nose, throat:		
Sore throat, fever.	Infrequent	3
Digestive:		
• Swallowing difficulty.	Infrequent	3
• Appetite loss, nausea, vomiting, diarrhea.	Common	4
Heart & lungs:	None expected.	
Blood vessels:		
Unusual bruising.	Infrequent	3
Muscles, bones, joints:		
Aching joints, muscles.	Infrequent	3
Genital, urinary:		
Painful urination.	Rare	3
Kidneys:		
Low back pain.	Rare	3
Liver:		
Jaundice (yellow skin and eyes).	Infrequent	3
Allergic:	None expected.	
Blood:	None expected.	
Others:	None expected.	

1 - Life-threatening. Seek emergency treatment immediately.
2 - Discontinue. Seek emergency treatment.
3 - Discontinue. Call doctor right away.
4 - Continue. Call doctor when convenient.

WARNINGS & PRECAUTIONS

Don't take if:
You are allergic to any sulfa drug.

Before you start, consult your doctor:
- If you are allergic to carbonic anhydrase inhibitors, oral antidiabetics or thiazide diuretics.
- If you are allergic by nature.
- If you have liver or kidney disease.
- If you have porphyria.
- If you have developed anemia from use of any drug.

Over age 60:
Adverse reactions and side effects may be more frequent and severe than in younger persons.

Pregnancy:
Risk to unborn child outweighs drug benefits. Don't use.

Breast-feeding:
Drug passes into milk. Avoid drug or discontinue nursing until you finish medicine. Consult doctor for advice on maintaining milk supply.

Infants & children:
Don't give to infants younger than 1 month.

Prolonged use:
- May enlarge thyroid gland.
- You may become more susceptible to infections caused by germs not responsive to this drug.
- Request frequent blood counts, liver- and kidney-function studies.

Skin & sunlight:
May cause rash or intensify sunburn in areas exposed to sun or sunlamp.

Driving, piloting or hazardous work:
Avoid if you feel dizzy. Otherwise, no problems expected.

Airplane passengers:
No problems expected.

Discontinuing:
Don't discontinue without doctor's advice until you complete prescribed dose, even though symptoms diminish or disappear.

Others:
- Drink 2 quarts of liquid each day to prevent adverse reactions.
- If you require surgery, tell anesthetist you take sulfa. Pentothal anesthesia should not be used.

INTERACTION WITH OTHER DRUGS

GENERIC NAME OR DRUG CLASS	COMBINED EFFECT
Anticoagulants (oral)	Increased anticoagulant effect.
Anticonvulsants (hydantoin)	Toxic effect on brain.
Aspirin	Increased sulfa effect.
Isoniazid	Possible anemia.
Methenamine	Possible kidney blockage.
Methotrexate	Increased methotrexate effect.
Oxyphenbutazone	Increased sulfa effect.
Para-aminosalicylic acid (PAS)	Decreased sulfa effect.
Penicillins	Decreased penicillin effect.
Phenylbutazone	Increased sulfa effect.
Probenecid	Increased sulfa effect.
Sulfinpyrazone	Increased sulfa effect.
Trimethoprim	Increased sulfa effect.
Vitamin C	Possible kidney damage. Avoid large doses of vitamin C.

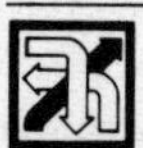

INTERACTION WITH OTHER SUBSTANCES

INTERACTS WITH	COMBINED EFFECT
Alcohol:	Increased alcohol effect.
Beverages: Less than 2 quarts of fluid daily.	Kidney damage.
Cocaine:	None expected.
Foods:	None expected.
Marijuana:	None expected.
Tobacco:	None expected.

SULINDAC

BRAND NAMES

Clinoril

Habit forming? No
Prescription needed? Yes

GENERAL INFORMATION

Available as generic? Yes
Drug class: Antiinflammatory (non-steroid)

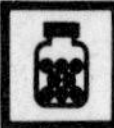

USES

- Treatment for joint pain, stiffness, inflammation and swelling of arthritis and gout.
- Pain reliever.

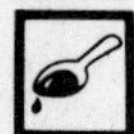

DOSAGE & USAGE INFORMATION

How to take:
Tablet—Swallow with liquid or food to lessen stomach irritation. If you can't swallow whole, crumble tablet and take with liquid or food.

When to take:
At the same times each day.

If you forget a dose:
Take as soon as you remember up to 2 hours late. If more than 2 hours, wait for next scheduled dose (don't double this dose).

What drug does:
Reduces tissue concentration of prostaglandins (hormones which produce inflammation and pain).

Time lapse before drug works:
Begins in 4 to 24 hours. May require 3 weeks regular use for maximum benefit.

Don't take with:
See Interaction column and consult doctor.

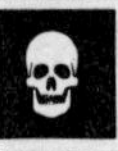

OVERDOSE

Symptoms:
Confusion, agitation, incoherence, convulsions, possible hemorrhage from stomach or intestine, coma.

What to do:
- Dial 0 (operator) or 911 (emergency) for an ambulance or medical help. Then give first aid immediately.
- Additional emergency information on page 886.

POSSIBLE ADVERSE REACTIONS OR SIDE EFFECTS

SYMPTOMS	FREQUENCY	WHAT TO DO
Brain & nervous system:		
• Depression, drowsiness.	Infrequent	4
• Convulsions, confusion.	Rare	3
• Dizziness	Common	4
• Headache	Common	5
Skin:		
Rash, hives or itch.	Rare	3
Eyes:		
Blurred vision.	Rare	3
Ears, nose, throat:		
Ringing in ears.	Infrequent	4
Digestive:		
• Bloody or black, tarry stools.	Rare	3
• Nausea, pain.	Common	4
• Constipation or diarrhea, vomiting.	Infrequent	4
Heart & lungs:		
Breathing difficulty, tightness in chest, rapid heartbeat.	Rare	3
Blood vessels:		
Unusual bleeding or bruising.	Rare	3
Muscles, bones, joints:		
Swollen feet, legs.	Infrequent	4
Genital, urinary:		
• Bloody urine.	Rare	3
• Difficult, painful or frequent urination.	Rare	4
Kidneys, allergic, blood:	None expected.	
Liver:		
Jaundice (yellow skin and eyes).	Rare	3
Others:		
Fatigue, weakness.	Rare	4

1- Life-threatening. Seek emergency treatment immediately.
2- Discontinue. Seek emergency treatment.
3- Discontinue. Call doctor right away.
4- Continue. Call doctor when convenient.
5- Continue. Tell doctor at next visit.

SULINDAC

WARNINGS & PRECAUTIONS

Don't take if:

- You are allergic to aspirin or any non-steroid, antiinflammatory drug.
- You have gastritis, peptic ulcer, enteritis, ileitis, ulcerative colitis, asthma, heart failure, high blood pressure or bleeding problems.
- You have had recent rectal bleeding and suppository form has been prescribed.
- Patient is younger than 15.

Before you start, consult your doctor:

- If you have epilepsy.
- If you have Parkinson's disease.
- If you have been mentally ill.
- If you have had kidney disease or impaired kidney function.

Over age 60:
Adverse reactions and side effects may be more frequent and severe than in younger persons.

Pregnancy:
Studies inconclusive on harm to unborn child. Decide with your doctor whether drug benefits justify risk to unborn child.

Breast-feeding:
May harm child. Avoid.

Infants & children:
Not recommended for those younger than 15. Use only under medical supervision.

Prolonged use:

- Eye damage.
- Reduced hearing.
- Sore throat, fever.
- Weight gain.

Skin & sunlight:
No problems expected.

Driving, piloting or hazardous work:
Don't drive or pilot aircraft until you learn how medicine affects you. Don't work around dangerous machinery. Don't climb ladders or work in high places. Danger increases if you drink alcohol or take medicine affecting alertness and reflexes, such as antihistamines, tranquilizers, sedatives, pain medicine, narcotics and mind-altering drugs.

Airplane passengers:
No problems expected.

Discontinuing:
Don't discontinue without consulting doctor. Dose may require gradual reduction if you have taken drug for a long time. Doses of other drugs may also require adjustment.

Others:
No problems expected.

INTERACTION WITH OTHER DRUGS

GENERIC NAME OR DRUG CLASS	COMBINED EFFECT
Anticoagulants (oral)	Increased risk of bleeding.
Aspirin	Increased risk of stomach ulcer.
Cortisone drugs	Increased risk of stomach ulcer.
Furosemide	Decreased diuretic effect of furosemide.
Oxyphenbutazone	Possible stomach ulcer.
Phenylbutazone	Possible stomach ulcer.
Probenecid	Increased sulindac effect.
Thyroid hormones	Rapid heartbeat, blood-pressure rise.

INTERACTION WITH OTHER SUBSTANCES

INTERACTS WITH	COMBINED EFFECT
Alcohol:	Possible stomach ulcer or bleeding.
Beverages:	None expected.
Cocaine:	None expected.
Foods:	None expected.
Marijuana:	Increased pain relief from sulindac.
Tobacco:	None expected.

TALBUTAL (BUTALBITAL)

BRAND NAMES

Fiorinal
Lotusate
Plexonal
Sandoptal

GENERAL INFORMATION

Habit forming? Yes
Prescription needed? Yes
Available as generic? Yes
Drug class: Sedative, hypnotic (barbiturate)

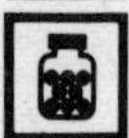

USES

- Reduces anxiety or nervous tension (low dose).
- Relieves insomnia (higher bedtime dose).

DOSAGE & USAGE INFORMATION

How to take:
Tablet or capsule—Swallow with liquid or food to lessen stomach irritation. If you can't swallow whole, crumble tablet or open capsule and take with liquid or food.

When to take:
At the same times each day.

If you forget a dose:
Take as soon as you remember up to 2 hours late. If more than 2 hours, wait for next scheduled dose (don't double this dose).

What drug does:
May partially block nerve impulses at nerve-cell connections.

Time lapse before drug works:
60 minutes.

Don't take with:
- Non-prescription drugs without consulting doctor.
- See Interaction column and consult doctor.

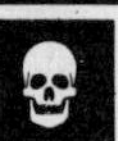

OVERDOSE

Symptoms:
Deep sleep, weak pulse, coma.

What to do:
- Dial 0 (operator) or 911 (emergency) for an ambulance or medical help. Then give first aid immediately.
- Additional emergency information on page 886.

POSSIBLE ADVERSE REACTIONS OR SIDE EFFECTS

SYMPTOMS	FREQUENCY	WHAT TO DO
Brain & nervous system:		
• Dizziness, drowsiness, "hangover effect."	Common	4
• Depression, confusion, slurred speech.	Infrequent	4
• Agitation	Rare	3
Skin:		
• Rash or hives.	Infrequent	3
• Face, lip swelling.	Infrequent	3
Eyes:		
Eyelid swelling.	Infrequent	3
Ears, nose, throat:		
Sore throat, fever.	Infrequent	3
Digestive:		
Diarrhea, nausea, vomiting.	Infrequent	4
Heart & lungs:		
• Slow heartbeat.	Rare	3
• Breathing difficulty.	Rare	3
Blood vessels:		
Unexplained bleeding or bruising.	Rare	4
Muscles, bones, joints:		
Joint or muscle pain.	Infrequent	4
Genital, urinary:	None expected.	
Kidneys:	None expected.	
Liver:		
Jaundice (yellow skin and eyes).	Rare	3
Allergic:	None expected.	
Blood:	None expected.	
Others:	None expected.	

1- Life-threatening. Seek emergency treatment immediately.
2- Discontinue. Seek emergency treatment.
3- Discontinue. Call doctor right away.
4- Continue. Call doctor when convenient.

WARNINGS & PRECAUTIONS

Don't take if:
- You are allergic to any barbiturate.
- You have porphyria.

Before you start, consult your doctor:
- If you have epilepsy.
- If you have kidney or liver damage.
- If you have asthma.
- If you have anemia.
- If you have chronic pain.
- If you will have surgery within 2 months, including dental surgery, requiring general or spinal anesthesia.

Over age 60:
Adverse reactions and side effects may be more frequent and severe than in younger persons. Use small doses.

Pregnancy:
Risk to unborn child outweighs drug benefits. Don't use.

Breast-feeding:
Drug passes into milk. Avoid drug or discontinue nursing until you finish medicine. Consult doctor for advice on maintaining milk supply.

Infants & children:
Use only under doctor's supervision.

Prolonged use:
- May cause addiction, anemia, chronic intoxication.
- May lower body temperature, making exposure to cold temperatures hazardous.

Skin & sunlight:
May cause rash or intensify sunburn in areas exposed to sun or sunlamp.

Driving, piloting or hazardous work:
Don't drive or pilot aircraft until you learn how medicine affects you. Don't work around dangerous machinery. Don't climb ladders or work in high places. Danger increases if you drink alcohol or take medicine affecting alertness and reflexes.

Airplane passengers:
No problems expected.

Discontinuing:
May be unnecessary to finish medicine. Follow doctor's instructions. If you develop withdrawal symptoms of hallucinations, agitation or sleeplessness after discontinuing, call doctor right away.

Others:
No problems expected.

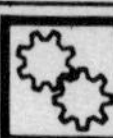

INTERACTION WITH OTHER DRUGS

GENERIC NAME OR DRUG CLASS	COMBINED EFFECT
Anticoagulants (oral)	Decreased anticoagulant effect.
Anticonvulsants	Changed seizure patterns.
Antidepressants (tricyclic)	Decreased antidepressant effect.
Antidiabetics (oral)	Increased talbutal (butalbital) effect.
Antihistamines	Dangerous sedation. Avoid.
Antiinflammatory drugs (non-steroidal)	Decreased antiinflammatory effect.
Aspirin	Decreased aspirin effect.
Beta-adrenergic blockers	Decreased effect of beta-adrenergic blocker.
Contraceptives (oral)	Decreased contraceptive effect.
Cortisone drugs	Decreased cortisone effect.
Digitoxin	Decreased digitoxin effect.
Doxycycline	Decreased doxycycline effect.
Griseofulvin	Decreased griseofulvin effect.

Additional interactions on page 843.

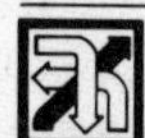

INTERACTION WITH OTHER SUBSTANCES

INTERACTS WITH	COMBINED EFFECT
Alcohol:	Possible fatal oversedation. Avoid.
Beverages:	None expected.
Cocaine:	Decreased talbutal (butalbital) effect.
Foods:	None expected.
Marijuana:	Excessive sedation. Avoid.
Tobacco:	None expected.

TEMAZEPAM

BRAND NAMES

Restoril

GENERAL INFORMATION

Habit forming? Yes
Prescription needed? Yes
Available as generic? No
Drug class: Tranquilizer (benzodiazepine)

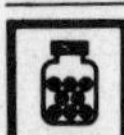

USES

Treatment for insomnia.

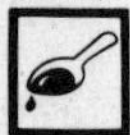

DOSAGE & USAGE INFORMATION

How to take:
Tablet or capsule—Swallow with liquid. If you can't swallow whole, crumble tablet or open capsule and take with liquid or food.

When to take:
At the same time each day, according to instructions on prescription label.

If you forget a dose:
Take as soon as you remember up to 2 hours late. If more than 2 hours, wait for next scheduled dose (don't double this dose).

What drug does:
Affects limbic system of brain—part that controls emotions. Induces near-normal sleep pattern.

Time lapse before drug works:
30 minutes.

Don't take with:
See Interaction column and consult doctor.

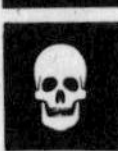

OVERDOSE

Symptoms:
Drowsiness, weakness, tremor, stupor, coma.

What to do:
- Dial 0 (operator) or 911 (emergency) for an ambulance or medical help. Then give first aid immediately.
- If patient is unconscious and not breathing, give mouth-to-mouth breathing. If there is no heartbeat, use cardiac massage and mouth-to-mouth breathing (CPR). Don't try to make patient vomit. If you can't get help quickly, take patient to nearest emergency facility.
- Additional emergency information on page 886.

POSSIBLE ADVERSE REACTIONS OR SIDE EFFECTS

SYMPTOMS	FREQUENCY	WHAT TO DO
Brain & nervous system:		
• Clumsiness, drowsiness, dizziness.	Common	4
• Hallucinations, confusion, depression, irritability.	Infrequent	3
Skin:		
Rash, itch.	Infrequent	3
Eyes:		
Vision changes.	Infrequent	3
Ears, nose, throat:		
Mouth, throat ulcers.	Rare	3
Digestive:		
Constipation or diarrhea, nausea, vomiting.	Infrequent	4
Heart & lungs:		
Slow heartbeat, breathing difficulty.	Rare	2
Blood vessels:	None expected.	
Muscles, bones, joints:	None expected.	
Genital, urinary:		
Urination difficulty.	Infrequent	4
Kidneys:	None expected.	
Liver:		
Jaundice (yellow eyes and skin).	Rare	3
Allergic:	None expected.	
Blood:	None expected.	
Others:	None expected.	

1- Life-threatening. Seek emergency treatment immediately.
2- Discontinue. Seek emergency treatment.
3- Discontinue. Call doctor right away.
4- Continue. Call doctor when convenient.
5- Continue. Tell doctor at next visit.
6- No action necessary.

WARNINGS & PRECAUTIONS

Don't take if:

- You are allergic to any benzodiazepine.
- You have myasthenia gravis.
- You are active or recovering alcoholic.
- Patient is younger than 6 months.

Before you start, consult your doctor:

- If you have liver, kidney or lung disease.
- If you have diabetes, epilepsy or porphyria.

Over age 60:
Adverse reactions and side effects may be more frequent and severe than in younger persons. May develop agitation, rage or "hangover effect."

Pregnancy:
Risk to unborn child outweighs drug benefits. Don't use.

Breast-feeding:
Drug passes into milk. Avoid drug or discontinue nursing until you finish medicine. Consult doctor for advice on maintaining milk supply.

Infants & children:
Use only under medical supervision for children older than 6 months.

Prolonged use:
May impair liver function.

Skin & sunlight:
No problems expected.

Driving, piloting or hazardous work:
Don't drive or pilot aircraft until you learn how medicine affects you. Don't work around dangerous machinery. Don't climb ladders or work in high places. Danger increases if you drink alcohol or take medicine affecting alertness and reflexes.

Airplane passengers:
No problems expected.

Discontinuing:
Don't discontinue without doctor's advice until you complete prescribed dose, even though symptoms diminish or disappear.

Others:

- Hot weather, heavy exercise and profuse sweat may reduce excretion and cause overdose.
- Blood sugar may rise in diabetics, requiring insulin adjustment.

INTERACTION WITH OTHER DRUGS

GENERIC NAME OR DRUG CLASS	COMBINED EFFECT
Anticonvulsants	Change in seizure frequency or severity.
Antidepressants	Increased sedative effect of both drugs.
Antihistamines	Increased sedative effect of both drugs.
Antihypertensives	Excessively low blood pressure.
Cimetidine	Excess sedation.
Disulfiram	Increased temazepam effect.
MAO inhibitors	Convulsions, deep sedation, rage.
Narcotics	Increased sedative effect of both drugs.
Sedatives	Increased sedative effect of both drugs.
Tranquilizers	Increased sedative effect of both drugs.

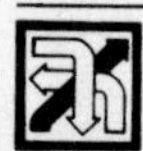

INTERACTION WITH OTHER SUBSTANCES

INTERACTS WITH	COMBINED EFFECT
Alcohol:	Heavy sedation. Avoid.
Beverages:	None expected.
Cocaine:	Decreased temazepam effect.
Foods:	None expected.
Marijuana:	Heavy sedation. Avoid.
Tobacco:	Decreased temazepam effect.

TERBUTALINE

BRAND NAMES

Brethine
Bricanyl

GENERAL INFORMATION

Habit forming? No
Prescription needed? Yes
Available as generic? No
Drug class: Sympathomimetic

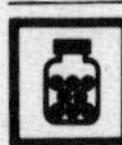

USES

Treatment of bronchial asthma, bronchitis and emphysema.

DOSAGE & USAGE INFORMATION

How to take:
Tablet or capsule—Swallow with liquid or food to lessen stomach irritation.

When to take:
At the same times each day.

If you forget a dose:
Take as soon as you remember up to 2 hours late. If more than 2 hours, wait for next scheduled dose (don't double this dose).

What drug does:
Dilates constricted bronchial tubes.

Time lapse before drug works:
30 minutes.

Don't take with:
See Interaction column and consult doctor.

OVERDOSE

Symptoms:
Rapid heartbeat, chest pain, tremors.

What to do:
- Dial 0 (operator) or 911 (emergency) for an ambulance or medical help. Then give first aid immediately.
- If patient is unconscious and not breathing, give mouth-to-mouth breathing. If there is no heartbeat, use cardiac massage and mouth-to-mouth breathing (CPR). Don't try to make patient vomit. If you can't get help quickly, take patient to nearest emergency facility.
- Additional emergency information on page 886.

POSSIBLE ADVERSE REACTIONS OR SIDE EFFECTS

SYMPTOMS	FREQUENCY	WHAT TO DO
Brain & nervous system:		
• Headache, nervousness, restlessness, trembling.	Common	4
• Drowsiness	Infrequent	3
Skin:	None expected.	
Eyes:	None expected.	
Ears, nose, throat:	None expected.	
Digestive:		
Nausea, vomiting.	Infrequent	3
Heart & lungs:		
Fast or pounding heartbeat.	Infrequent	3
Blood vessels:	None expected.	
Muscles, bones, joints:		
Cramps, weakness.	Infrequent	3
Genital, urinary:	None expected.	
Kidneys:	None expected.	
Liver:	None expected.	
Allergic:	None expected.	
Blood:	None expected.	
Others:		
Unusual sweating.	Infrequent	4

1- Life-threatening. Seek emergency treatment immediately.
2- Discontinue. Seek emergency treatment.
3- Discontinue. Call doctor right away.
4- Continue. Call doctor when convenient.
5- Continue. Tell doctor at next visit.
6- No action necessary.

WARNINGS & PRECAUTIONS

Don't take if:
You are allergic to any sympathomimetic.

Before you start, consult your doctor:
- If you have diabetes.
- If you have heart disease or high blood pressure.
- If you have overactive thyroid.
- If you have had seizures.
- If you take non-prescription amphetamines or other asthma medicines.

Over age 60:
Adverse reactions and side effects may be more frequent and severe than in younger persons.

Pregnancy:
No proven harm to unborn child. Avoid if possible. May prolong labor and delivery.

Breast-feeding:
No proven problems. Avoid if possible.

Infants & children:
Use only under medical supervision.

Prolonged use:
No problems expected.

Skin & sunlight:
No problems expected.

Driving, piloting or hazardous work:
Avoid if you feel drowsy. Otherwise, no problems expected.

Airplane passengers:
No problems expected.

Discontinuing:
May be unnecessary to finish medicine. Follow doctor's instructions.

Others:
If troubled breathing does not improve or worsens after using medicine, don't increase dose. Consult doctor.

INTERACTION WITH OTHER DRUGS

GENERIC NAME OR DRUG CLASS	COMBINED EFFECT
Beta-adrenergic blockers	Decreased terbutaline effect.
Ephedrine	Increased terbutaline effect. Excess heart stimulation.
Epinephrine	Increased terbutaline effect. Excess heart stimulation.
MAO inhibitors	Increased terbutaline effect. Dangerous. Avoid.
Sympathomimetics	Increased terbutaline effect.

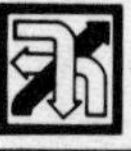

INTERACTION WITH OTHER SUBSTANCES

INTERACTS WITH	COMBINED EFFECT
Alcohol:	None expected.
Beverages:	None expected.
Cocaine:	Overstimulation.
Foods:	None expected.
Marijuana:	Possible increased therapeutic effect of terbutaline. May cause lung disorders to worsen.
Tobacco:	No interactions expected, but smoking may slow body's recovery. Avoid.

TERPIN HYDRATE

BRAND NAMES

Cotussis
Prunicodeine
SK-Terpin Hydrate w/Codeine
Terpin Hydrate and Codeine Syrup
Terpin Hydrate Elixir

GENERAL INFORMATION

Habit forming? Yes
Prescription needed? No
Available as generic? Yes
Drug class: Expectorant

USES

Decreases cough due to simple bronchial irritation.

DOSAGE & USAGE INFORMATION

How to take:
Follow each dose with 8 oz. water. Works better in combination with a cool-air vaporizer.

When to take:
3 to 4 times each day, spaced at least 4 hours apart.

If you forget a dose:
Take as soon as you remember. Wait 4 hours for next dose.

What drug does:
Loosens mucus in bronchial tubes to make mucus easier to cough up.

Time lapse before drug works:
10 to 15 minutes.

Don't take with:
See Interaction column and consult doctor.

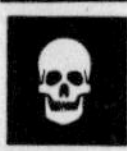

OVERDOSE

Symptoms:
Nausea, drowsiness.

What to do:
Overdose unlikely to threaten life. If person takes much larger amount than prescribed, call doctor, poison-control center or hospital emergency room for instructions.

POSSIBLE ADVERSE REACTIONS OR SIDE EFFECTS

SYMPTOMS	FREQUENCY	WHAT TO DO
Brain & nervous system:		
Symptoms of alcohol intoxication, especially in children.	Rare	3
Skin:	None expected.	
Eyes:	None expected.	
Ears, nose, throat:	None expected.	
Digestive:		
Nausea, vomiting, stomach pain.	Infrequent	4
Heart & lungs:	None expected.	
Blood vessels:	None expected.	
Muscles, bones, joints:	None expected.	
Genital, urinary:	None expected.	
Kidneys:	None expected.	
Liver:	None expected.	
Allergic:	None expected.	
Blood:	None expected.	
Others:	None expected.	

1- Life-threatening. Seek emergency treatment immediately.
2- Discontinue. Seek emergency treatment.
3- Discontinue. Call doctor right away.
4- Continue. Call doctor when convenient.
5- Continue. Tell doctor at next visit.
6- No action necessary.

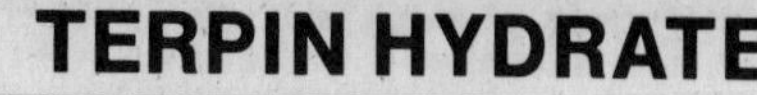

TERPIN HYDRATE

WARNINGS & PRECAUTIONS

Don't take if:
- You are allergic to terpin hydrate.
- You are a recovering or active alcoholic.

Before you start, consult your doctor:
If you plan to become pregnant within medication period.

Over age 60:
No problems expected.

Pregnancy:
Risk to unborn child outweighs drug benefits. Don't use.

Breast-feeding:
Drug filters into milk. May harm child. Avoid.

Infants & children:
Use only under medical supervision.

Prolonged use:
Habit forming.

Skin & sunlight:
No problems expected.

Driving, piloting or hazardous work:
Don't drive or pilot aircraft until you learn how medicine affects you. Don't work around dangerous machinery. Don't climb ladders or work in high places. Danger increases if you drink alcohol or take medicine affecting alertness and reflexes, such as antihistamines, tranquilizers, sedatives, pain medicine, narcotics and mind-altering drugs.

Airplane passengers:
No problems expected.

Discontinuing:
May be unnecessary to finish medicine. Follow doctor's instructions.

Others:
- Exceeding recommended doses may cause intoxication; drug is 42.5% alcohol.
- Frequently combined with codeine, which increases hazards.

INTERACTION WITH OTHER DRUGS

GENERIC NAME OR DRUG CLASS	COMBINED EFFECT
Antidepressants	Increased effect of terpin hydrate.
Antihistamines	Increased effect of terpin hydrate.
Muscle relaxants	Increased effect of terpin hydrate.
Narcotics	Increased effect of terpin hydrate.
Sedatives	Increased effect of terpin hydrate.
Sleep inducers	Increased effect of terpin hydrate.
Tranquilizers	Increased effect of terpin hydrate.

INTERACTION WITH OTHER SUBSTANCES

INTERACTS WITH	COMBINED EFFECT
Alcohol:	Increased sedative effect of both drugs. Avoid.
Beverages:	None expected.
Cocaine:	Unpredictable effect on nervous system. Avoid.
Foods:	None expected.
Marijuana:	Unpredictable effect on nervous system. Avoid.
Tobacco:	None expected.

TETRACYCLINES

BRAND AND GENERIC NAMES

Achromycin
Achrostatin V
Bio-Tetra
Bristacycline
Cyclopar
Medicycline
Neo-Tetrine
Nor-tet
Novotetra
Panmycin
Retet
Robitet
SK-Tetracycline
Tetrachel
Tetracyn
Tetracyrine
Tetrastatin
Tetrex

See complete brand and generic names list, page 832.

GENERAL INFORMATION

Habit forming? No
Prescription needed? Yes
Available as generic? Yes
Drug class: Antibiotic (tetracycline)

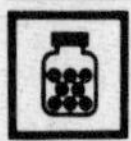

USES

- Treatment for infections susceptible to any tetracycline. Will not cure virus infections such as colds or flu.
- Treatment for acne.

DOSAGE & USAGE INFORMATION

How to take:
- Tablet or capsule—Take on empty stomach 1 hour before or 2 hours after eating. If you can't swallow whole, crumble tablet or open capsule and take with liquid or food.
- Liquid—Shake well. Take with measuring spoon.

When to take:
At the same times each day, evenly spaced.

If you forget a dose:
Take as soon as you remember up to 2 hours late. If more than 2 hours, wait for next scheduled dose (don't double this dose).

What drug does:
Prevents germ growth and reproduction.

Time lapse before drug works:
- Infections—May require 5 days to affect infection.
- Acne—May require 4 weeks to affect acne.

Don't take with:
- Non-prescription drugs without consulting doctor.
- See Interaction column and consult doctor.

OVERDOSE

Symptoms:
Severe nausea, vomiting, diarrhea.

What to do:
Overdose unlikely to threaten life. If person takes much larger amount than prescribed, call doctor, poison-control center or hospital emergency room for instructions.

POSSIBLE ADVERSE REACTIONS OR SIDE EFFECTS

SYMPTOMS	FREQUENCY	WHAT TO DO
Brain & nervous system:		
Headache	Infrequent	3
Skin:		
• Itching around rectum and genitals.	Common	3
• Rash	Infrequent	3
Eyes:		
Blurred vision.	Rare	3
Ears, nose, throat:		
• Dark tongue.	Common	5
• Sore mouth or tongue.	Common	2
• Excessive thirst.	Infrequent	4
Digestive:		
Nausea, vomiting, diarrhea, abdominal burning.	Common	2
Heart & lungs:	None expected.	
Blood vessels:	None expected.	
Muscles, bones, joints:	None expected.	
Genital, urinary:		
Increased urination.	Infrequent	4
Kidneys:	None expected.	
Liver:		
Jaundice (yellow eyes and skin) in pregnant women.	Rare	3
Allergic:	None expected.	
Blood:	None expected.	
Others:	None expected.	

1- Life-threatening. Seek emergency treatment immediately.
2- Discontinue. Seek emergency treatment.
3- Discontinue. Call doctor right away.
4- Continue. Call doctor when convenient.
5- Continue. Tell doctor at next visit.
6- No action necessary.

WARNINGS & PRECAUTIONS

Don't take if:
You are allergic to any tetracycline antibiotic.

Before you start, consult your doctor:
- If you have kidney or liver disease.
- If you have lupus.
- If you have myasthenia gravis.

Over age 60:
Dosage usually less than in younger adults. More likely to cause itching around rectum. Ask your doctor how to prevent it.

Pregnancy:
Risk to unborn child outweighs drug benefits. Don't use.

Breast-feeding:
Drug passes into milk. Avoid drug or discontinue nursing until you finish medicine. Consult doctor for advice on maintaining milk supply.

Infants & children:
May cause permanent teeth malformation or discoloration in children less than 8 years old. Don't use.

Prolonged use:
- You may become more susceptible to infections caused by germs not responsive to tetracycline.
- May cause rare problems in liver, kidney or bone marrow. Periodic laboratory blood studies, liver- and kidney-function tests recommended if you use drug a long time.

Skin & sunlight:
May cause rash or intensify sunburn in areas exposed to sun or sunlamp.

Driving, piloting or hazardous work:
No problems expected.

Airplane passengers:
No problems expected.

Discontinuing:
Don't discontinue without doctor's advice until you complete prescribed dose, even though symptoms diminish or disappear.

Others:
No problems expected.

INTERACTION WITH OTHER DRUGS

GENERIC NAME OR DRUG CLASS	COMBINED EFFECT
Antacids	Decreased tetracycline effect.
Anticoagulants (oral)	Increased anticoagulant effect.
Contraceptives (oral)	Decreased contraceptive effect.
Digitalis preparations	Increased digitalis effect.
Mineral supplements (iron, calcium, magnesium, zinc)	Decreased tetracycline absorption. Separate doses by 1 to 2 hours.
Lithium	Increased lithium effect.
Penicillins	Decreased penicillin effect.
Sodium bicarbonate	Decreased tetracycline effect.

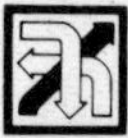

INTERACTION WITH OTHER SUBSTANCES

INTERACTS WITH	COMBINED EFFECT
Alcohol:	Possible liver damage. Avoid.
Beverages: Milk	Decreased tetracycline absorption. Take dose 2 hours after or 1 hour before drinking.
Cocaine:	No proven problems.
Foods: Dairy products	Decreased tetracycline absorption. Take dose 2 hours after or 1 hour before eating.
Marijuana:	No interactions expected, but marijuana may slow body's recovery. Avoid.
Tobacco:	None expected.

THEOPHYLLINE

BRAND NAMES

Accurbron
Aerolate
Asthmophylline
Bronkodyl
Elixicon
Elixophyllin
Physpan
Slophyllin
Somophyllin-T
Theobid
Theoclear
Theo-Dur
Theolair
Theolixir
Theophyl

See complete brand names list, page 832.

GENERAL INFORMATION

Habit forming? No
Prescription needed? Canada—No
U.S: High strength—Yes
Low strength—No
Available as generic? Yes
Drug class: Bronchodilator (xanthine)

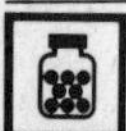

USES

Treatment for bronchial asthma symptoms.

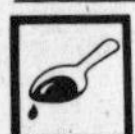

DOSAGE & USAGE INFORMATION

How to take:

- Tablet or capsule—Swallow with liquid.
- Extended-release tablets or capsules—Swallow each dose whole. If you take regular tablets, you may chew or crush them.
- Suppositories—Remove wrapper and moisten suppository with water. Gently insert larger end into rectum. Push well into rectum with finger.
- Syrup—Take as directed on bottle.
- Enema—Use as directed on label.

When to take:
Most effective taken on empty stomach 1 hour before or 2 hours after eating. However, may take with food to lessen stomach upset.

If you forget a dose:
Take as soon as you remember up to 2 hours late. If more than 2 hours, wait for next scheduled dose (don't double this dose).

What drug does:
Relaxes and expands bronchial tubes.

Time lapse before drug works:
15 to 30 minutes.

Don't take with:
See Interaction column and consult doctor.

OVERDOSE

Symptoms:
Restlessness, irritability, confusion, delirium, convulsions, rapid pulse, coma.

What to do:

- Dial 0 (operator) or 911 (emergency) for an ambulance or medical help. Then give first aid immediately.
- Additional emergency information on page 886.

POSSIBLE ADVERSE REACTIONS OR SIDE EFFECTS

SYMPTOMS	FREQUENCY	WHAT TO DO
Brain & nervous system:		
• Headache, irritability, nervousness, restlessness, insomnia.	Common	4
• Dizziness or lightheadedness.	Infrequent	4
Skin:		
• Rash or hives.	Infrequent	3
• Flushed face.	Infrequent	4
Eyes:	None expected.	
Ears, nose, throat:	None expected.	
Digestive:		
• Nausea, vomiting, stomach pain.	Common	4
• Diarrhea, appetite loss.	Infrequent	3
Heart & lungs:		
• Rapid breathing.	Infrequent	3
• Irregular heartbeat.	Infrequent	3
Blood vessels:	None expected.	
Muscles, bones, joints:	None expected.	
Genital, urinary:	None expected.	
Kidneys:	None expected.	
Liver:	None expected.	
Allergic:	None expected.	
Blood:	None expected.	
Others:	None expected.	

1-Life-threatening. Seek emergency treatment immediately.
2-Discontinue. Seek emergency treatment.
3-Discontinue. Call doctor right away.
4-Continue. Call doctor when convenient.
5-Continue. Tell doctor at next visit.
6-No action necessary.

WARNINGS & PRECAUTIONS

Don't take if:
- You are allergic to any bronchodilator.
- You have an active peptic ulcer.

Before you start, consult your doctor:
- If you have had impaired kidney or liver function.
- If you have gastritis.
- If you have a peptic ulcer.
- If you have high blood pressure or heart disease.
- If you take medication for gout.

Over age 60:
Adverse reactions and side effects may be more frequent and severe than in younger persons.

Pregnancy:
Risk to unborn child outweighs drug benefits. Don't use.

Breast-feeding:
Drug passes into milk. Avoid drug or discontinue nursing until you finish medicine. Consult doctor for advice on maintaining milk supply.

Infants & children:
Use only under medical supervision.

Prolonged use:
Stomach irritation.

Skin & sunlight:
No problems expected.

Driving, piloting or hazardous work:
Avoid if lightheaded or dizzy. Otherwise, no problems expected.

Airplane passengers:
No problems expected.

Discontinuing:
May be unnecessary to finish medicine. Follow doctor's instructions.

Others:
No problems expected.

INTERACTION WITH OTHER DRUGS

GENERIC NAME OR DRUG CLASS	COMBINED EFFECT
Allopurinol	Decreased allopurinol effect.
Ephedrine	Increased effect of both drugs.
Epinephrine	Increased effect of both drugs.
Erythromycin	Increased theophylline effect.
Furosemide	Increased furosemide effect.
Lincomycins	Increased theophylline effect.
Lithium	Decreased lithium effect.
Probenecid	Decreased effect of both drugs.
Propranolol	Decreased theophylline effect.
Rauwolfia alkaloids	Rapid heartbeat.
Sulfinpyrazone	Decreased sulfinpyrazone effect.
Troleandomycin	Increased theophylline effect.

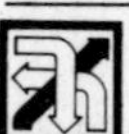

INTERACTION WITH OTHER SUBSTANCES

INTERACTS WITH	COMBINED EFFECT
Alcohol:	None expected.
Beverages: Caffeine drinks	Nervousness and insomnia.
Cocaine:	Excess stimulation. Avoid.
Foods:	None expected.
Marijuana:	Slightly increased antiasthmatic effect of theophylline.
Tobacco:	Decreased theophylline effect.

THIABENDAZOLE

BRAND NAMES

Foldan
Mintezol
Minzolum
Triasox

GENERAL INFORMATION

Habit forming? No
Prescription needed? Yes
Available as generic? No
Drug class: Antihelminthic (antiworm medication)

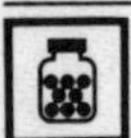

USES

Treatment of parasite infestations.

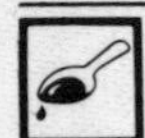

DOSAGE & USAGE INFORMATION

How to take:
Tablet or capsule—Swallow with liquid or food to lessen stomach irritation.

When to take:
According to instructions on prescription, after meals.

If you forget a dose:
Take as soon as you remember up to 2 hours late. If more than 2 hours, wait for next scheduled dose (don't double this dose).

What drug does:
Kills larvae and adult worms.

Time lapse before drug works:
Varies according to degree of infestation.

Don't take with:
See Interaction column and consult doctor.

OVERDOSE

Symptoms:
Aching, fever, blistered skin, seizures.

What to do:

- Dial 0 (operator) or 911 (emergency) for an ambulance or medical help. Then give first aid immediately.
- If patient is unconscious and not breathing, give mouth-to-mouth breathing. If there is no heartbeat, use cardiac massage and mouth-to-mouth breathing (CPR). Don't try to make patient vomit. If you can't get help quickly, take patient to nearest emergency facility.
- Additional emergency information on page 886.

POSSIBLE ADVERSE REACTIONS OR SIDE EFFECTS

SYMPTOMS	FREQUENCY	WHAT TO DO
Brain & nervous system:		
• Dizziness	Common	4
• Drowsiness	Common	4
• Headache	Common	4
Skin:		
• Redness, blistering, with fever.	Infrequent	3
• Rash with itching.	Infrequent	3
Eyes:		
Blurred or yellow vision.	Rare	3
Ears, nose, throat:		
Ringing or buzzing in ears.	Infrequent	4
Digestive:		
• Nausea, appetite loss.	Common	4
• Nausea/vomiting.	Common	3
• Abdominal pain.	Common	3
Heart & lungs:	None expected.	
Blood vessels:	None expected.	
Muscles, bones, joints:		
• Aching joints and muscles.	Infrequent	3
• Numbness/tingling feet & hands.	Infrequent	4
Genital, urinary:		
• Asparagus-like odor of urine.	Common	5
• Bed wetting.	Common	4
Kidneys, allergic, blood, liver:	None expected.	
Others:	None expected.	

1- Life-threatening. Seek emergency treatment immediately.
2- Discontinue. Seek emergency treatment.
3- Discontinue. Call doctor right away.
4- Continue. Call doctor when convenient.
5- Continue. Tell doctor at next visit.

WARNINGS & PRECAUTIONS

Don't take if:
You are allergic to thiabendazole.

Before you start, consult your doctor:
- If you have kidney disease.
- If you have liver disease.

Over age 60:
Adverse reactions and side effects may be more frequent and severe than in younger persons.

Pregnancy:
Risk to unborn child outweighs drug benefits. Don't use.

Breast-feeding:
Unknown effect. Consult doctor.

Infants & children:
Use only under medical supervision.

Prolonged use:
Request follow-up stool exams 2 to 3 weeks following treatment.

Skin & sunlight:
No problems expected.

Driving, piloting or hazardous work:
Don't drive or pilot aircraft until you learn how medicine affects you. Don't work around dangerous machinery. Don't climb ladders or work in high places. Danger increases if you drink alcohol or take medicine affecting alertness and reflexes, such as antihistamines, tranquilizers, sedatives, pain medicine, narcotics and mind-altering drugs.

Airplane passengers:
No problems expected.

Discontinuing:
May be unnecessary to finish medicine. Follow doctor's instructions.

Others:
To prevent reinfection: Deworm household pets regularly. Cover sand boxes. Cook all pork until well done.

INTERACTION WITH OTHER DRUGS

GENERIC NAME OR DRUG CLASS	COMBINED EFFECT
None expected.	

INTERACTION WITH OTHER SUBSTANCES

INTERACTS WITH	COMBINED EFFECT
Alcohol:	Decreased thiabendazole effect.
Beverages:	No problems expected.
Cocaine:	Decreased thiabendazole effect.
Foods:	Take with foods to decrease nausea.
Marijuana:	Decreased thiabendazole effect.
Tobacco:	May decrease absorption of medicine.

THIAMINE (VITAMIN B-1)

BRAND NAMES

Betalin S
Biamine
Betaxin
Pan-B-1
Bewon
Numerous other multiple vitamin-mineral supplements.

GENERAL INFORMATION

Habit forming? No
Prescription needed? No
Available as generic? Yes
Drug class: Vitamin supplement

USES

- Dietary supplement to promote normal growth, development and health.
- Treatment for beri-beri (a thiamine-deficiency disease).
- Dietary supplement for alcoholism, cirrhosis, overactive thyroid, infection, breast-feeding, absorption diseases, pregnancy, prolonged diarrhea, burns.

DOSAGE & USAGE INFORMATION

How to take:
Tablet or liquid—Swallow with beverage or food to lessen stomach irritation.

When to take:
At the same time each day.

If you forget a dose:
Take when remembered. Return to regular schedule.

What drug does:
- Promotes normal growth and development.
- Combines with an enzyme to metabolize carbohydrates.

Time lapse before drug works:
15 minutes.

Don't take with:
See Interaction column and consult doctor.

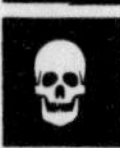

OVERDOSE

Symptoms:
Increased severity of adverse reactions and side effects.

What to do:
Overdose unlikely to threaten life. If person takes much larger amount than prescribed, call doctor, poison-control center or hospital emergency room for instructions.

POSSIBLE ADVERSE REACTIONS OR SIDE EFFECTS

SYMPTOMS	FREQUENCY	WHAT TO DO
Brain & nervous system:	None expected.	
Skin:		
Rash or itch.	Rare	3
Eyes:	None expected.	
Ears, nose, throat:	None expected.	
Digestive:	None expected.	
Heart & lungs:		
Wheezing	Rare	2
Blood vessels:	None expected.	
Muscles, bones, joints:	None expected.	
Genital, urinary:	None expected.	
Kidneys:	None expected.	
Liver:	None expected.	
Allergic:		
Life-threatening anaphylaxis may occur when given intravenously.	Rare	1 See Page 888.
Blood:	None expected.	
Others:	None expected.	

1- Life-threatening. Seek emergency treatment immediately.
2- Discontinue. Seek emergency treatment.
3- Discontinue. Call doctor right away.
4- Continue. Call doctor when convenient.
5- Continue. Tell doctor at next visit.
6- No action necessary.

THIAMINE (VITAMIN B-1)

WARNINGS & PRECAUTIONS

Don't take if:
You are allergic to any B vitamin.

Before you start, consult your doctor:
If you have liver or kidney disease.

Over age 60:
No problems expected.

Pregnancy:
No problems expected.

Breast-feeding:
No problems expected.

Infants & children:
No problems expected.

Prolonged use:
No problems expected.

Skin & sunlight:
No problems expected.

Driving, piloting or hazardous work:
No problems expected.

Airplane passengers:
No problems expected.

Discontinuing:
No problems expected.

Others:
A balanced diet should provide enough thiamine for healthy people to make supplement unnecessary. Best dietary sources of thiamine are whole-grain cereals and meats.

INTERACTION WITH OTHER DRUGS

GENERIC NAME OR DRUG CLASS	COMBINED EFFECT
Barbiturates	Decreased thiamine effect.

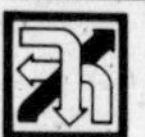

INTERACTION WITH OTHER SUBSTANCES

INTERACTS WITH	COMBINED EFFECT
Alcohol:	None expected.
Beverages: Carbonates, citrates (additives listed on many beverage labels).	Decreased thiamine effect.
Cocaine:	None expected.
Foods: Carbonates, citrates (additives listed on many food labels).	Decreased thiamine effect.
Marijuana:	None expected.
Tobacco:	None expected.

THIORIDAZINE

BRAND NAMES

Apo-Thioridazine
Mellaril
Novoridazine
SK-Thioridazine Hydrochloride
Thioril

GENERAL INFORMATION

Habit forming? No
Prescription needed? Yes
Available as generic? Yes
Drug class: Tranquilizer, antiemetic (phenothiazine)

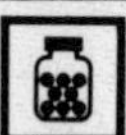

USES

- Stops nausea, vomiting.
- Reduces anxiety, agitation.

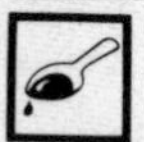

DOSAGE & USAGE INFORMATION

How to take:

- Tablet or capsule—Swallow with liquid or food to lessen stomach irritation.
- Suppositories—Remove wrapper and moisten suppository with water. Gently insert into rectum, large end first.
- Drops or liquid—Dilute dose in beverage.

When to take:

- Nervous and mental disorders—Take at the same times each day.
- Nausea and vomiting—Take as needed, no more often than every 4 hours.

If you forget a dose:

- Nervous and mental disorders—Take up to 2 hours late. If more than 2 hours, wait for next scheduled dose (don't double this).
- Nausea and vomiting—Take as soon as you remember. Wait 4 hours for next dose.

What drug does:

- Suppresses brain's vomiting center.
- Suppresses brain centers that control abnormal emotions and behavior.

Time lapse before drug works:

- Nausea and vomiting—1 hour or less.
- Nervous and mental disorders—4-6 weeks.

Don't take with:

- Antacid or medicine for diarrhea.
- Non-prescription drug for cough, cold or allergy.
- See Interaction column and consult doctor.

OVERDOSE

Symptoms:
Stupor, convulsions, coma.

What to do:

- Dial 0 (operator) or 911 (emergency) for an ambulance or medical help. Then give first aid immediately.
- Additional emergency information on page 886.

POSSIBLE ADVERSE REACTIONS OR SIDE EFFECTS

SYMPTOMS	FREQUENCY	WHAT TO DO
Brain & nervous system:		
• Restlessness, tremor.	Common	3
• Fainting	Infrequent	2
• Drowsiness	Common	3
Skin:		
• Rash	Infrequent	3
• Less perspiration.	Common	4
Eyes:		
Vision changes.	Rare	3
Ears, nose, throat:		
• Sore throat, fever.	Rare	3
• Dry mouth, nasal congestion.	Common	4
Digestive:		
Constipation	Common	4
Heart & lungs, blood vessels, kidneys, allergic, blood:	None expected.	
Muscles, bones, joints:		
Muscle spasms of face and neck, unsteady gait.	Common	2
Genital, urinary:		
Urination difficulty.	Infrequent	4
Liver:		
Jaundice (yellow eyes and skin).	Rare	3
Others:		
Less interest in sex, breast swelling, change in menstrual pattern.	Infrequent	4

1-Life-threatening. Seek emergency treatment immediately.
2-Discontinue. Seek emergency treatment.
3-Discontinue. Call doctor right away.
4-Continue. Call doctor when convenient.
5-Continue. Tell doctor at next visit.
6-No action necessary.

WARNINGS & PRECAUTIONS

Don't take if:
- You are allergic to any phenothiazine.
- You have a blood or bone-marrow disease.

Before you start, consult your doctor:
- If you will have surgery within 2 months, including dental surgery, requiring general or spinal anesthesia.
- If you have asthma, emphysema or other lung disorder.
- If you take non-prescription ulcer medicine, asthma medicine or amphetamines.

Over age 60:
Adverse reactions and side effects may be more frequent and severe than in younger persons. More likely to develop involuntary movement of jaws, lips, tongue, chewing. Report this to your doctor immediately. Early treatment can help.

Pregnancy:
Risk to unborn child outweighs drug benefits. Don't use.

Breast-feeding:
Drug passes into milk. Avoid drug or discontinue nursing until you finish medicine. Consult doctor for advice on maintaining milk supply.

Infants & children:
Don't give to children younger than 2.

Prolonged use:
May lead to tardive dyskinesia (involuntary movement of jaws, lips, tongue, chewing).

Skin & sunlight:
May cause rash or intensify sunburn in areas exposed to sun or sunlamp. Skin may remain sensitive for 3 months after discontinuing.

Driving, piloting or hazardous work:
Don't drive or pilot aircraft until you learn how medicine affects you. Don't work around dangerous machinery. Don't climb ladders or work in high places. Danger increases if you drink alcohol or take medicine affecting alertness and reflexes.

Airplane passengers:
No problems expected.

Discontinuing:
- Nervous and mental disorders—Don't discontinue without doctor's advice until you complete prescribed dose, even though symptoms diminish or disappear.
- Nausea and vomiting—May be unnecessary to finish medicine. Follow doctor's instructions.

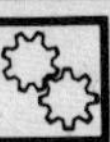

INTERACTION WITH OTHER DRUGS

GENERIC NAME OR DRUG CLASS	COMBINED EFFECT
Anticholinergics	Increased anticholinergic effect.
Antidepressants (tricyclic)	Increased thioridazine effect.
Antihistamines	Increased antihistamine effect.
Appetite suppressants	Decreased suppressant effect.
Levodopa	Decreased levodopa effect.
Mind-altering drugs	Increased effect of mind-altering drugs.
Narcotics	Increased narcotic effect.
Phenytoin	Increased phenytoin effect.
Quinidine	Impaired heart function. Dangerous mixture.
Sedatives	Increased sedative effect.
Tranquilizers (other)	Increased tranquilizer effect.

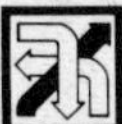

INTERACTION WITH OTHER SUBSTANCES

INTERACTS WITH	COMBINED EFFECT
Alcohol:	Dangerous oversedation.
Beverages:	None expected.
Cocaine:	Decreased thioridazine effect. Avoid.
Foods:	None expected.
Marijuana:	Drowsiness. May increase antinausea effect.
Tobacco:	None expected.

THIOTHIXENE

BRAND NAMES

Navane

GENERAL INFORMATION

Habit forming? No
Prescription needed? Yes
Available as generic? No

Drug class: Tranquilizer (thioxanthine), antiemetic

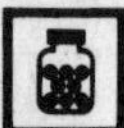

USES

- Reduces anxiety, agitation, psychosis.
- Stops vomiting.

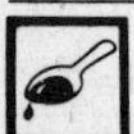

DOSAGE & USAGE INFORMATION

How to take:

- Capsule—Swallow with liquid. If you can't swallow whole, open capsule and take with liquid or food.
- Syrup—Dilute dose in beverage before swallowing.

When to take:
At the same time each day.

If you forget a dose:
Take as soon as you remember up to 2 hours late. If more than 2 hours, wait for next scheduled dose (don't double this dose).

What drug does:
Corrects imbalance of nerve impulses.

Time lapse before drug works:
3 weeks.

Don't take with:
See Interaction column and consult doctor.

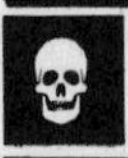

OVERDOSE

Symptoms:
Drowsiness, dizziness, weakness, muscle rigidity, twitching, tremors, confusion, dry mouth, blurred vision, rapid pulse, shallow breathing, low blood pressure, convulsions, coma.

What to do:

- Dial 0 (operator) or 911 (emergency) for an ambulance or medical help. Then give first aid immediately.
- If patient is unconscious and not breathing, give mouth-to-mouth breathing. If there is no heartbeat, use cardiac massage and mouth-to-mouth breathing (CPR). Don't try to make patient vomit. If you can't get help quickly, take patient to nearest emergency facility.
- Additional emergency information on page 886.

POSSIBLE ADVERSE REACTIONS OR SIDE EFFECTS

SYMPTOMS	FREQUENCY	WHAT TO DO
Brain & nervous system:		
• Fainting; restlessness; jerky, involuntary movements.	Common	3
• Dizziness, drowsiness.	Common	4
Skin:		
Rash	Infrequent	3
Eyes:		
Blurred vision.	Common	3
Ears, nose, throat:		
• Sore throat, fever.	Rare	3
• Dry mouth, nasal congestion.	Common	5
Digestive:		
Constipation	Common	4
Heart & lungs:		
Rapid heartbeat.	Common	3
Blood vessels, kidneys, allergic, blood:	None expected.	
Muscles, bones, joints:		
• Muscle spasms.	Common	4
• Shuffling walk.	Common	4
Genital, urinary:		
• Less sexual ability.	Infrequent	4
• Difficult urination.	Infrequent	4
Liver:		
Jaundice (yellow skin and eyes).	Rare	3
Others:		
• Less perspiration.	Common	4
• Menstrual changes.	Infrequent	5
• Breast swelling.	Infrequent	5

1 - Life-threatening. Seek emergency treatment immediately.
2 - Discontinue. Seek emergency treatment.
3 - Discontinue. Call doctor right away.
4 - Continue. Call doctor when convenient.
5 - Continue. Tell doctor at next visit.

WARNINGS & PRECAUTIONS

Don't take if:
- You are allergic to any thioxanthine or phenothiazine tranquilizer.
- You have serious blood disorder.
- You have Parkinson's disease.
- Patient is younger than 12.

Before you start, consult your doctor:
- If you have had liver or kidney disease.
- If you have epilepsy or glaucoma.
- If you have high blood pressure or heart disease (especially angina).
- If you use alcohol daily.
- If you will have surgery within 2 months, including dental surgery, requiring general or spinal anesthesia.

Over age 60:
Adverse reactions and side effects may be more frequent and severe than in younger persons.

Pregnancy:
No proven harm to unborn child. Avoid if possible.

Breast-feeding:
Studies inconclusive. Consult your doctor.

Infants & children:
Not recommended.

Prolonged use:
- Pigment deposits in lens and retina of eye.
- Involuntary movements of jaws, lips, tongue (tardive dyskinesia).

Skin & sunlight:
May cause rash or intensify sunburn in areas exposed to sun or sunlamp.

Driving, piloting or hazardous work:
Don't drive or pilot aircraft until you learn how medicine affects you. Don't work around dangerous machinery. Don't climb ladders or work in high places. Danger increases if you drink alcohol or take medicine affecting alertness and reflexes.

Airplane passengers:
No problems expected.

Discontinuing:
Don't discontinue without consulting doctor. Dose may require gradual reduction if you have taken drug for a long time. Doses of other drugs may also require adjustment.

Others:
Hot temperatures increase chance of heat stroke.

INTERACTION WITH OTHER DRUGS

GENERIC NAME OR DRUG CLASS	COMBINED EFFECT
Anticholinergics	Increased anticholinergic effect.
Anticonvulsants	Change in seizure pattern.
Antidepressants (tricyclic)	Increased thiothixene effect. Excessive sedation.
Antihistamines	Increased thiothixene effect. Excessive sedation.
Antihypertensives	Excessively low blood pressure.
Barbiturates	Increased thiothixene effect. Excessive sedation.
Bethanechol	Decreased bethanechol effect.
Guanethidine	Decreased guanethidine effect.
Levodopa	Decreased levodopa effect.
MAO inhibitors	Excessive sedation.
Mind-altering drugs	Increased thiothixene effect. Excessive sedation.
Narcotics	Increased thiothixene effect. Excessive sedation.

Additional interactions on page 843.

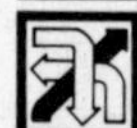

INTERACTION WITH OTHER SUBSTANCES

INTERACTS WITH	COMBINED EFFECT
Alcohol:	Excessive brain depression. Avoid.
Beverages:	None expected.
Cocaine:	Decreased thiothixene effect. Avoid.
Foods:	None expected.
Marijuana:	Daily use—Fainting likely, possible psychosis.
Tobacco:	None expected.

THYROGLOBULIN

BRAND NAMES

Proloid

GENERAL INFORMATION

Habit forming? No
Prescription needed? Yes
Available as generic? Yes
Drug class: Thyroid hormone

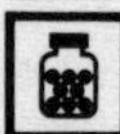

USES

Replacement for thyroid hormone deficiency.

DOSAGE & USAGE INFORMATION

How to take:

- Tablet or capsule—Swallow with liquid.
- Extended-release tablets or capsules—Swallow each dose whole. If you take regular tablets, you may chew or crush them.

When to take:
At the same time each day before a meal or on awakening.

If you forget a dose:
Take as soon as you remember up to 12 hours late. If more than 12 hours, wait for next scheduled dose (don't double this dose).

What drug does:
Increases cell metabolism rate.

Time lapse before drug works:
48 hours.

Don't take with:
See Interaction column and consult doctor.

OVERDOSE

Symptoms:
"Hot" feeling, heart palpitations, nervousness, sweating, hand tremors, insomnia, rapid and irregular pulse, headache, irritability, diarrhea, weight loss, muscle cramps.

What to do:
Overdose unlikely to threaten life. If person takes much larger amount than prescribed, call doctor, poison-control center or hospital emergency room for instructions.

POSSIBLE ADVERSE REACTIONS OR SIDE EFFECTS

SYMPTOMS	FREQUENCY	WHAT TO DO
Brain & nervous system: Tremor, headache, irritability, insomnia.	Common	3
Skin: Hives, rash.	Infrequent	3
Eyes:	None expected.	
Ears, nose, throat:	None expected.	
Digestive:		
• Appetite change.	Common	4
• Diarrhea	Common	4
• Vomiting	Infrequent	3
Heart & lungs: Chest pain, rapid and irregular heartbeat, shortness of breath.	Infrequent	3
Blood vessels:	None expected.	
Muscles, bones, joints: Leg cramps.	Common	4
Genital, urinary:	None expected.	
Kidneys:	None expected.	
Liver:	None expected.	
Allergic:	None expected.	
Blood:	None expected.	
Others:		
• Change in menstrual periods.	Common	4
• Fever, heat sensitivity, unusual sweating.	Common	4
• Weight loss.	Common	4

1- Life-threatening. Seek emergency treatment immediately.
2- Discontinue. Seek emergency treatment.
3- Discontinue. Call doctor right away.
4- Continue. Call doctor when convenient.
5- Continue. Tell doctor at next visit.
6- No action necessary.

WARNINGS & PRECAUTIONS

Don't take if:

- You have had a heart attack within 6 weeks.
- You have no thyroid deficiency, but use this to lose weight.

Before you start, consult your doctor:

- If you have heart disease or high blood pressure.
- If you have diabetes.
- If you have Addison's disease, have had adrenal gland deficiency or use epinephrine, ephedrine or isoproterenol for asthma.

Over age 60:
More sensitive to thyroid hormone. May need smaller doses.

Pregnancy:
Considered safe if for thyroid deficiency only.

Breast-feeding:
Present in milk. Considered safe if dose is correct.

Infants & children:
Use only under medical supervision.

Prolonged use:
No problems expected, if dose is correct.

Skin & sunlight:
No problems expected.

Driving, piloting or hazardous work:
No problems expected.

Airplane passengers:
No problems expected.

Discontinuing:
Don't discontinue without consulting doctor. Dose may require gradual reduction if you have taken drug for a long time. Doses of other drugs may also require adjustment.

Others:
Digestive upsets, tremors, cramps, nervousness, insomnia or diarrhea may indicate need for dose adjustment.

INTERACTION WITH OTHER DRUGS

GENERIC NAME OR DRUG CLASS	COMBINED EFFECT
Amphetamines	Increased amphetamine effect.
Anticoagulants (oral)	Increased anticoagulant effect.
Antidepressants (tricyclic)	Increased antidepressant effect.
Antidiabetics	Antidiabetic may require adjustment.
Aspirin (large doses, continuous use)	Increased thyroglobulin effect.
Barbiturates	Decreased barbiturate effect.
Cholestyramine	Decreased thyroglobulin effect.
Contraceptives (oral)	Decreased thyroglobulin effect.
Cortisone drugs	Requires dose adjustment to prevent cortisone deficiency.
Digitalis preparations	Increased digitalis effect.
Ephedrine	Increased ephedrine effect.
Epinephrine	Increased epinephrine effect.
Methylphenidate	Increased methylphenidate effect.
Phenytoin	Increased thyroglobulin effect.

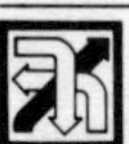

INTERACTION WITH OTHER SUBSTANCES

INTERACTS WITH	COMBINED EFFECT
Alcohol:	None expected.
Beverages:	None expected.
Cocaine:	Excess stimulation. Avoid.
Foods: Soybeans	Heavy consumption interferes with thyroid function.
Marijuana:	None expected.
Tobacco:	None expected.

THYROID

BRAND NAMES

Armour
Cytomel
Euthroid
Levothroid
Proloid
S-P-T
Synthroid
Thyrar
Thyrocrine

GENERAL INFORMATION

Habit forming? No
Prescription needed? Yes
Available as generic? Yes
Drug class: Thyroid hormone

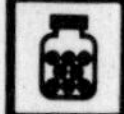

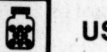

USES

Replacement for thyroid hormone deficiency.

DOSAGE & USAGE INFORMATION

How to take:
- Tablet or capsule—Swallow with liquid.
- Extended-release tablets or capsules—Swallow each dose whole. If you take regular tablets, you may chew or crush them.

When to take:
At the same time each day before a meal or on awakening.

If you forget a dose:
Take as soon as you remember up to 12 hours late. If more than 12 hours, wait for next scheduled dose (don't double this dose).

What drug does:
Increases cell metabolism rate.

Time lapse before drug works:
48 hours.

Don't take with:
See Interaction column and consult doctor.

OVERDOSE

Symptoms:
"Hot" feeling, heart palpitations, nervousness, sweating, hand tremors, insomnia, rapid and irregular pulse, headache, irritability, diarrhea, weight loss, muscle cramps.

What to do:
Overdose unlikely to threaten life. If person takes much larger amount than prescribed, call doctor, poison-control center or hospital emergency room for instructions.

POSSIBLE ADVERSE REACTIONS OR SIDE EFFECTS

SYMPTOMS	FREQUENCY	WHAT TO DO
Brain & nervous system:		
Tremor, headache, irritability, insomnia.	Common	3
Skin:		
Hives, rash.	Infrequent	3
Eyes:	None expected.	
Ears, nose, throat:	None expected.	
Digestive:		
• Appetite change.	Common	4
• Diarrhea	Common	4
• Vomiting	Infrequent	3
Heart & lungs:		
Chest pain, rapid and irregular heartbeat, shortness of breath.	Infrequent	3
Blood vessels:	None expected.	
Muscles, bones, joints:		
Leg cramps.	Common	4
Genital, urinary:	None expected.	
Kidneys:	None expected.	
Liver:	None expected.	
Allergic:	None expected.	
Blood:	None expected.	
Others:		
• Change in menstrual periods.	Common	4
• Fever, heat sensitivity, unusual sweating.	Common	4
• Weight loss.	Common	4

1- Life-threatening. Seek emergency treatment immediately.
2- Discontinue. Seek emergency treatment.
3- Discontinue. Call doctor right away.
4- Continue. Call doctor when convenient.
5- Continue. Tell doctor at next visit.
6- No action necessary.

WARNINGS & PRECAUTIONS

Don't take if:

- You have had a heart attack within 6 weeks.
- You have no thyroid deficiency, but use this to lose weight.

Before you start, consult your doctor:

- If you have heart disease or high blood pressure.
- If you have diabetes.
- If you have Addison's disease, have had adrenal gland deficiency or use epinephrine, ephedrine or isoproterenol for asthma.

Over age 60:
More sensitive to thyroid hormone. May need smaller doses.

Pregnancy:
Considered safe if for thyroid deficiency only.

Breast-feeding:
Present in milk. Considered safe if dose is correct.

Infants & children:
Use only under medical supervision.

Prolonged use:
No problems expected, if dose is correct.

Skin & sunlight:
No problems expected.

Driving, piloting or hazardous work:
No problems expected.

Airplane passengers:
No problems expected.

Discontinuing:
Don't discontinue without consulting doctor. Dose may require gradual reduction if you have taken drug for a long time. Doses of other drugs may also require adjustment.

Others:
Digestive upsets, tremors, cramps, nervousness, insomnia or diarrhea may indicate need for dose adjustment.

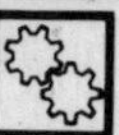

INTERACTION WITH OTHER DRUGS

GENERIC NAME OR DRUG CLASS	COMBINED EFFECT
Amphetamines	Increased amphetamine effect.
Anticoagulants (oral)	Increased anticoagulant effect.
Antidepressants (tricyclic)	Increased antidepressant effect.
Antidiabetics	Antidiabetic may require adjustment.
Aspirin (large doses, continuous use)	Increased thyroid effect.
Barbiturates	Decreased barbiturate effect.
Cholestyramine	Decreased thyroid effect.
Contraceptives (oral)	Decreased thyroid effect.
Cortisone drugs	Requires dose adjustment to prevent cortisone deficiency.
Digitalis preparations	Increased digitalis effect.
Ephedrine	Increased ephedrine effect.
Epinephrine	Increased epinephrine effect.
Methylphenidate	Increased methylphenidate effect.
Phenytoin	Increased thyroid effect.

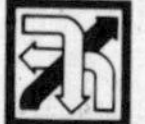

INTERACTION WITH OTHER SUBSTANCES

INTERACTS WITH	COMBINED EFFECT
Alcohol:	None expected.
Beverages:	None expected.
Cocaine:	Excess stimulation. Avoid.
Foods:	
Soybeans	Heavy consumption interferes with thyroid function.
Marijuana:	None expected.
Tobacco:	None expected.

THYROXINE (T-4, LEVOTHYROXINE)

BRAND NAMES

Choloxin
Cytolen
Elthroxin
Euthroid
Letter
Levoid
Levothroid
L-Thyroxine
L-T-S
Noroxine
Ro-Thyroxine
Synthroid
Thyrolar

GENERAL INFORMATION

Habit forming? No
Prescription needed? Yes
Available as generic? Yes
Drug class: Thyroid hormone

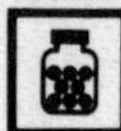

USES

Replacement for thyroid hormone deficiency.

DOSAGE & USAGE INFORMATION

How to take:

- Tablet or capsule—Swallow with liquid.
- Extended-release tablets or capsules—Swallow each dose whole. If you take regular tablets, you may chew or crush them.

When to take:
At the same time each day before a meal or on awakening.

If you forget a dose:
Take as soon as you remember up to 12 hours late. If more than 12 hours, wait for next scheduled dose (don't double this dose).

What drug does:
Increases cell metabolism rate.

Time lapse before drug works:
48 hours.

Don't take with:
See Interaction column and consult doctor.

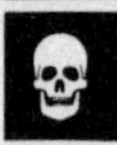

OVERDOSE

Symptoms:
"Hot" feeling, heart palpitations, nervousness, sweating, hand tremors, insomnia, rapid and irregular pulse, headache, irritability, diarrhea, weight loss, muscle cramps.

What to do:
Overdose unlikely to threaten life. If person takes much larger amount than prescribed, call doctor, poison-control center or hospital emergency room for instructions.

POSSIBLE ADVERSE REACTIONS OR SIDE EFFECTS

SYMPTOMS	FREQUENCY	WHAT TO DO
Brain & nervous system:		
Tremor, headache, irritability, insomnia.	Common	3
Skin:		
Hives, rash.	Infrequent	3
Eyes:	None expected.	
Ears, nose, throat:	None expected.	
Digestive:		
• Appetite change.	Common	4
• Diarrhea	Common	4
• Vomiting	Infrequent	3
Heart & lungs:		
Chest pain, rapid and irregular heartbeat, shortness of breath.	Infrequent	3
Blood vessels:	None expected.	
Muscles, bones, joints:		
Leg cramps.	Common	4
Genital, urinary:	None expected.	
Kidneys:	None expected.	
Liver:	None expected.	
Allergic:	None expected.	
Blood:	None expected.	
Others:		
• Change in menstrual periods.	Common	4
• Fever, heat sensitivity, unusual sweating.	Common	4
• Weight loss.	Common	4

1-Life-threatening. Seek emergency treatment immediately.
2-Discontinue. Seek emergency treatment.
3-Discontinue. Call doctor right away.
4-Continue. Call doctor when convenient.
5-Continue. Tell doctor at next visit.
6-No action necessary.

THYROXINE (T-4, LEVOTHYROXINE)

WARNINGS & PRECAUTIONS

Don't take if:
- You have had a heart attack within 6 weeks.
- You have no thyroid deficiency, but use this to lose weight.

Before you start, consult your doctor:
- If you have heart disease or high blood pressure.
- If you have diabetes.
- If you have Addison's disease, have had adrenal gland deficiency or use epinephrine, ephedrine or isoproterenol for asthma.

Over age 60:
More sensitive to thyroid hormone. May need smaller doses.

Pregnancy:
Considered safe if for thyroid deficiency only.

Breast-feeding:
Present in milk. Considered safe if dose is correct.

Infants & children:
Use only under medical supervision.

Prolonged use:
No problems expected, if dose is correct.

Skin & sunlight:
No problems expected.

Driving, piloting or hazardous work:
No problems expected.

Airplane passengers:
No problems expected.

Discontinuing:
Don't discontinue without consulting doctor. Dose may require gradual reduction if you have taken drug for a long time. Doses of other drugs may also require adjustment.

Others:
Digestive upsets, tremors, cramps, nervousness, insomnia or diarrhea may indicate need for dose adjustment.

INTERACTION WITH OTHER DRUGS

GENERIC NAME OR DRUG CLASS	COMBINED EFFECT
Amphetamines	Increased amphetamine effect.
Anticoagulants (oral)	Increased anticoagulant effect.
Antidepressants (tricyclic)	Increased antidepressant effect.
Antidiabetics	Antidiabetic may require adjustment.
Aspirin (large doses, continuous use)	Increased thyroxine effect.
Barbiturates	Decreased barbiturate effect.
Cholestyramine	Decreased thyroxine effect.
Contraceptives (oral)	Decreased thyroxine effect.
Cortisone drugs	Requires dose adjustment to prevent cortisone deficiency.
Digitalis preparations	Increased digitalis effect.
Ephedrine	Increased ephedrine effect.
Epinephrine	Increased epinephrine effect.
Methylphenidate	Increased methylphenidate effect.
Phenytoin	Increased thyroxine effect.

INTERACTION WITH OTHER SUBSTANCES

INTERACTS WITH	COMBINED EFFECT
Alcohol:	None expected.
Beverages:	None expected.
Cocaine:	Excess stimulation. Avoid.
Foods: Soybeans	Heavy consumption interferes with thyroid function.
Marijuana:	None expected.
Tobacco:	None expected.

TICARCILLIN

BRAND NAMES

Ticar

GENERAL INFORMATION

Habit forming? No
Prescription needed? Yes
Available as generic? Yes
Drug class: Antibiotic (penicillin)

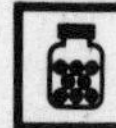

USES

Treatment of bacterial infections that are susceptible to ticarcillin.

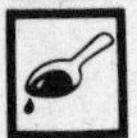

DOSAGE & USAGE INFORMATION

How to take:
By injection only.

When to take:
Follow doctor's instructions.

If you forget a dose:
Consult doctor.

What drug does:
Destroys susceptible bacteria. Does not kill viruses.

Time lapse before drug works:
May be several days before medicine affects infection.

Don't take with:
See Interaction column and consult doctor.

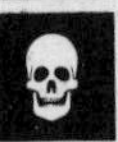

OVERDOSE

Symptoms:
Severe diarrhea, nausea, edema or vomiting.

What to do:
Overdose unlikely to threaten life. If person takes much larger amount than prescribed, call doctor, poison-control center or hospital emergency room for instructions.

POSSIBLE ADVERSE REACTIONS OR SIDE EFFECTS

SYMPTOMS	FREQUENCY	WHAT TO DO
Brain & nervous system:	None expected.	
Skin: Hives, rash, intense itch soon after a dose.	Rare	1
Eyes:	None expected.	
Ears, nose, throat: Dark or discolored tongue.	Common	5
Digestive: Mild nausea, vomiting, diarrhea.	Infrequent	4
Heart & lungs:	None expected.	
Blood vessels: Unexplained bleeding.	Rare	3
Muscles, bones, joints:	None expected.	
Genital, urinary:	None expected.	
Kidneys:	None expected.	
Liver:	None expected.	
Allergic: Life-threatening anaphylaxis may occur!	Rare	1 See page 888.
Blood:	None expected.	
Others:	None expected.	

1- Life-threatening. Seek emergency treatment immediately.
2- Discontinue. Seek emergency treatment.
3- Discontinue. Call doctor right away.
4- Continue. Call doctor when convenient.
5- Continue. Tell doctor at next visit.
6- No action necessary.

WARNINGS & PRECAUTIONS

Don't take if:
You are allergic to ticarcillin, cephalosporin antibiotics, other penicillins or penicillamine. Life-threatening reaction may occur.

Before you start, consult your doctor:
If you are allergic to any substance or drug.

Over age 60:
You may have skin reactions, particularly around genitals and anus.

Pregnancy:
Studies inconclusive on harm to unborn child. Animal studies show fetal abnormalities. Decide with your doctor whether drug benefits justify risk to unborn child.

Breast-feeding:
Drug passes into milk. Child may become sensitive to penicillins and have allergic reactions to penicillin drugs. Avoid ticarcillin or discontinue nursing until you finish medicine. Consult doctor for advice on maintaining milk supply.

Infants & children:
No problems expected.

Prolonged use:
You may become more susceptible to infections caused by germs not responsive to ticarcillin.

Skin & sunlight:
No problems expected.

Driving, piloting or hazardous work:
Usually not dangerous. Most hazardous reactions likely to occur a few minutes after taking ticarcillin.

Airplane passengers:
No problems expected.

Discontinuing:
Don't discontinue without doctor's advice until you complete prescribed dose, even though symptoms diminish or disappear.

Others:
No problems expected.

INTERACTION WITH OTHER DRUGS

GENERIC NAME OR DRUG CLASS	COMBINED EFFECT
Chloramphenicol	Decreased effect of both drugs.
Erythromycins	Decreased effect of both drugs.
Paromomycin	Decreased effect of both drugs.
Tetracyclines	Decreased effect of both drugs.
Troleandomycin	Decreased effect of both drugs.

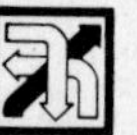

INTERACTION WITH OTHER SUBSTANCES

INTERACTS WITH	COMBINED EFFECT
Alcohol:	Occasional stomach irritation.
Beverages:	None expected.
Cocaine:	No proven problems.
Foods:	None expected.
Marijuana:	No proven problems.
Tobacco:	None expected.

TIMOLOL

BRAND NAMES

Blocadren
Timolide
Timoptic

GENERAL INFORMATION

Habit forming? No
Prescription needed? Yes
Available as generic? No
Drug class: Beta-adrenergic blocker

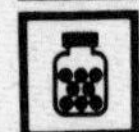

USES

- Reduces angina attacks.
- Stabilizes irregular heartbeat.
- Lowers blood pressure.
- Reduces frequency of migraine headaches. (Does not relieve headache pain.)
- Other uses prescribed by your doctor.

DOSAGE & USAGE INFORMATION

How to take:
Tablet or capsule—Swallow with liquid. If you can't swallow whole, crumble tablet or open capsule and take with liquid or food.

When to take:
With meals or immediately after.

If you forget a dose:
Take as soon as you remember. Return to regular schedule, but allow 3 hours between doses.

What drug does:
- Blocks certain actions of sympathetic nervous system.
- Lowers heart's oxygen requirements.
- Slows nerve impulses through heart.
- Reduces blood vessel contraction in heart, scalp and other body parts.

Time lapse before drug works:
1 to 4 hours.

Don't take with:
Non-prescription drugs or drugs in Interaction column without consulting doctor.

OVERDOSE

Symptoms:
Weakness, slow or weak pulse, blood-pressure drop, fainting, convulsions, cold and sweaty skin.

What to do:
- Dial O (operator) or 911 (emergency) for an ambulance or medical help. Then give first aid immediately.
- Additional emergency information on page 886.

POSSIBLE ADVERSE REACTIONS OR SIDE EFFECTS

SYMPTOMS	FREQUENCY	WHAT TO DO
Brain & nervous system:		
• Hallucinations, nightmares, insomnia, headache.	Infrequent	3
• Confusion, depression, reduced alertness.	Infrequent	4
• Drowsiness, numbness or tingling of fingers or toes, dizziness.	Common	4
Skin:		
Rash	Rare	3
Eyes:	None expected.	
Ears, nose, throat:		
Sore throat, fever.	Rare	3
Digestive:		
• Diarrhea, nausea.	Common	4
• Constipation	Infrequent	5
Heart & lungs:		
• Pulse slower than 50 beats per minute.	Common	3
• Breathing difficulty.	Infrequent	3
Blood vessels:		
Cold hands, feet.	Common	5
Muscles, bones, joints, genital, urinary, kidneys, liver, allergic:	None expected.	
Blood:		
Unusual bleeding and bruising.	Rare	4
Others:		
• Fatigue, weakness.	Common	4
• Dry mouth, eyes, skin.	Common	5

1- Life-threatening. Seek emergency treatment immediately.
2- Discontinue. Seek emergency treatment.
3- Discontinue. Call doctor right away.
4- Continue. Call doctor when convenient.
5- Continue. Tell doctor at next visit.

WARNINGS & PRECAUTIONS

Don't take if:
- You are allergic to any beta-adrenergic blocker.
- You have asthma.
- You have hay fever symptoms.
- You have taken MAO inhibitors in past 2 weeks.

Before you start, consult your doctor:
- If you have heart disease or poor circulation to the extremities.
- If you have hay fever, asthma, chronic bronchitis, emphysema.
- If you have overactive thyroid function.
- If you have impaired liver or kidney function.
- If you will have surgery within 2 months, including dental surgery, requiring general or spinal anesthesia.
- If you have diabetes or hypoglycemia.

Over age 60:
Adverse reactions and side effects may be more frequent and severe than in younger persons.

Pregnancy:
Risk to unborn child outweighs drug benefits. Don't use.

Breast-feeding:
Drug passes into milk. Avoid drug or discontinue nursing until you finish medicine. Consult doctor for advice on maintaining milk supply.

Infants & children:
Not recommended.

Prolonged use:
Weakens heart muscle contractions.

Skin & sunlight:
No problems expected.

Driving, piloting or hazardous work:
Don't drive or pilot aircraft until you learn how medicine affects you. Don't work around dangerous machinery. Don't climb ladders or work in high places. Danger increases if you drink alcohol or take medicine affecting alertness and reflexes.

Airplane passengers:
No problems expected.

Discontinuing:
Don't discontinue without consulting doctor. Dose may require gradual reduction if you have taken drug for a long time. Doses of other drugs may also require adjustment.

Others:
May mask hypoglycemia.

INTERACTION WITH OTHER DRUGS

GENERIC NAME OR DRUG CLASS	COMBINED EFFECT
Antidiabetics	Increased antidiabetic effect.
Antihistamines	Decreased antihistamine effect.
Antihypertensives	Increased antihypertensive effect.
Antiinflammatory drugs	Decreased antiinflammatory effect.
Barbiturates	Increased barbiturate effect. Dangerous sedation.
Digitalis preparations	Can either increase or decrease heart rate. Improves irregular heartbeat.
Narcotics	Increased narcotic effect. Dangerous sedation.
Phenytoin	Increased timolol effect.
Quinidine	Slows heart excessively.
Reserpine	Increased reserpine effect. Excessive sedation and depression.

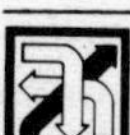

INTERACTION WITH OTHER SUBSTANCES

INTERACTS WITH	COMBINED EFFECT
Alcohol:	Excessive blood-pressure drop. Avoid.
Beverages:	None expected.
Cocaine:	Irregular heartbeat. Avoid.
Foods:	None expected.
Marijuana:	Daily use—Impaired circulation to hands and feet.
Tobacco:	Possible irregular heartbeat.

TOLAZAMIDE

BRAND NAMES

Tolinase

GENERAL INFORMATION

Habit forming? No
Prescription needed? Yes
Available as generic? No
Drug class: Antidiabetic (oral), sulfonurea

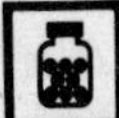

USES

Treatment for diabetes in adults who can't control blood sugar by diet, weight loss and exercise.

DOSAGE & USAGE INFORMATION

How to take:
Tablet—Swallow with liquid or food to lessen stomach irritation. If you can't swallow whole, crumble tablet and take with liquid or food.

When to take:
At the same times each day.

If you forget a dose:
Take as soon as you remember up to 2 hours late. If more than 2 hours, wait for next scheduled dose (don't double this dose).

What drug does:
Stimulates pancreas to produce more insulin. Insulin in blood forces cells to use sugar in blood.

Time lapse before drug works:
3 to 4 hours. May require 2 weeks for maximum benefit.

Don't take with:
See Interaction column and consult doctor.

OVERDOSE

Symptoms:
Excessive hunger, nausea, anxiety, cool skin, cold sweats, drowsiness, rapid heartbeat, weakness, unconsciousness, coma.

What to do:
- Dial 0 (operator) or 911 (emergency) for an ambulance or medical help. Then give first aid immediately.
- Additional emergency information on page 886.

POSSIBLE ADVERSE REACTIONS OR SIDE EFFECTS

SYMPTOMS	FREQUENCY	WHAT TO DO
Brain & nervous system:		
• Dizziness	Common	3
• Fatigue	Rare	3
Skin:		
Itching or rash.	Rare	3
Eyes:	None expected.	
Ears, nose, throat:		
• Sore throat, fever.	Rare	3
• Ringing in ears.	Rare	3
Digestive:		
Diarrhea, loss of appetite, nausea, stomach pain, heartburn.	Common	4
Heart & lungs, muscles, bones, joints, genital, urinary, kidneys, allergic, blood:	None expected.	
Blood vessels:		
Unusual bleeding or bruising.	Rare	3
Liver:		
Jaundice (yellow skin and eyes).	Rare	3
Others:		
Low blood sugar (ravenous hunger, nausea, anxiety, cold sweats, cool skin, chills, drowsiness, nervousness, headache, rapid heartbeat, weakness).	Infrequent	2

1- Life-threatening. Seek emergency treatment immediately.
2- Discontinue. Seek emergency treatment.
3- Discontinue. Call doctor right away.
4- Continue. Call doctor when convenient.

WARNINGS & PRECAUTIONS

Don't take if:
- You are allergic to any sulfonurea.
- You have impaired kidney or liver function.

Before you start, consult your doctor:
- If you have a severe infection.
- If you have thyroid disease.
- If you take insulin.
- If you have heart disease.

Over age 60:
Dose usually smaller than for younger adults. Avoid "low-blood-sugar" episodes because repeated ones can damage brain permanently.

Pregnancy:
No proven harm to unborn child. Avoid if possible.

Breast-feeding:
Drug filters into milk. May lower baby's blood sugar. Avoid.

Infants & children:
Don't give to infants or children.

Prolonged use:
None expected.

Skin & sunlight:
May cause rash or intensify sunburn in areas exposed to sun or sunlamp.

Driving, piloting or hazardous work:
No problems expected unless you develop hypoglycemia (low blood sugar). If so, avoid driving or hazardous activity.

Airplane passengers:
No problems expected.

Discontinuing:
Don't discontinue without consulting doctor. Dose may require gradual reduction if you have taken drug for a long time. Doses of other drugs may also require adjustment.

Others:
- Don't exceed 1500 mg. in 1 day.
- Hypoglycemia (low blood sugar) may occur, even with proper dose schedule. You must balance medicine, diet and exercise.

INTERACTION WITH OTHER DRUGS

GENERIC NAME OR DRUG CLASS	COMBINED EFFECT
Androgens	Increased tolazamide effect.
Anticoagulants (oral)	Unpredictable prothrombin times (see page 848).
Anticonvulsants (hydantoin)	Decreased tolazamide effect.
Antiinflammatory drugs (non-steroidal)	Increased tolazamide effect.
Aspirin	Increased tolazamide effect.
Beta-adrenergic blockers	Increased tolazamide effect.
Chloramphenicol	Increased tolazamide effect.
Clofibrate	Increased tolazamide effect.
Contraceptives (oral)	Decreased tolazamide effect.
Cortisone drugs	Decreased tolazamide effect.
Diuretics (thiazide)	Decreased tolazamide effect.
Epinephrine	Decreased tolazamide effect.
Estrogens	Increased tolazamide effect.
Guanethidine	Unpredictable tolazamide effect.

Additional interactions on page 844.

INTERACTION WITH OTHER SUBSTANCES

INTERACTS WITH	COMBINED EFFECT
Alcohol:	Disulfiram reaction (see page 846). Avoid.
Beverages:	None expected.
Cocaine:	No proven problems.
Foods:	None expected.
Marijuana:	Decreased tolazamide effect. Avoid.
Tobacco:	None expected.

TOLBUTAMIDE

BRAND NAMES

Apo-Tolbutamide
Mobenol
Neo-Dibetic
Novobutamide
Oramide
Orinase
SK-Tolbutamide
Tolbutone

GENERAL INFORMATION

Habit forming? No
Prescription needed? Yes
Available as generic? No
Drug class: Antidiabetic (oral), sulfonurea

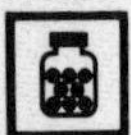

USES

Treatment for diabetes in adults who can't control blood sugar by diet, weight loss and exercise.

DOSAGE & USAGE INFORMATION

How to take:
Tablet—Swallow with liquid or food to lessen stomach irritation. If you can't swallow whole, crumble tablet and take with liquid or food.

When to take:
At the same times each day.

If you forget a dose:
Take as soon as you remember up to 2 hours late. If more than 2 hours, wait for next scheduled dose (don't double this dose).

What drug does:
Stimulates pancreas to produce more insulin. Insulin in blood forces cells to use sugar in blood.

Time lapse before drug works:
3 to 4 hours. May require 2 weeks for maximum benefit.

Don't take with:
See Interaction column and consult doctor.

OVERDOSE

Symptoms:
Excessive hunger, nausea, anxiety, cool skin, cold sweats, drowsiness, rapid heartbeat, weakness, unconsciousness, coma.

What to do:
- Dial 0 (operator) or 911 (emergency) for an ambulance or medical help. Then give first aid immediately.
- Additional emergency information on page 886.

POSSIBLE ADVERSE REACTIONS OR SIDE EFFECTS

SYMPTOMS	FREQUENCY	WHAT TO DO
Brain & nervous system:		
• Dizziness	Common	3
• Fatigue	Rare	3
Skin:		
Itching or rash.	Rare	3
Eyes:	None expected.	
Ears, nose, throat:		
• Sore throat, fever.	Rare	3
• Ringing in ears.	Rare	3
Digestive:		
Diarrhea, loss of appetite, nausea, stomach pain, heartburn.	Common	4
Heart & lungs, muscles, bones, joints, genital, urinary, kidneys, allergic, blood:	None expected.	
Blood vessels:		
Unusual bleeding or bruising.	Rare	3
Liver:		
Jaundice (yellow skin and eyes).	Rare	3
Others:		
Low blood sugar (ravenous hunger, nausea, anxiety, cold sweats, cool skin, chills, drowsiness, nervousness, headache, rapid heartbeat, weakness).	Infrequent	2

1- Life-threatening. Seek emergency treatment immediately.
2- Discontinue. Seek emergency treatment.
3- Discontinue. Call doctor right away.
4- Continue. Call doctor when convenient.

WARNINGS & PRECAUTIONS

Don't take if:
- You are allergic to any sulfonurea.
- You have impaired kidney or liver function.

Before you start, consult your doctor:
- If you have a severe infection.
- If you have thyroid disease.
- If you take insulin.
- If you have heart disease.

Over age 60:
Dose usually smaller than for younger adults. Avoid "low-blood-sugar" episodes because repeated ones can damage brain permanently.

Pregnancy:
No proven harm to unborn child. Avoid if possible.

Breast-feeding:
Drug filters into milk. May lower baby's blood sugar. Avoid.

Infants & children:
Don't give to infants or children.

Prolonged use:
None expected.

Skin & sunlight:
May cause rash or intensify sunburn in areas exposed to sun or sunlamp.

Driving, piloting or hazardous work:
No problems expected unless you develop hypoglycemia (low blood sugar). If so, avoid driving or hazardous activity.

Airplane passengers:
No problems expected.

Discontinuing:
Don't discontinue without consulting doctor. Dose may require gradual reduction if you have taken drug for a long time. Doses of other drugs may also require adjustment.

Others:
- Don't exceed 1500 mg. in 1 day.
- Hypoglycemia (low blood sugar) may occur, even with proper dose schedule. You must balance medicine, diet and exercise.

INTERACTION WITH OTHER DRUGS

GENERIC NAME OR DRUG CLASS	COMBINED EFFECT
Androgens	Increased tolbutamide effect.
Anticoagulants (oral)	Unpredictable prothrombin times (see page 848).
Anticonvulsants (hydantoin)	Decreased tolbutamide effect.
Antiinflammatory drugs (non-steroidal)	Increased tolbutamide effect.
Aspirin	Increased tolbutamide effect.
Beta-adrenergic blockers	Increased tolbutamide effect.
Chloramphenicol	Increased tolbutamide effect.
Clofibrate	Increased tolbutamide effect.
Contraceptives (oral)	Decreased tolbutamide effect.
Cortisone drugs	Decreased tolbutamide effect.
Diuretics (thiazide)	Decreased tolbutamide effect.
Epinephrine	Decreased tolbutamide effect.
Estrogens	Increased tolbutamide effect.
Guanethidine	Unpredictable tolbutamide effect.

Additional interactions on page 844.

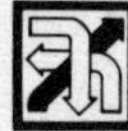

INTERACTION WITH OTHER SUBSTANCES

INTERACTS WITH	COMBINED EFFECT
Alcohol:	Disulfiram reaction (see page 846). Avoid.
Beverages:	None expected.
Cocaine:	No proven problems.
Foods:	None expected.
Marijuana:	Decreased tolbutamide effect. Avoid.
Tobacco:	None expected.

TOLMETIN

BRAND NAMES

Tolectin
Tolectin DS

GENERAL INFORMATION

Habit forming? No
Prescription needed? Yes
Available as generic? No
Drug class: Antiinflammatory (non-steroid)

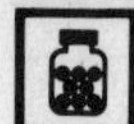

USES

- Treatment for joint pain, stiffness, inflammation and swelling of arthritis and gout.
- Pain reliever.

DOSAGE & USAGE INFORMATION

How to take:
Tablet or capsule—Swallow with liquid or food to lessen stomach irritation. If you can't swallow whole, crumble tablet or open capsule and take with liquid or food.

When to take:
At the same times each day.

If you forget a dose:
Take as soon as you remember up to 2 hours late. If more than 2 hours, wait for next scheduled dose (don't double this dose).

What drug does:
Reduces tissue concentration of prostaglandins (hormones which produce inflammation and pain).

Time lapse before drug works:
Begins in 4 to 24 hours. May require 3 weeks regular use for maximum benefit.

Don't take with:
See Interaction column and consult doctor.

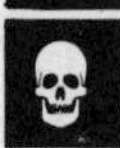

OVERDOSE

Symptoms:
Confusion, agitation, incoherence, convulsions, possible hemorrhage from stomach or intestine, coma.

What to do:
- Dial 0 (operator) or 911 (emergency) for an ambulance or medical help. Then give first aid immediately.
- Additional emergency information on page 886.

POSSIBLE ADVERSE REACTIONS OR SIDE EFFECTS

SYMPTOMS	FREQUENCY	WHAT TO DO
Brain & nervous system:		
• Depression, drowsiness.	Infrequent	4
• Convulsions, confusion.	Rare	3
• Dizziness	Common	4
• Headache	Common	5
Skin:		
Rash, hives or itch.	Rare	3
Eyes:		
Blurred vision.	Rare	3
Ears, nose, throat:		
Ringing in ears.	Infrequent	4
Digestive:		
• Bloody or black, tarry stools.	Rare	3
• Nausea, pain.	Common	4
• Constipation or diarrhea, vomiting.	Infrequent	4
Heart & lungs:		
Breathing difficulty, tightness in chest, rapid heartbeat.	Rare	3
Blood vessels:		
Unusual bleeding or bruising.	Rare	3
Muscles, bones, joints:		
Swollen feet, legs.	Infrequent	4
Genital, urinary:		
• Bloody urine.	Rare	3
• Difficult, painful or frequent urination.	Rare	4
Kidneys, allergic, blood:	None expected.	
Liver:		
Jaundice (yellow skin and eyes).	Rare	3
Others:		
Fatigue, weakness.	Rare	4

1- Life-threatening. Seek emergency treatment immediately.
2- Discontinue. Seek emergency treatment.
3- Discontinue. Call doctor right away.
4- Continue. Call doctor when convenient.
5- Continue. Tell doctor at next visit.

WARNINGS & PRECAUTIONS

Don't take if:

- You are allergic to aspirin or any non-steroid, antiinflammatory drug.
- You have gastritis, peptic ulcer, enteritis, ileitis, ulcerative colitis, asthma, heart failure, high blood pressure or bleeding problems.
- Patient is younger than 15.

Before you start, consult your doctor:

- If you have epilepsy.
- If you have Parkinson's disease.
- If you have been mentally ill.
- If you have had kidney disease or impaired kidney function.

Over age 60:
Adverse reactions and side effects may be more frequent and severe than in younger persons.

Pregnancy:
Studies inconclusive on harm to unborn child. Decide with your doctor whether drug benefits justify risk to unborn child.

Breast-feeding:
May harm child. Avoid.

Infants & children:
Not recommended for anyone younger than 15. Use only under medical supervision.

Prolonged use:

- Eye damage.
- Reduced hearing.
- Sore throat, fever.
- Weight gain.

Skin & sunlight:
No problems expected.

Driving, piloting or hazardous work:
Don't drive or pilot aircraft until you learn how medicine affects you. Don't work around dangerous machinery. Don't climb ladders or work in high places. Danger increases if you drink alcohol or take medicine affecting alertness and reflexes, such as antihistamines, tranquilizers, sedatives, pain medicine, narcotics and mind-altering drugs.

Airplane passengers:
No problems expected.

Discontinuing:
Don't discontinue without consulting doctor. Dose may require gradual reduction if you have taken drug for a long time. Doses of other drugs may also require adjustment.

Others:
No problems expected.

INTERACTION WITH OTHER DRUGS

GENERIC NAME OR DRUG CLASS	COMBINED EFFECT
Anticoagulants (oral)	Increased risk of bleeding.
Aspirin	Increased risk of stomach ulcer.
Cortisone drugs	Increased risk of stomach ulcer.
Furosemide	Decreased diuretic effect of furosemide.
Oxyphenbutazone	Possible stomach ulcer.
Phenylbutazone	Possible stomach ulcer.
Probenecid	Increased tolmetin effect.
Thyroid hormones	Rapid heartbeat, blood-pressure rise.

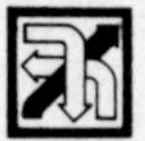

INTERACTION WITH OTHER SUBSTANCES

INTERACTS WITH	COMBINED EFFECT
Alcohol:	Possible stomach ulcer or bleeding.
Beverages:	None expected.
Cocaine:	None expected.
Foods:	None expected.
Marijuana:	Increased pain relief from tolmetin.
Tobacco:	None expected.

TRAZODONE

BRAND NAMES

Desyrel

GENERAL INFORMATION

Habit forming? No
Prescription needed? Yes
Available as generic? No
Drug class: Antidepressant (non-tricyclic)

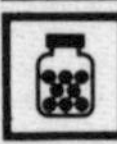

USES

- Treats mental depression.
- Treats anxiety.

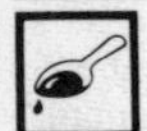

DOSAGE & USAGE INFORMATION

How to take:
Tablet or capsule—Swallow with liquid or food to lessen stomach irritation. If you can't swallow whole, crumble tablet or open capsule and take with liquid or food.

When to take:
According to prescription directions. Bedtime dose usually higher than other doses.

If you forget a dose:
Take as soon as you remember up to 2 hours late. If more than 2 hours, wait for next scheduled dose (don't double this dose).

What drug does:
Inhibits serotonin uptake in brain cells.

Time lapse before drug works:
2 to 4 weeks for full effect.

Don't take with:
See Interaction column and consult doctor.

OVERDOSE

Symptoms:
Fainting, irregular heartbeat, chest pain, seizures, coma.

What to do:
- Dial 0 (operator) or 911 (emergency) for an ambulance or medical help. Then give first aid immediately.
- If patient is unconscious and not breathing, give mouth-to-mouth breathing. If there is no heartbeat, use cardiac massage and mouth-to-mouth breathing (CPR). Don't try to make patient vomit. If you can't get help quickly, take patient to nearest emergency facility.
- Additional emergency information on page 886.

POSSIBLE ADVERSE REACTIONS OR SIDE EFFECTS

SYMPTOMS	FREQUENCY	WHAT TO DO
Brain & nervous system:		
• Tremors, incoordination.	Infrequent	3
• Dizziness on standing.	Infrequent	4
• Confusion, disorientation, drowsiness, excitement.	Infrequent	4
• Fatigue, headache, nervousness.	Infrequent	4
Skin:		
Rash, itching.	Infrequent	4
Eyes:		
Blurred vision.	Infrequent	4
Ears, nose, throat:		
• Ringing in ears.	Infrequent	4
• Dry mouth.	Infrequent	4
Digestive:		
• Bad taste.	Infrequent	4
• Diarrhea, nausea, vomiting.	Infrequent	4
• Constipation	Infrequent	4
Heart & lungs:		
• Blood pressure rise or drop.	Infrequent	3
• Rapid heartbeat.	Infrequent	3
• Shortness of breath.	Infrequent	3
Blood vessels:	None expected.	
Muscles, bones, joints:		
Aching	Infrequent	4
Genital, urinary:		
• Prolonged penile erections.	Infrequent	4
• Menstrual changes.	Infrequent	4
Kidneys, allergic, blood, liver:	None expected.	
Others:		
• Fainting	Infrequent	3
• Decreased sex drive.	Infrequent	4

3- Discontinue. Call doctor right away.
4- Continue. Call doctor when convenient.

WARNINGS & PRECAUTIONS

Don't take if:
- You are allergic to trazodone.
- You are thinking about suicide.

Before you start, consult your doctor:
- If you have heart rhythm problem.
- If you have any heart disease.
- If you will have surgery within 2 months, including dental surgery, requiring general or spinal anesthesia.

Over age 60:
Adverse reactions and side effects may be more frequent and severe than in younger persons.

Pregnancy:
Risk to unborn child outweighs drug benefits. Don't use.

Breast-feeding:
Drug passes into milk. Avoid drug or discontinue nursing until you finish medicine. Consult doctor for advice on maintaining milk supply.

Infants & children:
Not recommended.

Prolonged use:
Occasional blood counts, especially if you have fever and sore throat.

Skin & sunlight:
No problems expected.

Driving, piloting or hazardous work:
Don't drive or pilot aircraft until you learn how medicine affects you. Don't work around dangerous machinery. Don't climb ladders or work in high places. Danger increases if you drink alcohol or take medicine affecting alertness and reflexes, such as antihistamines, tranquilizers, sedatives, pain medicine, narcotics and mind-altering drugs.

Airplane passengers:
No problems expected.

Discontinuing:
Don't discontinue without consulting doctor. Dose may require gradual reduction if you have taken drug for a long time. Doses of other drugs may also require adjustment.

Others:
Electroshock therapy should be avoided.

INTERACTION WITH OTHER DRUGS

GENERIC NAME OR DRUG CLASS	COMBINED EFFECT
Antihypertensives	Too low blood pressure. Avoid.
Barbiturates	Too low blood pressure. Avoid.
Digitalis preparations	Increased digitalis level in blood.
Phenytoin	Increased phenytoin level in blood.
MAO inhibitors	May add to toxic effect of each.
Narcotics	Excess drowsiness.
Antihistamines	Excess drowsiness.
Sedatives	Excess drowsiness.
Antidepressants (other)	Excess drowsiness.
Tranquilizers	Excess drowsiness.

INTERACTION WITH OTHER SUBSTANCES

INTERACTS WITH	COMBINED EFFECT
Alcohol:	Excess sedation. Avoid.
Beverages:	
Caffeine	May add to heart-beat irregularity. Avoid.
Cocaine:	May add to heart-beat irregularity. Avoid.
Foods:	No problems expected.
Marijuana:	May add to heart-beat irregularity. Avoid.
Tobacco:	May add to heart-beat irregularity. Avoid.

TRETINOIN

BRAND NAMES

Retin-A
StieVAA
Vitamin A Acid

GENERAL INFORMATION

Habit forming? No
Prescription needed? Yes
Available as generic? No
Drug class: Antiacne (topical)

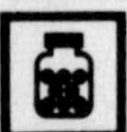

USES

Treatment for acne, psoriasis, ichthyosis, keratosis, folliculitis, flat warts.

DOSAGE & USAGE INFORMATION

How to use:
Wash skin with non-medicated soap, pat dry, wait 20 minutes before applying.
- Cream or gel—Apply to affected areas with fingertips and rub in gently.
- Solution—Apply to affected areas with gauze pad or cotton swab. Avoid getting too wet so medicine doesn't drip into eyes, mouth, lips or inside nose.

When to use:
At the same time each day.

If you forget an application:
Take as soon as you remember.

What drug does:
Increases skin-cell turnover so skin layer peels off more easily.

Time lapse before drug works:
2 to 3 weeks. May require 6 weeks for maximum improvement.

Don't use with:
- Benzoyl peroxide. Apply 12 hours apart.
- See Interaction column and consult doctor.

OVERDOSE

Symptoms:
None expected.

What to do:
If person swallows drug, call doctor, poison-control center or hospital emergency room for instructions.

POSSIBLE ADVERSE REACTIONS OR SIDE EFFECTS

SYMPTOMS	FREQUENCY	WHAT TO DO
Brain & nervous system:	None expected.	
Skin:		
• Blistering, crusting, severe burning, swelling.	Infrequent	3
• Pigment change in treated area, warmth or stinging, peeling.	Common	5
Eyes:	None expected.	
Ears, nose, throat:	None expected.	
Digestive:	None expected.	
Heart & lungs:	None expected.	
Blood vessels:	None expected.	
Muscles, bones, joints:	None expected.	
Genital, urinary:	None expected.	
Kidneys:	None expected.	
Liver:	None expected.	
Allergic:	None expected.	
Blood:	None expected.	
Others:		
Sensitivity to wind or cold.	Common	6

1- Life-threatening. Seek emergency treatment immediately.
2- Discontinue. Seek emergency treatment.
3- Discontinue. Call doctor right away.
4- Continue. Call doctor when convenient.
5- Continue. Tell doctor at next visit.
6- No action necessary.

WARNINGS & PRECAUTIONS

Don't take if:
- You are allergic to tretinoin.
- You are sunburned, windburned or have an open skin wound.

Before you start, consult your doctor:
If you have eczema.

Over age 60:
Not recommended.

Pregnancy:
No proven harm to unborn child. Avoid if possible.

Breast-feeding:
No problems expected.

Infants & children:
Not recommended.

Prolonged use:
No problems expected.

Skin & sunlight:
- May cause rash or intensify sunburn in areas exposed to sun or sunlamp.
- In some animal studies, tretinoin caused skin tumors to develop faster when treated area was exposed to ultraviolet light (sunlight or sunlamp). No proven similar effects in humans.

Driving, piloting or hazardous work:
No problems expected.

Airplane passengers:
No problems expected.

Discontinuing:
Don't discontinue without doctor's advice until you complete prescribed dose, even though symptoms diminish or disappear.

Others:
Acne may get worse before improvement starts in 2 or 3 weeks. Don't wash face more than 2 or 3 times daily.

INTERACTION WITH OTHER DRUGS

GENERIC NAME OR DRUG CLASS	COMBINED EFFECT
Antiacne topical preparations (other)	Severe skin irritation.
Cosmetics (medicated)	Severe skin irritation.
Skin preparations with alcohol	Severe skin irritation.
Soaps or cleansers (abrasive)	Severe skin irritation.

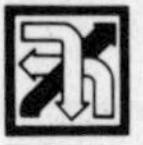

INTERACTION WITH OTHER SUBSTANCES

INTERACTS WITH	COMBINED EFFECT
Alcohol:	None expected.
Beverages:	None expected.
Cocaine:	None expected.
Foods:	None expected.
Marijuana:	None expected.
Tobacco:	None expected.

TRIAMCINOLONE

BRAND NAMES

Amcort
Aristocort
Aristospan
Cenocort Forte
Cino-40
Kenacort
Kenalog
Spencort
Tramacort
Triacet
Triacort
Triaderm

See complete brand names list, page 833.
Some of these brands are available as topical medicines (ointments, creams or lotions).
See ADRENOCORTICOIDS (TOPICAL), page 26.

GENERAL INFORMATION

Habit forming? No
Prescription needed? Yes
Available as generic? Yes
Drug class: Cortisone drug (adrenal corticosteroid)

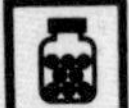

USES

- Reduces inflammation caused by many different medical problems.
- Treatment for some allergic diseases, blood disorders, kidney diseases, asthma and emphysema.
- Replaces corticosteroid deficiencies.

DOSAGE & USAGE INFORMATION

How to take:
Tablet or syrup—Swallow with liquid or food to lessen stomach irritation. If you can't swallow whole, crumble tablet.

When to take:
At the same times each day. Take once-a-day or once-every-other-day doses in mornings.

If you forget a dose:
- Several-doses-per-day prescription—Take as soon as you remember up to 2 hours late. If more than 2 hours, wait for next scheduled dose (don't double this dose).
- Once-a-day dose or less—Wait for next dose. Double this dose.

What drug does:
Decreases inflammatory responses.

Time lapse before drug works:
2 to 4 days.

Don't take with:
See Interaction column and consult doctor.

OVERDOSE

Symptoms:
Headache, convulsions, heart failure.

What to do:
- Dial 0 (operator) or 911 (emergency) for an ambulance or medical help. Then give first aid immediately.
- Additional emergency information on page 886.

POSSIBLE ADVERSE REACTIONS OR SIDE EFFECTS

SYMPTOMS	FREQUENCY	WHAT TO DO
Brain & nervous system:		
Mood changes, insomnia, restlessness.	Infrequent	4
Skin:		
• Acne	Common	4
• Rash	Rare	3
• Poor wound healing.	Common	4
Eyes:		
Blurred vision, halos around lights.	Infrequent	3
Ears, nose, throat:		
• Sore throat, fever.	Infrequent	3
• Thirst	Common	4
Digestive:		
• Indigestion, nausea, vomiting.	Common	4
• Bloody or black, tarry stool.	Infrequent	2
Heart & lungs:		
Irregular heartbeat.	Rare	2
Blood vessels, kidneys, liver, allergic, blood:	None expected.	
Muscles, bones, joints:		
Muscle cramps, swollen legs, feet.	Infrequent	3
Genital, urinary:		
Frequent urination.	Infrequent	4
Others:		
• Weight gain, round face.	Infrequent	4
• Fatigue, weakness.	Infrequent	4
• TB recurrence.	Infrequent	4
• Irregular menstrual periods.	Infrequent	4

2- Discontinue. Seek emergency treatment.
3- Discontinue. Call doctor right away.
4- Continue. Call doctor when convenient.

WARNINGS & PRECAUTIONS

Don't take if:
- You are allergic to any cortisone drug.
- You have tuberculosis or fungus infection.
- You have herpes infection of eyes, lips or genitals.

Before you start, consult your doctor:
- If you have had tuberculosis.
- If you have congestive heart failure.
- If you have diabetes.
- If you have peptic ulcer.
- If you have glaucoma.
- If you have underactive thyroid.
- If you have high blood pressure.
- If you have myasthenia gravis.
- If you have blood clots in legs or lungs.

Over age 60:
Adverse reactions and side effects may be more frequent and severe than in younger persons. Likely to aggravate edema, diabetes or ulcers. Likely to cause cataracts and osteoporosis (softening of the bones).

Pregnancy:
Risk to unborn child outweighs drug benefits. Don't use.

Breast-feeding:
Drug passes into milk. Avoid drug or discontinue nursing until you finish medicine. Consult doctor for advice on maintaining milk supply.

Infants & children:
Use only under medical supervision.

Prolonged use:
- Retards growth in children.
- Possible glaucoma, cataracts, diabetes, fragile bones and thin skin.
- Functional dependence.

Skin & sunlight:
No problems expected.

Driving, piloting or hazardous work:
No problems expected.

Airplane passengers:
No problems expected.

Discontinuing:
- Don't discontinue without doctor's advice until you complete prescribed dose, even though symptoms diminish or disappear.
- Drug affects your response to surgery, illness, injury or stress for 2 years after discontinuing. Tell about drug to anyone who takes medical care of you within 2 years.

Others:
Avoid immunizations if possible.

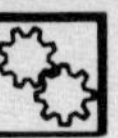

INTERACTION WITH OTHER DRUGS

GENERIC NAME OR DRUG CLASS	COMBINED EFFECT
Amphoterecin B	Potassium depletion.
Anticholinergics	Possible glaucoma.
Anticoagulants (oral)	Decreased anticoagulant effect.
Anticonvulsants (hydantoin)	Decreased triamcinolone effect.
Antidiabetics (oral)	Decreased antidiabetic effect.
Antihistamines	Decreased triamcinolone effect.
Aspirin	Increased triamcinolone effect.
Barbiturates	Decreased triamcinolone effect. Oversedation.
Beta-adrenergic blockers	Decreased triamcinolone effect.
Chloral hydrate	Decreased triamcinolone effect.
Chlorthalidone	Potassium depletion.
Cholinergics	Decreased cholinergic effect.
Contraceptives (oral)	Increased triamcinolone effect.
Digitalis preparations	Dangerous potassium depletion. Possible digitalis toxicity.
Diuretics (thiazide)	Potassium depletion.

Additional interactions on page 844.

INTERACTION WITH OTHER SUBSTANCES

INTERACTS WITH	COMBINED EFFECT
Alcohol:	Risk of stomach ulcers.
Beverages:	No proven problems.
Cocaine:	Overstimulation. Avoid.
Foods:	No proven problems.
Marijuana:	Decreased immunity.
Tobacco:	Increased triamcinolone effect. Possible toxicity.

TRIAMTERENE

BRAND NAMES

Dyazide
Dyrenium
Maxzide

GENERAL INFORMATION

Habit forming? No
Prescription needed? Yes
Available as generic? No
Drug class: Antihypertensive, diuretic

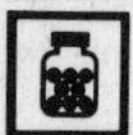

USES

- Reduces fluid retention (edema).
- Reduces potassium loss.

DOSAGE & USAGE INFORMATION

How to take:
Tablet or capsule—Swallow with liquid or food to lessen stomach irritation. If you can't swallow whole, crumble tablet or open capsule and take with liquid or food.

When to take:
- 1 dose per day—Take after breakfast.
- More than 1 dose per day—Take last dose no later than 6 p.m.

If you forget a dose:
Take as soon as you remember up to 6 hours late. If more than 6 hours, wait for next scheduled dose (don't double this dose).

What drug does:
Increases urine production to eliminate sodium and water from body while conserving potassium.

Time lapse before drug works:
2 hours. May require 2 to 3 days for maximum benefit.

Don't take with:
See Interaction column and consult doctor.

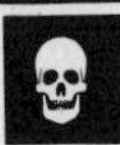

OVERDOSE

Symptoms:
Lethargy, irregular heartbeat, coma.

What to do:
- Dial 0 (operator) or 911 (emergency) for an ambulance or medical help. Then give first aid immediately.
- If patient is unconscious and not breathing, give mouth-to-mouth breathing. If there is no heartbeat, use cardiac massage and mouth-to-mouth breathing (CPR). Don't try to make patient vomit. If you can't get help quickly, take patient to nearest emergency facility.
- Additional emergency information on page 886.

POSSIBLE ADVERSE REACTIONS OR SIDE EFFECTS

SYMPTOMS	FREQUENCY	WHAT TO DO
Brain & nervous system:		
• Anxiety	Infrequent	5
• Drowsiness	Infrequent	3
• Headache	Rare	5
• Confusion	Infrequent	3
Skin:		
Rash	Rare	3
Eyes:	None expected.	
Ears, nose, throat:		
• Sore throat, fever.	Rare	3
• Dry mouth, thirst.	Infrequent	3
• Red, inflamed tongue.	Rare	3
Digestive:		
Diarrhea	Infrequent	4
Heart & lungs:		
Irregular heartbeat, shortness of breath.	Infrequent	3
Blood vessels:		
Unusual bleeding or bruising.	Rare	3
Muscles, bones, joints:	None expected.	
Genital, urinary:	None expected.	
Kidneys:	None expected.	
Liver:	None expected.	
Allergic:	None expected.	
Blood:	None expected.	
Others:		
Unusual tiredness, weakness.	Infrequent	3

1- Life-threatening. Seek emergency treatment immediately.
2- Discontinue. Seek emergency treatment.
3- Discontinue. Call doctor right away.
4- Continue. Call doctor when convenient.
5- Continue. Tell doctor at next visit.
6- No action necessary.

WARNINGS & PRECAUTIONS

Don't take if:
- You are allergic to triamterene.
- You have had severe liver or kidney disease.

Before you start, consult your doctor:
- If you have gout.
- If you have diabetes.
- If you will have surgery within 2 months, including dental surgery, requiring general or spinal anesthesia.

Over age 60:
- Warm weather or fever can decrease blood pressure. Dose may require adjustment.
- Extended use can increase blood clots.

Pregnancy:
No proven harm to unborn child. Avoid if possible.

Breast-feeding:
Present in milk. Avoid.

Infants & children:
Used infrequently. Use only under medical supervision.

Prolonged use:
Potassium retention which may lead to heart-rhythm problems.

Skin & sunlight:
May cause rash or intensify sunburn in areas exposed to sun or sunlamp.

Driving, piloting or hazardous work:
Avoid if you feel drowsy or confused. Otherwise, no problems expected.

Airplane passengers:
No problems expected.

Discontinuing:
Don't discontinue without consulting doctor. Dose may require gradual reduction if you have taken drug for a long time. Doses of other drugs may also require adjustment.

Others:
No problems expected.

INTERACTION WITH OTHER DRUGS

GENERIC NAME OR DRUG CLASS	COMBINED EFFECT
Antidiabetics (oral)	Decreased antidiabetic effect.
Antihypertensives (other)	Increased effect of other antihypertensives.
Digitalis preparations	Decreased digitalis effect.
Lithium	Increased lithium effect.
Spironolactone	Dangerous retention of potassium.

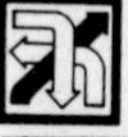

INTERACTION WITH OTHER SUBSTANCES

INTERACTS WITH	COMBINED EFFECT
Alcohol:	None expected.
Beverages:	None expected.
Cocaine:	Decreased triamterene effect.
Foods:	
Salt	Don't restrict unless directed by doctor.
Marijuana:	Daily use—Fainting likely.
Tobacco:	None expected.

TRIAZOLAM

BRAND NAMES

Halcion

GENERAL INFORMATION

Habit forming? Yes
Prescription needed? Yes
Available as generic? No
Drug class: Tranquilizer (benzodiazepine)

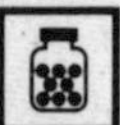

USES

Treatment of insomnia. Not recommended for more than 2 weeks maximum.

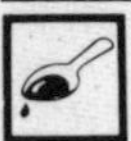

DOSAGE & USAGE INFORMATION

How to take:
Tablet or capsule—Swallow with liquid. If you can't swallow whole, crumble tablet or open capsule and take with liquid or food.

When to take:
At the same time each day, according to instructions on prescription label.

If you forget a dose:
Take as soon as you remember up to 2 hours late. If more than 2 hours, wait for next scheduled dose (don't double this dose).

What drug does:
Affects limbic system of brain—part that controls emotions.

Time lapse before drug works:
2 hours. May take 6 weeks for full benefit.

Don't take with:
See Interaction column and consult doctor.

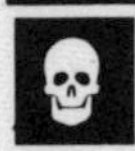

OVERDOSE

Symptoms:
Drowsiness, weakness, tremor, stupor, coma.

What to do:

- Dial 0 (operator) or 911 (emergency) for an ambulance or medical help. Then give first aid immediately.
- If patient is unconscious and not breathing, give mouth-to-mouth breathing. If there is no heartbeat, use cardiac massage and mouth-to-mouth breathing (CPR). Don't try to make patient vomit. If you can't get help quickly, take patient to nearest emergency facility.
- Additional emergency information on page 886.

POSSIBLE ADVERSE REACTIONS OR SIDE EFFECTS

SYMPTOMS	FREQUENCY	WHAT TO DO
Brain & nervous system:		
• Clumsiness, drowsiness, dizziness.	Common	4
• Hallucinations, confusion, depression, irritability.	Infrequent	3
Skin:		
Rash, itch.	Infrequent	3
Eyes:		
Vision changes.	Infrequent	3
Ears, nose, throat:		
Mouth, throat ulcers.	Rare	3
Digestive:		
Constipation or diarrhea, nausea, vomiting.	Infrequent	4
Heart & lungs:		
Slow heartbeat, breathing difficulty.	Rare	2
Blood vessels:	None expected.	
Muscles, bones, joints:	None expected.	
Genital, urinary:		
Urination difficulty.	Infrequent	4
Kidneys:	None expected.	
Liver:		
Jaundice (yellow eyes and skin).	Rare	3
Allergic:	None expected.	
Blood:	None expected.	
Others:	None expected.	

1- Life-threatening. Seek emergency treatment immediately.
2- Discontinue. Seek emergency treatment.
3- Discontinue. Call doctor right away.
4- Continue. Call doctor when convenient.
5- Continue. Tell doctor at next visit.
6- No action necessary.

WARNINGS & PRECAUTIONS

Don't take if:
- You are allergic to any benzodiazepine.
- You have myasthenia gravis.
- You are active or recovering alcoholic.
- Patient is younger than 6 months.

Before you start, consult your doctor:
- If you have liver, kidney or lung disease.
- If you have diabetes, epilepsy or porphyria.
- If you will have surgery within 2 months, including dental surgery, requiring general or spinal anesthesia.

Over age 60:
Adverse reactions and side effects may be more frequent and severe than in younger persons. You need smaller doses for shorter periods of time. May develop agitation, rage or "hangover effect."

Pregnancy:
Risk to unborn child outweighs drug benefits. Don't use.

Breast-feeding:
Drug passes into milk. Avoid drug or discontinue nursing until you finish medicine. Consult doctor for advice on maintaining milk supply.

Infants & children:
Use only under medical supervision for children older than 6 months.

Prolonged use:
May impair liver function.

Skin & sunlight:
No problems expected.

Driving, piloting or hazardous work:
Don't drive or pilot aircraft until you learn how medicine affects you. Don't work around dangerous machinery. Don't climb ladders or work in high places. Danger increases if you drink alcohol or take medicine affecting alertness and reflexes.

Airplane passengers:
No problems expected.

Discontinuing:
Don't discontinue without consulting doctor. Dose may require gradual reduction if you have taken drug for a long time. Doses of other drugs may also require adjustment.

Others:
- Hot weather, heavy exercise and profuse sweat may reduce excretion and cause overdose.
- Blood sugar may rise in diabetics, requiring insulin adjustment.

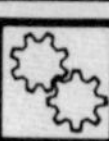

INTERACTION WITH OTHER DRUGS

GENERIC NAME OR DRUG CLASS	COMBINED EFFECT
Anticonvulsants	Change in seizure frequency or severity.
Antidepressants	Increased sedative effect of both drugs.
Antihistamines	Increased sedative effect of both drugs.
Antihypertensives	Excessively low blood pressure.
Cimetidine	Excess sedation.
Disulfiram	Increased triazolam effect.
MAO inhibitors	Convulsions, deep sedation, rage.
Narcotics	Increased sedative effect of both drugs.
Sedatives	Increased sedative effect of both drugs.
Sleep inducers	Increased sedative effect of both drugs.
Tranquilizers	Increased sedative effect of both drugs.

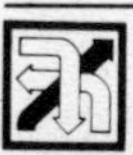

INTERACTION WITH OTHER SUBSTANCES

INTERACTS WITH	COMBINED EFFECT
Alcohol:	Heavy sedation. Avoid.
Beverages:	None expected.
Cocaine:	Decreased triazolam effect.
Foods:	None expected.
Marijuana:	Heavy sedation. Avoid.
Tobacco:	Decreased triazolam effect.

TRICHLORMETHIAZIDE

BRAND NAMES

Metahydrin
Metatensin
Naqua
Naquival

GENERAL INFORMATION

Habit forming? No
Prescription needed? Yes
Available as generic? Yes
Drug class: Antihypertensive, diuretic (thiazide)

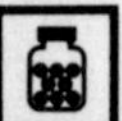

USES

- Controls, but doesn't cure, high blood pressure.
- Reduces fluid retention (edema) caused by conditions such as heart disorders and liver disease.

DOSAGE & USAGE INFORMATION

How to take:
Tablet or capsule—Swallow with liquid. If you can't swallow whole, crumble tablet or open capsule and take with liquid or food. Don't exceed dose.

When to take:
At the same time each day.

If you forget a dose:
Take as soon as you remember up to 2 hours late. If more than 2 hours, wait for next scheduled dose (don't double this dose).

What drug does:
- Forces sodium and water excretion, reducing body fluid.
- Relaxes muscle cells of small arteries.
- Reduced body fluid and relaxed arteries lower blood pressure.

Time lapse before drug works:
4 to 6 hours. May require several weeks to lower blood pressure.

Don't take with:
- See Interaction column and consult doctor.
- Non-prescription drugs without consulting doctor.

OVERDOSE

Symptoms:
Cramps, weakness, drowsiness, weak pulse, coma.

What to do:
- Dial 0 (operator) or 911 (emergency) for an ambulance or medical help. Then give first aid immediately.
- Additional emergency information on page 886.

POSSIBLE ADVERSE REACTIONS OR SIDE EFFECTS

SYMPTOMS	FREQUENCY	WHAT TO DO
Brain & nervous system:		
• Dizziness	Infrequent	4
• Mood changes.	Infrequent	4
• Headache	Infrequent	4
Skin:		
Rash or hives.	Rare	2
Eyes:		
Blurred vision.	Infrequent	3
Ears, nose, throat:		
• Sore throat, fever.	Rare	3
• Dry mouth, thirst.	Infrequent	5
Digestive:		
Severe abdominal pain, nausea, vomiting.	Infrequent	3
Heart & lungs:		
Irregular heartbeat, weak pulse.	Infrequent	3
Blood vessels:	None expected.	
Muscles, bones, joints:		
Weakness, tiredness.	Infrequent	4
Genital, urinary:	None expected.	
Kidneys:	None expected.	
Liver:		
Jaundice (yellow skin and eyes).	Rare	3
Allergic:	None expected.	
Blood:	None expected.	
Others:		
Weight changes.	Infrequent	4

1- Life-threatening. Seek emergency treatment immediately.
2- Discontinue. Seek emergency treatment.
3- Discontinue. Call doctor right away.
4- Continue. Call doctor when convenient.
5- Continue. Tell doctor at next visit.
6- No action necessary.

WARNINGS & PRECAUTIONS

Don't take if:
You are allergic to any thiazide diuretic drug.

Before you start, consult your doctor:
- If you are allergic to any sulfa drug.
- If you have gout.
- If you have liver, pancreas or kidney disorder.

Over age 60:
Adverse reactions and side effects may be more frequent and severe than in younger persons, especially dizziness and excessive potassium loss.

Pregnancy:
Risk to unborn child outweighs drug benefits. Don't use.

Breast-feeding:
Drug passes into milk. Avoid drug or discontinue nursing.

Infants & children:
No problems expected.

Prolonged use:
You may need medicine to treat high blood pressure for the rest of your life.

Skin & sunlight:
May cause rash or intensify sunburn in areas exposed to sun or sunlamp.

Driving, piloting or hazardous work:
Don't drive or pilot aircraft until you learn how medicine affects you. Don't work around dangerous machinery. Don't climb ladders or work in high places. Danger increases if you drink alcohol or take medicine affecting alertness and reflexes, such as antihistamines, tranquilizers, sedatives, pain medicine, narcotics and mind-altering drugs.

Airplane passengers:
No problems expected.

Discontinuing:
Don't discontinue without medical advice.

Others:
- Hot weather and fever may cause dehydration and drop in blood pressure. Dose may require temporary adjustment. Weigh daily and report any unexpected weight decreases to your doctor.
- May cause rise in uric acid, leading to gout.
- May cause blood-sugar rise in diabetics.

INTERACTION WITH OTHER DRUGS

GENERIC NAME OR DRUG CLASS	COMBINED EFFECT
Allopurinol	Decreased allopurinol effect.
Antidepressants (tricyclic)	Dangerous drop in blood pressure. Avoid combination unless under medical supervision.
Barbiturates	Increased trichlormethiazide effect.
Cholestyramine	Decreased trichlormethiazide effect.
Cortisone drugs	Excessive potassium loss that causes dangerous heart rhythms.
Digitalis preparations	Excessive potassium loss that causes dangerous heart rhythms.
Diuretics (thiazide)	Increased effect of other thiazide diuretics.
Lithium	Increased effect of lithium.
MAO inhibitors	Increased trichlormethiazide effect.
Probenecid	Decreased probenecid effect.

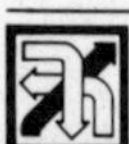

INTERACTION WITH OTHER SUBSTANCES

INTERACTS WITH	COMBINED EFFECT
Alcohol:	Dangerous blood-pressure drop.
Beverages:	None expected.
Cocaine:	None expected.
Foods:	
Licorice	Excessive potassium loss that causes dangerous heart rhythms.
Marijuana:	May increase blood pressure.
Tobacco:	None expected.

TRIDIHEXETHYL

BRAND NAMES

Milpath
Pathibamate
Pathilon

GENERAL INFORMATION

Habit forming? No
Prescription needed? Low strength: No
High strength: Yes
Available as generic? Yes
Drug class: Antispasmodic, anticholinergic

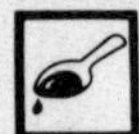

USES

Reduces spasms of digestive system, bladder and urethra.

DOSAGE & USAGE INFORMATION

How to take:
Tablet—Swallow with liquid or food to lessen stomach irritation.

When to take:
30 minutes before meals (unless directed otherwise by doctor).

If you forget a dose:
Take as soon as you remember up to 2 hours late. If more than 2 hours, wait for next scheduled dose (don't double this dose).

What drug does:
Blocks nerve impulses at parasympathetic nerve endings, preventing muscle contractions and gland secretions of organs involved.

Time lapse before drug works:
15 to 30 minutes.

Don't take with:
See Interaction column and consult doctor.

OVERDOSE

Symptoms:
Dilated pupils; rapid pulse and breathing; dizziness; fever; hallucinations; confusion; slurred speech; agitation; flushed face; convulsions; coma.

What to do:
- Dial 0 (operator) or 911 (emergency) for an ambulance or medical help. Then give first aid immediately.
- Additional emergency information on page 886.

POSSIBLE ADVERSE REACTIONS OR SIDE EFFECTS

SYMPTOMS	FREQUENCY	WHAT TO DO
Brain & nervous system:		
• Headache	Infrequent	4
• Confusion, delirium.	Common	3
Skin:		
Rash or hives.	Rare	3
Eyes:		
Pain, blurred vision.	Rare	3
Ears, nose, throat:		
Dryness	Common	6
Digestive:		
• Constipation	Common	5
• Nausea, vomiting.	Common	4
Heart & lungs:		
Rapid heartbeat.	Common	3
Blood vessels:	None expected.	
Muscles, bones, joints:	None expected.	
Genital, urinary:		
Difficult urination.	Infrequent	4
Kidneys:	None expected.	
Liver:	None expected.	
Allergic:	None expected.	
Blood:	None expected.	
Others:		
Less perspiration.	Common	4

1- Life-threatening. Seek emergency treatment immediately.
2- Discontinue. Seek emergency treatment.
3- Discontinue. Call doctor right away.
4- Continue. Call doctor when convenient.
5- Continue. Tell doctor at next visit.
6- No action necessary.

WARNINGS & PRECAUTIONS

Don't take if:
- You are allergic to any anticholinergic.
- You have trouble with stomach bloating.
- You have difficulty emptying your bladder completely.
- You have narrow-angle glaucoma.
- You have severe ulcerative colitis.

Before you start, consult your doctor:
- If you have open-angle glaucoma.
- If you have angina.
- If you have chronic bronchitis or asthma.
- If you have hiatal hernia.
- If you have liver disease.
- If you have enlarged prostate.
- If you have myasthenia gravis.
- If you have peptic ulcer.
- If you will have surgery within 2 months, including dental surgery, requiring general or spinal anesthesia.

Over age 60:
Adverse reactions and side effects may be more frequent and severe than in younger persons.

Pregnancy:
Studies inconclusive on harm to unborn child. Animal studies show fetal abnormalities. Decide with your doctor whether drug benefits justify risk to unborn child.

Breast-feeding:
Drug passes into milk and decreases milk flow. Avoid drug or discontinue nursing until you finish medicine. Consult doctor for advice on maintaining milk supply.

Infants & children:
Use only under medical supervision.

Prolonged use:
Chronic constipation, possible fecal impaction. Consult doctor immediately.

Skin & sunlight:
No problems expected.

Driving, piloting or hazardous work:
Use disqualifies you for piloting aircraft. Otherwise, no problems expected.

Airplane passengers:
No problems expected.

Discontinuing:
May be unnecessary to finish medicine. Follow doctor's instructions.

Others:
No problems expected.

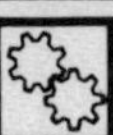

INTERACTION WITH OTHER DRUGS

GENERIC NAME OR DRUG CLASS	COMBINED EFFECT
Amantadine	Increased tridihexethyl effect.
Anticholinergics (other)	Increased tridihexethyl effect.
Antidepressants (tricyclic)	Increased tridihexethyl effect.
Antihistamines	Increased tridihexethyl effect.
Cortisone drugs	Increased internal-eye pressure.
Haloperidol	Increased internal-eye pressure.
MAO inhibitors	Increased tridihexethyl effect.
Meperidine	Increased tridihexethyl effect.
Methylphenidate	Increased tridihexethyl effect.
Orphenadrine	Increased tridihexethyl effect.
Phenothiazines	Increased tridihexethyl effect.
Pilocarpine	Loss of pilocarpine effect in glaucoma treatment.
Vitamin C	Decreased tridihexethyl effect. Avoid large doses of vitamin C.

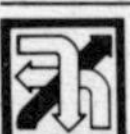

INTERACTION WITH OTHER SUBSTANCES

INTERACTS WITH	COMBINED EFFECT
Alcohol:	None expected.
Beverages:	None expected.
Cocaine:	Excessively rapid heartbeat. Avoid.
Foods:	None expected.
Marijuana:	Drowsiness and dry mouth.
Tobacco:	None expected.

TRIFLUOPERAZINE

BRAND NAMES

Clinazine
Novoflurazine
Pentazine
Solazine
Stelazine
Terfluzine
Triflurin
Tripazine

GENERAL INFORMATION

Habit forming? No
Prescription needed? Yes
Available as generic? Yes
Drug class: Tranquilizer, antiemetic (phenothiazine)

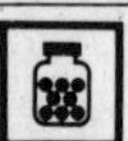

USES

- Stops nausea, vomiting.
- Reduces anxiety, agitation.

DOSAGE & USAGE INFORMATION

How to take:
- Tablet or capsule—Swallow with liquid or food to lessen stomach irritation.
- Suppositories—Remove wrapper and moisten suppository with water. Gently insert into rectum, large end first.
- Drops or liquid—Dilute dose in beverage.

When to take:
- Nervous and mental disorders—Take at the same times each day.
- Nausea and vomiting—Take as needed, no more often than every 4 hours.

If you forget a dose:
- Nervous and mental disorders—Take up to 2 hours late. If more than 2 hours, wait for next scheduled dose (don't double this).
- Nausea and vomiting—Take as soon as you remember. Wait 4 hours for next dose.

What drug does:
- Suppresses brain's vomiting center.
- Suppresses brain centers that control abnormal emotions and behavior.

Time lapse before drug works:
- Nausea and vomiting—1 hour or less.
- Nervous and mental disorders—4-6 weeks.

Don't take with:
- Antacid or medicine for diarrhea.
- Non-prescription drug for cough, cold or allergy.
- See Interaction column and consult doctor.

OVERDOSE

Symptoms:
Stupor, convulsions, coma.

What to do:
- Dial 0 (operator) or 911 (emergency) for an ambulance or medical help. Then give first aid immediately.
- Additional emergency information on page 886.

POSSIBLE ADVERSE REACTIONS OR SIDE EFFECTS

SYMPTOMS	FREQUENCY	WHAT TO DO
Brain & nervous system:		
• Restlessness, tremor.	Common	3
• Fainting	Infrequent	2
• Drowsiness	Common	3
Skin:		
• Rash	Infrequent	3
• Less perspiration.	Common	4
Eyes:		
Vision changes.	Rare	3
Ears, nose, throat:		
• Sore throat, fever.	Rare	3
• Dry mouth, nasal congestion.	Common	4
Digestive:		
Constipation	Common	4
Heart & lungs, blood vessels, kidneys, allergic, blood:	None expected.	
Muscles, bones, joints:		
Muscle spasms of face and neck, unsteady gait.	Common	2
Genital, urinary:		
Urination difficulty.	Infrequent	4
Liver:		
Jaundice (yellow eyes and skin).	Rare	3
Others:		
Less interest in sex, breast swelling, change in menstrual pattern.	Infrequent	4

1- Life-threatening. Seek emergency treatment immediately.
2- Discontinue. Seek emergency treatment.
3- Discontinue. Call doctor right away.
4- Continue. Call doctor when convenient.
5- Continue. Tell doctor at next visit.
6- No action necessary.

WARNINGS & PRECAUTIONS

Don't take if:
- You are allergic to any phenothiazine.
- You have a blood or bone-marrow disease.

Before you start, consult your doctor:
- If you will have surgery within 2 months, including dental surgery, requiring general or spinal anesthesia.
- If you have asthma, emphysema or other lung disorder.
- If you take non-prescription ulcer medicine, asthma medicine or amphetamines.

Over age 60:
Adverse reactions and side effects may be more frequent and severe than in younger persons. More likely to develop involuntary movement of jaws, lips, tongue, chewing. Report this to your doctor immediately. Early treatment can help.

Pregnancy:
Risk to unborn child outweighs drug benefits. Don't use.

Breast-feeding:
Drug passes into milk. Avoid drug or discontinue nursing until you finish medicine. Consult doctor for advice on maintaining milk supply.

Infants & children:
Don't give to children younger than 2.

Prolonged use:
May lead to tardive dyskinesia (involuntary movement of jaws, lips, tongue, chewing).

Skin & sunlight:
May cause rash or intensify sunburn in areas exposed to sun or sunlamp. Skin may remain sensitive for 3 months after discontinuing.

Driving, piloting or hazardous work:
Don't drive or pilot aircraft until you learn how medicine affects you. Don't work around dangerous machinery. Don't climb ladders or work in high places. Danger increases if you drink alcohol or take medicine affecting alertness and reflexes.

Airplane passengers:
No problems expected.

Discontinuing:
- Nervous and mental disorders—Don't discontinue without doctor's advice until you complete prescribed dose, even though symptoms diminish or disappear.
- Nausea and vomiting—May be unnecessary to finish medicine. Follow doctor's instructions.

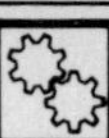

INTERACTION WITH OTHER DRUGS

GENERIC NAME OR DRUG CLASS	COMBINED EFFECT
Anticholinergics	Increased anticholinergic effect.
Antidepressants (tricyclic)	Increased trifluoperazine effect.
Antihistamines	Increased antihistamine effect.
Appetite suppressants	Decreased suppressant effect.
Levodopa	Decreased levodopa effect.
Mind-altering drugs	Increased effect of mind-altering drugs.
Narcotics	Increased narcotic effect.
Phenytoin	Increased phenytoin effect.
Quinidine	Impaired heart function. Dangerous mixture.
Sedatives	Increased sedative effect.
Tranquilizers (other)	Increased tranquilizer effect.

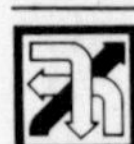

INTERACTION WITH OTHER SUBSTANCES

INTERACTS WITH	COMBINED EFFECT
Alcohol:	Dangerous oversedation.
Beverages:	None expected.
Cocaine:	Decreased trifluoperazine effect. Avoid.
Foods:	None expected.
Marijuana:	Drowsiness. May increase antinausea effect.
Tobacco:	None expected.

TRIFLUPROMAZINE

BRAND NAMES

Psyquil
Vesprin

GENERAL INFORMATION

Habit forming? No
Prescription needed? Yes
Available as generic? Yes
Drug class: Tranquilizer, antiemetic (phenothiazine)

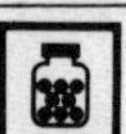

USES

- Stops nausea, vomiting.
- Reduces anxiety, agitation.

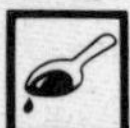

DOSAGE & USAGE INFORMATION

How to take:

- Tablet or capsule—Swallow with liquid or food to lessen stomach irritation.
- Suppositories—Remove wrapper and moisten suppository with water. Gently insert into rectum, large end first.
- Drops or liquid—Dilute dose in beverage.

When to take:

- Nervous and mental disorders—Take at the same times each day.
- Nausea and vomiting—Take as needed, no more often than every 4 hours.

If you forget a dose:

- Nervous and mental disorders—Take up to 2 hours late. If more than 2 hours, wait for next scheduled dose (don't double this).
- Nausea and vomiting—Take as soon as you remember. Wait 4 hours for next dose.

What drug does:

- Suppresses brain's vomiting center.
- Suppresses brain centers that control abnormal emotions and behavior.

Time lapse before drug works:

- Nausea and vomiting—1 hour or less.
- Nervous and mental disorders—4-6 weeks.

Don't take with:

- Antacid or medicine for diarrhea.
- Non-prescription drug for cough, cold or allergy.
- See Interaction column and consult doctor.

OVERDOSE

Symptoms:
Stupor, convulsions, coma.

What to do:

- Dial 0 (operator) or 911 (emergency) for an ambulance or medical help. Then give first aid immediately.
- Additional emergency information on page 886.

POSSIBLE ADVERSE REACTIONS OR SIDE EFFECTS

SYMPTOMS	FREQUENCY	WHAT TO DO
Brain & nervous system:		
• Restlessness, tremor.	Common	3
• Fainting	Infrequent	2
• Drowsiness	Common	3
Skin:		
• Rash	Infrequent	3
• Less perspiration.	Common	4
Eyes:		
Vision changes.	Rare	3
Ears, nose, throat:		
• Sore throat, fever.	Rare	3
• Dry mouth, nasal congestion.	Common	4
Digestive:		
Constipation	Common	4
Heart & lungs, blood vessels, kidneys, allergic, blood:	None expected.	
Muscles, bones, joints:		
Muscle spasms of face and neck, unsteady gait.	Common	2
Genital, urinary:		
Urination difficulty.	Infrequent	4
Liver:		
Jaundice (yellow eyes and skin).	Rare	3
Others:		
Less interest in sex, breast swelling, change in menstrual pattern.	Infrequent	4

1-Life-threatening. Seek emergency treatment immediately.
2-Discontinue. Seek emergency treatment.
3-Discontinue. Call doctor right away.
4-Continue. Call doctor when convenient.
5-Continue. Tell doctor at next visit.
6-No action necessary.

WARNINGS & PRECAUTIONS

Don't take if:
- You are allergic to any phenothiazine.
- You have a blood or bone-marrow disease.

Before you start, consult your doctor:
- If you will have surgery within 2 months, including dental surgery, requiring general or spinal anesthesia.
- If you have asthma, emphysema or other lung disorder.
- If you take non-prescription ulcer medicine, asthma medicine or amphetamines.

Over age 60:
Adverse reactions and side effects may be more frequent and severe than in younger persons. More likely to develop involuntary movement of jaws, lips, tongue, chewing. Report this to your doctor immediately. Early treatment can help.

Pregnancy:
Risk to unborn child outweighs drug benefits. Don't use.

Breast-feeding:
Drug passes into milk. Avoid drug or discontinue nursing until you finish medicine. Consult doctor for advice on maintaining milk supply.

Infants & children:
Don't give to children younger than 2.

Prolonged use:
May lead to tardive dyskinesia (involuntary movement of jaws, lips, tongue, chewing).

Skin & sunlight:
May cause rash or intensify sunburn in areas exposed to sun or sunlamp. Skin may remain sensitive for 3 months after discontinuing.

Driving, piloting or hazardous work:
Don't drive or pilot aircraft until you learn how medicine affects you. Don't work around dangerous machinery. Don't climb ladders or work in high places. Danger increases if you drink alcohol or take medicine affecting alertness and reflexes.

Airplane passengers:
No problems expected.

Discontinuing:
- Nervous and mental disorders—Don't discontinue without doctor's advice until you complete prescribed dose, even though symptoms diminish or disappear.
- Nausea and vomiting—May be unnecessary to finish medicine. Follow doctor's instructions.

INTERACTION WITH OTHER DRUGS

GENERIC NAME OR DRUG CLASS	COMBINED EFFECT
Anticholinergics	Increased anticholinergic effect.
Antidepressants (tricyclic)	Increased triflupromazine effect.
Antihistamines	Increased antihistamine effect.
Appetite suppressants	Decreased suppressant effect.
Levodopa	Decreased levodopa effect.
Mind-altering drugs	Increased effect of mind-altering drugs.
Narcotics	Increased narcotic effect.
Phenytoin	Increased phenytoin effect.
Quinidine	Impaired heart function. Dangerous mixture.
Sedatives	Increased sedative effect.
Tranquilizers (other)	Increased tranquilizer effect.

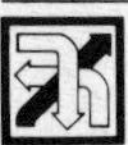

INTERACTION WITH OTHER SUBSTANCES

INTERACTS WITH	COMBINED EFFECT
Alcohol:	Dangerous oversedation.
Beverages:	None expected.
Cocaine:	Decreased triflupromazine effect. Avoid.
Foods:	None expected.
Marijuana:	Drowsiness. May increase antinausea effect.
Tobacco:	None expected.

TRIHEXYPHENIDYL

BRAND NAMES

Aparkane
Apo-Trihex
Artane
Artane Sequels
Novohexidyl
Tremin
T.H.P.
Trihexane
Trihexidyl
Trihexy

GENERAL INFORMATION

Habit forming? No
Prescription needed? Yes
Available as generic? No
Drug class: Antidyskinetic, antiparkinsonism

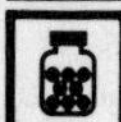

USES

- Treatment of Parkinson's disease.
- Treatment of adverse effects of phenothiazines.

DOSAGE & USAGE INFORMATION

How to take:
Tablets or capsules—Take with food to lessen stomach irritation.

When to take:
At the same times each day.

If you forget a dose:
Take as soon as you remember up to 2 hours late. If more than 2 hours, wait for next scheduled dose (don't double this dose).

What drug does:
- Balances chemical reactions necessary to send nerve impulses within base of brain.
- Improves muscle control and reduces stiffness.

Time lapse before drug works:
1 to 2 hours.

Don't take with:
- Non-prescription drugs for colds, cough or allergy.
- See Interaction column and consult doctor.

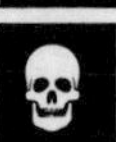

OVERDOSE

Symptoms:
Agitation, dilated pupils, hallucinations, dry mouth, rapid heartbeat, sleepiness.

What to do:
- Dial 0 (operator) or 911 (emergency) for an ambulance or medical help. Then give first aid immediately.
- If patient is unconscious and not breathing, give mouth-to-mouth breathing. If there is no heartbeat, use cardiac massage and mouth-to-mouth breathing (CPR). Don't try to make patient vomit. If you can't get help quickly, take patient to nearest emergency facility.
- Additional emergency information on page 886.

POSSIBLE ADVERSE REACTIONS OR SIDE EFFECTS

SYMPTOMS	FREQUENCY	WHAT TO DO
Brain & nervous system:		
Confusion, dizziness.	Rare	4
Skin:		
Rash	Rare	3
Eyes:		
• Pain	Rare	3
• Blurred vision, light sensitivity.	Common	4
Ears, nose, throat:		
Sore mouth or tongue.	Rare	4
Digestive:		
• Constipation	Common	4
• Nausea, vomiting.	Common	4
Heart & lungs:	None expected.	
Blood vessels:	None expected.	
Muscles, bones, joints:		
• Muscle cramps.	Rare	4
• Numbness, weakness in hands or feet.	Rare	4
Genital, urinary:		
Difficult or painful urination.	Common	5
Kidneys:	None expected.	
Liver:	None expected.	
Allergic:	None expected.	
Blood:	None expected.	
Others:	None expected.	

1- Life-threatening. Seek emergency treatment immediately.
2- Discontinue. Seek emergency treatment.
3- Discontinue. Call doctor right away.
4- Continue. Call doctor when convenient.
5- Continue. Tell doctor at next visit.
6- No action necessary.

WARNINGS & PRECAUTIONS

Don't take if:
You are allergic to any antidyskinetic.

Before you start, consult your doctor:
- If you have had glaucoma.
- If you have had high blood pressure or heart disease.
- If you have had impaired liver function.
- If you have had kidney disease or urination difficulty.

Over age 60:
More sensitive to drug. Aggravates symptoms of enlarged prostate. Causes impaired thinking, hallucinations, nightmares. Consult doctor about any of these.

Pregnancy:
Studies inconclusive on harm to unborn child. Animal studies show fetal abnormalities. Decide with your doctor whether drug benefits justify risk to unborn child.

Breast-feeding:
No problems expected.

Infants & children:
Not recommended for children 3 and younger. Use for older children only under doctor's supervision.

Prolonged use:
Possible glaucoma.

Skin & sunlight:
No problems expected.

Driving, piloting or hazardous work:
Don't drive or pilot aircraft until you learn how medicine affects you. Don't work around dangerous machinery. Don't climb ladders or work in high places. Danger increases if you drink alcohol or take medicine affecting alertness and reflexes, such as antihistamines, tranquilizers, sedatives, pain medicine, narcotics and mind-altering drugs.

Airplane passengers:
No problems expected.

Discontinuing:
Don't discontinue without consulting doctor. Dose may require gradual reduction if you have taken drug for a long time. Doses of other drugs may also require adjustment.

Others:
- Internal eye pressure should be measured regularly.
- Avoid becoming overheated.

INTERACTION WITH OTHER DRUGS

GENERIC NAME OR DRUG CLASS	COMBINED EFFECT
Amantadine	Increased amantadine effect.
Antidepressants (tricyclic)	Increased trihexyphenidyl effect. May cause glaucoma.
Antihistamines	Increased trihexyphenidyl effect.
Levodopa	Increased levodopa effect. Improved results in treating Parkinson's disease.
Meperidine	Increased trihexyphenidyl effect.
MAO inhibitors	Increased trihexyphenidyl effect.
Orphenadrine	Increased trihexyphenidyl effect.
Phenothiazines	Behavior changes.
Primidone	Excessive sedation.
Procainamide	Increased procainamide effect.
Quinidine	Increased trihexyphenidyl effect.
Tranquilizers	Excessive sedation.

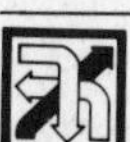

INTERACTION WITH OTHER SUBSTANCES

INTERACTS WITH	COMBINED EFFECT
Alcohol:	None expected.
Beverages:	None expected.
Cocaine:	Decreased trihexyphenidyl effect. Avoid.
Foods:	None expected.
Marijuana:	None expected.
Tobacco:	None expected.

TRIMEPRAZINE

BRAND NAMES

Panectyl
Temaril

GENERAL INFORMATION

Habit forming? No
Prescription needed? Yes
Available as generic? Yes
Drug class: Tranquilizer (phenothiazine), antihistamine

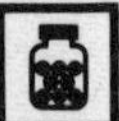

USES

Relieves itching of hives, skin allergies, chickenpox.

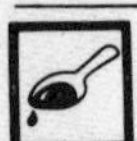

DOSAGE & USAGE INFORMATION

How to take:

- Tablet or syrup—Swallow with liquid or food to lessen stomach irritation.
- Extended-release capsules—Swallow each dose whole. If you take regular tablets, you may chew or crush them.

When to take:
At the same times each day.

If you forget a dose:
Take as soon as you remember up to 2 hours late. If more than 2 hours, wait for next scheduled dose (don't double this dose).

What drug does:
Blocks histamine action in skin.

Time lapse before drug works:
1 to 2 hours.

Don't take with:

- Antacid or medicine for diarrhea.
- Non-prescription drug for cough, cold or allergy.
- See Interaction column and consult doctor.

OVERDOSE

Symptoms:
Stupor, convulsions, coma.

What to do:

- Dial 0 (operator) or 911 (emergency) for an ambulance or medical help. Then give first aid immediately.
- Additional emergency information on page 886.

POSSIBLE ADVERSE REACTIONS OR SIDE EFFECTS

SYMPTOMS	FREQUENCY	WHAT TO DO
Brain & nervous system:		
• Restlessness, tremor, drowsiness.	Common	3
• Fainting	Infrequent	2
Skin:		
• Rash	Infrequent	3
• Less perspiration.	Common	4
Eyes:		
Vision changes.	Rare	3
Ears, nose, throat:		
• Sore throat, fever.	Rare	3
• Dry mouth, nasal congestion.	Common	4
Digestive:		
Constipation	Common	4
Heart & lungs:	None expected.	
Blood vessels:	None expected.	
Muscles, bones, joints:		
Muscle spasms of face and neck, unsteady gait.	Infrequent	3
Genital, urinary:		
Urination difficulty.	Infrequent	4
Kidneys:	None expected.	
Liver:		
Jaundice (yellow skin and eyes).	Rare	3
Allergic:	None expected.	
Blood:	None expected.	
Others:		
Less interest in sex, breast swelling, menstrual changes.	Infrequent	4

1 - Life-threatening. Seek emergency treatment immediately.
2 - Discontinue. Seek emergency treatment.
3 - Discontinue. Call doctor right away.
4 - Continue. Call doctor when convenient.

WARNINGS & PRECAUTIONS

Don't take if:

- You are allergic to any phenothiazine.
- You have a blood or bone-marrow disease.

Before you start, consult your doctor:

- If you will have surgery within 2 months, including dental surgery, requiring general or spinal anesthesia.
- If you have asthma, emphysema or other lung disorder.
- If you take non-prescription ulcer medicine, asthma medicine or amphetamines.

Over age 60:
Adverse reactions and side effects may be more frequent and severe than in younger persons. More likely to develop tardive dyskinesia (involuntary movement of jaws, lips, tongue, chewing). Report this to your doctor immediately. Early treatment can help.

Pregnancy:
Risk to unborn child outweighs drug benefits. Don't use.

Breast-feeding:
Drug passes into milk. Avoid drug or discontinue nursing until you finish medicine. Consult doctor for advice on maintaining milk supply.

Infants & children:
Don't give to children younger than 2.

Prolonged use:
May lead to tardive dyskinesia (involuntary movement of jaws, lips, tongue, chewing).

Skin & sunlight:
May cause rash or intensify sunburn in areas exposed to sun or sunlamp. Skin may remain sensitive for 3 months after discontinuing.

Driving, piloting or hazardous work:
Don't drive or pilot aircraft until you learn how medicine affects you. Don't work around dangerous machinery. Don't climb ladders or work in high places. Danger increases if you drink alcohol or take medicine affecting alertness and reflexes.

Airplane passengers:
No problems expected.

Discontinuing:
May be unnecessary to finish medicine. Follow doctor's instructions.

INTERACTION WITH OTHER DRUGS

GENERIC NAME OR DRUG CLASS	COMBINED EFFECT
Antacids	Decreased trimeprazine effect.
Anticholinergics	Increased anticholinergic effect.
Anticonvulsants (hydantoin)	Increased anticonvulsant effect.
Antidepressants (tricyclic)	Increased trimeprazine effect.
Antihistamines (other)	Increased antihistamine effect.
Appetite suppressants	Decreased suppressant effect.
Barbiturates	Oversedation.
Guanethidine	Decreased guanethidine effect.
Levodopa	Decreased levodopa effect.
MAO inhibitors	Increased trimeprazine effect.
Mind-altering drugs	Increased effect of mind-altering drugs.
Narcotics	Increased narcotic effect.
Sedatives	Increased sedative effect.
Tranquilizers	Increased tranquilizer effect. Avoid.

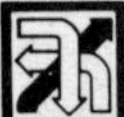

INTERACTION WITH OTHER SUBSTANCES

INTERACTS WITH	COMBINED EFFECT
Alcohol:	Dangerous oversedation.
Beverages:	None expected.
Cocaine:	Decreased effect of trimeprazine. Avoid.
Foods:	None expected.
Marijuana:	Drowsiness.
Tobacco:	None expected.

TRIMETHOBENZAMIDE

BRAND NAMES

Stemetic
Tigan
Tegamide

GENERAL INFORMATION

Habit forming? No
Prescription needed? Yes
Available as generic? Yes
Drug class: Antiemetic

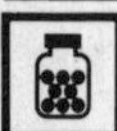

USES

Reduces nausea and vomiting.

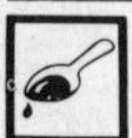

DOSAGE & USAGE INFORMATION

How to take:

- Capsule—Swallow with liquid. If you can't swallow whole, open capsule and take with liquid or food.
- Suppositories—Remove wrapper and moisten suppository with water. Gently insert larger end into rectum. Push well into rectum with finger.

When to take:
When needed, no more often than label directs.

If you forget a dose:
Take when you remember. Wait as long as label directs for next dose.

What drug does:
Possibly blocks nerve impulses to brain's vomiting centers.

Time lapse before drug works:
20 to 40 minutes.

Don't take with:
Non-prescription drugs or drugs in Interaction column without consulting doctor.

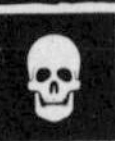

OVERDOSE

Symptoms:
Confusion, convulsions, coma.

What to do:

- Dial 0 (operator) or 911 (emergency) for an ambulance or medical help. Then give first aid immediately.
- If patient is unconscious and not breathing, give mouth-to-mouth breathing. If there is no heartbeat, use cardiac massage and mouth-to-mouth breathing (CPR). Don't try to make patient vomit. If you can't get help quickly, take patient to nearest emergency facility.
- Additional emergency information on page 886.

POSSIBLE ADVERSE REACTIONS OR SIDE EFFECTS

SYMPTOMS	FREQUENCY	WHAT TO DO
Brain & nervous system:		
• Dizziness, drowsiness, headache.	Infrequent	4
• Seizures, tremors, depression.	Rare	3
Skin:		
Rash	Infrequent	3
Eyes:		
Blurred vision.	Infrequent	3
Ears, nose, throat:		
Sore throat, fever.	Rare	3
Digestive:		
• Diarrhea	Infrequent	4
• Repeated vomiting.	Rare	3
Heart & lungs:	None expected.	
Blood vessels:		
Low blood pressure.	Infrequent	3
Muscles, bones, joints:		
• Muscle cramps.	Infrequent	4
• Back pain.	Rare	3
Genital, urinary:	None expected.	
Kidneys:	None expected.	
Liver:		
Jaundice (yellow skin and eyes).	Rare	3
Allergic:	None expected.	
Blood:	None expected.	
Others:		
Unusual tiredness.	Infrequent	4

1- Life-threatening. Seek emergency treatment immediately.
2- Discontinue. Seek emergency treatment.
3- Discontinue. Call doctor right away.
4- Continue. Call doctor when convenient.
5- Continue. Tell doctor at next visit.
6- No action necessary.

WARNINGS & PRECAUTIONS

Don't take if:
- You are allergic to trimethobenzamide.
- You are allergic to local anesthetics and have suppository form.

Before you start, consult your doctor:
If you have reacted badly to antihistamines.

Over age 60:
More susceptible to low blood pressure and sedative effects of this drug.

Pregnancy:
No proven harm to unborn child. Avoid if possible.

Breast-feeding:
No proven problems. Avoid if possible.

Infants & children:
- Injectable form not recommended.
- Avoid during viral infections. Drug may contribute to Reyes' syndrome.

Prolonged use:
- Damages blood-cell production of bone marrow.
- Causes Parkinson-like symptoms of tremors, rigidity.

Skin & sunlight:
Possible sun sensitivity. Use caution.

Driving, piloting or hazardous work:
- Use disqualifies you for piloting aircraft.
- Don't drive until you learn how medicine affects you. Don't work around dangerous machinery. Don't climb ladders or work in high places. Danger increases if you drink alcohol or take medicine affecting alertness and reflexes, such as antihistamines, tranquilizers, sedatives, pain medicine, narcotics and mind-altering drugs.

Airplane passengers:
No problems expected.

Discontinuing:
May be unnecessary to finish medicine. Follow doctor's instructions.

Others:
No problems expected.

INTERACTION WITH OTHER DRUGS

GENERIC NAME OR DRUG CLASS	COMBINED EFFECT
Antidepressants	Increased sedative effect.
Antihistamines	Increased sedative effect.
Barbiturates	Increased effect of both drugs.
Belladonna	Increased effect of both drugs.
Cholinergics	Increased effect of both drugs.
Mind-altering drugs	Increased effect of mind-altering drug.
Narcotics	Increased sedative effect.
Phenothiazines	Increased effect of both drugs.
Sedatives	Increased sedative effect.
Sleep inducers	Increased effect of sleep inducer.
Tranquilizers	Increased sedative effect.

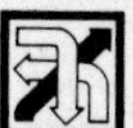

INTERACTION WITH OTHER SUBSTANCES

INTERACTS WITH	COMBINED EFFECT
Alcohol:	Oversedation. Avoid.
Beverages:	None expected.
Cocaine:	None expected.
Foods:	None expected.
Marijuana:	Increased antinausea effect.
Tobacco:	None expected.

TRIMETHOPRIM

BRAND NAMES

Apo-Sulfatrim
Bactrim
Cotrim
Novotrimel
Proloprim
Protrin
Rovbac
SMZ-TMP
Septra
Syraprim
Trimpex

GENERAL INFORMATION

Habit forming? No
Prescription needed? Yes
Available as generic? No
Drug class: Antimicrobial

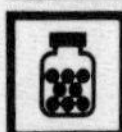

USES

- Treatment for urinary-tract infections susceptible to trimethoprim.
- Helps prevent recurrent urinary-tract infections if taken once a day.

DOSAGE & USAGE INFORMATION

How to take:
- Tablet or capsule—Swallow with liquid or food to lessen stomach irritation.
- Drops—Dilute dose in beverage before swallowing.

When to take:
Space doses evenly in 24 hours to keep constant amount in urine.

If you forget a dose:
Take as soon as possible. Wait 5 to 6 hours before next dose. Then return to regular schedule.

What drug does:
Stops harmful bacterial germs from multiplying. Will not kill viruses.

Time lapse before drug works:
2 to 5 days.

Don't take with:
See Interaction column and consult doctor.

OVERDOSE

Symptoms:
Nausea, vomiting, diarrhea.

What to do:
Overdose unlikely to threaten life. If person takes much larger amount than prescribed, call doctor, poison-control center or hospital emergency room for instructions.

POSSIBLE ADVERSE REACTIONS OR SIDE EFFECTS

SYMPTOMS	FREQUENCY	WHAT TO DO
Brain & nervous system:		
Headache	Infrequent	4
Skin:		
• Blue fingernails, lips, skin.	Rare	2
• Rash, itch.	Common	3
Eyes:	None expected.	
Ears, nose, throat:		
Sore throat, fever.	Rare	3
Digestive:		
Diarrhea, nausea, vomiting, abdominal pain.	Infrequent	3
Heart & lungs:		
Breathing difficulty.	Rare	2
Blood vessels:	None expected.	
Muscles, bones, joints:	None expected.	
Genital, urinary:	None expected.	
Kidneys:	None expected.	
Liver:	None expected.	
Allergic:	None expected.	
Blood:	None expected.	
Others:	None expected.	

1- Life-threatening. Seek emergency treatment immediately.
2- Discontinue. Seek emergency treatment.
3- Discontinue. Call doctor right away.
4- Continue. Call doctor when convenient.
5- Continue. Tell doctor at next visit.
6- No action necessary.

WARNINGS & PRECAUTIONS

Don't take if:
You are allergic to trimethoprim or any sulfa drug.

Before you start, consult your doctor:
If you have had liver or kidney disease.

Over age 60:
- Reduced liver and kidney function may require reduced dose.
- More likely to have severe anal and genital itch.
- Increased susceptibility to anemia.

Pregnancy:
Studies inconclusive on harm to unborn child. Animal studies show fetal abnormalities. Decide with your doctor whether drug benefits justify risk to unborn child.

Breast-feeding:
No proven harm to unborn child. Avoid if possible.

Infants & children:
Use under medical supervision only.

Prolonged use:
Anemia

Skin & sunlight:
May cause rash or intensify sunburn in areas exposed to sun or sunlamp.

Driving, piloting or hazardous work:
No problems expected.

Airplane passengers:
No problems expected.

Discontinuing:
Don't discontinue without doctor's advice until you complete prescribed dose, even though symptoms diminish or disappear.

Others:
No problems expected.

INTERACTION WITH OTHER DRUGS

GENERIC NAME OR DRUG CLASS	COMBINED EFFECT
Diuretics (thiazide)	Unusual bleeding or bruising.
Sulfamethoxazole	Beneficial increase of sulfamethoxazole effect.

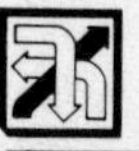

INTERACTION WITH OTHER SUBSTANCES

INTERACTS WITH	COMBINED EFFECT
Alcohol:	Increased alcohol effect with Bactrim or Septra.
Beverages:	None expected.
Cocaine:	No proven problems.
Foods:	None expected.
Marijuana:	None expected.
Tobacco:	None expected.

TRIMIPRAMINE

BRAND NAMES

Surmontil

GENERAL INFORMATION

Habit forming? No
Prescription needed? Yes
Available as generic? No
Drug class: Antidepressant (tricyclic)

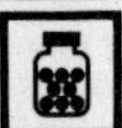

USES

Gradually relieves, but doesn't cure, symptoms of depression.

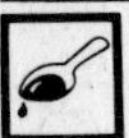

DOSAGE & USAGE INFORMATION

How to take:
Capsule—Swallow with liquid.

When to take:
At the same time each day, usually bedtime.

If you forget a dose:
Bedtime dose—If you forget your once-a-day bedtime dose, don't take it more than 3 hours late. If more than 3 hours, wait for next scheduled dose. Don't double this dose.

What drug does:
Probably affects part of brain that controls messages between nerve cells.

Time lapse before drug works:
Begins in 1 to 2 weeks. May require 4 to 6 weeks for maximum benefit.

Don't take with:
- Non-prescription drugs without consulting doctor.
- See Interaction column and consult doctor.

OVERDOSE

Symptoms:
Hallucinations, convulsions, coma.

What to do:
- Dial 0 (operator) or 911 (emergency) for an ambulance or medical help. Then give first aid immediately.
- If patient is unconscious and not breathing, give mouth-to-mouth breathing. If there is no heartbeat, use cardiac massage and mouth-to-mouth breathing (CPR). Don't try to make patient vomit. If you can't get help quickly, take patient to nearest emergency facility.
- Additional emergency information on page 886.

POSSIBLE ADVERSE REACTIONS OR SIDE EFFECTS

SYMPTOMS	FREQUENCY	WHAT TO DO
Brain & nervous system:		
• Hallucinations, shakiness, dizziness, fainting.	Infrequent	3
• Headache	Common	4
• Seizures	Rare	1
• Insomnia	Common	5
Skin:		
Rash, itch.	Rare	3
Eyes:		
Blurred vision, pain.	Infrequent	3
Ears, nose, throat:		
• Sore throat.	Rare	3
• Dry mouth or unpleasant taste.	Common	4
Digestive:		
• Constipation or diarrhea, nausea, indigestion.	Common	4
• Vomiting	Infrequent	3
• "Sweet tooth"	Common	5
Heart & lungs:		
Irregular heartbeat or slow pulse.	Infrequent	3
Blood vessels, muscles, bones, joints, kidneys, allergic, blood:	None expected.	
Genital, urinary:		
Difficulty urinating.	Infrequent	4
Liver:		
Jaundice (yellow skin and eyes).	Rare	3
Others:		
• Fever	Rare	3
• Fatigue, weakness.	Common	4

1- Life-threatening. Seek emergency treatment immediately.
2- Discontinue. Seek emergency treatment.
3- Discontinue. Call doctor right away.
4- Continue. Call doctor when convenient.
5- Continue. Tell doctor at next visit.

WARNINGS & PRECAUTIONS

Don't take if:

- You are allergic to any tricyclic antidepressant.
- You drink alcohol.
- You have had a heart attack within 6 weeks.
- You have glaucoma.
- You have taken MAO inhibitors within 2 weeks.
- Patient is younger than 12.

Before you start, consult your doctor:

- If you will have surgery within 2 months, including dental surgery, requiring general or spinal anesthesia.
- If you have an enlarged prostate.
- If you have heart disease or high blood pressure.
- If you have stomach or intestinal problems.
- If you have an overactive thyroid.
- If you have asthma.
- If you have liver disease.

Over age 60:
More likely to develop urination difficulty and side effects under *Brain & nervous system,* opposite.

Pregnancy:
Studies inconclusive on harm to unborn child. Animal studies show fetal abnormalities. Decide with your doctor whether drug benefits justify risk to unborn child.

Breast-feeding:
Drug passes into milk. Avoid drug or discontinue nursing until you finish medicine. Consult doctor on maintaining milk supply.

Infants & children:
Don't give to children younger than 12.

Prolonged use:
No problems expected.

Skin & sunlight:
May cause rash or intensify sunburn in areas exposed to sun or sunlamp.

Driving, piloting or hazardous work:
Don't drive or pilot aircraft until you learn how medicine affects you. Don't work around dangerous machinery. Don't climb ladders or work in high places. Danger increases if you drink alcohol or take medicine affecting alertness and reflexes.

Airplane passengers:
No problems expected.

Discontinuing:
Don't discontinue without consulting doctor. Dose may require gradual reduction if you have taken drug for a long time. Doses of other drugs may also require adjustment.

INTERACTION WITH OTHER DRUGS

GENERIC NAME OR DRUG CLASS	COMBINED EFFECT
Anticoagulants (oral)	Increased anticoagulant effect.
Anticholinergics	Increased sedation.
Antihistamines	Increased antihistamine effect.
Barbiturates	Decreased antidepressant effect.
Clonidine	Decreased clonidine effect.
Diuretics (thiazide)	Increased trimipramine effect.
Ethchlorvynol	Delirium
Guanethidine	Decreased guanethidine effect.
MAO inhibitors	Fever, delirium, convulsions.
Methyldopa	Decreased methyldopa effect.
Narcotics	Dangerous oversedation.
Phenytoin	Decreased phenytoin effect.
Quinidine	Irregular heartbeat.
Sedatives	Dangerous oversedation.
Sympathomimetics	Increased sympathomimetic effect.
Thyroid hormones	Irregular heartbeat.

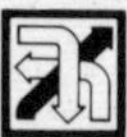

INTERACTION WITH OTHER SUBSTANCES

INTERACTS WITH	COMBINED EFFECT
Alcohol: Beverages or medicines with alcohol.	Excessive intoxication. Avoid.
Beverages:	None expected.
Cocaine:	Excessive intoxication. Avoid.
Foods:	None expected.
Marijuana:	Excessive drowsiness. Avoid.
Tobacco:	None expected.

TRIPELENNAMINE

BRAND NAMES

PBZ
PBZ-SR
Pyribenzamine
Ro-Hist

GENERAL INFORMATION

Habit forming? No
Prescription needed? High strength: Yes
Low strength: No
Available as generic? Yes
Drug class: Antihistamine

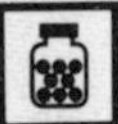

USES

- Reduces allergic symptoms such as hay fever, hives, rash or itching.
- Induces sleep.

DOSAGE & USAGE INFORMATION

How to take:
- Tablet or liquid—Swallow with liquid or food to lessen stomach irritation.
- Extended-release tablets—Swallow each dose whole.

When to take:
Varies with form. Follow label directions.

If you forget a dose:
Take as soon as you remember up to 2 hours late. If more than 2 hours, wait for next scheduled dose (don't double this dose).

What drug does:
Blocks action of histamine after an allergic response triggers histamine release in sensitive cells.

Time lapse before drug works:
30 minutes.

Don't take with:
See Interaction column and consult doctor.

OVERDOSE

Symptoms:
Convulsions, red face, hallucinations, coma.

What to do:
- Dial 0 (operator) or 911 (emergency) for an ambulance or medical help. Then give first aid immediately.
- If patient is unconscious and not breathing, give mouth-to-mouth breathing. If there is no heartbeat, use cardiac massage and mouth-to-mouth breathing (CPR). Don't try to make patient vomit. If you can't get help quickly, take patient to nearest emergency facility.
- Additional emergency information on page 886.

POSSIBLE ADVERSE REACTIONS OR SIDE EFFECTS

SYMPTOMS	FREQUENCY	WHAT TO DO
Brain & nervous system:		
• Nightmares, agitation, irritability.	Rare	3
• Drowsiness, dizziness.	Common	5
Skin:	None expected.	
Eyes:		
• Vision changes.	Infrequent	3
• Less tolerance for contact lenses.	Infrequent	4
Ears, nose, throat:		
• Sore throat, fever.	Rare	3
• Dry mouth, nose, throat.	Common	5
Digestive:		
• Nausea	Common	5
• Appetite loss.	Infrequent	5
Heart & lungs:		
Rapid heartbeat.	Rare	3
Blood vessels:		
Unusual bleeding or bruising.	Rare	3
Muscles, bones, joints, kidneys, liver, allergic, blood:	None expected.	
Genital, urinary:		
Urination difficulty.	Infrequent	4
Others:		
Fatigue, weakness.	Rare	3

1- Life-threatening. Seek emergency treatment immediately.
2- Discontinue. Seek emergency treatment.
3- Discontinue. Call doctor right away.
4- Continue. Call doctor when convenient.
5- Continue. Tell doctor at next visit.
6- No action necessary.

WARNINGS & PRECAUTIONS

Don't take if:
You are allergic to any antihistamine.

Before you start, consult your doctor:
- If you have glaucoma.
- If you have enlarged prostate.
- If you have asthma.
- If you have kidney disease.
- If you have peptic ulcer.
- If you will have surgery within 2 months, including dental surgery, requiring general or spinal anesthesia.

Over age 60:
Don't exceed recommended dose. Adverse reactions and side effects may be more frequent and severe than in younger persons, especially urination difficulty, diminished alertness and other brain and nervous-system symptoms.

Pregnancy:
No proven harm to unborn child. Avoid if possible.

Breast-feeding:
Drug passes into milk. Avoid drug or discontinue nursing until you finish medicine. Consult doctor for advice on maintaining milk supply.

Infants & children:
Not recommended for premature or newborn infants. Otherwise, no problems expected.

Prolonged use:
Avoid. May damage bone marrow and nerve cells.

Skin & sunlight:
May cause rash or intensify sunburn in areas exposed to sun or sunlamp.

Driving, piloting or hazardous work:
Don't drive or pilot aircraft until you learn how medicine affects you. Don't work around dangerous machinery. Don't climb ladders or work in high places. Danger increases if you drink alcohol or take medicine affecting alertness and reflexes, such as antihistamines, tranquilizers, sedatives, pain medicine, narcotics and mind-altering drugs.

Airplane passengers:
No problems expected.

Discontinuing:
No problems expected.

Others:
May mask symptoms of hearing damage from aspirin, other salicylates, cisplatin, paromomycin, vancomycin or anticonvulsants. Consult doctor if you use these.

INTERACTION WITH OTHER DRUGS

GENERIC NAME OR DRUG CLASS	COMBINED EFFECT
Anticholinergics	Increased anticholinergic effect.
Antidepressants	Excess sedation. Avoid.
Antihistamines (other)	Excess sedation. Avoid.
Hypnotics	Excess sedation. Avoid.
MAO inhibitors	Increased tripelennamine effect.
Mind-altering drugs	Excess sedation. Avoid.
Narcotics	Excess sedation. Avoid.
Sedatives	Excess sedation. Avoid.
Sleep inducers	Excess sedation. Avoid.
Tranquilizers	Excess sedation. Avoid.

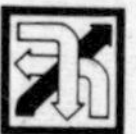

INTERACTION WITH OTHER SUBSTANCES

INTERACTS WITH	COMBINED EFFECT
Alcohol:	Excess sedation. Avoid.
Beverages: Caffeine drinks	Less tripelennamine sedation.
Cocaine:	Decreased tripelennamine effect. Avoid.
Foods:	None expected.
Marijuana:	Excess sedation. Avoid.
Tobacco:	None expected.

TRIPROLIDINE

BRAND NAMES

Actidil
Actifed
Eldafed
Triafed-C
Trifed
Tripodrine

GENERAL INFORMATION

Habit forming? No
Prescription needed? Yes
Available as generic? Yes
Drug class: Antihistamine

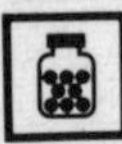

USES

- Reduces allergic symptoms such as hay fever, hives, rash or itching.
- Induces sleep.

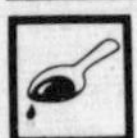

DOSAGE & USAGE INFORMATION

How to take:
Tablet or syrup—Swallow with liquid or food to lessen stomach irritation.

When to take:
Varies with form. Follow label directions.

If you forget a dose:
Take as soon as you remember up to 2 hours late. If more than 2 hours, wait for next scheduled dose (don't double this dose).

What drug does:
Blocks action of histamine after an allergic response triggers histamine release in sensitive cells.

Time lapse before drug works:
30 minutes.

Don't take with:
See Interaction column and consult doctor.

OVERDOSE

Symptoms:
Convulsions, red face, hallucinations, coma.

What to do:
- Dial 0 (operator) or 911 (emergency) for an ambulance or medical help. Then give first aid immediately.
- If patient is unconscious and not breathing, give mouth-to-mouth breathing. If there is no heartbeat, use cardiac massage and mouth-to-mouth breathing (CPR). Don't try to make patient vomit. If you can't get help quickly, take patient to nearest emergency facility.
- Additional emergency information on page 886.

POSSIBLE ADVERSE REACTIONS OR SIDE EFFECTS

SYMPTOMS	FREQUENCY	WHAT TO DO
Brain & nervous system:		
• Nightmares, agitation, irritability.	Rare	3
• Drowsiness, dizziness.	Common	5
Skin:	None expected.	
Eyes:		
• Vision changes.	Infrequent	3
• Less tolerance for contact lenses.	Infrequent	4
Ears, nose, throat:		
• Sore throat, fever.	Rare	3
• Dry mouth, nose, throat.	Common	5
Digestive:		
• Nausea	Common	5
• Appetite loss.	Infrequent	5
Heart & lungs: Rapid heartbeat.	Rare	3
Blood vessels: Unusual bleeding or bruising.	Rare	3
Muscles, bones, joints, kidneys, liver, allergic, blood:	None expected.	
Genital, urinary: Urination difficulty.	Infrequent	4
Others: Fatigue, weakness.	Rare	3

1- Life-threatening. Seek emergency treatment immediately.
2- Discontinue. Seek emergency treatment.
3- Discontinue. Call doctor right away.
4- Continue. Call doctor when convenient.
5- Continue. Tell doctor at next visit.
6- No action necessary.

WARNINGS & PRECAUTIONS

Don't take if:
You are allergic to any antihistamine.

Before you start, consult your doctor:
- If you have glaucoma.
- If you have enlarged prostate.
- If you have asthma.
- If you have kidney disease.
- If you have peptic ulcer.
- If you will have surgery within 2 months, including dental surgery, requiring general or spinal anesthesia.

Over age 60:
Don't exceed recommended dose. Adverse reactions and side effects may be more frequent and severe than in younger persons, especially urination difficulty, diminished alertness and other brain and nervous-system symptoms.

Pregnancy:
No proven harm to unborn child. Avoid if possible.

Breast-feeding:
Drug passes into milk. Avoid drug or discontinue nursing until you finish medicine. Consult doctor for advice on maintaining milk supply.

Infants & children:
Not recommended for premature or newborn infants. Otherwise, no problems expected.

Prolonged use:
Avoid. May damage bone marrow and nerve cells.

Skin & sunlight:
May cause rash or intensify sunburn in areas exposed to sun or sunlamp.

Driving, piloting or hazardous work:
Don't drive or pilot aircraft until you learn how medicine affects you. Don't work around dangerous machinery. Don't climb ladders or work in high places. Danger increases if you drink alcohol or take medicine affecting alertness and reflexes, such as antihistamines, tranquilizers, sedatives, pain medicine, narcotics and mind-altering drugs.

Airplane passengers:
No problems expected.

Discontinuing:
No problems expected.

Others:
May mask symptoms of hearing damage from aspirin, other salicylates, cisplatin, paromomycin, vancomycin or anticonvulsants. Consult doctor if you use these.

INTERACTION WITH OTHER DRUGS

GENERIC NAME OR DRUG CLASS	COMBINED EFFECT
Anticholinergics	Increased anticholinergic effect.
Antidepressants	Excess sedation. Avoid.
Antihistamines (other)	Excess sedation. Avoid.
Hypnotics	Excess sedation. Avoid.
MAO inhibitors	Increased triprolidine effect.
Mind-altering drugs	Excess sedation. Avoid.
Narcotics	Excess sedation. Avoid.
Sedatives	Excess sedation. Avoid.
Sleep inducers	Excess sedation. Avoid.
Tranquilizers	Excess sedation. Avoid.

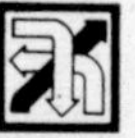

INTERACTION WITH OTHER SUBSTANCES

INTERACTS WITH	COMBINED EFFECT
Alcohol:	Excess sedation. Avoid.
Beverages: Caffeine drinks	Less triprolidine sedation.
Cocaine:	Decreased triprolidine effect. Avoid.
Foods:	None expected.
Marijuana:	Excess sedation. Avoid.
Tobacco:	None expected.

VALPROIC ACID (DIPROPYLACETIC ACID)

BRAND NAMES

Depakene
Depakote

GENERAL INFORMATION

Habit forming? No
Prescription needed? Yes
Available as generic? No
Drug class: Anticonvulsant

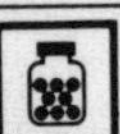

USES

Controls petit mal (absence) seizures in treatment of epilepsy.

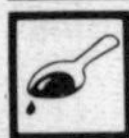

DOSAGE & USAGE INFORMATION

How to take:
Tablet or capsule—Swallow with liquid or food to lessen stomach irritation.

When to take:
Once a day.

If you forget a dose:
Take as soon as you remember. Don't ever double dose.

What drug does:
Increases concentration of gamma aminobutyric acid, which inhibits nerve transmission in parts of brain.

Time lapse before drug works:
1 to 4 hours.

Don't take with:
See Interaction column and consult doctor.

OVERDOSE

Symptoms:
Coma

What to do:

- Dial 0 (operator) or 911 (emergency) for an ambulance or medical help. Then give first aid immediately.
- If patient is unconscious and not breathing, give mouth-to-mouth breathing. If there is no heartbeat, use cardiac massage and mouth-to-mouth breathing (CPR). Don't try to make patient vomit. If you can't get help quickly, take patient to nearest emergency facility.
- Additional emergency information on page 886.

POSSIBLE ADVERSE REACTIONS OR SIDE EFFECTS

SYMPTOMS	FREQUENCY	WHAT TO DO
Brain & nervous system:		
Sleepy, weakness, easily upset emotionally, depression, psychic changes, headache, incoordination.	Infrequent	4
Skin:		
• Rash	Infrequent	3
• Bloody spots under skin.	Infrequent	3
• Hair loss.	Infrequent	3
Eyes:		
Double vision, unusual movements of eyes (nystagmus).	Rare	3
Ears, nose, throat:	None expected.	
Digestive:		
Nausea, vomiting, abdominal cramps, appetite change.	Infrequent	4
Heart & lungs:		
• Bleeding	Infrequent	3
• Easy bruising.	Infrequent	3
Blood vessels:	None expected.	
Muscles, bones, joints:	None expected.	
Genital, urinary:		
Irregular menstruation.	Common	4
Kidneys, allergic, blood, liver:	None expected.	
Others:		
Anemia	Rare	4

1-Life-threatening. Seek emergency treatment immediately.
2-Discontinue. Seek emergency treatment.
3-Discontinue. Call doctor right away.
4-Continue. Call doctor when convenient.
5-Continue. Tell doctor at next visit.
6-No action necessary.

VALPROIC ACID (DIPROPYLACETIC ACID)

WARNINGS & PRECAUTIONS

Don't take if:
You are allergic to valproic acid.

Before you start, consult your doctor:
- If you have blood, kidney or liver disease.
- If you will have surgery within 2 months, including dental surgery, requiring general or spinal anesthesia.

Over age 60:
Adverse reactions and side effects may be more frequent and severe than in younger persons.

Pregnancy:
No proven harm to unborn child. Avoid if possible.

Breast-feeding:
Unknown effect.

Infants & children:
Under close medical supervision only.

Prolonged use:
Request periodic blood tests, liver and kidney function tests.

Skin & sunlight:
No problems expected.

Driving, piloting or hazardous work:
Don't drive or pilot aircraft until you learn how medicine affects you. Don't work around dangerous machinery. Don't climb ladders or work in high places. Danger increases if you drink alcohol or take medicine affecting alertness and reflexes, such as antihistamines, tranquilizers, sedatives, pain medicine, narcotics and mind-altering drugs.

Airplane passengers:
No problems expected.

Discontinuing:
Don't discontinue without consulting doctor. Dose may require gradual reduction if you have taken drug for a long time. Doses of other drugs may also require adjustment.

INTERACTION WITH OTHER DRUGS

GENERIC NAME OR DRUG CLASS	COMBINED EFFECT
Central nervous system depressants: Antidepressants, Antihistamines, Narcotics, Sedatives, Sleeping pills, Tranquilizers. Other muscle relaxants	Increases sedative effect.
Anticoagulants	Increases chance of bleeding.
Aspirin	Increases chance of bleeding.
Dypiradamole	Increases chance of bleeding.
Sulfinpyrazone	Increases chance of bleeding.
Primidone	Increases chance of toxicity.
MAO inhibitors	Increases sedative effect.
Clonazepam	May prolong seizure.
Phenytoin	Unpredictable. May require increased or decreased dosage.

INTERACTION WITH OTHER SUBSTANCES

INTERACTS WITH	COMBINED EFFECT
Alcohol:	Deep sedation. Avoid.
Beverages:	No problems expected.
Cocaine:	Increased brain sensitivity. Avoid.
Foods:	No problems expected.
Marijuana:	Increased brain sensitivity. Avoid.
Tobacco:	Decreased valproic acid effect.

VERAPAMIL

BRAND NAMES

Calan
Isoptin

GENERAL INFORMATION

Habit forming? No
Prescription needed? Yes
Available as generic? No
Drug class: Calcium-channel blocker, antiarrhythmic, antianginal

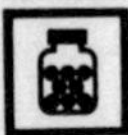

USES

- Prevents angina attacks.
- Stabilizes irregular heartbeat.

DOSAGE & USAGE INFORMATION

How to take:
Tablet—Swallow with liquid.

When to take:
At the same times each day 1 hour before or 2 hours after eating.

If you forget a dose:
Take as soon as you remember up to 2 hours late. If more than 2 hours, wait for next scheduled dose (don't double this dose).

What drug does:
- Reduces work that heart must perform.
- Reduces normal artery pressure.
- Increases oxygen to heart muscle.

Time lapse before drug works:
1 to 2 hours.

Don't take with:
See Interaction column and consult doctor.

OVERDOSE

Symptoms:
Unusually fast or unusually slow heartbeat, loss of consciousness, cardiac arrest.

What to do:
- Dial 0 (operator) or 911 (emergency) for an ambulance or medical help. Then give first aid immediately.
- If patient is unconscious and not breathing, give mouth-to-mouth breathing. If there is no heartbeat, use cardiac massage and mouth-to-mouth breathing (CPR). Don't try to make patient vomit. If you can't get help quickly, take patient to nearest emergency facility.
- Additional emergency information on page 886.

POSSIBLE ADVERSE REACTIONS OR SIDE EFFECTS

SYMPTOMS	FREQUENCY	WHAT TO DO
Brain & nervous system:		
• Dizziness	Infrequent	4
• Headache	Rare	5
• Fainting	Rare	3
Skin:	None expected.	
Eyes:	None expected.	
Ears, nose, throat:	None expected.	
Digestive:		
Nausea, constipation.	Infrequent	5
Heart & lungs:		
• Unusually fast or unusually slow heartbeat.	Infrequent	3
• Wheezing, cough, shortness of breath.	Infrequent	3
Blood vessels:	None expected.	
Muscles, bones, joints:		
• Numbness, tingling in hands and feet.	Infrequent	4
• Swelling of ankles, feet, legs.	Infrequent	4
Genital, urinary:		
Difficult urination.	Infrequent	4
Kidneys:	None expected.	
Liver:	None expected.	
Allergic:	None expected.	
Blood:	None expected.	
Others:		
Tiredness	Common	5

1-Life-threatening. Seek emergency treatment immediately.
2-Discontinue. Seek emergency treatment.
3-Discontinue. Call doctor right away.
4-Continue. Call doctor when convenient.
5-Continue. Tell doctor at next visit.
6-No action necessary.

WARNINGS & PRECAUTIONS

Don't take if:
- You are allergic to verapamil.
- You have very low blood pressure.

Before you start, consult your doctor:
- If you have kidney or liver disease.
- If you have high blood pressure.
- If you have heart disease other than coronary-artery disease.

Over age 60:
Adverse reactions and side effects may be more frequent and severe than in younger persons.

Pregnancy:
No proven harm to unborn child. Avoid if possible.

Breast-feeding:
Safety not established. Avoid if possible.

Infants & children:
Not recommended.

Prolonged use:
No problems expected.

Skin & sunlight:
No problems expected.

Driving, piloting or hazardous work:
Avoid if you feel dizzy. Otherwise, no problems expected.

Airplane passengers:
No problems expected.

Discontinuing:
Don't discontinue without doctor's advice until you complete prescribed dose, even though symptoms diminish or disappear.

Others:
Learn to check your own pulse rate. If it drops to 50 beats per minute or lower, don't take verapamil until your consult your doctor.

INTERACTION WITH OTHER DRUGS

GENERIC NAME OR DRUG CLASS	COMBINED EFFECT
Anticoagulants (oral)	Increased anticoagulant effect.
Anticonvulsants (hydantoin)	Increased anticonvulsant effect.
Antihypertensives	Dangerous blood-pressure drop.
Beta-adrenergic blockers	Possible irregular heartbeat.
Calcium (large doses)	Decreased verapamil effect.
Diuretics	Dangerous blood-pressure drop.
Digitalis preparations	Increased digitalis effect. May need to reduce dose.
Disopyramide	May cause dangerously slow, fast or irregular heartbeat.
Nitrates	Reduced angina attacks.
Quinidine	Increased quinidine effect.
Vitamin D (large doses)	Decreased verapamil effect.

INTERACTION WITH OTHER SUBSTANCES

INTERACTS WITH	COMBINED EFFECT
Alcohol:	Dangerously low blood pressure. Avoid.
Beverages:	None expected.
Cocaine:	Possible irregular heartbeat. Avoid.
Foods:	None expected.
Marijuana:	Possible irregular heartbeat. Avoid.
Tobacco:	Possible rapid heartbeat. Avoid.

VITAMIN A

BRAND NAMES

Acon
Afaxin
Alphalin
Aquasol A
Dispatabs
Sust-A
Numerous multiple vitamin-mineral supplements.

GENERAL INFORMATION

Habit forming? No
Prescription needed? No
Available as generic? Yes
Drug class: Vitamin supplement

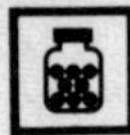

USES

Dietary supplement to ensure normal growth and health, especially eyes and skin.

DOSAGE & USAGE INFORMATION

How to take:
Tablet or capsule—Swallow with liquid. If you can't swallow whole, crumble tablet or open capsule and take with liquid or food.

When to take:
At the same time each day.

If you forget a dose:
Take as soon as you remember. Resume regular schedule.

What drug does:
- Prevents night blindness.
- Promotes normal growth and health.

Time lapse before drug works:
Requires continual intake.

Don't take with:
See Interaction column and consult doctor.

OVERDOSE

Symptoms:
Increased adverse reactions and side effects. Jaundice (yellow eyes and skin) rare, but may occur with large doses.

What to do:
Overdose unlikely to threaten life. If person takes much larger amount than prescribed, call doctor, poison-control center or hospital emergency room for instructions.

POSSIBLE ADVERSE REACTIONS OR SIDE EFFECTS

SYMPTOMS	FREQUENCY	WHAT TO DO
Brain & nervous system:		
• Bulging soft spot on baby's head.	Rare	3
• Confusion, dizziness, drowsiness, headache, irritability.	Infrequent	4
Skin:		
Dry lips, peeling skin, hair loss.	Infrequent	4
Eyes:		
Double vision.	Rare	3
Ears, nose, throat:	None expected.	
Digestive:		
Diarrhea, appetite loss, nausea, vomiting.	Rare	4
Heart & lungs:	None expected.	
Blood vessels:	None expected.	
Muscles, bones, joints:	None expected.	
Genital, urinary:	None expected.	
Kidneys:	None expected.	
Liver:	None expected.	
Allergic:	None expected.	
Blood:	None expected.	
Others:	None expected.	

1- Life-threatening. Seek emergency treatment immediately.
2- Discontinue. Seek emergency treatment.
3- Discontinue. Call doctor right away.
4- Continue. Call doctor when convenient.
5- Continue. Tell doctor at next visit.
6- No action necessary.

WARNINGS & PRECAUTIONS

Don't take if:
You have chronic kidney failure.

Before you start, consult your doctor:
If you have any kidney disorder.

Over age 60:
No problems expected.

Pregnancy:
Don't take more than 6,000 units daily.

Breast-feeding:
No problems expected.

Infants & children:
- Avoid large doses.
- Keep vitamin-mineral supplements out of children's reach.

Prolonged use:
No problems expected.

Skin & sunlight:
No problems expected.

Driving, piloting or hazardous work:
No problems expected.

Airplane passengers:
No problems expected.

Discontinuing:
Don't discontinue without doctor's advice until you complete prescribed dose, even though symptoms diminish or disappear.

Others:
- Don't exceed dose. Too much over a long time may be harmful.
- A balanced diet should provide all the vitamin A a healthy person needs and prevent need for supplements. Best sources are liver, yellow-orange fruits and vegetables, dark-green, leafy vegetables, milk, butter and margarine.

INTERACTION WITH OTHER DRUGS

GENERIC NAME OR DRUG CLASS	COMBINED EFFECT
Cholestyramine	Decreased vitamin A absorption.
Mineral oil (long term)	Decreased vitamin A absorption.
Vitamin E (excess dose)	Vitamin A depletion.

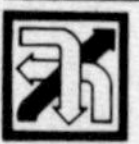

INTERACTION WITH OTHER SUBSTANCES

INTERACTS WITH	COMBINED EFFECT
Alcohol:	None expected.
Beverages:	None expected.
Cocaine:	None expected.
Foods:	None expected.
Marijuana:	None expected.
Tobacco:	None expected.

VITAMIN B-12 (CYANOCOBALAMIN)

BRAND NAMES

Alphamin
Alpha Redisol
Anocobin
Betalin 12
Betalin 12 Crystalline
Kaybovite
Neo-Betalin
Neo-Rubex
Redisol
Rubramin
Rubramin-PC
Sytobex

Numerous other multiple vitamin-mineral supplements.

GENERAL INFORMATION

Habit forming? No
Prescription needed? No
Available as generic? Yes
Drug class: Vitamin supplement

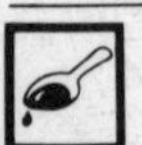

USES

- Dietary supplement for normal growth, development and health.
- Treatment for nerve damage.
- Treatment for pernicious anemia.
- Treatment and prevention of vitamin B-12 deficiencies in people who have had stomach or intestines surgically removed.
- Prevention of vitamin B-12 deficiency in strict vegetarians and persons with absorption diseases.

DOSAGE & USAGE INFORMATION

How to take:
- Tablets—Swallow with liquid.
- Injection—Follow doctor's directions.

When to take:
- Oral—At the same time each day.
- Injection—Follow doctor's directions.

If you forget a dose:
Take when remembered. Don't double next dose. Resume regular schedule.

What drug does:
Acts as enzyme to promote normal fat and carbohydrate metabolism and protein synthesis.

Time lapse before drug works:
15 minutes.

Don't take with:
See Interaction column and consult doctor.

OVERDOSE

Symptoms:
Increased adverse reactions and side effects.

What to do:
Overdose unlikely to threaten life. If person takes much larger amount than prescribed, call doctor, poison-control center or hospital emergency room for instructions.

POSSIBLE ADVERSE REACTIONS OR SIDE EFFECTS

SYMPTOMS	FREQUENCY	WHAT TO DO
Brain & nervous system:	None expected.	
Skin:		
Itching	Rare	3
Eyes:	None expected.	
Ears, nose, throat:	None expected.	
Digestive:		
Diarrhea	Rare	4
Heart & lungs:		
Wheezing	Rare	3
Blood vessels:	None expected.	
Muscles, bones, joints:	None expected.	
Genital, urinary:	None expected.	
Kidneys:	None expected.	
Liver:	None expected.	
Allergic:		
Life-threatening anaphylaxis may occur after injection.	Rare	1 See Page 888.
Blood:	None expected.	
Others:	None expected.	

1- Life-threatening. Seek emergency treatment immediately.
2- Discontinue. Seek emergency treatment.
3- Discontinue. Call doctor right away.
4- Continue. Call doctor when convenient.
5- Continue. Tell doctor at next visit.
6- No action necessary.

VITAMIN B-12 (CYANOCOBALAMIN)

WARNINGS & PRECAUTIONS

Don't take if:
You have Leber's disease (optic nerve atrophy).

Before you start, consult your doctor:
- If you have gout.
- If you have heart disease.

Over age 60:
No problems expected.

Pregnancy:
No problems expected.

Breast-feeding:
No problems expected.

Infants & children:
No problems expected.

Prolonged use:
No problems expected.

Skin & sunlight:
No problems expected.

Driving, piloting or hazardous work:
No problems expected.

Airplane passengers:
No problems expected.

Discontinuing:
Don't discontinue without doctor's advice until you complete prescribed dose, even though symptoms diminish or disappear.

Others:
- A balanced diet should provide all the vitamin B-12 a healthy person needs and make supplements unnecessary. Best sources are meat, fish, egg yolk and cheese.
- Tablets should be used only for diet supplements. All other uses of vitamin B-12 require injections.

INTERACTION WITH OTHER DRUGS

GENERIC NAME OR DRUG CLASS	COMBINED EFFECT
Anticonvulsants	Decreased absorption of vitamin B-12.
Aspirin	Decreased absorption of vitamin B-12.
Vitamin C (ascorbic acid)	Destroys vitamin B-12 if taken at same time. Take 2 hours apart.
Chloramphenicol	Decreased vitamin B-12 effect.
Colchicine	Decreased absorption of vitamin B-12.
Neomycin	Decreased absorption of vitamin B-12.
Potassium (extended-release forms)	Decreased absorption of vitamin B-12.

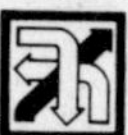

INTERACTION WITH OTHER SUBSTANCES

INTERACTS WITH	COMBINED EFFECT
Alcohol:	Decreased absorption of vitamin B-12.
Beverages:	None expected.
Cocaine:	None expected.
Foods:	None expected.
Marijuana:	None expected.
Tobacco:	None expected.

VITAMIN C (ASCORBIC ACID)

BRAND NAMES

Adenex	Cecon	Cevi-Bid	Megascorb
Arco-Cee	Cemill	Ce-Vi-Sol	Redoxon
Ascorbajen	Cenolate	Cevita	
Ascorbicap	Ceri-Bid	C-Ject	
Ascoril	Cetane	Flavorcee	
Calscorbate	Cevalin	Liqui-Cee	

Numerous other multiple vitamin-mineral supplements.

GENERAL INFORMATION

Habit forming? No
Prescription needed? No
Available as generic? Yes
Drug class: Vitamin supplement

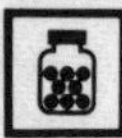

USES

- Prevention and treatment of scurvy and other vitamin-C deficiencies.
- Treatment of anemia.
- Maintenance of acid urine.

DOSAGE & USAGE INFORMATION

How to take:
- Tablets, capsules, liquid—Swallow with 8 oz. water.
- Extended-release tablets—Swallow whole.
- Drops—Squirt directly into mouth or mix with liquid or food.

When to take:
1, 2 or 3 times per day, as prescribed on label.

If you forget a dose:
Take as soon as you remember. Return to regular schedule.

What drug does:
- May help form collagen.
- Increases iron absorption from intestine.
- Contributes to hemoglobin and red-blood-cell production in bone marrow.

Time lapse before drug works:
1 week.

Don't take with:
See Interaction column and consult doctor.

OVERDOSE

Symptoms:
Diarrhea, vomiting, dizziness.

What to do:
Overdose unlikely to threaten life. If person takes much larger amount than prescribed, call doctor, poison-control center or hospital emergency room for instructions.

POSSIBLE ADVERSE REACTIONS OR SIDE EFFECTS

SYMPTOMS	FREQUENCY	WHAT TO DO
Brain & nervous system: Headache	Rare	5
Skin: Flushed face.	Infrequent	4
Eyes:	None expected.	
Ears, nose, throat:	None expected.	
Digestive: Mild diarrhea, nausea, vomiting.	Infrequent	3
Heart & lungs:	None expected.	
Blood vessels:	None expected.	
Muscles, bones, joints:	None expected.	
Genital, urinary:	None expected.	
Kidneys: Severe pain in lower abdomen (kidney stones).	Infrequent	3
Liver:	None expected.	
Allergic:	None expected.	
Blood: Anemia	Rare	3
Others:	None expected.	

1 - Life-threatening. Seek emergency treatment immediately.
2 - Discontinue. Seek emergency treatment.
3 - Discontinue. Call doctor right away.
4 - Continue. Call doctor when convenient.
5 - Continue. Tell doctor at next visit.
6 - No action necessary.

VITAMIN C (ASCORBIC ACID)

WARNINGS & PRECAUTIONS

Don't take if:
You are allergic to vitamin C.

Before you start, consult your doctor:
- If you have sickle-cell or other anemia.
- If you have had kidney stones.
- If you have gout.

Over age 60:
For daily doses of 1,000 mg. or more, drink at least 2 quarts of water daily.

Pregnancy:
No proven harm to unborn child. Avoid large doses.

Breast-feeding:
Avoid large doses.

Infants & children:
- Avoid large doses.
- Keep vitamin-mineral supplements out of children's reach.

Prolonged use:
Large doses for longer than 2 months may cause kidney stones.

Skin & sunlight:
No problems expected.

Driving, piloting or hazardous work:
No problems expected.

Airplane passengers:
No problems expected.

Discontinuing:
No problems expected.

Others:
- Store in cool, dry place.
- May cause inaccurate tests for sugar in urine or blood in stool.
- May cause crisis in patients with sickle-cell anemia.
- A balanced diet should provide all the vitamin C a healthy person needs and make supplements unnecessary. Best sources are citrus, strawberries, cantaloupe and raw peppers.

INTERACTION WITH OTHER DRUGS

GENERIC NAME OR DRUG CLASS	COMBINED EFFECT
Anticoagulants (oral)	Decreased anticoagulant effect.
Aspirin	Decreased vitamin C effect.
Anticholinergics	Decreased anticholinergic effect.
Barbiturates	Decreased vitamin C effect. Increased barbiturate effect.
Contraceptives (oral)	Decreased vitamin C effect.
Mineral oil	Decreased vitamin C effect.
Iron supplements	Increased iron effect.
Quinidine	Decreased quinidine effect.
Salicylates	Decreased vitamin C effect.
Sulfa drugs	Decreased vitamin C effect. Possible kidney stones.
Tetracyclines	Decreased vitamin C effect.

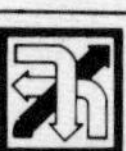

INTERACTION WITH OTHER SUBSTANCES

INTERACTS WITH	COMBINED EFFECT
Alcohol:	None expected.
Beverages:	None expected.
Cocaine:	None expected.
Foods:	None expected.
Marijuana:	None expected.
Tobacco:	Increased requirement for vitamin C.

VITAMIN D

BRAND NAMES

Calciferol
Calcifidiol
Calderol
Calcitriol
Deltalin
Dihydrotachysterol
Drisdol
Ergocalciferol
Hykaterol
Ostoforte
Radiostol
Radiostol Forte
Rocaltrol

Numerous other multiple vitamin-mineral supplements.

GENERAL INFORMATION

Habit forming? No
Prescription needed? Low strength: No
High strength: Yes
Available as generic? Yes
Drug class: Vitamin supplement

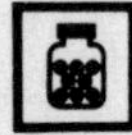

USES

- Dietary supplement.
- Prevention of rickets (bone disease).
- Treatment for hypocalcemia (low blood calcium) in kidney disease.
- Treatment for postoperative muscle contractions.

DOSAGE & USAGE INFORMATION

How to take:
- Tablet or capsule—Swallow with liquid.
- Drops—Dilute dose in beverage.

When to take:
As directed, usually once a day at the same time each day.

If you forget a dose:
Take up to 12 hours late. If more than 12 hours, wait for next dose (don't double this).

What drug does:
Maintains growth and health. Prevents rickets. Essential so body can use calcium and phosphate.

Time lapse before drug works:
2 hours. May require 2 to 3 weeks of continual use for maximum effect.

Don't take with:
Non-prescription drugs or drugs in Interaction column without consulting doctor.

OVERDOSE

Symptoms:
Severe stomach pain, nausea, vomiting, weight loss; bone and muscle pain; increased urination, cloudy urine; mood or mental changes (possible psychosis); high blood pressure, irregular heartbeat; eye irritation or light sensitivity; itchy skin.

What to do:
Overdose unlikely to threaten life. If person takes much larger amount than prescribed, call doctor, poison-control center or hospital emergency room for instructions.

POSSIBLE ADVERSE REACTIONS OR SIDE EFFECTS

SYMPTOMS	FREQUENCY	WHAT TO DO
Brain & nervous system: Headache	Infrequent	4
Skin:	None expected.	
Eyes:	None expected.	
Ears, nose, throat: Metallic taste in mouth, thirst, dry mouth.	Infrequent	4
Digestive: Constipation, appetite loss, nausea, vomiting.	Infrequent	4
Heart & lungs:	None expected.	
Blood vessels:	None expected.	
Muscles, bones, joints:	None expected.	
Genital, urinary:	None expected.	
Kidneys:	None expected.	
Liver:	None expected.	
Allergic:	None expected.	
Blood:	None expected.	
Others:	None expected.	

1- Life-threatening. Seek emergency treatment immediately.
2- Discontinue. Seek emergency treatment.
3- Discontinue. Call doctor right away.
4- Continue. Call doctor when convenient.
5- Continue. Tell doctor at next visit.
6- No action necessary.

WARNINGS & PRECAUTIONS

Don't take if:
You are allergic to medicine containing vitamin D.

Before you start, consult your doctor:
- If you plan to become pregnant while taking vitamin D.
- If you have epilepsy.
- If you have heart or blood-vessel disease.
- If you have kidney disease.

Over age 60:
Adverse reactions and side effects may be more frequent and severe than in younger persons.

Pregnancy:
Risk to unborn child outweighs drug benefits. Don't use.

Breast-feeding:
No problems expected, but consult doctor.

Infants & children:
- Avoid large doses.
- Keep vitamins out of children's reach.

Prolonged use:
No problems expected.

Skin & sunlight:
No problems expected.

Driving, piloting or hazardous work:
No problems expected.

Airplane passengers:
No problems expected.

Discontinuing:
Don't discontinue without doctor's advice until you complete prescribed dose, even though symptoms diminish or disappear.

Others:
- Don't exceed dose. Too much over a long time may be harmful.
- A balanced diet should provide all the vitamin D a healthy person needs and make supplements unnecessary. Best sources are fish and vitamin-D fortified milk and bread.

INTERACTION WITH OTHER DRUGS

GENERIC NAME OR DRUG CLASS	COMBINED EFFECT
Antacids (magnesium-containing)	Possible excess magnesium.
Anticonvulsants (hydantoin)	Decreased vitamin D effect.
Calcium (high doses)	Excess calcium in blood.
Calcium-channel blockers	Decreased effect of calcium-channel blockers.
Cholestyramine	Decreased vitamin D effect.
Digitalis preparations	Heartbeat irregularities.
Mineral oil	Decreased vitamin D effect.
Phenobarbital	Decreased vitamin D effect.
Phosphorous preparations	Accumulation of excess phosporous.
Vitamin D (other)	Possible toxicity.

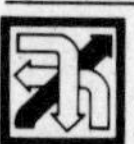

INTERACTION WITH OTHER SUBSTANCES

INTERACTS WITH	COMBINED EFFECT
Alcohol:	None expected.
Beverages:	None expected.
Cocaine:	None expected.
Foods:	None expected.
Marijuana:	None expected.
Tobacco:	None expected.

VITAMIN E

BRAND NAMES

Aquasol E
Chew-E
Daltose
Eferol
Eprolin
Pheryl-E
Numerous other multiple vitamin-mineral supplements.

GENERAL INFORMATION

Habit forming? No
Prescription needed? No
Available as generic? Yes
Drug class: Vitamin supplement

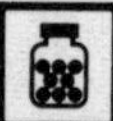

USES

- Dietary supplement to promote normal growth, development and health.
- Treatment and prevention of vitamin-E deficiency, especially in premature or low birth-weight infants.
- Treatment for fibrocystic disease of the breast.
- Treatment for circulatory problems to the lower extremities.
- Treatment for sickle-cell anemia.
- Treatment for lung toxicity from air pollution.

DOSAGE & USAGE INFORMATION

How to take:
- Tablet, capsule or chewable tablets—Swallow with liquid or food to lessen stomach irritation.
- Drops—Dilute dose in beverage before swallowing or squirt directly into mouth.

When to take:
At the same times each day.

If you forget a dose:
Take when you remember. Don't double next dose.

What drug does:
- Promotes normal growth and development.
- Prevents oxidation in body.

Time lapse before drug works:
Not determined.

Don't take with:
See Interaction column and consult doctor.

OVERDOSE

Symptoms:
Nausea, vomiting.

What to do:
Overdose unlikely to threaten life. If person takes much larger amount than prescribed, call doctor, poison-control center or hospital emergency room for instructions.

POSSIBLE ADVERSE REACTIONS OR SIDE EFFECTS

SYMPTOMS	FREQUENCY	WHAT TO DO
Brain & nervous system:	None expected.	
Skin:	None expected.	
Eyes:	None expected.	
Ears, nose, throat:	None expected.	
Digestive: Nausea, stomach pain.	Infrequent	4
Heart & lungs:	None expected.	
Blood vessels:	None expected.	
Muscles, bones, joints: Muscle aches, pain in lower legs.	Infrequent	4
Genital, urinary:	None expected.	
Kidneys:	None expected.	
Liver:	None expected.	
Allergic:	None expected.	
Blood:	None expected.	
Others: Fever, tiredness, weakness.	Infrequent	4

1-Life-threatening. Seek emergency treatment immediately.
2-Discontinue. Seek emergency treatment.
3-Discontinue. Call doctor right away.
4-Continue. Call doctor when convenient.
5-Continue. Tell doctor at next visit.
6-No action necessary.

WARNINGS & PRECAUTIONS

Don't take if:
You are allergic to vitamin E.

Before you start, consult your doctor:
- If you have had blood clots in leg veins (thrombophlebitis).
- If you have liver disease.

Over age 60:
No problems expected. Avoid excessive doses.

Pregnancy:
No problems expected with normal daily requirements. Don't exceed prescribed dose.

Breast-feeding:
No problems expected.

Infants & children:
Use only under medical supervision.

Prolonged use:
Toxic accumulation of vitamin E. Don't exceed recommended dose.

Skin & sunlight:
No problems expected.

Driving, piloting or hazardous work:
No problems expected.

Airplane passengers:
No problems expected.

Discontinuing:
No problems expected.

Others:
A balanced diet should provide all the vitamin E a healthy person needs and make supplements unnecessary. Best sources are vegetable oils, whole-grain cereals, liver.

INTERACTION WITH OTHER DRUGS

GENERIC NAME OR DRUG CLASS	COMBINED EFFECT
Iron supplements	Decreased effect of iron supplement in patients with iron-deficiency anemia. Decreased vitamin E effect in healthy persons.
Vitamin A	Recommended dose of vitamin E—Increased benefit and decreased toxicity of vitamin A. Excess dose of vitamin E—Vitamin A depletion.

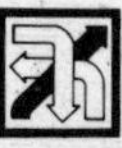

INTERACTION WITH OTHER SUBSTANCES

INTERACTS WITH	COMBINED EFFECT
Alcohol:	None expected.
Beverages:	None expected.
Cocaine:	None expected.
Foods:	None expected.
Marijuana:	None expected.
Tobacco:	None expected.

VITAMIN K

BRAND NAMES

AquaMEPHYTON
Kappadione
Konakion
Mephyton
Menadione
Menadiol
Phytonadione
Synkayvite

GENERAL INFORMATION

Habit forming? No
Prescription needed? No
Available as generic? Yes
Drug class: Vitamin supplement

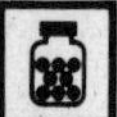

USES

- Dietary supplement.
- Treatment for bleeding disorders and malabsorption diseases due to vitamin K deficiency.
- Treatment for hemorrhagic disease of the newborn.
- Treatment for bleeding due to overdose of oral anticoagulants.

DOSAGE & USAGE INFORMATION

How to take:
Tablet—Swallow with liquid. If you can't swallow whole, crumble tablet or open capsule and take with liquid or food.

When to take:
At the same time each day.

If you forget a dose:
Take as soon as you remember up to 12 hours late. If more than 12 hours, wait for next scheduled dose (don't double this dose).

What drug does:
- Promotes growth, development and good health.
- Supplies a necessary ingredient for blood clotting.

Time lapse before drug works:
15 to 30 minutes to support blood clotting.

Don't take with:
See Interaction column and consult doctor.

OVERDOSE

Symptoms:
Nausea, vomiting.

What to do:
Overdose unlikely to threaten life. If person takes much larger amount than prescribed, call doctor, poison-control center or hospital emergency room for instructions.

POSSIBLE ADVERSE REACTIONS OR SIDE EFFECTS

SYMPTOMS	FREQUENCY	WHAT TO DO
Brain & nervous system:	None expected.	
Skin:	None expected.	
Eyes:	None expected.	
Ears, nose, throat:		
Unusual taste.	Infrequent	4
Digestive:	None expected.	
Heart & lungs:	None expected.	
Blood vessels:	None expected.	
Muscles, bones, joints:	None expected.	
Genital, urinary:	None expected.	
Kidneys:	None expected.	
Liver:	None expected.	
Allergic:	None expected.	
Blood:	None expected.	
Others:	None expected.	

1-Life-threatening. Seek emergency treatment immediately.
2-Discontinue. Seek emergency treatment.
3-Discontinue. Call doctor right away.
4-Continue. Call doctor when convenient.
5-Continue. Tell doctor at next visit.
6-No action necessary.

WARNINGS & PRECAUTIONS

Don't take if:
- You are allergic to vitamin K.
- You have G6PD deficiency.
- You have liver disease.

Before you start, consult your doctor:
If you are pregnant.

Over age 60:
No problems expected.

Pregnancy:
Don't exceed dose.

Breast-feeding:
No problems expected.

Infants & children:
Phytonadione is the preferred form for hemorrhagic disease of the newborn.

Prolonged use:
No problems expected.

Skin & sunlight:
No problems expected.

Driving, piloting or hazardous work:
No problems expected.

Airplane passengers:
No problems expected.

Discontinuing:
No problems expected.

Others:
- Tell all doctors and dentists you consult that you take this medicine.
- Don't exceed dose. Too much over a long time may be harmful.
- A balanced diet should provide all the vitamin K a healthy person needs and make supplements unnecessary. Best sources are green, leafy vegetables, meat or dairy products.

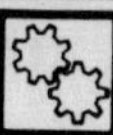

INTERACTION WITH OTHER DRUGS

GENERIC NAME OR DRUG CLASS	COMBINED EFFECT
Anticoagulants (oral)	Decreased anticoagulant effect.
Cholestyramine	Decreased vitamin K effect.
Mineral oil (long term)	Vitamin K deficiency.
Sulfa drugs	Vitamin K deficiency.

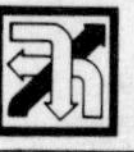

INTERACTION WITH OTHER SUBSTANCES

INTERACTS WITH	COMBINED EFFECT
Alcohol:	None expected.
Beverages:	None expected.
Cocaine:	None expected.
Foods:	None expected.
Marijuana:	None expected.
Tobacco:	None expected.

Additional Brand and Generic Names

The following drugs are alphabetized by generic name or drug class, shown in large capital letters. The brand and generic names that follow each title in this list are a more complete list than appears on the drug charts. Generic names are always capitalized in the lists.

ACETAMINOPHEN

A'Cenol
APAP
Aceta
Aceta w/Codeine
Acetaco
Acetaminophen w/Codeine
Actamin
Algisin
Amacodone
Amaphen
Amphenol
Anacin-3
Anapap
Anaphen
Anoquan
Anuphen
Apamide Tablets
Apo-Acetaminophen
Arthralgen
Atasol
Axotal
Bancap w/Codeine
Banesin Forte
Bayapap
Bromo-Seltzer
Campain
Capital
Capital w/Codeine
Chlorzone Forte
Coastaldyne
Coastalgesic
Codalan
Codap
Co-Gesic
Colrex
Compal
Comtrex
Conacetol
Congespirin
Co-Tylenol
Covangesic
D-Sinus
Dapa
Dapase
Darvocet-N
Datril
Dia-Gesic
Dialog
Dolacet
Dolanex
Dolene AP-65
Dolor
Dolprin
Dorcol
Dristan
Duadacin
Dularin
Duradyne DHC
Dynosal
Empracet w/Codeine
Endecon
Esgic
Excedrin
Exdol
Febrigesic
Febrinol
Febrogesic
Fendol
G-1
G-2
G-3
Gaysal
Guaiamine
Halenol
Hasacode
Hi-Temp
Hyco-Pap
Hycomine Compound
Korigesic
Liquiprin
Liquix-C
Lorcet
Lyteca
Metrogesic
Midol PMS
Midrin
Migralam
Minotal
NAPAP
Naldegesic
Nebs
Neopap
Oraphen-PD
Ornex
Ossonate-Plus
Pacaps
Panadol
Panex
Parafon Forte
Pavadon
Pedric
Percocet-5
Percogesic
Phenaphen
Phenaphen w/Codeine
Phendex
Phrenilin
Presalin
Prodolor
Protid
Proval
Repan
Rhinocaps
Robigesic
Ronuvex
Rovnox
S-A-C
SK-65 APAP
SK-APAP
SK-Oxycodone w/Acetaminophen
Salatin
Saleto
Salimeph Forte
Salphenyl
Sedapap
Sinarest
Sine-Aid
Sine-Off
Singlet
Sinubid
Sinulin
Sinutab
Stopayne
Strascogesic
Sudoprin
Supac
Suppap
Sylapar
T.P.I.
Talacen
Tapar
Temlo
Tempra
Tenlap
Tenol
Triaminicin
Trigesic
Trind Sryup
Two-Dyne
Tylenol
Tylenol w/Codeine
Tylox
Valadol
Valorin
Vanquish
Vicodin
Wygesic

ADRENOCORTICOIDS (TOPICAL)

Aeroseb-Dex
Aristocort
Benisone
Betacort
Betaderm
Betnovate
Celestoderm-V
Celestone
Cloderm
Cordran
Cort-Dome
Cortaid
Cortef
Corticreme
Corticosporin

Cortifoam
Cortisol
Cortril
Cyclocort
Decaderm
Decadron
Decaspray
Dermacort
Drenison
Florone
Fluoderm
Fluonid
Flurosyn
Halciderm
Halog
Hexadrol
Hyderm
Hydrocortone
Hytone
Kenalog
Lidemol
Lidex
Locorten
Medrol
Meti-Derm
Neo-Cortef
Neo-Decadron
Oxylone
Proctocort
Spencort
Synalar
Texacort
Topicort
Topsyn
Triacet
Triaderm
Tridesilon
Valisone
Vioform

ALUMINUM HYDROXIDE

ALternaGEL
Alu-Cap
Alu-Tab
Amphojel
Camalox
Chemgel
Creamalin
Delcid
Dialume
Di-Gel
Ducon
Gaviscon
Gelusil
Kolantyl
Maalox
Magnatril
Maxamag
Mygel
Mylanta
Mucotin
Pepsogel
Robalate
Rolaids
Sterazolidin
Vanquish

ANDROGENS

Anabolin
Anadrol-50
Anapolon 50
Anavar
Android
Androlone
Androyd
Danabol
Deca-Durabolin
Delatestryl
Depo-Testosterone
Dianabol
Durabolin
ETHYLESTRENOL
FLUOXYMESTERONE
Halotestin
Malogen
METHANDROSTENOLONE
METHYLTESTOSTERONE
Maxibolin
Metandren
NANDROLONE
OXANDROLONE
OXYMETHOLONE
Ora-Testryl
Oratestin
Oreton
STANOZOLOL
TESTOSTERONE
Testred
Winstrol

ANESTHETICS (TOPICAL)

Aero Caine
Americaine
Anbesol
Anestacon
Benzocaine
Benzocol
Burntame
BUTACAINE
BUTAMBEN
Butesin Picrate
Butyn Sulfate
Caine Spray
Cal-Vi-Nol
Cetacaine
Cetacine
Chiggerex
Cyclaine
CYCLOMETHYCAINE
Derma-Medicone
Dermo-Gen
Dibucaine
Diothane
DIPERODON
Dyclone
DYCLONINE
Ethyl Aminobenzoate
Foille
Hexathricin Aerospra
HEXYLCAINE
Hurricaine
Isotraine
Lida-Mantle
Lidocaine
Medicone
Morusan
Nupercainal
Panthocal A & D
Perifoam
Pontocaine
PRAMOXINE
Prax
Proctodon
Proctofoam
Quotane
Rectal Medicone
Solarcaine
Surfacaine
Tega-Dyne
TETRACAINE
Tronolane
Tronothane
Urolocaine
Xylocaine

APPETITE SUPPRESSANTS

Adipex-D
Adphen
Anorex
Bacarate
BENZPHETAMINE
B.O.F.
Bontril PDM
Chlorophen
CHLORPHENTERMINE
CLORTERMINE
Chlor-Tripolon
D.E.P.—75
Delcozine
Depletite
Dexatrim
Di-Ap-Trol
Didrex
Dietec
DIETHYLPROPION
Elephemet
Ex-Obese
Fastin
FENFLURAMINE
Ionamin
Limbitrol
Limit
Limitite
MASINDOL
Mazinor
Melfiat
Menrium
Minus
Nobesine-75
Nu-Dispoz
Obalan
Obe-Nil TR
Obephen
Obermine
Obestrin-30
Obestrol
Obeval
Obezine

Continued on page 822.

P.S.P.R.X. 1,2 &3
Parmine
Phendiet
PHENDIMETRAZINE
PHENMETRAZINE
PHENTERMINE
Phentrol
Phenzine
Plegine
Ponderal
Pondimin
Pre-Sate
Prelu-2
Preludin
Propion
Reducto
Regibon
Ro-Diet
Sanorex
Slim-Tabs
Span-RD
Statobex
Symetra
Tenuate
Tepanil
Trimstat
Trimtabs
Voranil
Weightrol
Wilpowr

ASPIRIN

4-Way Cold Tablets
A.P.C w/Codeine
A.P.C. Capsules
A.S.A.
A.S.A. Compound
A.S.A. & Codeine Compound
Acetophen
Alka Seltzer
Aluminum ASA
Amytal and Aspirin
Anacin
Anaphen
Ancasal
Anexsia w/Codeine
Apo-Asen
Arthritis Pain Formula
Ascodeen-30
Ascriptin
Ascriptin w/Codeine
Aspergum
Aspir-10
Aspirin Compound w/Codeine
Aspirjen Jr.
Astrin
Axotal
Bancap w/Codeine
Bayer
Bexophene
Buff-A
Buff-A-Comp
Buffered ASA
Bufferin
Calciphen
Cama Arthritis Pain Reliever
Cama Inlay
Causalin
Cefinal
Cirin
Codalan
Codasa
Congespirin
Coralsone
Coricidin D
Coryphen
Cosprin
Darvon Compound
Dasicon
Decagesic
Dia-Gesic
Dihydrocodein Compound
Dolene Compound-65
Dolor
Dolprn #3
Dynosal
Easprin
Ecotrin
Elder 65 Compound
Emagrin
Empirin
Empirin Compound
Empirin Compound w/Codeine
Emprazil
Encaprin
Entrophen
Equagesic
Excedrin
Fiorinal
Fiorinal w/Codeine
Hiprin
Histadyl and ASA Compound
Hyco-Pap
ICN 65 Compound
Kengesin
Lanorinal
Lemidyne w/Codeine
Measurin
Mepro Compound
Metrogesic
Mobidin
Norgesic
Nova-Phase
Novasen
P-A-C Compound
P-A-C Compound w/Codeine
Pabirin Buffered
Pargesic Compound 65
Percodan
Persistin
Phenodyne w/Codeine
Poxy Compound-65
Presalin
Progesic Compound-65
Propoxychel Compound
Propoxyphene HCl Compound
Repro Compound 65
Rhinocaps
Riphen-10
SK-65 Compound
St. Joseph
Sal-Adult
Sal-Infant
Salatin
Salatin w/Codeine
Saleto
Salimeph Forte
Salocol
Salsprin
Soma Compound
Soma Compound w/Codeine
Stero-Darvon
Supac
Supasa
Synalgos
Talwin Compound
Triaminic
Triaphen-10
Trigesic
Vanquish
Verin
Zorprin

ATROPINE

Almezyme
Amocine
Antrocol
Arco-Lase
Atrobarbital
Atromal
Atropine Bufopto
Atropisol
Atrosed
Bar-Cy-A-Tab
Bar-Cy-Amine
Bar-Don
Bar-Tropin
Barbella
Barbeloid
Barbidonna-CR
Belbutal
Belkaloids
Belladenal
Bellergal
Bioxatphen
Briabell
Briaspaz
Brobella
Buren
Butibel
Cerebel
Chardonna
Comhist
Contac
Copin
Dallergy
Ditropan
Donnacin
Donnagel
Donnamine
Donnatal
Donnazyme
Drinus
Eldonal
G.B.S.
HASP
Haponal
Harvitrate
Hyatal
Hybephen
Hycodan
Hyonal
Hyonatol
Hytrona

Isopto Atropine
Kalmedic
Kinesed
Koryza
Levamine
Magnased
Magnox
Maso-Donna
Neogel w/Sulfa
Nilspasm
Oxybutynin
P & A
PAMA
Palbar No. 2
Peece
Prydon
Renalgin
Ro Trim
Ru-Tuss
Sedamine
Sedapar
Sedatabs
Sedralex
Seds
SK-Diphenoxylate
SMP Atropine
Spabelin
Spasaid
Spasdel
Spasidon
Spasloids
Spasmate
Spasmolin
Spasquid
Spastolate
Spastosed
Stannitol
Thitrate
Trac
Unitral
Urised
Uriseptin
Urogesic
Zemarine

BELLADONNA

Amobel
Atrocap
Atrosed
B & O Supprettes
B-Sed
Barbidonna
Bebetab
Belap
Belatol
Belbarb
Bellachar
Belladenal
Bellafedrol
Bellergal
Bellkatal
Bello-phen
Belphen
Butabar
Butibel
Butibel-Zyme
Chardonna
Comhist
Coryztime
Decobel
Donabarb
Donnafed Jr.
Donnatal
Donnazyme
Fitacol
Gastrolic
Gelcomul
Hycoff Cold Caps
Hynaldyne
Kamabel
Kinesed
Lanothal
Mallenzyme
Medi-Spas
Nilspasm
Phebe
Phen-o-bel
Rectacort
Sedapar
Sedatromine
Spabelin
Spasnil
Trac 2X
U-Tract
Ultabs
Urilief
Urised
Wigraine
Woltac
Wyanoids

BENZOYL PEROXIDE

Acetoxyl
Allercreme Clear-Up
Alquan-X
Ben-Aqua
Benoxyl
Benzac
Benzagel
Buf-Oxal
Clear By Design
Clearasil
Dermodex
Dermoxyl
Desquam-X
Dry and Clean
Dry and Clear
Eloxyl
Epi-Clear
Fostex
H_2Oxyl
Intraderm-19
Loroxide
Oxy-10
Oxy-5
Oxyderm
Panoxyl
Persa-Gel
Persadox
Porox 7
Teen
Topex
Vanoxide
Vanoxide-HC
Xerac BP
Zeroxin

BETAMETHASONE

17-Valerate Celestone
17-Valerate Diprosone
Alphatrex
Beben
Beconase
Benzoate
Betacort
Beta-Val
Betnelan
Betnesol
Betratrex
B-S-P
Celestoderm
Celestoject
Celestone
Cel-U-Sec
Dipropinate Metaderm
Diprosone
Disodium Phosphate Betnovate
Lotrisone
Uticort
Valerate Novobetamet
Valerate Betaderm
Valerate Betaderm Scalp Loption
Valisone
Vancerace

BROMPHENIRAMINE

Brocon
Bromfed
Bromepath
Bromphen
Dimetane
Dimetapp
Disophrol Chronotabs
Drixoral
Dura Tap-PD
Eldatapp
E.N.T. Syrup
Histatapp
Poly-Histine
Ralabromophen
Rynatapp
S-T Decongestant
Symptom 3
Taltapp
Tamine S.R.
Tapp
Tolabromophen
Veltap

BUTABARBITAL

Broncholate
Brondilate
Butabell HMB
Butalan
Butatran
Butaserpazide
Butibel
Buticaps
Butisol
Butizide

Continued on page 824.

Cyclo-Bell
Cytospaz-SR
Day-Barb
Levamine
Neo-Barb
Numa-Dura-Tablets
Pyridium Plus
Quibron Plus
Sarisol No. 2
Scolate
Sidonna
Sinate-M
Tedral

CAFFEINE

A.P.C.
A.S.A. Compound
Amaphen
Amaphen w/Codeine #3
Anacin
Anaphen
Anexsia w/Codeine
Anoquan
Asphac-G
Aspirin Compound w/Codeine
Ban-Drow 2
Bexophene
Buff-A-Comp
Buffadyne
Butigetic
Cafacetin
Cafecon
Cafergot
Cafermine
Cafetrate
Cefinal
Cenagesic
Citrated Caffeine
Coastalgesic
Codalan #3
Colrex
Compal
Coryban D
Coryzaid
Darvon Compound
Dasicon
Dexatrim
Dia-Gesic
Dihydrocodeine Compound
Dolor
Duadacin
Dularin
Dynosal
Elder 65 Compound
Emagrin
Empirin Compound
Emprazil
Esgic
Excedrin Extra Strength
Fendol
Fiorinal
G-1 Capsules
Hista-Derfule
Histadyl Compound
ICN 65 Compound
Kengesin
Kirkaffeine
Korigesic
Lanorinal
Lemidyne w/Codeine
Midol
Migralam
Nodaca
Nodoz
P-A-C Compound w/Codeine
Pacaps
Pargesic Compound 65
Percodan
Phenodyne
Phenodyne w/Codeine
Phensal
Phrenilin
Poxy Compound-65
Prodolor
Progesic Compound-65
Propoxychel Compound-65
Propoxyphene Compound
Pyrroxate
Repro Compound 65
S-A-C
SK-65 Compound
Salatin
Salatin w/Codeine
Saleto
Salocol
Sinarest
Supac
Synalgos
Synalogo-DC
Tirend
Triaminic
Triaminicin
Trigesic
Two-Dyne
Vanquish
Vivarin
Wigraine

CALCIUM CARBONATE

Alka-2
Alkets
Amitone
Bio Cal
Calcet
Calcilac
Calglycine
Cal-Sup
Camalox
Chooz
Dicarbosil
Ducon
El-Da-Mint
Equilet
Fosfree
Gustalac
Iromin-G
Mallamint
Mission
Natacomp-FA
Natalins
Nu-Iron-V
Os-Cal
Pama No. 1
Pepto-Bismol
Pramet FA
Pramilet FA
Prenate 90
Ratio
Titracid
Titralac
Trialka
Tums
Zenate

CHLORPHENIRAMINE

4-Way Cold Tablets
AL-R
Acutuss Expectorant w/Codeine
Alermine
Alka-Seltzer Plus
Aller-chlor
Allerbid Tymcaps
Allerest
Allerform
Allergesic
Alumadrine
Anafed
Anamine
Anatuss
Antagonate
Brexin
Bronkotuss
Cerose Compound
Children's Allerest
Chlor-Histine
Chlor-Span
Chlor-Trimeton
Chlor-Trimeton w/Codeine
Chlorafed
Chloramate Unicelles
Chlormine
Chlortab
Ciramine
Ciriforte
Citra Forte
Codimal
Coldene
Colrex
Comhist
Comtrex
Conex w/Codeine
Conex-DA
Cophene-X
Co-Pyronil 2
Coricidin "D"
Corilin
Coryban-D
Coryzaid
Cosea
Co-Tylenol
Covanamine
Covangesic
DM Plus
Dallergy
Deconamine
Dehist
Demazin
Dextro-Tussin
Dextromal
Donatussin
Dorcol

Drinus
Dristan
Drize M
Duadacin
Duphrene
Dura-Vent/A
E.N.T.
Expectrosed
Extendryl
Fedahist
Fernhist
Ginsopan
Guaiahist TT
Guaiamine
Guistrey Fortis
Hista-Vadrin
Histalet
Histalon
Histamic
Histaspan
Histex
Historal
Histor-D Timecelles
Hycoff
Hycomine Compound
Iophen-C
Isoclor
Korigesic
Koryza
Kronofed-A
Kronohist Kronocaps
Lanatuss
Marhist
Naldecon
Naldetuss
Napril Plateau
Narine Gyrocaps
Narspan
Nasahist
Neo-Codenyl-M
Neotep Granucaps
Nilcol
Nolamine
Novafed A
Novahistine
Novopheniram
Omni-Tuss
Ornade Spansule
P-V-Tussin
P.R. Syrup
Palohist
Partuss T.D.
Pediacof
Phenacol-DM
Phenate
Phenetron
Polaramine
Probahist
Protid Improved Formula
Pseudo-Hist
Pyma
Pyrroxate
Pyrroxate w/Codeine
Quadrahist
Quelidrine
Queltuss
Resaid T.D.
Rhinex
Rhinolar
Rhinolar-EX
Ru-Tuss
Rynatan
Rynatuss
Salphenyl
Scot-Tussin
Sinarest
Singlet
Sinovan
Sinulin
T.P.I.
Tedral Anti-H
Teldrin Spansules
Triaminicin
Tusquelin
Tuss-Ornade
Tussar
Tussi-Organidin
U.R.I.
Wesmatic Forte

DEXAMETHASONE

Aeroseb-Dex
Dalalon L.A.
Decaderm
Decadron
Decadron Respihaler
Decadron Turbinaire
Decadron with Xylocaine
Decaspray
Deronil
Dexasone
Dexone
Hexandrol
Maxidex
SK-Dexamethasone

DEXTROMETHORPHAN

216 DM
2/C-DM
Anti-Tuss DM
Balminil DM
Benylin DM
Broncho-Grippol-DM
Cheracol
Contratuss
Cosanyl DM
Delsym Polistirex
Demo-Cincol
Dextro-Tussin GG
DM Syrup
Dormethan
Dristan
Duad Koff Balls
Endotussin-NN
Formula 44-D
Glycotuss-dM
Guiatuss D-M
Koffex
Lixaminol AT
Neo-DM
Novahistine DMX
Nyquil
Ornacol
Queltuss
Robidex
Robitussin
Romilar
St. Joseph
Sedatuss
Silence is Golden
Silexin
Sorbase
Sorbutuss
Trind DM
Trocal
Tussagesic
Tussaminic
Unproco
Vicks

DIPHENHYDRAMINE

Allerdryl
Ambenyl Expectorant
Benadryl
Bendylate
Benylin Cough Syrup
Caladryl
Diahist
Dihydrex
Diphen
Diphenadril
Eldadryl
Fenylhist
Hydril
Insomnal
Noradryl
Nytol
Phen-Amin
Rabalyn
SK-Diphenhydramine
Sominex
Tusstat
Valdrene
Wehydryl

DOCUSATE SODIUM

Afko-Lube
Bilax
Bu-Lax
Colace
Colax
Coloctyl
D-S-S
Di-Sosul
Dialose
Dilax
Dio-Sul
DioMedicone
Diocto
Dioctyl Sodium Sulfosuccinate
Dioeze
Diosuccin
Disonate
Doctate
Doss
Doxidan
Doxinate
Duosol
Ferro-sequels

Continued on page 826.

Geriplex-FS
Laxagel
Laxinate
Liqui-Doss
Modane Plus
Modane Soft
Molatoc
Neolax
Peri-Colase
Peritinic
Prenate 90
Regulex
Regutol
Senokot-S
Stulex
Trilax

EPHEDRINE

Acet-Am
Aladrine
Amesec
Amodrine
Asminyl
Benadryl w/Ephedrine
Broncholate
Brondilate
Bronkaid
Bronkolixir
Bronkotabs
Bronkotuss
Calcidrine
Co-Xan Elixir
Coryza Brengle
Dainite
Derma Medicone-HC
Duovent
Ectasule III
Ectasule Minus
Ephed-Organidin
Ephedrine and Amytal
Ephedrine and Nembutal-25
Ephedrine and Seconal
Ephedrol w/Codeine
Epragen
Iso-Asminyl
Isuprel
Luasmin
Lufyllin-EPG
Marax
Mudrane
Numa-Dura-Tablets
Nyquil
Phyldrox
Primatene
Pyribenazmine w/Ephedrine
Quadrinal
Quelidrine
Quibron Plus
Slo-Fedrin A-60
Tedfern
Tedral
T.E.H.
T-E-P
Thalfed
Theofedral
Theotabs
Theozine
Wesmatic
Wyanoids

EPINEPHRINE

Adrenalin
Asmolin
Asthma Haler
Asthma Nefrin
Ayerst Epitrate
Bronitin
Bronkaid
Dysne-Inhal
EpiPen-Epinephrine Auto-Injector
Epi-Pen Jr.
Epifrin
Epitrate
Eppy
Glaucon
Marcaine Hydrochloride w/Epinephrine
Medihaler-Epi
Murocoll
Mytrate
Primatene
Simplene
Sus-phrine
Vaponefrin
microNEFRIN

ERYTHROMYCINS

Apo-Erythro-S
A/T/S
Bristamycin
Dowmycin
E-Biotic
E-Mycin
E-Mycin E
E.E.S.
Eryc
Ery-derm
Erymax
Erypar
EryPed
Ery-Tab
Erythrocin
Erythrocin Ethyl Succinate
Erythromid
ERYTHROMYCIN
ERYTHROMYCIN ESTOLATE
ERYTHROMYCIN ETHYL-SUCCINATE
ERYTHROMYCIN GLUCEPTATE
ERYTHROMYCIN LACTOBIONATE
ERYTHROMYCIN STEARATE
Ethril
Ilosone
Ilosone Estolate
Ilotycin
Ilotycin Gluceptate
Kesso-mycin
Novorythro
Pediazole
Pendiamycin
Pfizer-E
RP-Mycin
Robimycin
SK-Erythromycin
Staticin
T-Star
Wyamycin
Wyamycin E

FERROUS FUMARATE

Cevi-Fer
Chromagen
Feco-T
Femiron
Feostat
Ferancee
Ferrofume
Ferro-sequels
Fersamal
Fetrin
Fumasorb
Fumerin
Hemocyte
Hemo-Vite
Ircon
Ircon-FA
Laud-Iron
Maniron
Natalins
Neo-Fer-50
Novofumar
Palafer
Poly-Vi-Flor
Pramilet FA
Prenate 90
Stuartinic
Toleron
Tolfrinic
Tolifer
Trinsicon
Vitron C
Zenate

GUAIFENESIN

2/G-DM
Actol
Ambenyl
Anti-Tuss
Asbron
Asma
Balminil
Breonesin
Brexin
Bromphen
Broncholate
Brondecon
Bronkolizir
Bronkotabs
Bronkotuss
Cetro Cirose
Cheracol
Chlor-Trimeton
Co-Xan
Codimal
Coditrate
Conar
Conex
Conex w/Codeine
Congess Jr. & Sr.

Corutol
Coryban-D
Cremacoat
Deproist w/Codeine
Detussin
Dilaudid
Dilor-G
Dimetane
Donatussin
Dorcol
Dristan
Duovent
Dura-Vent
Elixophyllin-GG
Emfaseen
Entex
Entuss-D
Fedahist
Formula 44-D
Glycotuss
Glytuss
Guaiahist
Guaifed
Guiatuss
Histalet X
Hycotuss
Hytuss
Luftodil
Lufyllin
Malotuss
Mudrane GG
Naldecon
Neo-Spec
Neospect
Neothyllin-G
Novahistine
Nucofed
P-V-Tussin
Poly-Histine
Queltuss
Quibron
Respaire-SR
Resyl
Robitussin
S-T Forte
Scot-Tussin Sugar-Free
Silexin
Sinufed Timecelles
Slo-Phyllin GG
Sorbase
Sorbutuss
Synophylate-GG
Tedral
Theo-Guaia
Theolair-Plus
Triafed-C
Triaminic
Triaminic w/Codeine
Trind
Tussar
Tussend
Uproco
Vicks
Zephrex

HYDROCHLOROTHIAZIDE

Aldactazide
Aldoril
Apo-Hydro
Apresazide
Apresoline-Esidrix
Butaserpazide
Butizide
Diuchlor H
Diupres
Dyazide
Esidrix
Esimil
H-H-R
Hydrid
Hydro-Aquil
HydroDIURIL
Hydropres
Hydroserp
Hydroserpine
Hydrotensin
Hydrozide-Z-50
Hyperetic
Inderide
Mallopress
Maxzide
Moduretic
Naquival
Natrimax
Nefrol
Neo-Codema
Novohydrazide
Oretic
Oreticyl
Reserpazide
Ser-Ap-Es
Serpasil-Esidrix
Singoserp-Esidrix
SK-Hydrochlorothiazide
Spironazide
Thiuretic
Timolide
Timolol and Hydrochlorothiazide
Tri-Hydroserpine
Unipres
Urozide
Zide

HYDROCORTISONE (CORTISOL)

Aeroseb-HC
A-hydroCort
Barseb
Biosone
Cort-Dome
Cortaid
Cortamed
Cortate
Cortef
Cortenema
Corticreme
Cortifoam
Cortiment
Cortisol
Cortoderm
Cortril
Dermacort
Emo-Cort
Fernisone
Hyderm
Hydro-Cortilean
Hydrocortone
Hytone
Microcort
Novohydrocort
Orabase HCA
Proctocort
Rectoid
Restocort
Solu-Cortef
Texacort
Unicort
Westcort

HYOSCYAMINE

Almezyme
Anaspa 3
Anaspaz PB
Arco-Lase Plus
Bar-Cy-A-Tab
Bar-Cy-Amine
Bar-Don
Barbella
Barbeloid
Barbidonna-CR
Belbutal
Belkaloids
Bellafoline
Brobella-PB
Buren
Cystospaz
Cytospa
De Tal
Donnacin
Donnagel
Donnamine
Donnatal
Donnazyme
Eldonal
Elixiril
Ergobel
Floramine
Gylanphen
Haponal
Hyatal
Hybephen
Hyonal
Hyonatol
Hytrona
Kinesed
Koryza
Kutrase
Levamine
Levsin
Levsinex
Maso-Donna
Neoquess
Nevrotase
Nilspasm
Omnibel
Peece
Pyridium Plus
Renalgin
Restophen
Ru-Tuss
Sedajen

Continued on page 828.

Sedamine
Sedapar
Sedatromine
Sedralex
Seds
Spabelin
Spasaid
Spasdel
Spasloids
Spasmolin
Spasquid
Spastolate
Trac 2X
Ultabs
Urised
Uriseptin
Urogesic
Zemarine

INSULIN

Actrapid
Globin Insulin
Humulin
Insulatard
Lentard
Lente
Mixtard
Monotard
Novolin
NPH
NPH Iletin I
NPH Iletin II
PZI
Protamine Zinc & Iletin
Protophane NPH
Regular (Concentrated) Iletin
Regular Iletin I
Regular Iletin II
Regular Insulin
Semilente
Semilente Iletin
Semitard
Ultralente
Ultratard
Velosulin

MEPROBAMATE

Arcoban
Bamate
Bamo 400
Coprobate
Deprol
Evenol
Equagesic
Equanil
Kalmn
Lan-Dol
Medi-Tran
Mep-E
Mepriam
Mepro Compound
Meprocon
Meprospan
Meprotabs
Meribam
Miltown
Neo-Tran
Neuramate
Novomepro
Pathibamate
Pax 400
PMB
Protran
Quietal
Robam
Robamate
Sedabamate
SK-Bamate
Tranmep

NARCOTIC ANALGESICS

A.P.C. w/Codeine Phosphate
Aceta w/Codeine
Acetaco
Acetaminophen w/Codeine
Actifed-C
Adatuss
Algodex
Ambenyl
Anaphen
Arthralgen
Ascriptin w/Codeine
Aspirin Compound w/Codeine
Axotal
Bancap w/Codeine
Banesin Forte
BUTORPHANOL
Calcidrine
Capital w/Codeine
Cetro Cirose
Cheracol
Co-Xan
Coastaldyne
Coastalgesic
Codalan
Codalex
Codap
CODEINE
Codeine Sulfate
Codimal PH
Coditrate
Codone
Colrex Compound
Copavin
Corutol DH
Cotussis
Dapase
Darvocet-N 100
Darvon
Demer-Idine
Demerol
Depronal-SA
Dialog
Dilaudid
Dimetane-DC
Dolene
Dolophine
Dolor
Dularin
Dynosal
Empirin w/Codeine
Empracet w/Codeine
Emprazil-C
Ephedrol w/Codeine
Esgic
FL-Tussex
Fiorinal w/Codeine
G-2
G-3
Gaysal
HYDROCODONE
HYDROMORPHONE
Hasacode
Hycodan
Hycotuss
Isoclor
LEVORPHANOL
Levo-Dromoran
Liquix-C
Lo-Tussin
MEPERIDINE
METHADONE
MORPHINE
Maxigesic
Mepergan Fortis
Methadose
Metrogesic
Minotal
M.O.S. Syrup
NALBUPHINE
Novahistine DH
Novopropoxyn
Nubain
Numorphan
OPIUM
Ossonate-Plus
OXYCODONE
OXYMORPHONE
Pantapon
PAREGORIC
Pargesic
Pavadon
Paveral
Pediacof
PENTAZOCINE
Percodan
Pethadol
Phenaphen w/Codeine
Phenergan
Phrenilin
Poly-Histine w/Codeine
Presalin
Pro-65
Prodolor
Profene
Promethazine HCl w/Codeine
PROPOXYPHENE
Proxagesic
Proxene
Prunicodeine
Robidone
Robitussin A-C
S-A-C
SK-65
SK-APAP w/Codeine
Salatin
Saleto
Salimeph Forte
Sedapap
Soma Compound w/Codeine

Sorbase II
Stadol
Strascogesic
Supac
Supevdol
Sylapar
Talwin
Terpin Hydrate w/Codeine
Triaminic w/Codeine
Trigesic
Tussar
Tussend
Tussi-Organidin
Tylenol w/Codeine
Tylox
Wygesic

PAPAVERINE

Cerebid
Cerespan
Copavin
Dipav
Durapav
Dylate
Hyobid
Kavrin
Lapav
Myobid
Octapav
P-200
P-A-V
Pavabid
Pavacap
Pavadon
Pavagen
Pavakey
Pavased
Pavasule
Pavatest
Pavatran
Pavatym
Paverolan
Payadur
Ro-Papan
Sustaverine
Therapav
Vasal
Vasospan

PHENIRAMINE

Citra Forte
Dri-Hist No. 2 Meta Caps
Dristan Nasal Spray
Fiogesic
Inhistor
Poly-Histine D
Robitussin-AC
Ru-Tuss
S-T Forte
Symptrol
Triaminic
Triaminicin
Triaminicol
Tussagesic
Tussaminic
Tussirex Sugar-Free
Ursinus

PHENOBARBITAL

Aminophylline-Phenobarbital
Anaspaz-PB
Antrocol
Asminyl
Banthine w/Phenobarbital
Bar-Tropin
Barbidonna
Bardase Filmseal
Belap
Belbarb
Belladenal
Bellergal
Bellkatal
Bentyl Phenobarbital
Bronkolixir
Bronkotabs
Cantil w/Phenobarbital
Chardonna
Cyclo-Bell
Dactil Phenobarbital
Dainite-KI
Daricon PB
Donna-Lix
Donnatal
Duovent
Eskabarb
Gardenal
Gastrolic
HASP
Hybephen
Hytrona
Iso-Asminyl
Isuprel Compound
Kinesed
Levsin PB
Levsin w/Phenobarbital
Luasmin
Luftodil
Lufyllin-EPG
Matropinal
Mesopin PB
Mudrane
Neospect
Nova-Pheno
Oxoids
Pamine PB
Pathilon w/Phenobarbital
Phyldrox
Primatene, P Formula
Pro-Banthine w/Phenobarbital
Probital
Pyrdonnal Spansules
Quadrinal
Robinul-PH
Sedadrops
SK-Phenobarbital
Solfoton
Spasdel
Spasticol
Tedral
T-E-P
Thalfed
Theofedral
Theotabs
Tral w/Phenobarbital
Valpin-PB

PHENYLBUTAZONE

Algoverine
Apo-Phenylbutazone
Azolid
Buffazone
Butagesic
Butazolidin
Intrabutazone
Malgesic
Nadozone
Neo-Zoline
Novobutazone
Phenbuff
Phenbutazone
Sterazolidin

PHENYLEPHRINE

4-Way Nasal Spray
4-Way Tablets
Albatussin
Alconefrin
Alka-Seltzer Plus
Anamine T.D.
Bromepaph
Bromphen Compound
Callergy
Cenagesic
Children's Allerest
Chlor-Histine
Chlor-Trimeton
Citra
Clistin D
Codalex
Codimal
Colrex
Comhist
Conar
Congespirin
Contac
Coricidin
Coryban-D
Coryzaid
Cosea-D
Co-Tylenol
Covanamine
Covangesic
Dallergy
Dehist
Demazin
Dimetapp
Donatussin DC
Dri-Hist No. Meta-Caps
Drinus Graduals
Dristan Advanced Formula
Dristan Nasal Spray
Drize M
Duadacin
Duo-Medihaler
Duphrene
Dura Tap-PD
Dura-Vent/DA
E.N.T.
Emagrin Forte
Entex
Extendryl
Fendol
Fernhist

Continued on page 830.

Ginospan
Guaiahist
Hista-Vadrin
Histabid Duracaps
Histalet
Histaspan
Histatapp
Historal No. 2
Histor-D Timecelles
Hycomine Compound
Isophrin
Korigesic
Koryza
Marhist
Mydrin
Naldecon
Napril Plateau
Narine Cyrocaps
Narspan
Nasahist
Neo-Mist
Neo-Synephrine
NeoSynephrin Compound
Neotep Granucaps
Novahistine
Palohist
Pediacof
Phenate
Phenergan VC
Phenergan VC w/Codeine
Prefrin
Protid Improved Formula
P-V-Tussin
Pyma Timed
Pyracort-D
Quelidrine
Rhinall
Rhinex
Rolabromophen
Rolahist
Ru-Tuss
Rynatan
Rynatapp
S-T Forte
Salphenyl
Singlet
Sinoran
Super Anahist
Synasal
T.P.I.
Taltapp
Tamine S.R.
Tapp
Tussar DM
Tussirex
Tympagesic
U.R.I.
Vacon
Veltar

PHENYLPROPANOLAMINE

4-Way Cold Tablets
4-Way Nasal Spray
Alka-Seltzer Plus
Allerest
Alumadrine
Asbron
Axon
Bayer Cold Tablets
Bayer Cough Syrup
Blu-Hist
Bromphen Compound
Caldecon
Children's Allerest
Cinsospan
Citra
Codimal
Coffee-Break
Colrex
Comtrex
Conex-DA
Congespirin
Conhist
Contac
Control
Coricidin "D" Decongestant
Cornex Plus
Coryban-D
Coryztime
CoTylenol Children's Liquid Cold Formula
Covanamine
Cremacoat
D-Sinus
Dal-Sinus
Dehist
Dexatrim
Dietac
Dieutrim
Dimetane
Dimetapp
Dri-Hist Meta-Kaps
Drinus Syrup
Dura Tap-PD
Dura-Vent, /A
Eldatapp
Endecon
Entex
E.N.T
Fiogesic
Formula 44-D
Help
Histalet Forte
Histapp
Histatapp
Hycomine
Korigesic
Koryza
Kronohist Kronocaps
MSC Triaminic
Naldecon
Naldecon
Napril Plateau
Nasahist
Nolamine
Novahistine
Obestat
Ornacol
Ornade
Ornex
Partuss T.D.
Phenate
Phenylin
Poly-Histine-D
Prolamine, Maximum Strength
Propadrine
Propagest
Quadrahist
Resaid T.D.
Rescaps-D T.D.
Rhindecon
Rhinex Ty-Med
Rhinidrin
Rhinocaps
Rhinolar
Robitussin-CF
Rolabromophen
Ru-Tuss
Rynatapp
S-T Decongestant
S-T Forte
Saleto-D
Sinarest
Sine-Aid
Sine-Off
Sinubid
Sinulin
Sinutab
Symtrol
T.P.I.
Taltapp
Tapp
Tavist-D
Triaminic
Triaminicin
Triaminicol
Tuss-Ade
Tuss-Ornade
Tussagesic
Tussaminic
U.R.I.
Ursinus
Veltap
Vernata Granucaps

PREDNISOLONE

Ak-Pred
Ak-Tate
Cortalone
Delta-Cortef
Econopred
Fernisolone-P
Hydeltrasol
Hydeltra-TBA
Inflamase
Metalone-TBA
Meticortelone
Meti-Derm
Metimyd
Metreton
Nor-Pred-TBA
Nova-Pred
Novaprednisolone
Predate
Pred Cor-TBA
Pred Forte
Pred Mild
Predulose
Savacort 50 & 100
Sterane

PSEUDOEPHEDRINE

Actifed
Afrinol
Ambenyl-D
Anafed
Anamine
Aramine
Brexin
Bromfed
Bronchobid
Cardec DM
Cenafed
Chlor-Trimeton
Chlorafed
Codimal
Co-Pyronil 2
Cosanyl
Cotrol-D
Co-Tylenol
D-Feda
Deconamine
Deproist w/Codeine
Detussin
Dimacol
Disobrom
Disophrol
Dorcol
Drixoral
Eltor
Emprazil
Entuss-D
Fedahist
Fedrazil
Guaifed
Hista-Clopane
Histalet DM
Histamic
Historal
Isoclor
Kronofed-A Kronocaps
Naldegesic
Neobid
Novafed
Novafed A
Novahistine DMX
Nucofed
Phenergan
Phenergan-D
Poly-Histine-DX
Probahist
Pseudo-Hist
Pseudofrin
Redahist Gyrocaps
Respaire-SR
Ro-Fedrin
Robidrine
Robitussin-DAC
Rondec
Sherafed
Sine-Aid Sinus Headache Tablets
Sinufed Timecelles
Suda-Prol
Sudafed
Sudahist
Sudolin
Sudrin
Triafed
Trifed
Trinalin Repetabs
Triphed
Tripodrine
Tussend
Tylenol Maximum Strength Sinus Medicine
Zephrex

PYRILAMINE

4-Way Nasal Spray
Albatussin
Allertoc
Allerstat
Citra Forte
Codimal DH, DM, PH
Covanamine
Dormarex
Duphrene
Excedrin P.M.
Fiogesic
Histalet Forte
Kronohist Kronocaps
Midol PMS
Napril Plateau
Panadyl
Poly-Histine D
Primatene, M Formula
P-V-Tussin
Relemine
Ru-Tuss
Rynatan
Somnicaps
Triaminic
Trihista-Phen-25
Tussanil
WANS

RAUWOLFIA ALKALOIDS

ALSEROXYLON
Alkarau
Bonapene
Broserpine
Butiserpazide-50 Prestabs
Buytizide-25 Prestabs
Chloroserpine
DESERPIDINE
Demi-Regroton
Diupres
Diutensin-R
Enduronyl
Harmonyl
H-H-R
Hydro-Fluserpine
Hydromox R
Hydropres
Hydroserp
Hydroserpine
Hydrotensin-50
Mallopress
Metatensin
Naquival
Novoreserpine
Oreticyl
RAUWOLFIA SERPENTINA
Rau-Sed
Raudixin
Raulfia
Raunormine
Raupoid
Rauraine
Rauserpa
Rautrax
Rauverid
Rauwiloid
Rauzide
Regroton
Renese-R
Reserfia
Reserpazide
RESERPINE
Reserpoid
Salutensin
Sandril
Ser-Ap-Es
Serpalan
Serpanray
Serpasil
Serpasil-Apresoline
Serpasil-Esidrix
Serpate
Singoserp-Eisdrix
SK-Reserpine
T-Serp
Unipres
Wolfina

SALICYLATES

Arcylate
Arthropan
CHOLINE AND MAGNESIUM SALICYLATES
CHOLINE SALICYLATE
DIFLUNISAL
Disalcid
Durasil
MAGNESIUM SALICYLATE
Magan
Mobidin
S-60
SALICYLAMIDE
SALSALATE
SODIUM SALICYLATE

SCOPOLAMINE

Allerspan
Almezyme
Aluscop
Bar-Cy-A-Tab
Bar-Cy-Amine
Bar-Don
Barbella
Barbeloid
Barbidonna-CR
Belbutal
Belkaloids
Bobid
Brobella-PB
Buren
Cenahist
Chlorpel
Conalsyn

Continued on page 832.

Dallergy
Donnacin
Donnagel
Donnamine
Donnatal
Donnazyme
Drinus
Drize
Eldonal
Eulcin
Extendryl
Haponal
Histaspan-D
Historal
Hyatal
Hybephen
Hydrochol-Plus
Hyonal
Hyonatol
Hytrona
Kinesed
Kleer
Kleer-Tuss
Koryza
Levamine
MSC Triaminic
Maso-Donna
Methnite
Narine
Narspan
Nilspasm
Omnibel
Pamine
Pamine PB
Paraspan
Renalgin
Ru-Tuss
Sanhist
Scoline
Scoline-Amobarbital
Scopolamine Trans-Derm
Scotnord
Sedamine
Sedapar
Sedralex
Seds
Sinaprel
Sinodec
Sinoran
Sinunil
Spabelin
Spasdel
Spasloids
Spasmid
Spasmolin
Spasquid
Spastolate
Symptrol
Transderm
Trisohist
Uriseptin
Urogesic
Vonnodonnal
Zemarine

TETRACYCLINES

Achromycin
Achrostatin V
Apo-Tetra
Bicycline
Bio-Tetra
Bristacycline
Cefacycline
Centet
Comycin
Cyclopar
DEMECLOCYCLINE
DOXYCYCLINE
Declomycin
Desamycin
Doxy-Lemmon
Doxy-Tabs
Doxychel
Fed-Mycin
G-Mycin
Kesso-Tetra
Lemtrex
METHACYCLINE
MINOCYCLINE
Maytrex-BID
Medicycline
Minocin
Muracine
Mysteclin F
Neo-Tetrine
Nor-Tet
Novotetra
OXYTETRACYCLINE
Oxlopar
Oxy-Kesso-Tetra
Paltet
Panmycin
Piracaps
PMS Tetracycline
Q'Dtet
Retet
Ro-Cycline
Robitet
Rondomycin
SK-Tetracycline
Sarocyclin
Scotrex
Sumycin
T-Caps
TETRACYCLINE
Terramycin
Tet-Cy
Tetet
Tetra-Co
Tetrachel
Tetracrine
Tetracyn
Tetracyrine
Tetralean
Tetram
Tetramax
Tetramine
Tetrastatin.(M)
Tetrex
Topicycline
Trexin
Ultramycin
Urobiotic
Vibramycin
Vibratabs

THEOPHYLLINE

Accurbron
Aerolate
Amesec
Aminophylline and Amytal
Aminophylline-Phenobarbital
Amodrine
Aquaphyllin
Asbron
Asma
Asminyl
Asthmophylline
Bronchobid Duracaps
Broncholate
Brondecon
Brondilate
Bronkodyl
Bronkolixir
Bronkotabs
Choledyl
Co-Xan
Constant-T
Dilor G
Duovent
Elixicon
Elixophyllin
Emfaseem
G-Bron
Iso-Asminyl
Isuprel Compound
Klophyllin
LABID
Lixaminol AT
Lodrane
Luasmin
Luftodil
Lufyllin
Marax
Marax DF
Mersalyl-Theophylline
Mudrane
Neospect
Neothylline-G
Numa-Dura-Tabs
Orthoxine & Aminophylline
Phenylin
Phyldrox
Physpan
PMS Theophylline
Primatene, M Formula
Primatene, P Formula
Pulmophylline
Quadrinal
Quibron
Quibron Plus
Respbid
Slo-Phyllin GG
Slo-bid Gyrocaps
Slophyllin
Somophyllin-T
Sudolin
Sustaire
Synophylate-GG
Tedfern
Tedral
T.E.H.
Thalfed

Theo-24
Theobid
Theoclear
Theo-Dur
Theo-Guaia
Theofedral
Theolair
Theolair-Plus
Theolixir
Theon
Theo-Nar 100
Theo-Organidin
Theophyl
Theospan
Theostate 80
Theotabs
Theozine
Uniphyl

TRIAMCINOLONE

Amcort
Aristocort
Aristospan
Azmacort
Cenocort Forte
Cinalone 40
Cino-40
Cinonide 40
Cremocort
Kenacort
Kenalog
Kenalog in Orabase
Kenalog-E
Mycolog
Myco-Triacet
Mytrex
Nust-Olone
Spencort
Tramacort
Triacet
Triacort
Triaderm
Trialean Acetonide
Triamcinair
Trimalone
Trymex

Additional Drug Interactions

The following lists of drugs and their interactions with other drugs are continuations of lists found in the alphabetized drug charts beginning on page 18. These lists are alphabetized by generic name or drug class name, shown in large capital letters. Only those lists too long for the drug charts are included in this section. For complete information about any generic drug, see the alphabetized charts.

GENERIC NAME OR DRUG CLASS	COMBINED EFFECT	GENERIC NAME OR DRUG CLASS	COMBINED EFFECT

ACETOHEXAMIDE

GENERIC NAME OR DRUG CLASS	COMBINED EFFECT	GENERIC NAME OR DRUG CLASS	COMBINED EFFECT
Isoniazid	Decreased acetohexamide effect.	**Probenecid**	Increased acetohexamide effect.
MAO inhibitors	Increased acetohexamide effect.	**Pyrazinamide**	Decreased acetohexamide effect.
Oxyphenbutazone	Increased acetohexamide effect.	**Sulfa drugs**	Increased acetohexamide effect.
Phenylbutazone	Increased acetohexamide effect.	**Sulfaphenazole**	Increased acetohexamide effect.
Phenyramidol	Increased acetohexamide effect.	**Thyroid hormones**	Decreased acetohexamide effect.

ALLOPURINOL

GENERIC NAME OR DRUG CLASS	COMBINED EFFECT	GENERIC NAME OR DRUG CLASS	COMBINED EFFECT
Metolazone	Decreased allopurinol effect.	**Probenecid**	Increased allopurinol effect.

AMOBARBITAL

GENERIC NAME OR DRUG CLASS	COMBINED EFFECT	GENERIC NAME OR DRUG CLASS	COMBINED EFFECT
MAO inhibitors	Increased amobarbital effect.	**Sedatives**	Dangerous sedation. Avoid.
Mind-altering drugs	Dangerous sedation. Avoid.	**Sleep inducers**	Dangerous sedation. Avoid.
Narcotics	Dangerous sedation. Avoid.	**Tranquilizers**	Dangerous sedation. Avoid.
Pain relievers	Dangerous sedation. Avoid.	**Valproic acid**	Increased amobarbital effect.

ANTICOAGULANTS (ORAL)

GENERIC NAME OR DRUG CLASS	COMBINED EFFECT	GENERIC NAME OR DRUG CLASS	COMBINED EFFECT
Barbiturates	Decreased anticoagulant effect.	**Carbamazepine**	Decreased anticoagulant effect.
Benzodiazepines	Unpredictable increased or decreased anticoagulant effect.		

ASPIRIN

GENERIC NAME OR DRUG CLASS	COMBINED EFFECT	GENERIC NAME OR DRUG CLASS	COMBINED EFFECT
Probenecid	Decreased probenecid effect.	**Spironolactone**	Decreased spironolactone effect.
Propranolol	Decreased aspirin effect.	**Sulfinpyrazone**	Decreased sulfinpyrazone effect.
Rauwolfia alkaloids	Decreased aspirin effect.	**Vitamin C (large doses)**	Possible aspirin toxicity.
Salicylates (other)	Likely aspirin toxicity.		

ADDITIONAL DRUG INTERACTIONS

GENERIC NAME OR DRUG CLASS	COMBINED EFFECT	GENERIC NAME OR DRUG CLASS	COMBINED EFFECT

BETAMETHASONE

GENERIC NAME OR DRUG CLASS	COMBINED EFFECT
Ephedrine	Decreased betamethasone effect.
Estrogens	Increased betamethasone effect.
Ethacrynic acid	Potassium depletion.
Furosemide	Potassium depletion.
Glutethimide	Decreased betamethasone effect.
Indomethacin	Increased betamethasone effect.
Insulin	Decreased insulin effect.
Isoniazid	Decreased isoniazid effect.
Oxyphenbutazone	Possible ulcers.
Phenylbutazone	Possible ulcers.
Rifampin	Decreased betamethasone effect.
Sympathomimetics	Possible glaucoma.

BUTABARBITAL

GENERIC NAME OR DRUG CLASS	COMBINED EFFECT
MAO inhibitors	Increased butabarbital effect.
Mind-altering drugs	Dangerous sedation. Avoid.
Narcotics	Dangerous sedation. Avoid.
Pain relievers	Dangerous sedation. Avoid.
Sedatives	Dangerous sedation. Avoid.
Sleep inducers	Dangerous sedation. Avoid.
Tranquilizers	Dangerous sedation. Avoid.
Valproic acid	Increased butabarbital effect.

CALCIUM CARBONATE

GENERIC NAME OR DRUG CLASS	COMBINED EFFECT
Quinidine	Increased quinidine effect.
Salicylates	Increased salicylate effect.
Sulfa drugs	Decreased sulfa effect.
Tetracyclines	Decreased tetracycline effect.
Vitamins A and C	Decreased vitamin effect.

CHLORPROPAMIDE

GENERIC NAME OR DRUG CLASS	COMBINED EFFECT
Isoniazid	Decreased chlorpropamide effect.
MAO inhibitors	Increased chlorpropamide effect.
Oxyphenbutazone	Increased chlorpropamide effect.
Phenylbutazone	Increased chlorpropamide effect.
Phenyramidol	Increased chlorpropamide effect.
Probenecid	Increased chlorpropamide effect.
Pyrazinamide	Decreased chlorpropamide effect.
Sulfa drugs	Increased chlorpropamide effect.
Sulfaphenazole	Increased chlorpropamide effect.
Thyroid hormones	Decreased chlorpropamide effect.

CHLORPROTHIXENE

GENERIC NAME OR DRUG CLASS	COMBINED EFFECT
Narcotics	Increased chlorprothixene effect. Excessive sedation.
Sedatives	Increased chlorprothixene effect. Excessive sedation.
Sleep inducers	Increased chlorprothixene effect. Excessive sedation.
Tranquilizers	Increased chlorprothixene effect. Excessive sedation.

ADDITIONAL DRUG INTERACTIONS

GENERIC NAME OR DRUG CLASS	COMBINED EFFECT	GENERIC NAME OR DRUG CLASS	COMBINED EFFECT

CIMETIDINE

GENERIC NAME OR DRUG CLASS	COMBINED EFFECT
Digitalis preparations	Increased digitalis effect.
Penicillins	Increased penicillin effect.
Propranolol	May increase propranolol effect.
Quinidine	Increased quinidine effect.
Theophylline	Increased theophylline effect.

CONTRACEPTIVES (ORAL)

GENERIC NAME OR DRUG CLASS	COMBINED EFFECT
Phenothiazines	Increased phenothiazine effect.
Rifampin	Decreased contraceptive effect.
Tetracyclines	Decreased contraceptive effect.

CORTISONE

GENERIC NAME OR DRUG CLASS	COMBINED EFFECT
Ephedrine	Decreased cortisone effect.
Estrogens	Increased cortisone effect.
Ethacrynic acid	Potassium depletion.
Furosemide	Potassium depletion.
Glutethimide	Decreased cortisone effect.
Indomethacin	Increased cortisone effect.
Insulin	Decreased insulin effect.
Isoniazid	Decreased isoniazid effect.
Oxyphenbutazone	Possible ulcers.
Phenylbutazone	Possible ulcers.
Rifampin	Decreased cortisone effect.
Sympathomimetics	Possible glaucoma.

DEXAMETHASONE

GENERIC NAME OR DRUG CLASS	COMBINED EFFECT
Diuretics (thiazide)	Potassium depletion.
Ephedrine	Decreased dexamethasone effect.
Estrogens	Increased dexamethasone effect.
Ethacrynic acid	Potassium depletion.
Furosemide	Potassium depletion.
Glutethimide	Decreased dexamethasone effect.
Indomethacin	Increased dexamethasone effect.
Insulin	Decreased insulin effect.
Isoniazid	Decreased isoniazid effect.
Oxyphenbutazone	Possible ulcers.
Phenylbutazone	Possible ulcers.
Rifampin	Decreased dexamethasone effect.
Sympathomimetics	Possible glaucoma.

ADDITIONAL DRUG INTERACTIONS

ETHACRYNIC ACID

GENERIC NAME OR DRUG CLASS	COMBINED EFFECT
Probenecid	Decreased probenecid effect.
Salicylates (including aspirin)	Dangerous salicylate retention.
Sedatives	Increased ethacrynic acid effect.

ETHOTOIN

GENERIC NAME OR DRUG CLASS	COMBINED EFFECT
Griseofulvin	Increased griseofulvin effect.
Isoniazid	Increased ethotoin effect.
Methadone	Decreased methadone effect.
Methotrexate	Increased methotrexate effect.
Methylphenidate	Increased ethotoin effect.
Oxyphenbutazone	Increased ethotoin effect.
Para-aminosalicylic acid (PAS)	Increased ethotoin effect.
Phenothiazines	Increased ethotoin effect.
Phenylbutazone	Increased ethotoin effect.
Propranolol	Increased propranolol effect.
Quinidine	Increased quinidine effect.
Sedatives	Increased sedative effect.
Sulfa drugs	Increased ethotoin effect.
Theophylline	Reduced anticonvulsant effect.

FLUPREDNISOLONE

GENERIC NAME OR DRUG CLASS	COMBINED EFFECT
Diuretics (thiazide)	Potassium depletion.
Ephedrine	Decreased fluprednisolone effect.
Estrogens	Increased fluprednisolone effect.
Ethacrynic acid	Potassium depletion.
Furosemide	Potassium depletion.
Glutethimide	Decreased fluprednisolone effect.
Indomethacin	Increased fluprednisolone effect.
Insulin	Decreased insulin effect.
Isoniazid	Decreased isoniazid effect.
Oxyphenbutazone	Possible ulcers.
Phenylbutazone	Possible ulcers.
Rifampin	Decreased fluprednisolone effect.
Sympathomimetics	Possible glaucoma.

FUROSEMIDE

GENERIC NAME OR DRUG CLASS	COMBINED EFFECT
Probenecid	Decreased probenecid effect.
Salicylates (including aspirin)	Dangerous salicylate retention.
Sedatives	Increased furosemide effect.

HEXOBARBITAL

GENERIC NAME OR DRUG CLASS	COMBINED EFFECT
MAO inhibitors	Increased hexobarbital effect.
Mind-altering drugs	Dangerous sedation. Avoid.
Narcotics	Dangerous sedation. Avoid.
Pain relievers	Dangerous sedation. Avoid.
Sedatives	Dangerous sedation. Avoid.
Sleep inducers	Dangerous sedation. Avoid.
Tranquilizers	Dangerous sedation. Avoid.
Valproic acid	Increased hexobarbital effect.

ADDITIONAL DRUG INTERACTIONS

HYDROCORTISONE (CORTISOL)

GENERIC NAME OR DRUG CLASS	COMBINED EFFECT	GENERIC NAME OR DRUG CLASS	COMBINED EFFECT
Ephedrine	Decreased hydrocortisone effect.	**Insulin**	Decreased insulin effect.
Estrogens	Increased hydrocortisone effect.	**Isoniazid**	Decreased isoniazid effect.
Ethacrynic acid	Potassium depletion.	**Oxyphenbutazone**	Possible ulcers.
Furosemide	Potassium depletion.	**Phenylbutazone**	Possible ulcers.
Glutethimide	Decreased hydrocortisone effect.	**Rifampin**	Decreased hydrocortisone effect.
Indomethacin	Increased hydrocortisone effect.	**Sympathomimetics**	Possible glaucoma.

INSULIN

GENERIC NAME OR DRUG CLASS	COMBINED EFFECT	GENERIC NAME OR DRUG CLASS	COMBINED EFFECT
Tetracyclines	Increased insulin effect.	**Thyroid hormones**	Decreased insulin effect.

KETOCONAZOLE

GENERIC NAME OR DRUG CLASS	COMBINED EFFECT	GENERIC NAME OR DRUG CLASS	COMBINED EFFECT
Propantheline	Decreased absorption of ketoconazole.	**Scopolamine**	Decreased absorption of ketoconazole.
Ranitidine	Decreased absorption of ketoconazole.		

MAGNESIUM CARBONATE

GENERIC NAME OR DRUG CLASS	COMBINED EFFECT	GENERIC NAME OR DRUG CLASS	COMBINED EFFECT
Sulfa drugs	Decreased sulfa effect.	**Vitamins A and C**	Decreased vitamin effect.
Tetracyclines	Decreased tetracycline effect.	**Vitamin D**	Too much calcium in blood.

MAGNESIUM HYDROXIDE

GENERIC NAME OR DRUG CLASS	COMBINED EFFECT	GENERIC NAME OR DRUG CLASS	COMBINED EFFECT
Sulfa drugs	Decreased sulfa effect.	**Vitamins A and C**	Decreased vitamin effect.
Tetracyclines	Decreased tetracycline effect.	**Vitamin D**	Too much calcium in blood.

MAGNESIUM TRISILICATE

GENERIC NAME OR DRUG CLASS	COMBINED EFFECT	GENERIC NAME OR DRUG CLASS	COMBINED EFFECT
Sulfa drugs	Decreased sulfa effect.	**Vitamins A and C**	Decreased vitamin effect.
Tetracyclines	Decreased tetracycline effect.	**Vitamin D**	Too much calcium in blood.

MEPHENYTOIN

GENERIC NAME OR DRUG CLASS	COMBINED EFFECT	GENERIC NAME OR DRUG CLASS	COMBINED EFFECT
Isoniazid	Increased mephenytoin effect.	**Methylphenidate**	Increased mephenytoin effect.
Methadone	Decreased methadone effect.	**Oxyphenbutazone**	Increased mephenytoin effect.
Methotrexate	Increased methotrexate effect.	**Para-aminosalicylic acid (PAS)**	Increased mephenytoin effect.

ADDITIONAL DRUG INTERACTIONS

MEPHENYTOIN continued

GENERIC NAME OR DRUG CLASS	COMBINED EFFECT
Phenothiazines	Increased mephenytoin effect.
Phenylbutazone	Increased mephenytoin effect.
Propranolol	Increased propranolol effect.
Quinidine	Increased quinidine effect.
Sedatives	Increased sedative effect.
Sulfa drugs	Increased mephenytoin effect.
Theophylline	Reduced anticonvulsant effect.

MEPHOBARBITAL

GENERIC NAME OR DRUG CLASS	COMBINED EFFECT
MAO inhibitors	Increased mephobarbital effect.
Mind-altering drugs	Dangerous sedation. Avoid.
Narcotics	Dangerous sedation. Avoid.
Pain relievers	Dangerous sedation. Avoid.
Sedatives	Dangerous sedation. Avoid.
Sleep inducers	Dangerous sedation. Avoid.
Tranquilizers	Dangerous sedation. Avoid.
Valproic acid	Increased mephobarbital effect.

METHARBITAL

GENERIC NAME OR DRUG CLASS	COMBINED EFFECT
MAO inhibitors	Increased metharbital effect.
Mind-altering drugs	Dangerous sedation. Avoid.
Narcotics	Dangerous sedation. Avoid.
Pain relievers	Dangerous sedation. Avoid.
Sedatives	Dangerous sedation. Avoid.
Sleep inducers	Dangerous sedation. Avoid.
Tranquilizers	Dangerous sedation. Avoid.
Valproic acid	Increased metharbital effect.

METHYLPREDNISOLONE

GENERIC NAME OR DRUG CLASS	COMBINED EFFECT
Contraceptives (oral)	Increased methylprednisolone effect.
Digitalis preparations	Dangerous potassium depletion. Possible digitalis toxicity.
Diuretics (thiazide)	Potassium depletion.
Ephedrine	Decreased methylprednisolone effect.
Estrogens	Increased methylprednisolone effect.
Ethacrynic acid	Potassium depletion.
Furosemide	Potassium depletion.
Glutethimide	Decreased methylprednisolone effect.
Indomethacin	Increased methylprednisolone effect.
Insulin	Decreased insulin effect.
Isoniazid	Decreased isoniazid effect.
Oxyphenbutazone	Possible ulcers.
Phenylbutazone	Possible ulcers.
Rifampin	Decreased methylprednisolone effect.
Sympathomimetics	Possible glaucoma.

ADDITIONAL DRUG INTERACTIONS

NICOTINE RESIN COMPLEX

GENERIC NAME OR DRUG CLASS	COMBINED EFFECT
Propoxyphene	Decreased blood level of propoxyphene.
Theophylline	Increased effect of theophylline.

PARAMETHASONE

GENERIC NAME OR DRUG CLASS	COMBINED EFFECT
Diuretics (thiazide)	Potassium depletion.
Ephedrine	Decreased paramethasone effect.
Estrogens	Increased paramethasone effect.
Ethacrynic acid	Potassium depletion.
Furosemide	Potassium depletion.
Glutethimide	Decreased paramethasone effect.
Indomethacin	Increased paramethasone effect.
Insulin	Decreased insulin effect.
Isoniazid	Decreased isoniazid effect.
Oxyphenbutazone	Possible ulcers.
Phenylbutazone	Possible ulcers.
Rifampin	Decreased paramethasone effect.
Sympathomimetics	Possible glaucoma.

PENTOBARBITAL

GENERIC NAME OR DRUG CLASS	COMBINED EFFECT
MAO inhibitors	Increased pentobarbital effect.
Mind-altering drugs	Dangerous sedation. Avoid.
Narcotics	Dangerous sedation. Avoid.
Pain relievers	Dangerous sedation. Avoid.
Sedatives	Dangerous sedation. Avoid.
Sleep inducers	Dangerous sedation. Avoid.
Tranquilizers	Dangerous sedation. Avoid.
Valproic acid	Increased pentobarbital effect.

PHENOBARBITAL

GENERIC NAME OR DRUG CLASS	COMBINED EFFECT
MAO inhibitors	Increased phenobarbital effect.
Mind-altering drugs	Dangerous sedation. Avoid.
Narcotics	Dangerous sedation. Avoid.
Pain relievers	Dangerous sedation. Avoid.
Sedatives	Dangerous sedation. Avoid.
Sleep inducers	Dangerous sedation. Avoid.
Tranquilizers	Dangerous sedation. Avoid.
Valproic acid	Increased phenobarbital effect.

PHENPROCOUMON

GENERIC NAME OR DRUG CLASS	COMBINED EFFECT
Benzodiazepines	Unpredictable increased or decreased anticoagulant effect.
Carbamazepine	Decreased phenprocoumon effect.
Chloral hydrate	Unpredictable increased or decreased anticoagulant effect.
Chloramphenicol	Increased phenprocoumon effect.
Chlorpromazine	Decreased phenprocoumon effect.
Cholestyramine	Unpredictable increased or decreased phenprocoumon effect.
Cimetidine	Increased phenprocoumon effect.
Clofibrate	Unpredictable increased or decreased phenprocoumon effect.

PHENPROCOUMON continued

GENERIC NAME OR DRUG CLASS	COMBINED EFFECT
Contraceptives (oral)	Unpredictable increased or decreased phenprocoumon effect.
Cortisone drugs	Unpredictable increased or decreased phenprocoumon effect.
Digitalis preparations	Decreased phenprocoumon effect.
Disulfiram	Increased phenprocoumon effect.
Estrogens	Decreased phenprocoumon effect.
Ethacrynic acid	Increased phenprocoumon effect.
Ethchlorvynol	Decreased phenprocoumon effect.
Furosemide	Decreased phenprocoumon effect.
Glucagon	Increased phenprocoumon effect.
Glutethimide	Decreased phenprocoumon effect.
Griseofulvin	Decreased phenprocoumon effect.
Guanethidine	Increased phenprocoumon effect.
Haloperidol	Decreased phenprocoumon effect.
Hydroxyzine	Increased phenprocoumon effect.
Indomethacin	Increased phenprocoumon effect.
Insulin	Increased insulin effect.
Isocarboxazid	Increased phenprocoumon effect.
Isoniazid	Increased phenprocoumon effect.
Mefenamic acid	Increased phenprocoumon effect.
Meprobamate	Decreased phenprocoumon effect.
Mercaptopurine	Increased phenprocoumon effect.
Methyldopa	Increased phenprocoumon effect.
Methylphenidate	Increased phenprocoumon effect.
Metronidazole	Increased phenprocoumon effect.
Nalidixic acid	Increased phenprocoumon effect.
Nortriptyline	Increased phenprocoumon effect.
Oxyphenbutazone	Increased phenprocoumon effect.
Para-aminosalicylic acid (PAS)	Increased phenprocoumon effect.
Phenelzine	Increased phenprocoumon effect.
Phenylbutazone	Unpredictable increased or decreased phenprocoumon effect.
Phenylpropanolamine	Decreased anticoagulant effect.
Phenyramidol	Increased phenprocoumon effect.
Probenecid	Increased phenprocoumon effect.
Propoxyphene	Increased phenprocoumon effect.
Propylthiouracil	Increased phenprocoumon effect.
Quinidine	Increased phenprocoumon effect.
Rauwolfia alkaloids	Unpredictable increased or decreased phenprocoumon effect.
Salicylates (including aspirin)	Increased phenprocoumon effect.
Sulfa drugs	Increased phenprocoumon effect.
Sulfinpyrazone	Increased phenprocoumon effect.
Tetracyclines	Increased phenprocoumon effect.
Thyroid hormones	Increased phenprocoumon effect.
Trimethoprim	Increased phenprocoumon effect.
Vitamin C (large doses)	Decreased phenprocoumon effect.
Vitamin E (large doses)	Increased phenprocoumon effect.

ADDITIONAL DRUG INTERACTIONS

PHENYTOIN

GENERIC NAME OR DRUG CLASS	COMBINED EFFECT
Griseofulvin	Increased griseofulvin effect.
Isoniazid	Increased phenytoin effect.
Methadone	Decreased methadone effect.
Methotrexate	Increased methotrexate effect.
Methylphenidate	Increased phenytoin effect.
Oxyphenbutazone	Increased phenytoin effect.
Para-aminosalicylic acid (PAS)	Increased phenytoin effect.
Phenothiazines	Increased phenytoin effect.
Phenylbutazone	Increased phenytoin effect.
Propranolol	Increased propranolol effect.
Quinidine	Increased quinidine effect.
Sedatives	Increased sedative effect.
Sulfa drugs	Increased phenytoin effect.
Theophylline	Reduced anticonvulsant effect.

PREDNISOLONE

GENERIC NAME OR DRUG CLASS	COMBINED EFFECT
Ephedrine	Decreased prednisolone effect.
Estrogens	Increased prednisolone effect.
Ethacrynic acid	Potassium depletion.
Furosemide	Potassium depletion.
Glutethimide	Decreased prednisolone effect.
Indomethacin	Increased prednisolone effect.
Insulin	Decreased insulin effect.
Isoniazid	Decreased isoniazid effect.
Oxyphenbutazone	Possible ulcers.
Phenylbutazone	Possible ulcers.
Rifampin	Decreased prednisolone effect.
Sympathomimetics	Possible glaucoma.

PREDNISONE

GENERIC NAME OR DRUG CLASS	COMBINED EFFECT
Ephedrine	Decreased prednisone effect.
Estrogens	Increased prednisone effect.
Ethacrynic acid	Potassium depletion.
Furosemide	Potassium depletion.
Glutethimide	Decreased prednisone effect.
Indomethacin	Increased prednisone effect.
Insulin	Decreased insulin effect.
Isoniazid	Decreased isoniazid effect.
Oxyphenbutazone	Possible ulcers.
Phenylbutazone	Possible ulcers.
Rifampin	Decreased prednisone effect.
Sympathomimetics	Possible glaucoma.

PRIMIDONE

GENERIC NAME OR DRUG CLASS	COMBINED EFFECT
Narcotics	Increased narcotic effect.
Oxyphenbutazone	Decreased oxyphenbutazone effect.
Phenylbutazone	Decreased phenylbutazone effect.
Sedatives	Increased sedative effect.
Sleep inducers	Increased effect of sleep inducer.
Tranquilizers	Increased tranquilizer effect.

ADDITIONAL DRUG INTERACTIONS

GENERIC NAME OR DRUG CLASS	COMBINED EFFECT	GENERIC NAME OR DRUG CLASS	COMBINED EFFECT

PROBENECID

GENERIC NAME OR DRUG CLASS	COMBINED EFFECT	GENERIC NAME OR DRUG CLASS	COMBINED EFFECT
Salicylates	Decreased probenecid effect.	**Sulfa drugs**	Slows elimination. May cause harmful accumulation of sulfa.

SALICYLATES

GENERIC NAME OR DRUG CLASS	COMBINED EFFECT	GENERIC NAME OR DRUG CLASS	COMBINED EFFECT
Phenytoin	Increased phenytoin effect.	**Salicylates (other)**	Likely salicylate toxicity.
Probenecid	Decreased probenecid effect.	**Spironolactone**	Decreased spironolactone effect.
Propranolol	Decreased salicylate effect.	**Sulfinpyrazone**	Decreased sulfinpyrazone effect.
Rauwolfia alkaloids	Decreased salicylate effect.	**Vitamin C (large doses)**	Possible salicylate toxicity.

SECOBARBITAL

GENERIC NAME OR DRUG CLASS	COMBINED EFFECT	GENERIC NAME OR DRUG CLASS	COMBINED EFFECT
MAO inhibitors	Increased secobarbital effect.	**Sedatives**	Dangerous sedation. Avoid.
Mind-altering drugs	Dangerous sedation. Avoid.	**Sleep inducers**	Dangerous sedation. Avoid.
Narcotics	Dangerous sedation. Avoid.	**Tranquilizers**	Dangerous sedation. Avoid.
Pain relievers	Dangerous sedation. Avoid.	**Valproic acid**	Increased secobarbital effect.

TALBUTAL (BUTALBITAL)

GENERIC NAME OR DRUG CLASS	COMBINED EFFECT	GENERIC NAME OR DRUG CLASS	COMBINED EFFECT
MAO inhibitors	Increased talbutal (butalbital) effect.	**Sedatives**	Dangerous sedation. Avoid.
Mind-altering drugs	Dangerous sedation. Avoid.	**Sleep inducers**	Dangerous sedation. Avoid.
Narcotics	Dangerous sedation. Avoid.	**Tranquilizers**	Dangerous sedation. Avoid.
Pain relievers	Dangerous sedation. Avoid.	**Valproic acid**	Increased talbutal (butalbital) effect.

THIOTHIXENE

GENERIC NAME OR DRUG CLASS	COMBINED EFFECT	GENERIC NAME OR DRUG CLASS	COMBINED EFFECT
Sedatives	Increased thiothixene effect. Excessive sedation.	**Tranquilizers**	Increased thiothixene effect. Excessive sedation.
Sleep inducers	Increased thiothixene effect. Excessive sedation.		

ADDITIONAL DRUG INTERACTIONS

TOLAZAMIDE

GENERIC NAME OR DRUG CLASS	COMBINED EFFECT
Isoniazid	Decreased tolazamide effect.
MAO inhibitors	Increased tolazamide effect.
Oxyphenbutazone	Increased tolazamide effect.
Phenylbutazone	Increased tolazamide effect.
Phenyramidol	Increased tolazamide effect.
Probenecid	Increased tolazamide effect.
Pyrazinamide	Decreased tolazamide effect.
Sulfaphenazole	Increased tolazamide effect.
Sulfa drugs	Increased tolazamide effect.
Thyroid hormones	Decreased tolazamide effect.

TOLBUTAMIDE

GENERIC NAME OR DRUG CLASS	COMBINED EFFECT
Isoniazid	Decreased tolbutamide effect.
MAO inhibitors	Increased tolbutamide effect.
Oxyphenbutazone	Increased tolbutamide effect.
Phenylbutazone	Increased tolbutamide effect.
Phenyramidol	Increased tolbutamide effect.
Probenecid	Increased tolbutamide effect.
Pyrazinamide	Decreased tolbutamide effect.
Sulfa drugs	Increased tolbutamide effect.
Sulfaphenazole	Increased tolbutamide effect.
Thyroid hormones	Decreased tolbutamide effect.

TRIAMCINOLONE

GENERIC NAME OR DRUG CLASS	COMBINED EFFECT
Ephedrine	Decreased triamcinolone effect.
Estrogens	Increased triamcinolone effect.
Ethacrynic acid	Potassium depletion.
Furosemide	Potassium depletion.
Glutethimide	Decreased triamcinolone effect.
Indomethacin	Increased triamcinolone effect.
Insulin	Decreased insulin effect.
Isoniazid	Decreased isoniazid effect.
Oxyphenbutazone	Possible ulcers.
Phenylbutazone	Possible ulcers.
Rifampin	Decreased triamcinolone effect.
Sympathomimetics	Possible glaucoma.

Glossary

The following medical terms are found in the drug charts.

A

Acute—Having a short and relatively severe course.

Addiction—Psychological or physiological dependence upon a drug.

Addison's Disease—Changes in the body caused by a deficiency of hormones manufactured by the adrenal gland. Usually fatal if untreated.

Adrenal Cortex—Center of the adrenal gland.

Adrenal Gland—Gland next to the kidney that produces cortisone and epinephrine (adrenalin).

Alkylating Agent—Chemical used to treat malignant diseases.

Allergy—Excessive sensitivity to a substance.

Amebiasis—Infection with amoeba, one-celled organisms. Causes diarrhea, fever and abdominal cramps.

Amphetamine—Drug that stimulates the brain and central nervous system, increases blood pressure, reduces nasal congestion and is habit-forming.

Analgesic—Agent that reduces pain without reducing consciousness.

Anaphylaxis—Severe allergic response to a substance. Symptoms are wheezing, itching, hives, nasal congestion, intense burning of hands and feet, collapse, loss of consciousness and cardiac arrest. Symptoms appear within a few seconds or minutes after exposure. Anaphylaxis is a severe medical emergency. Without appropriate treatment, it can cause death. Instructions for home treatment for anaphylaxis are on page 888.

Anemia—Not enough healthy red-blood cells in the bloodstream or too little hemoglobin in the red-blood cells. Anemia is caused by imbalance of blood loss and blood production.

Anemia, Hemolytic—Anemia caused by a shortened life span of red-blood cells. The body can't manufacture new cells fast enough to replace old cells.

Anemia, Iron-Deficiency—Anemia caused when iron necessary to manufacture red-blood cells is not available.

Anemia, Pernicious—Anemia caused by a vitamin B-12 deficiency. Symptoms include weakness, fatigue, numbness and tingling of the hands or feet, and degeneration of the central nervous system.

Anemia, Sickle-Cell—Anemia caused by defective hemoglobin that deprives red-blood cells of oxygen, making them sickle-shaped.

Anesthetic—Drug that eliminates the sensation of pain.

Angina (Angina Pectoris)—Chest pain with a sensation of suffocation and impending death. Caused by a temporary reduction in the amount of oxygen to the heart muscle through diseased coronary arteries.

Antacid—Chemical that neutralizes acid, usually in the stomach.

Antibiotic—Chemical that inhibits the growth of or kills germs.

Anticholinergic—Drug that chemically inhibits nerve impulses through the parasympathetic nervous system.

Anticoagulant—Drug that inhibits blood clotting.

Antiemetic—Drug that prevents or stops nausea and vomiting.

Antihypertensive—Medication to reduce blood pressure.

Appendicitis—Inflammation or infection of the appendix. Symptoms include loss of appetite, nausea, low-grade fever and tenderness in the lower right of the abdomen.

Artery—Blood vessel carrying blood away from the heart.

Asthma—Recurrent attacks of breathing difficulty due to spasms and contractions of the bronchial tubes.

B

Bacteria—Microscopic organism. Some bacteria contribute to health; others (germs) cause disease.

GLOSSARY

Basal Area of Brain—Part of the brain that regulates muscle control and tone.
Blood Count—Laboratory studies to count white-blood cells, red-blood cells, platelets and other elements of the blood.
Blood Pressure, Diastolic—Pressure (usually recorded in millimeters of mercury) in the large arteries of the body when the heart muscle is relaxed and filling for the next contraction.
Blood Pressure, Systolic—Pressure (usually recorded in millimeters of mercury) in the large arteries of the body at the instant the heart muscle contracts.
Blood Sugar (Blood Glucose)—Necessary element in the blood to sustain life.

C

Cataract—Loss of transparency in the lens of the eye.
Cell—Unit of protoplasm, the essential living matter of all plants and animals.
Cephalosporin—Antibiotic that kills many bacterial germs that penicillin and sulfa drugs can't destroy.
Cholinergic (also Parasympathomimetic)—Chemical that facilitates passage of nerve impulses through the parasympathetic nervous system.
Cirrhosis—Disease that scars and destroys liver tissue.
Cold Urticaria—Hives that appear in areas of the body exposed to the cold.
Colitis, Ulcerative—Chronic, recurring ulcers of the colon for unknown reasons.
Collagen—Support tissue of skin, tendon, bone, cartilage and connective tissue.
Colostomy—Surgical opening from the colon, the large intestine, to the outside of the body.
Congestive—Excess accumulation of blood. In congestive heart failure, congestion occurs in the lungs, liver, kidney and other parts to cause shortness of breath, swelling of the ankles and feet, rapid heartbeat and other symptoms.
Constriction—Tightness or pressure.
Contraceptive—Something that prevents pregnancy.
Convulsions—Violent, uncontrollable contractions of the voluntary muscles.
Corticosteroid (Adrenocorticosteroid)—Steroid hormones produced by the body's adrenal cortex or their synthetic equivalents.
Cystitis—Inflammation of the urinary bladder.

D

Delirium—Temporary mental disturbance characterized by hallucinations, agitation and incoherence.
Diabetes—Metabolic disorder in which the body can't use carbohydrates efficiently. This leads to a dangerously high level of glucose (a carbohydrate) in the blood.
Dialysis—Procedure to filter waste products from the bloodstream of patients with kidney failure.
Dilation—Enlarged.
Disulfiram Reaction—Disulfiram (Antabuse) is a drug to treat alcoholism. When alcohol in the bloodstream interacts with disulfiram, it causes a flushed face, severe headache, chest pains, shortness of breath, nausea, vomiting, sweating and weakness. Severe reactions may cause death.

A disulfiram reaction is the interaction of any drug with alcohol or another drug to produce these symptoms. See emergency first aid instructions, page 886.
Duodenum—The first 12 inches of the small intestine.

E

Eczema—Disorder of the skin with redness, itching, blisters, weeping and abnormal pigmentation.
Electrolyte—Substance that can transmit electrical impulses when dissolved in body fluids.
Embolism—Sudden blockage of an artery by a clot or foreign material in the blood.
Emphysema—Disease in which the lung's air sacs lose elasticity, and air accumulates in the lungs.
Endometriosis—Condition in which uterus tissue is found outside the uterus. Can cause pain, abnormal menstruation and infertility.
Enzyme—Protein chemical that can accelerate a chemical reaction in the body.
Epilepsy—Episodes of brain disturbance that cause convulsions and loss of consciousness.

Esophagitis—Inflammation of the lower part of the esophagus, the tube connecting the throat and the stomach.
Estrogens—Female sex hormones that stimulate female characteristics and prepare the uterus for fertilization.
Eustachian Tube—Small passage from the middle ear to the sinuses and nasal passages.
Extremity—Arm, leg, hand or foot.

F

Fecal Impaction—Condition in which feces become firmly wedged in the rectum.
Fibrocystic Breast Disease—Overgrowth of fibrous tissue in the breast, producing non-malignant cysts.
Fibroid Tumors—Non-malignant tumors of the muscular layer of the uterus.
Flu (Influenza)—A virus infection of the respiratory tract that lasts three to ten days. Symptoms include headache, fever, runny nose, cough, tiredness and muscle aches.
Folliculitis—Inflammation of a follicle.

G

G6PD—Deficiency of glucose 6-phosphate, necessary for glucose metabolism.
Gastritis—Inflammation of the stomach.
Gastrointestinal—Stomach and intestinal tract.
Gland—Cells that manufacture and excrete materials not required for their own metabolic needs.
Glaucoma—Eye disease in which increased pressure inside the eye damages the optic nerve, causes pain and changes vision.
Glucagon—Injectable drug that immediately elevates blood sugar by mobilizing glycogen from the liver.

H

Hangover Effect—The same feelings as a "hangover" after too much alcohol consumption. Symptoms include headache, irritability and nausea.
Hemochromatosis—Disorder of iron metabolism in which excessive iron is deposited in and damages body tissues, particularly liver and pancreas.
Hemoglobin—Pigment that carries oxygen in red-blood cells.
Hemorrhage—Heavy bleeding.
Hemosiderosis—Increase of iron deposits in body tissues without tissue damage.
Hepatitis—Inflammation of liver cells, usually accompanied by jaundice.
Hiatal Hernia—Section of stomach that protrudes into the chest cavity.
Histamine—Chemical in body tissues that dilates the smallest blood vessels, constricts the smooth muscle surrounding the bronchial tubes and stimulates stomach secretions.
History—Past medical events in a patient's life.
Hives—Elevated patches on the skin that are redder or paler than surrounding skin and often itch severely.
Hormone—Chemical substance produced in the body to regulate other body functions.
Hypertension—High blood pressure.
Hypocalcemia—Abnormally low level of calcium in the blood.
Hypoglycemia—Low blood sugar (blood glucose). A critically low blood-sugar level will interfere with normal brain function and can damage the brain permanently.

I

Ichthyosis—Skin disorder with dryness, scaling and roughness.
Ileitis—Inflammation of the ileum, the last section of the small intestine.
Ileostomy—Surgical opening from the ileum, the end of the small intestine, to the outside of the body.
Impotence—Male's inability to achieve or sustain erection of the penis for sexual intercourse.
Insomnia—Sleeplessness.
Interaction—Change in the body's response to one drug when another is taken. Interaction may increase effect of one or both drugs, decrease the effect of one or both drugs or cause toxicity.

J

Jaundice—Symptoms of liver damage, bile obstruction or red-blood-cell destruction. Includes yellowed whites of the eyes, yellow skin, dark urine and light stool.

K

Keratosis—Growth that is an accumulation of cells from the outer skin layers.
Kidney Stones—Small, solid stones made from calcium, cholesterol, cysteine and other body chemicals.

L

Lupus—Serious disorder of connective tissue that primarily affects women. Varies in severity with skin eruptions, joint inflammation, low white-blood cell count and damage to internal organs, especially the kidney.

Lymph Glands—Glands in the lymph vessels throughout the body that trap foreign and infectious matter and protect the bloodstream from infection.

M

Manic-Depressive Illness—Psychosis with alternating cycles of excessive enthusiasm and depression.

Mast Cell—Connective-tissue cell.

Menopause—The end of menstruation in the female, often accompanied by irritability, hot flushes, changes in the skin and bones and vaginal dryness.

Metabolism—Process of using nutrients and energy to build and break down wastes.

Migraine—Periodic headaches caused by constriction of arteries to the skull. Symptoms include severe pain, vision disturbances, nausea, vomiting and light sensitivity.

Mind-Altering Drugs—Any drug that decreases alertness, perception, concentration, contact with reality or muscular coordination.

Myasthenia Gravis—Disease of the muscles characterized by fatigue and progressive paralysis. It is usually confined to muscles of the face, lips, tongue and neck.

N

Narcotic—Drug, usually addictive, that produces stupor.

O

Osteoporosis—Softening of bones caused by a loss of chemicals usually found in bone.

Ovary—Female sexual gland where eggs mature and ripen for fertilization.

P

Palpitations—Rapid heartbeat noticeable to the patient.

Pancreatitis—Serious inflammation or infection of the pancreas that causes upper abdominal pain.

Parkinson's Disease—Disease of the central nervous system. Characteristics are a fixed, emotionless expression of the face, tremor, slower muscle movements, weakness, changed gait and a peculiar posture.

Pellagra—Disease caused by a deficiency of the water-soluble vitamin, thiamine (vitamin B-1). Symptoms include brain disturbance, diarrhea and skin inflammation.

Penicillin—Chemical substance (antibiotic) originally discovered as a product of mold, which can kill some bacterial germs.

Phlegm—Thick mucus secreted by glands in the respiratory tract.

Pinworms—Common intestinal parasite that causes rectal itching and irritation.

Pituitary Gland—Gland at the base of the brain that secretes hormones to stimulate growth and other glands to produce hormones.

Platelet—Disc-shaped element of the blood, smaller than red- or white-blood cells, necessary for blood clotting.

Polyp—Growth on a mucous membrane.

Porphyria—Inherited metabolic disorder characterized by changes in the nervous system and kidney.

Post-partum—Following delivery of a baby.

Potassium—Important chemical found in body cells.

Potassium Foods—Foods high in potassium content, including dried apricots and peaches, lentils, raisins, citrus and whole-grain cereals.

Prostate—Gland in the male that surrounds the neck of the bladder and the urethra.

Prothrombin—Blood substance essential in clotting.

Prothrombin Time—Laboratory study used to follow prothrombin activity and keep coagulation safe.

Psoriasis—Chronic, inherited skin disease. Symptoms are lesions with silvery scales on the edges.

Psychosis—Mental disorder characterized by deranged personality, loss of contact with reality and possible delusions, hallucinations or illusions.

Purine Foods—Foods that are metabolized into uric acid. Foods high in purines include anchovies, liver, brains, sweetbreads, sardines, kidney, oysters, gravy and meat extracts.

R

RDA—Recommended daily allowance of a vitamin or mineral.
Rebound Effect—Return of a condition, often with increased severity, once the prescribed drug is withdrawn.
Renal—Pertaining to the kidney.
Retina—Innermost covering of the eyeball on which the image is formed.
Reye's Syndrome—Rare, sometimes fatal, disease of children that causes brain and liver damage.
Rickets—Bone disease caused by vitamin-D deficiency. Bones become bent and distorted during infancy or childhood.

S

Sedative—Drug that reduces excitement or anxiety.
Seizure—Brain disorder causing changes of consciousness or convulsions.
Sinusitis—Inflammation or infection of the sinus cavities in the skull.
Streptococcus—Bacteria that causes infections in the throat, respiratory system and skin. Improperly treated, can lead to disease in the heart, joints and kidneys.
Stroke—Sudden, severe attack. Usually sudden paralysis from injury to the brain or spinal cord caused by a blood clot or hemorrhage in the brain.
Stupor—Near unconsciousness.
Sublingual—Under the tongue. Some drugs are absorbed almost as quickly this way as by injection.

T

Tardive Dyskinesia—Involuntary movements of the jaw, lips and tongue caused by an unpredictable drug reaction.
Thrombophlebitis—Inflammation of a vein caused by a blood clot in the vein.
Thyroid—Gland in the neck that manufactures and secretes several hormones.
Tic-douloureaux—Painful condition caused by inflammation of a nerve in the face.
Toxicity—Poisonous reaction to a drug that impairs body functions or damages cells.
Tranquilizer—Drug that calms a person without clouding consciousness.
Tremor—Involuntary trembling.
Trichomoniasis—Infestation of the vagina by *trichomonas,* an infectious organism. The infection causes itching, vaginal discharge and irritation.
Triglyceride—Fatty chemical manufactured from carbohydrates for storage in fat cells.
Tyramine—Normal chemical component of the body that helps sustain blood pressure. Can rise to fatal levels in combination with some drugs.

Tyramine is found in many foods:

Beverages—Alcoholic beverages, especially Chianti or robust red wines, vermouth, ale, beer.

Breads—Homemade bread with a lot of yeast and breads or crackers containing cheese.

Fats—Sour cream.

Fruits—Bananas, red plums, avocados, figs, raisins.

Meats and meat substitutes—Aged game, liver, canned meats, salami, sausage, cheese, salted dried fish, pickled herring.

Vegetables—Italian broad beans, green-bean pods, eggplant.

Miscellaneous—Yeast concentrates or extracts, marmite, soup cubes, commercial gravy, soy sauce, any protein food that has been stored improperly or is spoiled.

U

Ulcer, Peptic—Open sore on the mucous membrane of the esophagus, stomach or duodenum caused by stomach acid.
Urethra—Hollow tube through which urine (and semen in men) is discharged.
Urethritis—Inflammation or infection of the urethra.
Uterus—Also called *womb.* A hollow muscular organ in the female in which the embryo develops into a fetus.

V

Vascular—Pertaining to blood vessels.
Virus—Infectious organism that reproduces in the cells of the infected host.

Y

Yeast—A single-cell organism that can cause infections of the mouth, vagina, skin and parts of the gastrointestinal system.

Guide to Index

Alphabetical entries in the index include three categories—generic names, brand names and drug-class names.

1. Generic names appear in capital letters, followed by their chart page number:

   ASPIRIN, 64.

2. Brand names appear in *italic,* followed by their generic ingredient and chart page number.

   Bayer—See ASPIRIN, 64.

   Some brands contain two or more generic ingredients. These generic ingredients are listed in capital letters following the brand name:

   Cefinal —See
   ASPIRIN, 64
   CAFFEINE, 112

   Some brands contain generic ingredients that are not included in this book because of space limitations. These generics are designated by (NL), which means "not listed."

   Fedrazil—See
   CHLORCYCLIZINE (NL)
   PSEUDOEPHEDRINE, 670

3. Drug-class names appear in regular type, capital and lower-case letters. All generic drug names in this book that fall into a drug class are listed after the class name.

   Analgesics
   ACETAMINOPHEN, 18
   ASPIRIN, 64
   CARBAMAZEPINE, 118
   PHENACETIN, 582
   SALICYLATES, 700

A

INDEX

D

E

INDEX

J

K

L

M

N

O

P

Q

S

U

V

W

X

Y

Z

Emergency Guide for Overdose Victims

This section lists *basic* steps in recognizing and treating immediate effects of drug overdose.

Study the information before you need it. If possible, take a course in first aid and learn external cardiac massage and mouth-to-mouth breathing techniques, called *cardiopulmonary resuscitation* (CPR).

For quick reference, list emergency telephone numbers in the spaces provided on page 888 for fire department paramedics, ambulance, poison-control center and your doctor. These numbers, except for doctor, are usually listed on the inside cover of your telephone directory.

If Victim is Unconscious, *Not* Breathing:

1. Yell for help. Don't leave victim.
2. Begin mouth-to-mouth breathing immediately.
3. If there is no heartbeat, give external cardiac massage.
4. Have someone call O (operator) or 911 (emergency) for an ambulance or medical help.
5. Don't stop CPR until help arrives.
6. Don't try to make victim vomit.
7. If vomiting occurs, save vomit to take to emergency room for analysis.
8. Take medicine or empty bottles with you to emergency room.

If Victim is Unconscious *and* Breathing:

1. Dial 0 (operator) or 911 (emergency) for an ambulance or medical help.
2. If you can't get help immediately, take victim to the nearest emergency room.
3. Don't try to make victim vomit.
4. If vomiting occurs, save vomit to take to emergency room for analysis.
5. Watch victim carefully on the way to the emergency room. If heart or breathing stops, use cardiac massage and mouth-to-mouth breathing (CPR).
6. Take medicine or empty bottles with you to emergency room.

If Victim is Drowsy:

1. Dial 0 (operator) or 911 (emergency) for an ambulance or medical help.
2. If you can't get help immediately, take victim to the nearest emergency room.
3. Don't try to make victim vomit.
4. If vomiting occurs, save vomit to take to emergency room for analysis.
5. Watch victim carefully on the way to the emergency room. If heart or breathing stops, use cardiac massage and mouth-to-mouth breathing (CPR).
6. Take medicine or empty bottles with you to emergency room.

If Victim is Alert:

1. Dial 0 (operator) or 911 (emergency) for an ambulance or emergency medical help.
2. Call poison-control center or doctor for specific instructions.
3. If you can't get instructions, make victim swallow as much water as possible to dilute drug in the stomach. Don't use milk or other beverages.
4. If you are instructed to make victim vomit, use syrup of ipecac according to instructions from your doctor, poison-control center or ipecac label.
5. If you have no ipecac, induce vomiting by pushing your finger far back in victim's throat.
6. Save vomit for analysis.
7. If you can't get paramedic help quickly, take victim to nearest emergency room.
8. Take medicine or empty bottles with you to emergency room.

If Victim has No Symptoms but You Suspect Overdose:

1. Call poison-control center.
2. Describe the suspect drug with as much information as you can quickly gather. The center will give emergency instructions.
3. Or call victim's doctor or your doctor for instructions.
4. If you have no telephone, take victim to the nearest emergency room.
5. Take medicine or empty bottles with you to emergency room.

Emergency Guide for Anaphylaxis Victims

The following are *basic* steps in recognizing and treating immediate effects of severe allergic reaction, which is called *anaphylaxis.*

Some people may be highly sensitive to certain drugs. An anaphylactic reaction to a drug can be life-threatening! Persons suffering these allergic symptoms should receive immediate emergency treatment!

Study the information before you need it. If possible, take a course in first aid and learn external cardiac massage and mouth-to-mouth breathing techniques, called *cardiopulmonary resuscitation* (CPR).

Symptoms of Anaphylaxis:

- **Itching**
- **Rash**
- **Hives**
- **Runny nose**
- **Wheezing**
- **Paleness**
- **Cold sweats**
- **Low blood pressure**
- **Coma**
- **Cardiac arrest**

If Victim is Unconscious, *Not* Breathing:

1. Yell for help. Don't leave victim.
2. Begin mouth-to-mouth breathing immediately.
3. If there is no heartbeat, give external cardiac massage.
4. Have someone call O (operator) or 911 (emergency) for an ambulance or medical help.
5. Don't stop cardiopulmonary resuscitation (CPR) until help arrives.
6. Take medicine or empty bottles with you to the emergency room.

If Victim is Unconscious *and* Breathing:

1. Dial O (operator) or 911 (emergency) for an ambulance or emergency medical help.
2. If you can't get help immediately, take patient to nearest emergency room.
3. Take medicine or empty bottles with you to emergency room for analysis.

Emergency Telephone Numbers

____________________	____________________
Fire Department (Paramedic)	**Ambulance**
____________________	____________________
Doctor	**Poison-Control Center**

NOTES

NOTES

NOTES

NOTES

NOTES